REVISION NOTES IN PSYCHIATRY

THIRD EDITION

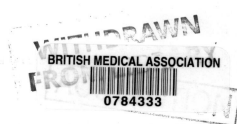

REVISION NOTES IN PSYCHIATRY

THIRD EDITION

BASANT K. PURI
ANNIE HALL
ROGER HO

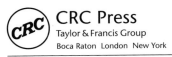 CRC Press
Taylor & Francis Group
Boca Raton London New York

CRC Press is an imprint of the
Taylor & Francis Group, an **informa** business

The authors acknowledge the following illustrators: Ms. Ja'naed Woods (for Chapter 1, "Descriptive Psychopathology"); Mr. Edwin Ng (for Chapter 7, "Cognitive Assessment and Neuropsychological Processes"); and Miss Anna Chua (for all other chapters).

CRC Press
Taylor & Francis Group
6000 Broken Sound Parkway NW, Suite 300
Boca Raton, FL 33487-2742

© 2014 by Basant K. Puri, Anne Hall and Roger Ho
CRC Press is an imprint of Taylor & Francis Group, an Informa business

No claim to original U.S. Government works

Printed on acid-free paper
Version Date: 20130916

Printed and bound in India by Replika Press Pvt. Ltd.

International Standard Book Number-13: 978-1-4441-7013-9 (Paperback)

Visit the Taylor & Francis Web site at
http://www.taylorandfrancis.com

and the CRC Press Web site at
http://www.crcpress.com

Contents

Preface

The preparation of the third edition of this book has involved a number of major changes. First, we have taken on a new co-author, Roger Ho. Roger has relatively recent experience of preparing for and sitting the examinations of the membership of the Royal College of Psychiatrists and is actively involved in teaching candidates based in Singapore. Second, we have added new chapters and, within existing chapters, we have included new material (including NICE guidelines), updated the DSM-IV-TR criteria to the new DSM-5, and cited more recent references. Finally, we have included many more figures. As with previous editions, we believe the third edition of *Revision Notes in Psychiatry* should prove useful not only for the membership of the Royal College of Psychiatrists but also for similar postgraduate examinations in psychiatry in other parts of the English-speaking world.

Basant K. Puri
Annie Hall
Roger Ho

Authors

Basant K. Puri, MA, PhD, MB, BChir, BSc (Hons) MathSci, DipStat, PG Dip Maths, MMath, FRCPsych, FSB, is based at Hammersmith Hospital and Imperial College London, United Kingdom. He read medicine at St. John's College, University of Cambridge. He also trained in molecular genetics at the MRC MNU, Laboratory of Molecular Biology, Cambridge. He has authored or co-authored more than 40 books, including the second edition of *Drugs in Psychiatry* (Oxford University Press, 2013), the third edition of *Textbook of Psychiatry* with Dr. Ian Treasaden (Churchill Livingstone, 2011) and, with the publisher of the present volume, the third edition of *Textbook of Clinical Neuropsychiatry and Neuroscience Fundamentals* with Professor David Moore (2012).

Annie Hall, BA, MB BCh, MRCPsych is a consultant psychiatrist at South Kensington and Chelsea Mental Health Centre and Chelsea and Westminster Hospital, London, United Kingdom. She read medicine at St Catherines' College, Oxford, and completed her clinical training at the Welsh National School of Medicine. She works in a busy NHS inner-city psychiatric service as a consultant general adult psychiatrist.

Dr. Roger Ho, MBBS, DPM, DCP, Gdip Psychotherapy, MMed (Psych), MRCPsych, FRCPC, is an assistant professor and consultant psychiatrist at the Department of Psychological Medicine, National University of Singapore. He graduated from the University of Hong Kong and received his training in psychiatry from the National University of Singapore. He is a general adult psychiatrist and in charge of the Mood Disorder Clinic, National University Hospital, Singapore. He is a member of the editorial board of *Advances of Psychiatric Treatment*, an academic journal published by the Royal College of Psychiatrists. His research focuses on mood disorders, psychoneuroimmunology, and liaison psychiatry. He is one of the key authors for the revision website, Exam doctor MRCPsych Paper 1 questions (http://examdoctor.co.uk/).

Abbreviations

5-HIAA	5-Hydroxyindoleacetic acid	CBT	Cognitive behavioural therapy
5-HT	Serotonin	CBT-Gp	Group-based CBT
5-HTT	Serotonin transporter	CBT-Mb	Mindfulness-based CBT
Aβ	Beta-amyloid	CBT-Tf	Trauma-focused CBT
AA	Alcoholics anonymous	CCBT	Computerized CBT
ACA	Anterior cerebral artery	CCK	Cholecystokinin
ACh	Acetylcholine	CD	Cluster of differentiation
AChE	Acetylcholinesterase	ChAT	Choline acetyltransferase
AChEI	Acetylcholinesterase inhibitor	CJD	Creutzfeldt–Jakob disease
ACT	Assertive community treatment	CK	Creatinine kinase
ACTH	Adrenocorticotrophic hormone	CMHT	Community mental health team
ADH	Antidiuretic hormone	CMV	Cytomegalovirus
ADHD	Attention-deficit hyperactivity disorder	CN	Cranial nerve
		CNS	Central nervous system
ADL	Activities of daily living	COMT	Catechol-O-methyl transferase
AED	Accident and emergency department	CPA	Care programme approach
AF	Atrial fibrillation	CPMS	Clozaril Patient Management System
ALDH	Acetaldehyde dehydrogenase	CPN	Community psychiatric nurse
AN	Anorexia nervosa	CR	Chronic release
APA	American Psychiatric Association	CRF	Chronic renal failure
ASPD	Antisocial personality disorder	CRP	C-reactive protein
ATP	Adenosine triphosphate	CSF	Cerebrospinal fluid
BCh	Butyrylcholinesterase	CT	Computed tomography
BDD	Body dysmorphic disorder	CVA	Cerebrovascular accident
BDNF	Brain-derived neurotrophic factor	CVS	Cardiovascular system
BMI	Body mass index	DBT	Dialectical behaviour therapy
BN	Bulimia nervosa	DDX	Differential diagnosis
BNF	British National Formulary	DLPFC	Dorsolateral prefrontal cortex
BPSD	Behavioural and psychological symptoms in dementia	DM	Diabetes mellitus
		DSH	Deliberate self-harm
BZD	Benzodiazepine	DST	Dexamethasone suppression test
CADASIL	Cerebral autosomal dominant arteriopathy with subcortical infarcts and leukoencephalopathy	DT	Delirium tremens
		DVLA	Drive and Vehicle Licensing Agency (United Kingdom)
CAMCOG	Cambridge Cognitive Examination	DZ	Dizygotic
CAMDEX	Cambridge Examination for Mental Disorder of the Elderly	ECG	Electrocardiogram
		ECT	Electroconvulsive therapy
CAMHS	Child and Adolescent Mental Health Services	ED	Erectile dysfunction
		EE	Expressed emotion
cAMP	Cyclic adenosine monophosphate	EEG	Electroencephalogram
CASC	Clinical Assessment of Skills & Competencies	EPI	Eysenck Personality Inventory
		EPSE	Extrapyramidal side effects
CAT	Cognitive analytic therapy	ERP	Exposure and response prevention
CBF	Cerebral blood flow	ESR	Erythrocyte sedimentation rate

FAS	Foetal alcohol syndrome	MDMA	Methylenedioxymethamphetamine
FBC	Full blood count	MDT	Multidisciplinary team
FRS	First-rank symptoms	Mg	Magnesium
FSH	Follicle-stimulating hormone	MHA	Mental Health Act
FTD	Fronto-temporal dementia	MI	Myocardial infarction
GA	General anaesthesia	MLF	Medial longitudinal fasciculus
GABA	γ-Aminobutyric acid	MMR	Measles, mumps, and rubella
GAD	Generalized anxiety disorder	MMSE	Mini-mental state examination
GAF	Global assessment of functioning	MRCPsych	Member of the Royal College of Psychiatrists
GDS	Geriatric Depression Scale		
GFR	Glomerular filtration rate	MRI	Magnetic resonance imaging
GH	Growth hormone	MS	Multiple sclerosis
GI/GIT	Gastrointestinal/gastrointestinal tract	MSE	Mental state examination
GMC	General Medical Council	MSU	Midstream urine
GP	General practitioner	MSW	Medical social worker
HCG	Human chorionic gonadotropin	^{99m}Tc-HMPAO	Tc99m hexamethylpropyleneamine oxime
HMSN	Hereditary motor and sensory neuropathies		
		MVP	Mitral valve prolapse
HPA	Hypothalamic–pituitary–adrenal	MZ	Monozygotic
HSV	Herpes simplex virus	NA	Noradrenaline
HVA	Homovanillic acid	NAI	Nonaccidental injury
HVS	Hyperventilation syndrome	NART	National Adult Reading Test
IBS	Irritable bowel syndrome	NAS	Neonate abstinence syndrome
ICP	Intracranial pressure	NF	Neurofibromatosis
IDDM	Insulin-dependent diabetes mellitus	NFT	Neurofibrillary tangle
IHD	Ischaemic heart disease	NHS	National Health Service (United Kingdom)
IM	Intramuscular		
IMR	Inmate record	NICE	National Institute for Health and Care Excellence (United Kingdom)
IPT	Interpersonal therapy		
IUGR	Intrauterine growth retardation	NMDA	N-methyl-D-aspartate
IV	Intravenous	nocte	Every night
K	Potassium	NPH	Normal pressure hydrocephalus
K-SADS-PL	Kiddie-Schedule for Affective Disorders and Schizophrenia-Present and Lifetime Version	NRT	Nicotine replacement therapy
		NSAID	Nonsteroidal anti-inflammatory drug
LBD	Lewy body dementia	OCD	Obsessive–compulsive disorder
LC	Locus coeruleus	OCPD	Obsessive–compulsive personality disorder
LD	Learning disability		
LFT	Liver function test	ODD	Oppositional defiant disorder
LH	Luteinizing hormone	OM	Every morning
LMBBS	Laurence–Moon–Biedl syndrome	OT	Occupational therapist
LMNL	Lower motor neurone lesion	PANDAS	Paediatric autoimmune neuropsychiatric disorders associated with streptococcal infections
LOC	Loss of consciousness		
LOCF	Last observation carried forward		
LP	Lumbar puncture	PANSS	Positive and Negative Syndrome Scale
LTM	Long-term memory		
MAOI	Monoamine oxidase inhibitor	PCA	Posterior cerebral artery
MCA	Middle cerebral artery	PCOS	Polycystic ovary syndrome
MCQ	Multiple-choice question	PCP	Phencyclidine
MCI	Mild cognitive impairment	PCS	Postconcussion syndrome
M:F	Male-to-female ratio	PDD	Pervasive development disorder

PE	Physical examination	SNRI	Serotonin–noradrenaline reuptake inhibitor
PFC	Prefrontal cortex		
PI	Projective identification	SPECT	Single-proton emission computed tomography
PK	Pharmacokinetics		
PKD	Parkinson's disease	SSRI	Selective serotonin reuptake inhibitor
PKU	Phenylketonuria	STD	Sexually transmitted disease
PMC	Premotor cortex	STM	Short-term memory
PMH	Past medical history	SWS	Slow-wave sleep
PMS	Premenstrual syndrome	$t_{1/2}$	Half-life
PNS	Peripheral nervous system	TCA	Tricyclic antidepressant
PPG	Penile plethysmography	TD	Tardive dyskinesia
PPH	Past psychiatric history	TFT	Thyroid function test
PROM	Premature rupture of membrane	TI	Therapeutic index
PrP	Prion protein	TIA	Transient ischaemic attack
PSP	Progressive supranuclear palsy	TLE	Temporal lobe epilepsy
PT	Physiotherapist	TMS	Transcranial magnetic stimulation
PTA	Posttraumatic amnesia	TNF	Tumour necrosis factor
PTSD	Posttraumatic stress disorder	TNR	Trinucleotide repeat
PWS	Prader–Willi syndrome	TRD	Treatment-resistant depression
QoL	Quality of life	TRH	Thyrotropin-releasing hormone
RCT	Randomized controlled trial	TRS	Treatment-resistant schizophrenia
RFLP	Restriction fragment length polymorphism	TSH	Thyroid-stimulating hormone
		U&E	Urea and electrolytes
RFT	Renal function test	UMNL	Upper motor neurone lesion
RTA	Road traffic accident	UTI	Urinary tract infection
SDH	Subdural haemorrhage	VaD	Vascular dementia
SIDS	Sudden infant death syndrome	VDRL	Venereal Disease Research Laboratory
SLE	Systemic lupus erythematosus		
SMR	Standardized mortality ratio	VIP	Vasoactive intestinal peptide
SMS	Smith–Magenis syndrome	VNS	Vagus nerve stimulation
SNECO	Special education needs coordinator	WBC	White blood cell
		WCST	Wisconsin card sorting test

1 Descriptive Psychopathology

1.1 DISORDERS OF GENERAL BEHAVIOUR

1.1.1 UNDERACTIVITY

1.1.1.1 Stupor

The key features of stupor, when the term is used in its psychiatric sense, include

- Mutism
- Immobility
- Occasional periods of excitement and overactivity

Stupor is seen in

- Catatonic stupor
- Depressive stupor
- Manic stupor
- Epilepsy
- Hysteria

In neurology, the term 'stupor' refers to a person who responds to pain and loud sounds and may exhibit brief monosyllabic utterances, and some spontaneous motor activity takes place.

1.1.1.2 Depressive Retardation

This is a lesser form of psychomotor retardation occurring in depression that, in its extreme form, merges with depressive stupor.

1.1.1.3 Obsessional Slowness

This may occur secondary to repeated doubts and compulsive rituals.

1.1.2 OVERACTIVITY

1.1.2.1 Psychomotor Agitation

A person with psychomotor agitation manifests

- Excessive overactivity, which is usually unproductive
- Restlessness

1.1.2.2 Hyperkinesis

In hyperkinesis, which may be seen in children and adolescents, the following features occur:

- Overactivity
- Distractibility
- Impulsivity
- Excitability

1.1.2.3 Somnambulism (Sleep Walking)

A complex sequence of behaviours is carried out by a person who rises from sleep and is not fully aware of his or her surroundings.

1.1.2.4 Compulsion (Compulsive Ritual)

This is a repetitive and stereotyped seemingly purposeful behaviour. It is the motor component of an obsessional thought. Examples of compulsions include

- Checking rituals
- Cleaning rituals
- Counting rituals
- *Dipsomania*: a compulsion to drink alcohol
- Dressing rituals
- *Kleptomania*: a compulsion to steal
- *Nymphomania*: a compulsive need in the female to engage in sexual intercourse
- *Polydipsia*: a compulsion to drink water
- *Satyriasis*: a compulsive need in the male to engage in sexual intercourse
- *Trichotillomania*: a compulsion to pull out one's hair

1.1.2.5 Abnormal Posture and Movements

Particularly in schizophrenia, but sometimes also in other disorders such as catatonia and some learning disabilities, the following abnormal movements may occur: ambitendency, echopraxia, mannerisms, negativism, posturing, stereotypies, and waxy flexibility.

- *Ambitendency*. The person makes a series of tentative incomplete movements when expected to carry out a voluntary action. For example, a woman offers a handshake, then withdraws and

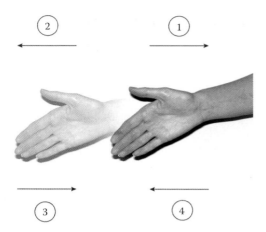

FIGURE 1.1   Ambitendency.

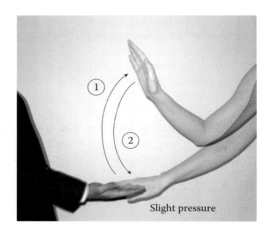

FIGURE 1.2   Mitgehen.

then offers again for 10 times. The examiner cannot make a handshake with her at the end (Figure 1.1).

- *Automatic obedience.* This refers to a condition where the person follows the examiner's instructions blindly without judgement and resistance. For example, the examiner asks the person to move his or her arm in different direction, and the person is unable to resist even if it is against his or her will.
- *Catalepsy.* This refers to abnormal maintenance of postures. For example, a person holds his or her arm in the air for a long time like a wax statue.
- *Cataplexy.* This refers to the temporary loss of muscle tone in narcolepsy. For example, a person develops temporary paralysis after emotional excitement.
- *Echopraxia.* This refers to the automatic imitation by the person of another person's movements. It occurs even when the person is asked not to. For example, when the consultant touches his or her spectacles with his or her right hand, the patient performs the same action even if he or she does not wear spectacles.
- *Mannerisms.* These are repeated involuntary movements that appear to be goal directed. For example, a person repeatedly moving his or her hand when he or she talks and tries to convey his or her message to the examiner.
- *Mitgehen.* This is the excessive limb movement in response to slight pressure of an applied force even when the person is told to resist movement. For example, the examiner wants to move the

person's arm upward and asks the person to resist movement. Even with a slight touch, the person continues to move his or her arm upward and then returns to the original position after the test (Figure 1.2).

- *Mitmachen.* This refers to the limb movement in response to an applied force to any direction without resistance. For example, the examiner wants to move the person's arm upward and asks the person not to move his or her limb and resist. The person's arm moves upward. When the examiner wants to move his or her arm downward, the person's arm moves downward without any resistance. At the end of examination, his or her arm returns to the original position (Figure 1.3).
- *Negativism.* This is a motiveless resistance to commands and to attempts to be moved.

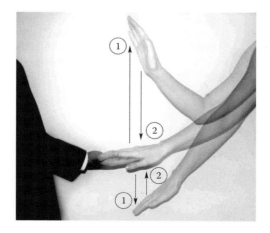

FIGURE 1.3   Mitmachen.

For example, the examiner asks the person to open his or her fist but he closes it tightly instead.

- *Posturing.* The person adopts an inappropriate or bizarre bodily posture continuously for a long time.
- *Stereotypies.* These are repeated regular fixed patterns of movement (or speech) that are not goal directed. For example, a person keeps on rubbing his or her right elbow with his or her left hand during the interview.
- *Waxy flexibility* (cerea flexibilitas). There is a feeling of plastic resistance resembling the bending of a soft wax rod as the examiner moves part of the person's body; that body part then remains 'moulded' by the examiner in the new position. For example, the examiner wants to move the person's arm upward. The person's arm moves in upward direction but stays in the same position for 3 h after the examination (Figure 1.4).
- *Tics.* These are repeated irregular movements involving a muscle group and may be seen following encephalitis, for example, in Huntington's disease and in Gilles de la Tourette's syndrome.
- *Parkinsonism.* The features of parkinsonism include
  - A resting tremor
  - Cogwheel rigidity
  - Postural abnormalities
  - A festinant gait

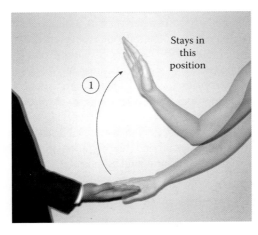

FIGURE 1.4 Waxy flexibility.

1.2 DISORDERS OF SPEECH

1.2.1 DISORDERS OF RATE, QUANTITY, AND ARTICULATION

- *Dysarthria.* This is difficulty in the articulation of speech.
- *Dysprosody.* This is speech with the loss of its normal melody.
- *Logorrhoea* (volubility). The speech is fluent and rambling with the use of many words.
- *Mutism.* This is the complete loss of speech.
- *Poverty of speech.* There is a restricted amount of speech. If the person replies to questions, he or she may do so with monosyllabic answers.
- *Pressure of speech.* There is an increase in both the quantity and rate of speech, which is difficult to interrupt.
- *Stammering.* The flow of speech is broken by pauses and the repetition of parts of words.
- *Verbigeration.* This refers to a form of stereotypy consisting of morbid repetition of words, phrases, or sentences.

1.2.2 DISORDERS OF THE FORM OF SPEECH

- *Approximate answer* (vorbeireden). This refers to an approximate answer that, although clearly incorrect, demonstrates the answer is known. For example, when asked 'how many legs does a duck have?' the person may reply 'three legs'. It is seen in the Ganser syndrome, first described in criminals awaiting trial.
- *Cryptolalia.* The speech is in a language that no one can understand.
- *Circumstantiality.* Thinking appears slow with the incorporation of unnecessary trivial details. The goal of thought is finally reached, however.
- *Echolalia.* This is the automatic imitation by the person of another person's speech. It occurs even when the person does not understand the speech (which may be in e.g. another language).
- *Flight of ideas.* The speech consists of a stream of accelerated thoughts with abrupt changes from topic to topic and no central direction. The connections between the thoughts may be based on the following:
  - Chance relationships.
  - *Clang associations.* A syllable of one word is associated with another word by sound (e.g. manic, garlic).

- Distracting stimuli.
- *Punning.* A humorous play of words.
- Verbal associations (e.g. alliteration and assonance).
- *Metonym.* Approximate but related term is used in an idiomatic way. For example, a person with schizophrenia refers cloud as 'sky sheep'.
- *Neologism.* A new word is constructed by the person or an everyday word used in a special way by the person.
- *Passing by the point* (vorbeigehen). The answers to questions, although clearly incorrect, demonstrate that the questions are understood. For example, when asked 'what colour is grass?' the person may reply 'blue'. It is seen in the Ganser syndrome.
- *Perseveration.* In perseveration (of both speech and movement), mental operations are continued beyond the point at which they are relevant. Particular types of perseveration of speech are
  - *Palilalia.* The person repeats a word with increasing frequency.
  - *Logoclonia.* The person repeats the last syllable of the last word.
- *Thought blocking.* There is a sudden interruption in the train of thought, before it is completed, leaving a 'blank'. After a period of silence, the person cannot recall what he or she had been saying or had been thinking of saying.

1.2.3 DISORDERS (LOOSENING) OF ASSOCIATION (FORMAL THOUGHT DISORDER)

These occur particularly in schizophrenia and may be considered to be a schizophrenic language disorder. Examples include knight's move thinking. The knight can go two squares forward, backward, left, or right and turn at a right angle. If the knight is blocked by another piece, the knight can jump over, and this refers to the abrupt change in schizophrenia speech (Figure 1.5).

In schizophrenia, there are odd tangential associations between ideas, leading to disruptions in the smooth continuity of the speech. Schizophasia, is, also called 'word salad' or 'speech confusion', in which the speech is an incoherent and incomprehensible mixture of words and phrases. Schneider described the following features of formal thought disorder:

- *Asyndesis.* Juxtaposition of elements without adequate linkage between them.
- *Condensation.* Combining ideas to make it incomprehensible.

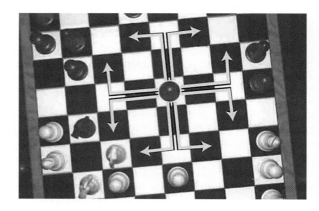

FIGURE 1.5   Knight's move thinking.

- *Derailment.* The thought derails onto a subsidiary thought.
- *Drivelling.* There is a disordered intermixture of the constituent parts of one complex thought.
- *Fusion.* Heterogeneous elements of thought are interwoven with each other.
- *Omission.* A thought or part of a thought is senselessly omitted.
- *Substitution.* A major thought is substituted by a subsidiary thought.

1.3   DISORDERS OF EMOTION

1.3.1 DISORDERS OF AFFECT

Affect is a pattern of observable behaviours that is the expression of a subjectively experienced feeling state (emotion) and is variable over time, in response to changing emotional states (DSM-IV-TR).

- *Blunted affect.* In a person with a blunted affect, the externalized feeling tone is severely reduced.
- *Flat affect.* This consists of a total or almost total absence of signs of expression of affect.
- *Inappropriate affect.* This is an affect that is inappropriate to the thought or speech it accompanies.
- *Labile affect.* A person with a labile affect has a labile externalized feeling tone that is not related to environmental stimuli.

1.3.2 DISORDERS OF MOOD

Mood is a pervasive and sustained emotion that, in the extreme, markedly colours the person's perception of the world (DSM-IV-TR).

- *Dysphoria.* This is an unpleasant mood.
- *Depression.* This is a low or depressed mood. It may be accompanied by anhedonia, in which the ability to enjoy pleasurable activities is lost. In normal grief or mourning, the sadness is appropriate to the loss.
- *Elation.* This is an elevated mood or exaggerated feeling of well-being that is pathological. It is seen in mania.
- *Euphoria.* This is a personal and subjective feeling of unconcern and contentment, usually seen after taking opiates or as a late sequel to head injury.
- *Irritability.* This is a liability to outbursts or a state of reduced control over aggressive impulses towards others. It may be a personality trait or may accompany anxiety. It also occurs in premenstrual syndrome.
- *Apathy.* There is a loss of emotional tone and the ability to feel pleasure, associated with detachment or indifference.
- *Alexithymia.* This is difficulty in the awareness of or description of one's emotions.

1.3.3 Disorders Related to Anxiety

- *Anxiety.* This is a feeling of apprehension, tension, or uneasiness owing to the anticipation of an external or internal danger. Types of anxiety include
  - *Phobic anxiety.* The focus of the anxiety is avoided (phobias are a disorder of thought content).
  - *Free-floating anxiety.* The anxiety is pervasive and unfocused.
  - *Panic attacks.* Anxiety is experienced in acute, episodic, intense attacks and may be accompanied by physiological symptoms.
  - *Fear.* This is anxiety caused by a realistic danger that is recognized at a conscious level.
  - *Agitation.* There is excessive motor activity associated with a feeling of inner tension.
  - *Tension.* There is an unpleasant increase in psychomotor activity.

1.4 DISORDERS OF THOUGHT CONTENT

1.4.1 Preoccupations

- *Hypochondriasis.* This is a preoccupation with a fear of having a serious illness that is not based on real organic pathology but instead on an unrealistic interpretation of physical signs or sensations as being abnormal.
- *Monomania.* This is a pathological preoccupation with a single object.
- *Egomania.* This is a pathological preoccupation with oneself.

1.4.2 Obsessions

Obsessions are repetitive senseless thoughts that are recognized as irrational by the person and that are unsuccessfully resisted. Themes include

- Aggression
- Dirt and contamination
- Fear of causing harm
- Religion
- Sex

1.4.3 Phobias

A phobia is a persistent irrational fear of an activity, object, or situation leading to avoidance. The fear is out of proportion to the real danger and cannot be reasoned away, being out of voluntary control. Some types of phobia are as follows:

- *Acrophobia.* The fear of heights.
- *Agoraphobia.* This literally means the fear of the marketplace. It is a syndrome with a generalized high anxiety level about, or avoidance of, places or situations from which escape might be difficult, or embarrassing, or in which help may not be available in the event of having a panic attack or panic-like symptoms. Objects of fear may include crowds, open and closed spaces, shopping, social situations, and travelling by public transport.
- *Algophobia.* The fear of pain
- *Claustrophobia.* The fear of closed spaces
- *Social phobia.* The fear of personal interactions in a public setting, such as public speaking, eating in public, and meeting people
- *Specific (simple) phobia.* The fear of discrete objects (e.g. snakes) or situations
- *Xenophobia.* The fear of strangers
- *Zoophobia.* The fear of animals
- *Phobias of internal stimuli.* These include obsessive phobias and illness phobias, which overlap with hypochondriasis

1.5   ABNORMAL BELIEFS AND INTERPRETATIONS OF EVENTS

1.5.1   OVERVALUED IDEAS

An overvalued idea is an unreasonable and sustained intense preoccupation maintained with less than delusional intensity, that is, the person is able to acknowledge the possibility that the belief may not be true. The idea or belief held is demonstrably false and is not one that is normally held by others of the person's subculture. There is a marked associated emotional investment.

1.5.2   DELUSIONS

A delusion is a false belief based on incorrect inference about external reality that is firmly sustained despite what almost everyone else believes and despite what constitutes incontrovertible and obvious proof or evidence to the contrary. The belief is not one ordinarily accepted by other members of the person's culture or subculture (e.g. it is not an article of religious faith). When a false belief involves a value judgement, it is regarded as a delusion only when the judgement is so extreme as to defy credibility (DSM-IV-TR).

- *Mood-congruent delusion.* The content of the delusion is appropriate to the mood of the person.
- *Mood-incongruent delusion.* The content of the delusion is not appropriate to the mood of the person.
- *Primary delusion.* A delusion that arises fully formed without any discernible connection with previous events. It may be preceded by a delusional mood in which the person is aware of something strange and threatening happening.
- *Bizarre delusion.* A delusion involving a phenomenon that the person's culture would regard as totally implausible.
- *Delusional jealousy* (pathological jealousy, Othello syndrome, delusion of infidelity). A delusion that one's sexual partner is unfaithful.
- *Delusion of being controlled.* Feelings, impulses, thoughts, or actions of the person are experienced as being under the control of some external force rather than under his or her own control.
- *Delusion of doubles* (l'illusion de sosies). A delusion that a person known to the person has been replaced by a double. It is seen in Capgras' syndrome. In contrast, l'illusion de Fregoli refers

to a delusion that a person known to the patient has been in disguise of different people.
- *Delusion of infestation* (Ekbom's syndrome). A delusion that one is infested by parasites.
- *Delusion of poverty.* A delusion that one is in poverty.
- *Delusion of pregnancy* (couvade syndrome). A delusion that one is pregnant (usually the husband of a pregnant wife).
- *Delusion of reference.* The theme is that events, objects, or other people in one's immediate environment have a particular and unusual significance. These delusions are usually of a negative or pejorative nature but also may be grandiose in content (DSM-IV). When similar thoughts are held with less than delusional intensity, they are ideas of reference.
- *Delusion of self-accusation.* A delusion of one's own guilt.
- *Doppelganger.* A delusion that a double of a person or place exists somewhere else.
- *Erotomania* (de Clérambault's syndrome). A delusion that another person, usually of higher status, is deeply in love with the individual.
- *Grandiose delusion.* A delusion of inflated worth, power, knowledge, identity, or special relationship to a deity or famous person.
- *Nihilistic delusion* (Cotard's syndrome). A delusion of death, disintegration of organs, and nonexistence.
- *Persecutory (querulant) delusion.* The central theme is that one (or someone to whom one is close) is being attacked, harassed, cheated, persecuted, or conspired against (DSM-IV-TR).
- *Somatic delusion.* A delusion whose main content pertains to the appearance or functioning of one's body (DSM-IV-TR).

1.5.3   PASSIVITY PHENOMENON

This is a delusional belief that an external agency is controlling aspects of the self that are normally entirely under one's own control. Passivity phenomena include the following:

- *Thought alienation.* The person believes that his or her thoughts are under the control of an outside agency or that others are participating in his or her thinking. This includes the following:
  - *Thought insertion.* The delusion that certain of one's thoughts are not one's own but rather are inserted into one's mind by an external agency.

- *Thought withdrawal.* The delusion that one's thoughts are being removed from one's mind by an external agency.
- *Thought broadcasting.* The delusion that one's thoughts are being broadcast out loud so that they can be perceived by others.
- *Made feelings.* This is the delusional belief that one's own free will has been removed and that an external agency is controlling one's feelings.
- *Made impulses.* This is the delusional belief that one's own free will has been removed and that an external agency is controlling one's impulses.
- *Made actions.* This is the delusional belief that one's own free will has been removed and that an external agency is controlling one's actions.
- *Somatic passivity.* This is the delusional belief that one is a passive recipient of somatic or bodily sensations from an external agency.

1.5.4 DELUSIONAL PERCEPTION

In a delusional perception, the person attaches a new and delusional significance to a familiar real perception without any logical reason.

1.6 ABNORMAL EXPERIENCES

1.6.1 SENSORY DISTORTIONS

- *Hyperesthesias.* These are changes in sensory perception in which there is an increased intensity of sensation. Hyperacusis is an increased sensitivity to sounds.
- *Hypoesthesias.* These are changes in sensory perception in which there is a decreased intensity of sensation. *Hypoacusis* is a decreased sensitivity to sounds.
- *Changes in quality.* Changes in quality of sensations occur particularly with visual stimuli, giving rise to visual distortions. Colourings of visual perceptions include
  - Chloropsia—green
  - Erythropsia—red
  - Xanthopsia—yellow
- *Dysmegalopsia.* Changes in spatial form include
  - *Macropsia.* Objects are seen larger or nearer than is actually the case.
  - *Micropsia.* Objects are seen smaller or farther away than is actually the case.

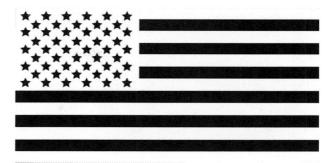

FIGURE 1.6   Afterimage.

1.6.2 SENSORY DECEPTIONS

1.6.2.1 Illusions

An illusion is a false perception of a real external stimulus.

- *Afterimage.* A visual illusion that refers to an image continuing to appear in one's vision after the exposure to the original image has ceased. Afterimage occurs after prolonged exposure to an unchanging visual stimulus such as inverted colour American flag due to the fatigue of cone cells in the retina (Figure 1.6).
- *Palinopia.* Prolonged afterimage.

1.6.2.2 Hallucinations

A hallucination is a false sensory perception in the absence of a real external stimulus. A hallucination is perceived as being located in objective space and as having the same realistic qualities as normal perceptions. It is not subject to conscious manipulation and only indicates a psychotic disturbance when there is also impaired reality testing. Hallucinations can be mood congruent or mood incongruent. Types of hallucination include the following:

- *Auditory.*
- *Simple auditory.* Sounds or musical.
- *Mood congruent complex auditory hallucination*:
  Stating depressive or manic themes in second person, for example, 'You are useless'.
  Command hallucination: 'Since you are useless, you should hurt yourself'.
- *Mood incongruent complex auditory hallucination*:
  Voices discussing the person in third person.
  Voices giving a running commentary on a person's behaviour.
  Thoughts spoken out loud (thought echo/écho de la pensée).

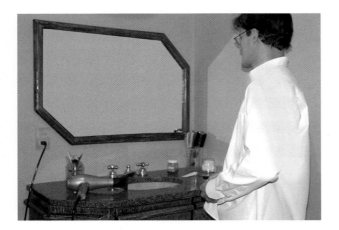

FIGURE 1.7   Negative autoscopy.

- *Autoscopy* (phantom mirror image). The person sees himself or herself and knows that it is he or she. Negative autoscopy occurs when a person looks into the mirror and cannot see one's image (Figure 1.7).
- *Cenesthesia*. The person feels that there is a change in tone in a part of the body.
- *Extracampine*. The hallucination occurs outside the person's sensory field.
- *Functional*. The stimulus causing the hallucination is experienced in addition to the hallucination itself.
- *Gustatory*. Taste hallucination.
- *Hallucinosis*. Hallucinations (usually auditory) occur in clear consciousness.
- *Hypnagogic*. The hallucination (usually visual or auditory) occurs while falling asleep.
- *Hypnopompic*. The hallucination (usually visual or auditory) occurs while waking from sleep.
- *Kinesthetic*. The hallucination occurs when there is a false sensation of body movement.
- *Lilliputian hallucination* (usually visual). Hallucinated objects appear greatly reduced in size.
- *Olfactory*.
- *Peduncular*. Vivid hallucinations (usually visual) in organic diseases.
- *Reflex*. A stimulus in one sensory field leads to a hallucination in another sensory field.
- *Somatic*. Somatic hallucinations include
  - *Tactile (haptic) hallucinations*. Superficial and usually involving sensations on or just under the skin in the absence of a

real stimulus; these include the sensation of insects crawling under the skin (*formication*).
  - *Visceral*. Hallucinations of deep sensations.
- *Trailing phenomenon*. Moving objects are seen as a series of discrete discontinuous images.
- *Visual*. Simple (e.g. flashlight) or complex (e.g. Charles de Bonnet syndrome). Charles de Bonnet syndrome refers to vivid and persisting hallucinations in people with central or peripheral reduction in vision.

1.6.2.3 Pseudohallucinations (Coined by Kandinsky in 1885)

A pseudohallucination is a form of imagery arising in the subjective inner space of the mind. It lacks the substantiality of normal perceptions and occupies subjective space rather than objective space. It is not subject to conscious manipulation. An *eidetic image* is a vivid and detailed reproduction of a previous perception. In *pareidolia*, vivid imagery occurs without conscious effort while looking at a poorly structured background (Figure 1.8 and Table 1.1).

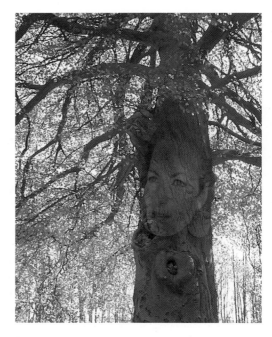

FIGURE 1.8   Pareidolia: seeing a woman's face when looking at the tree.

TABLE 1.1

Characteristics of Sensory Deceptions

Characteristics	Imagination (Fantasy)	Illusion	Pseudohallucination	Hallucination	Real Perception
Voluntary or involuntary	Voluntary	Involuntary	Involuntary (except eidetic imagery)	Involuntary	Involuntary
Vividness	Not vivid	Vivid	Vivid	Vivid	Vivid
Space	Inner subjective space	Inner subjective space	Inner subjective space	Outer space	Outer space
Insight	Intact	Intact	Intact	Impaired	Intact
Examples	Normal experience	Delirium	Depression	Schizophrenia	Normal experience

1.7 DISORDERS OF SELF-AWARENESS (EGO DISORDERS)

These include disturbances of

- Awareness of self-activity, including
  - *Depersonalization.* One feels that one is altered or not real in some way
  - *Derealization.* The surroundings do not seem real
- The immediate awareness of self-unity
- The continuity of self
- The boundaries of the self

1.8 COGNITIVE DISORDERS

1.8.1 DISORIENTATION

This is a disturbance of orientation in time, place, or person.

1.8.2 DISORDERS OF ATTENTION

- *Distractibility.* A distractible subject's attention is drawn too frequently to unimportant or irrelevant external stimuli.
- *Selective inattention.* In selective inattention, anxiety-provoking stimuli are blocked out.

1.8.3 DISORDERS OF MEMORY

- *Amnesia.* This is the inability to recall past experiences.
  - *Anterograde amnesia.* This refers to inability to form new memories due to failure to consolidate or inability to retrieve.
  - *Posttraumatic amnesia.* This refers to memory loss from the time of accident to the time that the person can give a clear account of the recent events. It tends to remain unchanged.

- *Psychogenic amnesia.* This is a part of the dissociative disorder consisting of a sudden inability to recall important personal data. It is associated with 'la belle indifference' (lack of concerns) with highly unpredictable course.
- *Retrograde amnesia.* This refers to loss of memory for events that occurred prior to the event (e.g. intoxication and head injury). It tends to improve with more distant events in the past recover first. In general, the retrograde amnesia is shorter than posttraumatic amnesia.
- *Transient global amnesia.* The person presents with abrupt onset of disorientation, loss of ability to encode recent memories, and retrograde amnesia for variable durations. This episode usually lasts for a few hours and is never repeated. The aetiology is due to transient ischaemia of the hippocampus–fornix–hypothalamus system.
- *Hypermnesia.* In hypermnesia, the degree of retention and recall is exaggerated.
- *Paramnesia.* A paramnesia is a distorted recall leading to falsification of memory. Paramnesias include the following:
  - *Confabulation.* Gaps in memory are unconsciously filled with false memories.
  - *Déjà vu.* The *subject* feels that the current situation has been seen or experienced before.
  - *Déjà entendu.* The *illusion* of auditory recognition.
  - *Déjà pensé.* The *illusion* of recognition of a new thought.
  - *Jamais vu.* The *illusion* of failure to recognize a familiar situation.
  - *Retrospective falsification.* False details are added to the recollection of an otherwise real memory.

1.8.4 DISORDERS OF INTELLIGENCE

- *Learning disability* (mental retardation). Learning difficulty or mental retardation is classified by DSM-IV-TR and ICD-10 according to the intelligence quotient (IQ) of the subject:
  $50 \leq IQ \leq 70$ ($50 \leq IQ \leq 69$ in ICD-10): mild mental retardation
  $35 \leq IQ \leq 49$: moderate mental retardation
  $20 \leq IQ \leq 34$: severe mental retardation
  $IQ \leq 20$: profound mental retardation
- *Dementia.* This is a global organic impairment of intellectual functioning without impairment of consciousness.
- *Pseudodementia.* This resembles dementia clinically, but is not organic in origin.

1.8.5 DISORDERS OF CONSCIOUSNESS

1.8.5.1 Levels of Consciousness

The neurological terms used to describe progressively more unconscious levels are as follows:

- *Somnolence* (drowsiness). A subject who is drowsy or somnolent can be awoken by mild stimuli and will be able to speak comprehensibly, albeit perhaps for only a little while before falling asleep again.
- *Stupor.* A stuporous person responds to pain and loud sounds. Brief monosyllabic utterances and some spontaneous motor activity may occur.
- *Semicoma.* A semicomatose person will withdraw from the source of pain, but spontaneous motor activity does not take place.
- *Deep coma.* No response can be elicited, and there is no response to deep pain nor is there any spontaneous movement. Tendon, pupillary, and corneal reflexes are usually absent.
- *Death.*

1.8.5.2 Clouding of Consciousness

The person is drowsy and does not react completely to stimuli. There is a disturbance of attention, concentration, memory, orientation, and thinking.

1.8.5.3 Delirium

The person is bewildered, disoriented, and restless. There may be associated fear and hallucinations. Variations include the following:

- *Oneiroid state.* A dreamlike state in a person who is not asleep
- *Torpor.* The person is drowsy and easily falls asleep
- *Twilight state*: A prolonged oneiroid state of disturbed consciousness with hallucinations

1.8.5.4 Fugue

This is a state of wandering from the usual surroundings in which there is also loss of memory.

1.8.5.5 Aphasias

- *Receptive (sensory) aphasia* (Wernicke's fluent aphasia). Difficulty is experienced in comprehending the meaning of words. Types include the following:
  Agnostic alexia: Words can be seen but cannot be read.
  Pure word deafness: Words that are heard and cannot be comprehended.
  Visual asymbolia: Words can be transcribed but cannot be read.
- *Intermediate aphasia.* Types of intermediate aphasia include
  Central (syntactical) aphasia: There is difficulty in arranging words in their proper sequence.
  Nominal aphasia (anomia): There is difficulty in naming objects. The person may use circumlocutions (speaking in a roundabout way) to express certain words (e.g. the person cannot name the 'clock' but labels the clock as 'the thing which tells time').
- *Expressive (motor) aphasia* (Broca's nonfluent aphasia). This refers to difficulty in expressing thoughts in words while comprehension remains.
- *Global aphasia.* Both receptive aphasia and expressive aphasia are present at the same time.
- *Jargon aphasia*: The person utters incoherent meaningless neologistic speech.
- *Semantic aphasia.* This refers to errors in using the target words due to deficits in semantic memory. It is associated with left temporal lobe tumours (e.g. orange is named as apple) (Table 1.2).

1.9 DYSLEXIA

Dyslexia refers to pure word blindness. Developmental dyslexia involves difficulty in reading, erratic spelling, and lack of capacity to apply written language. Half of the people with dyslexia also have achromatopsia (colour blindness).

TABLE 1.2
Summary of Aphasic Syndromes

Types of Aphasia	Fluency	Repetition	Comprehension	Naming
Anomic	Fluent	☑	☑	☒
Conduction	Fluent	☒	☑	☒
Broca's	Nonfluent	☒	☑	☒
Lesion in arcuate fasciculus	Fluent	☒	☑	☒
Wernicke's	Fluent	☒	☒	☒
Transcortical motor	Nonfluent	☑	☑	☒
Transcortical sensory	Fluent	☑	☒	☒
Global	Nonfluent	☒	☒	☒

☑: Intact ☒: Impaired

- *Surface dyslexia.* This is due to lesions in left temporoparietal region. The person breaks down the whole word (lexical reading) and has difficulty to deal with the irregularly spelt words. Reliance is placed on subword correspondence between letters and sounds but not the normal way: spelling to sound (e.g. big is read as dig).
- *Deep dyslexia.* This is due to extensive left hemisphere lesions. This occurs when the person produces verbal response based on the meaning of the word but not based on sound-based reading (e.g. sister is read as auntie**).**
- *Neglect dyslexia.* This usually occurs when the left half of the word is being ignored due to right parietal lobe lesion (e.g. bicycle is read as cycle). If the lesion is found in the left hemisphere, then the right half of the word is affected.

1.10   AGRAPHIA

Agraphia refers to impaired writing ability.

- *Lexical agraphia.* This is due to lesions in the left temporoparietal region. The person breaks down the word's spelling and has difficulty in writing irregular words (e.g. 'cough' is written as 'coff' as phonologically similar).
- *Neglect agraphia.* This is due to the right hemispheric lesions and leads to misspelling of the initial part of a word.
- *Dyspraxic agraphia.* This is due to dominant frontal or parietal lobe lesions. This leads to

defective copying although the person can spell correctly. The person has difficulty in writing the smooth part of a letter. Letter may be inverted or reversed (e.g. 'A' is written as '∀').

1.11   ALEXIA

Alexia refers to reading disorder that affects learning and academic skills.

- *Alexia with agraphia.* The person cannot read, write, or connect letters due to lesions of the angular or supramarginal gyrus.
- *Alexia without agraphia.* The person cannot comprehend any written material but he can write. This is due to occlusion of left posterior cerebral artery leading to infarction of the medial aspect of the left occipital lobe and the splenium of the corpus callosum.

1.12   ACALCULIA

Acalculia refers to a disturbance in the ability to comprehend or write numbers properly. This is due to lesion in the left angular gyrus.

1.13   APRAXIAS AND AGNOSIAS

1.13.1   Apraxias

Apraxia is an inability to perform purposive volitional acts, which does not result from paresis, incoordination, sensory loss, or involuntary movements. It may be considered to be the motor equivalent of agnosia.

- *Constructional apraxia.* There is difficulty in constructing objects or copying drawings (e.g. double pentagon). It is associated with non-dominant parietal lobe. This is closely associated with visuospatial agnosia, with some authorities treating the two as being essentially the same.
- *Dressing apraxia.* There is difficulty in putting on one's clothes correctly. It is associated with nondominant parietal lobe.
- *Ideomotor apraxia.* There is difficulty in carrying out progressively more difficult tasks, for example, involving touching parts of the face with specified fingers and in demonstrating the use of household items (e.g. toothbrush). It is associated with left parietal and frontal lobe lesions.
- *Ideational apraxia.* There is difficulty in carrying out a coordinated sequence of actions, but the individual components of the sequence can be successfully performed (e.g. a person cannot work in a café as he or she cannot make tea and serve the others. If you ask him or her to put a tea bag into the cup, he or she is able to do it). It is associated with lesions in corpus callosum.
- *Orobuccal apraxia.* There is difficulty in performing skilled movements of the face, lips, tongue, cheek, larynx, and pharynx (e.g. when a person is asked to pretend to blow out a match or suck a straw, he or she makes incorrect movements). It is associated with lesions in left inferior frontal lobe and insula.

1.13.2 AGNOSIAS AND DISORDERS OF BODY IMAGE

Agnosia is an inability to interpret and recognize the significance of sensory information, which does not result from impairment of the sensory pathways, mental deterioration, disorders of consciousness and attention, or, in the case of an object, a lack of familiarity with the object.

- *Visuospatial agnosia.* See 'constructional apraxia' earlier.
- *Visual (object) agnosia.* A familiar object, which can be seen though not recognized by sight, can be recognized through another modality such as touch or hearing.

- *Apperceptive visual agnosia.* The person is unable to copy shapes or discriminate two versions of the same object. Further details are considered in Chapter 7.
- *Associative visual agnosia.* The person is unable to recognize visually presented objects but able to copy objects that they cannot recognize. Further details are considered in Chapter 7.
- *Prosopagnosia.* This is an inability to recognize faces. In the *mirror sign*, which may occur in advanced Alzheimer's disease, a person may misidentify his or her own mirrored reflection.
- *Agnosia for colours.* The person is unable correctly to name colours, although colour sense is still present.
- *Simultanagnosia.* The person is unable to recognize the overall meaning of a picture, whereas its individual details are understood.
- *Agraphognosia or agraphesthesia.* The person is unable to identify, with closed eyes, numbers or letters traced on his or her palm.
- *Anosognosia.* There is a lack of awareness of disease, particularly of hemiplegia (most often following a right parietal lesion).
- *Coenestopathic state.* There is a localized distortion of body awareness.
- *Autotopagnosia.* This is an inability to name, recognize, or point on command to parts of the body.
- *Astereognosia.* Objects cannot be recognized by palpation.
- *Finger agnosia.* The person is unable to recognize individual fingers, be they his or her own or those of another person.
- *Topographical disorientation.* This can be tested by using a locomotor map-reading task in which the person is asked to trace out a given route by foot.
- *Distorted awareness of size and shape.* For example, a limb may be felt to be growing larger.
- *Hemisomatognosis or hemidepersonalization.* The person feels that a limb (which in fact is present) is missing.
- *Phantom limb.* The continued awareness occurs of the presence of a limb that has been removed.
- *Reduplication phenomenon.* The person feels that part or all of the body has been duplicated.

CLINICAL ASSESSMENT OF SKILLS AND COMPETENCIES (CASC)
STATION 1: A MAN WITH VISUAL HALLUCINATIONS

A 60-year-old man admitted to the orthopaedic ward was found to have a fractured tibia. He was brought in by the police prior to admission and told them he saw Spanish guerrillas. He also complains of seeing small animals and spiders around him.

Tasks: Assess his psychopathology and perform a risk assessment.

CASC Grid
The person can be frightened by his seeing Spanish guerrilla and be anticipated that your interview will be disrupted. Candidates are required to empathize with his fear from time to time.

A. Visual hallucinations	A1. 'Have you seen things that other people can't see?'	A2. 'What do you see? Can you give me an example? Are they very small?'	A3. 'How long have you been seeing those things? When do those things you saw appear? Do they usually come at night?'	A4. 'How do you feel when you see them?' Empathize with the patient: 'I can imagine that this is a frightening experience for you'. 'Do you feel that they are real? Can you stop them?'	A5. 'Do you have any explanation of above experience? Do you need help?'
B. Auditory hallucinations	B1. 'Do you hear sounds or voices others do not hear?'	B2. If there are voices, then ask 'How many voices are there?'	B3. 'What do they say?'	B4. 'How do you feel when you hear them?'	B5. 'Are you alert at that time when you hear those voices?'
C. Other hallucinations, persecutory ideas, and jealousy	C1. Olfactory: 'Is there anything wrong about the way you smell? Can you tell me more about it? Who sent the gas to you?'	C2. Gustatory: 'Have you noticed that food or drink seems to have a different taste recently?'	C3. Somatic: 'Have you had any strange feelings in your body? How about people touching you? How about insects crawling?'	C4. Persecutory ideas: 'Do you think someone is trying to harm you? How about watching or spying on you?'	C5. Jealousy: 'Can you tell me about your relationship? Do you feel that your partner is unfaithful? If so, what's your evidence?'
D. Alcohol and drug history	D1. 'Do you drink alcohol? If so, how often do you drink?'	D2. 'When did you start to drink? Have you increased your alcohol intake recently?'	D3. 'When was your last drink? You have told me that you started to see those things for 2 days. Did you drink a lot on that day?'	D4. 'Have you tried to quit alcohol? What was the outcome?'	D5. 'Do you use other drugs? Do you have other medical problems such as fit or head injury?'
E. Risk/ comorbidity/ social support	E1. Suicide risk: 'I can imagine that you are frightened and stressed? Some people may want to give up. Do you have thought of ending your life?'	E2. Risk on others: 'How about taking revenge on those small people? How about the other people?'	E3. Comorbidity: 'Some people started to drink to overcome depression and anxiety. Do you have such problems? How is your sleep at night?'	E4. Forensic history: 'Have you been involved with the justice system? Do you drive? Can you tell me more about your driving record?'	E5. Social history: 'Where do you stay at this moment?' 'Are you staying alone?' 'Do you get any support from others?'

CASC STATION 2: A PATIENT WITH DELUSION OF LOVE

Mr. P comes to the clinic and requests to see a female psychiatric trainee called Eva. He came to the clinic 1 week ago and she treated him. He firmly believes Eva is in love with him and he wants to make love with her. He hid a knife in his bag and prepared to attack someone if he is not allowed to see Eva.

Task: (1) Explore his belief and psychopathology. (2) Assess his risks.

CASC Grid

The patient may be aggressive and hostile. You need to spend time to build rapport. Be prepared that he will shout for the name of his love, 'Eva, Eva, Eva'. Pay attention to nonverbal cues as the patient may hold a bag with a knife in it. Inform the examiner that you will disarm the patient in real practice.

A. Establish rapport	A1. 'What is your relationship with Eva?'	A2. 'She is off duty now. Can I pass a message to her?'	A3. Acknowledge his eagerness to see Eva but no false promise.	A4. 'In the meantime, I was asked by Eva to talk to you?'	A5. 'I am here to help you. I want to hear your views in your own words.'
B. Delusion of love	B1. Onset: 'When did Eva start to love you?'	B2. Precipitant: 'What happened before that?'	B3. Evidence: 'How do you know that Eva loves you?'	B4. Intensity: 'From a scale of 1–10 (1 = unlikely, 10 = very likely), can you tell me how likely that Eva loves you?'	B5. Shake his delusion: 'Based on the information provided, Eva only met you once. How can you be so certain that she likes you? Is there any other explanation?'
C. Other symptoms and substance misuse	C1. Mood: 'How do you feel at this moment? Can you tell me more about your mood?'	C2. Biological symptoms: Sleep Appetite sexual drive, sexual activity, and unprotected sex 'Besides Eva, have you made a lot of new friends lately?'	C3. Grandiose thought: 'When compared to the others, are you superior? How would you feel if Eva rejects you?'	C4. Hallucinations/passivity: 'Do you hear voices? Are you in control in yourself?'	C5. Substance misuse: 'Do you use any recreational drugs? How about alcohol?'
D. Risk assessment	D1. Explore the bag: 'What is inside your bag?' Mr. P: 'There is a knife inside'.	D2. 'What are you going to do with the knife?' Inform the examiner that you will call in the security to disarm the patient.	D3. Risk on Eva: 'Do you know where Eva stays? Have you followed her before? Have you sent e-mail to her?'	D4. Self-harm: 'Do you have thought of harming yourself?'	D5. Risk to others: 'If someone stops you from seeing Eva, what would you do?'
E. Background history	E1. Forensic history: 'Were you involved with the justice system before?'	E2. Occupational history: 'Are you employed at this moment?' 'May I know the nature of your work?'	E3. Social history: 'Where do you stay at this moment?' 'Are you staying alone?'	E4. Relationship history: 'Can you tell me more about your relationship in the past?'	E5. Willingness for treatment: 'I can imagine that you are quite stressed when searching for Eva, can I offer you some help such as medication?'

BIBLIOGRAPHY

American Psychiatric Association. 2000: *DSM-IV-TR: Diagnostic and Statistical Manual of Mental Disorders*, 4th edn, text revision. Washington, DC: American Psychiatric Association Publishing Inc.

Campbell RJ. 1996: *Psychiatric Dictionary*. Oxford, U.K.: Oxford University Press.

Hamilton M. (ed.) 1985: *Fish's Clinical Psychopathology*, 2nd edn. Bristol, U.K.: Wright.

Hodges J. 2002: *Cognitive Assessment for Clinicians*. Oxford, U.K.: Oxford University Press.

Institute of Psychiatry. 1973: *Notes on Eliciting and Recording Clinical Information*. Oxford, U.K.: Oxford University Press.

Leff JP and Isaacs AD. 1990: *Psychiatric Examination in Clinical Practice*, 3rd edn. Oxford, U.K.: Blackwell Scientific.

Sadock BJ and Sadock VA. 2007: *Kaplan & Sadock's Synopsis of Psychiatry. Behavioural Sciences/Clinical Psychiatry*, 10th edn. Philadelphia, PA: Lippincott Williams & Wilkins.

Sims ACP. 1985: *Symptoms in the Mind*. London, U.K.: Baillière Tindall.

2 Classification

The main classification systems in use at the time of writing are as follows:

- Mental and behavioural disorders of the *International Classification of Diseases*, 10th edn. (ICD-10) of the World Health Organization (WHO), published in 1992
- *The Diagnostic and Statistical Manual of Mental Disorders*, 4th edn., text revision (DSM-IV-TR) of the American Psychiatric Association (APA), published in 2000

2.1 HISTORY OF CLASSIFICATION SCHEMES

2.1.1 ANCIENT GREEKS

The classification of mental illness proposed by Hippocrates (circa 460 BCE to circa 370 BCE) and his Hippocratic School of Medicine included the following categories:

- Mania
- Melancholia
- Paranoia
- Phobias
- Scythian disease (i.e. transvestism)

These were believed to be based on abnormalities in the levels and balance of the following four humours or cambia:

- Blood
- Yellow bile
- Black bile
- Phlegm

2.1.2 ANCIENT ROMANS

An ancient Roman (of Greek ancestry), Galen of Pergamon (CE 129 to circa 216), identified the following human temperaments based on the aforementioned humours or cambia, in which combinations of four qualities (warm, cold, moist, and dry) were said to occur:

- *Blood*. sanguine (extroverted, social)—warm and moist
- *Yellow bile*. choleric (charismatic, passionate, energy)—warm and dry

- *Black bile*. melancholic (considerate, creative, kind)—cold and dry
- *Phlegm*. phlegmatic (affectionate, dependable, kind)—cold and moist

2.1.3 CULLEN

William Cullen (1710–1790) of Edinburgh published a classification of diseases that was widely used in the English-speaking world (Doig et al., 1993). His classification of the neuroses was fourfold:

- Adynamias
- Coma
- Spasms
- Vesanias, which included amentia, mania, melancholia, and oneirodynia

2.2 ICD

A classification section for mental disorders first appeared in ICD-6 (1949) (WHO, 1990). At the time of writing, ICD-11 is being prepared and parts of it are undergoing field testing. It is probably due to be published by 2015.

2.3 DSM

DSM-I (1952) was essentially based on the mental disorders section of ICD-6 (Grob, 1991). There was a strong psychodynamic influence evident in DSM-I; for example, the widespread use of the term 'reaction' was based on Adolf Meyer's psychobiological viewpoint. The term reaction was removed from DSM-II (1968) (Kirk and Kutchins, 1994).

1. DSM-III (1980) was an innovative psychiatric classification system that tried not to appear favourably disposed to competing etiological theories and that introduced the following (APA, 1985):
   a. Operational diagnostic criteria
   b. A multiaxial classification

17

DSM-III was revised (and corrected) and published as DSM-III-R in 1987 (Wilson, 1993).

2. DSM-IV and DSM-IV-TR was published in 1994 and 2000 respectively. DSM-5 is essentially the version in use at the time of writing.

2.4   ICD-10 (WHO, 1992)

2.4.1   Organic, Including Symptomatic, Mental Disorders

F00	Dementia in Alzheimer's disease
F01	Vascular dementia
F02	Dementia in other diseases classified elsewhere
F03	Unspecified dementia
F04	Organic amnesic syndrome, not induced by alcohol and other psychoactive substances
F05	Delirium, not induced by alcohol and other psychoactive substances
F06	Other mental disorders caused by brain damage and dysfunction and by physical disease
F07	Personality and behavioural disorders caused by brain disease, damage, and dysfunction
F09	Unspecified organic or symptomatic mental disorder

Mental and behavioural disorders caused by psychoactive substance use

F10	Mental and behavioural disorders caused by the use of alcohol
F11	Mental and behavioural disorders caused by the use of opioids
F12	Mental and behavioural disorders caused by the use of cannabinoids
F13	Mental and behavioural disorders caused by the use of sedatives or hypnotics
F14	Mental and behavioural disorders caused by the use of cocaine
F15	Mental and behavioural disorders caused by the use of other stimulants, including caffeine
F16	Mental and behavioural disorders caused by the use of hallucinogens
F17	Mental and behavioural disorders caused by the use of tobacco
F18	Mental and behavioural disorders caused by the use of volatile solvents
F19	Mental and behavioural disorders caused by multiple drug use and the use of other psychoactive substances

2.4.2   Schizophrenia, Schizotypal, and Delusional Disorders

F20	Schizophrenia
F21	Schizotypal disorder
F22	Persistent delusional disorders
F23	Acute and transient psychotic disorders
F24	Induced delusional disorder
F25	Schizoaffective disorders
F28	Other nonorganic psychotic disorders
F29	Unspecified nonorganic psychosis

2.4.3   Mood (Affective) Disorders

F30	Manic episode
F31	Bipolar affective disorder
F32	Depressive episode
F33	Recurrent depressive disorder
F34	Persistent mood (affective) disorders
F35	Other mood (affective) disorders
F39	Unspecified mood (affective) disorder

2.4.4   Neurotic, Stress-Related, and Somatoform Disorders

F40	Phobic anxiety disorders
F41	Other anxiety disorders
F42	Obsessive–compulsive disorder
F43	Reaction to severe stress and adjustment disorders
F44	Dissociative (conversion) disorders
F45	Somatoform disorders
F48	Other neurotic disorders

2.4.5   Behavioural Syndromes Associated with Physiological Disturbances and Physical Factors

F50	Eating disorders
F51	Nonorganic sleep disorders
F52	Sexual dysfunction, not caused by organic disorder or disease
F53	Mental and behavioural disorders associated with the puerperium, not elsewhere classified
F54	Psychological and behavioural factors associated with disorders or diseases classified elsewhere
F55	Abuse of nondependence-producing substances
F59	Unspecified behavioural syndromes associated with physiological disturbances and physical factors

2.4.6 DISORDERS OF ADULT PERSONALITY AND BEHAVIOUR

F60 Specific personality disorders
F61 Mixed and other personality disorders
F62 Enduring personality changes, not attributable to brain damage and disease
F63 Habit and impulse disorders
F64 Gender identity disorders
F65 Disorders of sexual preference
F66 Psychological and behavioural disorders associated with sexual development and orientation
F68 Other disorders of adult personality and behaviour
F69 Unspecified disorder of adult personality and behaviour

2.4.7 MENTAL RETARDATION

F70 Mild mental retardation
F71 Moderate mental retardation
F72 Severe mental retardation
F73 Profound mental retardation
F78 Other mental retardation
F79 Unspecified mental retardation

2.4.8 DISORDERS OF PSYCHOLOGICAL DEVELOPMENT

F80 Specific developmental disorders of speech and language
F81 Specific developmental disorders of scholastic skills
F82 Specific developmental disorder of motor function
F83 Mixed specific developmental disorders
F84 Pervasive developmental disorders
F88 Other disorders of psychological development
F89 Unspecified disorder of psychological development

2.4.9 BEHAVIOURAL AND EMOTIONAL DISORDERS WITH ONSET USUALLY OCCURRING IN CHILDHOOD AND ADOLESCENCE

F90 Hyperkinetic disorders
F91 Conduct disorders
F92 Mixed disorders of conduct and emotions
F93 Emotional disorders with onset specific to childhood
F94 Disorders of social functioning with onset specific to childhood and adolescence
F95 Tic disorders

F98 Other behavioural and emotional disorders with onset usually occurring in childhood and adolescence
      Unspecified mental disorder
F99 Mental disorder, not otherwise specified

2.5 DSM-IV-TR AND DSM-5

This is a multiaxial classification with the following five axes:

Axis I Clinical disorders and other conditions that may be a focus of clinical attention
Axis II Personality disorders and mental retardation
Axis III General medical conditions
Axis IV Psychosocial and environmental problems
Axis V Global assessment of functioning

In the following summary, NOS stands for 'not otherwise specified'.

2.5.1 AXIS I: CLINICAL DISORDERS; OTHER CONDITIONS THAT MAY BE A FOCUS OF CLINICAL ATTENTION

2.5.1.1 DSM-IV-TR and DSM-5: Disorders Usually First Diagnosed in Infancy, Childhood, or Adolescence (Excluding Mental Retardation Which Is Diagnosed on Axis II)

Learning disorder
Motor skills disorder
Communication disorders
Pervasive developmental disorders

- Autistic disorder
- Rett's disorder
- Childhood disintegrative disorder
- Asperger's disorder
- NOS

Attention-deficit and disruptive behaviour disorders
Feeding and eating disorders of infancy and early childhood
Tic disorders
Elimination disorders

- Encopresis
- Enuresis

Other disorders of infancy, childhood, or adolescence

DSM-5 (APA, 2013)
Intellectual developmental disorders

- 319 Intellectual developmental disorder (mild, moderate, severe, and profound)
- 315.8 Global developmental delay

Communication disorders

- 315.39 Language disorder
- 315.39 Speech disorder
- 315.39 Social communication disorder
- 315.35 Childhood-onset fluency disorder

299 Autism spectrum disorder
314 Attention deficit/hyperactivity disorder

- 314.00 Attention deficit/hyperactivity disorder/combined type
- 314.01 Attention deficit/hyperactivity disorder not elsewhere classified

315 Specific learning disorder (reading, writing, and mathematics)

Motor disorders

- 315.4 Developmental coordination disorder
- 307.3 Stereotypic movement disorder
- 307.33 Tourette's disorder
- 307.22 Chronic motor or vocal tic disorder
- 307.21 Provisional tic disorder
- 307.20 Tic disorder not elsewhere classified

2.5.1.2 DSM-IV-TR and DSM-5: Delirium, Dementia, and Amnestic and Other Cognitive Disorders

- Delirium
- Dementia
- Amnestic disorders
- Other cognitive disorders

DSM-5 (APA, 2013)
292 Delirium

- Substance-induced delirium
- Delirium not elsewhere classified

Mild and major neurocognitive disorder

Subtypes of major and mild neurocognitive disorders

- 305 Neurocognitive disorder due to Alzheimer's disease
- 306 Frontotemporal neurocognitive disorder
- 310 Neurocogntive disorder due to traumatic brain injury
- 308 Neurocognitive disorder due to Lewy body dementia
- 316 Neurocognitive disorder due to Parkinson's disease
- 315 Neurocognitive disorder due to HIV infection
- 311 Substance-induced neurocognitive disorder
- 317 Neurocognitive disorder due to Huntington's disease
- 316 Neurocognitive disorder due to prion disease
- 318 Neurocognitive disorder due to another medical condition
- 320 Neurocognitive disorder not elsewhere classified

2.5.1.3 DSM-IV-TR and DSM-5: Substance-Related Disorders

- Alcohol-related disorders
- Amphetamine (or amphetamine-like)-related disorders
- Caffeine-related disorders
- Cannabis-related disorders
- Cocaine-related disorders
- Hallucinogen-related disorders
- Inhalant-related disorders
- Nicotine-related disorders
- Opioid-related disorders
- Phencyclidine (or phencyclidine-like)-related disorders
- Sedative-, hypnotic-, or anxiolytic-related disorders
- Polysubstance-related disorders
- Other (or unknown) substance-related disorders

DSM-5 (APA, 2013)
Alcohol-related disorders

- 305 Alcohol use disorder
- 303 Alcohol intoxication
- 291.81 Alcohol withdrawal
- 291.9 Alcohol-induced disorder not elsewhere classified

Caffeine-related disorders

- 305.9 Caffeine intoxication
- 292.0 Caffeine withdrawal
- 292.9 Caffeine-induced disorder not elsewhere classified

Cannabis-related disorders

- 305.2 Cannabis use disorder
- 292.89 Cannabis intoxication
- 292.0 Cannabis withdrawal
- 292.9 Cannabis-induced disorder not elsewhere classified

Hallucinogen-related disorders

- 305.9 Hallucinogen use disorder
- 292.89 Hallucinogen intoxication
- 292.89 Hallucinogen persisting perception disorder
- 292.9 Hallucinogen-induced disorder not elsewhere classified

Inhalant-related disorders

- 305.9 Inhalant use disorder
- 292.89 Inhalant intoxication
- 292.9 Inhalant-induced disorder not elsewhere classified

Opioid-related disorders

- 305.5 Opioid use disorder
- 292.89 Opioid intoxication
- 292.0 Opioid withdrawal
- 292.9 Opioid-induced disorder not elsewhere classified

Sedative/hypnotic-related disorders

- 305.4 Sedative/hypnotic use disorder
- 292.89 Sedative/hypnotic intoxication
- 292.0 Sedative/hypnotic withdrawal
- 292.9 Sedative/hypnotic-induced disorder not elsewhere classified

Stimulant-related disorders

- 305.7 Stimulant use disorder
- 292.89 Stimulant intoxication
- 292.0 Stimulant withdrawal
- 292.9 Stimulant-induced disorders not elsewhere classified

Tobacco-related disorders

- 305.1 Tobacco use disorder
- 292.0 Tobacco withdrawal

Unknown substance disorders

- 305.9 Unknown substance use disorder
- 292.89 Unknown substance intoxication
- 292.0 Unknown substance withdrawal
- 292.9 Unknown substance-induced disorder not elsewhere classified

312.31 Gambling disorder

Recommended for further study by DSM-5

- Caffeine use disorder
- Internet use disorder
- Neurobehavioural disorder associated with pre-natal alcohol exposure

2.5.1.4 DSM-IV-TR and DSM-5: Schizophrenia and Other Psychotic Disorders

- Schizophrenia
- Schizophreniform disorder
- Schizoaffective disorder
- Delusional disorder
- Brief psychotic disorder
- Shared psychotic disorder
- Psychotic disorder caused by a general medical condition
- Substance-induced psychotic disorder
- Psychotic disorder
- NOS

DSM-5 (APA, 2013)
    301.22 Schizotypal personality disorder
    297.1 Delusional disorder
    298.8 Brief psychotic disorder
        Substance-induced psychotic disorder

Psychotic disorder associated with another medical condition
293.89 Catatonic disorder associated with another medical condition
295.40 Schizophreniform disorder
295.70 Schizoaffective disorder
295.90 Schizophrenia
    Psychotic disorder not elsewhere classified
    Catatonic disorder not elsewhere classified

- Mood disorders

2.5.1.5   DSM-IV-TR and DSM-5: Depressive Disorders
DSM-5 (APA, 2013)
296.99 Disruptive mood dysregulation disorder
296.2 Major depressive disorder, single episode
296.3 Major depressive disorder, recurrent
300.4 Dysthymic disorder
625.4 Premenstrual dysphoric disorder
    Substance-induced depressive disorder
293.83 Depressive disorder associated with another medical condition
311 Depressive disorder not elsewhere classified

2.5.1.6   DSM-IV-TR and DSM-5: Bipolar Disorders
DSM-5 (APA, 2013)
296.4 Bipolar I disorder
296.89 Bipolar II disorder
301.13 Cyclothymic disorder
    Substance-induced bipolar disorder
293.83 Bipolar disorder associated with another medical condition
296.80 Bipolar disorder not elsewhere classified

2.5.1.7   DSM-IV-TR and DSM-5: Anxiety Disorders
- Panic disorder without agoraphobia
- Panic disorder with agoraphobia
- Agoraphobia without history of panic disorder
- Specific phobia
- Social phobia
- Obsessive–compulsive disorder
- Posttraumatic stress disorder
- Acute stress disorder
- Generalized anxiety disorder
- Anxiety disorder caused by a general medical condition
- Substance-induced anxiety disorder
- NOS

DSM-5 (APA, 2013)
309.21 Separation anxiety disorder

300.01 Panic disorder
300.22 Agoraphobia
300.29 Specific phobia
300.23 Social anxiety disorder (social phobia)
300.02 Generalized anxiety disorder
Substance-induced anxiety disorder
293.84 Anxiety disorder attributable to another medical condition
300.00 Anxiety disorder not elsewhere classified

2.5.1.8   DSM-IV-TR and DSM-5: Somatoform Disorders
Somatization disorder

- Undifferentiated somatoform disorder
- Conversion disorder
- Pain disorder
- Hypochondriasis
- Body dysmorphic disorder
- NOS

DSM-5 (APA, 2013)
300.82 Somatic symptom disorder
300.7 Illness anxiety disorder
300.11 Conversion disorder (functional neurological symptom disorder)
316 Psychological factors affecting medical condition
300.19 Factitious disorder
300.82 Somatic symptom disorder not elsewhere classified

2.5.1.9   DSM-IV-TR and DSM-5: Factitious Disorders
Dissociative disorders

- Dissociative amnesia
- Dissociative fugue
- Dissociative identity disorder
- Depersonalization disorder
- NOS

DSM-5 (APA, 2013)
300.6 Depersonalization–derealization disorder
300.12 Dissociative amnesia
300.14 Dissociative identity disorder
300.15 Dissociative disorder not elsewhere classified

2.5.1.10   DSM-IV-TR and DSM-5: Sexual and Gender Identity Disorders
Sexual dysfunctions

- Sexual desire disorders
- Sexual arousal disorders
- Orgasmic disorders

- Sexual pain disorders
- Sexual dysfunction caused by a general medical condition

Paraphilias

- Exhibitionism
- Fetishism
- Frotteurism
- Pedophilia
- Sexual masochism
- Sexual sadism
- Transvestic fetishism
- Voyeurism
- NOS

Gender identity disorders

DSM-5 (APA, 2013)
302.72 Erectile disorder
302.73 Female orgasmic disorder
302.74 Delayed ejaculation
302.75 Early ejaculation
302.73 Female orgasmic disorder
302.72 Female sexual interest/arousal disorder
302.71 Male hypoactive sexual desire disorder
302.76 Genito-pelvic pain/penetration disorder
Substance/medication-induced sexual dysfunction
302.80 Sexual dysfunction not elsewhere classified
302.6 Gender dysphoria in children
302.85 Gender dysphoria in adolescents or adults

2.5.1.11 DSM-IV-TR and DSM-5: Eating Disorders

Anorexia nervosa
Bulimia nervosa
NOS

DSM-5 (APA, 2013)
307.52 Pica
307.53 Rumination disorder
307.59 Avoidant/restrictive food intake disorder
307.1 Anorexia nervosa
307.51 Bulimia nervosa
307.51 Binge eating disorder
307.50 Feeding or eating disorder not elsewhere classified

2.5.1.12 DSM-IV-TR and DSM-5: Sleep Disorders

Primary sleep disorders

- Dyssomnias
- Parasomnias

Sleep disorders related to another medical disorder
Other sleep disorders

DSM-5 (APA, 2013)
780.52 Insomnia disorder
780.54 Hypersomnolence disorders
347.00 Narcolepsy/hypocretin deficiency
327.23 Obstructive sleep apnea hypopnea syndrome
      Central sleep apnea
      Sleep-related hypoventilation
      Circadian rhythm sleep-wake disorder
307.46 Sleepwalking disorder
307.46 Sleep terror disorder
307.47 Nightmare disorder
327.42 Rapid eye movement sleep behaviour disorder
333.94 Restless legs syndrome
      Substance-induced sleep disorder

2.5.1.13 DSM-IV-TR and DSM-5: Impulse-Control Disorders not Elsewhere Classified

DSM-5 (APA, 2013)
Disruptive, impulse-control, and conduct disorders
313.81 Oppositional defiant disorder
312.34 Intermittent explosive disorder
312.81 Conduct disorder
312.33 Pyromania
312.32 Kleptomania
312.9 Unspecified disruptive, impulse-control, and conduct disorders

2.5.1.14 Adjustment Disorders

Other conditions that may be a focus of clinical attention.

2.5.2 AXIS II: PERSONALITY DISORDERS; MENTAL RETARDATION

2.5.2.1 Personality Disorders

- Paranoid personality disorder
- Schizoid personality disorder
- Schizotypal personality disorder
- Antisocial personality disorder
- Borderline personality disorder
- Histrionic personality disorder
- Narcissistic personality disorder
- Avoidant personality disorder
- Dependent personality disorder
- Obsessive–compulsive personality disorder
- NOS

DSM-5 (2013)
Cluster A Personality disorders
301.0 Paranoid personality disorder

301.2 Schizoid personality disorder
301.22 Schizotypal personality disorder

Cluster B Personality disorders
301.7 Antisocial personality disorder
301.83 Borderline personality disorder
301.5 Histrionic personality disorder
301.81 Narcissistic personality disorder

Cluster C Personality disorders
301.82 Avoidant personality disorder
301.6 Dependent personality disorder
301.4 Obsessive–compulsive personality disorder

Other personality disorders
310.1 Personality change due to another medical condition
301.89 Other personality disorder

2.5.2.2 Mental Retardation

Mild mental retardation
Moderate mental retardation
Severe mental retardation
Profound mental retardation
Mental retardation, severity unspecified

2.5.3   AXIS III: GENERAL MEDICAL CONDITIONS

Infectious and parasitic diseases
Neoplasms
Endocrine, nutritional, and metabolic diseases and immunity disorders
Diseases of the blood and blood-forming organs
Diseases of the nervous system and sensory organs
Diseases of the circulatory system
Diseases of the respiratory system
Diseases of the digestive system
Diseases of the genitourinary system
Complications of pregnancy, childbirth, and the puerperium
Diseases of the skin and subcutaneous tissue
Diseases of the musculoskeletal system and connective tissue
Congenital anomalies
Certain conditions originating in the perinatal period
Symptoms, signs, and ill-defined conditions
Injury and poisoning

2.5.4   AXIS IV: PSYCHOSOCIAL AND ENVIRONMENTAL PROBLEMS

Problems with primary support group
Problems related to the social environment
Educational problems
Occupational problems
Housing problems
Economic problems
Problems with access to health-care services
Problems related to interaction with the legal system/crime
Other psychosocial and environmental problems

2.5.5   AXIS V: GLOBAL ASSESSMENT OF FUNCTIONING

The fifth axis allows for a global assessment of functioning of the individual.

REFERENCES

American Psychiatric Association. 1985: *DSM III: Diagnostic Statistical Manual*, 3rd edn., Washington, DC: American Psychiatric Association Press.

American Psychiatric Association. 2000: *Diagnostic and Statistical Manual of Mental Disorders,* 4th edn., Text Revision (DSM-IV-TR). Washington, DC: American Psychiatric Association.

American Psychiatric Association. 2013: *Desk Reference to the Diagnostic Criteria from DSM-5.* Washington, DC: American Psychiatric Association Press.

Doig A, Ferguson JPS, Milne IA, and Passmore R. 1993: *William Cullen and the Eighteenth Century Medical World*, pp. 34–55. Edinburgh University Press.

Grob GN. 1991: Origins of DSM-I: A study in appearance and reality. *American Journal of Psychiatry* 148(4):421–431.

Kirk SA and Kutchins H. 1994: The myth of the reliability of DSM. *Journal of Mind and Behavior* 15:1–2.

Wilson M. 1993: DSM-III and the transformation of American psychiatry: A history. *American Journal of Psychiatry* 150(3):399–410.

World Health Organization. 1990: History of the development of the ICD. http://www.who.int/classifications/icd/en/HistoryOfICD.pdf

World Health Organization. 1992: *The ICD-10 Classification of Mental and Behavioural Disorders.* Geneva, Switzerland: World Health Organization.

3 Basic Psychology

3.1 PRINCIPLES OF LEARNING THEORY

3.1.1 DEFINITION OF LEARNING

Learning is a change in behaviour as a result of prior experience. It does not include behaviour change caused by maturation or temporary conditions (e.g. drug effects or fatigue).

Learning may occur through associations being made between two or more phenomena. Two forms of such associative learning are recognized: classical conditioning and operant conditioning. Cognitive learning is a more complex process in which current perceptions are interpreted in the context of previous information in order to solve unfamiliar problems. Evidence that learning can also take place through the observation and imitation of others has led to the development of the observational learning theory.

3.1.2 CLASSICAL CONDITIONING

3.1.2.1 Definition and Introduction

Classical conditioning (respondent learning) was first described by the Russian physiologist Ivan Petrovich Pavlov (1849–1936) in 1927. (Although Pavlov was awarded a Nobel Prize, this was in 1904 for his work on digestion.) Following several repetitions of pairing of light (or a bell sounding) followed by the presentation of food to a dog, it was found that just switching on the light led to salivation. The dog had been conditioned to associate the light with food. Food was acting as the unconditioned stimulus (US), eliciting the reflex response of salivation without new learning being involved. The response to the US is known as the unconditioned response (UR). The light would not normally have elicited the response of salivation but was now a conditioned stimulus (CS) that had elicited the response through its association with a US. The conditioned response (CR) is the learned or acquired response to a CS. This is shown diagrammatically in Figure 3.1. Thus, in Pavlov's experiments, salivation was both a UR before conditioning and a CR after conditioning.

3.1.2.2 Acquisition Stage

The acquisition stage of conditioning is the period during which the association is being acquired between the CS and the US with which it is being paired.

3.1.2.3 Delayed Conditioning

In delayed conditioning, the onset of the CS precedes that of the US, and the CS continues until the response occurs. Delayed conditioning is optimal when the delay between the onsets of the two stimuli is around half a second.

3.1.2.4 Simultaneous Conditioning

In simultaneous conditioning, the onset of both stimuli is simultaneous, and the CS continues until the response occurs. It is less successful than delayed conditioning.

3.1.2.5 Trace Conditioning

In trace conditioning, the CS ends before the onset of the US, and the conditioning becomes less effective as the delay between the two increases.

3.1.2.6 Backward Conditioning

In backward conditioning, the presentation of the CS occurs after that of the US.

3.1.2.7 Higher-Order Conditioning

In higher-order conditioning, the CS is paired with a second (or third) CS, which on presentation by itself elicits the original CR. In other words, the original CS now acts as the US in the new pairing. If there is just a second CS, then this gives rise to second-order conditioning. A third CS gives rise to third-order conditioning. Higher-order (i.e. second-order or above) conditioning is weaker than first-order conditioning; in general, the higher the order, the weaker the conditioning.

3.1.2.8 Extinction

Extinction is the gradual disappearance of a CR and occurs when the CS is repeatedly presented without the US. It does not entail the complete loss of the condition stimulus. Following extinction, if an experimental

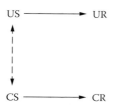

FIGURE 3.1 Diagram showing the processes associated with classical conditioning. US, unconditioned stimulus; UR, unconditioned response; CS, conditioned stimulus; CR, conditioned response.

animal is allowed to rest, a weaker CR reemerges; this is known as *partial recovery*.

3.1.2.9 Generalization

Generalization is the process whereby once a CR has been established to given stimulus, that response can also be evoked by other stimuli that are similar to the original CS.

3.1.2.10 Discrimination

Discrimination is the differential recognition of and response to two or more similar stimuli.

3.1.2.11 Incubation

Incubation is the increase in strength of CRs resulting from repeated brief exposure to the CS.

3.1.2.12 Stimulus Preparedness

Stimulus preparedness refers to the fact that some stimuli are more likely to become conditioned stimuli than are others.

3.1.2.13 Little Albert

In 1920, the American psychologist John Broadus Watson (1878–1958) and his research assistant Rosalie Rayner described the experimental induction of a phobia, using classical conditioning, in an 11-month-old boy known as Little Albert. Following several episodes of pairing in which the presentation of a white rat was accompanied by a loud noise caused by striking a steel bar, the boy developed a fear of the rat in the absence of the frightening noise. This was then repeated with a rabbit and then generalized to any furry mammal.

3.1.3 OPERANT CONDITIONING (INSTRUMENTAL LEARNING)

3.1.3.1 Definition and Introduction

Operant conditioning, or instrumental learning, is particularly associated with Skinner (see Skinner, 1953,

1969) although much of the groundwork for the underlying theory was carried out by Thorndike (1911); Burrhus Frederic Skinner (1904–1990) and Edward Lee Thorndike (1874–1949) were American psychologists. A voluntary behaviour is engaged in because its occurrence is reinforced by being rewarded. Such behaviour is independent of stimuli and was termed operant behaviour by Skinner. An alternative type of behaviour termed respondent behaviour by Skinner refers to behaviour that is dependent on known stimuli.

3.1.3.2 Trial-and-Error Learning/Behaviour

Thorndike described experiments in which hungry cats were placed in puzzle boxes. By chance, in time, a cat would effect an escape, for example, by pressing on a lever, and reach some visible food outside the box. Less time would be needed to carry out the same behaviour in later trials. This is trial-and-error learning or behaviour.

3.1.3.3 Law of Effect

Thorndike's law of effect holds that voluntary behaviour that is paired with subsequent reward is strengthened.

3.1.3.4 Skinner Box

Skinner developed the experimental procedures of Thorndike, creating the Skinner box. Operant conditioning can be demonstrated using a Skinner box in which, for example, every time the animal presses a lever, a pellet of food is released. If hungry rats are placed in it, random trial-and-error learning leads to the lever being pressed, the CR, to obtain the reinforcing stimulus of the reward of food pellets. If, after many repetitions of this pairing, the CR is no longer reinforced, then the CR abates, that is, extinction occurs. Following extinction, if the animal is allowed to rest, a weaker CR can reemerge; this is partial recovery. Discrimination (see preceding text) can also occur.

3.1.4 OBSERVATIONAL LEARNING (VICARIOUS LEARNING/MODELLING)

3.1.4.1 Definition and Introduction

Observational learning (or modelling), also known as vicarious learning (or modelling), is the learning of behaviours and skills that can occur by observation without direct reinforcement. The occurrence of the observational learning of aggressive behaviour in humans has been demonstrated by Bandura.

3.1.4.2 Bobo Doll Experiments

Albert Bandura (1925–present) is a Canadian psychologist (working at Stanford, United States) who carried out the Bobo doll experiments. (Bobo dolls are inflatable, balloon-like objects, shaped like eggs, which bob back up after being knocked down, owing to the presence of extra weighting in the dolls' 'bottoms'.) Bandura made a film of one of his female students verbally and physically attacking a Bobo doll, including hitting it with a hammer. This film was then shown to groups of kindergartners. The children liked the film and when let out to play in an area containing a new Bobo doll and some toy hammers, they proceeded verbally and physically to imitate the actions of the young woman in Bandura's film.

Bandura pointed out that a change in behaviour in the children had occurred without rewards being received for approximations to the new behaviour. He termed this phenomenon, which was clearly differed from classical and operant learning, observational learning or modelling; his theory is referred to as social learning theory.

To deal with the criticism that a Bobo doll is made to be hit, Bandura repeated the Bobo doll experiments, this time substituting a live clown for the doll. Again, the children imitated the actions of the young woman, to the extent of kicking and punching a live clown and hitting him with (toy) hammers.

3.1.4.3 Optimal Conditions for Observational Learning

1. The subject sees that the behaviour observed is being reinforced.
2. Perceived similarity—the subject must believe that they can emit the response necessary to obtain reinforcement (self-efficacy).

3.1.4.4 Steps Involved in the Modelling Process

According to Bandura (1973), the following steps are involved in the modelling process:

1. *Attention.* Successful observational learning is more likely to occur in association with the following factors:
   a. Optimal arousal
   b. An attractive model
   c. A prestigious model
   d. A colourful and dramatic model
   e. A model who appears to be like the observer
   In contrast, unsuccessful observational learning is more likely to occur in association with the following factors:
   a. Low arousal (e.g. sleepiness)
   b. Overarousal
   c. The presence of distracting stimuli
2. *Retention.*
3. *Reproduction.* The translation of what has been remembered into behaviour.
4. *Motivation.* See Section 3.1.6.

3.1.5 COGNITIVE LEARNING

3.1.5.1 Definition

The notion of a mental model of reality is central to the cognitive approach to psychology. Cognition involves the reception, organization, and utilization of information. Cognitive learning is an active form of learning in which mental cognitive structures (cognitive maps) are formed. These allow mental images to be formed, which allow meaning and structure to be given to the internal and external environment.

3.1.5.2 Mechanisms

Cognitive learning can occur in the following ways:

- *Insight learning*—the learning occurs apparently out of the blue, because of an understanding of the relationship between various elements relevant to a problem.
- *Latent learning*—cognitive learning takes place but is not manifested except in certain circumstances such as the need to satisfy a basic drive.

3.1.5.3 Assimilation Theory

The assimilation theory of cognitive learning is based on the following concepts:

1. Learning in humans is influenced by prior knowledge.
2. Human learning is manifested by a change in the meaning of experience rather than a purely behavioural change.
3. Those involved in teaching should help their students reflect on their experiences.
4. Those involved in teaching should construct new meanings.

3.1.6 Concepts of Extinction and Reinforcement in Explaining Behaviour

3.1.6.1 Extinction

Extinction has been defined earlier.

3.1.6.2 Reinforcement

A *positive reinforcer* is a reinforcing reward stimulus (e.g. food and water, money in humans), which increases the probability of occurrence of the operant behaviour, while a *negative reinforcer* is an aversive stimulus (e.g. an electric shock, fear) whose removal increases the probability of occurrence of the operant behaviour. For example, a Skinner box may be arranged so that in order to avoid an aversive stimulus, the animal must press a lever. Learning this response is called *avoidance conditioning*. *Escape conditioning* is a variety of negative reinforcement in which the response learnt provides complete escape from the aversive stimulus (very resistant to extinction).

3.1.6.3 Punishment

Punishment is the situation that occurs if an aversive stimulus is presented whenever a given behaviour occurs, thereby reducing the probability of occurrence of this response. The removal of the aversive stimulus then allows it to act as a negative reinforcer rather than a punisher.

3.1.6.4 Primary Reinforcement

This is reinforcement that is occurring through reduction of needs deriving from basic drives (e.g. food and drink).

3.1.6.5 Secondary Reinforcement

This is reinforcement deriving from association with primary reinforcers (e.g. money, tokens).

3.1.6.6 Schedules of Reinforcement

Different schedules of reinforcement can be used:

- In *continuous reinforcement*, reinforcement takes place following every CR. This leads to the maximum response rate.
- In *partial reinforcement*, only some of the CRs are reinforced.
  In a *fixed interval schedule*, reinforcement occurs after a fixed interval of time. It is poor at maintaining the CR; the maximum response rate typically occurs only when the reinforcement is expected.
  In a *variable interval schedule*, reinforcement occurs after variable intervals. It is very good at maintaining the CR.

In a *fixed ratio schedule*, reinforcement occurs after a fixed number of responses. It is good at maintaining a high response rate.
In a *variable ratio schedule*, reinforcement occurs after a variable number of responses. It is very good at maintaining a high response rate.

3.1.6.7 Motivation

In observational learning theory, Bandura has put forward the following motives that encourage observational learning:

- *Past reinforcement.* This is similar to the types of reinforcement that are recognized in classical and operant learning theory.
- *Promised reinforcements.* These are incentives that can be imagined.
- *Vicarious reinforcement.* This refers to the sight and recollection of the model that is being reinforced.

Negative motivations that inhibit observational learning include

- *Past punishment*
- *Promised punishment*, that is, threats
- *Vicarious punishment*

Bandura contends that punishment is less effective than reinforcement.

3.1.7 Clinical Applications of Behavioural Treatments

3.1.7.1 Reciprocal Inhibition

This holds that relaxation inhibits anxiety so that the two are mutually exclusive (Wolpe, 1958) and in fact does not hold true. It can be used in treating conditions associated with anticipatory anxiety (e.g. phobias). Patients identify increasingly greater anxiety-evoking stimuli, to form an anxiety hierarchy. During systematic desensitization, the patient is successfully exposed (in reality or in imagination) to these stimuli in the hierarchy, beginning with the least anxiety-evoking one, each exposure being paired with relaxation.

3.1.7.2 Habituation

Habituation is an important component of the behavioural treatment of obsessive–compulsive disorder using exposure and response prevention. The ultimate aim of exposure techniques is to reduce the discomfort associated with the eliciting stimuli through habituation.

For example, Vaughan and Tarrier (1992) have described the use of *image habituation training* in the therapy of patients suffering from post-traumatic stress disorder. Image habituation training involved the generation by the patient of verbal descriptions of the traumatic event, which were recorded onto audiotape. After the initial training session with the therapist, homework sessions of self-directed exposure in which the patient visualized the described event in response to listening to the audiotape recordings were carried out. There were significant decreases in anxiety between and within homework sessions, suggesting that habituation did occur and was responsible for improvement. Treatment gains were maintained at 6 month follow-up.

3.1.7.3 Chaining

In (response) chaining, the components of a more complex desired behaviour are first taught and then connected in order to teach the latter. Chaining may be conceptualized in the following two different ways:

1. Responses function as discriminative stimuli for subsequent responses.
2. Responses produce stimuli that function as discriminative stimuli for subsequent responses.

Chaining can be used in, for example, people with learning difficulties. Thvedt et al. (1984) described studied stimulus functions in chaining. Twenty-four adults with learning difficulties learned a chain of circuit board assembly responses consisting of placing resistors in the board and pressing switches. Lights came on after switch responses. After learning the chain, each subject was exposed to three experimental conditions (counterbalanced):

- Altered stimulus location
- Altered stimulus sequence
- Missing stimulus

This study lent some support for the second conceptual position given earlier (i.e. that responses produce stimuli that function as discriminative stimuli for subsequent responses).

3.1.7.4 Shaping

In shaping, successively closer approximations to the desired behaviour are reinforced in order to achieve the latter. It finds application clinically in the management of behavioural disturbances in people with learning difficulties and in the therapy of patients suffering from psychoactive substance use disorder.

For example, Preston et al. (2001) have used shaping to attempt to bring about cocaine abstinence by successive approximation. Cocaine-using methadone-maintenance patients were randomized to standard contingency management (abstinence group of size 49) or to a contingency designed to increase contact with reinforcers (shaping group of size 46). For 8 weeks, both groups earned escalating-value vouchers based on thrice-weekly urinalyses: the abstinence group earned vouchers for cocaine-negative urines only; the shaping group earned vouchers for each urine specimen with a 25% or greater decrease in cocaine metabolite (during the first 3 weeks) and then for negative urines only (during the final 5 weeks). Cocaine use was found to be lower in the shaping group but only in the last 5 weeks, when the response requirement was identical. Thus, the shaping contingency appeared to better prepare patients for abstinence. (A second phase of the study showed that abstinence induced by escalating-value vouchers can be maintained by a nonescalating schedule, suggesting that contingency management can be practical as a maintenance treatment.)

3.1.7.5 Cueing

Cueing is the process of helping the learner to focus their attention on the important or relevant stimuli to render the essential learning characteristics distinct from the other stimuli; it consists of any action that separates figure from ground (see succeeding text). The use of cueing can decrease learning times. For example, in reading matter and pictorial presentations, visual cues can be given using any of the following strategies:

- Highlighting
- Underlining
- Arrows
- Contrasting colours
- Animation
- Explosions
- Implosions
- Bordering
- Texture
- Novelty
- Size
- Labelling

A famous example is that of *Clever Hans*. Hans was a horse, belonging to Mr. Wilhelm von Osten, which appeared capable of carrying out a range of intellectual tasks normally associated with humans, such as the arithmetic operations of addition, subtraction, multiplication, and division of natural numbers and fractions; reading; and spelling. Answers were communicated by means of tapping out the answer with one of his feet. For example, if asked to calculate '2 + 3', Clever Hans would tap his foot five times and then stop. Pfungst (1907/1911), in conjunction with the Berlin psychologist Carl Stumpf, designed a set of experiments that showed that Clever Hans was, in fact, being cued to give the correct answer by the questioner. The questioner, consciously or unconsciously, would provide Clever Hans with visual cues, such as subtle changes in facial expression and posture. For example, in the earlier example, as Clever Hans reached five foot taps, he could pick up visual cues showing how the tension in the questioner was rising. As soon as the fifth tap was executed, the sense of relief in the questioner was also apparent in visual cues, and the horse knew this was when to stop tapping.

A clinical example of the therapeutic use of cueing is in unilateral neglect, following a cerebral lesion. Robertson et al. (1992) based their therapeutic intervention on the experimental finding that limb activation contralateral to a cerebral lesion appears to reduce visual neglect. (There is controversy as to whether this is the result of perceptual cueing or of hemispheric activation.) In the treatment of unilateral left neglect, Robertson et al. (1992) found that treatment focused on cueing for left arm activation, without explicit instructions for perceptual anchoring, gave positive results.

3.1.7.6 Escape Conditioning

As mentioned earlier, in escape conditioning, the animal learns to escape from an unpleasant or punishing stimulus by making a new response. For example, rodents can be trained to escape from electric shocks by pressing a button.

It is a form of negative reinforcement, in which the reinforcement is getting away from an aversive stimulus. It is a special form of operant conditioning, consisting of a conditioning procedure in which successive occurrences of a response repeatedly terminate a negative reinforcing stimulus.

Escape conditioning may be used in the treatment of alcoholism. For example, Glover and McCue (1977) found that a group of patients with alcoholism, when treated with partially reinforced electric escape conditioning, had a significantly better outcome on follow-up than a control group who showed a parallel level of motivation and were treated by conventional methods. No sex differences in outcome were found for either group. In the experimental group treated with escape conditioning,

better prognosis was associated with higher social class and older age, and poorer prognosis with single marital status. There were no variations in outcome for age in the control group. In the age range 20–40 years, escape conditioning did not show better results than conventional therapies, but with subjects above this age range, it was significantly superior.

3.1.7.7 Avoidance Conditioning

As mentioned earlier, in avoidance conditioning, the animal learns to avoid an unpleasant or punishing stimulus by making a new response. For example, rodents can be trained to avoid electric shocks by pressing a button.

Like escape conditioning, avoidance conditioning is a form of negative reinforcement, in which the reinforcement is getting away from an aversive stimulus. Avoidance conditioning may be considered to be a special case of operant conditioning under intermittent reinforcement.

Avoidance conditioning, and indeed also escape conditioning, may be used in the treatment of enuresis. For example, Hansen (1979) described a twin-signal device that provided both escape and avoidance conditioning in enuresis control.

3.1.7.8 Self-Control Therapy

Bandura helped to develop the therapeutic technique of self-control therapy, based on concepts of self-regulation. It may be used as part of a treatment package for the cessation of smoking, in countering overeating, and in helping students to improve their ability to study.

The components are as follows:

1. *Behavioural charts.* This involves keeping a record of one's behaviour based on self-observation. For example, in attempting to improve study habits prior to an examination, a student may make a record of how much time is spent studying each day, how many books are (re) read, and how many past or sample examination papers are fully attempted. Such a record could be graphical or in the form of a behavioural diary. In the case of the latter, further relevant details should be noted, which may offer insight into cues associated with the desired (or undesired) behaviour, for example, the student may find that they accomplish more when in a library compared with being at home and accomplish least when in a room with a television switched on.

2. *Environmental planning.* Based on the behavioural chart and diary, changes to one's environment

can be planned. For example, to continue with the example of the student, he or she may plan to spend more time in a library and in study groups with others also sitting the same examination and less time at home with the television switched on.

3. *Self-contracts.* A contract can be written down (perhaps witnessed by the therapist), stipulating the reward to oneself for accomplishing certain tasks and the punishment for not doing so. For example, in the case of the student, their contract might state 'If I fully revise chapters 1 to 4 from my revision book next week, then I shall reward myself by buying my favourite recording of Beethoven's 5th Piano Concerto; if I fail to achieve this goal, then I shall …[state some unpleasant but necessary task or chore]'.

3.1.7.9 Modelling Therapy
Bandura also developed modelling therapy. Here, a patient suffering from a difficulty coping with a certain situation watches somebody else cope perfectly easily with the same situation and then in turn is able to cope by means of observational learning. An example of the use of modelling therapy is in the treatment of phobias.

3.2 PHENOMENA OF VISUAL AND AUDITORY PERCEPTION

3.2.1 PERCEPTION

3.2.1.1 Definition
Perception is an active process involving the awareness and interpretation of sensations received through sensory organs.

3.2.1.2 Absolute Threshold
This is the minimum energy required to activate the sensory organ.

3.2.1.3 Difference Threshold
The difference threshold of two sources of a sensory modality is the minimum difference that has to exist between the intensities of the two sources to allow them to be perceived separately.

3.2.1.4 Weber's Law
The increase in stimulus intensity needed to allow two sources of intensity to be perceived as being different is directly proportional to the value of the baseline intensity.

3.2.1.5 Fechner's Law
Weber's law is only an approximation that fails to hold over a large range of stimulus intensity. A better, though again not perfect, approximation is provided by Fechner's law that holds that sensory perception is a logarithmic function of stimulus intensity.

3.2.1.6 Signal Detection Theory
This holds that perception does not depend solely on stimulus intensity but is also a function of biophysical factors and psychological factors such as motivation, previous experiences, and expectations.

3.2.2 PERCEPTUAL ORGANIZATION
Perception is an active process in which there is a search for meaning. A number of perceptual phenomena are described in Gestalt psychology:

- The whole perception is different from the sum of its parts.
- Law of simplicity—the percept corresponds to the simplest stimulation interpretation.
- Law of continuity—for example, interrupted lines seen as continuous.
- Law of similarity—like items are grouped together.
- Law of proximity—adjacent items are grouped together.
- Figure-ground differentiation.

Note that gestalt is a German word meaning shape or form.

3.2.2.1 Figure-Ground Differentiation
Patterns are perceived as figures differentiated from their background with contours and boundaries, thus simulating objects. Thus, the relevant perceptual system needs to make a 'decision' as to how to differentiate correctly between the figure that is being perceived and its background. In doing so, the following features characterize figure and ground, particularly in respect of visual stimuli:

- The figure is more conspicuous than the ground.
- The figure appears more like an object in its own right.
- The ground does not appear to be an object but rather generally formless.
- The ground extends past the figure.
- The perception is of the figure being 'in front of' the ground.
- The contour or outline that differentiates figure from ground is perceived as belonging to the figure rather than the ground.

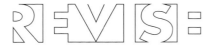

FIGURE 3.2   Visual example of a figure-ground relationship.

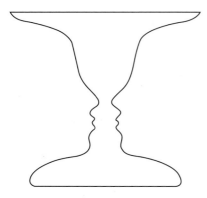

FIGURE 3.3   Visual example of a reversible figure-ground relationship—the Rubin vase.

An example of a visual figure-ground relationship is shown in Figure 3.2. (It may not be obvious, the first time it is looked at, what information it conveys. In fact, the figure consists of the spaces between the objects [the ground]. Armed with this knowledge, it is immediately clear that a word of importance to examination candidates is depicted.)

An example of an ambiguous, reversible, visual figure-ground relationship is that of the Rubin vase, shown in Figure 3.3. (This was devised by the Danish psychologist Edgar Rubin.) Here, the figure may be the face and the ground the vases. Alternatively, the two vases may be considered to be the figure and the facial shape in between them the ground.

Figure-ground differentiation is not confined to visual stimuli. An example involving auditory stimuli is that of hearing a particular conversation over background noise.

3.2.2.2   Object Constancy

This is the tendency to perceive objects as unchanged under different conditions:

- *Shape constancy*—the perception of an object's shape is constant regardless of the viewing angle.
- *Size constancy*—the perception of an object's size is constant regardless of the viewing distance.

- *Lightness/colour constancy*—the perception of an object's shade/colour is constant regardless of the lighting conditions.
- *Location constancy*—the perception of an object's spatial position is constant regardless of the viewer's movement.

For example, when walking or running through a room, all the walls and the ceiling and floor are perceived as each having a rectangular shape, in spite of the fact that the shapes projected on the retina are those of nonstatic nonrectangles.

3.2.2.3   Depth Perception

A 3D visual perception is formed from 2D retinal images as a result of multiple cues such as binocular vision and convergence, relative size and brightness, motion parallax, object interposition, and linear perspective.

3.2.2.4   Perceptual Set

Perceptual set is a motivational state of mind in which certain aspects of stimuli are perceived according to expectation. This can be associated with a change in the perception threshold. The way in which stimuli are perceived is influenced by personality and individual values and past experiences. Perceptual set was described in his book *Becoming* in 1955 by the American psychologist Gordon Willard Allport (1897–1967).

3.2.3   RELEVANCE OF VISUAL PERCEPTUAL THEORY TO PSYCHOPATHOLOGY

3.2.3.1   Illusions

Illusions are misperceptions of real stimuli that are influenced by the perceptual set and suggest an active search for meaning. With respect to visual perceptual theory, illusions can arise from the following phenomena:

- *Difficulties in figure-ground differentiation*—for example, ambiguous figures such as the Rubin vase.
- *Changes in object constancy*—for example, perceptual constancy may change as a result of different lighting conditions, giving rise to visual illusions.
- *Difficulties in depth perception*—for example, owing to ocular problems, abnormal ocular lens accommodation can give rise to abnormalities in monocular cueing, while defects in the ability of the eyes properly to converge can cause abnormalities in binocular cueing.

3.2.3.2 Hallucinations

Hallucinations are false sensory perceptions occurring in the absence of real external stimuli. They are perceived as being located in objective space and as having the same realistic qualities as normal perceptions.

According to visual perceptual theory, the majority of the processing that comprises perception takes place within the brain rather than in the sense organs themselves. Therefore, any factors that adversely affect neuronal processing within the brain may cause the subject to experience hallucinations. Such factors (described in Chapters 31 and 32) include cerebral lesions, psychoactive substances, and toxic states.

Furthermore, on the basis of visual perceptual theory, it would also be predicted that abnormalities in the sense organs themselves or in primary perceptual functioning could also give rise to hallucinations. Evidence exists to support this contention. For instance, visual hallucinations, in the absence of other psychopathology, have been reported in association with ocular disease with visual loss in Charles Bonnet syndrome ('visual hallucinations of the blind'). An auditory analogue to visual perceptual theory also exists; an example of auditory impairment being associated with auditory hallucinations is the report of the association of musical hallucinations with hearing impairment.

3.2.3.3 Other Psychopathologies

An agnosia is an inability to interpret and recognize the significance of sensory information, which does not result from impairment of the sensory pathways, mental deterioration, disorders of consciousness and attention, or, in the case of an object, a lack of familiarity with the object. Abnormalities in the way in which visual perceptual systems (functioning according to visual perceptual theory) interact with systems of the brain associated with functions such as learning and memory can give rise to agnosias.

In schizophrenia, depersonalization, derealization, temporal lobe epilepsy, and acute brain syndromes, there is disturbance of perception, particularly depth perception and perceptual constancy.

3.2.4 Development of Visual Perception

The development of human visual perception is an illustration of a constitutional–environmental interaction. In general complex, visual stimuli, such as human faces, are preferred. The early developmental stages are as follows:

- Birth—there is the ability to discriminate brightness and to carry out eye tracking; visual acuity is impaired and focusing is fixed at 0.2 m.

- 2 months—depth perception (as evidenced by visual cliff experiments).
- 4 months—accommodation and colour vision.
- 6 months—6:6 acuity.

The following visual processes appear to be innate:

- Visual scanning
- Tracking
- Fixating
- Figure-ground discrimination

In contrast, the following visual processes appear to be learnt:

- Size constancy
- Shape constancy
- Depth perception
- Shape discrimination

3.2.5 Culturally Sanctioned Distress States

Reports of cultural and ethnic variation in the experience of hallucinations (Al-Issa, 1977; Schwab, 1977) suggest that hallucinations are not necessarily pathological phenomena, while reports of hallucinatory experiences in the general population provide additional evidence that psychosis is on a continuum with normality (Johns et al., 2002); cognitive psychological models have attempted to explain how anomalous experiences are transformed into psychotic symptoms (Garety et al., 2001). Visual and auditory phenomena can occur in culturally sanctioned distress states without necessarily being pathognomonic of mental disorder. A few examples follow.

3.2.5.1 Nocturnal Hallucinations in Ultra-Orthodox Jewish Israeli Men

Greenberg and Brom (2001) reported that hallucinations that occur predominantly at night were found in 122 out of a sample of 302 ultra-orthodox Jewish Israeli men referred for psychiatric evaluation. Most of those with nocturnal hallucinations were in their late teens, were seen only once or twice, were brought in order to receive an evaluation letter for the Israeli army, and had a reported history of serious learning difficulties. The nocturnal hallucinatory experiences were predominantly visual, and the images were frightening figures from daily life or from folklore. Many of the subjects were withdrawn, monosyllabic, reluctant interviewees. Greenberg and Brom suggested that this cultural group's value on study at Yeshivas away from home places significant pressure on teenage boys with mild or definite subnormality, possibly precipitating the phenomenon at this age in this sex. Although malingering had to be considered as a possible explanation in many cases owing to the circumstances of the evaluation, short-term and long-term follow-up on a limited sample allowed this explanation to be dismissed in a significant number of cases. They therefore suggested that these nocturnal hallucinations are a culture-specific phenomenon.

3.2.5.2 Isolated Sleep Paralysis with Visual Hallucinations among Nigerian Students

Ohaeri et al. (1992) reported the results of a cross-sectional study of the pattern of isolated sleep paralysis among the entire population of nursing students at the Neuropsychiatric Hospital in Abeokuta, Nigeria, consisting of 58 males and 37 females. Forty-four percentage of the students (both male and female) admitted having experienced this phenomenon. The findings largely supported the results of a similar study of Nigerian medical students, except that there was a slight male preponderance among those who had the experience. Visual hallucination was the most common perceptual problem associated with the episodes, and all the affected subjects were most distressed by the experience. The popular, culturally sanctioned, view in Africa is that this distress state associated with visual phenomena is caused by witchcraft.

3.2.5.3 Mu-Ghayeb

Mu-Ghayeb is a traditional bereavement reaction that occurs in Oman following a sudden unexpected death. The deceased relative or friend may be seen as an unearthly figure at night. During the daytime, the deceased may be seen, normally clothed, in circumstances that are difficult to authenticate, for instance, sitting in a motor vehicle that passes by at speed. These visual phenomena are consistent with the belief in traditional Omani society that after such a sudden untimely 'death', the 'deceased' continue to be alive; they are expected to be resurrected to a strange, ghostly existence, with nocturnal wanderings and interleaved episodes of sleeping naked in caves during the day. This belief in the return of the dead persists even after an elaborate ritual of burial and a prescribed period of mourning. The deceased are expected to leave the grave after burial and join their families when the spell placed on them by a sorcerer is broken or counteracted. Although the Mu-Ghayeb belief is inconsistent with their Islamic religion, this culture-specific response to bereavement may be explained in terms of sudden and untimely death, which used to be rife in the seafaring Omani society (Al-Adawi et al., 1997).

3.2.5.4 Auditory and Visual Hallucinations Related to Bereavement in the Caribbean

Long-lasting auditory and visual hallucinations may occur in individuals living in, or originally from, the Caribbean, following the death of a relative, such that these auditory and visual phenomena may not be pathognomonic of mental disorder. An example is given in a case report by Boran and Viswanathan (2000) relating to an American patient originally from Jamaica:

> Mrs. G, a 28-year-old woman who was eight weeks pregnant, was hospitalized on an obstetrics-gynaecology unit of a university hospital with a diagnosis of mild hyperemesis gravidarum. The patient had no prior psychiatric history, including no history of alcohol or substance abuse, and no significant medical history. She lived with her mother and sister. A psychiatric consultation was requested because the patient had auditory and visual hallucinations.

> The patient was hearing someone knocking at the door and was seeing a man sitting in the chair next to her bed when there was nobody else in the room. When asked about the hallucinations, she said that she and her family believed that after death the spirit of the dead person was still among them. If the dead one was somebody who had always helped them in difficult moments of their life, then he or she continued to do so by 'showing up' and being of comfort. Such was 'Uncle Pete', the man the patient saw when she was admitted, and who appeared to the family on several other difficult occasions.

> Mrs. G's mental status examination was unremarkable except for the hallucinations. The medical workup did not reveal any organic causes for her symptoms. She showed no distress or impairment of functioning as a result of the belief. With the patient's permission, we spoke to her mother and sister by telephone. They reported that Uncle Pete had also appeared to them and confirmed that neither Mrs. G nor others in the family had any prior psychiatric history.

> The nurse assigned by the medical staff to watch the patient in the hospital also told the psychiatric consultant about her own family spirit, who was similar to Uncle Pete in many ways. The patient and the nurse were both from Jamaica and came to the United States with their families as children. The patient's symptoms were determined to be culturally based beliefs, and there was no evidence of psychosis. No psychiatric sequelae appeared in the patient's subsequent hospital course.

3.3 INFORMATION PROCESSING AND ATTENTION

3.3.1 Information Processing

Information processing is concerned with the way in which external signals arriving at the sense organs are converted into meaningful perceptual experiences.

3.3.1.1 Data-Driven Processing

The processing is initiated by the arrival of data. The simplest scheme for classifying and recognizing patterns is template matching, in which recognition is achieved by matching the external signal against the internal template.

3.3.1.2 Conceptually Driven Processing

This applies when data input is incomplete. The processing starts with the conceptualization of what might be present and then looks for confirmatory evidence, thereby biasing the processing mechanisms to give the expected results. Conceptually driven data (schema) are essential to perception. However, they can lead to misperceptions.

3.3.2 Attention

Attention is an intensive process in which information selection takes place. Types include the following:

- *Selective/focused attention*—one type of information is attended to while additional distracting information is ignored, for example, cocktail party effect. In dichotic listening studies in which subjects attend to one channel, evidence indicates that the unattended channel is still being processed and the listener can switch rapidly if appropriate.
- *Divided attention*—at least two sources of information are attended simultaneously. Performance is inefficient. Loss of performance is called dual-task interference.
- *Sustained attention*—the environment is monitored over a long period of time. Performance deteriorates with time.

- *Controlled attention*—effort is required. It has been suggested that a defect of controlled attention might underlie symptoms of schizophrenia.
- *Automatic attention*—the subject becomes skilled at a task, and therefore little conscious effort is required.
- *Stroop effect*—automatic process is so ingrained that it interferes with controlled processing.

3.4 FACTORS AFFECTING MEMORY

3.4.1 Memory

Memory comprises encoding/registration, storage, and retrieval of information.

3.4.1.1 Encoding/Registration

This is the transformation of physical information into a code that memory can accept.

3.4.1.2 Storage

This is the retention of encoded information. According to the multistore model of Atkinson and Shriffrin (1968), which has now been superseded, memory storage can be considered to be made up of

- Sensory memory
- Short-term memory
- Long-term memory

This modal model is shown in Figure 3.4.

3.4.1.3 Retrieval

This is the recovery of information from memory when needed.

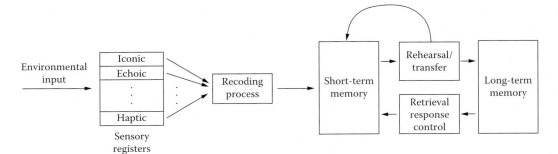

FIGURE 3.4 The multistore modal model of memory. (After Atkinson, R.C. and Shriffrin, R.M., Human memory: A proposed system and its control processes, in Spence, K.W. and Spence, J.T. (eds.), *The Psychology of Learning and Memory*, Vol. 2, Academic Press, New York, 1968, pp. 90–191.)

3.4.2 Influences upon Memory

According to the multistore modal model, sensory memory has a large capacity; sensory information is retained here in an unprocessed form in peripheral receptors. Sensory memory is a very short-lived (fade time 0.5 s) trace of the sensory input. Visual input is briefly retained as a mental image called an icon; this is known as an iconic memory. The sensory memory for auditory information is called an echoic memory, while that for information from touch is called a haptic memory. Sensory memory is considered to give an accurate account of the environment as experienced by the sensory system. It holds a representation of the stimulus so that parts of it can be attended to, processed, and transferred into more permanent memory stores.

Those aspects of sensory information that are the object of active attention are transferred into a temporary working memory called the short-term memory. Encoding is mainly acoustic; visual encoding rapidly fades. This is the memory used temporarily to hold a telephone number, for example, until dialled. It is lost in 20 s unless rehearsed. Short-term (primary or working) memory consists of a small finite number (seven ± two) of registers that can be filled only by data entering one at a time. According to the *displacement principle*, when the registers are full, the addition of a new datum leads to the displacement and loss of an existing one. The probability of correctly recalling an item of information is greater if it is one of the first items to be encountered, even if more than seven items have been presented; this is known as the *primacy effect*. Similarly, the *recency effect* refers to the finding that the probability of correctly recalling an item of information is increased if it is one of the most recent items to be encountered. Those items having an intermediate serial position are least likely to be recalled accurately, and this overall phenomenon is referred to as the *serial position effect*. Whereas the recency effect can be accounted for in terms of the comparatively short interval of time elapsing before recall, the primary effect is more difficult to explain and may be caused by greater rehearsal of these first items. Retrieval from short-term memory is considered to be effortless and error free.

Rehearsal is not as necessary in approximately 5% of children possessing a photographic memory, known in psychology as *eidetic imagery*, in whom a detailed visual image can be retained for over half a minute.

Long-term memory stores information more or less permanently and theoretically may have unlimited capacity, although there may be limitations on retrieval. Input and retrieval take longer and are more effortful than for short-term memory. Some motivation is required to encode information into long-term memory. Schizophrenia and depression affect memory at this level.

3.4.3 Optimal Conditions for Encoding, Storage, and Retrieval of Information

3.4.3.1 Encoding/Registration

Conrad (1964) showed that confusion occurs between acoustically similar letters presented against background noise. For example, the letter P is more likely to be incorrectly recalled as V (which is acoustically similar) than as the letter R (which is visually similar). Baddeley (1966a) then went on to demonstrate that acoustically similar words are also more difficult to recall immediately (a test of short-term memory) than are semantically similar words. For example, the sequence rat, mat, cat, cap (which is acoustically similar) is more difficult to recall immediately than the sequence large, big, huge, grand (which is semantically similar). However, in a test of long-term memory, Baddeley (1966b) found a semantic similarity effect rather than a phonological similarity effect. So, in terms of the parameters studied, it appeared that encoding or registration for short-term memory is better for semantically similar word sequences than for phonologically (acoustically) similar words, while encoding or registration for long-term memory is better for phonologically (acoustically) similar word sequences than for semantically similar words.

Semantic encoding has been shown to aid short-term memory in respect of trigrams (three-letter sequences). Increased memory span has been demonstrated for meaningful trigrams, such as CNN, CIA, NBC, than for meaningless trigrams, such as AUM, GLB, CDX (Bower and Springston, 1970).

With respect to iconic memory encoding, a preceding or subsequent visual sensory presentation of data at a similar energy level (i.e. brightness) to that of the index presentation leads to a masking of the index presentation so that it is not registered. The term for this phenomenon is *energy masking* and occurs at the level of the retina. Another form of masking that has been described is *pattern masking*, in which the preceding or subsequent visual presentation is of data visually similar to that of the index presentation. Pattern masking occurs at a deeper level of visual information processing than the retinal level. The deduction of the relative depth of level of visual processing at which energy masking and pattern masking occur followed from the finding that whereas the former can only take place when the index presentation and the masking presentation are both to the same eye, the latter can take place even when the index presentation is to one eye and the corresponding masking presentation is to the other eye (Turvey, 1973). With respect to rapidly changing picture presentations, it appears to take about 100 ms for a scene to be understood and no longer be susceptible to ordinary visual masking and a further 300 ms or so to no longer be susceptible to conceptual masking (e.g. from a succeeding picture representation) (Potter, 1976).

So far, as the registration of two auditory stimuli is concerned, experiments in which two sounds are presented to subjects and in which the just noticeable interval between noise pulses is compared with the level of second noise pulse demonstrate that confusion occurs between the echoic image of the first auditory presentation and the onset of the second auditory presentation, unless either a sufficient time interval is allowed for the echoic image of the first presentation to fade before presenting the second stimulus or increasing the volume of the second stimulus (Plomp, 1964).

As with visual masking (see aforementioned), *binaural masking* has also been demonstrated. A masking sound presented soon after an index sound interferes with detection; this interference is greater when both stimuli are presented to the same ear than when the masking sound is presented to the contralateral ear following the presentation of the index auditory stimulus (Deatherage and Evans, 1969).

In studies of auditory encoding of stimuli and their serial position, a *suffix effect* occurs. This refers to the auditory encoding error that occurs when there is a categorical similarity between the penultimate and ultimate speech-like sounds heard (Crowder, 1971; Ayres et al., 1979).

Elaborating meaning appears to improve encoding of the written word. For instance, your encoding of the text of each of the remaining chapters of this book is likely to be better if you look at some questions specifically related to these chapters before reading each of them. (Suitable questions may be found in the companion books of multiple choice questions [MCQs] and extended matching items [EMIs].) When you read the actual chapters after being primed with the need to search for the answers, you are more likely to elaborate parts of each of these chapters and encode the information better (Frase, 1975; Anderson, 1980).

3.4.3.2   Storage
One of many examples of findings that are not consistent with the multistore modal model of memory is that of the finding of positive recency effects in delayed free recall.

According to the model, a *continuous distraction procedure*, such as counting backward between the presentation of items such as unrelated words, should prevent the subject from rehearsing the items and should replace these items in short-term memory. However, in practice, the serial position curve shows both a primacy effect and a recency effect under such circumstances (Tzeng, 1973). There also does not appear to be a positive (or negative) relationship between the amount of rehearsal of presented items and how well they are recalled from short-term memory (Craik and Watkins, 1973; Glenberg et al., 1977).

Gillund and Shiffrin (1981) found that the free recall of complex pictures was better than that of words. Many further studies have confirmed a *picture superiority effect*. In general, pictures are remembered and recalled better than words, and nonverbal information storage of pictures and designs is found to be more stable over a period of hours and days than is the storage of words (e.g. Hart and O'Shanick, 1993). Simple pictures appear to be better remembered than complex pictures; the *asymmetric confusability effect* is manifested in the finding that there is a greater accuracy in recognition testing of same versus changed stimulus in simple rather than complex pictures (Pezdek and Chen, 1982).

3.4.3.3   Retrieval
Retrieval of information from the long-term memory is error prone but is improved if the information being stored is organized. *Hierarchical organization* is particularly useful in this regard, perhaps because it improves the search process within long-term memory (Bower et al., 1969).

Another optimal condition for retrieval of information is to arrange that the context within which the information is to be retrieved is similar to that within which it was encoded (Estes, 1972).

3.4.4   Memory Information Processing

3.4.4.1   Primary Working Memory Storage Capacity
Working memory refers to the temporary storage of information in connection with performing other, more complex, tasks (Baddeley, 2007). In the multistore modal model of memory, it is the short-term memory (or short-term store) that acts as a key working memory system to allow information to transfer into the long-term memory (or long-term store) and thereby allow learning to take place.

As mentioned earlier, a number of findings, such as the lack of a positive (or negative) relationship between the amount of rehearsal of presented items and how well they are recalled from short-term memory (Craik and Watkins, 1973), cast doubt on the validity of the multi-store modal model of memory and in particular on the assumption implicit in this model that holding information in short-term memory (or the short-term store) necessarily leads to information transfer into long-term memory (or the long-term store). Furthermore, since in this modal model the short-term memory (store) acts as the working memory that is essential for learning, it would be expected that patients with short-term memory (store) impairment should manifest impaired long-term learning. However, Shallice and Warrington (1970) described the case of a patient with a severely affected short-term memory (store) who nonetheless had a normal long-term learning capacity; this patient had a memory span of just two digits and almost no recency effect in the free recall task (in which the subject is asked to recall as many of a previously presented list of unrelated words as they can, in any order). Moreover, when a short-term memory (store) deficit is experimentally induced in normal subjects by giving them digits to rehearse concurrently with a grammatical reasoning task, even with eight digits, the reasoning time only increases by around 50% and the error rate remains around 5% (the same as with fewer digits to rehearse) (Baddeley and Hitch, 1974), and this in spite of the fact that a digit load of eight should have totally filled the short-term memory (store) according to the multistore modal model. Tasks using a similar digit load concurrent with comprehension and free recall learning also show that the long-term memory (store) can be impaired but that the recency effect still occurs, again contrary to the modal model prediction.

In response to these difficulties, Baddeley and Hitch formulated the working memory model shown diagrammatically in Figure 3.5. The *central executive* is an attentional controller, which is supported by two active slave systems, the *articulatory* or *phonological loop*, responsible for the maintenance of speech-based information, and the *visuospatial scratchpad* or *sketchpad*, which can hold and manipulate information in the visuospatial domain. This model was compatible with the findings mentioned in the previous paragraph. For example, concurrent verbal (articulatory) activity and visual or spatial activity appear to interfere with two different systems; subjects using a mnemonic based on spatial location to remember word lists have better recall of the lists than those who use a simple rote rehearsal procedure, but this advantage disappears if the former subjects are required to carry out a

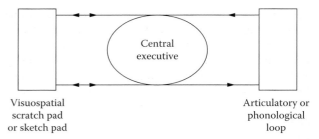

FIGURE 3.5   The working memory model of Baddeley and Hitch. (After Baddeley, A.D. and Hitch, G., Working memory, in Bower, G.A. (ed.), *The Psychology of Learning and Motivation*, Vol. 8, Academic Press, New York, 1974, pp. 47–89.)

visuospatial task concurrently (Baddeley and Lieberman, 1980). Again, a patient with gross impairment of digit span would be hypothesized to have a defect of their phonological loop functioning; if there were no coexistent impairment of the functioning of the central executive or visuospatial sketchpad, then normal learning would still be possible.

Working memory capacity can be measured using a task in which, after reading a series of sentences, the subject is required to recall the last word of each of these sentences (Daneman and Carpenter, 1980). This task therefore requires both comprehension and recall (as opposed to just recall in the simple word span task).

There is a strong positive correlation between working memory tests and intelligence quotient (IQ) tests. Furthermore, standard IQ appear to be more susceptible to the subject's previous knowledge, whereas working memory tests appear to have a greater relationship to the speed of processing (Kyllonen and Christal, 1990).

In terms of the model of working memory of Baddeley and Hitch (1974), the central executive is a limited-capacity system, which provides the link between the two slave systems (see Figure 3.5) and long-term memory; it is responsible for planning and selecting strategies (Baddeley, 2007). The visuospatial scratchpad or sketchpad appears to have a visual component, which is concerned with such factors as shape and colour, and a spatial component, which is concerned with location (Baddeley and Lieberman, 1980; Baddeley, 2007). The articulatory or phonological loop also appears to be made up of two components: a memory store that can hold phonological information for 1–2 s and an articulatory control process (or processor) (Paulesu et al., 1993; Baddeley, 2007). Memory traces in the phonological loop can be refreshed by means of subvocal articulation. (Subvocal or vocal articulation may also be used to provide an input into this slave system upon the visual presentation of objects by the subject articulating the names of those objects.) The phonological loop is held to provide the basis for digit span. In particular, the number of items retained in the digit span is believed to be a function of both the rate of fading of the memory trace in the phonological loop and the rate of refreshing of memory traces by means of subvocal articulation. The size of the storage capacity can be reduced in the following ways:

- *The phonological similarity effect*—trying to remember items with similar sounding names.
- *Presenting irrelevant spoken material*—this gains access to the store and corrupts the memory trace.
- *The word length effect*—as the length of the words increases, the memory span decreases, presumably because of the longer time required for longer words to be rehearsed, leading to a greater probability of memory trace decay.
- *Articulatory suppression*—requiring a subject repeatedly to articulate an irrelevant speech sound that interferes with subvocal rehearsal.

3.4.4.2   Principle of Chunking

Chunking increases the amount of information stored in 'short-term memory registers' (in the multimodal model) by allowing one entry to cover several items. While the number of chunks is restricted, their content is not. With the help of long-term memory, new material can be recoded, thereby increasing the content of chunks.

For example, British trainee and qualified psychiatrists are unlikely to require eight 'registers' in order to remember the letters MRCPSYCH. Similarly, the string DSMIVTRICDEEG can readily be split into the chunks DSM-IV-TR, ICD, and EEG.

It has been suggested that the acquisition of skills through practice may involve the grouping of sets of mental entities (be they motor or perceptual) as chunks (Newell and Rosenbloom, 1981).

3.4.4.3   Semantic Memory

Semantic memory refers to the subject's knowledge of facts, language, concepts, and the like and is an aspect of long-term/secondary memory that is consistent with the finding that verbal information is stored in terms of meaning rather than exact words (Tulving, 1972). It is easier to remember words paired with meanings (Bower, 1972) and to recall words synonymous to those in a given list (Sachs, 1967). Therefore, semantic encoding is a more efficient way than simple rehearsal of transferring information from the 'short-term memory' to the long-term/secondary one.

3.4.4.4   Episodic Memory

Episodic memory is an aspect of long-term/secondary memory that refers to the memory for events. It provides a continually changing and updated record of autobiographical material (Tulving, 1972).

3.4.4.5   Skills Memory

Skills memory, or procedural memory, is an aspect of long-term/secondary memory that supports skilled performance.

3.4.4.6   Other Aspects of Long-Term/ Secondary Memory

Ryle (1949) distinguished between procedural knowledge and *declarative knowledge*; whereas the former referred to knowledge that supported the performance of tasks, the latter referred to factual knowledge. Tulving (1985) distinguished between *autonoetic awareness* (or remembering) and *noetic awareness* (or knowing).

3.4.5   Process of Forgetting and the Influence of Emotional Factors on Retrieval

3.4.5.1   Forgetting

Forgetting from long-term/secondary memory is usually the result of retrieval failure rather than storage failure. This explains why forgotten memories can be recovered under hypnosis and also the 'tip of the tongue' experience.

3.4.5.2   Theories of Forgetting

Under the multimodal model of memory, forgetting from long-term memory could be caused by interference or trace decay.

According to the *interference theory*, forgetting by interference is item dependent. There are two main types:

- *Proactive interference/inhibition*—previous learning is likely to impair subsequent learning.
- *Retroactive interference/inhibition*—new learning is likely to impair previous learning.

According to the *decay theory*, memories fade with time. The longer the item remains in the memory system, the weaker is its strength. New material has a high trace strength, while older has a low trace strength. Forgetting by decay is time dependent.

3.4.5.3 Influence of Emotional Factors on Retrieval

Emotional factors can influence retrieval from long-term memory in the following ways:

- Emotionally charged situations are rehearsed and organized more than nonemotionally charged ones. Retrieval is facilitated.
- Negative emotions and anxiety hinder retrieval.
- Retrieval of events and emotions is more likely to be successful if it occurs in the same context as that in which the original events and emotions occurred; this is known as *state-dependent learning.*
- Repression of emotionally charged material hinders retrieval.

3.4.6 Processes of Interference, Schemata, and Elaboration

3.4.6.1 Interference

Retroactive interference refers to the negative effect of new learning on retrieval of prior knowledge. It has been demonstrated in many experimental trials, for example, by Slamecka (1960). In contrast, proactive interference refers to the negative effect of prior knowledge on new learning.

3.4.6.2 Schemata

A schema (plural schemata) may be defined as a mental model or representation, built up through experience, about a person, an object, a situation, or an event (Searleman and Herrmann, 1994). The roles of schemata include (Morton and Bekerian, 1986)

- Interpretation of sensory data
- Retrieval of information from memory
- Organization of actions
- Determination of goals
- Determination of behaviour
- Allocation of processing resources
- Directing overall processing in attentional, perceptual, and memory systems

They help to integrate information that is currently being experienced with the subject's long-term past in a single representation (Groeger, 1997).

It has been suggested that their lack of the schemata needed to help organize episodic memory may help explain the origin of *infantile amnesia*, that is, the inability of humans to access their early childhood memories (Schachtel, 1947). In contrast, the organization of retrieval cues into stable *retrieval schemata* has been put forward as being part of the explanation of the occurrence of exceptional memory performance, in the *skilled memory theory* (Ericsson and Kintsch, 1995).

3.4.6.3 Elaboration

As mentioned in Section 3.4, elaboration appears to improve encoding of new information. Methods of elaboration include

- Semantic processing
- Forming complex images
- Attempting to answer questions based on the material to be learned

3.5 FACTORS AFFECTING THOUGHT

3.5.1 Relationship of Thought to Language

Early work in psychology suggested that thought could not occur independently of language. It was held that children, on learning to speak, simply articulated their thoughts until they learned to suppress the vocalization, whence thought simply became concealed speech. Watson (1913) argued that (unarticulated) thought consisted of laryngeal motor habits. This gained support from the electrophysiological finding of Jacobsen (1932) that mental activities ('thought') were accompanied by electric activity in the musculature of the throat.

There is much evidence that stands in opposition to this early theory. The following two examples are;

- Many infrahuman animals appear to be able to think but do not appear to possess language.
- Temporary paralysis of all voluntary muscles with *d*-tubocurarine is not associated with an inability to think (Smith et al., 1947).

3.5.1.1 Concepts

Concepts are the properties or relationships that given object classes or ideas have in common. They constitute a means of grouping what otherwise would form too wide a variety of disparate items or ideas for efficient thought and communication.

Concrete concepts refer to objects. For example, the concept 'book' refers to objects having properties shared by most books, such as having pages, containing information, having a title, and having authors.

Abstract concepts refer to abstract ideas, such as honesty, integrity, and justice. Concepts of activities include drinking, walking, and cycling.

3.5.1.2 Prototypes

Prototypes are idealized forms. For instance, the prototypical book might be considered to have the shape of this book with a front cover having a title; a back cover; multiple pages in between the covers mostly containing printed words arranged into sentences, paragraphs, subsections, sections, and chapters; some diagrams interspersed among the words; a title page and list of contents at the beginning; and an index at the end of the pages. According to the prototype theory, the acquisition of prototypes occurs through repeated exposure.

3.5.2 REASONING

3.5.2.1 Deductive Reasoning

This is reasoning based on deduction, the domains of which include

- Relational inferences
- Propositional inferences
- Syllogisms
- Multiply quantified inferences

Relational inferences are based on relations such as

- Is equal to, denoted by =
- Is greater than, denoted by >
- Is less than, denoted by <
- Is greater than or equal to, denoted by $\geq$
- Is less than or equal to, denoted by $\leq$
- After
- Before
- To the right of
- To the left of

Propositional inferences are based on relations such as

- Negation, denoted by −
- Conjunction, denoted by &
- Disjunction, denoted by $\vee$
- Implication, denoted by $\rightarrow$
- Bi-implication, denoted by $\leftrightarrow$

(Note that these are the symbols used in logic; in ordinary mathematics, other symbols are often used, for instance $\Rightarrow$ for implication.)

Syllogisms are based on pairs of statements or premises, each of which contains one quantifier, such as

- The universal quantifier ('for all'), denoted by $\forall$
- Some
- The existential quantifier ('there exist(s)'), denoted by $\exists$

Multiply quantified inferences are based on statements or premises that contain more than quantifier. (Such statements in turn can be converted into sets of statements that each contain only one quantifier.)

The arithmetic symbols used in formal reasoning statements can be reduced to just three:

- The zero symbol, denoted by 0
- The successor symbol, denoted by ′
- The addition symbol, denoted by +

In addition, it is convenient to include

- The multiplication symbol, denoted by ·

For example, the statement that every (real) number possesses a square root may be formally stated as

$$\forall x_0 \, \exists x_1 \, (x_1 \cdot x_1) = x_0$$

Some have argued that human cerebral deductive reasoning is dependent on the formal rules of inference, as used in formal logic (e.g. Braine et al., 1984); these are known as *formal rule theories*. In contrast, other cognitive scientists such as Johnson-Laird (1993) have argued that deductive reasoning (and indeed also inductive reasoning) is a semantic process rather similar to that carried out when searching for counterexamples; this is known as the *mental model theory*.

As an example, suppose that we consider the following deductive reasoning problem relating to the relative positions of various chapters of this book:

- The chapter on schizophrenia comes after the chapter on social sciences.
- The chapter on social psychology comes before the chapter on social sciences.
- What is the positional relationship between the chapter on schizophrenia and the chapter on social psychology?

The only model containing all three chapters that is consistent with these statements is

Social psychology
Social sciences
Schizophrenia

So the answer to the question is that the chapter on schizophrenia comes after the chapter on social psychology. There is just one model corresponding to the statements, and the problem has a valid answer, and so this is known as a *one-model problem with a valid answer*. Now, consider the following problem:

- The chapter on schizophrenia comes after the chapter on social psychology.
- The chapter on social sciences comes after the chapter on social psychology.
- What is the positional relationship between the chapter on schizophrenia and the chapter on social sciences?

There are now two models containing all three chapters that are consistent with these statements:

Social psychology
Social sciences
Schizophrenia

and

Social psychology
Schizophrenia
Social sciences

In this particular case, there are two models, and there is no positional relationship between the chapter on schizophrenia and the chapter on social sciences that is common to both models. We say that there is no valid answer. This case is a *multiple-model problem with no valid answers*.

Formal rule theories predict that one-model problems are more difficult than multiple-model problems with valid answers. In contrast, the mental model theory predicts that multiple-model problems with no valid answers are more difficult than multiple-model problems with valid answers, which in turn are themselves more difficult than one-model problems. Experimental evidence supports the mental model theory (e.g. Byrne and Johnson-Laird, 1989).

3.5.2.2 Inductive Reasoning
In inductive reasoning, a general statement is derived by inductive arguments from many instances. An elementary example is given from number theory in mathematics.

Consider the following (correct) equations:

- $1 = 1$
- $1 + 2 = 3$
- $1 + 2 + 2^2 = 7$
- $1 + 2 + 2^2 + 2^3 = 15$
- $1 + 2 + 2^2 + 2^3 + 2^4 = 31$
- $1 + 2 + 2^2 + 2^3 + 2^4 + 2^5 = 63$

Consider the values of the positive integers (whole numbers) on the right-hand side of each equation. We have

- $1 = 2 - 1 = 2^1 - 1$
- $3 = 2^2 - 1$
- $7 = 2^3 - 1$
- $15 = 2^4 - 1$
- $31 = 2^5 - 1$
- $63 = 2^6 - 1$

So here we have the following pattern that appears to be emerging:

$$1 + 2 + 2^2 + 2^3 + \cdots + 2^{n-1} = 2^n - 1 \tag{3.1}$$

(This may also be written as $2^0 + 2^1 + 2^2 + 2^3 + \cdots + 2^{n-1} = 2^n - 1$.)

We have six instances in which Equation 3.1 is true. What we shall now do is use inductive reasoning to prove that the general statement, Equation 3.1, is itself true.

Let S represent the set of positive integers (positive whole numbers, such as 1, 2, and 3) for which the formula given in Equation 3.1 is correct. Now, when $n = 1$, the left-hand side of this formula is 1, while the right-hand side is $2^1 - 1 = 2 - 1 = 1$. Since $1 = 1$, the formula is correct for $n = 1$. Therefore, the integer 1 belongs to the set S. Assume now that Equation 3.1 is true for a fixed positive integer k. Then we have

$$1 + 2 + 2^2 + \cdots + 2^{k-1} = 2^k - 1 \tag{3.2}$$

Now we need to show that our formula holds for the positive integer $k + 1$. If we add 2^k to each side of Equation 3.2, we obtain

$$1 + 2 + 2^2 + \cdots + 2^{k-1} + 2^k = 2^k - 1 + 2^k$$
$$= 2^k + 2^k - 1$$
$$= 2 \cdot 2^k - 1$$
$$= 2^1 \cdot 2^k - 1$$
$$= 2^{k+1} - 1$$

So this means that Equation 3.1 is true when $n = k+1$. Therefore, $k + 1$ belongs to S. Hence, whenever the positive integer k belongs to S, then $k + 1$ belongs to S. But we know that 1 belongs to S. Hence, by inductive reasoning, it follows that S must contain all positive integers. So the formula shown in Equation 3.1, initially hypothesized on just six instances, has been shown to hold for all positive integers (infinite in number) by inductive reasoning.

3.5.3 Problem-Solving Strategies

3.5.3.1 Alternative Representations

One method of problem solving is to represent the given data in a different way. For example, we have seen two different representations in the last two examples. In the first of these, in which a problem relating to the relative order of chapters of this book was set, a diagrammatic representation was used, in which the data were, as it were, visualized. In the most recent example, on the other hand, in which inductive reasoning was being used, it was more convenient to use symbolic representation. In a similar fashion, in elementary mathematics, problem-solving can also sometimes be carried out using a more geometric approach or a more algebraic approach.

3.5.3.2 Expertise

The way in which problems are represented by experts tends to differ from the representations used by inexperienced people. For instance, the way in which the reader (assumed to be clinically competent and qualified) might diagnose a central nervous system lesion in a patient would likely be different and more efficient (and more likely to be correct) than the methods employed by relatively inexperienced third-year medical students; the recall of the patient symptoms and signs would also tend to be better for the reader. In particular, compared with a beginner, an expert's memory would tend to have more potential representations of the problem that he or she can draw upon to solve it. Experts are also more likely to be able to invoke heuristics (see succeeding text) that are not available to novices.

3.5.3.3 Computer Simulation

Computer simulations may be used to study the way in which representations and heuristics are employed in problem solving.

3.5.4 Algorithms

In a general sort of way, an algorithm consists of a specific sequence of steps that need to be carried out according to precise instructions in order to solve a given problem. For example, suppose you were to stop reading right now and take a pencil and paper and calculate the value of 22 divided by 7 to 3 decimal places, using long division. The correct answer is 3.143. The method you used to carry out this calculation involved a mechanical use of the rules of long division; no deep thought is required but, rather, a simple adherence to the simple rules of this method of problem solving. This is a characteristic feature of algorithms.

More precisely, an algorithm is any process that can be carried out by a Turing machine. A Turing machine is a simple, mechanical calculating device invented by the British mathematician Alan Turing (1912–1954). At its most basic, a Turing machine can be imagined to be an infinitely long tape segmented into squares. Starting at any one square, the Turing machine can do the following:

1. Stop the computation
2. Move one square to the right
3. Move one square to the left
4. Write S_0 to replace whatever is in the square being scanned
5. Write S_1 to replace whatever is in the square being scanned

.
.
.

$n+4$. Write S_n to replace whatever is in the square being scanned

This may seem, at first sight, to be a rather primitive machine that can only handle addition and subtraction, say. In fact, however, it can carry out multiplication, division, and the calculation of square roots and other power functions. Indeed, it may be the case that, in principle, a Turing machine can carry out any calculation that a powerful modern supercomputer can.

3.5.5 Heuristics

As mentioned earlier, heuristics are strategies that can be applied to problems and that often give the correct answer (or 'goal state') more quickly than simple algorithms; they are not guaranteed to work, however. Such heuristic techniques are not usually available to novices, whereas experts can access these during problem-solving. As an example, at one stage of his career, the author of this chapter had cause to devise a method of accurately quantifying cerebral ventricular volumes in serial magnetic resonance scans that had been accurately matched using a subvoxel registration, a feat that had not hitherto been accomplished. A heuristic of the type 'consider an analogous problem that you know you can solve' was used first, and then this solution was generalized to allow the required equations to be arrived at.

3.6 FACTORS AFFECTING PERSONALITY

3.6.1 DERIVATION OF NOMOTHETIC AND IDIOGRAPHIC THEORIES

The terms nomothetic and idiographic in respect of the study of people were introduced by Wilhelm Windelband, the German philosopher who taught at Heidelberg and initiated axiological neo-Kantianism. He distinguished between the study of whole populations (the nomothetic approach) and the study of individuals (the idiographic approach).

The nomothetic approach to personality considers that personality theory should be at least partly based on the study of the common features and differences between people. For instance, personality has been defined by Wiggins (1979) as being

> …that branch of psychology which is concerned with providing a systematic account of the ways in which individuals differ from one another.

In contrast, the idiographic approach attempts to gain an understanding of personality in the context of each individual's unique existence. According to Tyrer and Ferguson (2000),

> The idiographic approach focuses on the uniqueness of the individual and as such can provide a rich, multifaceted description of subtle areas of personal attributes and behaviour. Numerous strands are brought together to build up a portrait which cannot be confused with any other. The case history is the most obvious example and has been used with effect to describe processes, which can then be generalized to explain similar psychological mechanisms in others.

An influential early proponent of the idiographic approach was Gordon Willard Allport (1937), but the nomothetic approach has prevailed.

3.6.2 TRAIT AND STATE APPROACHES

Traits are 'broad, enduring, relatively stable characteristics used to assess and explain behaviour' (Hirschberg, 1978).

The study of traits has a long history. Aristotle (in his *Nicomachean Ethics* of the fourth century BCE) regarded determinants of moral and immoral behaviour to include the following phenomena, which we might regard as being traits:

- Cowardice
- Modesty
- Vanity

As mentioned in Chapter 2, the Greek physician Galen of Pergamum (Greek: Claudios Galenos; Latin: Claudius Galenus) regarded the four Hippocratic humours as forming the basis for his four temperaments:

- Choleric
- Melancholic
- Phlegmatic
- Sanguine

The German philosopher Immanuel Kant (1724–1804) placed these four temperaments along the following two dimensions:

- Activity
- Feelings

Thus, a choleric temperament corresponded to strong activity, and a phlegmatic temperament corresponded to weak activity. Similarly, a sanguine temperament corresponded to strong feelings, and a melancholic temperament corresponded to weak feelings.

The German physiologist and psychologist Wilhelm Wundt (1832–1920), whom most regard as the father of experimental psychology, superimposed the following two dimensions on the four temperaments:

- Strong *versus* weak emotions
- Changeable (or rapid changes) *versus* unchangeable activity (or slow changes)

Thus, a choleric temperament was unstable (strong emotion) and changeable (rapid changes); a melancholic temperament was unstable and unchangeable; a phlegmatic temperament was stable (weak emotions) and unchangeable; and a sanguine temperament was stable and changeable.

A major impetus was given to the scientific study of the trait approach to personality research by developments in statistical techniques, particularly the use of systematic collection of data and the discovery of correlational and factor analytic techniques. Cattell et al. (1970) have developed the Sixteen Personality Factor

Questionnaire (16PF) that measures 16 primary factors along 16 dimensions. These are as follows:

- Trait A: Outgoing/warmhearted *versus* reserved/detached
- Trait B: Intelligence
- Trait C: Unemotional/calm *versus* emotional/changeable
- Trait E: Assertive/dominant *versus* humble/cooperative
- Trait F: Cheerful/lively *versus* sober/taciturn
- Trait G: Conscientious/persistent *versus* expedient/undisciplined
- Trait H: Venturesome/socially bold *versus* shy/retiring
- Trait I: Tough minded/self-reliant *versus* tender minded/sensitive
- Trait L: Suspicious/sceptical *versus* trusting/accepting
- Trait M: Imaginative/Bohemian *versus* practical/conventional
- Trait N: Shrewd/discreet *versus* forthright/straightforward
- Trait O: Guilt prone/worrying *versus* resilient/self-assured
- Trait Q1: Radical/experimental *versus* conservative/traditional
- Trait Q2: Self-sufficient/resourceful *versus* group dependent/affiliative
- Trait Q3: Controlled/compulsive *versus* undisciplined/lax
- Trait Q4: Tense/driven *versus* relaxed/tranquil

In contrast, Hans Eysenck's rating studies initially only yielded two dimensions and more recently the following three dimensions (following a factor analysis of items) (see Eysenck and Eysenck, 1991):

- Extraversion (i.e. extraversion *vs.* introversion)
- Neuroticism
- Psychoticism

The first two of these dimensions were derived by Eysenck (1944) following the study of 700 soldiers in a military hospital suffering from various 'neurotic' disorders and complaints (such as 'headaches', 'sex anomalies', and 'narrow interests'). Extraversion is associated with traits such as

- Sociable
- Lively

- Dominant
- Carefree
- Active
- Assertive
- Sensation seeking
- Venturesome
- Surgent

Introversion is associated with the opposite traits. Neuroticism is associated with traits such as

- Anxious
- Depressed
- Emotional
- Guilt feelings
- Irrational
- Low self-esteem
- Moody
- Shy
- Tense

Psychoticism, which is orthogonal to (and therefore independent of) extraversion and neuroticism in the revised Eysenck factor analysis-based model of personality, is associated with traits such as

- Aggressive
- Antisocial
- Cold
- Creative
- Egocentric
- Impersonal
- Impulsive
- Tough minded
- Unempathetic

In contrast to traits, which refer to stable phenomena related to behaviour and ideas relating to enduring dispositions, states are unstable short-term features of the individual. An example of a state variable is a temporary short-term feeling of anxiety in someone who normally scores highly on the extraversion dimension.

Trait and state approaches can be combined. For example, Figure 3.6 shows a model (based on Michael Eysenck, 1982) of the adverse effects of anxiety on information processing and performance; this model in turn is based on the more complex model of Spielberger (1962).

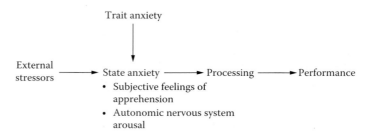

FIGURE 3.6 Eysenck's state–trait model showing the effects of anxiety on performance. (After Eysenck, M.W., *Attention and Arousal: Cognition and Performance*, Springer, New York, 1982.)

3.6.3 Construct Theory

The personal construct theory of George Kelly (an American engineer who went on to become a clinical psychologist) is based on the proposition that behaviour in humans is anticipatory rather than reactive (Kelly, 1955). Kelly considered every man to be a scientist, interpreting the world on the basis of past experience. Constructs are created and predictions made accordingly. A system of constructs results, unique in each individual, existing at various levels of consciousness, those formed at earlier developmental stages being unconscious. Each construct has a range of convenience; some are specific, for example, chewy versus tender; and others have a wider range of convenience. Constructs are arranged into hierarchies. Superordinate constructs are central to the individual's sense of identity, and subordinate constructs less so.

According to this theory, anxiety results when the individual is presented with events outside their range of personal constructs. Hostility comprises imposition of constructs upon another.

The main points relating to construct systems are as follows:

1. Individuals' construct systems make the world more predictable and thereby make it easier to negotiate one's way around.
2. Individuals' construct systems are not static but may grow and be modified in response to circumstances. For example, suppose you were under the impression that professors of psychiatry are honest, intelligent people of integrity who care deeply about the need to help discover the aetiology of various types of mental illness and who wish to help find the best treatments for such illnesses. If you were then to discover that a couple of such professors were in fact utterly dishonest, cruel, selfish, and psychopathic, with little or no real commitment to academic excellence but ready to steal the fruits of the work of others, then your

construct system in this regard would be challenged. In these circumstances, you could alter your construct system in one of following ways:
   a. Adaptation. Your construct system could be changed to reflect your new experience.
   b. Immunization. You could try to maintain your belief system by having thoughts such as 'There must be some important reason that I am not privy to which explains why they seemed to act in such an evil way'.
3. The construct system of an individual represents the truth as uniquely understood and experienced by that person.
4. A construct system is not necessarily internally consistent.
5. Since construct systems are partly a function of prior experience, they affect expectations and behaviour.
6. Constructs representing core values and the most important relationships of a person are more firmly held and of greater importance that those related to less important matters.
7. The degree to which one individual can relate to and understand the construct system of another person is a function to their empathy with the latter.

3.6.4 Humanist Approaches

Humanistic approaches pay particular attention to those qualities that differentiate humans from nonhuman animal species. The Association for Humanistic Psychology lists the following five basic postulates:

- Man, as man, supersedes the sum of his parts.
- Man has his being in a human context.
- Man is aware.
- Man has choice.
- Man is intentional.

Self-actualization is held to be a core individual motivational force.

3.6.4.1 Roger's Self Theory

Each individual has a drive to fulfil themselves and develop an *ideal self* within a *phenomenal field* of subjective experience. The most important aspect of personality is the congruence between the individual's view of himself or herself and reality and their view of themselves compared with the ideal self. If an individual acts at variance to their own self-image, anxiety, incongruence, and denial result. The congruent individual is able to grow (self-actualization) and achieve their potential both internally and socially.

3.6.4.2 Maslow

Abraham Maslow is considered to be another leading founder of the humanist approach. Maslow's hierarchy of needs is considered in Section 3.7.5. Transient episodes of self-actualization have been termed *peak experiences* by Maslow (1970); they are described in terms such as

- Aliveness
- Beauty
- Effortlessness
- Goodness
- Perfection
- Self-sufficiency
- Truth
- Uniqueness
- Wholeness

Characteristics of self-actualizers according to Maslow (1967) include the following:

- They accept themselves and other people for what they are.
- They are highly creative.
- They have a good sense of humour.
- They tend to be problem centred rather than self-centred.
- They are able to tolerate uncertainty.
- They exhibit spontaneous thought.
- They exhibit spontaneous behaviour.
- Even though they do not make an effort to be unconventional, nevertheless they are resistant to enculturation.
- They have the capacity to consider life objectively.
- They form deep and satisfying relationships with relatively few others.

Behaviours that Maslow (1967) considered that may lead to self-actualization include

- Being honest
- Assuming responsibility
- Working hard at the tasks decided upon
- Become fully absorbed and concentrate fully, experiencing life as a child does
- Identifying one's defences and giving them up
- Being prepared to try new things
- Evaluate experiences personally without being swayed by the opinions of others
- Being willing to be unpopular

3.6.5 Psychoanalytic Approaches

Behaviour and feelings are explained by unconscious drives and conflicts. The *id* is held to be derived from the libido. Irrational, impulsive instincts are unable to postpone gratification and are present at birth. The *ego* develops as the child grows. A conscious mind balances the demands of the id with the realities of the outside world. Anxiety results if ego is unable to control the energies of id. The *superego* comprises the internalization of the views of parents and society, like a conscience. The id, ego, and superego are in balance with each other.

3.6.5.1 Freud's Stages of Psychosexual Development

Oral stage

- Age 0–1 year.
- Gratification through sucking, biting.
- Failure to negotiate leads to oral personality traits: moodiness, generosity, depression and elation, talkativeness, greed, optimism, pessimism, wishful thinking, and narcissism.

Anal stage

- Age 1–3 years.
- The anus and defecation are sources of sensual pleasure.
- Failure to negotiate leads to anal personality traits: obsessive–compulsive personality, tidiness, parsimony, rigidity, and thoroughness.

Phallic stage

- Age 3–5 years.
- Genital interest relates to own sexuality. Oedipus/Electra complex.
- Failure to negotiate leads to hysterical personality traits: competitiveness and ambitiousness.

Latency stage

- Age 5–12 years.

Genital stage

- Age 12–20 years.
- Gratification from normal relations with people.
- Able to relate to a partner.

3.6.5.2 Erikson's Stages of Development

Age (Years)	Sense of
0–1	Trust/security
1–4	Autonomy
4–5	Initiative
5–11	Duty/accomplishment
11–15	Identity
15–adult	Intimacy
Adulthood	Generativity
Maturity	Integrity

Epigenesis is the process of development of the ego through these stages.

3.6.6 SITUATIONIST APPROACH

The external situation is considered the most powerful determinant of behaviour. Situationists maintain that traits *result* from differences in learning experiences. Behaviour changes according to the situation an individual finds themselves in. Proponents dismiss the trait theory. Mischel (1983) argues against the existence of any stable personality dimension because of poor correlation between behaviour or attitudes in one situation compared with another.

3.6.7 INTERACTIONIST APPROACH

Interactionism holds that behaviour depends upon both the situation and the person (or personality traits) as well as their mutual interaction. Endler (1983) was a prominent advocate of the interactionist approach, arguing that behaviour is

a function of a continuous multidirectional process of person-by-situation interactions; cognitive, motivational and emotional factors have important determining roles on behaviour, regarding the person side; and the perception or psychological meaning that the situation has for the person is an essential determining factor of behaviour.

3.6.8 INVENTORIES

Personality inventories are questionnaires in which the same questions are put to each person.

3.6.8.1 16PF

As mentioned earlier, Cattell et al. (1970) developed the 16PF that measures 16 primary factors along 16 dimensions. It was based on the use of factor analysis to identify these 16 basic personality traits, which are listed earlier, from an initial list of over 3000 personality trait names of Allport and Odbert (1936). Over 100 questions (with yes/no answers) were then selected to allow these traits to be measured. For example, the following question helps to assess trait E (assertive/dominant *vs*. humble/cooperative):

Do you tend to keep in the background on social occasions?

An affirmative reply would give the subject a point on the humble/cooperative end of the trait E scale, while a negative reply would give a point on the assertive/domain end.

The 16PF gives scores on various personality characteristics such as

- Dominance
- Emotional stability
- Self-control

3.6.8.2 MMPI

The opinions of experts (usually working in psychiatry) were garnered in generating the categories for subjects on whom the Minnesota Multiphasic Personality Inventory or MMPI was developed. The final version of the MMPI contains over 550 (567 in one recent version) statements (or questions), relating to

- Attitudes
- Emotional reactions
- Physical symptoms
- Psychological symptoms

The person being tested is asked to answer true, false, or cannot say to each statement.

An example of such a statement is as follows:

At times, my thoughts have raced ahead faster that I could speak them.

An affirmative to this statement would yield a higher score on the hypomania (Ma) scale. Scores are obtained for several scales from the MMPI as follows (with their abbreviations):

- Lie/social desirability (L)
- Frequency/distress (F)
- Correction/defensiveness (K)
- Hypochondriasis (Hs)
- Depression (D)
- Hysteria (Hy)
- Psychopathic deviancy (Pd)
- Paranoia (Pa)
- Psychasthenia (Pt)
- Schizophrenia (Sc)
- Hypomania (Ma)
- Social introversion–extraversion (Si)
- Masculinity–femininity (Mf)

The first three of these scales are used for validity purposes. They include the following statements:

1. L scale
   a. Once in a while, I think of things too bad to talk about.
   b. At times, I feel like swearing.
   c. I do not always tell the truth.
   d. Once in a while, I put off until tomorrow what I ought to do today.
   e. I would rather win than lose in a game.
   f. I do not like everyone I know.
2. F scale
   a. Evil spirits possess me at times.
   b. When I am with people, I am bothered by hearing very queer things.
   c. My soul sometimes leaves my body.
   d. Someone has been trying to poison me.
   e. Someone has been trying to rob me.
   f. Everything tastes the same.
   g. My neck spots with red often.
   h. Someone has been trying to influence my mind.
3. K scale
   a. Often, I can't understand why I have been so cross and grouchy.
   b. At times, my thoughts have raced ahead faster than I could speak them.
   c. Criticism or scolding hurts me terribly.
   d. I certainly feel useless at times.
   e. I have never felt better in my life than I do now.
   f. What others think of me does not bother me.

g. I find it hard to make talk when I meet new people.
h. I frequently find myself worrying about something.

Tyrer and Ferguson (2000) have made the following comment:

> …the individual scales … show a considerable degree of intercorrelation. The scales themselves have unfortunately been labelled using standard psychiatric nosology (e.g. paranoia, schizophrenia and hypomania) which can lead to confusion with Axis I diagnosis. They should more properly be regarded as indicative of the presence of specific personality attributes. Although the MMPI is currently used in candidate-selection procedures, its principal value would appear to be in the study of clinically abnormal personalities where interpretation by an experienced psychologist is required.

In addition to the problem of the intercorrelation of many scales, another problem with the MMPI is that responses may change over time. (This is a problem relating to reliability.) The same person taking the MMPI at baseline and then a few days later may score differently overall and on different scales.

3.6.8.3 CPI

The California Psychological Inventory or CPI employs some of the same statements as the MMPI. In the development of the CPI, the opinions of nonexperts, such as the peers of the test subjects, were used. The CPI is constructed to measure less 'abnormal' personality traits than the MMPI (in 'normal' people), such as

- Dominance
- Independence
- Responsibility
- Self-acceptance
- Socialization
- Flexibility
- Masculinity/femininity

In total, the CPI has over 450 (480 in one recent version) true/false items, of which many (178 in the same recent version) are from the MMPI, and yields 15 scales that measure personality and three scales that are used to eliminate response bias. Overall, the CPI yields the following three broad *vector scales*:

- Internality/externality
- Norm favouring/norm questioning
- Self-fulfilled/dispirited

The CPI was given to 13,000 individuals, and separate scores were obtained for males and females. The mean scores for each scale were obtained. The scores of subjects now taking the CPI can be compared with the mean scores for these original 13,000 individuals.

3.6.8.4   Other Inventories

Other personality inventories include

- Children's Personality Questionnaire
- Differential Personality Inventory
- Edwards Personality Inventory
- Eysenck Personality Inventory (EPI)
- Eysenck Personality Questionnaire (EPQ)
- Maudsley Personality Inventory (MPI)
- NEO Personality Inventory
- Omnibus Personality Inventory

The MPI was superseded by the EPI, which in turn was superseded by the EPQ that measures psychoticism and contains a lie scale.

3.6.8.5   Limitations

There are several limitations on the use of personality inventories. These include the following:

- There are limitations imposed by the cultural origins of the questionnaires. For example, in assessing the answers to the MMPI and the CPI, it needs to be borne in mind that these questionnaires were created for American subjects. One of the statements on the F scale of the MMPI is that 'Evil spirits possess me at times'; in some cultures, it is accepted as perfectly normal that 'evil spirits' should 'possess' a person, while in other cultures, such terminology might be normal but not to be taken literally.
- Deliberate faking. Subjects may deliberately try to come across as possessing (or not possessing) a particular personality trait. Lie scales are often included to try to detect for this.
- Questionnaires are susceptible to response sets—subjects may exhibit a systematic tendency to respond to test questions.
- The inventories tend to have a low validity, particularly in respect of predictive validity.
- A social desirability bias may occur, in which subjects may have an unconscious tendency to give socially desirable responses that make them look good.

- The inventories only rarely allow an assessment of the underlying reasons for the responses to questions.
- The responses depend on an accurate knowledge, on the part of the subject, of their beliefs, behaviour, abilities, and feelings.
- The responses depend on a willingness, on the part of the subject, to make known their beliefs, behaviour, abilities, and feelings.
- Questionnaires are susceptible to contamination by reliability minor changes in the mental state of the subject.
- The dimensions chosen by psychologists in creating questionnaires may be difficult to relate to personality disorder categories used by psychiatrists.

3.6.9   RATING SCALES

There are several rating scales that may be used for the assessment of personality disorder. The following are all structured interview schedules.

3.6.9.1   SAP

The Standardized Assessment of Personality or SAP is carried out by a trained clinical interviewer. A personality profile is obtained from an informant. An ICD-10 diagnosis is obtained.

3.6.9.2   SCID II

The Structured Clinical Interview for DSM-III-R Personality Disorders or SCID II is carried out by a clinician and yields DSM diagnoses.

3.6.9.3   SIDP

The Structured Interview for DSM-III Personality Disorders or SIDP is carried out by a psychologist or psychiatrist and yields DSM-III-R diagnoses.

3.6.9.4   PAS

The Personality Assessment Schedule or PAS yields five diagnostic categories:

- Sociopathic
- Schizoid
- Passive dependent
- Anankastic
- Normal

It assesses 24 dimensions of personality and should be carried out by a trained clinical interviewer.

3.6.9.5 PDE

The Personality Disorder Examination or PDE yields DSM diagnoses.

3.6.9.6 IPDE

The International Personality Disorder Examination for DSM-IV and ICD-10 personality disorders or IPDE is carried out by trained interviewers and covers DSM-IV(-TR) and ICD-10 operational criteria.

3.6.10 REPERTORY GRID

George Kelly devised the repertory grid or role construct repertory (REP) test. This grid assesses personality based on an individual's personal constructs. A typical grid might consist of 10 rows (excluding rows containing headings), which need to be filled in by the subject. The subject begins by naming specific people who fit into given categories, such as a happy person and a successful person. These form columns that cross the rows. Other columns correspond to other people, such as the subject's father and mother, the subject himself or herself, their children, and their spouse or partner. There is now a grid of, say, 10 rows and around 10 columns. On each row, three cells are circled; no two rows contain the same three circles. These correspond to three different individuals. Row by row, the subject must now decide for the three individuals concerned what description shows how two of these three individuals are similar and how they differ from the third individual. The former description is placed in a column (column 1) on the left-hand side of the grid, while the latter description is similarly placed in a column (column 2) on the right-hand side of the grid. A code is used to fill in the circles (e.g. 1 for similarity, as in the column 1 description; 2 for difference, as in column 2; and 0 if neither column 1 nor column 2 applies). Then the rest of the grid is filled in. There are many scoring systems available, although the grid itself overall gives an indication of how the subject views others.

3.6.11 Q-SORT SCHEDULE

This is an *ipsative method*, that is, one which compares alternatives within an individual, in which the rater (or coder) sorts statements into a standard distribution. Jack Block (1961, 1971) used it in his research on childhood development. A deck of cards was produced in which each card contained a word or phrase. An individual was described by sorting this deck into piles corresponding to how closely the card descriptions were deemed to apply to the subject. The Q-sort schedule is designed to apply across different individuals and over time, over different ages.

3.7 FACTORS AFFECTING MOTIVATION

3.7.1 EXTRINSIC THEORIES AND HOMEOSTASIS

Theories based on instincts were replaced by a drive reduction theory in which the motivation of behaviour is to reduce the level of arousal associated with a basic drive (biological drive, e.g. hunger and thirst) in order to maintain homeostatic control of the internal somatic environment.

Hull developed a theory in which *primary biological drives* are activated by needs that arise from homeostatic imbalance acting via brain receptors.

Mowrer developed the notion of *secondary drives* (e.g. anxiety), which result from generalization and conditioning.

3.7.2 HYPOTHALAMIC SYSTEMS AND SATIETY

An example of a primary biological drive is provided by hypothalamic systems and satiety. In rat experiments, the hypothalamic ventromedial nucleus acts as a satiety centre, with hyperphagia occurring if it is ablated, while the lateral hypothalamus contains a hunger centre, with aphagia occurring if it is ablated.

3.7.3 INTRINSIC THEORIES

Whereas extrinsic theories require reduction of drive externally, intrinsic theories propose that the activity engaged in has its own intrinsic reward.

3.7.3.1 Optimal Arousal

An example is offered by optimal arousal, in which the subject attains an optimal level of arousal to achieve optimal performance. In general, a moderate level of arousal leads to an optimum degree of alertness and interest and therefore to a comparatively high efficiency of performance. High and low arousals lead to reduced performance and are described in the inverted U shape of the Yerkes–Dodson curve.

3.7.3.2 Cognitive Dissonance

According to this theory, first formulated by Festinger, discomfort occurs when two or more cognitions are held but are inconsistent with each other. The individual is motivated to achieve cognitive consistency and may change one or more of the cognitions.

3.7.3.3 Attitude-Discrepant Behaviour

When attitude and behaviour are inconsistent (attitude-discrepant behaviour), alteration of attitude helps bring about cognitive consistency.

3.7.3.4 Need for Achievement

McClelland formulated a need for achievement (nAch) to explain pleasure resulting from mastery.

3.7.4 CURIOSITY DRIVE

Whereas the homeostatic model predicts that once physiological needs such as thirst and hunger have been satisfied, or aversive stimuli such as pain have successfully been avoided, and the body returned to its normal state, the organism should no longer be motivated and should be quiescent; in practice, this is not the case. Humans and other mammals, for example, have been noted actively to seek stimulation. A curiosity drive has been proposed to help explain this phenomenon, in which the organism has drives to

- Explore new environments
- Investigate objects
- Manipulate objects (if appropriate)
- Seek changing sensory stimulation (and avoid sensory deprivation)
- Seek sensation

3.7.5 MASLOW'S HIERARCHY OF NEEDS

This unified theory, relating to self-actualization, integrates both extrinsic and intrinsic theories of motivation. A hierarchy of needs is described in which those with survival importance take precedence over others:

- Self-actualization needs (highest)
- Aesthetic needs
- Cognitive needs
- Self-esteem needs
- Love and belonging needs
- Safety needs
- Physical/physiological needs (lowest)

3.8 FACTORS AFFECTING EMOTION

3.8.1 TYPES OF EMOTION

An emotion is a mental feeling or affection having cognitive, physiological, and social concomitants. Plutchik has classified them into eight primary emotions:

- Disgust
- Anger
- Anticipation
- Joy
- Acceptance
- Fear
- Surprise
- Sadness

Any two adjacent emotions can give rise to a secondary emotion. For example, the secondary emotion of love is derived from the primary emotions of joy and acceptance. Similarly, submission results from acceptance and fear, disappointment from surprise and sadness, contempt from disgust and anger, and so on.

3.8.2 COMPONENTS OF EMOTIONAL RESPONSE

The main components of emotional response are

- Subjective awareness
- Physiological changes
- Behaviour

3.8.3 JAMES–LANGE THEORY

According to this theory, the experience of emotion is secondary to the somatic responses (e.g. sweating, increased cardiac rate, increased arousal) to the perception of given emotionally important events. For example, if an arachnophobe becomes aroused, experiences increased activity of the sympathetic nervous system, and runs away after seeing a spider, the feelings of anxiety and fear are the result of the increased sympathetic activity and running away and not primarily because of the emotion-evoking stimulus.

Cannon criticized this theory. It was argued that similar physiological changes can accompany different emotions. Also, pharmacologically induced simulation of such physiological changes is usually not accompanied by these emotions. The experience of emotions can be shown to be independent of somatic responses, sometimes occurring before the somatic responses.

3.8.4 CANNON–BARD THEORY

This holds that following the perception of an emotionally important event, both the somatic responses and the experience of emotion occur together. In neurophysiological terms, the perceived stimulus undergoes thalamic processing, and signals are then relayed to both the cerebral cortex, leading to the experience of emotion, and other parts of the body, such as the autonomic nervous system, leading to somatic responses.

This theory can be criticized on the basis of the observation that there are stimuli, for example, sudden danger, which can lead to increased sympathetic activity before the emotion is experienced. Conversely, the experience of emotions sometimes occurs before the somatic response.

3.8.5 SCHACHTER'S COGNITIVE LABELLING THEORY AND COGNITIVE APPRAISAL

According to this theory, the conscious experience of an emotion is a function of the stimulus, of somatic or physiological responses, and of cognitive factors such as the cognitive appraisal of the situation and input from long-term memory. The influence of cognitive factors on the conscious experience of emotion was demonstrated in an experiment by Schachter and Singer (1962) in which subjects were injected with adrenaline. Their cognitive appraisal of the current situation, based on observation of others, influenced the conscious experience of emotion. Thus, cognitive cues were important in their interpretation of arousal.

3.9 STRESS

Stress results when demand exceeds resources. An individual's response to a stressful situation is affected by biological susceptibility and personality characteristics.

3.9.1 PHYSIOLOGICAL AND PSYCHOLOGICAL ASPECTS

Physiological effects of stress include physical disorders (ulcers, cardiac disease, and hypertension) and immune response changes. Other physical disorders have also been attributed to emotional stress, for example, migraine, eczema, asthma, and allergies.

3.9.2 SITUATIONAL FACTORS

These include life events, daily hassles/uplifts, conflict, and trauma (see Chapter 28).

3.9.2.1 Life Events

These are changes in a person's life that require readjustment. They are ranked in order from most to least stressful. The most stressful include death of spouse, divorce, marital separation, jail term, death of close family member, personal illness, and marriage. The scale has been found to be universally applicable to people in both underdeveloped and Western countries. Many conditions, both physical and mental, show an excess of life events in the months preceding onset.

3.9.3 VULNERABILITY AND INVULNERABILITY

Type A behaviour is related to increased proneness to heart disease. Such behaviour includes competitiveness, striving for achievement, time urgency, difficulty relaxing, impatience, and anger. It is possible to modify such behaviour.

Type B individuals do not exhibit the earlier characteristics; for example, they can relax more easily and are slow to anger.

Stress-resistant people are those who view change as a challenge and feel they have more control over events.

3.9.4 COPING MECHANISMS

Although the following mechanisms, used to cope with stress, are conscious, they relate to unconscious defence mechanisms too (given in parentheses):

- Concentration only on the current task (denial)
- Empathy (projection)
- Logical analysis (rationalization)
- Objectivity (isolation)
- Playfulness (regression)
- Substitution of other thoughts for disturbing ones (reaction formation)
- Suppression of inappropriate feelings (repression)

3.9.5 LEARNED HELPLESSNESS

Seligman found that dogs given unavoidable electric shocks suffered a number of phenomena, which he considered were similar to depression, such as reduced appetite, disturbed sleep, and reduced sex drive. He called this learned helplessness.

The cognitive theory of depression is based largely on this concept. Further work has found that individuals who believe that they have no personal control over events much more likely to develop learned helplessness, whereas those believing that nobody could have controlled the outcome are unlikely to do so. Thus, a person's attribution of what is occurring influences the likelihood of developing major depression in cognitive terms.

3.9.6 LOCUS OF CONTROL

Rotter differentiated those who see their lives as being under their own control (internal locus of control) from those who see their lives as being controlled externally (external locus of control).

REFERENCES

Al-Adawi S, Burjorjee R, and Al-Issa I. 1997: Mu-Ghayeb: A culture-specific response to bereavement in Oman. *International Journal of Social Psychiatry* 43:144–151.

Al-Issa I. 1977: Social and cultural aspects of hallucinations. *Psychological Bulletin* 84:570–587.

Allport GW. 1937: *Personality: A Psychological Interpretation.* New York: Holt, Rinehart & Winston.

Allport GW and Odbert HS. 1936: Trait names: A psycholexical study. *Psychological Monographs* 47:211.

Anderson JR. 1980: *Cognitive Psychology and Its Implications.* San Francisco, CA: Freeman.

Atkinson RC and Shriffrin RM. 1968: Human memory: A proposed system and its control processes. In Spence KW and Spence JT (eds.) *The Psychology of Learning and Motivation*, Vol. 2, pp. 90–191. New York: Academic Press.

Ayres TJ, Jonides J, Reitman JS, Egan JC, and Howard DA. 1979: Differing suffix effects for the same physical suffix. *Journal of Experimental Psychology: Human Learning and Memory* 5:315–321.

Baddeley AD. 1966a: Short-term memory for word sequences as a function of acoustic, semantic and formal similarity. *Quarterly Journal of Experimental Psychology* 18:362–365.

Baddeley AD. 1966b: The influence of acoustic and semantic similarity on long-term memory for word sequences. *Quarterly Journal of Experimental Psychology* 18:302–309.

Baddeley AD. 2007: *Working Memory, Thought, and Action.* Oxford, U.K.: Oxford University Press.

Baddeley AD and Hitch G. 1974: Working memory. In Bower GA (ed.) *The Psychology of Learning and Motivation*, Vol. 8, pp. 47–89. New York: Academic Press.

Baddeley AD and Lieberman K. 1980: Spatial working memory. In Nickerson RS (ed.) *Attention and Performance VIII*, pp. 521–538. Hillsdale, NJ: Erlbaum.

Bandura, A. 1973: *Aggression: A Social Learning Analysis.* Englewood Cliffs, NJ: Prentice-Hall.

Block J. 1961: *The Q-Sort Method in Personality Assessment and Psychiatric Research.* Springfield, IL: Charles C. Thomas.

Block J. 1971: *Lives Through Time.* Berkeley, CA: Bancroft Books.

Boran M and Viswanathan R. 2000: Separating subculture from psychopathology. *Psychiatric Services* 51:678

Bower GH. 1972: Mental imagery and associative learning. In Gregg LW (ed.) *Cognition in Learning and Memory.* New York: Wiley.

Bower GH, Clark M, Winzenz D, and Lesgold A. 1969: Hierarchical retrieval schemes in recall of categorical word lists. *Journal of Verbal Learning and Verbal Behavior* 8:323–343.

Bower GH and Springston F. 1970: Pauses as recoding points in letter series. *Journal of Experimental Psychology* 83:421–430.

Braine MDS, Reiser BJ, and Rumain B. 1984: Some empirical justification for a theory of natural propositional logic. In *The Psychology of Learning and Motivation*, Vol. 18. New York: Academic Press.

Byrne RMJ and Johnson-Laird PN. 1989: Spatial reasoning. *Journal of Memory and Language* 28:564–575.

Cattell RB, Eber HW, and Tatsuoka MM. 1970: *Handbook for the Sixteen Personality Factor Questionnaire.* Champaign, IL: Institute for Personality and Ability Testing.

Conrad R. 1964: Acoustic confusion in immediate memory. *British Journal of Psychology* 55:75–84.

Craik FIM and Watkins MJ. 1973: The role of rehearsal in short-term memory. *Journal of Verbal Learning and Verbal Behavior* 12:599–607.

Crowder RG. 1971: The sound of vowels and consonants in immediate memory. *Journal of Verbal Learning and Verbal Behavior* 10:587–596.

Daneman M and Carpenter PA. 1980: Individual differences in working memory and reading. *Journal of Verbal Learning and Verbal Behavior* 19:450–466.

Deatherage BH and Evans TR. 1969: Binaural masking: Backward, forward and simultaneous effects. *Journal of the Acoustical Society of America* 46:362–371.

Endler NS. 1983: Interactionism: A personality model but not yet a theory. In Page MM (ed.) *Nebraska Symposium on Motivation 1982: Personality—Current Theory and Research*, pp. 167–193. Lincoln, NE: University of Nebraska Press.

Ericsson KA and Kintsch W. 1995: Long-term working memory. *Psychological Review* 102:211–245.

Estes WK. 1972: An associative basis for coding and organization in memory. In Melton AW and Martin E (eds.) *Coding Processes in Human Memory*, pp. 161–177. Washington, DC: Winston.

Eysenck HJ. 1944: Types of personality—A factorial study of 700 neurotic soldiers. *Journal of Mental Science* 90:851–961.

Eysenck MW. 1982: *Attention and Arousal: Cognition and Performance.* New York: Springer.

Eysenck HJ and Eysenck SBG. 1991: *The Eysenck Personality Questionnaire – Revised.* Sevenoaks, Kent: Hodder & Stoughton.

Frase LT. 1975: Prose processing. In Bower GH (ed.) *The Psychology of Learning and Motivation*, Vol. 9, pp. 1–47. New York: Academic Press.

Garety P, Kuipers E, Fowler D et al. 2001: A cognitive model of the positive symptoms of psychosis. *Psychological Medicine* 31:189–195.

Gillund G and Shiffrin RM. 1981: Free recall of complex pictures and abstract words. *Journal of Verbal Learning and Verbal Behavior* 20:575–592.

Glenberg AM, Smith SM, and Green C. 1977: Type I rehearsal: Maintenance and more. *Journal of Verbal Learning and Verbal Behavior* 16:339–352.

Glover JH and McCue PA. 1977: Electrical aversion therapy with alcoholics: A comparative follow-up study. *British Journal of Psychiatry* 130:279–286.

Greenberg D and Brom D. 2001: Nocturnal hallucinations in ultra-orthodox Jewish Israeli men. *Psychiatry* 64:81–90.

Groeger JA. 1997: *Memory and Remembering: Everyday Memory in Context*. Edinburgh, Scotland: Longman.

Hansen GD. 1979: Enuresis control through fading, escape, and avoidance training. *Journal of Applied Behavioural Analysis* 12:303–307.

Hart RP and O'Shanick GJ. 1993: Forgetting rates for verbal, pictorial, and figural stimuli. *Journal of Clinical and Experimental Neuropsychology* 15:245–265.

Hirschberg N. 1978: A correct treatment of traits. In London H (ed.) *Personality: A New Look at Metatheories*, pp. 45–63. New York: Macmillan.

Jacobsen E. 1932: The electrophysiology of mental activities. *American Journal of Psychology* 44:677–694.

Johns LC, Nazroo JY, Bebbington P, and Kuipers E. 2002: Occurrence of hallucinatory experiences in a community sample and ethnic variations. *British Journal of Psychiatry* 180:174–178.

Johnson-Laird PN. 1993: *Human and Machine Thinking*. Hillsdale, NJ: Erlbaum.

Kelly GA. 1955: *The Psychology of Personal Constructs*. New York: Norton.

Kyllonen PC and Christal RE. 1990: Reasoning ability is (little more than) working-memory capacity. *Intelligence* 14:389–433.

Maslow AH. 1967: Self-actualization and beyond. In Bugental JFT (ed.) *Challenges of Humanistic Psychology*, pp. 275–284. New York: McGraw Hill.

Maslow AH. 1970: *Motivation and Personality*, 2nd edn. Philadelphia, PA: Saunders.

Mischel W. 1983: Alterations in the pursuit of predictability and consistency of persons: Stable data that yield unstable interpretations. *Journal of Personality* 51:578–604.

Morton J and Bekerian DA. 1986: Three ways of looking at memory. In Sharkey NE (ed.) *Advances in Cognitive Science 1*. Chichester, U.K.: Ellis Horwood.

Newell A and Rosenbloom PS. 1981: Mechanisms of skill acquisition and the law of practice. In Anderson JR (ed.) *Cognitive Skills and Their Acquisition*, pp. 1–56. Hillsdale, NJ: Erlbaum.

Ohaeri JU, Adelekan MF, Odejide AO, and Ikuesan BA. 1992: The pattern of isolated sleep paralysis among Nigerian nursing students. *Journal of the National Medical Association* 84:67–70.

Paulesu E, Frith CD, and Frackowiak RSJ. 1993: The neural correlates of the verbal component of working memory. *Nature* 362:342–345.

Pezdek K and Chen HC. 1982: Developmental differences in the role of detail in picture recognition memory. *Journal of Experimental Child Psychology* 33:207–215.

Pfungst O. 1907: *Das Pferd des Herrn von Osten (Der Kluge Hans). Ein Beitrag zur experimentellen Tier—und Menschen-Psychologie*. Leipzig, Germany: Johann Ambrosius Barth; the book was translated into English by C.L. Rahn, with a prefatory note by J.R. Angell as Pfungst O. 1911: *Clever Hans (The Horse of Mr. von Osten). A Contribution to Experimental Animal and Human Psychology*. New York: Henry Holt.

Plomp R. 1964: Rate of decay of auditory sensation. *Journal of the Acoustical Society of America* 36:277–282.

Potter MC. 1976: Short-term conceptual memory for pictures. *Journal of Experimental Psychology: Human Learning and Memory* 2:509–522.

Preston KL, Umbricht A, Wong CJ, and Epstein DH. 2001: Shaping cocaine abstinence by successive approximation. *Journal of Consulting and Clinical Psychology* 69:643–654

Robertson IH, North NT, and Geggie C. 1992: Spatiomotor cueing in unilateral left neglect: Three case studies of its therapeutic effects. *Journal of Neurology, Neurosurgery and Psychiatry* 55:799–805.

Ryle G. 1949: *The Concept of the Mind*. London, U.K.: Hutchinson.

Sachs JDS. 1967: Recognition memory for syntactic and semantic aspects of connected discourse. *Perception and Psychophysics* 2:437.

Schachtel EG. 1947: On memory and childhood amnesia. *Psychiatry* 10:1–26.

Schachter S and Singer JE. 1962: Cognitive, social and physiological determinants of emotional state. *Psychological Review* 69:379–399.

Schwab ME. 1977: A study of reported hallucinations in a southeastern county. *Mental Health and Society* 4:344–354.

Searleman A and Herrmann D. 1994: *Memory from a Broader Perspective*. New York: McGraw-Hill.

Shallice T and Warrington EK. 1970: Independent functioning of verbal memory stores: A neuropsychological study. *Quarterly Journal of Experimental Psychology* 22:261–273.

Skinner BF. 1953: *Science and Human Behavior*. New York: Macmillan.

Skinner BF. 1969: *Contingencies of Reinforcement*. New York: Appleton-Century-Crofts.

Slamecka NJ. 1960: Retroactive inhibition of connected discourse as a function of practice level. *Journal of Experimental Psychology* 59:104–108.

Smith SM, Brown HO, Thomas JEP, and Goodman LS. 1947: The lack of cerebral effects of d-tubocurarine. *Anesthesiology* 8:1–14.

Spielberger CD. 1962: The effects of manifest anxiety on the academic achievement of college students. *Mental Hygiene* 46:420–426.

Thorndike EL. 1911: *Animal Intelligence*. New York: Macmillan.

Thvedt JE, Zane T, and Walls RT. 1984: Stimulus functions in response chaining. *American Journal of Mental Deficiency* 88:661–667.

Tulving E. 1972: Episodic and semantic memory. In Tulving E and Donaldson W (eds.) *The Organization of Memory*, pp. 385–401. New York: Academic Press.

Tulving E. 1985: Memory and consciousness. *Canadian Psychology* 26:1–12.

Turvey MT. 1973: On peripheral and central processes in vision: Inferences from an information-processing analysis of masking with patterned stimuli. *Psychological Review* 80:1–52.

Tyrer P and Ferguson B. 2000: Classification of personality disorder. In Tyrer P (ed.) *Personality Disorders: Diagnosis, Management and Course*, pp. 13–127. Oxford, U.K.: Butterworth-Heinemann.

Tzeng OJL. 1973: Positive recency effects in delayed free recall. *Journal of Verbal Learning and Verbal Behavior* 12:436–439.

Vaughan K and Tarrier N. 1992: The use of image habituation training with post-traumatic stress disorders. *British Journal of Psychiatry* 161:658–664.

Watson JB. 1913: Psychology as the behaviorist views it. *Psychological Review* 20:158–177.

Wiggins JS. 1979: A psychological taxonomy of trait-descriptive terms: The interpersonal domain. *Journal of Personality and Social Psychology* 37:395–412.

Wolpe J. 1958: *Psychotherapy by Reciprocal Inhibition*. Palo Alto, CA: Stanford University Press.

4 Social Psychology

Note that intergroup behaviour, including stigma, is considered in Chapter 8.

4.1 ATTITUDES AND HOW THEY ARE AFFECTED

4.1.1 DEFINITION

The definition of an attitude has been given variously as 'a mental and neural state of readiness, organized through experience, exerting a directive or dynamic influence upon the individual's response to all objects and situations with which it is related' (Katz, 1979), and 'an enduring organization of motivational, emotional, perceptual, and cognitive processes with respect to some aspect of the individual's world' (Krech et al., 1962). They are mutually consistent and internally consistent.

4.1.2 COMPONENTS

Attitudes are based on *beliefs*, a tendency to *behave in an observable way*, and also have *affective* components that are the most resistant to change. A change in one of these three components leads to changes in the other two.

When predicting behaviour, situational variables must be taken into account. Otherwise, measured attitudes are poor predictors of behaviour.

4.1.3 MEASUREMENT

4.1.3.1 Thurstone Scale

This is a dichotomous scale indicating agreement/disagreement with presented and previously ranked statements. Disadvantages of this scale include the following:

- Different response patterns may result in the same mean score.
- The set-up is unwieldy.
- The ranking may be biased.

4.1.3.2 Likert Scale

This is a five-point scale indicating level of agreement with presented statements. Its advantages include the fact that it has increased sensitivity compared with the dichotomous Thurstone scale and that it is more easily administered. A disadvantage is that different response patterns may result in the same mean score.

4.1.3.3 Semantic Differential Scale

This is a bipolar visual analogue scale.

Its advantages include

- Ease of use
- Good test–retest reliability

Its disadvantages include the following:

- Positional response bias may occur
- No consistent meaning is attributed to a mid-point mark

4.1.4 ATTITUDE CHANGE

A change in one of the three components of attitude leads to changes in the other two.

The origin of attitudes can be by means of the processes of learning: classical conditioning, operant conditioning, and observational learning. Superimposed on these are cognitive processes such as appraisal and modification in the light of new information.

Attitudes can be modified either by central pathways, entailing the consideration of new information, or by peripheral pathways involving the presentation of cues. Advertising uses both pathways.

The *balance theory* of Heider (1946) holds that each individual attempts to organize his or her attitudes, perceptions, and beliefs so that they are in harmony or balance with each other.

4.1.5 PERSUASIVE COMMUNICATION

The factors to consider are those concerned with the communicator, the recipient, and the message being communicated.

4.1.5.1 Communicator

Characteristics of persuasive communicators include

- Attractiveness
- Audience identification with the communicator

- Credibility
- Expertise
- Genuine motivation
- Being an opinion leader
- Nonverbal communication
- Views of reference groups

4.1.5.2 Recipient

High self-esteem and intelligence of the recipient increase the likelihood that complex communications will be persuasive.

4.1.5.3 Message

Key aspects relating to the message and attitude change include the following:

- Message repetition can be a persuasive influence leading to attitude change.
- Explicit messages are more persuasive for the less intelligent and implicit messages for the more intelligent recipient.
- Interactive personal discussions are more persuasive than mass media communication.
- One-sided communications are more persuasive for those who are less intelligent and/or already favourably disposed to the message.
- Two-sided presentations are more effective with intelligent and neutral recipients.
- A low anxiety recipient is more influenced by a high fear message, and vice versa.

4.1.6   Cognitive Consistency and Dissonance

When cognitive dissonance occurs, the individual feels uncomfortable, may experience increased arousal, and is motivated to achieve cognitive consistency. This may occur by changing one or more of the cognitions involved in the dissonant relationship, changing the behaviour that is inconsistent with the cognition(s), or adding new cognitions that are consonant with preexisting ones. Cognitive consistency can also be achieved, when attitude and behaviour are inconsistent (attitude discrepant behaviour), by altering attitude.

4.2   SELF-PSYCHOLOGY

4.2.1   Self-Concept

This is a set of attitudes that the individual holds about himself or herself. It does not necessarily correspond to reality. Self-theory was developed by Rogers (1951).

4.2.1.1   Self-Esteem

This is one's own evaluation of self-worth and feeling accepted by others. Those lacking in self-esteem have feelings of worthlessness, alienation, and lack of acceptance by others, whereas those with high self-esteem are more socially active, less prejudiced, more risk-taking, and warmer in social relationships. It is learned and so may change with experience.

Self-esteem may be raised by identification with a group. For example, deaf individuals who identify with other deaf people have a higher self-esteem, on average, than those who do not. In turn, the raised self-esteem can help to compensate for problems relating to *personal identity*.

4.2.1.2   Self-Image

Self-image is a set of beliefs held about oneself, based on achievements and social interactions, which influences personal meaning and behaviour.

4.2.2   Self-Perception Theory

An individual infers what his or her attitude must be by observation of his or her own behaviour, in a similar way to how other people infer his or her behaviour.

Self-perception theory provides a better explanation than cognitive dissonance theory for behaviour that lies within the general range of behaviours acceptable to the individual.

4.3   INTERPERSONAL ISSUES

4.3.1   Interpersonal Attraction

In general, humans seek the company of others, to whom they are attracted. In difficult situations, this may allow assessment by social comparisons, taking note of the opinions of others (*social comparison theory* [Festinger, 1954]). An alternative theory is that seeking the company of others leads to *arousal reduction* (Eppley et al., 1989).

Theories of interpersonal attraction include the following:

- *Reinforcement theory*—reciprocal reinforcement of the attractions occurs with rewards in both directions (Newcomb). Conversely, punishments diminish the probability of interpersonal attraction.
- *Social exchange theory*—people prefer relationships that appear to offer an optimum cost-benefit ratio (Homans, 1958).

- *Equity theory*—the preferred relationships are those in which each feels that the cost-benefit ratio of the relationship for each person is approximately equal (Hatfield et al., 1978).
- *Proxemics*—relates to interpersonal space/body buffer zone.

Factors predisposing to interpersonal attraction include proximity, familiarity, similarity of interests and values, exposure, perceived competence, reciprocal liking, and self-disclosure and physical attractiveness. Similarity is more important than complementarity although the latter increases in importance with time.

According to the *matching hypothesis*, pairing occurs such that individuals seek others who have a similar level of physical attractiveness.

4.3.2 ATTRIBUTION THEORY (HEIDER)

This deals with the rules people use to infer the causes of observed behaviour.

4.3.2.1 Internal or Dispositional Attribution

This is the inference that the person is primarily responsible for their behaviour.

4.3.2.2 External or Situational Attribution

This is the inference that the cause of a behaviour is external to the person.

4.3.2.3 Primary (Fundamental) Attribution Error

When inferring the cause of other people's behaviour, there is a bias towards dispositional rather than situational attribution.

4.3.3 THEORY OF MIND

In primate research, theory of mind refers to the ability of primates to *mentalize* their fellows. In humans, the ('cold') theory of mind refers to the ability of most normal people to comprehend the thought processes (such as their attention, feelings, beliefs, false beliefs, and knowledge) of others.

Research into children would tend to suggest that at the age of 3 years, normal human children do not acknowledge false belief as they have difficulty in differentiating belief from world. Formulating a theory of mind appears not to be inevitable, but relies on cognitive changes that occur at around the age of 4. It has been suggested that a failure to acquire a theory of mind is associated with disorders such as autism.

A 'hot' theory of mind entails constructing the meaningful intentions and evaluative attitudes (such as fear, surprise, and pleasure) of others. The latter can be inferred from facial expressions.

4.4 LEADERSHIP, SOCIAL INFLUENCE, POWER, AND OBEDIENCE

4.4.1 LEADERSHIP

Lewin et al. distinguished between the following leadership styles:

- Autocratic—abandon task in leader's absence; good for situations of urgency
- Democratic—yields greater productivity unless a highly original product is required
- *Laissez-faire*—appropriate for creative, open-ended, person-oriented tasks

4.4.2 SOCIAL FACILITATION

This refers to the way in which tasks and responses are facilitated when carried out in the presence of others (Allport; Harlow). To occur, the others do not necessarily have to be engaging in the same task. Facilitation also occurs if the others are simply observing; this has been called the *audience effect* (Dashiell, 1930).

4.4.3 SOCIAL POWER

French and Raven described the following five types of social power:

- Authority—power derived from role
- Reward—power derived from ability to allocate resources
- Coercive—power to punish
- Referent—charismatic and liked by others
- Expert—power derived from skill, knowledge, and experience

4.4.4 CONFORMITY

Two types of conformity to the actions and opinions of others have been identified (Deutsch and Gerard, 1955):

- *Informational social influence*—an individual conforms to the consensual opinion and behaviour of the group both publicly and in his or her own thoughts (evident with ambiguous stimuli).

- *Normative social influence*—situations in which an individual publicly conforms to the consensual opinion and behaviour of the group but has a different view in his or her own mind. The individual conforms to the group under social pressure to avoid *social rejection*.

Self-reliance, intelligent, expressive, socially effective individuals are least vulnerable to group pressure.

4.4.5   Obedience to Authority

Milgram found that most subjects would obey an experimenter's orders to administer what they believed to be increasingly powerful electrical shocks to others, right up to the maximum voltage available. Factors that increased the rate of obedience included

- The presence of the experimenter
- The belief that the prior agreement was binding on the subject
- Increasing distance from the apparently suffering person

4.5   PHENOMENON OF AGGRESSION

Aggression is behaviour intended to harm others. We may distinguish between the following:

- Hostile aggression—the sole intent is to inflict injury.
- Instrumental aggression—the intention is to obtain reward or inflict suffering.

4.5.1   Explanations

4.5.1.1   Psychoanalytic

Aggression is viewed as a basic instinct.

4.5.1.2   Social Learning Theory

Aggression is viewed as a learned response. It is learned through observation, imitation, and operant conditioning.

4.5.1.3   Operant Conditioning

Positive reinforcers can include victim suffering and material gains. The consequences of aggression play an important role in shaping future behaviour.

4.5.1.4   Ethology

Some ethologists believe that humans and animals are innately aggressive. Animal studies show that certain behaviours inhibit aggression:

- Maintaining a distance
- Evoking a social response incompatible with aggression
- Familiarity

4.5.1.5   Frustration–Aggression Hypothesis

This proposes that preventing a person reaching their goal induces an aggressive drive resulting in behaviour intended to harm the one causing the frustration. Expressing this aggression reduces the aggressive drive.

4.5.1.6   Arousal

Emotional arousal can increase aggression.

4.5.2   Influence of Television

It is known that children imitate observed aggression. Some studies suggest a relationship between exposure to violence on television and aggressive behaviour in boys, but not in girls. It may be that this is because aggressive behaviour in boys, but not in girls, is socially reinforced.

Ways in which filmed violence may increase aggressive behaviour include

- Teaching aggressive styles of conduct
- Increasing arousal
- Desensitizing people to violence
- Reducing restraint on aggressive behaviour
- Distorting views about conflict resolution

4.6   CONCEPT OF ALTRUISM

The concept of the type of interpersonal cooperation known as altruism refers to an act (or acts) that is motivated by the desire to benefit another person (or persons) rather than oneself.

Altruism may be considered to be a higher defence mechanism in which the individual deals with emotional conflict or internal or external stressors by dedication to meeting the needs of others. Unlike self-sacrifice, sometimes characteristic of reaction formation, the individual receives gratification either vicariously or from the response of others (APA, 1994).

Altruism can also be explained on the basis of social exchange theory (see Section 4.3.1).

It has been suggested that failure to exclude an ulterior motive means that, strictly speaking, altruism cannot be said to have occurred under these circumstances. Indeed, there may be personal rewards of a private nature that occur as a result of acting in this way; for instance, a person may feel virtuous.

BIBLIOGRAPHY

American Psychiatric Association. 1994: *Diagnostic and Statistical Manual of Mental Disorders*, 4th edn., Washington, DC: American Psychiatric Association.

Bandura A and Walters RH. 1963: *Social Learning and Personality Development*. New York: Holt, Rinehart & Winston.

Dashiell JF. 1930: An experimental analysis of some group effects. *Abnormal Social Psychology*, 25:190–199.

Deutsch M, Gerard HB. 1955: A study of normative and informational social influences upon individual judgment. *The Journal of Abnormal and Social Psychology*, 51(3):629–636.

Eppley KR, Shear J, and Abrams AJ. 1989: Differential effects of relaxation techniques on trait anxiety: A meta-analysis. *Journal of Clinical Psychology*, 45:957–974.

Festinger L. 1954: A theory of social comparison processes. *Human Relations* 7(2):117–140.

Hatfield E, Traupmann J, and Walster GW. 1978: Equity and extramarital sexuality. *Archives of Sexual Behavior*, 7:127–141.

Heider F. 1946: Attitudes and cognitive organization. *The Journal of Psychology* 21:107–112.

Homans GC. 1958: Social behavior as exchange. *American Journal of Sociology*, 63:597–606.

Katz D. 1979: Floyd H. Allport (1890-1978). *American Psychologist* 34:351–353.

Krech D, Crutchfield RS, and Ballachey EL. 1962: *Individual in Society*. New York, NY: McGraw Hill.

Nolen-Hoeksema S, Fredrickson BL, Loftus GR, and Wagenaar WA. 2009: *Atkinson & Hilgard's Introduction to Psychology*, 15th edn. Hampshire, U.K.: Cengage Learning EMEA.

Persaud R. 2010: Social psychology. In Puri BK and Treasaden IH (eds.) *Psychiatry: An Evidence-Based Text*, pp. 285–296. London, U.K.: Hodder Arnold.

Rogers C. 1951: *Client-Centered Therapy: Its Current Practice, Implications and Theory*. London, U.K.: Constable.

Smith JR and Haslam SA (eds.). 2012: *Social Psychology: Revisiting the Classic Studies*. Thousand Oaks, CA: Sage.

Spear PD, Penrod SD, and Baker TB. 1988: *Psychology: Perspectives on Behaviour*. New York: John Wiley.

5 Human Growth and Development

5.1 CONCEPTUALIZING DEVELOPMENT

5.1.1 BASIC CONCEPTS

Human development involves an interaction between nature and nurture.

Stage theories propose that development occurs in a progressive sequence reflecting maturation. Examples include Piaget's cognitive stages, Freud's psychosexual stages, and Kohlberg's stage theory. Maturation refers to the orderly changes in behaviour that result from biological development and whose timing and form are relatively independent of external experience. Maturational tasks are influenced by biological growth, the drive for independence, and other people's general expectations.

5.1.2 GENE–ENVIRONMENT INTERACTIONS

These interactions determine all psychological characteristics, such as intelligence. Genetic factors determine the inherited potential, while environmental factors determine the degree to which this potential is fulfilled.

With respect to intelligence, while it is generally agreed that there is a genetic component to intelligence, there is disagreement about the degree of environmental influence on it. The correlation coefficient for IQ between MZ twins is 0.86 compared with 0.60 for DZ twins. Using factor analysis, Spearman identified a general factor, g, and a specific factor, s, of intelligence; it was proposed that the level of g was associated with how intelligent the individual was.

5.1.3 HISTORICAL MODELS

The historical developmental models of Freud and Erikson are described in Chapter 29. Social-learning models lay emphasis on the way in which environmental influences affect subsequent behaviour. The most influential theory of cognitive development is that of Piaget (see the succeeding text).

5.2 ATTACHMENT AND BONDING

5.2.1 ATTACHMENT THEORY

This comes from the work of Bowlby (1969). *Attachment* refers to the tendency of infants to remain close to certain people (attachment figures) with whom they share strong positive emotional ties. Monotropic attachment is when the attachment is to one individual, usually the mother. Polytropic attachment is less common. Attachment usually takes place from infant to mother. In contrast, neonatal–maternal *bonding* takes place in the opposite direction. Both processes can start immediately after birth.

Some behaviourists consider attachment to result from the mother acting as a conditioned reinforcer.

This theory was challenged by Harlow who, using cuddly and wire artificial surrogate mothers and infant rhesus monkeys, found that attachment is a function of the requirement to be in contact with a soft object (contact comfort), which provides security. Other studies have found that warm or rocking artificial surrogate mothers are preferred to colder or still surrogates, respectively.

Lorenz considered attachment to result from imprinting whereby geese, during a critical period soon after hatching, persistently follow the first nearby moving object encountered. There is no evidence that imprinting occurs in primates.

Bowlby (1969) considered infant attachment to take place in the context of a warm, intimate, and continuous relationship with the caregiver in which there is reciprocal satisfaction. The attachment process takes an average of 6 months to become fully established. Bonding is stronger if there is tactile contact as soon as possible after birth. The mother's attachment behaviour is reinforced by infant smiling, movement, and crying. *Attachment behaviours* are the signs of distress shown by the child when separated from their attachment figure and include

- Crying when the caregiver (usually mother) leaves the room
- Attempting to follow her
- Clinging hard when distressed
- Hugging her
- Being more playful and talkative in her company
- Using her as a secure base from which exploration can take place

These start to occur at about the age of 6 months and decrease visibly by 3 years. Prior to this, age separation is tolerated without distress.

5.2.2 ATTACHMENT ABNORMALITIES

5.2.2.1 Insecure Attachment

There is chronic clinginess and ambivalence towards the mother. Clinically, this may be relevant, as it may be a precursor to

- Childhood emotional disorders (including school refusal)
- Disorders (such as agoraphobia) starting in adolescence and adulthood

5.2.2.2 Avoidant Attachment

A distance is kept from the mother, who may sometimes be ignored. Clinically, avoidant attachment caused by rejection by the mother may be relevant as it may be a precursor to

- Poor social functioning in later life (including aggression)

5.2.3 SEPARATION ANXIETY

This is the fear an infant shows of being separated from his or her caregiver. Holding a comfort object or transitional object (Winnicott, 1965) may help with separation.

The rate of disappearance of separation anxiety varies with the child's

- Experiences of previous separations (real or threatened)
- Handling by mother
- Perception of whether mother will die or depart
- Temperament

5.2.4 ACUTE SEPARATION REACTION

After starting to form attachments, around 6 months to 2 years of age, separation from mother leads to the following reaction:

- First, *protest*—including crying and searching behaviour
- Second, *despair*—apathy and misery with an apparent belief that mother may not return
- Finally, *detachment*—emotionally distant from (and indifferent to) mother

5.2.5 STRANGER ANXIETY

This refers to a fear of strangers shown by infants usually between the ages of 8 months and 1 year. It is not necessarily part of attachment behaviour and may occur independently of separation anxiety.

5.2.6 MATERNAL DEPRIVATION

Following a failure to form adequate attachments, for example, because of prolonged maternal separation or rejecting parents, the effects of maternal deprivation may include

- Developmental language delay
- Indiscriminate affection seeking
- Shallow relationships
- Enuresis
- Aggression
- Lack of empathy
- Social disinhibition
- Attention seeking and overactivity in school
- *Poor growth*—deprivation dwarfism

5.3 FAMILY RELATIONSHIPS AND PARENTING PRACTISE

5.3.1 CHILD-REARING PRACTISE

Table 5.1 (after Baumrind, 1967) shows how the parents of three groups of children have been found to score on the four dimensions of

- *Control*—by the parents of the child's activities and behaviour
- *Maturity demands*—of the child to act at his or her ability level
- *Communication*—clarity of parent–child communication
- *Nurturance*—parental nurturance towards the child

TABLE 5.1

Way in Which Parents of Three Groups of Children Score on the Dimensions of Control, Maturity Demands, Communication, and Nurturance

	Control	Maturity Demands	Communication	Nurturance
Group I	↑↑	↑↑	↑↑	↑↑
Group II	↑	→	↓	↓↓
Group III	↓↓	↓↓	↓↓	↑

The three groups of children were

- *Group I*—the most mature and competent
- *Group II*—moderately self-controlled and self-reliant but somewhat withdrawn and distrustful
- *Group III*—the most immature and dependent

5.3.2 FAMILY STRUCTURE

In the United Kingdom and the United States, around 25% of children are not living with both biological parents by the age of 16 years. If orthodox families are defined as those nuclear families in which there are two parents with a small number of children, then nonorthodox family structures may or may not be relevant so far as healthy psychosocial development of the child is concerned.

Single parents
↑ Behavioural and emotional problems (particularly if no other support)

Extended family
Not harmful

Two lesbian parents
Not harmful

Large family size
↑ Behavioural and educational problems
↓ Intelligence

5.3.3 ORDINAL POSITION IN FAMILY

The oldest child has a slight advantage in intellectual development. This also applies to only children. Twins show delayed language development.

5.3.4 DISTORTED FAMILY FUNCTION

Dysfunctional families may manifest the following:

- Discord.
- Overprotection of the child(ren) by the parents.
- Rejection of the child(ren).
- *Enmeshment*—parents may be overinvolved in their children's feelings and lives.
- *Disengagement*—parents may be underinvolved in their children's feelings and lives.
- *Triangulation*—exclusive alliances are formed within the family, for example, father/daughter alliance (although this may, e.g. be helpful in preventing father from leaving home).

- *Communication difficulties*—for example, ambiguous or incongruous communications.
- *Myths*—created within the families.

Marital conflicts may cause the parents to need to have a child with a problem who can act as a scapegoat (until he or she leaves home).

5.3.5 IMPACT OF BEREAVEMENT

The death of a parent leads to initial bereavement reactions, which may include prolonged sadness, crying and irritability during childhood, and

- *Young children*—↑ functional enuresis
  ↑ Temper tantrums
- *Older children (especially girls)*—↑ sleep disturbance
  ↑ Clear-cut depressive reactions
- *School performance*—impaired (may be only temporary)

5.3.6 IMPACT OF PARENTAL DIVORCE

Parental divorce is associated with an increased rate of disturbance in children (greater than following parental bereavement). Protective factors include

- Amicable arrangements for access following the divorce
- Good parental relationship with the child
- Good relationships of the child with other siblings
- The child's temperament

5.3.7 IMPACT OF INTRAFAMILIAL ABUSE

5.3.7.1 Sexual Abuse

Child sexual abuse is 'the involvement of dependent, developmentally immature children and adolescents in sexual activities that they do not fully comprehend, are unable to give informed consent to, and that violate the social taboos of family roles' (Schechter and Roberge, 1976).

The findings of a study by Cosentino et al. (1995) suggest that sexual abuse in preadolescent girls is associated with sexual behaviour problems. This study compared a group of sexually abused girls, aged 6–12 years, with two demographically comparable control groups, girls from a child psychiatry outpatient department and girls from a general paediatric clinic. Compared to both control groups, sexually abused girls manifested more sexual behaviour problems: masturbating openly and excessively, exposing their genitals, indiscriminately hugging and kissing strange adults and children, and attempting to insert objects into their genitals. Abuse by fathers or stepfathers involving intercourse was associated with particularly marked sexual behaviour disturbances. There was a subgroup of sexually abused girls who tended to force sexual activities on siblings and peers. All of these girls had experienced prolonged sexual abuse (>2 years) involving physical force that was perpetrated by a parent.

Recognized sequelae of sexual abuse include

- Anxiety states and anxiety-related symptoms (e.g. sleep disturbance, nightmares, psychosomatic complaints, and hypervigilance), reenactments of the victimization, and post-traumatic stress disorder (Green, 1978; Goodwin, 1988)
- Depression (Gaensbauer and Sands, 1979; Sgroi, 1982)
- Dissociation (Kluft, 1985; Putnam, 1985)
- Paranoid reactions and mistrust (Green, 1978; Herman, 1981)
- Excessive reliance on primitive defence mechanisms (e.g. denial, projection, dissociation, and splitting) (Green, 1978)
- Borderline personality disorder (especially in females) (Herman et al., 1989)
- Inability to control sexual impulses (precocious sexual play with high sexual arousal) (Yates, 1982; Friedrich and Reams, 1987; Cosentino et al., 1995)
- Weakened gender identity (a tendency to reject their maleness or femaleness) (Aiosa-Karpas et al., 1991)
- ↑ Incidence of homosexuality (Finkelhor, 1984)
- ↑ Incidence of molesting children (the cycle of abuse may continue—there is a high incidence of sexual abuse in the backgrounds of male and female child molesters) (Mccarty, 1986; Seghorn et al., 1987)
- Drug and alcohol abuse (Herman, 1981)
- Eating disorders (Oppenheimer et al., 1985)

5.3.7.2 Physical Abuse/Nonaccidental Injury

Nonaccidental injury can be defined as occurring 'when an adult inflicts a physical injury on a child more severe than that which is culturally acceptable' (Graham, 1991).

Recognized sequelae of physical abuse (which overlap with those of sexual abuse) include

- Anxiety states and anxiety-related symptoms (e.g. sleep disturbance, nightmares, psychosomatic complaints, and hypervigilance), reenactments of the victimization, and post-traumatic stress disorder (Green, 1978; Goodwin, 1988)
- Depression (Gaensbauer and Sands, 1979; Sgroi, 1982)
- Dissociation (Kluft, 1985; Putnam, 1985)
- Paranoid reactions and mistrust (Green, 1978; Herman, 1981)
- Excessive reliance on primitive defence mechanisms (e.g. denial, projection, dissociation, and splitting) (Green, 1978)
- Borderline personality disorder (especially in females) (Herman et al., 1989)
- Aggressive and destructive behaviour at home and school (Green, 1978; George and Main, 1979)
- Cognitive and developmental impairment (Elmer and Gregg, 1967; Oates, 1986)
- Delayed language development (Martin, 1972)
- Neurological impairment (Green et al., 1981)
- Abusive behaviour with their own children (the cycle of abuse may continue) (Steele, 1983)

5.4 TEMPERAMENT

Temperament can be defined as early appearing, biologically rooted, basic personality dimensions (Zuckerman, 1991).

5.4.1 Individual Temperamental Differences

In the New York Longitudinal Study, Thomas and Chess (1977) (Chess and Thomas, 1984) identified the following nine categories of temperament describing how children behave in daily life situations:

1. Activity level
2. Rhythmicity (regularity of biological functions)
3. Approach or withdrawal to new situations
4. Adaptability in new or altered situations
5. Sensory threshold of responsiveness to stimuli
6. Intensity of reaction
7. Quality of mood
8. Distractibility
9. Attention span/persistence

In terms of the impact of individual temperamental differences on parent–child relationships, the previously mentioned nine categories have been found to cluster as follows:

- *Easy child* pattern—characterized by regularity, positive approach responses to new stimuli, high adaptability to change, and expressions of mood that are mild/moderate in intensity and predominantly positive
- *Difficult child* pattern—characterized by irregularity in biological functions, negative withdrawal responses to new situations, non-adaptability or slow adaptability to change, and intense, frequently negative expressions of mood
- *Slow-to-warm-up child*—characterized by a combination of negative responses of mild intensity to new situations with slow adaptability after repeated contact

5.4.2 ORIGINS, TYPOLOGIES, AND STABILITY OF TEMPERAMENT

Medieval personality theorists relied on a temperament typology based on the balance of the humours, but twentieth and twenty-first century theorists have put the strongest emphasis on environmental causation models. Acceptance of the concept of biologically rooted personality dimensions is a fairly recent stage in the history of scientific psychology and psychiatry (Bates et al., 1995); important points to note are as follows:

- Temperament is a theoretical construct—it is more useful to think of specific dimensions of temperament, for example, activity level, sociability, negative emotionality, or distractibility. Temperament concepts can be defined at the following three levels (Bates, 1989):
  1. As patterns of surface behaviour
  2. As a pattern of nervous system responses
  3. As having inborn genetic roots
- There is an increased understanding of the biological processes involved in temperament. Since concepts of temperament typically focus on individual differences in emotion, attention, and activity (Bates, 1989), the neural basis of temperament can be thought of as emerging from the brain systems supporting emotion, attention, and activity:
  1. Limbic structures
  2. Association cortex
  3. Motor cortical areas
- Environmental influences affect how the biological bases of temperament are expressed. For example, Gunnar (1992) showed how sensitive, responsive caregivers could enhance otherwise highly inhibited preschoolers' likelihood of approaching novel stimuli.
- Concepts of temperament can be useful in helping people solve problems. When the processes of linkage between temperament and the evolution of character and personality are understood better, this should assist prevention and treatment.

The stability of temperament and its relationship to the evolution of character and personality have been demonstrated in a number of studies. Characteristics of temperament in infants and preschool-age children predict adjustment in middle childhood and adolescence. For example, Caspi and Silva (1995) showed how temperamental qualities at the age of 3 years predict personality traits in young adulthood. In an unselected sample of over 800 subjects, the following five temperament groups were identified when the children were aged 3 years:

- Undercontrolled
- Inhibited
- Confident
- Reserved
- Well adjusted

These groups were reassessed at the age of 18 years. The findings in the young adults were as follows:

- Undercontrolled children scored high on measures of impulsivity, danger seeking, aggression, and interpersonal alienation (as young adults).
- Inhibited children scored low on measures of impulsivity, danger seeking, aggression, and social potency.
- Confident children scored high on impulsivity.
- Reserved children scored low on social potency.
- Well-adjusted children continued to exhibit normative behaviours.

5.5 PIAGET'S MODEL OF COGNITIVE DEVELOPMENT

Piaget believed that infantile and childhood intellectual development involves interactions with the outside world (e.g. through play). These lead to the following:

1. New cognitive structures (*schemes*) are constructed incorporating new information.
2. In the presence of suitable existing schemes
   a. *Assimilation*: New information is incorporated into appropriate existing schemes.
   b. *Accommodation*: Modification of existing scheme(s).

Piaget identified the following four stages of cognitive development:

* Sensorimotor
* Preoperational
* Concrete operational
* Formal operational

5.5.1 Sensorimotor Stage

This is the first stage and occurs from birth to 2 years of age.

Circular reactions are repeated voluntary motor activities, for example, shaking a toy, occurring from around 2 months. They are classified as follows:

* Primary circular reactions—from 2 to 5 months (approximately), when they have no apparent purpose.
* Secondary circular reactions—from 5 to 9 months (approximately), experimentation and purposeful behaviour are gradually manifested.
* Tertiary circular reactions—from 1 year to 18 months (approximately), include the creation of original behaviour patterns and the purposeful quest for novel experiences.

During this stage, the infant comes to distinguish himself or herself from the environment. Thought processes exhibit *egocentrism*, in which the infant believes that everything happens in relation to him or her. Until around 6 months, the infant believes that an object hidden from view no longer exists. *Object permanence* is fully developed after around the age of 18 months.

5.5.2 Preoperational Stage

This is the second stage and occurs from age 2 to 7 years. During this stage, the child learns to use the symbols of language.

Thought processes exhibited during this stage include the following:

* *Animism*—life, thoughts, and feelings are attributed to all objects, including inanimate ones.
* *Artificialism*—natural events are attributed to the action of people.
* *Authoritarian morality*—it is believed that wrongdoing, including breaking the rules of a game, should be punished according to the degree of the damage caused, whether accidental or not, rather than according to motive; negative events are perceived as punishments.
* *Creationism*—a teleological approach is taken in which, for example, the stars and the moon exist in order to provide light at night.
* *Egocentrism*—as in the sensorimotor stage.
* *Finalism*—all things have a purpose.
* *Precausal reasoning*—based on internal schemes rather than the results of observation so that, for example, the same volume of liquid poured from one container to another with a different height and diameter may be considered to have changed volume.
* *Syncretism*—everything is believed to be connected with everything else.

5.5.3 Concrete Operational Stage

This is the third stage and occurs from age 7 to around 12–14 years of age. During this stage, the child demonstrates logical thought processes and more subjective moral judgements.

An understanding of the *laws of conservation* of, initially, number and volume, and then weight, is normally achieved. Reversibility and some aspects of classification are mastered.

5.5.4 Formal Operational Stage

This is the final stage and occurs from the age of around 12–14 years of age onward.

It is characterized by the achievement of being able to think in the *abstract*, including the ability systematically to test hypotheses.

5.6 LANGUAGE DEVELOPMENT

Language can be defined as the sum of the skills required to communicate verbally (Graham, 1991).

5.6.1 NORMAL CHILDHOOD DEVELOPMENT

In the first hours postnatally, the baby learns to distinguish his or her mother's voice:

- By 3–4 months, babbling occurs.
- By 8 months, repetitive babbling occurs.
- By 1 year, the baby has usually acquired the equivalent designations 'Mama', 'Dada' (no matter what language the parent speaks), and one additional word.
- By 18 months, a 20–50-word vocabulary is expressed in single-word utterances.
- By 2 years, two- or three-word utterances can be strung together with some understanding of grammar. These are telegraphic utterances omitting grammatical morphemes (e.g. small units of meaning signifying the plural).
- At an average age of 3 years, the child can usually understand a request containing three parts.

5.6.2 ENVIRONMENTAL INFLUENCES AND COMMUNICATIVE COMPETENCE

Bilingual home

Being brought up in a home in which two languages are spoken is not a disadvantage unless there is another cause of slowed language development.

Family size

Larger family size is associated with slower speech development.

Pregnancy

Intrauterine growth retardation is associated with slower language development.

Prolonged second stage labour is associated with slower language development.

Sex

Early language development in girls is slightly greater than in boys.

Social class

Being middle class is associated with relatively faster language development.

Stimulation

Although the capacity for language and grammar may be built-in, speech and language are not achieved in the usual manner if children are deaf or are not spoken to.

Twins

Being a twin is associated with slower speech development.

5.7 MORAL DEVELOPMENT

5.7.1 KOHLBERG'S STAGE THEORY

Kohlberg presented a set of stories, each containing a moral dilemma, to various individuals of various ages and backgrounds. Questions were posed concerning the moral dilemmas. On the basis of the reasons given for the answers, Kohlberg formulated a theory of moral development consisting of six developmental stages of moral judgement categorized into three levels (I–III).

5.7.1.1 Preconventional Morality (Level I)

This is the level at which the moral judgements of children up to the age of 7 years mainly lie:

- *Stage 1: Punishment orientation*—rules are obeyed in order to avoid punishment.
- *Stage 2: Reward orientation*—rules are conformed to in order to be rewarded.

5.7.1.2 Conventional Morality (Level II)

This is the level at which most moral judgements of children lie by the age of 13 years:

- *Stage 3: Good-boy/good-girl orientation*—rules are conformed to in order to avoid the disapproval of others.
- *Stage 4: Authority orientation*—laws and social rules are upheld in order to avoid the censure of authorities and because of guilt about not doing one's duty.

5.7.1.3 Postconventional Morality (Level III)

This level, which may never be reached even in adulthood, requires individuals to have achieved the later stages of Piaget's formal operational stage:

- *Stage 5: Social contract orientation*—actions are guided by principles generally agreed to be essential for public welfare. These principles are upheld in order to maintain the respect of peers and self-respect.

- *Stage 6: Ethical principle orientation*—actions are guided by principles chosen by oneself, usually emphasizing dignity, equality, and justice. These principles are upheld in order to avoid self-condemnation.

5.7.2 RELATIONSHIP TO THE DEVELOPMENT OF SOCIAL PERSPECTIVE TAKING

Social perspective taking is the ability to take the perspective of others. It is a skill that may be seen at the following levels:

- Perceptual role taking—the ability to take into account how a perceptual array appears to another person when their perspective differs from that of oneself
- Cognitive role taking—the ability to take into account the thoughts of another person when they differ from those of oneself
- Affective role taking—the ability to take into account the feelings of another person when they differ from those of oneself

In addition to being necessary to being able to empathize with others, social perspective taking was considered by Kohlberg as being necessary to develop higher stages of moral reasoning.

5.8 DEVELOPMENT OF FEARS IN CHILDHOOD AND ADOLESCENCE

5.8.1 DEFINITION

Fear is an unpleasant emotional state (a feeling of apprehension, tension, or uneasiness) caused by a realistic current or impending danger that is recognized at a conscious level. It differs from anxiety in that in the latter the cause is vague or not as understandable. However, fear and anxiety are terms that are often used interchangeably.

5.8.2 DEVELOPMENT WITH AGE

The types of fear that develop in childhood and adolescence differ with age (Marks, 1987):

- 6 Months: Fear of novel stimuli begins (such as fear of strangers), reaching a peak at 18 months–2 years.

- 6–8 Months: Fear of heights begins and becomes worse when walking starts.
- 3–5 Years: Common fears are those of animals, the dark, and 'monsters'.
- 6–11 Years: Fear of shameful social situations (such as ridicule) begins.
- Adolescence: Fear of death, failure, social gatherings (such as parties), and thermonuclear war may be particularly evident.

5.8.3 POSSIBLE ETIOLOGICAL AND MAINTENANCE MECHANISMS

5.8.3.1 Unconscious Conflict

Sigmund Freud (1926/1959) suggested that psychological anxiety is a signal phenomenon and that neurotic anxiety starts as the remembrance of realistic anxiety/fear related to a real danger. Each stage of life was considered to have age-appropriate determinants of anxiety/fear, including, with increasing age

- Fear of birth
- Fear of separation from the mother
- Fear of castration
- Fear of the superego—fear of its anger or punishment
- Fear of the superego—fear of its loss of love
- Fear of the superego—fear of death

5.8.3.2 Learned Response

Fear/anxiety may become associated with particular situations by means of learning.

5.8.3.3 Lack of Control

Fear/anxiety may occur when an individual feels helpless in a situation beyond his or her control.

5.9 SEXUAL DEVELOPMENT

5.9.1 SEX DETERMINATION

Sex determination is primarily as a result of the sex chromosomes (XX female and XY male). Gonad formation is first indicated in the embryo by the appearance of an area of thickened epithelium on the medial aspect of the mesonephric ridge during week 5. Factors affecting subsequent differentiation of the genital organs into male ones (epididymis, ductus [vas] deferens, ejaculatory ducts, penis, and scrotum) or female ones (fallopian tubes, clitoris, and vagina) during ontogeny include the following:

- *Y chromosome*—in mammals, testis determination is under the control of the testis-determining factor borne by the Y chromosome. SRY, a gene cloned from the sex-determining region of the human Y chromosome, has been equated with the testis-determining factor in humans.
- *Degree of ripeness of the ovum at fertilization*—overripeness of the ovum at fertilization is associated with a reduced number of primordial germ cells. This in turn leads to a masculinizing effect on genetic females.
- *Endocrine actions*—androgens and oestrogens can modify the process of sexual differentiation, while in twin pregnancy with fetuses of opposite sex and anastomosed placental circulations, the genetically male fetus may have a masculinizing effect on the genetically female fetus. A genetically female fetus may also be masculinized (and be born with either ambiguous or male genitalia) by fetal androgen from another source (e.g. in congenital adrenal [suprarenal] hyperplasia). Similarly, a genetically male fetus with a Y chromosome and testes may develop female genitalia in the absence of fetal androgen (e.g. in enzyme deficiency) or if androgen receptors are defective (e.g. in testicular feminization).

5.9.2 CHANGES AT PUBERTY

Puberty consists of a series of physical and physiological changes that convert a child into an adult who is capable of sexual reproduction.

5.9.2.1 Physical Changes

These include

- Growth spurt
- Change in body proportion
- Development of sexual organs
- Development of secondary sexual characteristics

Tanner described a standardized system for recording breast, pubic hair, and genital maturation. An example of a Tanner growth chart for height for boys is shown in Figure 5.1.

5.9.2.2 Onset in Girls

In 95%, onset occurs between 9 and 13 years. The first sign is

- Breast formation—in 80%
- Pubic hair growth—in 20%

In Western countries, menarche occurs at a mean age of 13.5 years.

5.9.2.3 Onset in Boys

In 95%, onset occurs between 9.5 and 13.5 years. The first sign is usually testicular and scrotal enlargement, followed by growth of the penis and pubic hair. On average, the first ejaculation occurs at around 13 years.

5.9.2.4 Physiological Changes

A raising of the threshold for gonadohypothalamic negative feedback precedes the onset of puberty. An increase in suprarenal androgen release (adrenarche) usually begins between the ages of 6 and 8 years; these hormones lead to the growth of sexual hair and skeletal maturation.

5.9.3 GENDER IDENTITY

This is an individual's perception and self-awareness with respect to gender. It is usually established by the age of 3 or 4 years and usually remains firmly established thereafter.

5.9.4 GENDER/SEX TYPING

This is the process by which individuals acquire a sense of gender and gender-related cultural traits appropriate to the society and age into which they are born. It usually begins at an early age with male and female infants being treated differently, for example, with respect to the choice of their clothing.

5.9.5 GENDER ROLE

This is the type of behaviour that an individual engages in that identifies him or her as being male or female, for example, with respect to the type of clothes worn and the use of cosmetics.

5.9.6 SEXUAL BEHAVIOUR

5.9.6.1 Sexual Drive

This is the need to achieve sexual pleasure through genital stimulation. It exists from birth to middle childhood and increases again during adolescence as a result of increased androgen secretion.

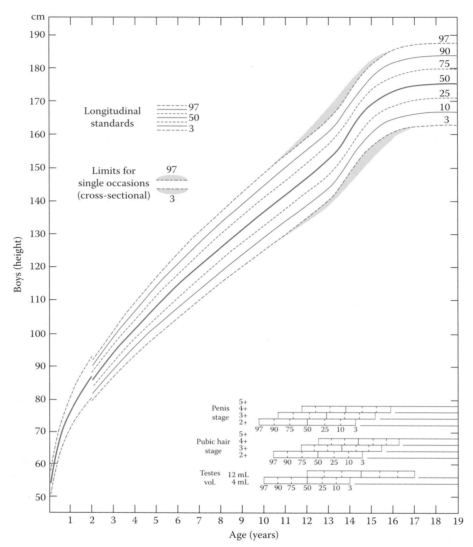

FIGURE 5.1 Example of Tanner growth chart for height. A series of charts of longitudinal growth standards for physical development (including parameters for height, weight, skin folds) were developed for children according to age, sex, and sexual maturity. (From Tanner, J.M. and Whitehouse, R.H., *Arch. Dis. Child.*, 51, 170, 1976.)

5.9.6.2 Childhood Sexuality

This may manifest itself in normal children as

- Sex play in infancy
- Erections in boys
- Vaginal lubrication in girls
- Masturbation—which may involve orgasm
- Exploratory encounters with other children

5.9.6.3 Masturbation

This is the predominant mode of sexual expression for most adolescent males and probably fewer adolescent females.

5.9.7 SEXUAL ORIENTATION

This is the erotic attraction that an individual feels. Its shaping is a developmental process associated with certain patterns of childhood experience and activity. Superimposed on this, there are arguments for and against the theory that human sexual orientation is biologically determined.

5.9.7.1 Homosexuality

This term is associated with the following behavioural dimensions:

- Sexual fantasy
- Sexual activity
- Sense of identity
- Social role

The first of these is the most important dimension in assessing homosexual orientation. If present, it does not necessarily imply sexual activity with others, as in individuals who are homosexual in orientation and celibate.

It should be noted that there is no nonhuman mammalian species in which predominant or exclusive homosexuality occurs in the way it does in humans.

5.9.7.2 Modern Arguments in Favour of Biological Determinism

- *Endocrine.* On the basis of rat and human experiments, Dorner (1986, 1989) has hypothesized that 21-hydroxylase deficiency represents a genetic predisposition to female homosexuality in heterozygous forms (homozygous forms lead to congenital adrenal hyperplasia), while in males 21-hydroxylase deficiency and/or prenatal stress leads to an overall inhibition in the effects of androgen on brain differentiation and to male homosexuality. Among their experiments on humans, Dorner et al. studied the effects of oestrogen infusion on LH secretion and reported that in contrast to heterosexual men, homosexual men manifest a positive oestrogen feedback effect on LH secretion, which was said to provide evidence that homosexual men have a predominantly female-differentiated brain. Furthermore, as a result of ACTH provocation tests on the suprarenal (adrenal) glands, Dorner reported that female homosexuals display significantly increased ratios of 17a-hydroxyprogesterone/cortisol and androstenedione/cortisol after ACTH stimulation compared with female heterosexual control subjects.
- *Neuroanatomical.* LeVay (1991) reported histological differences in the interstitial nuclei of the anterior hypothalamus (INAH) between homosexual and heterosexual men, suggesting that sexual orientation may be mediated by the central nervous system. The anterior hypothalamus of the brain is known to participate in the regulation of male-typical sexual behaviour. The volumes of four cell groups in this region (INAH 1, 2, 3, and 4) were measured in postmortem tissue from three subject groups: women, men who were presumed to be heterosexual, and

homosexual men. No differences were found between the groups in the volumes of INAH 1, 2, or 4. As had been previously reported, INAH 3 was found to be more than twice as large in the heterosexual men as in the women. It was also, however, more than twice as large in the heterosexual men as in the homosexual men. This finding indicates that INAH is dimorphic with sexual orientation, at least in men. A second neuroanatomical difference was reported by Allen and Gorski (1992): On the basis of the examination of 90 postmortem brains, it was found that the midsagittal plane of the anterior commissure in homosexual men was 18% larger than in heterosexual women and 34% larger than in heterosexual men. This finding of a difference in a structure not known to be related to reproductive functions supports the hypothesis that factors operating early in development differentiate sexually dimorphic structures and functions of the brain in a global fashion.

- *Genetic.* Bailey and Pillard (1991) found evidence of heritability of homosexuality in a study of monozygotic and dizygotic twins. Homosexual male probands with monozygotic co-twins, dizygotic co-twins, or adoptive brothers were recruited. Of the relatives whose sexual orientation could be rated, 52% (29/56) of monozygotic co-twins, 22% (12/54) of dizygotic co-twins, and 11% (6/57) of adoptive brothers were homosexual. Childhood gender nonconformity did not appear to be an indicator of genetic loading for homosexuality. In a second genetic study, Hamer et al. (1993) reported a linkage between DNA markers on the X chromosome and male sexual orientation. Pedigree and linkage analyses on 114 families of homosexual men were carried out. Increased rates of homosexual orientation were found in the maternal uncles and male cousins of these subjects but not in their fathers or paternal relatives, suggesting the possibility of sex-linked transmission in a portion of the population. DNA linkage analysis of a selected group of 40 families in which there were two gay brothers and no indication of nonmaternal transmission revealed a correlation between homosexual orientation and the inheritance of polymorphic markers on the X chromosome in approximately 64% of the sib-pairs tested. The linkage to markers on Xq28 had a multipoint lod score of 4.0.

5.9.7.3 Arguments against Biological Determinism

- *Endocrine.* Gooren et al. (1990) have argued that oestrogen feedback cannot be used to assess the status of brain differentiation in primates in the same way as it can in the rat. For example, sexual differentiation of the control of LH secretion occurs in the mouse, hamster, and guinea pig but not in primates. Among their experiments on humans, Gooren et al. studied directly the control of LH secretion in homosexuals and transsexuals compared with heterosexuals. Following oestrogen exposure, the response of LH to LHRH was not positive in male homosexuals, transsexuals, and heterosexuals; it was positive in female homosexuals, transsexuals (prior to treatment), and heterosexuals; moreover, a positive LH response to oestrogen infusion in homosexual men was not found.
- *Neuroanatomical.* LeVay (1991) pointed out that his sample contained no homosexual women and that AIDS patients may constitute an unrepresentative sample of homosexual men. Moreover, some presumed heterosexual men had relatively small INAH 3 nuclei (within the homosexual range), and some presumed homosexual men had relatively large INAH 3 nuclei (within the heterosexual range). The effect might have resulted from AIDS (although there was no effect of AIDS on the volume of the three other INAH nuclei examined and the size difference in INAH 3 was present when the homosexual men were compared with heterosexual AIDS patients).
- *Genetic.* King (1993) has pointed out that the result of Hamer et al. (1993) is preliminary. Their evidence is based on a small, highly selected group of homosexual men. The result is purely statistical. The gene is hypothetical and has not been cloned, and the linkage has been observed in only one series of families.

5.10 ADOLESCENCE

Adolescence is a time of transitions, representing a developmental phase between middle childhood/latency and adulthood, but its boundaries are difficult to demarcate clearly. In his model of cognitive development, Piaget viewed adolescence as the final, formal operational stage of development; the adolescent has a greater capacity to focus on himself or herself.

The pubertal changes of adolescence have been considered earlier.

5.10.1 Conflict with Parents and Authority

Theories of why conflict between adolescents and parents and other authority figures often occurs include

- Cognitive developmental models
- Erikson's stages of psychosocial development
- Ethological and sociobiological models
- Social-learning theory
- Equity theory
- Separation–individuation

5.10.1.1 Cognitive Developmental Models

The adolescent has newly acquired powers of hypothetical reasoning that enable him or her to consider and articulate alternatives to the *status quo.*

5.10.1.2 Erikson's Stages of Psychosocial Development

In his fifth psychosocial developmental stage (identity vs. role confusion), Erikson considered adolescence to be a time of identity formation during which the individual pursues personal autonomy. This pursuit is associated with the potential for conflict with parents and other authority figures.

5.10.1.3 Ethological and Sociobiological Models

Conflict at the time of pubertal changes is considered to be adaptive, prompting the individual to spend more time with his or her peers. It forms part of the status realignments of entry into adulthood.

5.10.1.4 Social-Learning Theory

Adolescents may be considered to have experienced vicarious exposure to problem-solving occurring via conflict. Witnessing their parents giving in to their children's conflicting demands may be considered to provide intermittent reinforcement to the children.

5.10.1.5 Equity Theory

According to equity theory, the preferred relationships, particularly those of an intimate nature, between any two given people are those in which each feels that the cost–benefit ratio of the relationship for each person is approximately equal. It has been argued that the amount of emotional investment of both the adolescent and the parent(s) in their relationship means they both want to preserve it. As the adolescent pursues autonomy, this can lead to occasional conflicts, but these are usually not fervent enough to destroy the relationship.

5.10.1.6 Separation–Individuation

It has been argued that adolescence can be considered to represent a second separation–individuation phase, in which continued biological, motor, and social developments now allow the adolescent to move away from a dependent relationship with the parent(s) to take his or her own place in society. However, social and psychological pulls towards dependency mean that the separation–individuation may entail ambivalence and conflict.

5.10.2 AFFECTIVE STABILITY AND 'TURMOIL'

Successive developments in the psychological understanding of affective stability and 'turmoil' in adolescence have been provided by Anna Freud, Erikson, and Offer and Offer.

5.10.2.1 Anna Freud

A rapid oscillation between excess and asceticism during adolescence was described by Anna Freud (1936/1946). Affective instability and behaviour swings were considered to be caused by

- The drives stimulated by sexual maturity
- Pubertal endocrine changes
- Instability of the newly stressed defences of the ego against these drives

5.10.2.2 Erikson

Erikson (1959) characterized adolescence as manifesting 'adolescent turmoil' and a maladaptive, temporary state of 'identity diffusion', which he implied all adolescents passed through.

5.10.2.3 Offer and Offer

Offer and Offer (1975) showed that, in general, adolescence is a time of less turmoil and upheaval than previously thought. They studied a cohort of American males who had been aged 14 years in 1962. Sixty-one of these adolescents were studied intensively and followed up into adulthood. They came mainly from intact families, and there were no serious drug problems or major delinquent activity. Seventy-four per cent went to college during the 1 year after high school graduation. They showed no significant difference in basic values from that of their parents.

5.10.3 NORMAL AND ABNORMAL ADOLESCENT DEVELOPMENT

5.10.3.1 Offer and Offer

Offer and Offer (1975) identified the following three adolescent developmental routes (the percentages given are those of the sample of adolescents they studied; the remaining 21% could not be classified easily but were closer to the first two categories than to the third one):

- *Continuous growth* (23%). Eriksonian intimacy was achieved, and shame and guilt could be displayed. Major separation, death, and severe illness were less frequent. Their parents encouraged independence.
- *Surgent growth* (35%). The adolescents in this group were 'late bloomers'. They were more likely than the first group to have frequent depressive and anxious moments. Although often successful, they were less introspective and not as action oriented as the first group. There were more areas of disagreement with their parents.
- *Tumultuous growth* (21%). Recurrent self-doubt and conflict with their families occurred in this group. Their backgrounds were less stable than in the first two groups. The arts, humanities, and social sciences were preferred to professional and business careers.

5.10.3.2 Block and Haan

Block and Haan (1971) used factor analysis to isolate the following groups among a cohort of 84 male adolescents studied longitudinally to adulthood:

- Ego-resilient adolescents
- Belated adjustors—similar to the surgent group of Offer and Offer
- Vulnerable overcontrollers
- Anomic extroverts—less inner life and relatively uncertain values
- Unsettled undercontrollers—given to impulsivity

A similar cohort of 86 females was divided into

- Female prototype
- Cognitive type—individuals tend to be intellectualized in the way problems are negotiated
- Hyperfeminine repressors—similar to hysterical personality disorder
- Dominating narcissists
- Vulnerable undercontrollers
- Lonely independents

5.11 ADAPTATIONS IN ADULT LIFE

5.11.1 Pairing

Even in Western countries, it appears that there are a number of constraints that govern the choice of mate in much the same way as elders or parents do in arranged marriages.

5.11.1.1 Homogamous Mate Selection

Pairing tends to occur within the same socioeconomic, religious, and cultural group (Eshelman, 1985).

5.11.1.2 Reinforcement Theory

People are attracted to those who reinforce the attraction with rewards. This process is a reciprocal one with rewards also passing in the opposite direction and further reinforcing the interpersonal attraction (Newcomb, 1956).

5.11.1.3 Social Exchange Theory

People have a preference for relationships that appear to offer an optimum cost–benefit ratio—maximum benefits such as love with minimum costs such as time spent with each other (Homans, 1961).

5.11.1.4 Equity Theory

As mentioned earlier, this is a modification of the social exchange theory in which the preferred relationships, particularly of an intimate nature, between two people are those in which each feels that the cost–benefit ratio of the relationship for each person is approximately equal (Hatfield et al., 1978).

5.11.1.5 Matching Hypothesis

According to this hypothesis, heterosexual pairing tends to occur in such a way that, although ideally a person would prefer to pair with the most attractive people (Huston, 1973), in practice individuals seek to pair with others who have a similar level of physical attractiveness rather than the most attractive (Berscheid and Walster, 1974). This is felt by the individual to lead to a greater probability of acceptance by the other person, a lower probability of rejection, and a lower probability of losing the partner to another person in the future.

5.11.1.6 Cultural Differences

People in Asian and African countries tend to value home-keeping potential and a desire for home and children in mate selection, while people in Western countries tend to value love, character, and emotional maturity. Chastity is rated very highly in some countries (such as India and China) and cultures (such as orthodox/traditional Jewish, Christian, and Islamic communities) and very low in others (such as Australia, New Zealand, North America, South America, and Scandinavia—excluding their traditional observant religious groups) (Buss et al., 1990).

5.11.1.7 Cross-Cultural Constancies

Across cultures, men prefer mates who are physically attractive, while women prefer mates who show ambition, industriousness, and other signs of earning power potential (Buss et al., 1990).

5.11.2 Parenting

Parenting is a complex, dyadic process that is influenced by a range of factors, including

- Cultural beliefs of the parent about child rearing (Maccoby and Martin, 1983)
- Genetic-temperamental characteristics of the parent (i.e. genetic factors influencing the provision of parenting) (Perusse et al., 1994)
- Genetic-temperamental characteristics of the child (i.e. genetic factors influencing the elicitation of parenting) (Bell, 1968)

Furthermore, reporting bias is likely, with parents stressing the similarity with which they treat their children and children emphasizing the differences in parental treatment that they perceive (Plomin et al., 1994).

Abusive parenting is a strong predictor of later psychopathology. On the other hand, parental warmth and support buffers children against externalizing and antisocial behaviour (Hetherington and Clingempeel, 1992) and is positively associated with a child's self-esteem (Bell and Bell, 1983).

5.11.3 Grief, Mourning, and Bereavement

5.11.3.1 Definitions

- *Grief*—those psychological and emotional processes, expressed both internally and externally, that accompany bereavement.
- *Mourning*—those culture-bound social and cognitive processes through which one must pass in order that grief is resolved, allowing one to return to more normal functioning; it is often used, less strictly, as being synonymous with grief.
- *Bereavement*—a term that can apply to any loss event, from the loss of a relative by death to unemployment, divorce, or loss of a pet; it refers to being in the state of mourning.

5.11.3.2   Normal Grief

The symptomatology of normal grief may include the following:

- Initial shock and disbelief—'a feeling of numbness'.
- Increasing awareness of the loss is associated with painful emotions of sadness and anger.
- Anger may be denied.
- Irritability.
- Somatic distress—may include sleep disturbance, early morning waking, tearfulness, loss of appetite, weight loss, loss of libido, and anhedonia.
- Identification phenomena—the mannerisms and characteristics of the deceased may be taken on.

In 1944, Lindemann read to the centenary meeting of the American Psychiatric Association the results of his study of 101 bereaved individuals, many of whom had lost loved ones in the tragic Cocoanut Grove nightclub fire in Boston, MA. He identified the following five points as being pathognomonic of acute grief:

- Somatic distress
- Preoccupation with the image of the deceased
- Guilt
- Hostile reactions
- Loss of patterns of conduct

Note that grief is not seen in babies if a parent/caregiver dies prior to the development of attachment behaviour.

5.11.3.3   Bereavement

Parkes described the following five stages of bereavement:

- Alarm
- Numbness
- Pining for the deceased—illusions or hallucinations of the deceased may occur
- Depression
- Recovery and reorganization

5.11.3.4   Morbid Grief Reactions

Lindemann described the following morbid grief reactions:

1. Delay of reaction
2. *Distorted reactions*—subclassified into
   a. Overactivity without a sense of loss
   b. The acquisition of symptoms belonging to the last illness of the deceased

   c. A recognized medical disease
   d. Alteration in relationship to friends and relatives
   e. Furious hostility against specific persons
   f. Loss of affectivity
   g. A lasting loss of patterns of social interaction
   h. Activities attain a colouring detrimental to social and economic existence
   i. Agitated depression

5.11.3.5   Differentiating between Bereavement and a Depressive Episode

The diagnosis of major depressive disorder in DSM-IV-TR is generally not given unless the symptoms are still present 2 months after the loss. However, the presence of certain symptoms that are not characteristic of a normal grief reaction may be helpful in differentiating bereavement from a major depressive episode:

- Guilt about things other than actions taken or not taken by the survivor at the time of the death
- Thoughts of death other than the survivor feeling that he or she would be better off dead or should have died with the deceased person
- Morbid preoccupation with worthlessness
- Marked psychomotor retardation
- Prolonged and marked functional impairment
- Hallucinatory experiences other than thinking that he or she hears the voice of, or transiently sees the image of, the deceased person

Freud (1917/1957) differentiated between normal grief and the depressive response by the presence of shame and guilt in the latter. Yearning for the lost object was considered to be part of the normal response to loss. It was overcome gradually as the mental representation was decathected.

5.12   NORMAL AGEING

5.12.1   Physical Aspects

5.12.1.1   Health

In general, most elderly people in Western countries enjoy good health, in spite of the changes that occur in body systems with increasing age.

5.12.1.2   Cerebral Changes

Blessed et al. (1968) found no histological evidence of dementia in the brains of 28 nondemented individuals.

Evidence of cerebral atrophy was absent or slight in the majority, and brain mass and ventricular size did not differ significantly from those of younger adults (Tomlinson et al., 1968). Terry and Hanson (1988) found that the neuronal loss per unit volume of the normal brain in the elderly was much less than that previously reported.

5.12.2 Social Aspects

5.12.2.1 Stereotyping

Old age is generally a stigmatized period. For instance, people are complimented for looking younger than their chronological age.

5.12.2.2 Empty Nest Syndrome

Prior to the onset of old age, parents usually witness their children leaving home, particularly in Western countries. The difficulties some parents encounter on being left on their own have been described as the empty nest syndrome.

5.12.3 Ego Integrity versus Despair

This is Erikson's eighth and final stage of psychosocial development, occurring in old age.

5.12.3.1 Ego Integrity

Successful resolution of the psychosocial crisis of this age leads to an integrated view of one's life, its meaning, its achievements (both for the self and others, including future generations), and the ways in which difficulties were coped with. There is an acceptance of one's mortality, a feeling that one's life has been lived in a satisfactory way, and a readiness to face death.

5.12.3.2 Despair

The alternative is despair, both on reflection of how life has been lived and the way in which others have been treated and also on looking to the future and the sense of transience that is felt on facing the end of life. Rather than having a sense of contentment and completion, there is despair at the prospect of death.

5.12.4 Cognitive Aspects

Prior to the late 1960s, it was generally believed that the normal ageing brain degenerates and that this is accompanied by intellectual deterioration. By the 1970s, this view had been challenged on the basis of new research. Thus, Schaie (1974) wrote:

The presumed universal decline in adult intelligence is at best a methodological artifact and at worst a popular misunderstanding of the relation between individual development and sociocultural change... the major finding...in the area of intellectual functioning is the demolishing of [the belief in] serious intellectual decrement in the aged.

Although the elderly do not generally perform as well as younger subjects on cognitive tasks dependent on processing speed, old age is not necessarily associated with a large decline in intellectual ability (Durkin, 1995). Reasons for this include the following:

- Different abilities contribute to intellectual behaviour, so that a reduction in one (e.g. processing speed) may be compensated for by an increase in another (such as experience-based judgement).
- Cross-sectional comparisons of different age groups may confound age differences with cohort effects.
- Changes in performance with age may be offset by practice.
- Crystallized intelligence (the ability to store and manipulate learned information) increases through adulthood and often remains high into old age.

5.13 DEATH AND DYING

5.13.1 Definitions

5.13.1.1 Timely Death

This refers to the situation in which the expected life expectancy is approximately equal to the actual length of time lived.

5.13.1.2 Untimely Death

This refers to the situation in which the actual length of time lived is significantly less than the expected life expectancy, as a result of one of the following:

- Premature death at a young age
- Sudden unexpected death
- Violent/accidental death

5.13.1.3 Unintended Death

This refers to the situation in which death is unintended, usually occurring as a result of pathological processes or trauma.

5.13.1.4 Intended Death

This refers to the situation in which death is intended by the deceased, who played a part in his or her suicide.

5.13.1.5 Subintended Death

This refers to the situation in which the deceased may have manifested an unconscious desire to bring about his or her death, for example, by facilitating the onset of death through psychoactive substance abuse.

5.13.2 IMPENDING DEATH

If it is believed that one's death is near, an individual may pass through the following five stages that are similar to those recognized as occurring in the terminally ill (Kübler-Ross, 1969):

- *Shock and denial*—the diagnosis may be disbelieved and another opinion sought; this first stage may never be passed.
- *Anger*—the person may be angry and wonder why this has happened to him or her.
- *Bargaining*—the person may, for example, try to negotiate with God.
- *Depression*—the symptomatology of a depressive episode is manifested.
- *Acceptance*—the person may finally come to terms with his or her mortality and understand the inevitability of death.

REFERENCES

Aiosa-Karpas CJ, Karpas R, Pelcovitz D et al. 1991: Gender identification and sex role attribution in sexually abused adolescent females. *Journal of the American Academy of Child and Adolescent Psychiatry* 30:266–271.

Allen LS and Gorski RA. 1992: Sexual orientation and the size of the anterior commissure in the human brain. *Proceedings of the National Academy of Sciences* 85:7199–7202.

Bailey JM and Pillard RC. 1991: A genetic study of male sexual orientation. *Archives of General Psychiatry* 48:1089–1096.

Bates JE. 1989: Concepts and measures of temperament. In Kohnstamm GA, Bates JE, and Rothbart MK (eds.) *Temperament in Childhood*, pp. 3–69. New York: Wiley.

Bates JE, Wachs TD, and VandenBos GR. 1995: Trends in research on temperament. *Psychiatric Services* 46:661–663.

Baumrind D. 1967: Child care practices anteceding three patterns of pre-school behavior. *Genetic Psychology Monographs* 75:43–88.

Bell RQ. 1968: A reinterpretation of the direction of effects in studies of socialization. *Psychological Review* 75:81–95.

Bell DC and Bell LG. 1983: Parental validation and support in the development of adolescent daughters. In Grotevant HD (ed.) *Adolescent Development in the Family*, pp. 27–41. San Francisco, CA: Jossey Bass.

Berscheid E and Walster E. 1974: Physical attractiveness. In Berkowitz L (ed.) *Advances in Experimental Social Psychology*, pp. 285–290. New York: Academic Press.

Blessed G, Tomlinson BE, and Roth M. 1968: The association between quantitative measures of dementia and of senile change in the cerebral grey matter of elderly subjects. *British Journal of Psychiatry* 114:797–811.

Block J and Haan N. 1971: *Lives Through Time*. Berkeley, CA: Bancroft Books.

Bowlby J. 1969: *Attachment and Loss, Vol. 1: Attachment*. New York: Basic Books.

Buss DM et al. 1990: International preferences in selecting mates: A study of 37 cultures. *Journal of Cross-Cultural Psychology* 21:5–47.

Caspi A and Silva PA. 1995: Temperamental qualities at age three predict personality traits in young adulthood: Longitudinal evidence from a birth cohort. *Child Development* 66:486–498.

Chess S and Thomas A. 1984: *Origins and Evolution of Behavior Disorders: From Infancy to Early Adult Life*. New York: Brunner/Mazel.

Cosentino CE, Meyer-Bahlburg HFI, Nat DR et al. 1995: Sexual behavior problems and psychopathology symptoms in sexually abused girls. *Journal of the American Academy of Child and Adolescent Psychiatry* 34:1033–1042.

Dorner G. 1986: Hormone-dependent brain development and preventative medicine. *Monographs in Neural Sciences* 12:17–27.

Dorner G. 1989: Hormone-dependent brain development and neuroendocrine prophylaxis. *Experimental and Clinical Endocrinology* 94:4–22.

Durkin K. 1995: *Developmental Social Psychology*. Cambridge, MA: Blackwell.

Elmer E and Gregg CS. 1967: Developmental characteristics of abused children. *Pediatrics* 40:596–602.

Erikson E. 1959: *Growth and Crises of the Healthy Personality*. New York: International Universities Press.

Eshelman JR. 1985: One should marry a person of the same religion, race, ethnicity, and social class. In Feldman H and Feldman M (eds.) *Current Controversies in Marriage and the Family*, pp. 57–68. Newbury Park, CA: Sage.

Finkelhor D. 1984: *Child Sexual Abuse: New Theory and Research*. New York: Free Press.

Freud S. 1917/1957: Mourning and melancholia. In Translated and edited by Strachey J *Standard Edition of the Complete Psychological Works of Sigmund Freud*, Vol. 14. London, U.K.: Hogarth.

Freud S. 1926/1959: Inhibitions, symptoms and anxiety. In Translated and edited by Strachey J *Standard Edition of the Complete Psychological Works of Sigmund Freud*, Vol. 20. London, U.K.: Hogarth.

Freud A. 1936/1946: *The Ego and the Mechanisms of Defense* (Translated by Baines C). New York: International Universities Press.

Friedrich W and Reams R. 1987: Course of psychological symptoms in sexually abused young children. *Psychotherapy* 24:160–171.

Gaensbauer T and Sands K. 1979: Regulation of emotional expression in infants from two contrasting environments. *Journal of the American Academy of Child Psychiatry* 21:167–171.

George C and Main M. 1979: Social interactions and young abused children: Approach, avoidance, and aggression. *Child Development* 50:306–319.

Goodwin J. 1988: Post-traumatic symptoms in abused children. *Journal of Traumatic Stress* 1(4):475–488.

Gooren L, Fliers E, and Courtney K. 1990: Biological determinants of sexual orientation. *Annual Review of Sex Research* 1:175–196.

Gowers S.G. (ed.) 2001: *Adolescent Psychiatry in Clinical Practice*. London, U.K.: Arnold.

Graham P. 1991: *Child Psychiatry: A Developmental Approach*, 2nd edn. Oxford, U.K.: Oxford University Press.

Green AH. 1978: Psychiatric treatment of abused children. *Journal of the American Academy of Child Psychiatry* 17:356–371.

Green AH, Voeller K, Gaines R et al. 1981: Neurological impairment in battered children. *Child Abuse and Neglect* 5:129–134.

Gunnar M. 1992: Reactivity of the hypothalamic–pituitary–adrenocortical system to stressors in normal infants and children. *Pediatrics* 90:491–497.

Hamer DH, Hu S, Magnuson VL, Hu N, and Pattatucci AM. 1993: A linkage between DNA markers on the X chromosome and male sexual orientation. *Science* 261:321–327.

Hatfield E, Traupmann J, and Walster GW. 1978: Equity and extramarital sexuality. *Archives of Sexual Behaviour*, 7:127–141.

Hatfield E and Traupmann J. 1981: Intimate relationships: A perspective from equity theory. In Duck S and Gilmour R (eds.) *Personal Relationships,* Vol. 1, pp. 109–124. New York: Academic Press.

Herman J. 1981: *Father-Daughter Incest*. Cambridge, MA: Harvard University Press.

Herman J, Perry JC, and van der Kolk B. 1989: Childhood trauma in borderline personality disorder. *American Journal of Psychiatry* 146:490–495.

Hetherington EM and Clingempeel WG. 1992: Coping with marital transitions: A family systems perspective. *Monographs of the Society of Research into Child Development* 57 (serial no. 227).

Homans GC. 1961: *Social Behavior: Its Elementary Forms*. New York: Harcourt Brace.

Huston TL. 1973: Ambiguity of acceptance, social desirability and dating choice. *Journal of Experimental Social Psychology* 9:32.

King M-C. 1993: Human genetics: Sexual orientation and the X [news and views]. *Nature* 364:288–289.

Kluft R. 1985: *Childhood Antecedents of Multiple Personality*. Washington, DC: American Psychiatric Press.

Kübler-Ross E. 1969: *On Death and Dying*. New York: Macmillan.

LeVay S. 1991: A difference in hypothalamic structure between heterosexual and homosexual men. *Science* 253:1034–1037.

Maccoby EE and Martin JA. 1983: Socialization in the context of the family: Parent–child interaction. In Mussen PH (ed.) *Handbook of Child Psychology*, Vol. IV: *Socialization, Personality, and Social Development*, pp. 3–97. New York: John Wiley.

Marks I. 1987: The development of normal fear: A review. *Journal of Child Psychology and Psychiatry* 28:667–698.

Martin HP. 1972: The child and his development. In Kempe CH and Helfer RE (eds.) *Helping the Battered Child and His Family*, pp. 97–109. Philadelphia, PA: Lippincott.

McCarty L. 1986: Mother–child incest: Characteristics of the offender. *Child Welfare* 65:447–458.

Munafò M and Attwood A. 2010: Human development. In Puri BK and Treasaden IH (eds.) *Psychiatry: An Evidence-Based Text*, pp. 103–126. London, U.K.: Hodder Arnold.

Newcomb T. 1956: The prediction of interpersonal attraction. *American Psychologist* 11:575.

Oates K. 1986: *Child Abuse and Neglect: What Happens Eventually?* New York: Brunner/Mazel.

Offer B and Offer JB. 1975: *From Teenage to Young Manhood: A Psychological Study*. New York: Basic Books.

Oppenheimer R, Howells K, Palmer L et al. 1985: Adverse sexual experiences in childhood and clinical eating disorders: A preliminary description. *Journal of Psychosomatic Research* 19:157–161.

Perusse D, Neale MC, Heath AC, and Eaves LJ. 1994 Human parental behavior: Evidence for genetic influence and potential implication for gene-culture transmission. *Behavioral Genetics* 24:327–335.

Plomin R, Reiss D, Hetherington EM, and Howe GW. 1994: Nature and nurture: Genetic contributions to measures of the family environment. *Developmental Psychology* 30:32–43.

Schaie KW. 1974: Translations in gerontology – From lab to life. Intellectual functioning. *American Psychologist* 29:802–807.

Schechter MD and Roberge L. 1976: Sexual exploitation. In Helfer RE and Kempe CH (eds.) *Child Abuse and Neglect: The Family and the Community*, pp. 129–141. Cambridge, MA: Ballinger.

Seghorn TK, Prentky RA, and Boucher RJ. 1987: Child sexual abuse in the lives of sexually aggressive offenders. *Journal of the American Academy of Child and Adolescent Psychiatry* 26:262–267.

Sgroi S. 1982: *Handbook of Clinical Intervention in Child Sexual Abuse*. Lexington, MA: Lexington Books.

Steele BF. 1983: The effect of abuse and neglect on psychological development. In Call JD, Galenson E, and Tyson RL (eds.) *Frontiers of Infant Psychiatry*, pp. 235–244. New York: Basic Books.

Tanner JM and Whitehouse RH. 1976: Clinical longitudinal standards for height, weight, height velocity, weight velocity, and stages of puberty. *Archives of Disease in Childhood* 51:170–179.

Thomas A and Chess S. 1977: *Temperament and Development.* New York: Brunner/Mazel.

Tomlinson BE, Blessed G, and Roth M. 1968. Observations on the brains of non-demented old people. *Journal of the Neurological Science*s 7:331–356.

Winnicott DW. 1965: *The Maturational Process and the Facilitating Environment.* New York, NY: International Universities Press.

Yates A. 1982: Children eroticized by incest. *American Journal of Psychiatry* 139:482–485.

Zuckerman M. 1991: *Psychobiology of Personality.* New York: Cambridge.

6 Description and Measurement

6.1 DESCRIPTION

6.1.1 TYPES OF DATA

6.1.1.1 Qualitative

Qualitative variables refer to attributes that can be categorized such that the categories do not have a numerical relationship with each other, for example, eye colour.

6.1.1.2 Quantitative

Quantitative variables refer to numerically represented data. These can be of the following types:

- *Discrete* quantitative variables—can only take on known fixed values, for example, the number of new patients seen each week in a psychiatric outpatient department
- *Continuous* quantitative variables—can only take on any value in a defined range, for example, the height of psychiatric inpatients

6.1.2 SCALES OF MEASUREMENT

Table 6.1 summarizes the properties of different types of measurement scale.

6.1.3 SAMPLING METHODS

6.1.3.1 Simple Random Sampling

A *simple random sample* is one chosen from a given population such that every possible sample of the same size has the same probability of being chosen.

6.1.3.2 Systematic Sampling

This type of sampling saves time and effort. Common examples include the following:

- *Periodic sampling*—very nth member of the population is chosen. This may not always lead to a random choice because of an unforeseen underlying pattern.
- *Using random numbers*—using random numbers can be a better method than periodic sampling for ensuring random choice. Random numbers, obtained, for example, from a computer program, a scientific calculator with a (pseudo) random number generator, or a table of random numbers, can be used to choose every nth member of the population.
- *Stratified random sampling*—a given population is stratified before random samples are chosen from each stratum. This can be useful when studying a disease that varies with respect to sex and age, for example.

6.1.4 FREQUENCY DISTRIBUTIONS

6.1.4.1 Frequency Distribution

This is a systematic way of arranging data, with frequencies being given for categories of a qualitative or quantitative variable. For continuous quantitative variables, the categories should be contiguous and mutually exclusive and are known as *class intervals*.

6.1.4.2 Frequency Table

This is a frequency distribution arranged in the form of a table, with the first column giving contiguous mutually exclusive values (which may be class intervals) of a variable and the adjoining column giving the corresponding frequencies.

6.1.4.3 Relative Frequency

The relative frequency of a category/class interval/variable is the proportion of the total frequency corresponding to that category/class interval/variable:

$$\text{Relative frequency} = \frac{\text{Frequency of category}}{\text{Total frequency}}$$

6.1.4.4 Cumulative Frequency

The cumulative frequency of a given value of a variable is the total frequency up to that value.

6.1.4.5 Cumulative Frequency Table

This is a cumulative frequency distribution arranged in the form of a table, with the first column giving contiguous mutually exclusive values (which may be class intervals) of a variable and the adjoining column giving the corresponding cumulative frequencies.

TABLE 6.1
Types of Measurement Scale

Property	Nominal	Ordinal	Interval	Ratio
Categories mutually exclusive	✓	✓	✓	✓
Categories logically ordered		✓	✓	✓
Equal distance between adjacent categories			✓	✓
True zero point				✓

Source: Reproduced from Puri, B.K., *Statistics for the Health Sciences*, WB Saunders, London, U.K., 1996. With permission.

6.1.4.6 Cumulative Relative Frequency

The cumulative relative frequency of a given value of a variable is the total relative frequency up to that value.

6.1.4.7 Cumulative Relative Frequency Table

This is a cumulative relative frequency distribution arranged in the form of a table, with the first column giving contiguous mutually exclusive values (which may be class intervals) of a variable and the adjoining column giving the corresponding cumulative relative frequencies.

6.1.5 DISCRETE PROBABILITY DISTRIBUTIONS

6.1.5.1 Bernoulli Trial

This is a trial or experiment having two and only two alternative outcomes.

6.1.5.2 Bernoulli Distribution

This is the probability distribution for a discrete binary variable (range = 0, 1), which is a special case of the binomial distribution $B(1, p)$, where p is the probability of 'success':

$$\text{Mean} = p$$

$$\text{Variance} = p(1-p)$$

6.1.5.3 Binomial Distribution

The binomial distribution, $B(n, p)$, is the probability distribution for a discrete finite variable (range = 0, 1, 2, …, n):

$$\text{Mean} = np$$

$$\text{Variance} = np(1-p)$$

6.1.5.4 Poisson Distribution

The Poisson distribution, Poisson (μ), is the probability distribution for a discrete infinite variable (range = 0, 1, 2, …), where $\mu = np$:

$$\text{Mean} = \mu$$

$$\text{Variance} = \mu$$

The Poisson distribution can be used in situations in which the following criteria are fulfilled:

- Events occur randomly in time or space (length, area, or volume).
- The events are independent (i.e. the outcome of any given event does not affect the outcome of any other).
- Two or more events cannot take place simultaneously.
- The mean number of events per given unit of time or space is constant.

6.1.6 CONTINUOUS PROBABILITY DISTRIBUTIONS

6.1.6.1 Normal Distribution

The normal (or Gaussian) distribution, $N(\mu, \sigma^2)$, is the probability distribution for a continuous variable (range = ∞):

$$\text{Mean} = \mu$$

$$\text{Variance} = \sigma^2$$

Properties of the normal distribution probability density function curve include the following:

- It is unimodal.
- It is continuous.
- It is symmetrical about its mean.

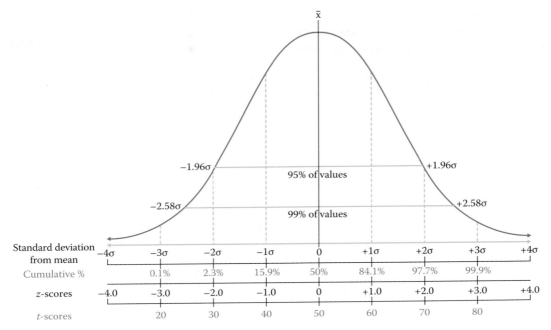

FIGURE 6.1   Normal or Gaussian distribution. (From Stahl, D. and Leese, M., Research methods and statistics, in Puri, B.K. and Treasaden, I.H. (eds.), *Psychiatry: An Evidence-Based Text*, Hodder Arnold, London, U.K., 2010, pp. 34–71.)

- Its mean, median, and mode are all equal.
- The area under the curve is one.
- The curve tends to zero as the variable moves in either direction from the mean (Figure 6.1).

The interval one standard deviation either side of the mean of the probability density function of a normal distribution encloses 68.27% of the total area under the curve.

The interval two standard deviations either side of the mean of the probability density function of a normal distribution encloses 95.45% of the total area under the curve.

The interval three standard deviations either side of the mean of the probability density function of a normal distribution encloses 99.73% of the total area under the curve.

If $X \sim N(\mu, \sigma^2)$, then the standard normal variate Z is given by

$$Z = \frac{(X - \mu)}{\sigma}$$

For $Z \sim N(0, 1)$

$$\text{Mean} = 0$$

$$\text{Variance} = 1$$

The cumulative distribution function, $P(Z < z)$, is given by $\Phi(z)$.

For $N(\mu, \sigma^2)$, the two-tailed 5% points are given by

$$\mu - 1.96\sigma$$

$$\mu + 1.96\sigma$$

6.1.6.2   *t* Distribution

When $n < 30$, the t distribution, $t(\nu)$ or t_ν, is used in making inferences about the mean of a normal population when its variance is unknown. The t distribution is symmetrical about the mean but has longer tails than the normal distribution.

ν is the number of degrees of freedom and is given by

$$\nu = n - 1$$

For $n \geq 30$, $t(\nu) \approx N(0, 1)$.

6.1.6.3 χ^2 Distribution

The chi-squared distribution with ν degrees of freedom, $\chi^2(\nu)$, is obtained from the sum of the squares of ν independent variables, Z_1 to Z_ν, where each $Z \sim N(0, 1)$:

If $W = \sum Z_i^2$, where $i = 1$ to ν, and $Z_i \sim N(0, 1)$,

then $W \sim \chi^2(\nu)$

The chi-squared distribution is asymmetrical.

6.1.6.4 *F* Distribution

The *F* distribution is related to the χ^2 distribution and is asymmetrical. A given *F* distribution is described in terms of ν_1 and ν_2, each of which gives a number of degrees of freedom. This is usually abbreviated to $F(\nu_1, \nu_2)$.

6.1.7 SUMMARY STATISTICS: MEASURES OF LOCATION

6.1.7.1 Measures of Central Tendency

The *(arithmetic) mean* (or average) of a sample with *n* items $(x_1, x_2, x_3, \ldots x_n)$, $\bar{x}$, is given by

$$\bar{x} = \frac{\Sigma x}{n}$$

The population mean, μ, of a population of size *N* is given by

$$\mu = \frac{\Sigma x}{N}$$

The arithmetic mean is suitable for use with data measured on at least an interval scale. A major disadvantage is that it can be unduly influenced by an extreme value.

The *median* is the middle value of a set of observations ranked in order. If the number of observations is odd,

Median = Middle value

If the number of observations is even,

Median = Arithmetic mean of the two middle values

The median is suitable for use with data measured on at least an ordinal scale. It gives a better measure of central tendency than the mean for skewed (asymmetrical) distributions.

The *mode* of a distribution is the value of the observation occurring most frequently. The category/interval occurring most frequently is the modal category. It can be used with all measurement scales.

6.1.7.2 Quantiles

Quantiles are cutoff points that split a continuous distribution into equal groups. They include the following:

- The median splits a distribution into 2 equal parts.
- The 3 quartiles split the distribution into 4 equal parts.
- The 4 quintiles split the distribution into 5 equal parts.

- The 9 deciles split the distribution into 10 equal parts.
- The 99 percentiles split the distribution into 100 equal parts.

The *k*th quantile of *n* observations ranked in increasing order from the first to the *n*th is calculated by interpolating between the two observations adjacent to the *q*th, where *q* is given by

$$q = \frac{k(n+1)}{Q}$$

where *Q* is the number of groups into which the quantiles divide the distribution.

6.1.8 SUMMARY STATISTICS: MEASURES OF DISPERSION

6.1.8.1 Range

The range is the difference between the smallest and largest values in a distribution:

$$\text{Range} = (\text{Largest value}) - (\text{Smallest value})$$

It can be used with data that are measured on at least an interval scale.

6.1.8.2 Measures Relating to Quantiles

The most commonly used measures relating to quantiles include

- The interquartile range = the difference between the third and first quartiles
- The semiquartile range = half the interquartile range
- The 10–90 percentile range = the difference between the 90th and 10th (per)centiles, or equivalently, between the ninth and first deciles
- The interdecile range = the difference between the 90th and 10th (per)centiles, or equivalently, between the ninth and first deciles

The median and interquartile or 10–90 percentile range can be more useful summary statistics than the mean and standard deviation for skewed distributions.

6.1.8.3 Standard Deviation

The standard deviation of a distribution is based on deviations from the mean and has the same units as the original observations.

For a population of size N and mean μ, the population standard deviation, σ, is given by

$$\text{Population standard deviation}, \sigma = \sqrt{\frac{\sum(x-\mu)^2}{N}}$$

For a sample of size n and mean $\bar{x}$, the sample standard deviation, s, is given by

$$\text{Sample standard deviation}, s = \sqrt{\frac{\sum(x-\bar{x})^2}{n-1}}$$

The standard deviation can be used for data measured on at least an interval scale.

6.1.8.4   Variance

The variance is the square of the standard deviation and has units that are the square of those of the observations. For a population of size N and mean μ, the population variance, σ^2, is given by

$$\text{Population variance}, \sigma^2 = \frac{\sum(x-\mu)^2}{N}$$

For a sample of size n and mean $\bar{x}$, the sample variance, s^2, is given by

$$\text{Sample variance}, s^2 = \frac{\sum(x-\bar{x})^2}{n-1}$$

The variance can be used for data measured on at least an interval scale.

6.1.9   GRAPHS

6.1.9.1   Definition

The graph of a function f is the set of points $(x, f(x))$.

6.1.9.2   Drawing Graphs

A properly drawn graph should have the following properties:

1. Clearly labelled axes.
2. The independent variable is usually represented on the horizontal axis.
3. A clear heading/caption or reference in the accompanying text.
4. The units for both axes are clearly stated.
5. The scales for both axes are given; these may, for example, be
   a. Linear
   b. Logarithmic
   c. Broken (which can be represented by a break in the axis)

6.1.9.3   Linear Relationship

If the graph of variable y against variable x is a straight line, these variables are related by the equation

$$y = mx + c$$

in which m and c are constants:

- m is the gradient of the line.
- c is the intercept of the line on the vertical axis (y-axis).

6.1.9.4   Power Law Relationship

If the graph of y against x is a straight line, where

$$y = \log Y$$

$$x = \log X$$

(the logarithm is to any base, so long as it is the same one in both cases), then variables X and Y are related by the equation

$$Y = CX^m$$

in which m and C are constants such that

- m is the gradient of the line
- $\log C$ is the intercept of the line on the vertical axis (y-axis)

6.1.9.5   Exponential Relationship

If the graph of y against x is a straight line, where

$$y = \ln Y$$

$$x = X$$

($\ln Y$ is the logarithm of Y to base e, i.e. $\log_e Y$), then variables X and Y are related by the equation

$$Y = Ce^{mx}$$

in which m and C are constants such that

- m is the gradient of the line
- $\ln C$ is the intercept of the line on the vertical axis (y-axis)

This exponential relationship also holds if

- e is replaced by 10
- $\ln Y$ is replaced by $\log_{10} Y$
- $\ln C$ is replaced by $\log_{10} C$

6.1.9.6   Other Relationships Involving Expressions

If the graph of y against x is a straight line, where

$$y = g(Y)$$

$$x = f(X)$$

($f(X)$ is an expression involving X and $g(Y)$ is an expression involving Y), then variables X and Y are related by the equation

$$g(Y) = mf(X) + c$$

in which m and c are constants:

- m is the gradient of the line.
- c is the intercept of the line on the vertical axis (y-axis).

6.1.10   Outliers

Outliers are extreme values.

6.1.10.1   Measures of Central Tendency

Outliers can exert an extreme effect on the arithmetic mean, particularly when the total number of values is small. The median is less affected in such a case and may therefore be preferred.

6.1.10.2   Measures of Dispersion

Outliers exert an extreme effect on the range. Measures relating to quantiles are less affected in such a case and may therefore be preferred. Since it takes into account all the values in a distribution, the standard deviation (or variance) may be affected by outliers, although less so than the range.

6.1.10.3   Correlation and Linear Regression

Outliers may exert an extreme effect on the results of correlation and linear regression. In such cases, it may be necessary to consider excluding outliers from the calculations.

6.1.11   Stem-and-Leaf Plots

Stem-and-leaf plots can be used to represent a continuous variable. Their advantage over histograms is that they allow the representation of all the individual data. The stems consist of a vertical column of numbers on the left-hand side of the plot. The leaves are numbers to the right of the stems, which may, for example, represent tenths. All the individual data can then be derived by combining the individual leaves with their corresponding stems, while the shape of the overall plot indicates the shape of the distribution. They are particularly easy to represent in computer printouts. For instance, the distribution 13.5, 13.7, 14.5, 14.6, 14.6, 14.7, 15.2, 15.9, and 16.4 (arbitrary units) may be represented as the following stem-and-leaf plot:

13	5 7
14	5 6 6 7
15	2 9
16	4

6.1.12   Boxplots (Box-and-Whisker Plots)

Boxplots (box-and-whisker plots) can be used to represent a continuous variable. A boxplot consists of a box whose longer sides are placed vertically, with vertical lines (whiskers) extending vertically. Boxplots for two differently distributed samples are shown in Figure 6.2.

The boxplot has the following features:

- The upper boundary of the box is the upper (third) quartile.
- The lower boundary of the box is the lower (first) quartile.
- The length of the box is the interquartile range.
- A thick horizontal line inside the box is the median (second quartile).
- The lower whisker extends to the smallest observation, excluding outliers.
- The upper whisker extends to the largest observation, excluding outliers.
- Outliers are indicated by the symbol O.

The earlier arrangement is sometimes represented horizontally (the whole plot being rotated through $-\pi/2$) if more convenient. Boxplots can be useful for comparing two or more sets of observations diagrammatically, before or in addition to more formal statistical analyses.

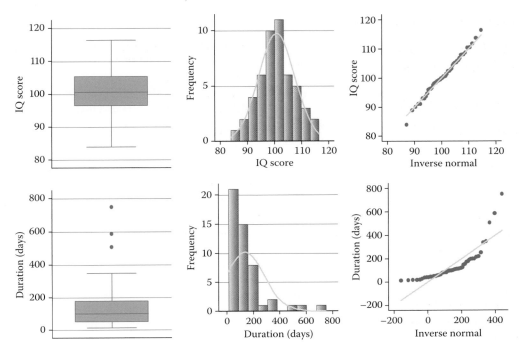

FIGURE 6.2 Boxplots for two differently distributed samples. (From Stahl, D. and Leese, M., Research methods and statistics, in Puri, B.K. and Treasaden, I.H. (eds.), *Psychiatry: An Evidence-Based Text*, Hodder Arnold, London, U.K., 2010, pp. 34–71.)

6.1.13 SCATTER PLOT (SCATTERGRAMS, SCATTER DIAGRAMS, OR DOT GRAPHS)

Scatter plots can be used to represent two continuous variables. Two orthogonal axes divide 2D space into a coordinate system, in which each pair of observations is plotted. The two variables can then be compared diagrammatically, before or in addition to more formal statistical analyses. Figure 6.3 shows a scatter plot for a dataset, with a superimposed linear regression line of best fit.

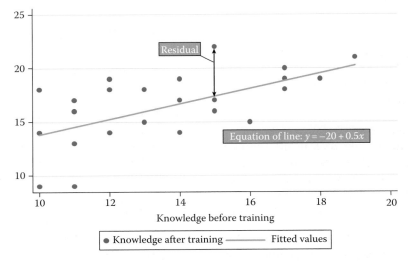

FIGURE 6.3 Scatter plot showing linear regression line. (From Stahl, D. and Leese, M., Research methods and statistics, in Puri, B.K. and Treasaden, I.H. (eds.), *Psychiatry: An Evidence-Based Text*, Hodder Arnold, London, U.K., 2010, pp. 34–71.)

6.2 PRINCIPLES OF MEASUREMENT

6.2.1 INTERVIEWS

Sources of error include the following:

- Response set—the tendency always to agree or to disagree with the questions asked.
- Bias towards the centre—the tendency always to avoid extreme responses. As a result, there is an excess choice of middle responses.
- Extreme responding—the opposite tendency of selecting extreme responses.
- Social desirability—the choice of responses that the subject believes the interviewer desires. May be reduced through the inclusion of lie scales or the forced-choice technique.
- Defensiveness—the subject avoids giving too much self-related information.
- Halo effect—the observer allows his or her pre-conception to influence the responses.
- Hawthorne effect—interviewer alters the situation by their presence.

6.2.2 SELF-PREDICTIONS

A direct method of measuring behaviour in which the subject is asked to give their own prediction concerning the behaviour under question. It can be combined with self-recording.

6.2.3 PSYCHOPHYSIOLOGICAL TECHNIQUES

These involve the direct use of physiological measurements in assessing behaviour.

6.2.4 NATURALISTIC OBSERVATIONS

These involve the assessment of behaviour as it occurs with minimum interference by the observer. In time-sampling techniques, the subject is observed during given time intervals at given times of the day or night.

Naturalistic observations are used in the functional analysis of problem behaviours. This method is sometimes referred as ABC (for antecedents, behaviours, and consequences).

6.2.5 SCALING

This refers to the conversion of raw data into types of scores more readily understood, for example, ranks, (per) centiles, and standardized scores.

6.2.6 NORM REFERENCING

A norm is an average, common, or standard performance under specified conditions. A test may be standardized to this norm.

6.2.7 CRITERION REFERENCING

A criterion is a set of scores against which the success of a predictive test can be compared.

6.3 INTELLIGENCE

6.3.1 APTITUDE

This is the raw or potential ability of an individual.

6.3.2 ATTAINMENT

This is the result of learning.

6.3.3 COMPONENTS OF INTELLIGENCE

Charles Spearman, who discovered factor analysis, put forward the notion that all individuals possess, to varying extents, general abilities; this general intelligence factor is known as g. The main determinant of intelligence test scores was held to be g by Spearman (1904).

A separate component of intelligence comprised specific abilities, known as s. Different intelligence subtests were held to index different s factors.

Overall, a person would be considered bright (high g factor) or not-so-bright (low g factor), but their actual overall intelligence would be comprised as follows:

$$\text{Intelligence} = g + (\text{Sum of the magnitudes of the various } s \text{ factors})$$

For example, arithmetic performance would be a function of g plus the individual's aptitude for arithmetic (specific s).

Louis Thurstone (1938) criticized Spearman's g and instead suggested that intelligence consisted of several primary abilities. On the basis of the factor analysis of a large database of intelligence test scores, he found the following seven primary abilities (Thurstone and Thurstone, 1963):

- Verbal comprehension
- Word fluency
- Number
- Space

- Memory
- Perceptual speed
- Reasoning

6.3.4 MENTAL AGE SCALE

The concept of the mental age (MA) was devised by Binet as the average intellectual ability, as measured by the level of problem-solving and reasoning. The scale was devised such that the average range of scores corresponds to the chronological age (CA).

For children with a higher than average level of intelligence, MA > CA. In contrast, for children with a lower than average level of intelligence, MA < CA.

The Stanford–Binet test can be applied to each year, up to the age of 15 years. Its reliability and validity are acceptable.

6.3.5 INTELLIGENCE QUOTIENT

This is the ratio of the MA to the CA, expressed as a percentage:

$$IQ = \left(\frac{MA}{CA}\right) \times 100$$

By convention, intelligence has a normal distribution with a mean of 100 and a standard deviation of 15.

There is a natural decline in intellectual ability with age. Performance IQ falls off with age more quickly than verbal IQ—the verbal–performance discrepancy. This decline is taken into account when raw scores are converted into IQ equivalents. Thus, although raw abilities decline with age, measured IQ remains constant.

6.3.6 WECHSLER ADULT INTELLIGENCE SCALE

The Wechsler Adult Intelligence Scale (WAIS)-IV was released in 2008 and allows the following four index scores to be derived:

- Verbal comprehension index (VCI)
- Perceptual reasoning index (PRI)
- Working memory index (WMI)
- Processing speed index (PSI)

The VCI is derived from the following four tests:

- Similarities (assesses abstract verbal reasoning)
- Vocabulary (the subject is asked to give the meaning of words)

- Information (particularly related to that derived from culture, such as being able to name the Prime Minister of the United Kingdom or the President of the United States of America)
- Comprehension (including questions evaluating the subject's ability to explain the meaning of conventions and proverbs)

The PRI is derived from the following five tests:

- Block design
- Matrix reasoning (solving nonverbal abstract problems)
- Visual puzzles
- Picture completion
- Figure weights

The WMI is derived from the following three tests:

- Digit span
- Arithmetic
- Letter–number sequencing

The PSI is derived from the following three tests:

- Symbol search
- Coding (tests visuomotor coordination)
- Cancellation

The general ability index (GAI) is derived from the VCI and PRI. The full scale IQ (FSIQ) is derived from the VCI, PRI, WMI, and PSI. The FSIQ follows a normal (Gaussian) distribution with a mean of 100 and a standard deviation of 15.

6.3.7 WECHSLER INTELLIGENCE SCALE FOR CHILDREN: REVISED

This is a modified version of the WAIS for children between the ages of 5 and 15 years.

6.3.8 WECHSLER PRESCHOOL AND PRIMARY SCALE OF INTELLIGENCE

This is a modified version of the WAIS for children between the ages of 4 and 6 years and 6 months.

6.3.9 GROUP ABILITY TESTS

Unlike the aforementioned, these can be used by one examiner to assess the intellectual ability and aptitude of a group of people, for example, the Armed Services Vocational Aptitude Battery (ASVAB).

6.3.10 NATURE–NURTURE

Potential intelligence (aptitude) is inherited, but environmental factors influence the fulfillment of potential (attainment).

6.3.11 CULTURAL INFLUENCES

Tests of attainment can give rise to discrepant results when applied to people from different cultures. It is thought that tests measuring aptitude are less prone to such influences.

6.4 TECHNIQUES USED IN NEUROPSYCHOLOGICAL ASSESSMENT

6.4.1 COMPREHENSIVE TEST BATTERIES

6.4.1.1 Halstead–Reitan Battery

This comprehensive test battery can detect damage to the brain and whether such damage is

- Lateralized—and, if so, to which hemisphere it is lateralized
- Associated with an acute or chronic disorder
- Focal or diffuse

The Halstead–Reitan Battery (HRB) is available in the following three age-related versions, for

- Adults (aged 15 years and older)
- Older children (aged between 9 and 14 years)
- Young children (aged between 5 and 8 years)

The core test procedures of the Halstead–Reitan Neuropsychological Test Battery include the following:

- *Aphasia Test*—naming common objects; spelling simple words; identifying individual numbers and letters; reading, writing, enunciating, and understanding spoken language; identifying body parts; calculating simple arithmetic problems; differentiating between right and left; and copying simple geometric shapes.
- *Category Test*—testing for learning, cognitive flexibility, and the ability to form abstract concepts.
- *Finger-Tapping Test*—the subject taps as many times as possible over 10 trial intervals.
- *Fingertip Number-Writing Perception Test*—a tactile perception test.

- *Lateral Dominance Examination*—a laterality examination.
- *(Seashore) Rhythm Test*—assesses the ability to discriminate nonverbal auditory stimuli.
- *Speech-Sounds Perception Test (SSPT)*—the subject is asked to match a spoken sound (from a recording) to the correct choice among similar printed sounds; tests for focused attention.
- *Tactile Form Recognition Test*—tests tactile perception and therefore parietal lobe functioning; the total time required to perform this test is a good screen for brain impairment.
- *Tactile Performance Test (TPT)*—involves tactile form discrimination, kinesthesis, upper limb movement coordination, manual dexterity, an appreciation of spatial configuration, and tactile memory.
- *Trail Making Test*—see succeeding text.

Data from the HRB, particularly from the Finger-Tapping Test and TPT, can help differentiate frontal from non-frontal involvement.

6.4.1.2 Luria–Nebraska Neuropsychological Battery

This test battery is designed for use in individuals aged 15 years and older. It may typically take between 1½ h and 2½ h to administer, depending on the subject's condition. The administration does not have to be in one sitting; it can be broken down into a series of short administrations. It is suitable for bedside use.

The Luria–Nebraska neuropsychological battery (LNNB) assesses a wide range of functions on

- Clinical scales
- Localization scales
- Optional scales
- Summary scales

The clinical scales assess

- Motor functions
- Rhythm
- Tactile functions
- Visual functions
- Receptive speech
- Expressive speech
- Writing
- Reading

- Arithmetic
- Memory
- Intellectual processes
- Intermediate memory (in the second of two forms of the LNNB)

The localization scales assess

- Left frontal functioning
- Left sensorimotor functioning
- Left parieto-occipital functioning
- Left temporal functioning
- Right frontal functioning
- Right sensorimotor functioning
- Right parieto-occipital functioning
- Right temporal functioning

The optional scales assess

- Spelling
- Motor writing

The summary scales are

- Pathognomonic—containing items best discriminating those with brain impairment from those without
- Left hemisphere
- Right hemisphere
- Profile elevation
- Impairment

Furthermore, 28 factor analysis-derived scales may reflect more specific cognitive and sensory functions.

6.4.1.3 Repeatable Battery for the Assessment of Neuropsychological Status

The repeatable battery for the assessment of neuropsychological status (RBANS) can be used to test the neuropsychological status of adults aged from 20 to 89 years. It takes approximately half an hour to administer. It gives scores on the following subtests:

- List learning
- Story memory
- Figure copy
- Line orientation
- Picture naming
- Semantic fluency
- Digit span
- Coding
- List recall

- List recognition
- Story recall
- Figure recall

These scores can be used to calculate a variety of indices.

6.4.2 LANGUAGE TESTS

6.4.2.1 Boston Diagnostic Aphasia Examination, 3rd Edition

The Boston Diagnostic Aphasia Examination, 3rd Edition (BDAE-3) is a test battery for the assessment of aphasic syndromes in adults (Goodglass et al., 2000). The short form takes around 35–45 min to administer. The long version contains 34 subtests and may take up to 4 h to administer. The BDAE-3 tests the following domains:

1. Auditory comprehension
   a. Word discrimination
   b. Body-part identification
   c. Complex ideational material
2. Oral expression
   a. Verbal and nonverbal agility
   b. Automatized sequences
   c. Recitation
   d. Repetition
   e. Word reading
   f. Responsive naming
   g. Animal naming
   h. Visual confrontation naming
   i. Oral sentence reading
3. Written language comprehension
   a. Symbolic and word discrimination
   b. Phonetic association
   c. Word–picture matching
   d. Reading sentences and paragraphs
4. Writing
   a. Writing mechanics
   b. Written symbol recall
   c. Written word finding
   d. Written formulation

6.4.2.2 Boston Naming Test

In the second edition of this language test, the subject is asked to name 60 line drawings (Goodglass and Kaplan, 2001). Adults are supposed to start at item number and progress towards item 60 unless a mistake is made in the first 8 items (from 30 to 37) in which case the test is proceeded with in the reverse order until the subject correctly responds to 8 consecutive items.

6.4.2.3   Graded Naming Test

In this language test, the subject is asked to name 30 line drawings (McKenna and Warrington, 1983).

6.4.2.4   Token Test

A number of tokens, such as differently coloured rectangles and circular discs, are used in this test. The subject is asked to carry out progressively more complicated verbal instructions using these tokens (De Renzi and Vignolo, 1962). The Token Test is sensitive to minor impairment in language comprehension, and performance tends to be more impaired in aphasia than in patients who are nonaphasic.

6.4.2.5   Speed and Capacity of Language Processing Test

The Speed and Capacity of Language Processing Test (Baddeley et al., 1992) consists of two parts. The first part is the Speed of Comprehension Test, in which the subject is asked to decide, as quickly as possible, whether each of a series of statements is true/sensible or false/not sensible (silly). The second part is the Spot-the-Word Test, in which 60 pairings of words with nonwords are presented and the subject must decide which of each pair, in turn, is a real word. The Spot-the-Word Test controls for poor verbal skills and has been found to give a robust estimate of verbal intelligence and therefore premorbid intelligence. (In this respect, it is rather like the NART.)

6.4.3   PERCEPTION TESTS

6.4.3.1   Bender–Gestalt Test/Bender Visual Motor Gestalt Test

The subject is asked to copy nine designs in this test (Bender, 1938, 1946).

6.4.3.2   Visual Object and Space Perception Battery

This battery tests visual perception (Warrington and James, 1991) and consists of the following nine tests:

- Screening test for visual impairment
- Incomplete letters
- Silhouettes
- Object decision
- Progressive silhouettes
- Dot counting
- Position discrimination
- Number location
- Cube analysis

The last four of these tests are concerned with spatial perception.

6.4.3.3   Behavioural Inattention Test

This battery tests for unilateral visual neglect (Wilson et al., 1987). The first six tests deal with visual neglect in the usual way:

- Line crossing
- Letter cancellation
- Star cancellation
- Figure copying and shape copying
- Line bisection
- Free drawing (clock, person, butterfly)

These are followed by nine behavioural tests:

- Picture scanning
- Telephone dialling
- Menu reading
- Article reading
- Clock face—telling the time and setting the time
- Coin sorting
- Address copying and sentence copying
- Map navigation
- Card sorting

These nine behavioural tests include tasks that are activities of daily living and so help in rehabilitation assessments.

6.4.4   MEMORY TESTS

6.4.4.1   Benton Visual Retention Test

In the fifth edition of this visual recall test, the subject is serially presented with 10 designs, which he or she has to reproduce from memory (Sivan, 1992). It may be used in subjects aged 8 years and over. Fifteen–twenty min may typically be required for administration, followed by another 5 min for scoring. It may be used to test for brain damage and early cognitive decline.

6.4.4.2   Graham–Kendall Memory for Designs Test

This is another visual recall test in which the subject is asked to draw from immediate recall designs that are presented for 5 s each (Graham and Kendall, 1960).

6.4.4.3   Rey–Osterrieth Test

In this visual memory test, the subject is presented with a complex design. The subject is asked to copy this design, and then, 40 min later, without previous notification that this will occur, the subject is asked to draw the same design again from memory (Rey, 1941; Osterrieth, 1944). Nondominant temporal lobe damage can lead to impaired performance on this test, whereas domain temporal lobe damage tends not to (but is associated with verbal memory difficulties).

6.4.4.4 Paired Associate Learning Tests

In these tests, the subject is given paired associates to learn and then must respond appropriately (e.g. by stating the paired word) when the first, stimulus, words are given. Different forms of these tests, of varying difficulty, have been produced (e.g. Inglis, 1959; Isaacs and Walkey, 1964). These tests may be used to assess memory disorder in old age, independently of verbal intelligence.

6.4.4.5 Synonym Learning Test

This is a modified version of the Walton–Black Modified Word Learning Test, specifically for use in the differential diagnosis of dementia from depression in the elderly (particularly if combined with the Digit Copying Test). In the Synonym Learning Test, 10 words with which the subject is not familiar are first identified and then the subject is asked to learn their meanings (Kendrick et al., 1965).

6.4.4.6 Object Learning Test

This test has similar aims to those of the Synonym Learning Test but is less stressful to take for elderly patients. As with the Synonym Learning Test, the results of the Object Learning Test combined with those of the Digit Copying Test can aid in the differential diagnosis of dementia from depression in the elderly. In the Object Learning Test, the subject is exposed to drawings of familiar items on sections of cards and asked to recall them (Kendrick et al., 1979).

6.4.4.7 Rey Auditory Verbal Learning Test

This is a word list learning test involving 5 presentations of a list containing 15 words, which the subject is asked to recall. The same then occurs with a second list of 15 words. Finally, the subject is asked to recall words from the first list, both immediately after completing the second recall task (involving the second list) and some time later (say, after 30 min). Information is obtained about immediate recall, learning curve, primacy and recency effects, and learning strategies used.

6.4.4.8 California Verbal Learning Test

This is a word list learning test involving 16 words from 4 known categories. As with the Rey Auditory Verbal Learning Test, the California Verbal Learning Test gives information about immediate recall, learning curve, and learning strategies used.

6.4.4.9 Wechsler Memory Scale-IV

The fourth edition of the Wechsler Memory Scale, WMS-IV, was released in 2009. It is a memory test battery that contains the following subtests:

- Spatial addition
- Symbol span
- Design memory
- General cognitive screener
  - Temporal orientation
  - Mental control
  - Clock drawing
  - Memory
  - Inhibitory control
  - Verbal productivity
- Logical memory
- Verbal paired associates
- Visual reproduction

6.4.4.10 Rivermead Behavioural Memory Test

This is another memory test battery (Wilson, 1987; Wilson et al., 1991). It lays emphasis on tests that are related to skills required in daily living. The subtests of the Rivermead Behavioural Memory Test include

- Orientation—for time, date, and place
- Name recall—of a forename and surname associated with a given photograph
- Picture recognition
- Face recognition
- Story recall—immediate recall and recall after a quarter of an hour
- Route memory
- Prospective memory

6.4.4.11 Adult Memory and Information Processing Battery

This is also a memory test battery (Coughlan and Hollows, 1985). It contains the following four memory subtests:

- Short story recall
- Figure copy and recall
- List learning
- Design learning

The Adult Memory and Information Processing Battery also contains the following two information-processing tests:

- Number cancellation
- Digit cancellation

The norms used in this battery are age stratified.

6.4.5 INTELLIGENCE TESTS

6.4.5.1 WAIS and Similar Tests

The intelligence tests based on the WAIS are considered earlier in Section 6.3.3.

6.4.5.2 National Adult Reading Test

The National Adult Reading Test or NART (Nelson and McKenna, 1975; Nelson, 1982) is a reading test consisting of phonetically irregular words that have to be read aloud by the subject. If a patient suffers deterioration in intellectual abilities, their premorbid vocabulary may remain less affected (or unaffected). The NART can therefore be used to estimate the premorbid IQ.

6.4.5.3 Raven's Progressive Matrices

This test of nonverbal intelligence consists of a series of printed designs from each of which a part is missing (Raven, 1958, 1982). The subject is required correctly to choose the missing part for each design from the alternatives offered. The test requires the perception of relations between abstract items.

6.4.6 EXECUTIVE FUNCTION (FRONTAL LOBE) TESTS

6.4.6.1 Stroop

There exist several types of Stroop test. A typical Stroop test involves asking a subject is given a card containing columns of colour names, printed in black on white, and asked to read aloud as many of the words as possible in 2 min. The words might be in columns, as follows:

Red	Green	Blue	Green
Blue	Tan	Red	Green
...	...	...	...

The correct answer to this part of the test, with the subject reading across rows, would be 'red, green, blue, green, blue, tan, red, green, …'. The score is the total number of words correctly named in the 2 min period. This part of the test checks that the patient is capable of following the directions and of reading such words (in the given print size) out aloud. In the second part of the test, a similar card of columns of words is presented to the subject and the same instructions of reading out what the words say are given. This time, however, the words are not in black but instead are printed in different colours. These colours are those described by some of the words but such that no given word is printed in its own colour. For example, green may be printed in blue the first time it occurs and then in red the second time. (In each case, the correct answer is 'green'.) Again, the score is the total number of words correctly named in the 2 min period. Finally, a card constructed in a similar way to that used for the second part of the test is again presented to the subject, and this time they are asked to name the *colour* in which each word is printed and to ignore the actual colour names printed. This is the Stroop interference test. For instance, if green is printed in blue the first time it occurs and then in red the second time, then the correct answers for these two occasions would be 'blue' and 'red' and *not* 'green' and 'green'.

This tests the (Stroop) interference that may occur between reading words and naming colours (Stroop, 1935; Trenerry et al., 1989; Lezak, 1995). Left (dominant) frontal lobe lesions are associated with poor performance on the Stroop test. The anterior cingulate cortex is particularly involved in carrying out this test (Pardo et al., 1990). However, activation of the anterior cingulate cortex does not invariably accompany the interference task. Another region of the brain that appears to be associated with this task is the left inferior precentral sulcus (at the border between the inferior frontal gyrus, the pars opercularis, and the ventral premotor area); this region appears to be involved with the mediation of competing articulatory demands during the interference condition of the Stroop test (Mead et al., 2002).

6.4.6.2 Verbal Fluency

A typical verbal fluency test involves asking the subject to articulate as many words as possible, during 2 min intervals, starting with the letters F, A, and S, in turn. Proper nouns (such as the name Forsythe) and derivatives such as plurals and different verb endings are not allowed to count together with the root words. For instance, one cannot count both 'font' and 'fonts' or 'float' and 'floated' and 'floating'. The score is the total number of allowable words achieved. Verbal fluency is impaired in left (dominant) frontal lobe lesions.

6.4.6.3 Tower of London Test

The Tower of London Test (Shallice, 1982) is based on the Tower of Hanoi game and test planning. The subject is asked to move coloured discs of varying sizes between three columns, either using a model or via a computer program (preferably with a touch screen), in order to achieve a given result. Left frontal lobe lesions are associated with poor performance on this test.

6.4.6.4 Wisconsin Card Sort Test

The Wisconsin Card Sort Test consists of a number of cards (64 in the original and 24 in the Modified Wisconsin Card

Sort Test) that contain different shapes (circles, crosses, stars, and triangles). Other variables include the number of shapes on a card and the colour of the shapes on a given card (there are four possible colours for each card). Following the presentation of index cards, the subject has to sort the remaining cards corresponding to the index cards. They are not given the variable(s) by means of which this sorting should occur but are told if they are right or wrong each time. For instance, the first indexing variable might be colour. After a certain number of consecutive correct responses, the rule suddenly changes, without the subject being warned in advance. These days, this test is more conveniently administered via a computer program, preferably using a touch screen. The Wisconsin Card Sort Test picks up perseverative errors (such as continuing for too long to sort cards by number, well after the indexing rule has changed to colour) and nonperseverative errors. Poor performance on this task is particularly associated with dysfunction of the left dorsolateral (pre-) frontal cortex.

6.4.6.5 Cognitive Estimates Test

In the absence of a reduction of intelligence quotient (IQ), some frontal lobe-damaged patients may give outrageously incorrect cognitive estimates of commonly known phenomena. For instance, asked to estimate the length of an adult elephant, such a patient might venture a reply of 100 yards. This abnormality is exploited in the Cognitive Estimates Test, in which the subject is asked to give a series of cognitive estimates, such as estimating the height of the average man.

6.4.6.6 Six Elements Test

This is a strategy application test that attempts to uncover evidence of the organizational difficulty that may occur as a result of frontal lobe damage. The subject is asked to carry out six different tasks (in two groups of three) during a quarter of an hour. In order to maximize their score, the subject needs adequately to plan and schedule these tasks while also monitoring the time that has elapsed.

6.4.6.7 Multiple Errands Task

This is another strategy application test that attempts to uncover evidence of the organizational difficulty that may occur as a result of frontal lobe damage. It is rather more difficult than the Six Elements Test. The subject is asked to carry out multiple errands, usually in a shopping centre that is not known to them.

6.4.6.8 Trail Making Test

There are two parts to this test (Trail A and Trail B). In the first part, a piece of paper is presented to the subject.

On the paper are a number (say, 25) of circles, each labelled with a different number (from 1 to 25, say). The subject is asked to draw a trail, as quickly as possible, that passes through all the circles, starting with the lowest numbered one (say, 1) and ending with the highest number (25, say). In the second part of the test (Trail B), both numbers and letters are contained in the circles, and this time the subject is asked to draw a trail, as quickly as possible, that passes through all the circles, starting with the lowest numbered one (say, one) and then passing to the circle with the lowest letter (A, say) and continuing to alternate between number and letter in increasing order, ending with the highest number and highest letter. So the two trails should be between circles labelled as follows:

Trail A: $1 \rightarrow 2 \rightarrow 3 \rightarrow 4 \rightarrow \ldots$
Trail B: $1 \rightarrow A \rightarrow 2 \rightarrow B \rightarrow 3 \rightarrow C \rightarrow \ldots$

The Trail Making Test tests the following abilities:

- Sequencing
- Cognitive flexibility
- Visual scanning
- Spatial analysis
- Motor control
- Alertness
- Concentration

Difficulties with cognitive flexibility or with complex conceptual tracking may manifest as much longer times being required for Trail B than would be expected from the Trail A time score.

6.4.7 Personality Tests

Personality inventories have been considered in Chapter 3. Here, psychometric methods of assessing personality are summarized.

6.4.7.1 Objective Tests

The items presented have limited responses. Objective tests include the following:

- 16PF (Sixteen Personality Factor Questionnaire) —see Chapter 3.
- MMPI (Minnesota Multiphasic Personality Inventory)—see Chapter 3.
- CPI (California Psychological Inventory)—see Chapter 3.
- EPQ (Eysenck Personality Questionnaire)—this contains 90 items in true/false format. Subjects are rated on the following dimensions: extraversion, introversion, and neuroticism

- HDHQ (Hostility and Direction of Hostility Questionnaire)—this is used to measure relationships that could be affected by personality status.

In general, because of evidence that mental state markedly affects scoring of questionnaires, they have been replaced by interview schedules and other observer ratings.

6.4.7.2 Projective Tests

The presented items have no one correct answer, instead taking the form of ambiguous stimuli, upon which the subject projects their personality. Their reliability and validity have not been established. Examples include the

- Rorschach Inkblot Test
- Thematic Apperception Test (TAT)
- Sentence Completion Test (SCT)

6.4.8 Dementia Tests and Related Tests

6.4.8.1 Mini-Mental State Examination

The Mini-Mental State Examination or MMSE (Folstein et al., 1975) is a brief test that can be routinely used rapidly to detect possible dementia, to estimate the severity of cognitive impairment, and to follow the course of cognitive changes over time. It can be used to differentiate between delirium and dementia (Anthony et al., 1982). The combination of cognitive testing and an informant questionnaire has not been found to result in any advantage over the use of the MMSE alone in screening for dementia (Knafelc et al., 2003). The MMSE includes the following assessments:

- Orientation
- Attention—serial subtraction or spelling a word (such as 'world' backward)
- Immediate recall
- Short-term memory
- Naming common objects
- Following simple verbal commands
- Following simple written commands
- Writing a sentence spontaneously
- Copying a figure

The total score that may be achieved is 30. Age and MMSE scores appear to be inversely related, from a median of 29 for Americans aged between 18 and 24 years to a median of 25 in those aged over 80 years. A total MMSE score of less than 24 tends to be considered as indicating cognitive impairment, in the absence of any other cause for such a low score (such as no more than 4 years of schooling or learning disability).

6.4.8.2 Cambridge Neuropsychological Test Automated Battery

The Cambridge Neuropsychological Test Automated Battery or CANTAB is an automated computerized battery that offers sensitive and specific cognitive assessment, preferably using a touch screen. The standard CANTAB consists of the following 13 computerized tasks:

- Motor screening—this screening task is administered before the other tasks and introduces the subject to the touch screen and checks that the subject can touch this properly and that he or she can hear, comprehend, and follow instructions appropriately.
- Big/little circle—this tests that a subject can follow an explicit instructional rule and that he or she can then reverse this rule.
- Delayed matching to sample.
- ID/ED shift—this tests the ability to attend to specific attributes of compound stimuli and then to shift that attention as required.
- Matching to sample visual search—this is a speed/accuracy trade-off visual search task.
- Paired associates learning—this delayed response procedure tests list memory and then list learning (or visuospatial conditional learning).
- Pattern recognition memory.
- Rapid visual information processing—this tests vigilance (sustained attention) and working memory.
- Reaction time.
- Spatial recognition memory.
- Spatial span—this tests spatial memory span.
- Spatial working memory—this tests both spatial working memory and strategy performance.
- Stockings of Cambridge—this has replaced the Tower of London test in earlier versions of CANTAB and is somewhat similar to the Tower of London test described earlier.

6.4.8.3 Gresham Ward Questionnaire

In the Gresham Ward Questionnaire (Post, 1965), questions are asked that cover the following abilities:

- Orientation in time
- Orientation in place
- Memory for past personal events
- Memory for recent personal events
- General information
- Topographical orientation

6.4.8.4 Blessed's Dementia Scale

This questionnaire (Blessed et al., 1968) is administered to a relative or friend of the subject who is asked to answer the questions on the basis of performance over the previous 6 months. There are three sets of questions. The first set deals with activities of daily living such as

- Ability to cope with small sums of money
- Ability to remember a short list of items such as a shopping list
- Ability to find their way indoors
- Ability to find their way around familiar streets
- Ability to grasp situations or explanations
- Ability to recall recent events
- Tendency to dwell in the past

The second set of questions deals with further activities of daily living including

- Ability to feed oneself
- Ability to dress oneself
- Level of incontinence, if any

The third set of questions is concerned with changes in

- Personality
- Interest
- Drive

6.4.8.5 Information–Memory–Concentration Test

This is a relatively straightforward set of questions that may be tried even by those with medium to severe levels of dementia.

6.4.8.6 Geriatric Mental State Schedule

The Geriatric Mental State Schedule or GMS is a semistructured interview that assesses the subject's mental state.

6.4.8.7 Cambridge Examination for Mental Disorders

The Cambridge Examination for Mental Disorders of the Elderly or CAMDEX is an interview schedule consisting of three sections (Roth et al., 1986, 1988):

- A structured clinical interview with the patient to obtain systematic information about the present state, past history, and family history.
- A range of objective cognitive tests that constitute a mini-neuropsychological battery, known as the CAMCOG (Cambridge Cognitive Examination).
- A structured interview with a relative or other informant to obtain independent information about the respondent's present state, past history, and family history.

The assessment also includes a brief physical and neurological examination and recording the results of investigations.

6.4.8.8 Crichton Geriatric Behaviour Rating Scale

This is a retrospective nursing-rated assessment.

6.4.8.9 Clifton Assessment Schedule

This is also a nursing-rated assessment.

6.4.8.10 Stockton Geriatric Rating Scale

This is also a nursing-rated assessment.

6.4.8.11 Present Behavioural Examination

The Present Behavioural Examination or PBE involves interviewing carers and rates psychopathological and behavioural changes in dementia.

6.4.8.12 Manchester and Oxford Universities Scale for the Psychopathological Assessment of Dementia

The Manchester and Oxford Universities Scale for the Psychopathological Assessment of Dementia or MOUSEPAD also involves interviewing carers and rates psychopathological and behavioural changes in dementia.

6.4.8.13 Sandoz Clinical Assessment

The Sandoz Clinical Assessment—Geriatric or SCAG consists of 18 symptom areas and an overall global assessment, each being rated on a seven-point scale (from zero, not present, to seven, severe) (Shader et al., 1974):

- Mood depression
- Confusion
- Mental alertness
- Motivation initiative
- Irritability
- Hostility
- Bothersome
- Indifference to surroundings
- Unsociability
- Uncooperativeness
- Emotional liability
- Fatigue
- Self-care
- Appetite
- Dizziness
- Anxiety
- Impairment of recent memory
- Disorientation
- Overall impression of the patient

6.4.8.14   Vineland Social Maturity Scale

The Vineland Social Maturity Scale consists of 117 items that assess different aspects of social maturity and social ability. Although it can be used for the assessment of dementia, the Vineland Social Maturity Scale is primarily designed to be used in the assessment of childhood development and learning disability.

6.4.8.15   Performance Test of Activities of Daily Living

The Performance Test of Activities of Daily Living or PADL is a simple performance test that assesses the self-care capacity of the subject by asking him or her to carry out certain essential activities of daily living.

REFERENCES

Anthony JC, Le Resche L, Niaz U, Von Korf MR, and Folstein MF. 1982: Limits of the 'Mini-Mental State' as a screening test for dementia and delirium among hospital patients. *Psychological Medicine* 12:397–408.

Baddeley A, Emslie H, and Nimmo-Smith I. 1992: *The Speed and Capacity of Language Processing Test.* Bury St Edmunds, U.K.: Thames Valley Test Company.

Bender L. 1938: *A Visual Motor Gestalt Test and its Clinical Uses.* New York: American Orthopsychiatric Association.

Bender L. 1946: *Instructions for the Use of Visual Motor Gestalt Test.* New York: American Orthopsychiatric Association.

Blessed G, Tomlinson BE, and Roth M. 1968: The association between quantitative measures of dementia and of senile change in the cerebral grey matter of elderly subjects. *British Journal of Psychiatry* 114:797–811.

Coughlan AK and Hollows SE. 1985: *The Adult Memory and Information Processing Battery.* Leeds, U.K.: A.K. Coughlan, Psychology Department, St James University Hospital.

De Renzi E and Vignolo LA. 1962: The token test: A sensitive test to detect receptive disturbances in aphasics. *Brain* 85:665–678.

Folstein MF, Folstein SE, and McHugh PR. 1975: 'Mini-mental state'. A practical method for grading the cognitive state of patients for the clinician. *Journal of Psychiatric Research* 12:189–198.

Goodglass H and Kaplan E. 2001: *Boston Naming Test.* Philadelphia, PA: Lippincott Williams & Wilkins.

Goodglass H, Kaplan E, and Barresi B. 2000: *The Boston Diagnostic Aphasia Examination, 3rd edn. (BDAE-3).* Philadelphia, PA: Lippincott Williams & Wilkins.

Graham FK and Kendall BS. 1960: Memory-for-designs test: Revised general manual. *Perceptual and Motor Skills* 11:147–188.

Inglis J. 1959: A paired-associate learning test for use with elderly psychiatric patients. *Journal of Mental Science* 105:440–443.

Isaacs B and Walkey FA. 1964: A simplified paired-associate test for elderly hospital patients. *British Journal of Psychiatry* 110:80–83.

Kendrick DC, Gibson AJ, and Moyes ICA. 1979: The revised Kendrick battery: Clinical studies. *British Journal of Social and Clinical Psychology* 18:329–340.

Kendrick DC, Parboosingh R-C, and Post F. 1965: A synonym learning test for use with elderly psychiatric subjects: a validation study. *British Journal of Social and Clinical Psychology* 4:63–71.

Knafelc R, Lo Giudice D, Harrigan S, Cook R, Flicker L, Mackinnon A, and Ames D. 2003: The combination of cognitive testing and an informant questionnaire in screening for dementia. *Age and Ageing* 32:541–547.

Lezak MD. 1995: *Neuropsychological Assessment,* 3rd edn. New York: Oxford University Press.

McKenna P and Warrington EK. 1983: *Graded Naming Test.* Windsor, U.K.: NFER-Nelson.

Mead LA, Mayer AR, Bobholz JA, Woodley SJ, Cunningham JM, Hammeke TA, and Rao SM. 2002: Neural basis of the Stroop interference task: Response competition or selective attention? *Journal of the International Neuropsychological Society* 8:735–742.

Nelson HE. 1982: *The National Adult Reading Test Manual.* Windsor, U.K.: NFER-Nelson.

Nelson HE and McKenna P. 1975: The use of current reading ability in the assessment of dementia. *British Journal of Social and Clinical Psychology* 14:259–267.

Osterrieth P-A. 1944: Le test depression copie d'une figure complexe. Contribution à l'étude de la perception et de la mémoire. *Archives de Psychologie* 30:206–353.

Pardo JV, Pardo PJ, Janer KW, and Raichle ME. 1990: The anterior cingulate cortex mediates processing selection in the Stroop attention of conflict paradigm. *The Proceedings of the National Academy of Sciences of the United States of America* 87:256–259.

Post F. 1965: *The Clinical Psychiatry of Late Life.* Oxford, U.K.: Pergamon Press.

Raven JC. 1958: *Guide to Using the Mill Hill Vocabulary Scale and the Progressive Matrices Scales.* London, U.K.: H.K. Lewis.

Raven JC. 1982: *Revised Manual for Raven's Progressive Matrices and Vocabulary Scale.* Windsor, U.K.: NFER-Nelson.

Rey A. 1941: L'examen psychologique dans les cas d'encéphalopathie traumatique. *Archives de Pathologie* 28:286–340.

Roth M, Huppert FA, Tym E, and Mountjoy CQ. 1988: *CAMDEX. The Cambridge Examination for Mental Disorders of the Elderly.* Cambridge, U.K.: Cambridge University Press.

Roth M, Tym E, Mountjoy CQ, Huppert FA, Hendrie H, Verma S, and Goddard R. 1986: CAMDEX. A standardised instrument for the diagnosis of mental disorder in the elderly with special reference to the early detection of dementia. *British Journal of Psychiatry* 149:698–709.

Shader RI, Harmatz JS, and Salzman C. 1974: A new scale for clinical assessment in geriatric populations: Sandoz Clinical Assessment—Geriatric (SCAG). *Journal of the American Geriatrics Society* 22:107–113.

Shallice T. 1982: Specific impairments of planning. In Broadbent DE and Weiskrantz L (eds). *The Neuropsychology of Cognitive Function*. London, U.K.: The Royal Society.

Sivan AB. 1992: *Benton Visual Retention Test,* 5th edn. San Antonio, TX: Psychological Corporation.

Spearman C. 1904: General intelligence, objectively determined and measured. *The American Journal of Psychology*, 15(2):201–292.

Stahl D and Leese M. 2010: Research methods and statistics. In Puri BK and Treasaden IH (eds.) *Psychiatry: An Evidence-Based Text*, pp. 34–71. London, U.K.: Hodder Arnold.

Stroop JR. 1935: Studies of interference in serial verbal reactions. *Journal of Experimental Psychology* 18:643–662.

Thurstone LL. 1938: Primary mental abilities. *Psychometric Monographs* No. 1. Chicago, IL: University of Chicago Press.

Thurstone LL and Thurstone TG. 1963: *SRA Primary Abilities*. Chicago, IL: Science Research Associates.

Trenerry MR, Crossan B, Deboe J, and Leber WR. 1989: *Stroop Neuropsychological Screening Test Manual*. Lutz, FL: Psychological Assessment Resources Inc.

Warrington EK and James M. 1991: *The Visual Object and Space Perception Battery*. Bury St Edmunds, U.K.: Thames Valley Test Company.

Wilson BA. 1987: *Rehabilitation of Memory*. New York: Guildford Press.

Wilson BA, Cockburn J, and Baddeley A. 1991: *The Rivermead Behavioural Memory Test*, 2nd edn. Bury St Edmunds, U.K.: Thames Valley Test Company.

Wilson BA, Cockburn J, and Halligan P. 1987 *Behavioural Inattention Test*. Fareham, U.K.: Thames Valley Test Company.

7 Cognitive Assessment and Neuropsychological Processes

7.1 MEMORY

7.1.1 SENSORY MEMORY

The anatomical correlate of iconic memory is probably visual association cortex, while that of echoic memory is probably auditory association cortex.

7.1.1.1 Short-Term Memory

The anatomical correlate of auditory verbal short-term memory is the left (dominant) parietal lobe, while that of visual verbal short-term memory is possibly the left temporo-occipital area. That of nonverbal short-term memory is possibly the right (nondominant) temporal lobe.

7.1.1.2 Explicit Memory

This requires a deliberate act of recollection and can be reported verbally. It includes declarative memory and episodic memory, which are probably stored separately, since it is possible to lose one type of memory while retaining the other. Declarative memory involves knowledge of facts, whereas episodic memory involves memory of autobiographical events. Explicit memory involves the medial temporal lobes, particularly the hippocampus, entorhinal cortex, subiculum, and parahippocampal cortex. Damage to these structures results in an inability to store new memory; they have been termed bottleneck structures. Memory probably passes from medial temporal lobe structures after a few weeks/months to longer-term storage in the cortex.

The amygdala may be involved in the emotional charging of information. It may also be a bottleneck structure.

7.1.1.3 Implicit Memory

This is recalled automatically without effort and is learned slowly through repetition. It is not readily amenable to verbal reporting. It comprises procedural knowledge, that is, knowing how. Its storage requires functioning of the cerebellum, amygdala, and specific sensory and motor systems used in the learned task. For example, the basal ganglia are involved in learning motor skills. Classical and operant learnings involve implicit memory.

7.2 AMNESIA

Amnesia is defined as the inability to recall past experience or the loss of memory (Table 7.1).

7.3 LANGUAGE

7.3.1 CEREBRAL DOMINANCE

Cerebral dominance for language is as follows:

- In 99% of right-handers, the left cerebral hemisphere is dominant.
- In 60% of left-handers, the left cerebral hemisphere is dominant.

In early life, there is plasticity for cerebral dominance for language before the functions are established.

7.3.1.1 Speech and Language Areas

7.3.1.1.1 Broca's Area

This is the motor speech area, occupying the opercular and triangular zones of the inferior frontal gyrus (BA 44 and 45). It is involved in coordinating the organs of speech to produce coherent sounds. In lesions confined to this area in the dominant hemisphere, speech comprehension is intact and muscles involved in speech production work normally, but production of speech is affected.

7.3.1.1.2 Wernicke's Area

This is the sensory speech and language area, occupying the posterior part of the auditory association cortex (BA 42 and 22) of the superior temporal gyrus. It is usually larger in the left hemisphere. It is involved in making sense of speech and language.

7.3.1.1.3 Angular Gyrus

This part of the brain (BA 39) has abundant connections with the somatosensory, visual, and auditory association cortices. Lesions here produce inability to read or write.

TABLE 7.1
Summary of Various Types of Amnesia

Anterograde amnesia	Anterograde amnesia refers to inability to form new memories, either because of failure to consolidate what is perceived into permanent memory storage or because of inability to retrieve memory from the storage
Retrograde amnesia	Retrograde amnesia refers to loss of memory for events that occurred prior to an event or condition (e.g. intoxication or head injury). Such event is presumed to have caused the memory disturbance in the first place. Retrograde memory related to public events is more likely to be subjected to a greater memory loss than personal events
	In head injury, retrograde amnesia is sometimes referred as pre-traumatic amnesia, which is composed of events the person remembers up to the immediate time of an accident. The pre-traumatic amnesia usually lasts less than 1 week. Retrograde amnesia tends to improve with more distant events in the past
	Depressed patients with preexisting cognitive impairment are more likely to develop post-ECT retrograde amnesia.
Post-traumatic amnesia	Post-traumatic amnesia is defined as the memory loss from the time of accident to the time that the patient can give a clear account of the recent events. In general, the retrograde amnesia is shorter than post-traumatic amnesia. Post-traumatic amnesia, once present, tends to remain unchanged. Post-traumatic amnesia is confounded by sedatives given after admission and prolonged sleep. Post-traumatic amnesia does not necessarily correlate with the duration of consciousness loss
Psychogenic amnesia	Psychogenic amnesia is part of the dissociative disorder consisting of a sudden inability to recall important personal data. The amnesia may be localized (for several hours) or generalized (for entire life is lost). The amnesia may be selective (involving certain memories) or continuous (loss of all memories subsequent to a specific time). The clinical presentation is usually atypical and cannot be explained by ordinary forgetfulness (e.g. loss of biographical memory in dissociative fugue). Psychogenic amnesia is associated with 'la belle indifference' (lack of concerns) and has a highly unpredictable course
	Differential diagnosis includes situational amnesia, PTSD, Ganser's syndrome (vorbeireden or approximate answers), dissociative fugue, pseudodementia (associated with sudden onset and depressive disorder), and multiple personality disorder
False memory	False memory involves confabulation, report of false events (e.g. childhood sexual abuse), and false confessions
	The false-memory syndrome is a condition in which a person's identity and interpersonal relationships are centred around a memory of a traumatic experience, which is objectively false, but the person strongly believes that such experience did take place. False confessions may not have a psychiatric cause because the person falsely confesses to enhance publicity and to conceal evidence in criminal offence
	Differential diagnosis includes organic amnesias and frontal lobe syndrome
Transient global amnesia	The person presents with abrupt onset of disorientation, loss of ability to encode recent memories, and retrograde amnesia for variable durations. The patient has a remarkable degree of alertness and responsiveness. This episode usually lasts for a few hours and is never repeated. The pathophysiology is a result of transient ischaemia of the hippocampus–fornix–hypothalamic system. Functional neuroimaging may show transient reduction in metabolic and functional activities in the mesial temporal lobes
	For example, a 59-year-old man came to the emergency department at 9 pm and complains of memory loss for a few hours. He claims that he cannot remember what he did in the afternoon
Amnestic syndrome	Amnestic syndrome is closely related to Wernicke–Korsakoff syndrome. The person has impairment of short-term memory (i.e. unable to recall items 30 min after presentation), but immediate memory (immediate three items recall) is intact. Hence, anterograde amnesia is more prominent because memories cannot be consolidated and stored. Confabulation may occur
Amnesia involving episodic memory	Episodic memory is time and context specific. In contrast, semantic memory that involves vocabulary and facts is not time or context specific. The neuroanatomical areas involved in episodic memory and semantic memory are the limbic system and temporal neocortex, respectively. Semantic memory is assessed by the National Adult Reading Test
	Acute causes of episodic memory impairment include transient global amnesia, temporal lobe epilepsy, closed head injury, drugs (benzodiazepine and alcohol), and psychogenic fugues
	Causes of chronic episodic memory impairment include hippocampal and diencephalic damages. Hippocampal damage is caused by *herpes simplex virus* (*HSV*) encephalitis, anoxia, surgical removal of temporal lobes, bilateral posterior cerebral artery occlusion, closed head injury, and early Alzheimer's disease. The causes of diencephalic damage include Korsakoff's syndrome, third ventricle tumours and cysts, bilateral thalamic infarction, and post-subarachnoid haemorrhage

7.3.1.2　Pathways

- Understanding spoken language (hearing): spoken word → auditory cortex → auditory association cortex → Wernicke's area → hear and comprehend speech
- Understanding written language (reading): written word → visual cortex → visual association cortex → angular gyrus → Wernicke's area → read and comprehend
- Speaking: thought/cognition → Wernicke's area → Broca's area → motor speech areas → speech
- Writing: thought/cognition → Wernicke's area → angular gyrus → motor areas → write

7.3.2　DYSPHASIAS

Dysphasia, paraphasia, or aphasia refers to any disturbance in the comprehension and expression of speech as a result of brain lesions. For example, a person says, 'murder of two companies' instead of 'merger of two companies'.

Aetiology: middle cerebral artery (MCA) infarct/haemorrhage, tumour, abscess, other space occupying lesions, Alzheimer's disease, and Pick's disease.

Pathophysiology: Damage to brain areas involved with speech and language results in dysphasia; the type of dysphasia is determined by the areas of the brain involved.

7.3.2.1　Receptive Dysphasia

Damage to Wernicke's area disrupts the ability to comprehend language, either written or spoken. In addition to loss of comprehension, the person also is unaware that his or her dysphasic speech is difficult for others to follow. Speech is normal in rhythm and intonation (because Broca's area is intact), but the content is abnormal. Words used have lost their meaning; empty words (e.g. 'thing', 'it') and paraphrasias are used liberally. Thus, damage to Wernicke's area results in a fluent receptive dysphasia.

7.3.2.2　Expressive Dysphasia

Damage to Broca's area results in loss of rhythm, intonation, and grammatical aspects of speech. Comprehension is normal (because Wernicke's area is intact) and the person is aware that his or her speech is difficult for others to follow, resulting in distress and frustration. Speech is slow and hesitant, often lacking connecting words. Speech sounds agrammatical and articulation may be crude, probably because of the close proximity of Broca's area to motor areas. Thus, damage to Broca's area results in dysfluent expressive dysphasia.

7.3.2.3　Conduction Dysphasia

Damage to the arcuate fasciculus results in a conduction dysphasia in which the person cannot repeat what is said by another. Comprehension and verbal fluency remain intact.

7.3.2.4　Global Dysphasia

This results from global left hemispheric dysfunction and shows a combination of all the aforementioned (Table 1.2).

7.3.3　MUTISM

Mutism refers to a statue of silence or voicelessness.

Aetiology: MCA infarct/haemorrhage, Broca's aphasia, bulbar palsy (lower motor neuron lesions), pseudobulbar palsy (upper motor neuron lesions), catatonic schizophrenia, severe depression, and elective mutism

7.4　PERCEPTION

Perception relates to the means by which the brain makes representations of the external environment.

Agnosia is the inability to interpret and recognize the significance of sensory information, which does not result from impairment of the sensory pathways, mental deterioration, disorders of consciousness and attention, or, in the case of an object, a lack of familiarity with the object.

7.4.1　VISUAL PERCEPTION

- Shape, colour, and spatial orientation are recognized in the occipital lobes. A lesion at this level results in pseudoagnosia.
- Visuospatial elements are drawn together into complete percepts (objects seen as a whole) in the right parietal lobe. Meaning is not yet attributed to the objects. A lesion at this level results in apperceptive agnosia. A person with apperceptive agnosia is unable to copy shapes or discriminate two versions of the same object. The person cannot name the object when he or she sees it but is able to name it when he or she touches it. The person has preserved elementary visual abilities (e.g. acuity or brightness discrimination). The lesion is found in the bilateral posterior occipitoparietal regions. Apperceptive agnosia is caused by carbon monoxide or mercury poisoning, bilateral posterior watershed strokes, and penetrating head injury (Figure 7.1).

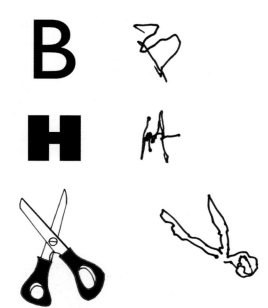

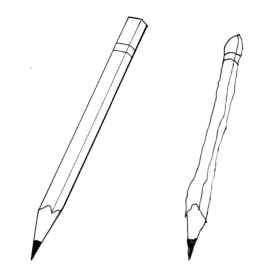

FIGURE 7.2   Associative visual agnosia.

FIGURE 7.1   Apperceptive visual agnosia.

- The meaning of objects is then accessed from the left parietal lobe (which itself accesses meaning from semantic memory) and processed in parieto-occipital areas. A lesion at this level results in associative agnosia. A person with associative agnosia is unable to recognize visually presented objects. In contrast to apperceptive agnosia, the person has a high level of perceptual processing. Preservation of the high-level perceptual processing is demonstrated by the normal copying of objects that the person cannot recognize (e.g. fountain pen in this case). The person has preserved ability to match pairs of similar stimuli. Furthermore, patients with apperceptive agnosia are unable to identify objects by any modality (e.g. touching). Aetiology includes moderate Alzheimer's disease, Pick's disease, and HSV encephalitis (Figure 7.2).

7.4.1.1 Other Agnosias
- Prosopagnosia is an inability to recognize faces. In advanced Alzheimer's disease, a person may misidentify his or her own mirrored reflection—the mirror sign (autoprosopagnosia). Prosopagnosia is associated with bilateral inferior occipitotemporal lesions.
- Achromatopsia is an acquired disorder characterized by a loss of ability to discriminate between colours. On the other hand, people with colour agnosia are able to perceive and distinguish

between colours but are impaired on tasks requiring the retrieval of colour information (e.g. 'What colour is an apple?'). Colour anomia (e.g. showing the red colour but unable to name the colour) is associated with alexia and right hemianopia as a result of disconnection between the left hemisphere language centre and visual information.
- In simultanagnosia, the person is unable to recognize the overall meaning of a picture, whereas its individual details are understood. Simultanagnosia is associated with lesion in the anterior part of occipital lobe or children suffering from generalized brain dysfunction.
- Agraphognosia or agraphesthesia is tested by asking the person to identify, with closed eyes, numbers or letters traced on his or her palm; this disorder is present if the person is unable to identify such writing.
- In anosognosia, there is a lack of awareness of disease, particularly of hemiplegia (most often following a right parietal lesion).
- Autotopagnosia is the inability to name, recognize, or point on command to parts of the body.
- In astereognosia, objects cannot be recognized by palpation.
- In finger agnosia, the person is unable to recognize individual fingers.
- Topographical disorientation can be tested using a locomotor map-reading task in which the person is asked to trace out a given route by foot.

- In hemisomatognosis or hemidepersonalization, the person feels that a limb (which in fact is present) is missing.

7.4.1.1.1 Anomia (Nominal Aphasia)

Anomia is a type of aphasia characterized by problems recalling words or names. The person may use circumlocutions (speaking in a roundabout way, e.g. the thing that tells time) in order to express a certain word for which they cannot remember the name (e.g. clock in this case). Sometimes, the person can recall the name when clues are given. Anomia may lead to frustration.

Aetiology: Anomia is caused by damage to the parietal lobe or the temporal lobe.

7.4.1.1.2 Dysnomia

Dysnomia refers to the marked difficulty in remembering names or recalling a word needed for oral or written language. It is often a 'tip-of-the-tongue' phenomenon.

7.4.1.1.3 Dysnomic Dysphasia

Dysnomic dysphasia refers to the profound word finding difficulties.

7.5 DYSLEXIA AND DYSGRAPHIA

7.5.1 DYSLEXIA

Dyslexia refers to pure word blindness. In developmental dyslexia, a young child initially manifests difficulty in learning to read. Later, the child exhibits erratic spelling and lack of capacity to manipulate written language. People with developmental dyslexia have symmetrical planum temporale (leftward asymmetry in people without dyslexia). Verbal language skills seem to be intact. In general, the affected persons have problems with perception of the shapes of words. 50% of people with dyslexia also have achromatopsia (colour blindness).

Types of dyslexia are as follows:

1. *Central dyslexia*: Linguistically based and spelling is affected:
   a. Surface dyslexia is caused by lesions in left temporoparietal region. The person breaks down the whole word (lexical reading) and has difficulty to deal with irregularly spelt words.
   b. Deep dyslexia is caused by extensive left hemisphere lesions. There is a loss of sound-based (phonological) reading. The person has difficulty to deal with abstract words.

2. *Peripheral dyslexia*: Oral and written spelling is preserved:
   a. Alexia without agraphia.
   b. Neglect dyslexia: Errors in reading the initial part of words. It is caused by a right parietal lobe lesion affecting the left half of words. Left hemisphere lesions affecting the right half of words are rare.

7.5.2 DYSGRAPHIA

Dysgraphia refers to impaired writing ability.

Types of dysgraphia are as follows:

1. *Central dysgraphia*: Written and oral spelling is affected:
   a. Lexical dysgraphia is caused by lesions in the left temporoparietal region. The person breaks down the word's spelling and has difficulty in writing irregular words.
   b. Deep dysgraphia is caused by extensive left hemisphere lesions and a breakdown of the sound-based route for spelling. The person cannot spell nonexistent words.

2. Neglect dysgraphia is caused by right hemispheric lesions and leads to misspelling of the initial part of words.

3. Dyspraxic dysgraphia is caused by dominant frontal or parietal lobe lesions. This leads to defective copying although the person can spell correctly (Table 7.2).

7.6 ALEXIA AND AGRAPHIA

Alexia refers to reading disorder that affects learning and academic skills. Agraphia refers to writing impairment.

7.6.1 ALEXIA WITHOUT AGRAPHIA

1. *Clinical example*: A 58-year-old man suffered from acute stroke. At first, he developed acute impairment in comprehending written materials including his own works although he could write. When the words were spelt out loud by his wife, he recognized the word immediately. After 3 months, he develops a new technique to help himself recognize words. He reads letter by letter and spells the word out loud. Then he recognizes the word after hearing himself spell it out.

TABLE 7.2
Examples of Dysphasia, Dyslexia, and Dysgraphia

Examples	Diagnosis
Orange is named as apple.	Semantic paraphasia occurs when there is an error in using the target word because of deficits in semantic memory. It is associated with left temporal lobe tumours
Big is read as dig.	Surface dyslexia occurs when reliance is placed on sub-word correspondence between letters and sounds but not the normal way, which is spelling to sound
Bicycle is read as cycle.	Neglect dyslexia occurs when the left half of the word is being ignored as a result of the right parietal lobe lesion
Sister is read as auntie.	Deep dyslexia occurs when the person produces verbal response based on the meaning of the word but not based on sound-based reading
'A' is written as 'Ɐ'.	Dyspraxic dysgraphia has the following manifestations: disturbance in writing the smooth part of a letter, letter may be inverted or reversed, abnormal letter, and illegible handwriting. Oral spelling is preserved
'Cough' is written as 'coff'.	Lexical dysgraphia: The person has difficulty to write irregular words 'cough' in this case and produces an error that is phonologically similar

2. *Neuroanatomical areas involved*: The occlusion of left posterior cerebral artery leads to infarction of the medial aspect of the left occipital lobe and the splenium of the corpus callosum.

3. *Pathophysiology*: The explanation for the clinical presentation is as follows: After the stroke, the patient starts off with right hemianopia and he cannot read in the right visual field. Then, the words have to be seen on the left side, which are projected onto the right hemisphere. There is a lesion in the splenium that prevents the transfer of visual information from the right to the left side. The primary language area is disconnected from incoming visual information. As a result, he cannot comprehend any written material although he can write. As time goes by, he develops a strategy of identifying the individual letters in the right hemisphere. Saying each letter aloud enables him to access the pronunciation of word in the left hemisphere.

4. *Comorbidity*: Defects in colour naming (although with intact colour vision) or actual impairment of colour perception (achromatopsia) may occur.

7.6.2 ALEXIA WITH AGRAPHIA

1. *Clinical features*: The person cannot read, write, or connect letters.
2. *Neuroanatomical area involved*: Lesions of the angular or supramarginal gyrus.

7.7 APRAXIAS

Apraxia is an inability to perform purposive volitional acts, which does not result from paresis, incoordination, sensory loss, or involuntary movements (Table 7.3).

Dressing apraxia: A person is unable to wear clothes properly, for example, putting on a jacket upside down. Dressing apraxia is associated with nondominant parietal lobe lesions (Figure 7.3).

7.7.1 ACALCULIA AND ANARITHMETRIA

Acalculia refers to a disturbance in the ability to comprehend or write numbers properly. This condition is seen in people with aphasia. Lesion is found in the angular gyrus of the left hemisphere.

Anarithmetria refers to the inability to perform number manipulation. This disorder is common in people with dementia of Alzheimer type.

TABLE 7.3

Summary of Various Types of Apraxia

Type	Definition	Lesion	Example
Ideational apraxia	The patient has an inability to carry out a complex sequence, but the individual components of the sequence can be successfully performed	Corpus callosum, extensive left hemisphere lesion, and advanced Alzheimer's disease	A person cannot work in a café because he or she cannot make tea and serve the others. If you ask him or her to put a tea bag into the cup, he or she is able to do so
Ideomotor apraxia	The patient has difficulty with selection, sequencing, and spatial orientation. There are problems in gestures (e.g. waving) and in demonstrating the use of imagined household items (e.g. toothbrush)	Left parietal or frontal lobe. There is damage in the motor programmes (e.g. cortically stored movement patterns) or disconnection in the flow of information necessary for initiating complex motor acts	A person does not know how to use a hammer
Orobuccal apraxia	The patient has difficulty in performing learned, skilled movements of the face, lips, tongue, cheek, larynx, and pharynx on command	Left inferior frontal lobe and insula	When a person is asked to pretend to blow out a match or suck a straw, he or she makes incorrect movements
Construction apraxia	The patient has difficulty in reproducing simple geometric patterns and an inability to connect the separate parts	Nondominant parietal lobe	Failure to draw interconnected double pentagon

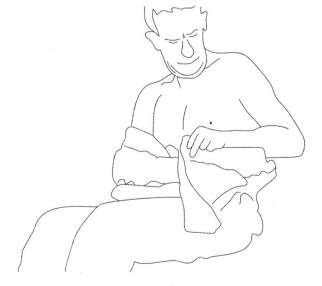

FIGURE 7.3   Dressing apraxia.

7.8   FRONTAL LOBE FUNCTIONS

7.8.1   PREFRONTAL CORTEX

This is probably involved in the following functions:

- Problem-solving
- Perceptual judgement
- Memory
- Programming and planning of sequences of behaviour
- Verbal regulation
- Level of response emission
- Adaptability of response pattern
- Tertiary level of motor control

7.8.2   FRONTAL EYE FIELDS

These are involved in voluntary eye movements.

7.8.3 Motor and Premotor Cortex

These are probably involved in the following functions:

- Primary and secondary levels of motor control
- Design fluency

7.8.4 Broca's Area

This is involved in expressive speech.

7.8.5 Orbital Cortex

This is probably involved in the following functions:

- Personality
- Social behaviour

Orbital cortex damage may lead to abnormal sexual behaviour.

7.8.6 Frontal Lobe Lesions

These may cause the following:

- Personality change—disinhibition, reduced social and ethical control, sexual indiscretions, poor judgement, elevated mood, lack of concern for the feelings of other people, and irritability.
- Perseveration.
- Utilization behaviour.
- Palilalia.
- Impairment of attention, concentration, and initiative.
- Aspontaneity, slowed psychomotor activity.
- Motor Jacksonian fits.
- Urinary incontinence.
- Contralateral spastic paresis.
- Aphasia.
- Primary motor aphasia.
- Motor agraphia.
- Anosmia.
- Ipsilateral optic atrophy.
- The left frontal lobe is involved in controlling language-related movement (Broca's area) and the right frontal lobe is involved in nonverbal abilities. Left frontal lobe damage leads to nonfluent speech (expressive dysphasia) and depression. Right frontal

lobe damage may lead to disinhibition and antisocial behaviour (Table 7.4; Figures 7.4 through 7.6).

CASC STATION: ASSESS FRONTAL LOBE FUNCTIONS (TABLE 7.6)

A 23-year-old man was involved in a fight in the pub and suffered head injuries. He was taken to the hospital and treated for subdural hematoma. His mother has noticed a change in his personality after the injury.

Task: Assess his frontal lobe functions.

Candidates are advised to familiarise with assessment of parietal and temporal lobe functions in the CASC exam (Table 7.6).

7.8.7 Assessment of Temporal Lobe Functions

1. *Language function*: Repeat 'No ifs, and, or, buts'.
2. *Visual recognition*: Show a pen or a watch to the person and ask the person to name it.
3. *Semantic memory*: Test the person knowledge on landmarks (e.g. Great Wall, Eiffel Tower) or the names of famous people (current Prime Minister of United Kingdom, current president of the United States) and knowledge of famous people (e.g. John Lennon, Tony Blair).
4. *Registration and recall after few minutes*: Tell the person three objects, ask them what the three objects are immediately, and recall after a few minutes.
5. *Assessment of visual field*: Look for upper quadratic field defect.

7.9 LEFT AND RIGHT CEREBRAL HEMISPHERES

If a person suffers damages in the left hemisphere, the intact right hemisphere can take over the task of attending to the right side (Tables 7.6 and 7.7). On the other hand, if a person suffers damages in the right hemisphere, it will cause right-sided neglect because the left hemisphere cannot compensate. In this case, the person neglected the right side of the flower in the drawing (see Figure 7.7).

TABLE 7.4
Neuropsychological Assessments of Frontal Lobe Functions

Neurological Tests	Methodology and Interpretation
Wisconsin card sorting task (WCST)	Methodology: Patients are given a pack of cards with symbols on them, which differ in form, colour, and numbers. Four stimulus cards are available and the patient has to place each response card in front of one of the four stimulus cards. The psychologist then tells the person if he or she is right or wrong. The person has to use the feedback from the psychologist to place the next card in front of the next stimulus card. The sorting is done arbitrarily into colour, form, or number. The person is required to shift the set from one type of stimulus response to another as indicated by the psychologist Interpretation: People with frontal lobe lesions cannot overcome previously established responses and show a high frequency of preservative errors
Tower of London task	Methodology: The person needs to rearrange the beads on vertical rods to match a template, using as few moves as possible. This task assesses the person's planning skills Interpretation: People with frontal lobe impairment have difficulty with planning and organization. They take many more moves compared to people without frontal lobe impairment

Stroop task	Methodology: The Stroop task assesses the person's attention and ability to inhibit inappropriate response. People have the ability to read words more quickly and automatically than naming colour. For example, if the word 'red' is printed or displayed in 'black' ink, people will say the word 'red' more readily than naming the colour, 'black' in which it is displayed. The Stroop test involves words in different colours, and there are three levels:
	    Level 1: Choose the word that matches the stated colour
	    Level 2: Choose the word that matches the stated word
	    Level 3: Choose the colour that matches the colour of a stated word
	Interpretation: People with frontal lobe impairment have difficulty in dividing their attention and fail to suppress the tendency to name the words rather than the printed colour. As a result, they will make more mistakes in the tasks compared to people without frontal lobe impairment

Hayling and Brixton tests	Methodology of the Hayling test: The first part measures the speed of response initiation. The assessor reads each sentence and the subject has to simply complete the sentences The second part measures response suppression. The subject completes a sentence with a nonsense ending word and suppresses the sensible ending word Interpretation: People with frontal lobe impairment have poor response initiation and suppression. Methodology of the Brixton test: The Brixton test is a visuospatial sequencing test with changes in rule in between. It is useful to assess people with speech difficulties, with rule change Interpretation: People with frontal lobe impairment have poor visuospatial sequencing

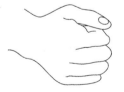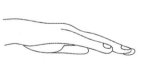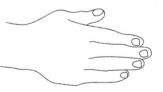

FIGURE 7.4   Luria's hand test (hand position test).

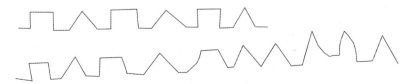

FIGURE 7.5   Alternating sequence test.

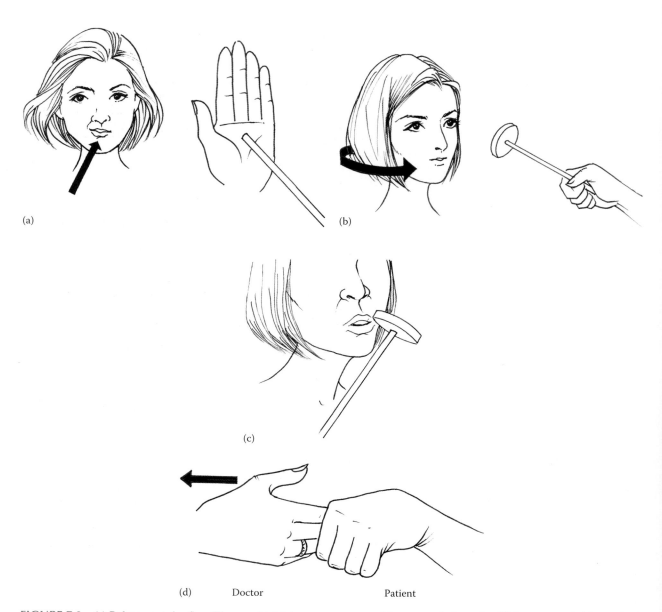

FIGURE 7.6 (a) Palmomental reflex: The psychiatrist uses an orange stick to scratch the palm. If there are wrinkles or folds appear on the ipsilateral chin, palmomental reflex is present. (b) Visual rooting reflex: The psychiatrist uses a tendon hammer to approach the patient. If she turns to the tendon hammer with her mouth open, the visual rooting reflex is present. (c) Snout reflex: A tendon hammer is tapped lightly on the patient's lip. If she forms small folds and wrinkles on the lip and around the mouth, the pout reflex is present. This resembles the sucking reflex. (d) Grasp reflex: The psychiatrist places two fingers in the open palm of each of the patient's hands. If the patient grasps the psychiatrist's fingers and resists the attempts of removal, grasp reflex is present.

TABLE 7.5

CASC Grid

Tasks and Instructions to Patient	Findings in People without Frontal Lobe Impairment	Findings in People with Frontal Lobe Impairment
Word fluency *Instruction:* 'Name as many English words as possible starting with letter "F","A", and "S"'. Category fluency is for non-English speaking patients: *Instruction:* 'Name as many animals as possible in 1 min'	Expected response: Able to say 12–15 words in 1 min Some people may develop strategies to help them to find words. A person may think of a category of items starting with 'F' and then move to other categories. For example, a medical student will think of diseases started with 'F' and then move onto household items started with 'F'	The person can only mention a few words. Very often, they repeat those words that have already been mentioned. Finally, the person stops and cannot provide more words or items
Abstract thinking Instruction: 'Can you interpret the following proverb, a rolling stone gathers no moss?' For non-English speaking patients, the examiner may ask similarity between an apple and an orange and a table and a chair.	Expected response: 'People who are always moving with no roots in one place. They avoid responsibilities and cares. They cannot achieve much' Expected response: 'Both apples and oranges are fruits. They have skin. People can make juice from them. They have seeds and contain nutrients'	Response: 'Stone is stone. Moss is moss'. The patient cannot appreciate the deeper meanings but just focuses on the words superficially Response: 'Apple is red. Orange is orange'. It is not uncommon to find a patient talking about the differences as it seems to be easier than talking about the similarities
Cognitive estimation Instruction: 'How tall is an average British woman?' Instruction: 'How many elephants are there in Sheffield or Hong Kong?'	Expected response: 'An average British woman is 1.6–1.8 m tall' Expected response: 'I guess 5–10 elephants'	Response: '10 feet tall' Response: '900 elephants' Candidates may not know the exact number of elephants in Sheffield or Hong Kong, but the answer given by the patient is obviously beyond the normal estimates
Judgement Instruction: 'If you find a letter on the floor and there is a stamp attached to it, what will you do?' This task assesses the orbitofrontal lobe function.	Expected response: 'I will put in the mail box and post it'	Response: 'I will bring it home and hide it' The patient may give various responses but not conform with the logical actions proposed by people without frontal lobe impairment
Luria's hand test The candidate needs to demonstrate the Luria's hand test to the subject being examined. After the subject has mastered the technique, he or she has to do it with one hand for at least five times. Then the subject has to repeat with the other hand. (See Figure 7.4.)	Expected response: A subject without frontal lobe impairment can appreciate the three different hand positions	Patients with frontal lobe impairment may not appreciate that there are three different hand positions and cannot alternate from one to another as a result of motor preservation
Alternative sequence test The candidate draws the alternating shapes and asks the person being examined to continue without telling them that there is a pattern.	Expected response: People without frontal lobe impairment will recognize and continue the three alternating shapes	Patients with frontal lobe impairment will continue with the last shape (a triangle in this case) The failure to appreciate the alternative pattern is a result of preservation (See Figure 7.5.)
Elicit primitive reflexes (See Figure 7.6.)	Expected response: no primitive reflex	Patients with frontal lobe impairment show emergence of primitive reflexes

TABLE 7.6

Assessment of Parietal Lobe Functions

Assessment of Dominant Parietal Lobe

1. (Gerstmann's syndrome)
   a. Finger agnosia: inability to recognize the name of the finger
   b. Left and right orientation: inability to recognize left and right
   c. Acalculia: inability to recognize number and calculation
   d. Dysgraphia
2. Astereoagnosia: inability to recognize the size, shape, and texture of an object by palpation
3. Dysgraphesthesia: inability to recognize letters or numbers written on the hand
4. Ideomotor apraxia
5. Wernicke's or Broca's aphasia
6. Impairment in two-point discrimination (e.g. a patient cannot recognize the presence of two sharp stimuli by placing a divider on the finger pulp)

Assessment of Nondominant Parietal Lobe

1. Asomatognosia: lack of awareness of the condition of all or parts of the body
2. Constructional dyspraxia: inability to copy double interlocking pentagons

TABLE 7.7

Summary of the Neuropsychological Impairments of the Left and Right Cerebral Hemispheres

Lesions in the Left Cerebral Hemisphere (Dominant)

1. Gerstmann's syndrome: finger agnosia, left and right orientation, acalculia, and dysgraphia (lexical and deep)
2. Astereoagnosia
3. Dysgraphesthesia
4. Ideomotor apraxia
5. Dyslexia: surface or deep
6. Apraxia: ideation, ideomotor, and orobuccal

Lesions in the Right Cerebral Hemisphere (Nondominant)

1. Neglect phenomena (one side of body, sensation, reading, writing)
2. Apraxia: depressing and constructional
3. Agnosia: apperceptive

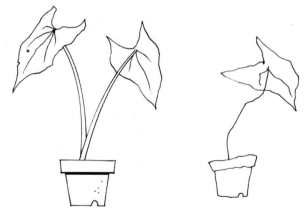

FIGURE 7.7   Unilateral neglect in a person with damage in the right hemisphere.

BIBLIOGRAPHY

Brandon S, Boakes J, Glaser D, and Green R. 1998: Recovered memories of childhood sexual abuse. Implications for clinical practice. *British Journal of Psychiatry* 172:296–307.

Brown J and Hillam J. 2004: *Dementia: Your Questions Answered*. Edinburgh, U.K.: Churchill Livingstone.

Burgess P and Shallice T. 1997: *The Hayling and Brixton Tests. Test Manual*. Bury St. Edmunds, U.K.: Thames Valley Test Company.

Campanella F, Mondani M, Skrap M, and Shallice T. 2009: Semantic access dysphasia resulting from left temporal lobe tumours. *Brain* 132(1):87–102.

Campbell RJ. 1996: *Psychiatric Dictionary*. New York: Oxford University Press.

Hodges J. 2002: *Cognitive Assessment for Clinicians*. Oxford, U.K.: Oxford University Press.

Smith EE, Nolen-Hoeksema S, Fredrickson BL et al. (eds.) 2003: *Atkinson and Hilgard's Introduction to Psychology (with Lecture Notes and InfoTrac)*, 14th edn. Florence, KT: Wadsworth.

Trimble M. 2004: *Somatoform Disorders—A Medico-Legal Guide*. Cambridge, U.K.: Cambridge University Press.

Yudofsky SC and Hales RE. 2007: *The American Psychiatric Publishing Textbook of Neuropsychiatry and Behavioural Neuroscience*, 5th edn. Washington, DC: American Psychiatric Press Inc.

8 Social Sciences and Stigma

8.1 DESCRIPTIVE TERMS

8.1.1 SOCIAL CLASS

A social class is a segment of the population sharing a broadly similar type and level of resources, with a broadly similar style of living and some shared perception of its common condition.

8.1.1.1 Determinants

The determinants of social class include

- Education
- Financial status
- Occupation
- Type of residence
- Geographic area of residence
- Leisure activities

8.1.1.2 Occupational Classification

In British psychiatry, the following occupationally based classification given by the Office of Population Censuses and Surveys has traditionally been used:

- Social class I—professional, higher managerial, landowners
- Social class II—intermediate
- Social class III—skilled, manual, clerical
- Social class IV—semiskilled
- Social class V—unskilled
- Social class 0—unemployed, students

Members of the same household are assigned to the social class of the head of the household.

8.1.2 SOCIOECONOMIC STATUS

The socioeconomic status of an individual is his or her position in the social hierarchy. It is related to social class and may increase, for example, through educational achievement, or decrease, for example, through unemployment or mental illness.

8.1.3 RELEVANCE TO PSYCHIATRIC DISORDER AND HEALTH-CARE DELIVERY

8.1.3.1 Psychiatric Disorder

The incidence and prevalence of many psychiatric disorders have been found to vary with social class. In particular, the following disorders are more likely to be diagnosed in the lower social classes:

- Schizophrenia
- Alcohol dependence
- Organic psychosis
- Depressive episodes in women
- Parasuicide/deliberate self-harm
- Personality disorder

The following disorders are more likely to be diagnosed in the upper social classes:

- Anorexia nervosa in females
- Bulimia nervosa in females
- Bipolar mood disorder

8.1.3.2 Relationship between Social Class and Psychiatric Disorder

The existence of a relationship between social class and a given psychiatric disorder does not necessarily imply causation, from social class to the disorder. In general, the possible explanations of such a relationship may include the following:

- *Downward social drift*—for example, the increased representation of schizophrenia in lower social classes may be partly a result of social drift.
- *Environmental stress*—lower social class is associated with adverse life situations, material deprivation, and the lower self-esteem that manual jobs entail; women in lower social classes are more likely to experience severe life events and vulnerability factors.
- *Differential labelling*—for example, it may be that some people in Britain of Afro-Caribbean

origin are more likely to be detained under mental health legislation and diagnosed as suffering from schizophrenia (although this may in fact reflect genuine differences in prevalence and incidence rates).

- *Differential treatment*—for example, there is a difference in the type of psychiatric treatment likely to be received by those from different social classes (see the succeeding text).

8.1.3.3   Health-Care Delivery

Those with a psychiatric disorder who are from lower social classes are more likely to

- Be admitted to hospital as psychiatric inpatients
- Remain as psychiatric inpatients for longer
- Receive physical treatments, for example, electroconvulsive therapy

Those with a psychiatric disorder who are from upper social classes are more likely to

- Spend a shorter period of time as psychiatric inpatients
- Be treated as psychiatric outpatients without inpatient admission
- Receive psychological treatments, for example, individual psychotherapy

8.1.3.4   Pathways to Psychiatric Care

Goldberg and Huxley (1980) described the existence of filters to psychiatric care, each of which depends on

- *Social factors*—such as age, sex, ethnic background, socioeconomic status
- *Service organization and provision*—for example, time and location of clinics, length of waiting list
- *Aspects of the disorder itself*—for example, its severity and chronicity

These filters include

- The decision to consult the general practitioner
- Recognition of the disorder by the general practitioner
- The decision by the general practitioner as to whether or not to refer the patient to a specialist

8.1.4   BLACK REPORT ON SOCIOECONOMIC INEQUALITIES IN HEALTH

According to the Black Report of 1980 exploring the difference in health and mortality in Britain between the social classes, compared with those in social class I, individuals in social class V

- Have twice the neonatal mortality
- Are twice as likely to die before retirement
- Have an increased rate of almost all diseases

8.1.4.1   Explanations

The following explanations for the relationship between social class and illness found in the Black Report on socioeconomic inequalities in health have been suggested:

- *Artefactual*—the health inequalities found are artificial.
- *Natural and social selection*—good health is associated with an improvement in social class, while poor health is associated with social drift downward.
- *Materialist/structural*—poor health is primarily a function of material deprivation; inequalities in wealth and income distribution are associated with inequalities in health.
- *Cultural/behavioural*—certain unhealthy behaviour patterns are more common in lower social classes (e.g. smoking, unhealthy diets), leading to health inequalities.

8.1.4.2   Changes after 10 Years

A decade after the publication of the Black Report, Smith et al. (1990) found

- Social class differences in mortality had widened.
- Better measures of socioeconomic position showed greater inequalities in mortality.
- Inequalities in health had been found in all countries that collect relevant data.
- Measurement artefacts and social selection did not account for mortality differences.
- Social class differences existed for health during life as well as for the length of life.
- Trends in income distribution suggested a further likely widening of mortality differences.

8.2 HISTORICAL SOCIOLOGICAL THEORIES

8.2.1 WEBER

Max Weber was born in Erfurt, Prussia, in 1864 and died in Munich, Germany, in 1920.

8.2.1.1 Bureaucracy

Weber studied bureaucracy, starting with his 1908 studies on *Economies of Antiquity* (Love, 1991). He started by outlining the development of modern forms of administration and put forward the notion that states in which the political machinery was centred around officialdom formed the basis of modern bureaucratic structures. (He considered that ancient societies were not bureaucratic in the same way.) He suggested that there existed the following types of bureaucracy:

- Religious communities
- States
- Economies
- The judiciary
- The modern agency
- The military

8.2.1.2 Rationalization

Rationalization was the term used to denote the way in which nature, society, and the actions of individuals were oriented towards planning, technical procedures, and rational actions.

8.2.1.3 Religion

According to Weber et al. (2002), social change can be caused by religious belief. He suggested that change can both cause and be caused by ideas. His thesis of *The Protestant Ethic and the Spirit of Capitalism* related capitalism to Protestantism. He had noted that, in his native Germany, that there was a positive association between success in capitalist ventures and being of the Protestant faith or background. This association was caused, according to Weber, by the consequences of Puritan theology (as a reaction to the severity of Calvinism). For example, the combination of the work ethic (based on the Fourth Commandment), the belief that gain of wealth was a sign of being blessed, and an ascetic unwillingness of Puritans to enjoy the fruits of such labour themselves would lead overall to yet further accumulation of capital.

8.2.2 MARX

Karl Heinrich Marx was born in Trier, Prussia, in 1818 and died in London, England, in 1883.

8.2.2.1 Communism

After he and his wife (newlywed) moved to Paris in 1843, Marx became a communist, authoring *Economic and Philosophic Manuscripts of 1844* (which was not published for about a century; Marx et al., 2011). In collaboration with Engels, he coauthored *The German Ideology* in 1845–1846 (published in 1932), in which it was argued that historically nation states and societies generally had developed in such a way that the interests of the economically dominant class were favoured (Marx et al., 1987). (Such arguments might account for the difficulty that Marx and Engels encountered in trying to find a publisher for this work.) Some of the unpublished ideas contained in this work were summarized by Marx and Engels in their 1848 pamphlet *The Communist Manifesto* (Marx and Engels, 2004). Here, they also argued that all history had fundamentally been a history of class struggle.

8.2.2.2 Crime

Marx argued that powerful entities, such as corporations, could influence the definition of crime. Thus, while white collar crime was deemed punishable, acts by more privileged members of society, such as fraud and tax evasion, might go unpunished. Furthermore, corporate crimes might be carried out in order to increase company profits, even if they involved engaging in activities that may harm people (for instance, not paying heed to laws on health and safety or disposing of toxic waste inappropriately).

8.2.2.3 Religion

Arguing that religion was 'an opiate of the masses', Marx held that religion came from the oppressed but benefited those at the top in society. He thought that organized religion

- Helped to anaesthetize the pain caused by oppression
- Promised a reward in heaven or the afterlife for those who endured oppression in their current lives
- Provided justification for the current social order, including the position in this that a believer found themselves in
- Promised that good behaviour would be rewarded
- Suggested to the population that the current problems on the planet would be solved through divine intervention

8.2.3 DURKHEIM

Emile Durkheim was born in Epinal, France, in 1858 and died in Paris, France, in 1917.

8.2.3.1 Anomie

Durkheim introduced the term anomie to refer to social disconnectedness or a lack of social norms, which may be caused by a change in an individual's relationship with their social group, in which norms for conduct are absent, weak, or conflicting. Two types of anomie may be distinguished (Boulton, 1998):

1. *Acute anomie*—this is caused by a sudden change or crisis that leaves the individual in an unfamiliar situation.
2. *Chronic anomie*—this refers to circumstances in which the rules of a social group have become unclear to the individual or do not provide the means of meeting his or her aspirations.

Causes of acute anomie include

- Migration
- Bereavement
- Redundancy

Causes of chronic anomie include

- Homelessness
- Long-term unemployment

Widespread anomie may lead to a breakdown in social order; Durkheim considered that science (in particular, social science), educational reform, and religion were ways of avoiding this.

8.2.3.2 Suicide

In his 1897 work *Suicide*, Durkheim suggested that there appeared to be an inverse relationship between, on the one hand, how integrated individuals were in their society and culture and, on the other hand, the rate of suicide (Durkheim, 1966). A major cause of suicide, then, could be seen in terms of social forces. According to Durkheim, there were, in fact, three types of suicide:

1. *Altruistic suicide*—this results from social integration in a culture that accepts suicide as way of expiating shame or blame.
2. *Egoistic suicide*—this results in the context of the individual being socially further distanced from social norms and restraints, such that meaning is questioned.
3. *Anomic suicide*—this also results in the context of the individual being socially further distanced from social norms and restraints, in which anomie exists.

8.2.4 Foucault

Michel Foucault was born in Poitiers, France, in 1926 and died in Paris, France, in 1984.

8.2.4.1 Principles of Exclusion

In books such as his 1975 work *Discipline and Punish: The Birth of the Prison*, Foucault put forward his thesis that society uses institutions to carry out social exclusion (Foucault and Sheridan, 1991). Such institutions included, he argued, the following:

- Asylums
- Hospitals
- Prisons

In respect to mental illness, Foucault argued that one of the principles of exclusion that society uses to define itself is the distinction between sanity and insanity.

8.2.4.2 Sexuality

Foucault made a study of the history of sexuality from ancient times. This was published in his 1976–1984 three-volume work *History of Sexuality* (Foucault and Hurley, 1998).

8.2.5 Parsons

Talcott Parsons was born in Colorado Springs, the United States of America, in 1902 and died in Munich, West Germany, in 1979. Aspects of his contribution to sociological theories are given in Section 8.2.7.

8.2.6 Goffman

Erving Goffman was born in Canada in 1922 and died in Philadelphia, the United States of America, in 1982. Aspects of his contribution to sociological theories are given in Section 8.2.6.

8.2.7 Habermas

Jürgen Habermas was born in 1929 in Düsseldorf, Germany.

In his two-volume magnum opus, *The Theory of Communicative Action* (Habermas and McCarthy, 1989), Habermas built on the sociological theories of Max Weber, George Herbert Mead, Emile Durkheim, and Talcott Parsons to suggest reasoning capacities, besides traditional cognitive–instrumental reasoning, which carry out subjective and intersubjective functions within the framework of societal interactions. He has gone on to defend modern society and civil society.

8.3 SOCIAL ROLES OF DOCTORS AND ILLNESS

8.3.1 SOCIAL ROLE

The social role of an individual in social is the pattern of behaviour in given social situations expected of him or her in relation to his or her social status. It consists of

- *Obligations*—behaviours towards others expected of the individual
- *Rights*—behaviours from others expected in return for obligations

8.3.2 SOCIAL ROLE OF DOCTORS

In the model proposed by Parsons (1951), the role of the doctor includes

- Defining illness
- Legitimizing illness
- Imposing an illness diagnosis if necessary
- Offering appropriate help

Doctors therefore control access to the sick role and they and patients have reciprocal obligations and rights.

8.3.3 SICK ROLE

The sick role was defined by Parsons (1951) as the role given by society to a sick individual and was considered to carry rights or privileges and obligations.

8.3.3.1 Rights (Privileges)

According to Parsons (1951), the sick role carries the following two rights for the sick individual:

- Exemption from blame for the illness
- Exemption from normal responsibilities while sick, such as the need to go to work

8.3.3.2 Obligations

The sick individual has the following obligations:

- The wish to recover as soon as possible, including seeking appropriate help from the doctor
- Cooperation with medical investigations and acceptance of medical advice and treatment

8.3.4 ILLNESS BEHAVIOUR

Illness behaviour is a set of stages describing the behaviour adopted by sick individuals (Mechanic, 1978). It describes the way in which individuals respond to somatic symptoms and signs and the conditions under which they come to view them as abnormal. Illness behaviour therefore involves the manner in which individuals

- Monitor their bodies
- Define and interpret their symptoms and signs
- Take remedial action
- Utilize sources of help

8.3.4.1 Stages

Illness behaviour includes the following stages:

- Initially well.
- Symptoms of the illness begin to be experienced.
- The opinion of immediate social contacts is sought.
- Contact is made with a doctor (or doctors).
- The illness is legitimized by the doctor(s).
- The individual adopts the sick role.
- On recovery (or death), the dependent stage of the sick role is given up.
- A rehabilitation stage is entered if the individual recovers.

8.3.4.2 Determinants

The determinants of illness behaviour, according to Mechanic (1978), are

- The visibility, recognizability, or perceptual salience of deviant signs and symptoms
- The extent to which symptoms are seen as being serious
- The extent to which symptoms disrupt the family, work, and other social activities
- The frequency of appearance of deviant signs or symptoms, their persistence, and the frequency of recurrence
- The tolerance threshold of exposed deviant signs and symptoms
- Available information, knowledge, and cultural understanding of exposed deviant signs and symptoms
- Basic needs leading to denial

- The competition between needs and illness responses
- Competing interpretations assigned to recognized symptoms
- The availability and physical proximity of treatment resources and the costs in terms of time, money, effort, and stigma

8.4 FAMILY LIFE IN RELATION TO MAJOR MENTAL ILLNESS

Family life is guided by the explicit and implicit relationship rules that prescribe and limit the behaviour of members of the family and provide expectations within the family with respect to the roles, actions, and consequences of individuals.

8.4.1 ELEMENTS OF FAMILY FUNCTIONING

Elements of family functioning of importance in relation to major mental illness (after Dare, 1985) include

- *Interactional patterns*—family members and relationships, communication patterns, hierarchical structure, control/authority systems, relationship with the outside world
- *Sociocultural context of the family*—socioeconomic status, social mobility, migration status
- *Location of the family in the life cycle*—number of transitions, adaptation requirements
- *Intergenerational structure*—experiences of parents as children, influences of grandparents and extended family
- Significance of symptoms of mental illness for the family
- *Family problem-solving skills*—family style, previous experience

8.4.2 SCHIZOPHRENIA

Historically, the following types of family dysfunction were at various times believed to be a cause of schizophrenia:

- Schizophrenogenic mother
- Double bind
- Marital skew and marital schism
- Abnormal family communication

These theories are now out of favour, but there is evidence for the more recent theory relating to the effects of expressed emotion with respect to relapse in schizophrenia.

8.4.2.1 Schizophrenogenic Mother

This concept was put forward by Fromm-Reichmann in 1948 (Hoff, 1982). Schizophrenia was said to be a consequence of an inadequate relationship between the future sufferer from schizophrenia, as a child, and his or her mother. Characteristics of the schizophrenogenic mother were said to include her being

- Rejecting
- Aloof
- Overly protective
- Overtly hostile

8.4.2.2 Double Bind

This concept was put forward by Bateson et al. (1956). The parents communicated with the child (the future sufferer from schizophrenia) in abnormal ways leading to feelings of ambivalence and ambiguity, with messages that were typically

- Vague
- Ambiguous
- Confusing

Schizophrenia developed as a result of exposure to such double-bind situations.

8.4.2.3 Marital Skew and Marital Schism

This concept was put forward by Lidz et al. (1957):

- *Marital skew*—dominant and eccentric mother; passive and dependent father
- *Marital schism*—parental conflict, argument, and hostility leading to divided loyalties to mother and father on the part of the child (the future sufferer from schizophrenia)

8.4.2.4 Abnormal Family Communication

This concept was put forward by Wynne and colleagues in 1958 and suggested that disordered communication took place between the parents of schizophrenics.

8.4.2.5 Expressed Emotion

In an outcome study of 200 patients, mainly with schizophrenia, Brown et al. (1958) found that those discharged to their families had a poor outcome, with the highest relapse rate occurring in those families having close and frequent contact with the patients.

Subsequent follow-up studies have confirmed the association of high expressed emotion in families, characterized by the frequent, intense expression of emotion and a pushy and critical attitude by relatives to the patient, with an increased relapse rate in family members with schizophrenia.

In assessing expressed emotion, the five relevant scales of the Camberwell Family Interview (CFI) are

- *Critical comments*—indicating unambiguous dislike or disapproval
- *Hostility*—expressed towards the person rather than his or her behaviour
- *Emotional overinvolvement*—exaggerated self-sacrificing or overprotective concern
- *Warmth*—based on sympathy, affection, and empathy
- *Positive remarks*—expressing praise or approval of the patient

The first three of these are associated with high expressed emotion and predict relapse (Vaughn and Leff, 1976):

	Relapse Rate in 9 Months Following Discharge (%)
Antipsychotic medication, low expressed emotion family	12
Antipsychotic medication, high expressed emotion family, <35 h/week face-to-face contact	42
No antipsychotic medication, high expressed emotion family, >35 h/week face-to-face contact	92

8.4.3 MOOD DISORDERS

8.4.3.1 Expressed Emotion

As with schizophrenia, high expressed emotion at home is associated with an increased risk of relapse of depression.

8.4.3.2 Vulnerability Factors

Two of the four vulnerability factors found by Brown and Harris (1986) to make women more susceptible to suffer from depression following life events (see the following) were

- A lack of a confiding relationship
- Having three or more children under the age of 15 years at home

8.4.4 PROBLEM DRINKING AND ALCOHOL DEPENDENCE

Family life often suffers as a result of excessive alcohol consumption, with the breakdown of relationships, marriages, and families being common. This may result from the following consequences of excessive alcohol consumption:

- Mood changes
- Personality deterioration
- Verbal abuse
- Physical violence
- Psychosexual disorders
- Pathological jealousy
- Associated gambling
- Associated abuse of other psychoactive substances

8.4.5 LEARNING DISABILITY/MENTAL RETARDATION

Psychological processes that may occur in families with an impaired or disabled member (after Bicknell, 1983) include

- Shock → panic → denial
- Denial → shopping around
- Denial → overprotection/rejection
- Grief → projection of grief
- Guilt
- Anger
- Bargaining → late rejection
- Acceptance → infantilization
- Ego-centred work → 'other'-centred work
- Overidentification

8.5   LIFE EVENTS

8.5.1   DEFINITION

Life events are sudden changes, which may be positive or negative, in an individual's social life, which disrupt its normal course.

8.5.2   LIFE-CHANGE SCALE

The following table gives some life-change values for life events in the Holmes and Rahe Social Readjustment Rating Scale (after Holmes and Rahe, 1967):

Life Event	Life-Change Value
Death of spouse	100
Divorce	73
Marital separation	65
Gaol term	63
Death of close family member	63
Personal injury or illness	53
Marriage	50
Being sacked from job	47
Retirement	45
Marital reconciliation	45
Pregnancy	40
Birth of child	39
Death of close friend	37
Child leaving home for good	29
Problems with in-laws	29
Problems with boss	23
Change in sleeping habits	16
Change in eating habits	15
Minor legal violation	11

The full Holmes and Rahe Social Readjustment Rating Scale, which was introduced in 1967, consists of a self-report questionnaire containing 43 classes of life event.

8.5.3   AETIOLOGY OF PSYCHIATRIC DISORDERS

In order to demonstrate that life events have an aetiological role in a given psychiatric disorder, the following criteria should be fulfilled:

- The occurrence of life events should correlate with onset of the disorder.
- The life events should precede the onset of the disorder and not the other way round.
- A hypothetical construct should exist with confounded variables excluded.

- The relationship between life events and the psychiatric disorder should be found to occur in different populations and at different times.

8.5.4   DIFFICULTIES IN THE EVALUATION OF LIFE EVENTS

Methodological problems in the evaluation of life events include the following:

1. Assessments tend to be retrospective, which can lead to difficulties such as
   a. Biased recall
   b. Falloff in recall with time
   c. Retrospective contamination
   d. Effort after meaning
2. Causation and association need to be separated
3. Contextual evaluation
4. Subjective evaluation

A widely used instrument for current research into life events and psychiatric disorder is the Life Events and Difficulties Schedule (LEDS) of Brown and Harris (1978, 1989), which has the following features:

- Semistructured interview schedule
- 38 areas probed
- Detailed narratives collected about events, including their circumstances
- High reliability
- High validity

8.5.5   CLINICAL SIGNIFICANCE

8.5.5.1   Depression

Many studies have found a relationship between life events and the onset of depression. In 6–12 months prior to the onset, compared with normal controls, patients have a three to five times greater chance of having suffered at least one life event with major negative long-term implications (involving threat or loss). However, most people who experience adverse life events do not develop depression; as mentioned earlier, Brown and Harris (1978) identified four vulnerability factors that make women more susceptible to suffer from depression following life events:

- Loss of mother before the age of 11 years
- Not working outside the home
- A lack of a confiding relationship
- Having three or more children under the age of 15 years at home

8.5.5.2 Schizophrenia

The evidence tends to suggest that independent life events are more likely to occur prior to relapse rather than prior to first onset of schizophrenia (Brown and Birley, 1968; Tennant, 1985).

8.5.5.3 Anxiety

There is some evidence that life events are more likely to occur prior to anxiety (Finlay-Jones and Brown, 1981; Miller and Ingham, 1985). From their study of life events occurring in the year before the onset of three types of cases of psychiatric disorder of recent onset (depression, anxiety, and mixed depression/anxiety) in young women and normal controls, Finlay-Jones and Brown (1981) argued that life events involving severe loss were a causal agent in the onset of depression and life events involving severe danger were a causal agent in the onset of anxiety states. Cases of mixed depression/anxiety were more likely to report both a severe loss and a severe danger before onset.

8.5.5.4 Mania

In general, the results of life event studies of mania are conflicting.

8.5.5.5 Parasuicide/Deliberate Self-Harm

There is strong evidence that threatening life events are more common prior to self-poisoning attempts (e.g. Morgan et al., 1975; Farmer and Creed, 1989).

8.5.5.6 Functional Disorders

Threatening life events have been found to be more likely to precede functional disorders presenting physically such as abdominal pain without an organic cause (Creed, 1981; Craig and Brown, 1984) and menorrhagia (Harris, 1989).

8.6 RESIDENTIAL INSTITUTIONS

8.6.1 SOCIAL INSTITUTIONS

8.6.1.1 Definition

A social institution is an established and sanctioned form of relationship between social beings.

8.6.1.2 Examples

Examples of social institutions include

- The family
- Political parties
- Religious groups

8.6.2 TOTAL INSTITUTIONS

8.6.2.1 Definition

A total institution is an organization in which a large number of like-situated individuals, cut off from the wider social for an appreciable period of time, together lead an enclosed formally administered round of life (Goffman, 1961).

8.6.2.2 Examples

Examples of total institutions include

- Older large psychiatric hospitals
- Prisons
- Monasteries
- Large ships

8.6.3 GOFFMAN

From his study of the large St. Elizabeth's Hospital, in Washington, DC, Goffman (1961) was one of the first to suggest that institutions may be harmful. Concepts introduced by Goffman include the following:

- *Total institution.*
- *Binary management*—the daily lives of patients were highly regulated by staff who appeared to live in a different world to the patients.
- *Binary living.*
- *Batch living*—whereas normally life consists of a balance between work, home life, and leisure time, these three distinct entities did not exist in the total institution studied.
- *Institutional perspective*—the existence of an institutional perspective leads to the assumption that there exists an overall rational plan.
- *Mortification process*—the process whereby an individual becomes an inhabitant of a total institution.
- *Betrayal funnel*—the start of the mortification process through which relatives, via doctors, send the individual into a psychiatric hospital.
- *Role stripping*—the patient is processed through the admissions procedure, which would also usually include being physically stripped naked for the purposes of a physical examination.
- *Patient/inmate role*—patients or inmates could be considered to be metaphorically baptized into this role through the admissions procedure,

which would usually include bathing before being given institutional clothing.
- *Moral career*—gradual changes in perception of patients about themselves and others, occurring as a result of institutionalization.

8.6.3.1 Reactions to the Mortification Process

According to Goffman, patients were said to show various possible reactions to the mortification process, including

- Withdrawal
- Open rebellion
- Colonization—the patient pretends to show acceptance
- Conversion
- Institutionalization—actual acceptance both outwardly and inwardly

8.6.4 INSTITUTIONAL NEUROSIS

Barton (1959) used the term institutional neurosis to describe a syndrome he considered to be caused by institutions in which the individual shows

- Apathy
- Inability to plan for the future
- Submissiveness
- Withdrawal
- Low self-esteem

8.6.5 SECONDARY HANDICAP

Wing (1967, 1978) used the term secondary handicap to include both institutional neurosis and similar features occurring in individuals living outside total institutions.

8.6.5.1 Primary Handicap

This may be psychiatric illness, somatic illness, or social difficulties that the individual has to contend with.

8.6.5.2 Secondary Handicap

This results from the unfortunate way in which other people may react to the primary handicap, both inside and outside total institutions.

8.6.6 THREE MENTAL HOSPITALS STUDY

Wing and Brown (1961, 1970) carried out an important comparative study in the 1960s of three British mental hospitals (Netherne Hospital, South London; Severalls

Hospital, Essex; and Mapperley Hospital, Nottingham). These hospitals were chosen because they had different social conditions but otherwise were similar in that they had patients with schizophrenia who suffered illnesses of similar severity and similar catchment area populations, and all such patients were accepted for admission. Thus, it was hoped to test the hypothesis that social environment could influence schizophrenic symptoms and behaviour. A strong association was found between poverty of the social environment and severity of clinical poverty; clinical poverty consists of

- Blunted affect
- Poverty of speech
- Social withdrawal

8.7 ETHNIC MINORITIES, ADAPTATION, AND MENTAL HEALTH

8.7.1 PREVALENCE OF SCHIZOPHRENIA

In Britain, there is a higher rate of diagnosis of schizophrenia in Afro-Caribbean and Irish populations, compared with the indigenous population, and a lower rate in those of South Asian origin.

8.7.2 CAUSES OF DIFFERENT PREVALENCE RATES

Explanations of the different prevalence rates of schizophrenia in ethnic minorities in Britain include the following:

- Those who migrate from their countries of origin have a greater likelihood of having schizophrenia or a predisposition for schizophrenia (social selection)—however, there is a reduced rate in Asians and an increased rate in second-generation Afro-Caribbeans.
- Migration is associated with increased stress leading to an increased precipitation of schizophrenia in those with an underlying predisposition—however, there is a reduced rate in Asians and an increased rate in second-generation Afro-Caribbeans.
- Discrimination and deprivation lead to an increased rate of schizophrenia or an increased precipitation of schizophrenia in those with an underlying predisposition (social causation)—however, there is a reduced rate in Asians.
- Schizophrenia is overdiagnosed in Afro-Caribbeans.

8.7.3 Depression and Anxiety

Those from ethnic minorities may not tell their doctor they feel depressed or anxious. For example,

- Afro-Caribbean men when depressed may instead complain of erectile dysfunction or reduced libido
- South Asians may somatize depression
- South Asians may somatize anxiety

8.8 PROFESSIONS

8.8.1 Characteristics of Professions

The characteristics of professional status include

- The possession of practical skills based on theoretical knowledge
- Requiring an extended period formal training and education
- Assessments of competence carried out by the profession
- Belonging to an organization
- Recognition by the state of the professional organization
- Adherence to a code of conduct
- Providing altruistic service
- The possession of a monopoly of practice in their field

8.8.2 Professional Groups Involved in Patient Care

Long-established professions in health-care services include

- Doctors
- Pharmacists
- Dentists

Newer 'semiprofessions' or 'subprofessions' include

- Psychiatric nurses
- Clinical psychologists
- Nonmedically trained psychotherapists
- Occupational therapists

'Semiprofessions' or 'subprofessions' may increase their 'professionalization' over time, for instance, by increasing the length of training and training requirements. Conversely, professional groups involved in patient care may decrease their 'professionalization' over time, for instance, by going on strike even if this adversely affects patient care.

8.9 INTERGROUP BEHAVIOUR AND STIGMA

8.9.1 Stereotypes

A stereotype is an overgeneralized inference about a person or group of people in which they are all assumed to possess particular traits or characteristics.

The use of schemata (working stereotypes) is inevitable until further experience either refines or discredits them. Many stereotypes are benign but may be resistant to change. However, stereotypes can become self-perpetuating and self-fulfilling.

8.9.2 Stigma

8.9.2.1 Definition

Sigma is an attribute of an individual that marks him or her as being unacceptable, inferior, or dangerous and 'spoils' identity.

8.9.2.2 Example

Psychiatric disorders are highly stigmatized in societies that value rationality.

8.9.2.3 Enacted Stigma

This is the experience of discrimination of an individual who bears a stigma.

8.9.2.4 Felt Stigma

This is the fear of discrimination of an individual who bears a stigma.

8.9.2.5 Development

Stigma first appears during the psychoanalytic stage of latency, approximately corresponding with Erikson's stage of industry versus inferiority, during which children develop a strong awareness of the ways in which they are similar to and differ from others.

8.9.3 Prejudice

8.9.3.1 Definition

Prejudice is a preconceived set of beliefs held about others who are 'prejudged' on this basis; the negative meaning of the term is the one usually used. It is not amenable to discussion and is resistant to change. Prejudiced individuals may behave in ways that create stereotyped behaviour that sustains their prejudice.

8.9.3.2 Example

Racism or racial prejudice is the dogmatic belief that one 'race' is superior to another one and that there exist identifiable 'racial characteristics' that influence cognition, achievement, behaviour, etc.

8.9.3.3 Discrimination

This is the enactment of prejudice. (In the case of racism, the enactment is also termed racialism.)

8.9.3.4 Causes

Causes of prejudice may include the following:

- The person holding the prejudice is rigid in his or her beliefs and does not tolerate weaknesses in others; this is sometimes referred to by sociologists as an authoritarian personality.
- Scapegoating of the victims of the prejudice.
- Stereotyping of the victims of the prejudice.

8.9.3.5 Reducing Prejudice

Cook showed that the following conditions need to be satisfied in order to reduce prejudice:

- Equal status
- The potential for personal acquaintance
- Exposure to nonstereotypic individuals
- Social environment favours equality
- Cooperative effort

REFERENCES

Bateson G, Jackson DD, Haley J, and Weakland J. 1956: Towards a theory of Schizophrenia. *Behavioral Science* 1:251–264.

Barton WR. 1959: *Institutional Neurosis*. Bristol, U.K.: Wright.

Bicknell J. 1983: The psychopathology of handicap. *British Journal of Medical Psychology* 56:167–178.

Boulton M. 2010: Social science and sociocultural psychiatry. In Puri BK and Treasaden IH (eds.) *Psychiatry: An Evidence-Based Text*. London, U.K.: Hodder Arnold.

Brown GW and Birley JL. 1968: Crises and life changes and the onset of schizophrenia. *Journal of Health Social Behaviour* 9:203–214.

Brown GW, Carstairs GM, and Topping GC. 1958: The post-hospital adjustment of chronic mental patients. *Lancet* 2:658–659.

Brown GW and Harris T. 1986: Stressor, vulnerability and depression: A question of replication. *Psychological Medicine* 16(4):739–744.

Brown GW and Harris TO. (eds.) 1978: *Social Origins of Depression: A Study of Psychiatric Disorder in Women*. London, U.K.: Tavistock.

Brown GW and Harris TO. (eds.) 1989: *Life Events and Illness*. New York: Guilford Press.

Craig TKJ and Brown GW. 1984: Goal frustration and life events in the etiology of painful gastrointestinal disorder. *Journal of Psychosomatic Research* 28:411–421.

Creed F. 1981: Life events and appendectomy. *Lancet* 1:1381–1385.

Creed F. 1992: Life-events. In Weller M and Eysenck M (eds.) *The Scientific Basis of Psychiatry*, 2nd edn. London, U.K.: W.B. Saunders.

Dare C. 1985: Family therapy. In Rutter M and Hersov L (eds.) *Child and Adolescent Psychiatry: Modern Approaches*. Oxford, U.K.: Blackwell Scientific.

Durkheim E. 1966: *Suicide*. New York, NY: Free Press.

Farmer R and Creed F. 1989: Life events and hostility in self-poisoning. *British Journal of Psychiatry* 154:390–395.

Finlay-Jones R and Brown GW. 1981: Types of stressful life event and the onset of anxiety and depressive disorders. *Psychological Medicine* 11:803–815.

Foucault M and Hurley R. 1998: *The History of Sexuality: The Will to Knowledge*, Vol. 1. London, U.K.: Penguin.

Foucault M and Sheridan A. 1991: *Discipline and Punish: The Birth of the Prison*. London, U.K.: Penguin.

Goffman E. 1961: *Asylums: Essays on the Social Situation of Mental Patients and Other Inmates*. New York: Doubleday.

Goldberg D and Huxley P. 1980: *Mental Illness in the Community: The Pathways to Psychiatric Care*. London, U.K.: Tavistock Publications.

Habermas J and McCarthy R. 1989: *The Theory of Communicative Action*. Cambridge, MA: Polity Press.

Harris TO. 1989: Disorders of menstruation. In Brown GW and Harris TO (eds.) *Life Events and Illness*. New York: Guildford Press.

Hoff SG. 1982: Frieda Fromm-Reichmann, the early years. *Psychiatry* 45(2):115–120.

Holmes TH and Rahe RH. 1967: The social readjustment rating scale. *Journal of Psychosomatic Research* 11:213–217.

Lidz T, Cornelison AR, Fleck S, and Terry D. 1957: The intrafamilial environment of schizophrenic patients: II. Martial schism and marital skew. *American Journal of Psychiatry* 114:241–248.

Love JR. 1991: *Antiquity and Capitalism: Max Weber and the Sociological Foundations of Roman Civilization*. New York, NY: Routledge.

Marx K and Engels F. 2004: *The Communist Manifesto*. London, U.K.: Penguin.

Marx K, Engels F, and Arthur CJ. 1987: *The German Ideology: Introduction to a Critique of Political Economy*. London, U.K.: Lawrence & Wishart Ltd.

Marx K, Engels F, and Milligan M. 2011: *Economic and Philosophic Manuscripts 1844*. New York, NY: Wilder Publications.

Mechanic D. 1978 *Medical Sociology*, 2nd edn. Glencoe, IL: Free Press.

Miller PM and Ingham JG. 1985: Dimensions of experience and symptomatology. *Journal of Psychosomatic Research* 29:475–488.

Morgan HG, Burns-Cox CJ, Pocock H et al. 1975: Deliberate self-harm: Clinical and socio-economic characteristics of 368 patients. *British Journal of Psychiatry* 127:564–574.

Nolen-Hoeksema S, Fredrickson BL, Loftus GR, and Wagenaar WA. 2009: *Atkinson & Hilgard's Introduction to Psychology*, 15th edn. Hampshire, U.K.: Cengage Learning EMEA.

Parsons T. 1951: *The Social System*. Glencoe, Scotland: Free Press.

Persaud R. 2010: Social psychology. In Puri BK and Treasaden IH (eds.) *Psychiatry: An Evidence-Based Text*. London, U.K.: Hodder Arnold.

Scrambler G. (ed.) 2008: *Sociology as Applied to Medicine*, 6th edn. Edinburgh, U.K.: Saunders Elsevier.

Smith GD, Bartley M, and Blane D. 1990: The Black report on socioeconomic inequalities in health 10 years on. *British Medical Journal* 301:373–377.

Tantum D and Birchwood M. (eds.) 1994: *Psychiatry and the Social Sciences*. London, U.K.: Gaskell.

Tennant CC. 1985: Stress and schizophrenia: A review. *Integrative Psychiatry* 3:248–261.

Vaughn CE and Leff JP. 1976: The influence of family and social factors on the course of schizophrenic illness. *British Journal of Psychiatry* 129:125–137.

Weber M, Baehr PR, and Wells GC. 2002: *The Protestant Ethic and The "Spirit" of Capitalism and Other Writings*. London, U.K.: Penguin.

Wing JK. 1967: Social treatment, rehabilitation and management. In Coppen A and Walker A (eds.) *Recent Developments in Schizophrenia*. *British Journal of Psychiatry*, Special Publication No. 1.

Wing JK. 1978: *Schizophrenia: Towards A New Synthesis*. London, U.K.: Academic Press.

Wing JK and Brown GW. 1961: Social treatment of chronic schizophrenia: A comparative survey of three mental hospitals. *Journal of Mental Science* 107:847–861.

Wing JK and Brown GW. 1970: *Institutionalism and Schizophrenia: A Comparative Study of Three Mental Hospitals 1960–1968*. London, U.K.: Cambridge University Press.

9 Dynamic Psychopathology and Psychoanalytic Theories

9.1 BASIC PRINCIPLES OF DYNAMIC PSYCHOTHERAPY

Malan (2001) has summarized the basic principles of dynamic psychotherapy as follows:

> Within an atmosphere of unconditional acceptance, the therapist establishes a relationship with the patient, the aim of which—usually unspoken—is to enable the patient to understand his true feelings and to bring them to the surface and experience them. For this purpose, the therapist uses theoretical knowledge, guided wherever possible by his own self-knowledge, to identify himself with the patient and puts his understanding to the patient in the form of *interpretations*, which constitute his main therapeutic tool.

9.2 SIGMUND FREUD (1856–1939)

9.2.1 Early Influences

Those who had an important early influence on Freud, and his pre-psychoanalytic theories, included

- *Helmholtz* and *Brücke*—the physicochemical basis of brain function, concepts of energy and conservation, the Helmholtz School of Medicine
- *Meynert*—neuroanatomy and behaviour
- *Charcot*—hysteria and hypnosis

Freud also gained important ideas from the writings of

- *Darwin*—the theory of evolution by natural selection
- *Hughlings Jackson*—the relationship of brain structure and function

9.2.2 Protopsychoanalytic Phase (1887 to c.1897)

9.2.2.1 Studies on Hysteria

In 1895, Josef Breuer and Sigmund Freud published *Studies on Hysteria* (Freud, 1962). This included the case of Anna O. (Bertha Pappenheim) who had been treated by Breuer for hysterical symptomatology, including limb paralysis, associated with her father's illness. The development of hysteria in general was considered to take the following course:

- The cause consisted of real experiences, which were usually traumatic.
- The (traumatic) event(s) gave rise to painful/ unpleasant memories and represented ideas incompatible with conscious belief structures.
- These memories and ideas were then repressed.
- However, the powerful affects associated with them gave rise to somatic hysterical manifestations, sometimes including reenactments of the (traumatic) event(s).
- In consciousness, there remain mnemonic symbolic representations of the event(s).
- Bringing the event(s) to consciousness leads to a discharge or release of the associated affects ('psychic pus') and resolution of the hysterical symptomatology (*abreaction*).

9.2.2.2 Technical Development

The techniques employed by Freud progressed gradually through the following major phases:

- The use of *hypnosis*.
- The *concentration method*—the patient, lying on a couch with closed eyes, was asked leading questions, and Freud would press his hands on the patient's forehead.
- *Free association*—the patient, with open eyes but lying on a couch, was encouraged to articulate, without censorship, all thoughts that came to mind.

9.2.2.3 Project for a Scientific Psychology

This was mostly written by Freud in 1895 and published after his death in 1950 (Freud, 1950). It consists essentially of an attempt to link psychological processes with neurophysiology.

9.2.3 Topographical Model of the Mind

This was set out in Freud's *The Interpretation of Dreams* (1900) and developed during the following two decades until its eventual replacement by the structural model (Freud, 2010). In this model, the mind is considered to consist of the following three parts:

- The unconscious
- The preconscious
- The conscious

9.2.3.1 Unconscious

This contains memories, ideas, and affects that are repressed. Characteristic features include

1. Outside awareness
2. Operating system—*primary process* thinking
3. Motivating principle—the pleasure principle
4. Access—access to its repressed contents is difficult, occurring when the censor gives way, for instance, by becoming:
   a. Relaxed, for example, in dreaming
   b. Fooled, for example, in jokes
   c. Overpowered, for example, in neurotic symptomatology
5. System position:
   a. No negation
   b. Timelessness (reference to time is bound up in unconsciousness)
   c. Image oriented
   d. Connotative
   e. Symbolic
   f. Nonlinear

9.2.3.2 Preconscious

This part of the mind develops during childhood and serves to maintain repression and censorship. Characteristic features include

1. Outside awareness
2. Operating system—*secondary process* thinking
3. Motivating principle—the reality principle
4. Access—access can occur through focused attention
5. System position:
   a. Bound by time
   b. Word oriented
   c. Denotative
   d. Linear

9.2.3.3 Conscious

This can be considered to be an attention sensory organ. Characteristic features include

1. Within awareness
2. Operating system—*secondary process* thinking
3. Motivating principle—the reality principle
4. Access—easy
5. System position:
   a. Bound by time
   b. Word oriented
   c. Declarative
   d. Linear

9.2.3.4 Censorship

Freud described the censorship process in the following way (Galison, 2012):

> Let us compare the system of the unconscious to a large entrance hall, in which the mental impulses jostle one another like separate individuals. Adjoining this entrance hall there is a second narrow room, a kind of drawing room, in which consciousness also resides but on the threshold between these two rooms a watchman performs his function; he examines the different mental impulses, acts as a censor, and will not admit them into the drawing room if they displease him. It does not make much difference if the watchman turns away from a particular impulse at the threshold itself or if he pushes it back across the threshold after it has entered the drawing room. If they have already pushed their way forward to the threshold and have been turned back by the watchman then they are inadmissible to the consciousness; we speak of them as *repressed* but even the impulses which the watchman has allowed to cross the threshold are not on that account necessarily conscious as well; they can only become so if they succeed in catching the eye of consciousness. They are therefore justified in calling the second room the system of the *preconscious*.

9.2.3.5 Primary Process

This is the operating system of the unconscious. Its attributes include the following:

- *Displacement*—an apparently insignificant idea is invested with all the psychical depth of meaning and intensity originally attributed to another idea.
- *Condensation*—all the meanings and several chains of association converge onto a single idea standing at their point of intersection.
- *Symbolization*—symbols are used rather than words.

Characteristics of primary process thinking include the following (Sklar, 1989):

- *Timelessness*—the concept of time only develops after a period in the mind of a child in connection to conscious reality, for example, periodicity or chaos of feeding.
- *Disregard of reality* of the conscious world.
- *Psychical reality*—memories of a real event and of imagined experience are not distinguished; abstract symbols are treated concretely.
- *Absence of contradiction*—opposites have a psychic equivalence.
- Absence of negation.

9.2.3.6 Secondary Process

This is the operating system of the preconscious and the conscious. Characteristics of secondary process thinking include the following:

- *Time* flows forward linearly.
- *Reality* is regarded—the content and logical basis of ideas is important.
- Verbal word—presentations are used.
- *Contradictions* are recognized and should not exist.

9.2.3.7 Pleasure Principle

This is the motivating principle of primary process. It is mainly inborn. Pain/'unpleasure' is avoided and pleasure is sought through tension discharge. This leads to

- Wish fulfillment
- The discharge of instinctual drives

9.2.3.8 Reality Principle

This is the motivating principle of secondary process. It is the result of external reality. It leads to

- Delayed gratification

9.2.4 DREAMING

In his *The Interpretation of Dreams* (1900), Freud referred to dreams as 'the Royal Road to the Unconscious'.

9.2.4.1 Dream Composition

Dreams were considered to be composed of

- *The day residue*—memories of the waking hours before the dream that are particularly emotionally charged

- *Nocturnal stimuli*—external stimuli, for example, noise, moisture, touch, and internal stimuli, for example, pain and urinary bladder distension
- Unconscious wishes
- *Latent dream*—the day residue, nocturnal stimuli, and unconscious wishes

9.2.4.2 Dream Work

This refers to the process whereby the latent dream is converted into the manifest dream. Operations that contribute to dream work can include

- Displacement
- Condensation
- Symbolization
- *Secondary elaboration (secondary revision)*—the process of revising and/or elaborating the dream after awakening in order to make it more consistent with the rules of secondary process

9.2.5 STRUCTURAL MODEL OF THE MIND

This was set out in Freud's *The Ego and the Id* (1923) and replaced the topographical model. In this model, the mind is considered to consist of the following three parts:

- The *id*
- The *ego*
- The superego

9.2.5.1 Id

Most of the id is unconscious. It contains primordial energy reserves derived from instinctual drives. Its aim is to maximize pleasure by fulfilling these drives.

9.2.5.2 Ego

According to Freud (1984), the principal characteristics of the ego are as follows:

In consequence of the preestablished connection between sense and perception and muscular action, the ego has voluntary movement at its command. It has the task of self-preservation. As regards external events, it performs that task by becoming aware of stimuli by storing up experiences about them (in the memory), by avoiding excessively strong stimuli (through adaptation), and finally by learning to bring about expedient changes in the external world to its own advantage (through activity). As regards internal events in relation to the id, it performs that task by gaining control over the demands of the instinct, by deciding whether they are to be allowed satisfaction, by postponing that satisfaction to times and circumstances favourable in the external world, or by suppressing their excitations entirely. It is guided in its activity by consideration of the tension produced by stimuli, whether these tensions are present in it or introduced into it.

Although much of the ego is conscious, most of its activity occurs without consciousness. Owing to its direct access to perception, reality testing takes place in the ego. However, the ego can be said to serve the following 'three harsh masters':

- The superego
- Reality
- The id

9.2.5.3 Superego

The superego is concerned with issues of morality. It develops initially as a result of the imposition of parental restraint. Although more of the superego is conscious than is the case for the id, most of its activity occurs without consciousness.

9.2.5.4 Relationship between the Id, Ego, and Superego

Freud (1984) described this relationship in the following way:

We were justified… in dividing the ego from the id… [But] the ego is identical with the id, and is merely a specially differentiated part of it…. if a real split has occurred between the two, the weakness of the ego becomes apparent. But if the ego remains bound up with the id and indistinguishable from it, then it displays its strength. The same is true of the relation between the ego and the super-ego. In many situations the two are merged; and as a rule we can only distinguish one from the other when there is a tension or conflict between them. In repression the decisive fact is that the ego is an organization and the id is not. The ego is, indeed, the organized portion of the id. We should be quite wrong if we pictured the ego and the id as two opposing camps….

9.2.6 Resistance

This is everything, in words and actions of the analysand, that obstructs him or her gaining access to their unconscious. It can be used in psychoanalysis as a means to reach the repressed; indeed, the forces at work in resistance and repression are the same.

9.2.7 Transference

Sklar (1989) described the important features of the transference:

The transference is an unconscious process in which the patient transfers to the therapist feelings, emotions and attitudes that were experienced and/or desired in the patient's childhood, usually in relation to parents and siblings. It can be a passionate demand for love and hate in past relationships between the child and the adult. This is a complex field that includes the unconscious splitting of the therapist into masculine and feminine and locating unconscious affect and thinking of the 'child' part of the patient in relation to the maternal and paternal aspects of the therapist (i.e. oedipal transference). Furthermore, the direction of such a transference can be both positive and negative. Thus, Freud encountered transference in many variations and certainly also in its hidden form, transformed by resistance. The therapist's transference represents on the one hand the most powerful ally but, on the other, in terms of transference's resistance, a therapeutic difficulty.

9.2.8 Countertransference

Sklar (1989) described the important features of the countertransference:

The countertransference is the therapist's own feelings, emotions and attitudes to his patient. In the treatment mode, the therapist needs to screen out those that are mediated only by the therapist, and take note of those generated in the therapist from emotional contact with the patient. The latter can be an interesting aspect of the patient, e.g. the therapist may have the feelings of the patient as child in relation to the patient enacting the parent. Thus, in the reverse transference, an aspect of the patient is located in the therapist *as a communication*.

9.2.9 Instinctual Drives

Freud used the German word trieb to refer to an instinctual drive. Unfortunately, this has often been translated into the word 'instinct', a concept different from a 'drive'. Important instinctual drives identified by Freud were

- *Libido*—sexual 'instinct' and energy of the eros
- *Eros*—life preservation 'instinct'
- *Thanatos*—death 'instinct'

9.2.10 Psychosexual Development

The stages of psychosexual development identified by Freud were the

- Oral phase
- Anal phase
- Phallic phase
- Latency phase
- Genital phase

9.2.10.1 Oral Phase

From birth to around 15–18 months of age. Erotogenic pleasure is derived from sucking. In addition to the mother's breast, the infant has a desire to place other objects in his or her mouth.

9.2.10.2 Anal Phase

From around 15–18 months to 30–36 months of age. Erotogenic pleasure is derived from stimulation of the anal mucosa, initially through faecal excretion and later also through faecal retention.

9.2.10.3 Phallic Phase

From around 3 years of age to around the end of the fifth year. Boys pass through the Oedipal complex. Girls develop penis envy and pass through the Electra complex.

9.2.10.4 Latency Stage

From around 5–6 years to the onset of puberty. The sexual drive remains relatively latent during this period.

9.2.10.5 Genital Stage

From the onset of puberty to young adulthood a strong resurgence in the sexual drive takes place. Successful resolution of conflicts from this and previous psychosexual stages leads to a mature well-integrated adult identity.

9.3 CARL JUNG (1875–1961)

Jung founded the psychoanalytic school of *analytic psychology*.

9.3.1 Early Influences

Jung was originally an important member of Sigmund Freud's inner circle and indeed at one time his designated successor.

9.3.2 Differences between Jungian and Freudian Theory

Jung came to different conclusions to Freud on a number of issues, including the following.

9.3.2.1 Libido Theory

Jung did not believe that libido was confined to being sexual, but considered the libido as being the unitary force of every manifestation of psychic energy.

9.3.2.2 Nature of the Unconscious

Jung believed in the *collective unconscious*, later referred to as the *objective psyche*, which he considered contained latent memories of our cultural, racial, and phylogenetic past. In Jungian theory, the objective psyche gives rise to consciousness.

9.3.2.3 Causality

Rather than explaining present events in terms of Freudian psychic determinism, Jungian theory employs

- *Causality*—offers an explanation in terms of the past
- *Teleology*—offers an explanation in terms of the future potential
- *Synchronicity*—offers an explanation in terms of causation at the boundary of the physical world with the psychical ('mystic') world

9.3.2.4 Dreaming

Jungian theory views the contents of dreams within a phylogenetic framework in which archetypes may be projected onto others.

9.3.3 Archetypes

The archetypes of the objective psyche are energy-field configurations manifesting themselves as representational images having universal symbolic meaning and typical emotional and behavioural patterns. Five important types of archetype are identified in Jungian theory.

9.3.3.1 Anima

The feminine prototype within each person.

9.3.3.2 Animus

The masculine prototype within each person.

9.3.3.3 Persona

The outward mask covering the individual's personality and allowing social demands to be balanced with internal needs. Both a public and a private persona may be possessed by a person. The persona may be represented in terms of clothing in dreams.

9.3.3.4 Shadow

This represents repressed animal instincts arising from phylogenetic development and in dreams manifests itself as another person of the same sex.

9.3.3.5 Self

A central archetype holding together conscious and unconscious aspects, including future potential, archetypes, and complexes.

9.3.4 COMPLEXES

Complexes surround archetypes and can be defined as feeling-toned ideas. They develop from an interaction of personal experiences and archetypal models.

9.3.5 MENTAL OPERATIONS

Jungian theory postulates four operations of the mind:

- Feeling
- Intuition
- Sensation
- Thinking

9.3.5.1 Feeling

This allows feelings:

- Anger and joy
- Love and loss
- Pleasure and pain

Judgements regarding good and evil also use this operation.

9.3.5.2 Intuition

This is perception through unconscious processes.

9.3.5.3 Sensation

This allows the acquisition of factual data.

9.3.5.4 Thinking

This is composed of logic and reasoning. It is verbal and ideational.

9.3.6 EXTROVERSION AND INTROVERSION

9.3.6.1 Extroversion

The individual's concerns and mental operations are directed to the objective reality in the external world.

9.3.6.2 Introversion

The individual's concerns and mental operations are directed to the subjective reality of the inner world.

9.3.7 INDIVIDUATION

This is the process of personality growth leading to the development of a unique realization of what one intrinsically is.

9.4 MELANIE KLEIN (1882–1960)

9.4.1 BACKGROUND

Klein, who lacked any formal higher education and never developed a full theory of development, was a controversial figure in the British Psychoanalytical Society. When she began developing her theories, Sigmund Freud viewed her as potentially challenging the work in child analysis of his daughter Anna Freud.

It is now known that Klein analysed her three children and wrote them up as disguised clinical cases. She proposed that the aim of child psychoanalysis was to 'cure' all children of their 'psychoses'.

9.4.2 DIFFERENCES BETWEEN KLEINIAN AND FREUDIAN THEORY

Among the important differences between the theories of Klein and Freud were the following.

9.4.2.1 Object Relations

Klein believed that the infant was capable of object relations.

9.4.2.2 Paranoid-Schizoid Position

Rejecting the critical importance of autoeroticism for the infant, Klein believed instead that the *paranoid position*, later, under the influence of Fairburn, renamed the *paranoid-schizoid position*, developed as a result of frustration during the first year of life with pleasurable contact with objects such as the *good breast*. The paranoid-schizoid position, characterized by isolation and persecutory fears, developed as a result of the infant viewing the world as *part objects*, using the following defence mechanisms:

- Introjection (internalization)
- Projective identification
- Splitting

Objects viewed by the infant as good are believed to be introjected, while those viewed as bad are split or projected.

9.4.2.3 Aggression

A strong emphasis was placed on aggression, occurring particularly during the paranoid-schizoid position.

9.4.2.4 Depressive Position

This is said to develop by the age of 6 months when the child no longer views the world in terms of part objects but realizes that objects are whole and the world is not perfect.

9.4.2.5 Development of the Ego and Superego

The ego and a primitive superego are present, according to Klein, during the first year of life.

9.4.3 EARLY DEVELOPMENT

The stages of development during the first year were considered to include, in chronological order,

- Oral frustration
- *Oral envy* (of parental 'oral' sex) and *oral sadism*, leading to Oedipal impulses
- A longing for the *oral incorporation of father's penis*, by *aggressive desires* to bring about the destruction of mother's body (which contains father's penis)
- *Castration anxiety* in boys and fear of destruction of her own body in girls
- Emergence of the *primitive superego*
- *Introjection* of pain-causing objects
- Development of a *cruel superego*
- Ejection of the superego

9.4.4 ANALYTIC PLAY TECHNIQUE

The analysis of children's play was considered to be the homologue, for children, of the free association technique and dream interpretation for adults.

9.5 DONALD WINNICOTT (1897–1971)

9.5.1 BACKGROUND

Winnicott was a British paediatrician who became a psychoanalyst. He was a contemporary of Anna Freud and Melanie Klein, between whom he at one time tried to mediate. He made important contributions to object relations theory and his reputation has grown steadily since his death.

9.5.2 MOTHER–BABY DYAD

Winnicott believed it was wrong to consider the baby in isolation, noting that there was

> no such thing as an infant (apart from the maternal provision).

9.5.3 COUNTERTRANSFERENCE

9.5.3.1 Objective Countertransference

Winnicott broadened the understanding of the countertransference from that of Freud, speaking of the *objective countertransference*. The objectivity derived from his belief that the countertransference was an understandable and normal reaction to the personality and behaviour of the analysand.

9.5.3.2 Countertransference Hate

Winnicott normalized the existence of countertransference hate. He gave reasons why a mother hates her infant (male or female) even from the start of their relationship. He then drew an analogy from this mother–infant dyad to the therapist–patient relationship. Winnicott suggested that the countertransference hate should be articulated to the analysand at the end of therapy, but most analysts would tend not to go this far.

9.5.4 MOTHERHOOD

9.5.4.1 Good-Enough Mother

The good-enough mother is a mother who responds to her baby's communications and meets his or her needs within an optimal zone of frustration and gratification.

9.5.4.2 Pathological Mother

This is a mother who imposes her own needs over those of her baby, causing her baby to create a *false self* in order to protect his or her *true self*.

9.5.4.3 Capacity to Be Alone

Good parenting by the mother, allowing her child to become increasingly autonomous while at the same time being dependent on her, results in the child being able to be himself or herself in the presence of his or her mother, and vice versa. This was termed the *capacity to be alone* in the presence of another.

9.5.5 TRANSITIONAL OBJECT

This is an object, which is neither oneself nor another person (including mother), that is selected by an infant between 4 and 18 months of age for self-soothing and anxiety reduction. Examples include a blanket or toy that helps the infant go to sleep. It helps during the process of separation–individuation. In adults, transitional phenomena that may allow us to cope with loneliness and separation can include music, religion, and scientific creativity.

9.5.6 OTHER CONCEPTS

Other important concepts associated with Winnicott include

- The *holding environment*—a therapeutic ambiance or setting allowing the patient to experience safety, and so facilitating psychotherapy
- The *potential space*—an area of experiencing identified as existing between the baby and the object; it subsequently underlies all play, imagination, dreams, and the interdependence of transference and countertransference
- The *squiggle game*—a play therapy technique
- At-one-ment
- Primary maternal preoccupation
- Regression to dependence
- Going on being
- Impingement
- Object usage

9.6 PSYCHODYNAMIC THEORY OF DEFENCE MECHANISMS

9.6.1 REPRESSION

The basic defence mechanism, repression is the pushing away (*verdrängung*) of unacceptable ideas, affects, emotions, memories, and drives, relegating them to the unconscious. When successful, no trace remains in consciousness but some affective excitation does remain.

9.6.2 REACTION FORMATION

Psychological attitude diametrically opposed to an oppressed wish and constituting a reaction against it. Often seen in patients with obsessive–compulsive disorder.

9.6.3 ISOLATION

Thoughts/affects/behaviours are isolated so that their links with other thoughts or memories are broken. Often seen in patients with obsessive–compulsive disorder.

9.6.4 UNDOING (WHAT HAS BEEN DONE)

An attempt is made to negate or atone for forbidden thoughts, affects, or memories. This defence mechanism is seen, for example, in the compulsion of magic in patients with obsessive–compulsive disorder.

9.6.5 PROJECTION

Unacceptable qualities, feelings, thoughts, or wishes are projected onto another person or thing. Often seen in paranoid patients.

9.6.6 PROJECTIVE IDENTIFICATION

The subject not only sees the other as possessing aspects of the self that have been repressed but constrains the other to take on those aspects. It is a primitive form of projection.

9.6.7 IDENTIFICATION

Attributes of others are taken into oneself.

9.6.8 INTROJECTION

In fantasy, the subject transposes objects and their qualities from external world into themselves.

9.6.9 INCORPORATION

Another's characteristics are taken on.

9.6.10 TURNING AGAINST THE SELF

An impulse meant to be expressed to another is turned against oneself.

9.6.11 REVERSAL INTO THE OPPOSITE

The polarity of an impulse is reversed in the transition from activity to passivity.

9.6.12 RATIONALIZATION

An attempt to explain in a logically consistent or ethically acceptable way, ideas, thoughts, and feelings whose true motive is not perceived. It operates in everyday life and in delusional symptoms.

9.6.13 SUBLIMATION

A process that utilizes the force of a sexual instinct in drives, affects, and memories in order to motivate creative activities having no apparent connection with sexuality.

9.6.14 IDEALIZATION

The object's qualities are elevated to the point of perfection.

9.6.15 REGRESSION

Transition, at times of stress and threat, to moods of expression and functioning that are on a lower level of complexity, so that one returns to an earlier level of maturational functioning.

9.6.16 DENIAL

Denying the external reality of an unwanted or unpleasant piece of information.

9.6.17 SPLITTING

Dividing 'good' objects, affects, and memories from 'bad' ones. Often seen in patients with borderline personality disorder.

9.6.18 DISTORTION

Reshaping external reality to suit inner needs.

9.6.19 ACTING OUT

Expressing unconscious emotional conflicts or feelings directly in actions without being consciously aware of their meaning.

9.6.20 DISPLACEMENT

Emotions, ideas, or wishes are transferred from their original object to a more acceptable substitute.

9.6.21 INTELLECTUALIZATION

Excessive abstract thinking occurs in order to avoid conflicts or disturbing feelings.

BIBLIOGRAPHY

Freud A. 1936: *The Ego and the Mechanisms of Defence*. London, U.K.: Hogarth Press.

Freud S. 1950: Project for a scientific psychology (1950 [1895]). *The Standard Edition of the Complete Psychological Works of Sigmund Freud, Vol. I (1886–1899)*, pp. 281–391. Pre-Psycho-Analytic Publications and Unpublished Drafts.

Freud S. 1953–1966: *The Standard Edition of the Complete Psychological Works of Sigmund Freud*, Vols. 1–24. London, U.K.: Hogarth Press.

Freud S. 1962: *The Standard Edition of the Complete Psychological Works of Sigmund Freud: Vol. III (1893–1899)*, pp. 11–23. London, U.K.: Hogarth Press.

Freud S. 1984: *On Metapsychology - The Theory of Psychoanalysis: 'Beyond the Pleasure Principle', 'The Ego and the Id' and Other Works*. London, U.K.: Penguin Books.

Freud S. 2010: *The Interpretation of Dreams the Illustrated Edition*. London, U.K.: Sterling Press.

Galison P. 2012: Blacked-out spaces: Freud, censorship and the re-territorialization of mind. *British Journal for the History of Science* 45 (165):235–266.

Hall CS. 1956: *A Primer of Freudian Psychology*. London, U.K.: George Allen & Unwin.

Jung CG. 1961: *Memories, Dreams, Reflections*. New York: Random House.

Jung CG. 1964: *Man and His Symbols*. New York: Doubleday.

Klein M. 1948: *Contributions to Psycho-Analysis, 1921–1945*. London, U.K.: Hogarth Press.

Klein M. 1949: *The Psycho-Analysis of Children*, 3rd edn. London, U.K.: Hogarth Press.

Malan DH. 2001: *Individual Psychotherapy and the Science of Psychodynamics*, 2nd edn. London, U.K.: Arnold.

Ogden TH. 1992: The dialectically constituted/decentred subject of psychoanalysis, II: The contributions of Klein and Winnicott. *International Journal of Psycho-Analysis* 73:613–626.

Segal H. 1980: *Melanie Klein*. New York: Viking Press.

Sklar J. 1989: Dynamic psychopathology. In Puri BK and Sklar J (eds.) *Examination Notes for the MRCPsych Part I*. London, U.K.: Butterworth/Heinemann.

Storr A. 1990: *The Art of Psychotherapy*, 2nd edn. London, U.K.: Hodder Education.

Winnicott DW. 1949: Hate in the counter-transference. *International Journal of Psycho-Analysis* 30:69–74.

Winnicott DW. 1958: *Collected Papers: Through Paediatrics to Psycho-Analysis*. New York: Basic Books.

Winnicott DW. 1965: *The Maturational Processes and the Facilitating Environment*. New York: International Universities Press.

Winnicott DW. 1971: *Playing and Reality*. New York: International Universities Press.

10 History of Psychiatry

10.1 BEFORE COMMON ERA (BCE)

Mental illnesses were perceived as originated from God in the ancient world. There were references to mental disorders in Egyptian papyri in 1500 BCE and in the Old Testament.

In 400 BCE, *Plato* thought that the brain is the seat of mental disorders. *Hippocrates* considered mental disorders to be bodily conditions requiring medical treatment. Hippocrates was the first person to describe mental disturbances as mania and melancholia.

10.2 COMMON ERA

Melancholia was described by a Roman physician, Celsus, as depression caused by black bile.

10.3 MIDDLE AGES

Mental disorders were considered to be spiritual issues rather than medical illnesses. This concept was prominent throughout the Middle Ages.

10.4 1247–1320

In 1247, the *Bethlem hospital* was the first mental hospital in Great Britain to offer care for people who were insane. *The first lunacy (insanity) legislation* was passed in England in 1320.

10.5 1700s

King George III suffered from recurrent mental disorder (possible porphyria) in Great Britain. As a result of the King's mental illness, a committee was appointed by the House of Lords. The committee considered the mental illness of the King and mental illnesses in general. The King was looked after by Francis Willis who ordered physical restraints on the King.

10.6 1790–1830

Popularization of psychiatric treatment included the proposal of removing physical restraints. In 1793, *Philippe Pinel* advised the removal of chain from people who were considered to be mad in Great Britain.

Moral treatment of insanity was promoted after the *Retreat in York*.

In 1811, *Wilhelm Griesinger* established the modern model of the department of psychiatry in Germany. He thought psychiatric illness was a brain disease. He was the first psychiatrist to establish the model of general hospital psychiatry.

In 1812, Benjamin Rush and Samuel Merritt published the first textbook in psychiatry, *Medical inquiries and observations upon the diseases of the mind* (Rush and Merritt, 1812).

Based on Pinel's work, *Esquirol* set up a series of lectures in psychological medicine to teach medical students in Edinburgh in 1823.

In 1827, *Johann Heinroth* was appointed as the first professor in psychological therapy in Leipzig.

Paul Briquet coined the term *hysteria or Briquet syndrome*, which refers to multiple somatization disorder.

10.7 1830–1914

During the *first wave of biological treatments*, the following drugs were discovered: chloral hydrate (a hypnotic) in 1832 and barbiturates in 1903.

10.8 1830s

In 1835, *Phineas Gage* was the first patient to be reported to suffer from frontal lobe syndrome in the medical literature. He suffered from an injury after an iron rod went through his frontal lobe. He was noted to have a personality change but no changes in memory and intelligence. Through his case, the neuroscientists started to have a better understanding of the frontal lobe functions.

10.9 1840s

In 1847, *Wilhelm Griesinger* (1817–1868) defined mental disorder as a disease of the brain by using the *general paralysis of the insane* as an example.

The Association of Medical Officers of Asylums and Hospitals for the Insane was formed in Great Britain. It evolved into the Medico Psychological Association that was the former organization before the establishment of the Royal College of Psychiatrists.

10.10   1850s

Jean-Martin Charcot (1825–1893) is the founder of modern neurology. He coined at least 15 medical eponyms including Charcot–Marie–Tooth disease and amyotrophic lateral sclerosis (Lou Gehrig's disease).

In 1854, *Jules Falret*, a French psychiatrist, described alternating mood and depression as *folie circulaire*.

10.11   1860s

Down syndrome was first described by *Langdon Down* in 1866.

Benedict Morel proposed the *degeneration theory* that stated that mental illness affecting one generation could be passed on to the next in ever-worsening degrees.

Jacob Mendes Da Costa coined the term *Da Costa's syndrome* or 'soldier's heart' during the American Civil War. This condition is a functional heart disease and the soldiers presented with left-sided chest pain, palpitation, breathlessness, sweating, and fatigue during exertion.

10.12   1870s

The following terminologies were coined in schizophrenia during this period: *hebephrenia* by *Ewald Hecker* and *catatonia* by *Karl Ludwig Kahlbaum*.

Paul Broca (1824–1888) coined *Broca's aphasia*, which involves a lesion in the ventroposterior region of the frontal lobe. This leads to Broca's aphasia that affects speech production but not comprehension.

Carl Wernicke (1848–1905) coined *Wernicke's aphasia*. Lesion in the left posterior and superior temporal gyrus leads to impairment in language comprehension.

Sir William Gull (1816–1890) published his work *Anorexia Nervosa* (*Apepsia Hysterica, Anorexia Hysterica*) in 1873 by describing three women presenting with extreme emaciation and amenorrhoea (Silverman, 1997).

10.13   1880s AND 1890s

Psychiatrists at that time were *pessimistic* about the possibilities of cure.

There were developments in neuroanatomy during this period. *Theodor Meynert* was involved in the pioneering work on the microscopic structure of the brain and spinal cord. *Paul Flechsig* studied the basic functional aspects of the cerebral cortex. Wernicke tried to establish specific symptom complex and its association with specific areas of the brain.

Joseph Breuer and *Sigmund Freud* published two books, *Studies on Hysteria* (Freud and Breuer, 1955) and *Interpretation of Dreams* (Marinelli and Mayer, 2003).

In 1882, *Karl Kahlbaum*, a German psychiatrist, coined the term *cyclothymia*.

In 1885, *Georges Gilles de la Tourette* (1857–1904) diagnosed a patient with multiple motor tics, coprolalia and echolalia, to suffer from *Tourette's syndrome*.

In 1897, *Alois Alzheimer* gave a report of neurofibrillary tangles and plaques in a 51-year-old woman with cognitive impairment.

In 1899, *Emil Kraepelin* coined two terms, *dementia praecox* (schizophrenia in modern psychiatry) and *manic–depressive psychosis* (bipolar disorder in modern psychiatry, absence of a dementia, and deteriorating course).

Magnan coined the term *bouffee delirante*, which is an acute delusional psychosis precipitated by stress such as exhaustion. The person may exhibit cyclical mood disturbance. This phenomenon is related to acute and transient psychosis in modern psychiatry.

10.14   1900s

Sigmund Freud was initially studying cases of hysteria using hypnosis. Then he began to develop the technique of *psychoanalysis*, which was later used to explain the psychological causes of symptoms. He helped psychiatrists to establish themselves as an office-based specialty and to wrest *psychotherapy* from the neurologists.

Carl Jung (1916), *Alfred Adler* (1912), and *Pierre Janet* (1903) gave emphasis to the unconscious mind and to underlying sexual motives. They formed the *International Psychoanalytic Association*.

Henry Maudsley (1835–1918) was the first person to propose the abolishment of physical restraints in England. He went on to become one of the best-known psychiatrists during the Victorian era. He believed psychiatric illness to be a physical disorder of the body, similar to other medical illnesses. To him, malformation on the face is a visible sign of underlying cerebral disorganization. He was the editor of the *Journal of Mental Science* that later became the *British Journal of Psychiatry*. He founded the Maudsley Hospital with London County Council.

The concept of *degeneration* emerged. In modern genetics, degeneration is related to the trinucleotide repeat mutations. The mutation causes an illness to descend in the family, and the subsequent generations will have earlier an onset or manifest a more severe form of the illness. Unfortunately, the idea of degeneration was misused and supported social policies such as sterilization, euthanasia, and the persecution of the Jews on the assumption that they were degenerated people.

In 1901, *Ivan Petrovich Pavlov (1849–1936)* proposed *classical conditioning* by demonstrating that the repeated pairing of a conditioned (neutral) stimulus (e.g. food) with an unconditioned stimulus (e.g. bell) will allow the presence of unconditioned stimulus alone to produce the same response (e.g. drooling of saliva) as conditioned stimulus.

In 1908, *Eugen Bleuler (1857–1939)* proposed the term 'schizophrenia'.

In 1909, *Emil Kraepelin (1856–1926)* coined the term *late paraphrenia*, which has a later onset than dementia praecox. This condition is more common in women with sensory impairment.

Pierre Janet (1859–1947) coined the term *psychasthenia* that is composed of anxiety, phobias, obsessions, and neurotic depression.

In the early 1900s, children suffering from encephalitis often developed impulsivity, disinhibition, and hyperactivity. This neuropsychiatric sequela is known as *hyperactive syndrome*.

10.15   1910s

Adolph Meyer (1866–1950) emphasized the need for an eclectic approach combining physical, social, and psychological aspects when treating people with mental illnesses.

The *Mental Deficiency Act* was passed in Great Britain.

William H. R. Rivers (1864–1922) coined the term 'shell shock'. During the First World War (1914–1917), shell shock reached a peak incidence following the Battle of the Somme in 1916. The patient may develop traumatic neurosis as a result of external source or transference neurosis as a result of internal source. As cowardice and desertion were capital offences in the British Army at that time, the military authorities tried to distinguish intentional from non-intentional symptoms. There was debate whether shell shock was an organic disease or a form of malingering. Mott considered that there was a pathological basis for shell shock, consisting of haemorrhages in the brain. Shell shock finally led to an acceptance among the general public that overwhelming stress could lead to illness even among soldiers of previously proven bravery.

The 'malarial fever cure for neurosyphilis' was discovered by *Julius Wagner-Jauregg* and became the first successful physical therapy in psychiatry. Wagner-Jauregg was awarded the Nobel Prize. During that time, there was a deliberate denial of treatment for African Americans with syphilis.

In 1916, *Alfred Binet (1857–1911)* and Lewis Terman from Stanford University proposed *the Stanford–Binet Intelligence Scale* that forms the basis of modern intelligence quotient (IQ) test.

In 1918, *Jean Piaget (1896–1980)* received a doctorate in biology at the age of 22. He proposed cognitive development stages.

The *Maudsley Hospital* was opened in 1919 by Sir Aubrey Lewis (1900–1975). The first academic department of psychiatry in the United Kingdom was opened in Edinburgh.

10.16   1920s

In 1921, the *Serbsky Institute* was founded in Moscow. This institute was used to house political prisoners during the Soviet era, and they were diagnosed to suffer from *progressively sluggish schizophrenia* based on their struggle for truth and justice.

Neurasthenia and related conditions were accepted as disorders for which military pensions could be drawn. In 1924, Mayer-Gross coined the term *oneirophrenia*, which is an acute form of illness characterized by a dreamlike state.

In 1927, *Wilhelm Reich (1897–1951)* was a pioneer of body psychotherapy and several emotion-based psychotherapies. He also laid the foundation for *Gestalt therapy* and *primal therapy*.

Otto Rank (1884–1939) coined the term 'primal anxiety'. Rank was an important figure to move psychotherapy away from psychoanalysis. He developed a more *active and egalitarian psychotherapy* focused on the here-and-now and conscious mind rather than past history, transference, and unconscious.

Development in psychology during this period included the following: *The Little Albert experiment* by *John Watson and Rosalie Rayner, Rorschach inkblot test, systematic desensitization, the theory of emotions* by *Cannon–Bard, psychodrama* by *Jacob Levy Moreno (1889–1974)*, and *Gestalt psychology and psychotherapy* by *Frederick Salomon Perls (1893–1970)*.

The Medico Psychological Association received its Royal Charter.

10.17   1930s

There were developments of new physical therapies during this period:

- *Hydrotherapy* was one of the common methods used to treat agitated patients. The actual spa therapy of psychoses and neuroses was conducted in the hydros.
- *Manfred Sakel (1900–1957)* introduced *insulin coma therapy* that was initially used to treat

drug addiction, but, later, it was widely used to treat schizophrenia. Patients were permitted to spend no more than 20 min in coma before being brought back to consciousness with a sugar solution.

- *Electroconvulsive treatment (ECT)* was introduced by *Ugo Cerletti* (1877–1963) who induced convulsions electronically rather than pharmacologically. *Lucio Bini* (1908–1964) was the first person to perform ECT using bilateral placement of electrodes. ECT was initially used to treat schizophrenia but more widely used for severe depressive illness in the later development.
- In 1935, *psychosurgery* was introduced by Egas Moniz (1874–1955). Moniz got the idea for psychosurgery from the observation that emotional changes occur in a chimpanzee following the ablation of its frontal lobes.

Jacob Kasanin introduced the concept of *schizoaffective illness*.

During the Second World War (1933–1945), the Nazi Germany launched the *operation T4* that killed around 70,000 people suffering from incurable illness (e.g. mental illnesses and learning disability).

In 1935, *Alcoholics Anonymous (AA)* was first established by *Bill Wilson* and *Robert Smith* in the United States with the aim to provide a meeting place and offer support to people with alcohol misuse.

William Herbert Sheldon (1899–1977) studied body types and characters. He classified people as ectomorph, mesomorph, and endomorph somatotypes.

John Bowlby (1907–1990), a British psychoanalyst, studied infant attachment and separation. He proposed the attachment theory.

10.18   1940s

The *National Health Service (NHS)* was formed in the United Kingdom in 1948 and the *Institute of Psychiatry* (IOP) was also established at the Maudsley. The NHS provided a comprehensive system of general practice allowing early treatment and permitting many milder cases of psychiatric disorders to be treated by general practitioners (GPs). Furthermore, the NHS enabled large epidemiology studies to be conducted.

John Cade (1912–1980) injected guinea pigs with urine from patients with mania to see if mania was caused by

a toxic product. *Lithium* was used to dissolve the uric acid prior to injection. Guinea pigs injected with lithium became very placid. In 1949, Cade decided to inject manic patients with lithium.

Paul Hoch and *Philip Polatin* described *pseudoneurotic schizophrenia* (pan-anxiety, pan-neurosis, and pansexuality) that later developed into the concept of *borderline personality disorder*.

In 1943, *Leo Kanner* coined the term *infantile autism* in his classic paper, 'Autistic Disturbances of Affective Contract' (Kanner, 1968).

In 1944, *Hans Asperger* described a syndrome applied to persons with normal intelligence who exhibits a qualitative impairment in reciprocal social interaction and behavioural oddities without delays in language development. He named his syndrome 'autistic psychopathy' that later became *Asperger's syndrome*.

The *ICD-1* was published by the World Health Organization (WHO, 1990).

10.18.1   DEVELOPMENT OF PSYCHOTHERAPIES IN THE 1940s

Maxwell Jones developed *therapeutic community*. The idea came from the Mill Hill Emergency Hospital (London, United Kingdom) that specialized in the treatment of military and civilian shell-shock cases. Doctors would bring patients together in a group to explain to them tactfully about their conditions. Unexpectedly, the discussion group began to affect the social structure of the ward.

Viktor Frankl (1905–1997) developed *existential therapy*. Frankl was a Holocaust survivor. His bestselling book, *Man's Search for Meaning*, described his experiences when he was a concentration camp inmate and the psychotherapeutic method of finding meaning in all forms of existence and the reasons to continue living (Frankl, 2006).

Carl Rogers (1902–1987) developed *client-centred psychotherapy*. This was a unique approach to understand personality and human relationships. It had wide application in psychotherapy and counselling (client-centred therapy), education (student-centred learning), organizations, and group settings.

Joseph Wolpe (1915–1997) enlisted himself in the South African army as a medical officer and he had to treat war neurosis among soldiers. The lack of successful treatment outcomes made him search for an effective treatment. This ultimately led to the concept of *systematic desensitization*.

10.19 1950s

The second wave of biological treatment included the following developments:

- *Donald Ewen Cameron* (1901–1967) conducted the 'depatterning' experiments with sleep therapy and high-dose ECT on people with mild mental illnesses. Unfortunately, Cameron's experiments caused damage to his patients.
- Charpentier synthesized chlorpromazine. Delay and Deniker applied chlorpromazine on patients.
- *Monoamine oxidase inhibitors* (*MAOI*) was introduced in 1957.
- *Imipramine* was introduced in 1958 by *Roland Kuhn* (1912–2005).
- *Haloperidol* and *diazepam* were synthesized.

In 1950, *Erik Erikson* (1902–1994) published a book, *Childhood and Society* (1965). In this book, he presented the *psychosocial theory of development*.

In 1951, *Richard Asher* coined the term 'Munchausen syndrome' in the *Lancet*, referring to a syndrome that patients fabricate symptoms in order to gain admission to the hospital (Asher, 1951). The term 'Munchausen' refers to Baron Münchhausen (1720–1797), a German nobleman who served in the Russian army and fabricated a number of outrageous stories that were not experienced by him but modified from preexisting folktales.

Kurt Schneider (1887–1967) coined the term 'first-rank symptoms' of schizophrenia.

The *Mental Health Act* (*1959*) was passed by the Parliament in England.

10.20 1960s

The mechanisms of action of *antidepressants and antipsychotics* were better understood. The *antipsychotic effect of clozapine* was recognized in the early 1960s. *Amitriptyline* was launched.

Aaron Beck (1921–) introduced cognitive behaviour therapy (CBT).

Token economy was developed during this period.

The movement of anti-psychiatry: People who are anti-psychiatry believed in the sociogenesis of severe mental illness, particularly for schizophrenia. Anti-psychiatry gained popularity in Europe and the United States.

Andreas Rett (1924–1997), an Austrian neurologist, coined the *Rett syndrome* based on 22 girls who developed normally for the first 6 months and followed by devastating developmental deterioration subsequently in their life.

10.21 1970s

The *Royal College of Psychiatrists* was established in 1971 and the *MRCPsych examination* was introduced.

In the United Kingdom, *Gottesman and Shields* performed twin studies in schizophrenia. *Sir Michael Rutter* (1934–) published the *Isle of Wight study* that reported the epidemiology of psychiatric disorders among children (Rutter et al., 1976).

Abraham Maslow (1908–1970) developed humanistic psychology, self-actualization, and the theory of hierarchy of needs.

In 1979, *Gerald Russell* (1928–) established the term *bulimia nervosa* and named the *Russell's sign* that refers to the calluses on the knuckles or dorsal part of the hand as a result of chronic self-induced vomiting.

Clozapine was withdrawn as a result of agranulocytosis.

10.22 1980s

In 1983, the *Mental Health Act* in the United Kingdom introduced consent and approved social workers and a Mental Health Act Commission.

In schizophrenia, *Andreasen* developed the Positive and Negative Syndrome Scale (*PANSS*), and *Liddle* described the three-symptom cluster of schizophrenia (*reality distortion, disorganization, and psychomotor poverty*).

Julian Leff and *Christine Vaughn* performed family studies on *expressed emotion* among relatives of schizophrenia patients.

Kane reintroduced clozapine in the treatment of treatment-resistant schizophrenia.

Fluvoxamine was introduced.

10.23 1990s

There were speculations that *fluoxetine* increased suicide risk in adults with depression but turned out to be a result of poor study design.

Citalopram, moclobemide, paroxetine, sertraline, nefazodone, mirtazapine, venlafaxine, risperidone, olanzapine, and donepezil were introduced during this period.

Marsha Linehan (1943–), an American psychologist, developed the *dialectical behaviour therapy* for people with borderline personality disorder.

Repression of *Falun Gong* took place in China. Ankangs are secure psychiatric hospitals in China where Falun Gong 'dissidents' are 'treated' for the qigong-related mental disorder.

10.24   2000s

'Black box warning' was issued to all *selective serotonin reuptake inhibitors (SSRIs)* (*except fluoxetine*) in causing suicide in adolescents with depression.

Risperidone depot injection, paliperidone, and aripiprazole (D_2 partial agonist) were introduced.

Thioridazine was withdrawn from the market as a result of cardiotoxicity.

There were advances in anti-dementia medication. *Rivastigmine, memantine, and galantamine* were introduced.

Bateman and Fonagy developed the *mentalization-based treatment* for treating people with borderline personality disorder.

In 2007, the *Revised Mental Health Act* in the United Kingdom introduced approved clinicians and mental health professionals.

In 2008, there were major reforms in the *MRCPsych examination*.

In 2013, the *DSM-5* is launched.

BIBLIOGRAPHY

Asher R. 1951: Munchausen's syndrome. *Lancet* 1(6650): 339–341.

Erikson E. 1965: *Childhood and Society*. London, U.K.: Hogarth Press.

Frankl V. 2006: *Man's Search for Meaning*. Boston, MA: Beacon Press.

Freud S and Breuer J. 1955: *Studies on Hysteria (English translation)*. London, U.K.: Hogarth Press.

Gull WW. 1997: Anorexia nervosa (apepsia hysterica, anorexia hysterica). 1868. *Obesity Research* 5(5):498–502.

Johnstone EC, Cunningham ODG, Lawrie SM, Sharpe M, and Freeman CPL. 2004: *Companion to Psychiatric Studies*, 7th edn, pp. 1–7. London, U.K.: Churchill Livingstone.

Kane J, Honigfeld G, Singer J, and Meltzer H. 1988: Clozapine for the treatment-resistant schizophrenic. A double-blind comparison with chlorpromazine. *Archives of General Psychiatry* 45(9):789–796.

Kanner L. 1968: Autistic disturbances of affective contact. *Acta Paedopsychiatrica* 35(4):100–136.

Lieberman EJ. 1985: *Acts of Will: The Life and Work of Otto Rank*. New York, NY: Free Press.

Macnaughton I. (ed.) 2004: *Body, Breath and Consciousness: A Somatics Anthology*. Berkeley, CA: North Atlantic Books.

Marinelli L and Mayer AA. 2003: *Dreaming by the Book: Freud's 'The Interpretation of Dreams' and the History of the Psychoanalytic Movement*, New York, NY: Other Press.

Rush B and Merritt S. 1812: *Medical Inquiries and Observations upon the Diseases of the Mind*. Philadelphia, PA: Kimber & Richardson.

Russell G. 1979: Bulimia nervosa: An ominous variant of anorexia nervosa. *Psychological Medicine* 9(3):429–448.

Rutter M, Tizard J, Yule W, Graham P, and Whitmore K. 1976: Research report: Isle of Wight Studies, 1964–1974. *Psychological Medicine* 6(2):313–332.

Sadock BJ and Sadock VA. 2007: *Kaplan & Sadock's Synopsis of Psychiatry. Behavioral Sciences/Clinical Psychiatry*, 10th edn. Philadelphia, PA: Lippincott Williams & Wilkins.

Shorter E. 1997: *A History of Psychiatry*. New York: John Wiley & Sons.

Silverman JA. 1997: Sir William Gull (1819–1890). Limner of anorexia nervosa and myxoedema. An historical essay and encomium. *Eating and Weight Disorders* 2(3):111–116.

Trevor T. 2010: History of psychiatry. In Puri BK and Treasaden IH (eds.) *Psychiatry: An Evidence-Based Text*, pp. 3–15. London, U.K.: Hodder Arnold.

Watson JB. 1913: Psychology as the behaviorist views it. *Psychological Review* 20:158–177.

Wolpe J and Wolpe D. 1981: *Our Useless Fears*. Boston, MA: Houghton Mifflin Company.

World Health Organization. 1990; History of the development of the ICD. http://www.who.int/classifications/icd/en/HistoryOfICD.pdf

11 Basic Ethics, Principles of Law, and Philosophy of Psychiatry

11.1 ETHICAL STANDARDS AND CODES OF PRACTISE

11.1.1 HIPPOCRATIC OATH

1. A doctor should apply dietetic measures for the benefit of the sick according to his or her ability and judgement.
2. A doctor should keep his or her patients from harm and injustice.
3. A doctor should never give a deadly drug to anyone even that person requests for it.
4. When it comes to patient's care, a doctor should be free of intentional injustice, mischief, and sexual relations with both female and male patients.

11.1.2 DECLARATION OF GENEVA (1948)

1. A doctor should give his or her teachers respects and treat colleagues as brothers or sisters.
2. A doctor should always give the health of his or her patients the first consideration.
3. A doctor should not permit considerations of religion, nationality, race, party politics, or social standing to intervene between his or her duty with patients.
4. A doctor should hold utmost respect for human life from the time of conception.

11.1.3 DECLARATION OF MADRID

1. A doctor should offer the best, evidence-based and the least restrictive treatment to his or her patients with fair allocation of health resources.
2. A doctor should accept his or her patients as partners. The patient should be informed on the purpose of assessment and the doctor should empower his or her patients to make free and informed decisions.
3. If a patient does not have the capacity to make decision, the doctor should consult his or her family or seek legal advice to preserve human dignity and legal rights.

4. A doctor should keep the information obtained from a patient as confidential. Breach of confidentiality is permitted if there is serious harm to the patient or third party. The doctor should inform the patient the actions to be taken if breach of confidentiality is required.
5. Psychiatric patients are vulnerable groups of patients and research should safeguard their autonomy and mental and physical integrity. The principal investigator should seek approval from research ethics committee before commencement of psychiatric research.

11.1.4 ROYAL COLLEGE OF PSYCHIATRISTS

The member should provide the highest standard of professional psychiatric service to patients and follow the College Guidance on Good Psychiatric Practice. The member is committed to the elimination of unlawful discrimination, the promotion of equality of opportunity, and the promotion of good race relations.

11.2 CLASSICAL ETHICAL THEORIES

11.2.1 UTILITARIAN THEORIES

The utilitarian theories emphasize on minimizing the risks and maximizing the benefits for the greatest number (not necessarily the patients). There are two types of utilitarian approach: act utilitarian and rule utilitarian. For example, a patient has thoughts of harming his or her family. In act utilitarian, the psychiatrist may consider disclosing confidential information (e.g. his or her intention to harm) to his or her family or police by providing good or avoiding harm to the greatest number who stay with him or her or near him or her. In rule utilitarian, the rule of confidentiality may act against the rule of protecting others. If the conflict cannot be resolved, it will fall back on the decision of act utilitarian.

There are four subprinciples:

1. Principles of utility: A doctor must maximize the act of doing good.
2. Standard of goodness: A doctor should provide good service to his or her patients and do not vary from patients to patients.
3. Consequentialism: An action is considered to be morally right if it leads to greatest human pleasure, happiness, and satisfaction.
4. Universalism: All parties must receive equal and impartial consideration.

11.2.2 DEONTOLOGICAL THEORIES (AKA THE KANTIAN THEORIES)

The deontological theories emphasize on a doctor's motive to provide morally correct care to his or her patients. The deontological theories focus on the rightness and wrongness of doctor's actions but not on the consequences of the actions. Kant also developed maxims to direct moral action. One example is the universalization of rules. He or she did not allow any exception to wrongful practice such as lying by doctors as this opposes the presupposed practice of truth telling.

11.2.3 VIRTUE THEORIES (PLATO AND ARISTOTLE)

The virtue theories emphasize on the qualities of a personality that make a doctor a caring, compassionate, committed, and conscientious person. Plato and Aristotle regarded the cultivation of virtuous traits such as conscientiousness as the central feature of moral life. For example, a psychiatrist in private practice advises patient to be admitted not for the patient's safety but to earn more money. One cannot find the psychiatrist's advice unethical, but this psychiatrist simply lacks moral character.

11.2.3.1 Ethical Principles

11.2.3.1.1 Autonomy

Autonomy refers to the obligation of a doctor to respect his or her patients' rights to make their own choices in accordance with their beliefs and responsibilities.

11.2.3.1.2 Nonmaleficence

Nonmaleficence refers to the obligation of a doctor to avoid harm to his or her patients.

11.2.3.1.3 Beneficence

Beneficence refers to the fundamental commitment of a doctor to provide benefits to patients and to balance benefits against risks when making such decisions.

11.2.3.1.4 Justice

Justice refers to fair distribution of medical services or resources.

11.2.3.2 Other Ethical Theories

11.2.3.2.1 Duty-Based Approach

The duty-based approach is mainly concerned with the clinicians' obligations under a set of rules.

11.2.3.2.2 Paternalism

The paternalism approach occurs when beneficence overrules autonomy, and it is the duty of a doctor to act in his or her patient's best interests. The word 'paternal' refers to the way that a parent would treat his or her child.

11.2.3.2.3 Prima Facie Duty and Actual Duty

A prima facie duty is a duty that is always to be acted upon unless it conflicts on a particular occasion with an equal or stronger duty. When there is conflict between different ethical principles, an actual duty will be performed by an examination of the respective weights of competing prima facie duties in a particular situation. For example, a psychiatrist always maintains his or her patient's confidentiality (a prima facie duty). One day, one of his patients mentions that he or she has a plan to harm his or her neighbours. Several ethical principles (e.g. the duty of maintaining confidentiality, nonmaleficence, and justice) are in operation. The psychiatrist must weigh in the balance of the competing ethical principles and decide whether to breach confidentiality or not.

11.2.3.2.4 Fiduciary Duty

The fiduciary duty refers to the duty of a doctor who should act in the patient's best interests.

A fiduciary duty exists when a patient places special trust and confidence on a doctor and relies upon the doctor or the fiduciary to exercise his or her discretion or expertise in acting for the patient.

11.2.3.3 Confidentiality and Privileges

Confidentiality refers to the process when a patient entrusts his or her doctor in keeping information private. The patient can consent to or not to release his or her confidential information to the third party. Confidentiality is a right owned by the patient. It is the obligation of the doctor to safeguard his or her patients' confidentiality. Confidentiality is a subset of privacy.

A patient has the privileges to control his or her clinical information and decides what happens to his or her clinical information.

It is the duty of a doctor to be aware of the local legislation safeguarding patients' confidentiality (e.g. the Mental Health Act, Children and Adolescents Act, Family Act, Human Rights Act, Infectious Disease Act, privacy legislation, transportation and criminal laws).

11.2.3.4 Exceptions to Confidentiality

11.2.3.4.1 Duty to Warn and Protect

1. The duty to warn and protect follows the Tarasoff's ruling. The Tarasoff-I (1974) refers to the duty to warn. The Tarasoff-II (1976) refers to the duty to protect.
2. The duty to warn and protect is indicated when
   a. There are sufficient factual grounds for high risk of harm (such as death or substantial bodily harm) to a third party, and the risk is sufficiently specified
   b. The risk of danger to the public is imminent
   c. The harm to a third party is not likely to be prevented unless the mental health professionals make a disclosure
   d. The third party cannot reasonably be expected to foresee or comprehend high risk of harm to himself or herself
3. The duties to community safety override confidentiality. This includes passing confidential information to a government department if public safety is at risk (e.g. homicide, passing communicable diseases such as AIDS or tuberculosis to others, and dangerous driving).

11.2.3.4.2 Mandatory Reporting

Confidence limited by legislation requires mandatory reporting when the protection of the community outweighs the duty to the patient. Indications for mandatory reporting include child protection, abuse of old people, firearm possession, unfit to drive, certain infectious diseases (e.g. HIV), professional–patient boundary violation, and occupational hazards (e.g. sick pilots).

11.2.3.4.3 Court Order

The court can subpoena information and override confidentiality. This can result in ethical dilemma.

A psychiatrist should balance the duty to inform the court and the duty to provide care to a patient. If the testimony is going to cause tremendous damage to the therapeutic relationship, the patient should be evaluated by an independent psychiatrist. Prior to forensic assessment, the psychiatrist should inform the patient regarding to the purpose of assessment and to whom information will be released to.

11.2.3.5 Approaches to Breach Confidentiality

1. Advance notice: The psychiatrist should alert his or her patient that information is to be released and discuss the basis for decision.
2. All limits to confidentiality should be discussed with the patient at the outset of treatment or when mental state becomes stable.

11.2.3.6 Confidentiality in Minors

1. If an informed consent is required from a parent or guardian, a doctor should provide adequate information to the parent or guardian.
2. If a minor undergoes psychotherapy, it is important to explain to the parent or guardian at outset that the information gathered from psychotherapy is confidential and the disclosure of such information will depend on the clinical judgement made by the therapist.
3. When parents divorce, a psychiatrist needs to work with the custodial parent and obtain legal permit when disclosure of information to noncustodial parents is required.

11.3 ETHICS AND PSYCHIATRIC RESEARCH

11.3.1 NUREMBERG CODE (1947)

The Nuremberg Code was developed by war crimes tribunal against Nazi German doctors, and the main objective is to protect human subjects during experiments and research. An experiment should avoid suffering and injury. Experiments leading to death and disability should not be conducted. Proper preparations should be performed to protect research subjects, and the experiments should be conducted by qualified personals. During the experiment, the research subjects have the liberty to withdraw at any time, and the investigators should stop the experiments if continuation results in potential injury or death of research subjects. The design should be based on results obtained from animal experiments and natural history of disease. Seeking consent from research subjects is absolutely necessary. Research should yield meaningful results for the good of mankind.

11.3.2 DECLARATION OF HELSINKI (1964)

The Declaration of Helsinki states the importance of formulation in research protocol and informs the subjects of the protocol details. The principal investigator should balance the predictable risks and foreseeable benefits, to respect integrity and privacy, to obtain consent with liberty and free from undue influence, and to preserve accuracy in publication of results. The principal investigator should obtain consent from the legal guardian if a research subject does not have capacity to give consent.

11.3.3 BELMONT REPORT (1979)

The Belmont Report (Jennifer, 2010) emphasizes on justice. Individual justice requires the researcher to offer beneficial research to all participants independent of his or her personal preference. Social justice requires an order of preference in selection of subjects (e.g. adults before children, less burdened class before burdened class such as institutionalized patients).

11.4 COMPETENCY AND CAPACITY

11.4.1 COMPETENCY

Competence is a legal concept and refers to the capacity to act and understand. Competence is determined by the legal system (e.g. the competence to adopt a child).

11.4.2 CAPACITY

Capacity is a clinical concept and refers to the mental ability to make a rational decision based on understanding and appreciating all relevant information (e.g. testimonial capacity—ability to be a witness).

11.4.2.1 Capacity for Informed Consent

A valid consent has the following properties:

1. A consent is classified as an implicit consent (e.g. verbal consent for blood taking) or an explicit consent (e.g. written consent to participate in a clinical trial).
2. The presence of capacity in a person so that he or she must be able to understand the information and appreciate the foreseeable consequence of a decision and be able to communicate such decision.
3. Informed with clear information (e.g. diagnosis, purpose of proposed treatment, risks and benefits, alternatives, and associated prognosis).
4. Voluntary and without coercion or persuasion.
5. Specific to the issue involved.

It is the responsibility of a doctor to judge whether a patient has the capacity to give a valid consent. The doctor has a duty to provide information in a language understandable by a lay person about a condition, the benefits and risks of a proposed treatment, and alternatives to a treatment. The High Court has held that an adult has capacity to consent to a medical or surgical treatment if he or she can

1. Understand and retain the information relevant to the decision in question.
2. Believe in the information.
3. Weigh the information in balance to arrive at a choice. The person has the right to refuse treatment even though the refusal is contrary to the views of most other people. The decision should be consistent with the individual value system.

11.4.2.1.1 Testamentary Capacity

To make a will, a person must be of *sound disposing mind*. This means that the person must

- Understand to whom he or she is giving personal property
- Understand and recollect the extent of that personal property
- Understand the nature and extent of the claims upon the person, both of those included and of those excluded from the will

A valid will is not invalidated by the subsequent impairment of testamentary capacity.

11.4.2.1.2 Advocacy

An advocate enters into a relationship with the patient, to speak on his or her behalf and to represent the patient's wishes or stand up for his or her rights. An advocate has no legal status—the patient should have an idea of personal preferences so that the advocate truly represents the patient's wishes.

11.4.2.1.3 Appointeeship

An appointee is someone authorized by the Department of Social Security to receive and administer benefits on behalf of someone else, who is not able to manage his or her affairs. It can be used solely to administer money derived from social security benefits and cannot be used to administer any other income or assets. If benefits accumulate, application may need to be made to the Public Trust Office or the Court of Protection to gain access to the accumulated capital.

11.4.2.1.4 Powers of Attorney

A power of attorney is a means whereby one person (the donor) gives legal authority to another person (the attorney) to manage his or her affairs. The donor has sole responsibility for the decision as to whether power of attorney is given, provided the donor fully understands the implications of what he or she is undertaking.

An ordinary power of attorney allows the attorney to deal with the donor's financial affairs generally, or it can be limited to specific matters. An ordinary power of attorney is automatically revoked by law when the donor loses his or her mental capacity to manage personal affairs.

An enduring power of attorney allows a person to decide who should manage his or her affairs if the person becomes mentally incapable. This has been possible since 1985. An enduring power of attorney continues in force after the donor has lost the mental capacity to manage his or her affairs, provided it is registered with the Public Trust Office. It is thus of use for people with early dementia who can set their affairs in order early in the illness provided the illness has not already progressed to a point where the person is unable to manage personal affairs. Once the donor is unable to manage personal affairs, the attorney must apply to the Public Trust Office for registration of the enduring power of attorney to allow the attorney authority to continue to act.

11.4.2.1.5 Court of Protection

This is an office of the Supreme Court. It exists to protect the property and affairs of persons who, through mental disorder, are incapable of managing personal financial affairs. The court's powers are limited to dealing with the financial and legal affairs of the person concerned. Only one medical certificate is required, from a registered medical practitioner who has examined the patient. Guidance to medical practitioners accompanies the certificate of incapacity.

The court appoints somebody to manage the patient's affairs on his or her behalf. This person is called the *receiver*. It may be a relative, friend, solicitor, or other persons. The receiver must keep accounts and spend the patient's money on things that will benefit the patient. The court must give permission before the disposal of capital assets such as property.

11.4.2.1.6 Capacity to Drive

Assessment of capacity to drive should include the following: driving patterns, driving frequency and distances, changes in driving patterns in the past year, number of road traffic accidents, use of seat belt, presence of driving-impairing medical conditions, use of medications known to impair driving, and alcohol use. Basic examination should include mini-mental state examination, neurological examination for gait and balance, Snellen eye chart for vision, whisper test for hearing, and go-and-no-go test for response control.

The responsibility for making the decision about whether or not a person should continue to drive is that of the Driver and Vehicle Licensing Authority (DVLA), with a doctor acting only as a source of information and advice. The driver has a duty to keep the DVLA informed of any condition that may impair the ability to drive. The doctor is responsible for advising the patient to inform the DVLA of a condition likely to make driving dangerous. If the patient fails to take this advice, the doctor may then contact the DVLA directly. Tables 11.1 through 11.3 summarize the advice of the DVLA to British doctors with respect to fitness to drive in patients with psychiatric disorders. In this table, two types of licence are referred to:

- *Group 1 licence.* A driver with a mobility allowance may drive from the age of 16 years. Licences are normally issued until age 70, unless restricted to a shorter duration for medical reasons. There is no upper age limit, but after the age of 70, licences are renewable every 3 years.
- *Group 2 licence.* These licences can be issued at the age of 21 years and are valid until the age of 45. They are then issued every 5 years to the age of 65 unless restricted to a shorter duration for medical reasons. From the age of 65, the licence is issued annually.

11.5 PRINCIPLES OF LAW

11.5.1 Mental Capacity Act (2005) (England and Wales)

Although each country has its own mental health legislation and it is impossible to discuss here, candidates are advised to be familiar with the Mental Capacity Act (2005) in England and Wales that serves as a basic framework for similar legislation. The Mental Capacity Act (2005) provides the legal framework for acting and making decisions on behalf of people who lack the capacity to make specific decisions for themselves in relation to personal welfare, health care, and financial matters. It applies to persons aged 16 and over in England and Wales. The relevant legislation in Scotland is called the Adults with Incapacity Act (2000). The Act draws on the common law principles that have been established through judicial decisions in previous legal cases.

TABLE 11.1

Advice of the DVLA to Doctors with Respect to Fitness to Drive in Patients with Psychiatric Disorders

Psychiatric Disorder	Group 1 Entitlement	Group 2 Entitlement
Neurosis, e.g. anxiety state/depression	DVLA need not be notified. Driving need not cease. Patients must be warned about the possible effects of medication which may affect fitness. However, serious psychoneurotic episodes affecting or likely to affect driving should be notified to DVLA and the person advised not to drive	Driving should cease with serious acute mental illness from whatever cause. Driving may be permitted when the person is symptom free and stable for a period of 6 months. Medication must not cause side effects that would interfere with alertness or concentration. Driving may be permitted also if the mental illness is long standing but maintained symptom-free on small doses of psychotropic medication with no side effects likely to impair driving performance. Psychiatric reports may be required.
Psychosis Schizoaffective Acute psychosis Schizophrenia	Six months off the road after an acute episode requiring hospital admission. Licence restored after freedom from symptoms during this period, and the person demonstrates that he or she complies safely with recommended medication and shows insight into the condition. A 1, 2 or 3 year licence with medical review on renewal. Loss of insight or judgement will lead to recommendation to refusal/revocation of licence.	Recommended refusal or revocation. At least 3 years off driving, during which must be stable and symptom-free and not on major psychotropic or neuroleptic medication, except lithium. Consultant psychiatric examination required before restoration of licence, to confirm that there is no residual impairment; the applicant has insight and would be able to recognize if he or she became unwell. There should be no significant likelihood of recurrence. Any psychotropic medication necessary must be of low dosage and not interfere with alertness or concentration or in any way impair driving performance.
Manic–depressive psychosis	Six to twelve months off the road after an acute episode of hypomania requiring hospital admission, depending upon the severity and frequency of relapses. Licence restored after freedom from symptoms during this period and safe compliance with medication. A 1, 2 or 3 year licence with medical review on renewal. Loss of insight or judgement will lead to recommendation to refusal/revocation of licence.	As aforementioned for psychosis.
Dementia Organic brain disorders, e.g. Alzheimer's disease NB: There is no single marker to determine fitness to drive, but it is likely that driving may be permitted if there is retention of ability to cope with the general day-to-day needs of living, together with adequate levels of insight and judgement.	If early dementia, driving may be permitted if there is no significant disorientation in time and space, and there is adequate retention of insight and judgement. Annual medical review required. Likely to be recommended to be refused or revoked if disorientated in time and space and especially if insight has been lost or judgement is impaired.	Recommended permanent refusal or revocation if the condition is likely to impair driving performance.
Severe mental handicap A state of arrested or incomplete development of mind, which includes severe impairment of intelligence and social functioning	Severe mental handicap is a prescribed disability; licence must be refused or revoked. If stable, mild, to moderate mental handicap, it may be possible to hold a licence, but he or she will need to demonstrate adequate functional ability at the wheel and be otherwise stable.	Recommended permanent refusal or revocation if severe. Minor degrees of mental handicap when the condition is stable with no medical or psychiatric complications may be able to have a licence. Will need to demonstrate functional ability at the wheel.

TABLE 11.1 (continued)

Advice of the DVLA to Doctors with Respect to Fitness to Drive in Patients with Psychiatric Disorders

Psychiatric Disorder	Group 1 Entitlement	Group 2 Entitlement
Personality disorder Including post-head injury syndrome and psychopathic disorders	If seriously disturbed such as evidence of violent outbreaks or alcohol abuse and likely to be a source of danger at the wheel, licence would be refused or revoked. Licence restricted after medical reports that behaviour disturbances have been satisfactorily controlled.	Recommended refusal or revocation if associated with serious behaviour disturbance likely to be a source of danger at the wheel. If the person matures and psychiatric reports confirm stability supportive, licence may be permitted/restored. Consultant psychiatrist report required.

Note: A person holding entitlement to Group I (i.e. motor car/motor bike) or Group II (i.e. LGV/PCV), who has been relicenced following an acute psychotic episode, of whatever type, should be advised as part of follow-up that if the condition recurs, driving should cease and DVLA be notified. General guidance with respect to psychotropic/neuroleptic medication is contained under the appropriate section in the text. Alcohol and illicit drug misuse/dependency are dealt with under his or her specific sections. Reference is made in the introductory page to the current GMC guidance to doctors concerning disclosure in the public interest without the consent of the patient.

11.5.1.1 Principles of the Mental Capacity Act (2005)

The five main principles are as follows:

1. A person must be assumed to have capacity unless it is established that he or she lacks capacity.
2. A person is not to be treated as unable to make a decision unless all practicable steps to help him to do so have been taken without success.
3. A person is not to be treated as unable to make a decision merely because he or she makes an unwise decision.
4. An act done, or decision made, under this Act for or on behalf of a person who lacks capacity must be done, or made, in his best interests.
5. Before the act is done, or the decision is made, regard must be had to whether the purpose for which it is needed can be as effectively achieved in a way that is less restrictive of the person's rights and freedom of action.

11.5.1.2 Three Parts of the Mental Capacity Act (2005)

1. Part 1 contains the main regulatory framework.
2. Part 2 mentions the establishment of a new court to deal with matters arising from the Act (the Court of Protection) and a new office of the Public Guardian. The Court of Protection has the same powers, rights, privileges, and authority as the High Court. The Court of Protection has the powers to

a. Decide whether a person has capacity to make a particular decision for themselves
b. Make declarations, decisions, or orders on financial or welfare matters affecting people who lack capacity to make such decisions
c. Appoint deputies to make decisions for people lacking capacity to make those decisions
d. Decide whether an enduring or lasting power of attorney is valid
e. Remove deputies or attorneys who fail to carry out their duties

3. Part 3 deals with a range of miscellaneous issues relating to the Act (Table 11.4).

11.5.2 Mental Health Act (MHA, 2007) in England and Wales

The MHA (2007) has made the following amendments to the MHA (1983):

1. Mental disorder is defined as any disorder or disability of the mind. The categories of 'mental impairment' and 'psychopathic disorder' were removed.
2. Replacement of 'treatability' and 'care tests' by 'appropriate medical treatments (to alleviate, or prevent a worsening of, the disorder) must be available for the patients'.
3. Civil partners are given the status as nearest relatives.
4. Introduction of supervised community treatment.
5. Sections 2–4 under the MHA (1983) are valid.

TABLE 11.2

Advice of the DVLA to Doctors with Respect to Fitness to Drive in Patients with Alcohol Problems

Alcohol Problem	Group 1 Entitlement	Group 2 Entitlement
Alcohol misuse/alcohol dependency (See note)	Alcohol misuse Alcohol misuse, confirmed by medical inquiry and by evidence of otherwise unexplained abnormal blood markers, requires licence revocation or refusal for a minimum 6 month period, during which time controlled drinking should be attained with normalization of blood parameters. Alcohol dependency Including detoxification and/or alcohol-related fits. Alcohol dependency, confirmed by medical inquiry, requires a recommended 1 year period of licence revocation or refusal, to attain abstinence or controlled drinking and with normalization of blood parameters if relevant Licence restoration Will require satisfactory independent medical examination, arranged by DVLA, with satisfactory blood results and medical reports from own doctors. Patients are recommended to seek advice from medical or other sources during the period off the road.	Alcohol misuse Alcohol misuse, confirmed by medical inquiry and by evidence of otherwise unexplained abnormal blood markers, will lead to revocation or refusal of a vocational licence for at least 1 year, during which time controlled drinking should be attained with normalization of blood parameters. Alcohol dependency Vocational licensing will not be granted where there is a history of alcohol dependency within the past 3 years Licence restoration On reapplication, independent medical examination arranged by DVLA, with satisfactory blood results and medical reports from own doctors. Consultant support/referral may be necessary. If an alcohol-related seizure or seizures have occurred, the vocational Epilepsy Regulations apply.
Alcohol-related seizure(s)	A licence will be revoked or refused for a minimum 1 year period from the date of the event. Where more than one seizure occurs, consideration under the Epilepsy Regulations may be necessary Before licence restoration, medical inquiry will be required to confirm appropriate period free from alcohol misuse and/or dependency.	Vocational Epilepsy Regulations apply (see DVLA guidelines)
Alcohol-related disorders e.g. severe hepatic cirrhosis, Wernicke's encephalopathy, Korsakoff's psychosis	Licence recommended to be refused/revoked.	Recommended to be refused/revoked.

Note: There is no single definition that embraces all the variables in these conditions. But as a guideline, the following is offered: 'a state which because of consumption of alcohol, causes disturbance of behaviour, related disease or other consequences, likely to cause the patient, his family or society harm now or in the future and which may or may not be associated with dependency. In addition, assessment of the alcohol consumption with respect to current national advised guidelines is necessary'.

A person who has been relicenced following alcohol misuse or dependency must be advised as part of his or her follow-up that if his or her condition recurs, he or she should cease driving and notify DVLA medical branch.

High-risk offender scheme for drivers convicted of certain drink/driving offences:

1. One disqualification for drink/driving when the level of alcohol is 2.5 or more times the legal limit.
2. One disqualification that he or she failed, without reasonable excuse, to provide a specimen for analysis.
3. Two disqualifications within 10 years for being unfit through drink.
4. Two disqualifications within 10 years when the level of alcohol exceeds the legal limit. DVLA will be notified by courts. On application for licence, satisfactory independent medical examination with completion of structured questionnaire with satisfactory liver enzyme tests and MCV is required. If favourable, restore for Group I and can recommend issue Group II. For a high-risk offender associated with previous history of alcohol dependency or misuse, after earlier satisfactory examination and blood tests, short-period licence only for ordinary and vocational use is issued, depending on time interval between previous history and reapplication. A high-risk offender found to have current unfavourable alcohol misuse history and/or abnormal blood test analysis would have application refused.

TABLE 11.3

Advice of the DVLA to Doctors with Respect to Fitness to Drive in Patients with Drug Misuse and Dependency

Drug Misuse and Dependency	Group 1 Entitlement	Group 2 Entitlement
Cannabis, ecstasy, and other 'recreational' psychoactive substances, including LSD and hallucinogens	The regular use of these substances, confirmed by medical inquiry, will lead to licence revocation or refusal for a 6 month period. Independent medical assessment and urine screen, arranged by DVLA, may be required	Regular use of these substances will lead to refusal or revocation of a vocational licence for at least a 1-year period. Independent medical assessment and urine screen, arranged by DVLA, may be required
Amphetamines, heroin, morphine, methadone[a], cocaine, benzodiazepines	Regular use of, or dependency on, these substances, confirmed by medical inquiry, will lead to licence refusal or revocation for a minimum 1 year period. Independent medical assessment and urine screen, arranged by DVLA, may be required. In addition, favourable consultant or specialist report will be required on reapplication	Regular use of, or dependency on, these substances will require revocation or refusal of a vocational licence for a minimum 3 year period. Independent medical assessment and urine screen, arranged by DVLA, may be required. In addition, favourable consultant or specialist report will be required before relicensing
Seizure(s) associated with illicit drug usage	A seizure or seizures associated with illicit drug usage may require a licence to be refused or revoked for a 1 year period. Thereafter, licence restoration will require independent medical assessment, with urine analysis, together with favourable report from own doctor, to confirm no ongoing drug misuse. In addition, patients may be assessed against the Epilepsy Regulations	Vocational Epilepsy Regulations apply

NB: A person who has been relicenced following illicit drug misuse or dependency must be advised as part of his or her follow-up that if his or her condition recurs, he or she should cease driving and notify DVLA medical branch.

[a] Applicants or drivers on consultant-supervised oral methadone withdrawal programme may be licenced, subject to annual medical review and favourable assessment.

6. The MHA (2007) emphasizes that primary care trusts should have the responsibility to provide 'age-appropriate' services for children. This includes guidelines for good practice and the use of Child and Adolescent Mental Health Services (CAMHS) in the assessment process. The law on the admission to hospital and treatment of mental disorders of children (under 16) is based on parental responsibility and the Human Rights Act (1998).

7. The admission of young people (aged 16–17) is influenced by the Gillick competence when the young person has achieved a certain level of intelligence and consent for admission. The Family Law Reform Act (1969) indicates that the earlier process does not require parental consent. If an at-risk young person refuses admission, the parents, the legal guardians, or the court can override the young person's decision. If both the young person and parents refuse admission but the young person is at high psychiatric risk, the psychiatrist may consider applying for compulsory admission under the MHA (2007) or seeking an opinion from the court (Tables 11.5 through 11.9).

TABLE 11.4

Summary of the Relevant Sections of the Mental Capacity Act (2005) for Psychiatric Practice in England and Wales

Section Number	Main Principle	Details
Part I Sections 2 and 3	Determining capacity	These sections set out the legal requirement for assessing capacity. The concept builds on the common law test for capacity
Part I Section 4	The best interest principle	This section expands on the principle that any act or decision on behalf of a person who lacks capacity should be made in the person's best interests. This follows the common law principle, but the Act is more specific about the process and the best interest checklist must be followed
Part I Section 5	Connection with care or treatment	This section sets out the conditions under which a person caring for someone who lacks capacity will not incur liability for their actions in caring for that person
Section 6	Restraining a person who lacks capacity	This section sets out the additional conditions that must be fulfilled if a person who lacks capacity is to be restrained. This section considers the degree of harm that is likely to be suffered by the person if he or she is not restrained
Part I Section 9	Lasting powers of attorney	This section creates a new power, the lasting powers of attorney, by which a person who has capacity can confer authority on another person (the donee) to make decisions about his or her personal welfare, property, or affairs at a future date when he or she no longer has the capacity to make decisions. This is a new power in England and Wales and was not legally possible under the common law
Part I Sections 24–26	Advance decisions to refuse treatment	These sections set out the legal framework within which a person with capacity can make an advance decision to refuse treatment (including life-sustaining treatment) that is applicable when that person no longer has the capacity to make such decision. This clarifies and sets in statute the legal position on advance refusals of treatment
Part I Sections 30–34	Research	These sections set out the legal framework within which researchers must act if they are conducting research that involves persons who lack capacity to consent to the research being conducted
Part I Sections 35–41	Independent Mental Capacity Advocates (IMCAs)	These sections introduce and set out the role of IMCA. This is a new service created under the Act. Its aim is to provide independent safeguards for people who lack capacity when important decisions need to be made and there is no other person except the designated carer to represent the person who lacks capacity or to be consulted on his or her behalf
Part I Section 44	The offence of ill treatment or neglect	This section creates an offence of ill treatment or neglect. If a carer or donee of a lasting power of attorney is found guilty, he or she is liable to imprisonment of up to 5 years or a fine (or both)

11.6 PHILOSOPHY OF PSYCHIATRY

11.6.1 PHILOSOPHY AND SCIENCE

Philosophy is concerned with conceptual problems and science is concerned with empirical problems. Science and philosophy can work productively together and complement each other.

There are two types of logic. Formal logic is concerned with the form of arguments and it is context-free. A valid argument is independent of any specific context. Informal logic, on the other hand, cannot remove itself from the context where the arguments take place.

11.6.2 FORMAL AND INFORMAL LOGIC

Consider the following example:

1. If I have many years of life experience, I will be intelligent.
2. If I am an old person, I should have many years of experience.
3. Therefore, if I am an old person, I should be intelligent.

The earlier arguments are valid in formal logic. Informal logic is concerned with the context of an argument,

TABLE 11.5

Relevant Sections of the MHA (1983/2007) for Psychiatric Practice in England and Wales

Section Number	Purpose	Duration	Grounds
2	Admission for assessment or assessment followed by treatment	Up to 28 days from admission	1. Mental disorder that warrants detention in hospital for assessment. 2. Admission is necessary in interests of the patient's own health, or safety, or for the protection of others
3	Admission for treatment	Up to 6 months, renewable after 6 months and then annually	1. The mental disorder is of a nature or degree, which makes it appropriate for the patient to receive medical treatment in hospital 2. Admission is necessary for the health, or safety, of the patient or for the protection of others 3. Medical treatment is likely to alleviate or prevent deterioration in the patient's condition
4	Emergency admission for assessment	Up to 72 h from admission and Section 2 may apply after admission	1. Mental disorder that warrants detention in hospital for assessment 2. Admission is necessary in the interests of the patient's own health or safety or for the protection of others

TABLE 11.6

Consent to Treatment under MHA (1983). Consent to Treatment Should Be Informed and Voluntary (Implies Mental Illness, e.g. Dementia, Does Not Affect Judgement)

Type of Treatment	Informal	Detained
Urgent treatment	No consent	No consent
Section 57: Irreversible, hazardous, or nonestablished treatments (e.g. psychosurgery such as leucotomy), hormone implants (for sex offenders), surgical operations (e.g. castration)	Consent and second opinion	Consent and second opinion
Section 58: Psychiatric drugs, ECT	Consent	Consent or second opinion

Source: Reproduced from Puri, B.K. and Treasaden, I.H., *Textbook of Psychiatry*, 3rd edn., Churchill Livingstone, Edinburgh, U.K., 2011. With permission.

Notes: 1. For first 3 months of treatment, a detained patient's consent is not required for Section 58 medicines but is required for ECT.
2. Patients can withdraw voluntary consent at any time.

and this example suggests the context of an argument can have an important effect. Informally, we are doubtful of these arguments. It is unclear that the possession of many years of life experience refers to intelligence. Furthermore, it is not necessarily true that an old person having many years of life experience is correlated with intelligence and the old person may suffer from dementia. The fallacy of formal logic illustrates that all humans are prone to faults of reasoning.

11.6.3 PHILOSOPHY OF ANTI- AND PROPSYCHIATRY

11.6.3.1 Philosophy of Antipsychiatry (Fulford et al., 2006)

1. *The psychological model.* Mental illness is not a disorder but learned abnormalities of behaviour.
2. *The labelling model.* The clinical features of mental disorder are responses of an individual to being labelled as deviant. This model fails to explain the

TABLE 11.7
Civil Treatment Orders under MHA (1983)

Section	Grounds	Application by	Medical Recommendations	Maximum Duration	Eligibility for Appeal to Mental Health Review Tribunal
Section 2: Admission for assessment	Mental disorder	Nearest relative or approved social worker	Two doctors (one approved under Section 12)	28 days	Within 14 days
Section 3: Admission for treatment impairment, severe mental impairment (if psychopathic disorder or mental impairment, treatment must be likely to alleviate or prevent deterioration)	Mental illness, psychopathic disorder, mental disorder	Nearest relative or approved social worker	Two doctors (one approved under Section 12)	6 months	Within first 6 months. If renewed, within second 6 months, then every year. Mandatory every 3 years.
Section 25 Supervised discharge. Hospital managers cannot discharge.	Same as Section 3	CRMO	Social worker, one doctor	If renewed, 6 months	Within first 6 months. Renewable for 6 months, then every year.
Section 4 Emergency admission for assessment	Mental disorder (urgent necessity)	Nearest relative or approved social worker	Any doctor	72 h	
Section 5(2) Urgent detention of voluntary in-patient	Danger to self or to others	Doctor in charge	72 h of patient's care		
Section 5(4) Nurses holding power of voluntary in-patient	Mental disorder (danger to self, health or others)	Registered mental nurse or registered nurse for mental handicap	None	6 h	
Section 136 Admission by police	Mental disorder	Police officer	Allows patient in public place to be removed to 'place of safety'	72 h	
Section 135 entry to home and removal of patient to place of safety	Mental disorder	Magistrates	Allows power of	72 h	

Source: Reproduced from Puri, B.K. and Treasaden, I.H., *Textbook of Psychiatry*, 3rd edn., Churchill Livingstone, Edinburgh, U.K., 2011. With permission.

onset of psychiatric illness but explains maintaining factors that inhibit recovery.

3. *The hidden meaning model.* This model argues that the apparently meaningless or nonunderstandable symptoms of people with schizophrenia can be understood, once the origins and underlying context in the patient's past experiences are recognized. Psychiatric symptoms are not signs of illnesses but contain hidden meanings.

4. *The unconscious mind model.* Mental illness is not a disorder but a product of unconscious mental activities such as unconscious motives, reasons, desires, and fantasies.

5. *The political control model.* The boundary between mental illness and normality is debatable and often set by authority. For example, the authority wants to separate people with antisocial personality disorder and sexual deviance from the norm even in a democratic society. In some political regimes, political dissidence has been the basis of attributions of madness.

TABLE 11.8
Forensic Treatment Orders for Mental Abnormally Offenders

Section	Grounds	Made By	Medical Recommendations	Maximum Duration	Eligibility for Appeal to Mental Health Review Tribunal
Section 35: Remand to hospital for report Maximum 12 weeks	Mental disorder	Magistrates or Crown Court	Any doctor	28 days Renewable at 28 day intervals	
Section 36: Remand to hospital for treatment Maximum 12 weeks	Mental illness, severe mental impairment (not if charged with murder)	Crown Court	Two doctors: one approved under Section 12	28 days Renewable at 28 day intervals	
Section 37: Hospital and guardianship orders Accused of, or convicted for, an imprisonable offence	Mental disorder. (If psychopathic disorder or mental impairment must be likely to alleviate or prevent deterioration.)	Magistrates or Crown Court	Two doctors, one approved under Section 12 and then annually	6 months Renewable for further 6 months	During second 6 months, then every year. Mandatory every 3 years
Section 41: Restriction order. Effect: leave, transfer, or discharge only with consent of Home Secretary	Added to Section 37 To protect public from serious harm	Crown Court	Oral evidence from one doctor	Usually without limit of time	As Section 37
Section 38: Interim hospital order Section 12: Maximum 6 months	Mental disorder For trial of treatment intervals	Magistrates or Crown Court	Two doctors: one approved under	12 weeks Renewable at 28 day intervals	None
Section 47: Transfer of a sentenced prisoner to hospital	Mental disorder	Home Secretary	Two doctors: one approved under Section 12	Until earliest date of release from sentence	Once in the first 6 months, then once in the next 6 months. Thereafter, once a year.
Section 48: Urgent transfer to hospital of remand prisoner	Mental disorder	Home Secretary	Two doctors: one approved under Section 12	Until date of trial	Once in the first 6 months, then once in the next 6 months. Thereafter, once a year.
Section 49: Restriction direction. Effect: leave, transfer, or discharge only with consent of Home Secretary	Added to Section 47 or 48	Home Secretary	—	Until end of Section 47 or 48	As for Sections 47 and 48 to which applied.

Source: Reproduced from Puri, B.K. and Treasaden, I.H., *Textbook of Psychiatry*, 3rd edn., Churchill Livingstone, Edinburgh, U.K., 2011. With permission.

Thomas Szasz (1920–2012), a prominent anti-psychiatrist, identifies mental illness as problematic and somatic illnesses as unproblematic. In a society, bodily illness is a genuine illness, and genuine illness is defined by deviation from normal anatomy and physiology of a body organ. On the other hand, Szasz believes that mental illnesses are defined by deviation from social norms in terms of acceptable behaviours. Hence, mental illness is very different in its meaning and nature from a physical illness. Robert Kendell (1935–2002), a prominent pro-psychiatrist, argued that the value ladenness of mental illness can be translated into value-free factual norms. Hence, mental illness is essentially no different from physical illness.

TABLE 11.9
Other Legislations Relevant to Mental Health Services in the United Kingdom

Legislations	Details of the Legislation	Influence on Psychiatric Practice
The Human Rights Act (1998)	Article 8: Rights to respect for private and family life. Everyone has the rights to respect for his or her private and family life, his or her home, and his or her correspondence There shall be no interference by a public authority with the exercise of these rights except in the threat of national security and public safety, for the prevention of disorder or crime, for the protection of health or morals	Clinical decisions must be proportional and balance the severity of the effect of an intervention with the severity of the presenting clinical problem The Mental Health Review Tribunals should refer to the Human Rights Act when deciding the time limit of involuntary hospitalization For children, their consent for treatment is viewed from the human rights perspective and should be taken into consideration when a decision is made between the psychiatrist and their parents or legal guardian
The Disability Discrimination Act (2005)	1. Definition of disability: A disabled person suffers from physical or mental impairment, with substantial and long-term adverse effect on a person's ability to carry out normal day-to-day activities. 2. Protection of disabled people from discrimination in employment. 3. Protection of disabled people from discrimination in the provision of goods, services, and facilities. 4. Protection of disabled people from discrimination in education.	This law offers protections for mental health service users against discrimination in employment and purchasing insurance Psychiatrists should inform people with mental health problems on their rights and support them in job application
The Children Act (2004)	The Children Act (2004) places a duty on health services to ensure that every child, whatever their background or circumstances, to 1. Be healthy. 2. Stay safe. 3. Enjoy and achieve through learning.	If a child is suspected to be a victim or abused or in danger as a result of parental psychiatric illnesses, the social worker can apply the Children Act for Emergency Placement order to remove the child and place the child in a safe environment. The duration of the emergency order ranges from 7 to 14 days.

BIBLIOGRAPHY

Appelbaum PS and Gutheil TG. 2007: *Clinical Handbook of Psychiatry and the Law*, 3rd edn. Philadelphia, PA: Lippincott Williams & Wilkins.

Beauchamp TL. 1998: The philosophical basis of psychiatric ethics. In Bloch S, Chodoff P, and Green SA (eds.) *Psychiatric Ethics*, 3rd edn, pp. 25–48. Oxford, U.K.: Oxford University Press.

Bloch S, Chodoff P, and Green SA. 1998: *Psychiatric Ethics*, 3rd edn. Oxford, U.K.: Oxford University Press.

Bloch S and Green SA. 2006: An ethical framework for psychiatry. *The British Journal of Psychiatry* 188:7–12.

Curtice M. 2009: Article 8 of the Human Rights Act 1998: Implications for clinical practice. *Advances in Psychiatric Treatment* 15:23–31.

Forciea MA, Schwab EP, Raziano DB, and Lavizzo-Mourey RJ. 2004: *Geriatric Secrets*. Philadelphia, PA: Hanley & Belfus.

Fulford B, Thornton T, and Graham G. 2006: *Oxford Textbook of Philosophy and Psychiatry*. Oxford, U.K.: Oxford University Press.

Gelder M, Mayou R, and Cowen P. 2001: *Shorter Oxford Textbook of Psychiatry*. Oxford, U.K.: Oxford University Press.

Green SA. 1998: The ethics of managed mental health care. In Bloch S, Chodoff P, and Green SA (eds.) *Psychiatric Ethics*, 3rd edn, pp. 401–422. Oxford, U.K.: Oxford University Press.

Jennifer S. 2010: A brief review of the Belmont report. *Dimensions of Critical Care Nursing* 29(4):173–174.

Joseph DI and Onet J. 1998: Confidentiality in psychiatry. In Bloch S, Chodoff P, and Green SA (eds.) *Psychiatric Ethics*, 3rd edn. Oxford, U.K.: Oxford University Press.

Office of Public Sector Information, U.K. http://www.opsi.gov.uk (accessed on 20 June 2012).

Sayce L and Boardman J. 2003: The disability discrimination act 1995: Implications for psychiatrists. *Advances in Psychiatric Treatment* 9:397–404.

The U.K. Clinical Ethics Network. http://www.ethics-network.org.uk/educational-resources/mental-capacity-act-2005 (accessed on 20 June 2012).

12 Neurology and Neurological Examination

12.1 CRANIAL NERVES (CNs II, III, IV, AND VI) AND THE VISUAL SYSTEM

12.1.1 CENTRAL VISUAL PATHWAY AND VISUAL FIELD DEFICITS

The examination of visual field is performed by asking the patient to cover one eye and fixate on the examiner's opposite eye. Then the examiner tries to map the visual field by bringing his or her finger from the periphery to the boundary of the visual field. This will repeat for the four quadrants (i.e. from upper right, upper left, lower right, and lower left to the centre) (Figure 12.1).

12.1.1.1 Common Lesions in the Central Visual Pathway

1. The axons of retinal ganglion cells assemble at the optic disc and pass into the optic nerve (CN II). Lesion in the optic nerve at this location is associated with unilateral visual field loss (i.e. monocular blindness).
2. The two optic nerves converge to form the optic chiasma at the base of the brain. Lesion at the optic chiasma is associated with bitemporal hemianopia.
3. The optic nerves from nasal hemiretinae decussate and pass into the contralateral optic tract. The optic nerves from the temporal hemiretinae remain ipsilateral. Lesion of the optic nerves at this location is associated with incongruent homonymous hemianopia.
4. Most optic tract fibres pass around the cerebral peduncle to terminate in the lateral geniculate body of the thalamus. Some of the optic tract fibres involving in papillary light reflex terminate in the pretectal area and superior colliculus. Lesion in the Meyer's loop is associated with superior homonymous quadrantanopia.
5. The optic radiations are the projection from the internal capsule to the primary visual cortex that locates on the medical surface of the occipital lobe below the calcarine sulcus. Lesion in the optic rations is associated with inferior homonymous quadrantanopia.

An object produces a visual image upon the nasal hemiretina of the ipsilateral eye and the temporal hemiretina of the contralateral eye. The upper half of the visual field forms images upon the lower halves of the retinae and the lower visual field upon the upper hemiretinae.

12.2 CRANIAL NERVES (CNs III, IV, AND VI) AND DOUBLE VISION

After examining the visual field, the examiner can ask the patient (without covering the eye) to follow his or her finger to the left, upper left corner, lower left corner, right, upper right corner, and lower right corner of the visual field. The examiner needs to observe the eye movements and the patient is asked to report any double vision. Weakness of the extraocular muscles results in double vision in the direction of movement of that muscle. Ask the patient to cover each eye in turn to identify the eye that can see the outer image. This will indicate the location of lesion. If double vision does not confirm to originate from a single cranial nerve (CN), differential diagnoses such as myasthenia gravis and thyroid eye disease should be considered.

If the double images are horizontally displaced and parallel, this indicates a weakness in the lateral or medial muscles (see Figure 12.2a).

If the double images are at an angle, the other muscles such as inferior oblique/superior rectus or superior oblique/inferior rectus are affected (see Figure 12.2b).

12.2.1 OCULOMOTOR NERVE (CN III)

The oculomotor nerve nucleus is located in the midbrain. The autonomic components involve in focusing of vision and pupillary constriction.

Oculomotor nerve palsy is caused by tumour or aneurysm. Ptosis occurs with failure to elevate the eyelids. The pupil is dilated and remains unresponsive to light

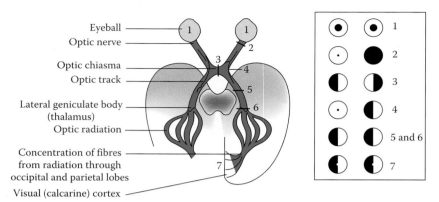

FIGURE 12.1 Optic nerve and pathways to the visual cortex: 1, pathology in the eye (e.g. glaucoma)—tunnel vision (damage to peripheral field); 2, damage to optic nerve—unilateral blindness; 3, damage to optic chiasma (e.g. pituitary tumour)—bitemporal hemianopia; 4, damage to lateral chiasma (e.g. aneurysms)—nasal blindness on same side; 5 and 6, tumours and trauma to unilateral optic tract—blindness of opposite visual field (homonymous hemianopia); 7, cortical damage may not destroy macular vision. (From Abrahams, P.H. et al., *Illustrated Clinical Anatomy*, CRC Press, Oxford, U.K., 2005, p. 328.)

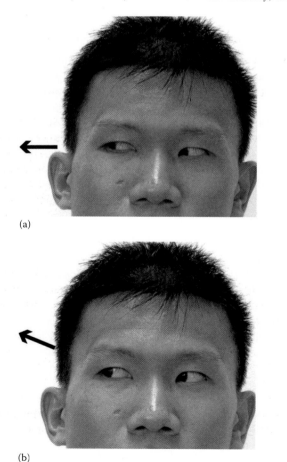

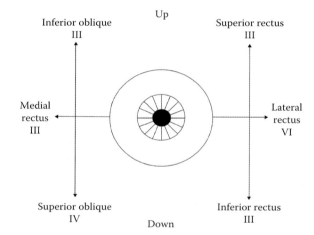

FIGURE 12.3 The motor functions of CNs III, IV, and VI.

and accommodation. Extraocular muscle palsies are found in the upward, downward, and inward gaze (i.e. failure in adduction) (Figure 12.3).

12.2.2 TROCHLEAR NERVE (CN IV)

The trochlear nerve nucleus is found in the midbrain.

Trochlear nerve palsy is caused by tumour or aneurysm and results in difficulty in moving the eye downward and medially.

12.2.3 ABDUCENS NERVE (CN VI)

The abducens nerve nucleus is found in the pons.

Abducens nerve palsy is caused by tumour or aneurysm and leads to extraocular muscle palsy in outward gaze (i.e. failure in abduction).

FIGURE 12.2 The relative position of the images in diplopia and location of lesions. (a) Double images are horizontally displaced and parallel. (b) Double images are at an angle.

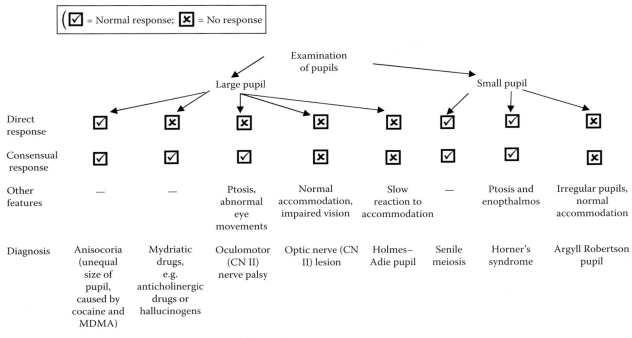

FIGURE 12.4   Summary of the examination of the pupils.

12.2.4   MEDIAL LONGITUDINAL FASCICULUS

Lesion in the medial longitudinal fasciculus (MLF) does not produce double vision but produces upgaze, downgaze, and lateral gaze paresis. This lesion is associated with internuclear ophthalmoplegia (INO). In lateral gaze, the ipsilateral eye can abduct but the contralateral eye cannot adduct. INO is associated with ataxic nystagmus.

The combined CN III, IV, and VI palsies lead to ptosis and dilation of the pupil, which is unresponsive to light and accommodation. The combined palsies may lead to paralysis of all eye movement.

12.2.4.1   Examination of the Pupils and Related Conditions

12.2.4.1.1   *Three-Step Approach When Assessing the Pupils*

1. Assess the size of the two pupils: large, normal, or small size.
2. Ask the patient to look into the distance and shine the torch twice in each eye in turn:
   a. The response of the eye where the torch is directly shone into is known as the *direct response*.
   b. The response of the other eye is known as the *consensual response*.

3. Ask the patient to look at your finger held at 15 cm from the patient's face. The presence of constriction is known as *accommodation response*. If there is no response in step 2 but a normal response in step 3, this is known as an *afferent pupillary defect*, which involves the optic nerve (CN II) (Figure 12.4).

12.2.4.1.2   *Pathologies of the Pupils and Optic Disc*
12.2.4.1.2.1   *Holmes–Adie Pupil*
Clinical features: Unilateral (80% of cases), moderately dilated, poor reaction to light, and slow reaction to accommodation. It is associated with diminished and absent knee jerk.

12.2.4.1.2.2   *Hutchison's Pupil*
Aetiology: Caused by rapidly rising unilateral intracranial pressure (e.g. intracerebral haemorrhage).

Clinical features: Dilated and unreactive on the side of an intracranial mass lesion as a result of compression of the oculomotor nerve (CN IIII) on the ipsilateral side.

12.2.4.1.2.3   *Argyll Robertson Pupil*
Aetiology: Neurosyphilis and diabetes mellitus.

Clinical features: Constricted pupils, unreactive to light but reactive to accommodation.

12.2.4.1.2.4 Horner's Syndrome

Aetiology: Brain stem stroke, Pancoast tumour at the lung apex, and carotid dissection.

Pathology: Lesion to the sympathetic supply to the eye at the central brain stem (e.g. medulla), cervical spine, cervical ganglion, and carotid body.

Clinical features: Meiosis (a constricted pupil), anhidrosis, and partial ptosis.

12.2.4.1.2.5 Papilloedema

Aetiology: Increased in intracranial pressure (tumour, abscess, encephalitis, hydrocephalus, benign intracranial hypertension) and retro-orbital lesion (e.g. cavernous sinus thrombosis).

Clinical features: Swelling of the optic discs is identified during the fundoscopy examination.

12.2.4.1.2.6 Nystagmus

Nystagmus refers to rhythmic to-and-fro movement of the eyes. Different types of nystagmus are listed as follows:

12.2.4.1.2.7 Different Types of Nystagumus

Ataxic Nystagmus

Cause: Internuclear ophthalmoplegia (INO)

Multidirectional jerk nystagmus

Cause: Central vestibular syndrome (e.g. phenytoin toxicity)

Unidirectional jerk nystagmus

Cause: Central or peripheral vestibular syndromes

Pendular nystagmus (symmetrical in primary gaze)

Cause: Albinism, coal miners

12.2.5 TRIGEMINAL NERVE (CN V)

1. *The ophthalmic branch.* This supplies from the tip of the nose to the forehead and vertex, including the cornea. If a cotton wool touches the cornea, it will lead to a brisk contraction of both orbicularis oculi. This response is known as the corneal reflex. A lesion in this branch leads to loss of the corneal reflex.
2. *The maxillary branch.* This supplies the cheek to the angle of the jaw (including the inner aspect of the mouth and the upper palate).

3. *Physical examination.* Trigeminal nerve can be tested by asking the patient to clench their teeth and feel the masseter and temporalis (Figure 12.5).
4. *The mandibular branch.* This supplies the lower jaw but not the angle of the jaw.
5. *Sensory function.* Cutaneous sensation from the anterior part of the head including teeth, cornea, sinuses, meninges, and mouth. In *herpes zoster*, the sensory root is infected and leads shingles (i.e. pain and eruption of vesicles located on a dermatome).
6. The cell bodies of afferents are located in the *semilunar (trigeminal) ganglion* where the convergence of ophthalmic, maxillary, and mandibular nerves lies. The sensory information will be sent to the *trigeminal sensory nucleus*, which is distributed throughout the brain stem. There is a separation of affect fibres: fibres conveying touch and pressure terminate in the principal nucleus, while those carrying pain and temperature terminate in the spinal nucleus.
7. Then the nerves will decussate to the contralateral trigeminothalamic tract and terminate in the contralateral *ventral posterior nucleus of*

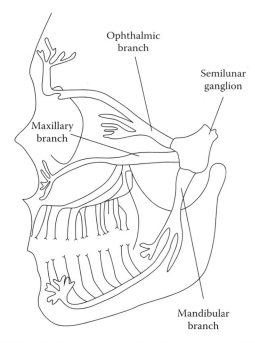

FIGURE 12.5   The anatomy of the trigeminal nerve (CN V).

the thalamus. The sensory information will be sent to the sensory cortex of parietal lobe. In *syringobulbia*, there is a compressive destruction of the decussating trigeminothalamic tract that leads to selective loss of pain and temperature in the face.

8. *Motor function*: Mastication and movement of the soft palate. The motor cell bodies are located in the mesencephalic nucleus of the trigeminal, which sends fibres to the cerebellum to facilitate movement coordination.

12.2.6 Facial Nerve

1. The facial nerve has three components (Figure 12.6):
   a. *Sensory component*: to detect taste on the anterior 2/3 of the tongue.
   b. *Motor component*: facial expression, elevation of hyoid tension of stapes muscle, and corneal reflex. Lesion affects reflex on the ipsilateral side of the face.

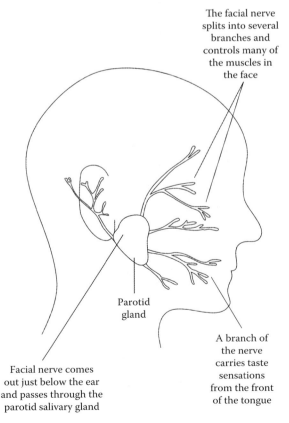

The facial nerve splits into several branches and controls many of the muscles in the face

Parotid gland

A branch of the nerve carries taste sensations from the front of the tongue

Facial nerve comes out just below the ear and passes through the parotid salivary gland

FIGURE 12.6   The anatomy of facial nerve (CN VII).

   c. *Autonomic component*: causing lacrimation and salivation from the sublingual and submandibular glands.

2. The facial nerve joins the brain stem at the cerebellopontine angle.

   Cell bodies of primary afferent lie in the *geniculate ganglion* in the facial canal of the petrous temporal bone. The fibres terminate in the nucleus solitarius of the medulla and project to the ventral posterior nucleus of the thalamus. The information will be sent to the parietal lobe.

3. The corticobulbar fibres from the motor cortex innervate the facial motor nucleus, which supplies the muscles of the bilateral upper face (frontalis, orbicularis oculi), while the lower face is supplied by contralateral fibres. Hence, upper motor and lower motor neuron lesions (UMNL and LMNL) lead to different consequences as illustrated in Figure 12.7.

4. Postganglionic fibres from the pterygopalatine ganglion innervate the lacrimal gland and the nasal and oral mucous membrane.

Figure 12.7a shows the facial features of the right-sided UMNL. The signs include sparing of the forehead muscles, weakness of the lower face, loss of nasolabial fold, and drooping of the mouth.

Figure 12.7b shows that facial features of the right-sided LMNL or Bell's palsy. All facial muscles are affected. Other signs include loss of eyebrow lines, inability to close the eyes, loss of nasolabial fold, and drooping of the mouth. Patients suffering from Bell's palsy also complain of pain behind the ear, altered taste on one side of the tongue, and hyperacusis. Bell's palsy is associated with herpes zoster virus, which causes vesicular rash in the external auditory canal. This phenomenon is known as the Ramsay Hunt syndrome. The treatment of the Bell's palsy includes steroid and artificial tears.

12.2.7 Vestibulocochlear Nerve (CN VIII)

12.2.7.1 Weber's Test

12.2.7.1.1 *Instructions for Weber's Test*

1. Place the tuning fork on the vertex.
2. Ask the patient where the sound is heard.
3. Normally, the sound is heard at the centre of the head (Figure 12.8).

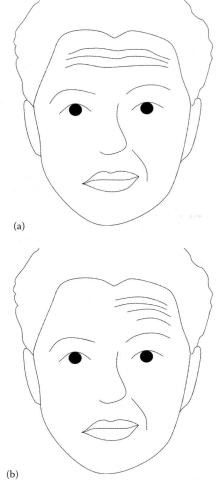

(a)

(b)

FIGURE 12.7 Upper and lower motor neuron lesions of the facial nerve (CN VII). (a) Right-sided upper motor neuron lesion (UMNL) and (b) right-sided lower motor neuron lesion (LMNL) or Bell's palsy.

12.2.7.2 Rinne's Test

12.2.7.2.1 Instruction

1. Hold a tuning fork (512 Hz) in front of the patient's ear.
2. Transfer the fork to the mastoid process behind the ear.
3. Ask which sound is louder.
4. Conduction in air should be louder than that in bone (Figure 12.9 and Table 12.1).

12.2.7.3 Anatomy of the Auditory System

The vestibulocochlear nerve (CN VIII) conveys sensory impulses from the inner ear. It has two components: (1) the *vestibular nerve*, which carries information

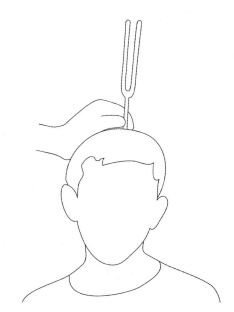

FIGURE 12.8 Weber's test.

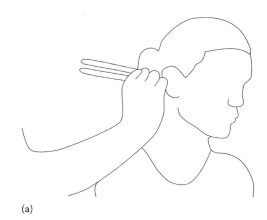

(a)

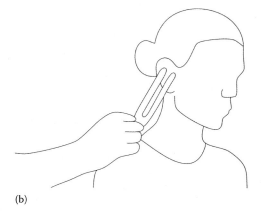

(b)

FIGURE 12.9 Rinne's test. Conduction in (a) bone and (b) air.

TABLE 12.1

Interpretation of the Results of Weber's and Rinne's Tests

Conditions	Weber's Test	Rinne's Test
Normal	The sound is heard in the centre of the head.	Conduction in air should be louder than that in bone.
Conductive hearing loss	Lateralization to the affected ear	Bone conduction is better than air conduction.
Sensorineural deafness	Lateralization to the good ear	Air conduction is better than bone conduction.

related to position and movement of the head, and (2) the *cochlear nerve*, which carries auditory information:

1. The vestibular nuclei contribute fibres to the MLF, which connects with nuclei of CNs III, IV, and VI to coordinate head and eye movements. It is also connected to the cerebellum to maintain equilibrium.
2. The cochlear nerve makes dendritic contact with the hair cells of the *organ of Corti*.

3. The cochlear nerve connects to the cochlear nuclei, which lie in the *inferior cerebellar peduncle*. Acoustic neuroma in the cerebello-pontine angle leads to dizziness with deafness by compression on the nerve. In severe case, it leads to ataxia and paralysis.
4. From the cochlear nuclei, the cochlear nerve decussates to the contralateral superior olivary nucleus in the pons and the inferior colliculus in the midbrain.
5. The fibres will send from the inferior colliculus to the *medial geniculate nucleus* of the thalamus.
6. The auditory information will finally reach the primary auditory cortex in the *Heschl's gyri on the superior temporal gyrus*. The primary auditory cortex is surrounded by Wernicke's area where the auditory information is interpreted and given contextual significance.

12.3 OTHER CRANIAL NERVES (TABLE 12.2)

12.3.1 SPINAL CORD

Note that diagrams of the ascending and descending white column tracts are considered in Chapter 13.

TABLE 12.2

Summary of Other Cranial Nerves (CN)

CN/Physical Examination Technique	Motor Component	Sensory Component	Autonomic Component	Clinical Significance
Olfactory nerve (CN I) Ask the patient for the quality of smell	—	Olfactory sensation	—	Olfaction
Glossopharyngeal nerve (CN IX) It is tested by gag reflex.	Stylopharyngeus muscle	Pharynx, posterior third of tongue, Eustachian tube, middle ear, carotid body, and carotid sinus	Stimulates the parotid salivary gland via the parasympathetic fibres	Motor: swallowing and salivation Sensory: general sensation, chemo- and baroreception
Vagus nerve (CN X)	Soft palate, pharynx, larynx, and upper oesophagus	Pharynx, larynx, oesophagus, and external ear	Parasympathetic in thoracic and abdominal viscera	Motor: swallowing and speech
Accessory nerve (CN XI) Ask the patient to shrug the shoulders.	Sternocleidomastoid and trapezius muscles	—	—	Movement of head and shoulder
Hypoglossal nerve (CN XII) It is tested by asking the patient to move the tongue and look for wasting or fasciculation	Intrinsic and extrinsic muscles of the tongue	—	—	Movement of the tongue LMNL: wasting and weakness of the tongue

12.3.1.1 Spinothalamic Tracts

Function: The spinothalamic tract carries information related to pain and temperature via the *lateral spinothalamic tracts*. Information related to the nondiscriminative touch and pressure is carried by the ventral *spinothalamic tracts* of the contralateral side of the body. The *spinoreticulothalamic tract* involves in the dull pain transmission.

Lesion of the spinothalamic tract is associated with the loss of contralateral sensation of pain, thermosensations, nondiscriminative touch, and pressure. The spinothalamic tract is selectively damaged in syringomyelia (Table 12.3).

The dorsal root ganglion consists of the slow-conducting (C and A delta) fibres. Pain has two components: the first pain, a well-localized sharp sensation, is carried by small myelinated fibres and the second pain, an unlocalized burning sensation, is carried by unmyelinated fibres. After leaving the dorsal root ganglion, the spinothalamic axons decussate to the opposite side of the cord by passing through the ventral white commissure and then enter the contralateral spinothalamic tract. The lateral spinothalamic tract decussates within one segment of the origin, and the ventral spinothalamic tract decussates several segments after crossing.

TABLE 12.3
Summary of the Spinal Cord Lesions

Lesions	Clinical Features
Central cord lesions	1. Early sphincter disturbance 2. Spinothalamic loss (unilateral or bilateral) 3. Loss of pain and temperature sensation 4. Weakness, wasting, and areflexia in the affected segment with spasticity below the level of lesion
Anterior cord syndrome	1. Preservation of dorsal column functions (i.e. proprioception of movement, joint position sense, and discriminative touch) 2. Loss of all other functions
Dorsal column loss	1. Ataxia 2. Loss of proprioception and vibration sense
Brown–Sequard syndrome	1. Ipsilateral spasticity and pyramidal signs 2. Posterior column sensory loss 3. Contralateral spinothalamic loss
Total spinal transection	1. Loss of all function below the level of the lesion (paraplegia or tetraplegia) 2. Urinary retention 3. Constipation

---

In *syringomyelia*, there is an enlargement in the central canal that compresses the lateral spinothalamic tract at the decussation, and the ventral spinothalamic tract is not affected. This leads to *dissociated sensory loss*. The loss of sensation in pain and temperature makes the patient injure his or her hands without awareness. This leads to the *Charcot's joint*.

12.3.1.2 Second-Order Neurons

In the brain stem, the spinothalamic fibres run in proximity to the medial lemniscus and form the spinal lemniscus.

12.3.1.3 Third-Order Neurons

The majority of the fibres terminate in the ventral posterior nucleus of the thalamus and then projects to the somatosensory cortex.

12.3.2 DORSAL COLUMN

Functions: The dorsal column carries sensory information concerning proprioception (movement and joint position sense) and discriminative touch.

Aetiologies: There are several conditions that affect the dorsal columns:

- *Tabes dorsalis* (*tertiary syphilis*) is associated with sensory ataxia (high steppage and unsteady gait) with *Romberg's sign*.
- *The combined subacute degeneration of the cord* is caused by vitamin B12 deficiency and leads to sensory ataxia (lesions of the dorsal column) and spasticity of the limbs (lesions in the lateral columns). This condition is associated with pernicious anaemia.
- *Multiple sclerosis* leads to the loss of proprioception in hands and fingers and causes astereognosis.

There are two tracts in the dorsal column:

1. The cuneate fasciculus lies in the medial tract and fibres join at the upper thoracic levels or cervical dorsal roots. Multiple sclerosis damages this area and leads to astereognosis.
2. The gracilis fasciculus lies in the lateral tract and fibres join at sacral, lumber, and lower thoracic levels.

12.3.2.1 Ascending Dorsal Columns

The sensation reaches the spinal cord via the fast conducting myelinated axons. There is no decussation until the fibres reach the medulla oblongata. Hence, the dorsal column carries the ipsilateral sensory information before it reaches the brain stem.

12.3.2.2 Decussation in the Medulla

The axons of second-order neurons decussate in the medulla. The internal arcuate fibres ascent through the brain stem as the medial lemniscus.

12.3.2.3 Third-Order Neurons

The medial lemniscus terminates in the ventral posterior nucleus of the thalamus and projects to the somatosensory cortex.

12.3.4 CORTICOSPINAL AND CORTICOBULBAR TRACTS

Functions: The corticospinal tracts are involved with voluntary and skilled movement of the limbs.

Lesions

1. Lesion in the *corticospinal tract* causes weakness, unsteadiness, and stiffness in walking with spontaneous spasms of the legs. Physical examination reveals increased tone, reflexes, and extensor plantar responses.
2. Lesion in the *bilateral lateral corticospinal* tract is associated with incontinence.
3. *Hereditary spastic paraparesis* is an autosomal dominant disorder that involves the degeneration of the lateral corticospinal tracts. This causes a spastic paraparesis with hyperreflexia and extensor plantar responses but spares the bladder function.
4. *Motor neuron disease* (*MND*) is a chronic degenerative disorder seen in patients aged over 50 years. MND involves degeneration of the corticobulbar tracts projecting to the nucleus ambiguous and hypoglossal nucleus. MND is associated with the following conditions (Table 12.4):
   a. *Bulbar palsy* is an LMNL that leads to flaccid, fasciculating tongue with normal jaw jerk and quiet and nasal speech. It also occurs in syringobulbia, central pontine myelinolysis (due to alcohol misuse), and brain stem tumours.
   b. *Pseudobulbar palsy* is a UMNLs and commoner than bulbar palsy. Clinical features include a spastic tongue, increase in jaw jerk, Donald Duck speech, emotional incontinence, and hollow laugher. It is caused by head injury, stroke, and multiple sclerosis (Table 12.5).

TABLE 12.4

Compare and Contrast LMNLs and UMNLs

	LMNL	UMNL
Weakness	Weakness or paralysis of individual muscles	Weakness or paralysis of individual movements
Muscles	Wasting of muscles	No wasting of muscles
Reflexes	Loss of deep tendon reflexes/hypotonia	Hyperactivity of deep tendon reflexes/hyperreflexia
Tone	Hypotonia (reduced resistance to passive stretching)	Hypertonia (increased resistance to passive stretching)
Fasciculation	Fasciculation (spontaneous contractions)	No fasciculation

TABLE 12.5

Compare and Contrast Bulbar and Pseudobulbar Palsy

	Bulbar Palsy	Pseudobulbar Palsy
Lesions	Lower motor neuron	Upper motor neuron
Causes	MNDs, Guillain–Barré syndrome, polio, syringobulbia, brain stem tumours, central pontine myelinolysis in people with alcohol misuse	Bilateral lesions above the midpons. For example, in the corticobulbar tracts in multiple sclerosis, MND, and stroke. It is commoner than bulbar palsy.
Tongue	Flaccid and fasciculating	Spastic
Jaw jerk	Normal	Increased
Speech	Quiet, hoarse, and nasal	Donald Duck speech Inappropriate laughter or emotional incontinence

Anatomy

1. The neurons of the corticospinal tract neuron arise from cell bodies in the precentral gyrus or primary motor cortex.
2. The corticospinal tract passes through the corona radiata and internal capsule and enters the crus cerebri of the midbrain.
3. 75%–90% of the fibres decussate and enter the contralateral lateral corticospinal tract. The sphincter function is supplied by bilateral lateral corticospinal tracts.

4. 10%–25% of the fibres remain ipsilateral and enter the ventral corticospinal tract and decussate near termination.
5. Corticospinal neurons terminate at the following sites:
   a. The cervical levels: 55%
   b. The thoracic levels: 20%
   c. The lumbosacral levels: 25%

12.4   MYOTOMES AND NEUROLOGICAL EXAMINATION IN THE CASC

12.4.1   MYOTOMES OF THE UPPER LIMB

1. Shoulder abduction and adduction (Figure 12.10)
   Muscle: Deltoid
   Nerve: Axillary nerve
   Myotome: C5
2. Internal and external rotation (Figure 12.11)
   Muscle: Supraspinatus muscle (abduction), the infraspinatus and teres minor (external rotation), and the subscapularis (internal rotation)
   Nerve: Suprascapular nerve
   Myotomes: C5, C6
3. Elbow flexion (Figure 12.12)
   Muscle: Biceps
   Nerve: Musculocutaneous nerve
   Myotomes: C5, C6
   Reflex at biceps: C5, C6

4. Elbow extension (Figure 12.13)
   Muscle: Triceps
   Nerve: Radial nerve
   Myotomes: C6, C7, C8
   Reflex at triceps: C7, C8

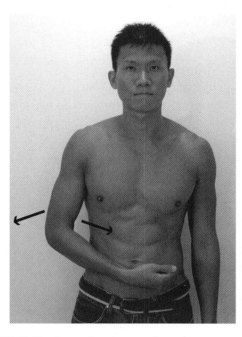

FIGURE 12.11   Internal and external rotation.

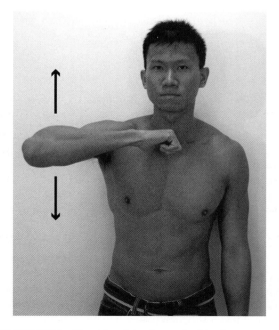

FIGURE 12.10   Shoulder abduction and adduction.

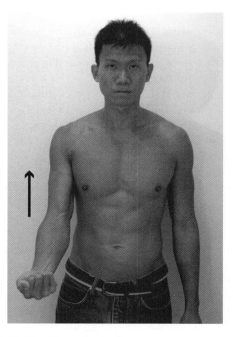

FIGURE 12.12   Elbow flexion.

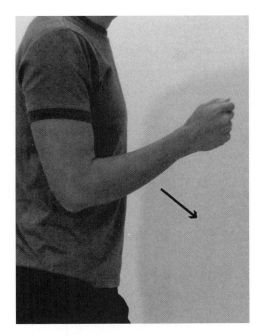

FIGURE 12.13   Elbow extension.

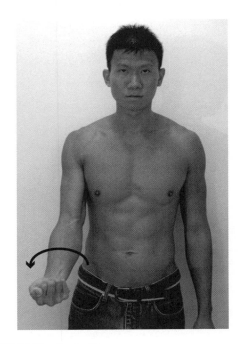

FIGURE 12.14   Supination.

5. Supination (Figure 12.14)
   Muscle: Biceps
   Nerve: Musculocutaneous nerve
   Myotomes: C6, C7
   Reflex at supinator: C5, C6

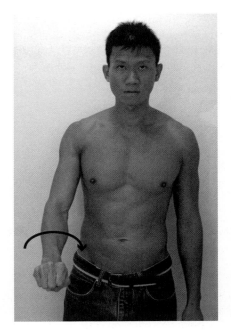

FIGURE 12.15   Pronation.

6. Pronation (Figure 12.15)
   Muscle: Pronator teres and quadratus
   Nerve: Median nerve
   Myotomes: C6, C7 (Tables 12.6 and 12.7)

12.4.2   MYOTOMES OF THE LOWER LIMB

1. Hip flexion (Figure 12.16)
   Muscle: Iliopsoas
   Nerve: Lumbar plexus and femoral nerve
   Myotome: L1 and L2

TABLE 12.6
Summary of Other Movements of the Upper Limbs

Movements	Muscles	Nerves	Myotomes
Wrist extension	Extensors carpi radialis and ulnaris	Radial nerve	C6 and C7
Wrist flexion	Flexors carpi radialis and ulnaris	Median and ulnar nerve	C7 and C8
Finger extension	Extensor digitorum	Radial nerve	C7
Finger flexion	Flexors digitorum profundus and superficialis	Median and ulnar nerves	C8 and T1
Thumb abduction	Abductor pollicis brevis	Median nerve	T1
Index finger abduction	Dorsal interossei	Ulnar nerve	T1

TABLE 12.7

Summary of the Medical Research Council (United Kingdom) Grades for Muscle Power

Grade	0	1	2	3	4	5
Clinical features	No movement	Flicker of movement	Moves when gravity is eliminated	Moves against the gravity but not resistance	Some movement against resistance	Full power

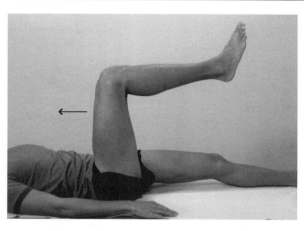

FIGURE 12.16   Hip flexion.

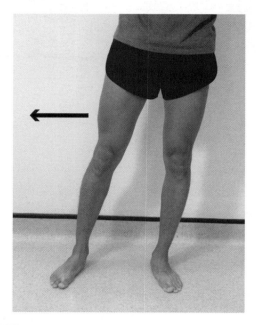

FIGURE 12.18   Hip abduction.

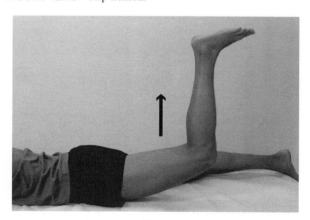

FIGURE 12.17   Hip extension.

2. Hip extension (Figure 12.17)
   Muscle: Gluteus maximus
   Nerve: Inferior gluteal nerve
   Myotomes: L5 and S1
3. Hip abduction (Figure 12.18)
   Muscle: Gluteus medius
   Nerve: Lumbosacral plexus
   Myotomes: L5
4. Hip adduction (Figure 12.19)
   Muscle: Hip adductors
   Nerve: Lumbosacral plexus
   Myotomes: L2–L4

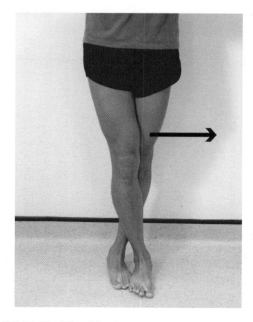

FIGURE 12.19   Hip adduction.

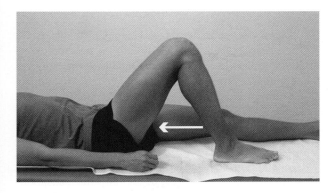

FIGURE 12.20   Knee flexion.

5. Knee flexion (Figure 12.20)
   Muscle: Hamstrings
   Nerve: Sciatic nerve
   Myotomes: S1 and S2
6. Knee extension
   Muscle: Quadriceps femoris
   Nerve: Femoral nerve
   Myotomes: L3 and L4
7. Knee jerk: L3, L4
8. Ankle dorsiflexion (Figure 12.21)
   Muscle: Tibialis anterior
   Nerve: Deep peroneal nerve
   Myotomes: L4 and L5
9. Ankle plantar flexion
   Muscle: Gastrocnemius and soleus
   Nerve: Sciatic nerve
   Myotomes: S1 and S2
10. Ankle jerk: S1, S2

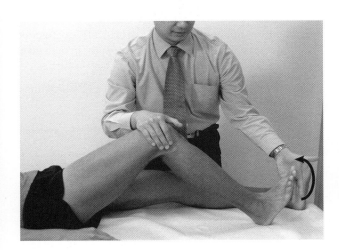

FIGURE 12.21   Ankle dorsiflexion.

12.5   DERMATOMES

Dermatome is the area of the skin or cutaneous distribution that is supplied by a particular spinal nerve (Table 12.8). Dermatomes are arranged as a succession of bands encircling the trunk in a manner that reflects the segmentation of the spinal cord (Figures 12.22 and 12.23).

TABLE 12.8
Summary of Plexuses and Innervations

Plexus	Nerves	Functions
Cervical plexus	C1–C4	Innervation of the diaphragm, shoulder, and neck
Brachial plexus	C5–T1	Innervation of the upper limbs
Lumbar plexus	T12/L1–L4	Innervation of the thigh
Sacral plexus	L4–S4	Innervation of the leg and foot

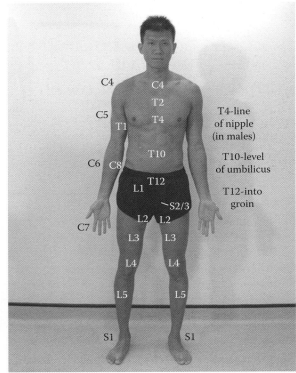

FIGURE 12.22   Dermatomes from the anterior view.

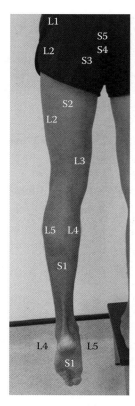

FIGURE 12.23 Dermatomes from the posterior view.

12.6 COMPRESSION AND ENTRAPMENT NEUROPATHIES (TABLE 12.9)

12.7 OTHER NEUROLOGICAL CONDITIONS

12.7.1 HEADACHE

12.7.1.1 Types of Headache

12.7.1.1.1 Migraine Headache
Causes: Vascular causes

12.7.1.1.1.1 Clinical Features
- Throbbing unilateral or occipital pain.
- Preceded by or associated with nausea, vomiting, and photophobia.
- Migraine aura precedes the headache, and patients may see teichopsia (wavy lines or fortification spectra) or scotoma.
- Motor deficits may be present.

12.7.1.1.1.2 Treatment
- Prophylaxis includes β-blockers and clonidine.
- Acute episode is treated by ergotamine and methysergide.

12.7.1.1.2 Cluster Headache
Involves severe headache or facial pain. Cluster headache is often described by patients as red-hot poker sticking in the face. This headache occurs in cluster that appears quickly and lasts for 1–3 h. It is associated with unilateral lacrimation and local erythema of skin. Treatments include NSAIDs and antimigraine medications.

12.7.1.1.3 Tension Headache
This bitemporal headache is like a circumstantial band around the head. It gives rise to pressure-like sensation. Treatment includes relaxation therapy and β-blockers.

12.7.2 PELLAGRA

Aetiology: Nicotinic acid deficiency.

Clinical triad: Diarrhoea, dermatitis, and dementia.

12.7.3 BLEPHAROSPASM

Definition: An adult-onset focal dystonia involving spasm of the orbicularis oculi.

Aetiology: Associated with Parkinson's disease, demyelinating disease, and brain stem infarction.

Epidemiology: Onset in the fifth decade; M/F = 1:2.

Clinical features: Bilateral forced eye closure, exacerbated by bright lights but improved by relaxation, yawning, singing, and talking.

Comorbidity: 75% of patients have other form of dystonia (usually facial).

Treatment: Anticholinergics or surgical treatments involving the muscle involved. Botulinum toxin may give benefits to 70% of the patients.

Prognosis: Spontaneous remission in 10%; 50% are functionally blind.

12.7.4 OTHER DYSTONIA

Spasmodic torticollis: Commonest focal dystonia involving sudden contraction of the neck and leads to deviation of the head to one side. Treatment is similar to blepharospasm.

Writer's cramp: Dystonia involving hand movement when controlling a pen.

TABLE 12.9

Summary of the Compression and Entrapment Neuropathies

Nerves	Site of Compression	Muscles Affected	Distribution of Sensory Impairment
Radial nerve	Compression in the spiral groove of the humerus	Finger dorsiflexors Thumb dorsiflexors and abductors Wrist dorsiflexors Brachioradialis	
Median nerve	Compression at the wrist	Abductor pollicis brevis	
Ulnar nerve	Compression at the elbow	Small muscles of the hand except abductor pollicis brevis Ulnar half of flexor Digitorum profundus Flexor carpi ulnaris	
Common peroneal nerve	Compression at the head of the fibula of the lower limb	Toe dorsiflexors Foot dorsiflexors Foot evertors	

12.7.4.1 Gait Abnormalities

Shuffling gait: Short paced, stooped, poor arm swing, difficulty in starting and stopping, and trying to catch up (festinant gait); associated with Parkinson's disease

Marche à petit pas: Associated with hydrocephalus

Broad-based gait: As a result of loss of proprioception and coordination and associated with lesion in the dorsal column

High stepping gait: As a result of bilateral foot drop caused by peripheral neuropathy

12.7.4.2 Ekbom's Syndrome (Restless Leg Syndrome)

Aetiology: Most cases are idiopathic; secondary causes include iron deficiency, uraemia, gestational diabetes, polyneuropathy, and rheumatoid arthritis.

Clinical features: Irresistible desire to move the legs when in bed with unpleasant leg sensations.

Treatment: Dopamine agonist and benzodiazepines such as clonazepam.

12.7.4.3 Peripheral Neuropathies

12.7.4.3.1 *Pathogenesis*

1. Axon degeneration (as a result of toxic, metabolic, nutritional, physical insults, genetic conditions).
2. Demyelination (as a result of inflammatory and metabolic neuropathies).
3. Vascular nerve damage.

12.7.4.3.1.1 *Clinical Features*

1. *Distal symmetrical neuropathy*: the most common presentation of axonal neuropathies.
2. *Multifocal/asymmetrical neuropathies*: as a result of demyelinating or vasculitic neuropathy.
3. *Mononeuropathies*: affecting an individual nerve.
4. *Mononeuritis multiplex*: affecting multiple named muscles including vasculitis, diabetes, lupus, sarcoidosis, and leprosy.
5. Demyelination produces weakness but not wasting.

12.7.4.4 Guillain–Barré Syndrome

Epidemiology: 2/100,000 per year

Aetiology: Campylobacter jejuni, cytomegalovirus, and Epstein–Barr virus infection. H1N1 vaccine

Clinical course: From days to a month

Clinical features: This syndrome affects the limbs and CNs. Clinical features range from mild weakness to complete paralysis. Ten to twenty percentage of patients require ventilatory support. This syndrome leads to cardiac arrhythmias and hypo- or hypertension.

Diagnosis: Acellular CSF with raised protein

Treatment: Plasma exchange and intravenous immunoglobulins shorten the duration of illness.

Prognosis: Mortality rate is 5%. Twenty per cent of patients suffer from motor deficits at 1 year and 3% of patients have recurrence of the syndrome.

Huntington's disease, Parkinson's disease, epilepsy, and multiple sclerosis are considered in Chapter 31.

ACKNOWLEDGMENTS

The authors of this book would like to acknowledge Dr. Anselm Mak *M.D. (HK), FRCP (Edin)* Assistant Professor and Consultant Physician, Department of Medicine, Yong Loo Lin School of Medicine, National University of Singapore for his contribution to this chapter.

BIBLIOGRAPHY

Abrahams PH, Craven JL, Lumley JSP. 2005: *Illustrated Clinical Anatomy*, p. 328. Oxford, U.K.: CRC Press.

Butler S. 1993: Functional neuroanatomy. In Morgan G and Butler S (eds.) *Seminars in Basic Neurosciences*, pp. 1–41. London, U.K.: Gaskell.

Crossman AR and Neary D. 2000: *Neuroanatomy: An Illustrated Colour Text*, 2nd edn. Edinburgh, U.K.: Churchill Livingstone.

Fuller G and Manford M. 2003: *Neurology: An Illustrated Colour Text*. Edinburgh, U.K.: Churchill Livingstone.

Longmore M, Wilkinson I, Turmezei T, and Cheung CK. 2007: *Oxford Handbook of Clinical Medicine*, 7th edn. Oxford, U.K.: Oxford University Press.

Logan S. 1993: Neurophysiology. In Morgan G and Butler S (eds.) *Seminars in Basic Neurosciences*, pp. 42–70. London, U.K.: Gaskell.

13 Neuroanatomy

13.1 ORGANIZATION OF THE NERVOUS SYSTEM

13.1.1 STRUCTURAL ORGANIZATION

The nervous system can be divided structurally into

- The central nervous system (CNS)
- The peripheral nervous system (PNS)

13.1.1.1 Central Nervous System

The CNS consists of

- The brain
- The spinal cord

It is well protected by the skull and vertebral column and the meninges (layers of connective tissue membrane):

- The dura mater—outermost layer
- The arachnoid mater—middle layer
- The pia mater—inner layer

Cerebrospinal fluid (CSF) in the subarachnoid space offers further protection of the CNS.

13.1.1.2 Peripheral Nervous System

The PNS consists of

- The cranial nerves
- The spinal nerves
- Other neuronal processes and cell bodies lying outside the CNS

It is not as well protected as the CNS.

13.1.2 FUNCTIONAL ORGANIZATION

The nervous system can be divided functionally into

- The somatic nervous system
- The autonomic nervous system

13.1.2.1 Somatic Nervous System

This is concerned primarily with the innervation of voluntary structures.

13.1.2.2 Autonomic Nervous System

This is concerned primarily with the innervation of voluntary structures. It is subdivided into two parts:

- The sympathetic
- The parasympathetic

13.1.3 DEVELOPMENTAL ORGANIZATION

During ontogeny, the midline neural tube differentiates into the following vesicles:

Prosencephalon, which differentiates into the *telencephalon*, gives rise to the cerebral hemispheres and contains the

1. Pallium
2. Rhinencephalon
3. Corpus striatum
4. Medullary centre

Diencephalon—consisting of the

1. Thalamus
2. Subthalamus
3. Hypothalamus
4. Epithalamus, consisting of the
   a. Habenular nucleus
   b. Pineal gland

Mesencephalon, consisting of the tectum, consisting of the corpora quadrigemina, made up of the

1. Superior colliculi
2. Inferior colliculi
   a. Basis pedunculi
   b. Tegmentum, containing
      i. The red nucleus
      ii. Fibre tracts
      iii. Grey matter surrounding the cerebral aqueduct

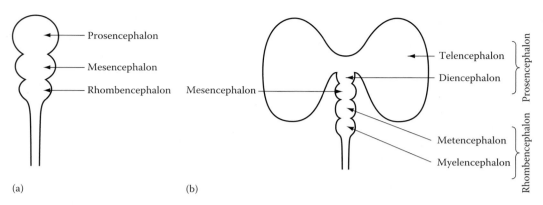

FIGURE 13.1   Ontological development of the cerebral vesicles. (a) At an early stage. (b) At a later stage.

Rhombencephalon, which differentiates into the *metencephalon*, consisting of the

1. Pons
2. Oral part of the medulla oblongata
3. Cerebellum

Myelencephalon—the caudal part of the medulla oblongata

The main ontological divisions are shown diagrammatically at an early stage and a later stage of neurodevelopment in Figure 13.1.

13.2   TYPES OF NERVOUS SYSTEM CELL

13.2.1   NEURONS

13.2.1.1   Classification by Morphology
On a morphological basis, neurons can be classified as follows:

- Unipolar—the perikaryon has one neurite.
- Bipolar—the perikaryon has two neurites.
- Multipolar—each neuron has one axon and more than one dendrite.

13.2.1.2   Classification by Size
An alternative classification is on the basis of size:

- Golgi type I—long axon
- Golgi type II—short axon terminating near the parent cell
- Amacrine—no axon

13.2.2   NEUROGLIA

13.2.2.1   Relative Numbers
Neuroglia, or interstitial cells, outnumber neurons by a factor of 5–10 times.

13.2.2.2   Central Nervous System
The main types of neuroglia in the CNS are

- Astrocytes
- Oligodendrocytes
- Microglia
- Ependyma

13.2.2.3   Peripheral Nervous System
The main types of neuroglia in the PNS are

- Schwann cells
- Satellite cells

13.2.2.4   Astrocytes
There are two types of astrocytes or astroglia:

- Fibrous astrocytes
- Protoplasmic astrocytes

They are multipolar and their functions include

- Structural support of neurons
- Phagocytosis
- Forming CNS neuroglial scar tissue
- Contributing to the blood–brain barrier

13.2.2.5 Oligodendrocytes

The functions of oligodendrocytes or oligodendroglia include

- CNS myelin sheath formation
- Phagocytosis

13.2.2.6 Microglia

They are the smallest neuroglial cells and are most abundant in the grey matter. One of their functions is

- Acting as scavenger cells at sites of CNS injury

13.2.2.7 Ependymal Cells

They line the cavities of the CNS. One of their functions is

- Aiding the flow of CSF (cilial beating)

Types of ependymal cell include

- Choroidal epithelial cells—cover the surfaces of the choroidal plexuses
- Ependymocytes—line the central canal of the spinal cord and ventricles
- Tanycytes—line the floor of the third ventricle over the hypothalamic median eminence

13.2.2.8 Schwann Cells

In addition to being part of myelinated peripheral nerves, Schwann cells encircle some unmyelinated peripheral nerve axons. Their functions include

- PNS myelin sheath formation
- Neurilemma formation

13.2.2.9 Satellite Cells

Satellite cells, or capsular cells, are found in

- Sensory ganglia
- Autonomic ganglia

One of their functions is

- Neuronal support in sensory and autonomic ganglia

13.3 FRONTAL LOBES

13.3.1 FRONTAL OPERCULUM

This consists of Brodmann areas 44, 45, and 47 (see Figure 13.2).

13.3.1.1 Broca's Area

This is the core of the frontal operculum on the dominant (usually left) side and consists of areas 44 and 45. A lesion in this region can lead to expressive (motor) aphasia (Broca's nonfluent aphasia). This is shown in Figure 13.3.

13.3.1.2 Right Side

Lesions in the nondominant frontal operculum can lead to dysprosody.

13.3.2 SUPERIOR MESIAL REGION

This contains

- *Supplementary motor area* (SMA) (mesial part of area 6)
- *Anterior cingulate* cortex (area 24)

Lesions of the left or right superior mesial region can lead to akinetic mutism.

13.3.3 INFERIOR MESIAL REGION

This consists of

- *Orbital cortex* (including areas 11, 12, and 32)
- *Basal forebrain*

13.3.3.1 Orbital Cortex

Lesions of the orbital cortex (either side) can lead to a form of acquired sociopathy.

13.3.3.2 Basal Forebrain

This includes the following nuclei:

- Diagonal band of Broca
- Nucleus accumbens
- Septal nuclei
- Substantia innominata

Lesions of the basal forebrain (either side) can lead to amnesia (retrograde and anterograde) and confabulation.

13.3.4 DORSOLATERAL PREFRONTAL CORTEX

The dorsolateral prefrontal cortex (DLPFC) contains areas 8, 9, 10, and 46. Lesions in this region can lead to abnormalities in cognitive executive functions, impairment of

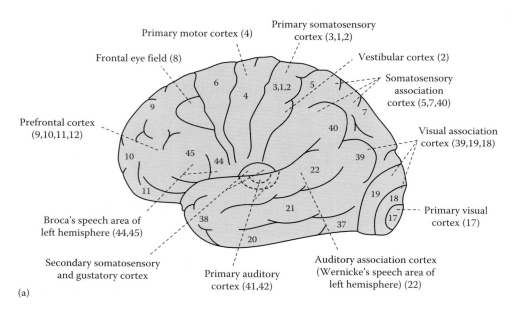

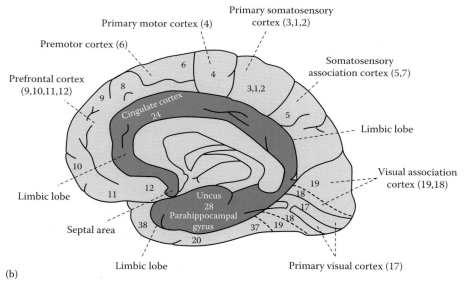

FIGURE 13.2 (a) Lateral and (b) medial aspects of the cerebral hemisphere, showing important Brodmann areas (numbered). (Reproduced from Graham, D.I. et al., *Adams & Graham's Introduction to Neuropathology*, 3rd edn., Hodder, London, U.K., 2006. With permission.)

verbal (left) or nonverbal (right) intellectual functions, memory impairments affecting recency and frequency judgements, poor organization, poor planning, poor abstraction, and disturbances in motor programming. Left-sided lesions may cause impaired verbal fluency, while right lesions may cause impaired nonverbal (design) fluency.

13.4 TEMPORAL LOBES

13.4.1 SUPERIOR TEMPORAL GYRUS

The posterior part of the superior temporal gyrus, area 22, forms Wernicke's area in the left hemisphere (see Figure 13.2). Lesions in this region can lead to a receptive (sensory) aphasia (Wernicke's fluent aphasia; see Figure 13.3).

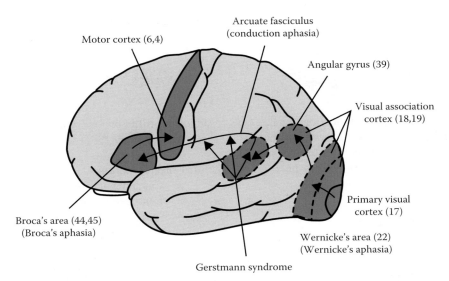

FIGURE 13.3 Left hemisphere: language, vision, and Gerstmann syndrome. (Reproduced from Graham, D.I. et al., *Adams & Graham's Introduction to Neuropathology*, 3rd edn., Hodder, London, U.K., 2006. With permission.)

13.4.2 POSTERIOR INFEROLATERAL REGION

This consists of

- Posterior portion of the *middle temporal gyrus* (part of area 37)
- Posterior portion of the *inferior temporal gyrus* (part of area 37)
- Posterior portion of the *fourth temporal gyrus* (part of area 37)

Lesions in this region, and in the adjoining occipitotemporal junction, can lead to prosopagnosia and impaired object recognition.

13.4.3 ANTERIOR INFEROLATERAL REGION

This consists of

- Anterior portion of the *middle temporal gyrus* (part of area 21)
- Anterior portion of the *inferior temporal gyrus* (part of area 20)
- Anterior portion of the *fourth temporal gyrus* (part of area 20)
- Temporal pole (area 38)

Lesions in the left side can lead to anomia and defects in accessing the reference lexicon. Lesions in the right side can lead to an inability to name facial expressions. Retrograde amnesia may result from bilateral lesions.

13.4.4 MESIAL TEMPORAL REGION

This consists of

- *Parahippocampal gyrus* (areas 27 and 28)
- *Amygdala*
- *Entorhinal cortex*
- *Hippocampus*

Left-sided lesions can lead to anterograde amnesia affecting verbal information, while right-sided lesions can lead to anterograde amnesia affecting nonverbal information. Bilateral lesions can lead to verbal and nonverbal anterograde amnesia.

13.5 PARIETAL LOBES

13.5.1 TEMPOROPARIETAL JUNCTION

The posterior part of the inferior parietal lobule together with the posterior part of the superior temporal gyrus (Wernicke's area) forms the greater Wernicke's area. Left-sided lesions can lead to a receptive (sensory) aphasia (Wernicke's fluent aphasia), while right-sided lesions can lead to phonagnosia (impairment in the ability to recognize familiar voices) and amusia (impaired ability to recognize and process music).

13.5.2 INFERIOR PARIETAL LOBULE

This consists of

- *Angular gyrus* (area 39)
- *Supramarginal gyrus* (area 40)

Lesions on the left can lead to conduction aphasia (see Figure 13.3) and tactile agnosia. Lesions on the right can lead to anosognosia, neglect, tactile agnosia, and anosodiaphoria (impaired concern with respect to neurological deficits).

13.6 OCCIPITAL LOBES

The occipital lobe contains

- Primary visual cortex (area 17)
- Visual association cortices (areas 18 and 19)

Lesions of the dorsal region (superior to the calcarine fissure) and adjoining parietal region (areas 7 and 39) can lead to partial (unilateral lesions) or a full-blown (bilateral lesions) Balint's syndrome, consisting of

- Simultanagnosia
- Ocular apraxia or psychic gaze paralysis
- Optic ataxia

Bilateral dorsal lesions can also lead to astereopsis and impaired visual motion perception. Lesions of the left ventral region (inferior to the calcarine fissure) can lead to contralateral (right) acquired (central) hemiachromatopsia (impaired visual colour perception) and acquired (pure) dyslexia. Lesions of the right ventral region can lead to contralateral (left) acquired (central) hemiachromatopsia and apperceptive visual agnosia. Bilateral lesions can lead to acquired (central) hemiachromatopsia affecting the whole visual field, associative visual agnosia, and prosopagnosia.

13.7 BASAL GANGLIA

13.7.1 COMPONENTS

Authorities differ on the components of the basal ganglia. According to Snell (1987), the basal ganglia consist of the

1. Corpus striatum
   a. Caudate nucleus
   b. Lentiform nucleus
2. Amygdala (amygdaloid nucleus or amygdaloid body)
3. Claustrum

The lentiform nucleus consists of the

1. Globus pallidus
2. Putamen

Some of these structures are shown in the diagrammatic sketch of Figure 13.4.

13.7.2 CONNECTIONS OF THE LENTIFORM NUCLEUS

13.7.2.1 Afferents

Afferents to the putamen come from the

- Caudate nucleus
- Cerebral cortex

Afferents to the globus pallidus come from the

- Caudate nucleus
- Putamen
- Substantia nigra

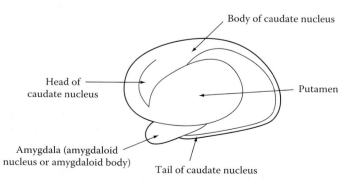

FIGURE 13.4   Sketch of the basal ganglia of the left adult cerebral hemisphere.

13.7.2.2 Efferents

Efferents from the putamen pass to the

- Globus pallidus

Efferents from the globus pallidus pass to the

- Hypothalamus
- Reticular formation
- Substantia nigra
- Subthalamus
- Ventroanterior nucleus of the thalamus
- Ventrolateral nucleus of the thalamus

13.7.3 Frontal–Subcortical Circuits

Alexander et al. (1986) have identified five parallel frontal–subcortical circuits that together form one of the main organizational networks of the brain and are central to brain–behaviour relationships. They connect specific regions of the frontal cortex with the basal ganglia and the thalamus in circuits that mediate

- Motor activity
- Eye movements
- Behaviour

The overall structure of each circuit is as follows:
Frontal lobe cortex → caudate nucleus → globus pallidus/substantia nigra → thalamus → frontal lobe cortex

13.7.3.1 Motor Circuit

This circuit originates in SMA and subserves motor function.

13.7.3.2 Oculomotor Circuit

This circuit originates in the frontal eye fields and subserves eye movements.

13.7.3.3 Dorsolateral Prefrontal Circuit

This circuit originates in DLPFC and subserves executive cognitive functions.

13.7.3.4 Lateral Orbitofrontal Circuit

This circuit originates in the lateral orbital cortex and subserves personality.

13.7.3.5 Anterior Cingulate Circuit

This circuit originates in the anterior cingulate cortex and subserves motivation.

13.8 LIMBIC SYSTEM

13.8.1 Limbic Lobe

This was described by Broca in 1878 as an arrangement of cortical structures around the diencephalon, forming a border on the medial side of each cerebral hemisphere between the neocortex and the remainder of the brain.

13.8.1.1 Cortical Areas

Cortical areas of the limbic lobe form the limbic cortex and include the

- Cingulate gyrus
- Parahippocampal gyrus
- Subcallosal gyrus

13.8.1.2 Nuclei

Subcortical nuclei that are part of the limbic lobe include the

- Amygdaloid nucleus
- Septal nucleus

13.8.2 Components

There is disagreement as to precisely which structures form part of the modern definition of the limbic system. A good guide is provided by both Snell (1987) and Trimble (1981).

13.8.2.1 Cortical Areas

Cortical areas that are generally considered to be part of the limbic system nowadays include the

1. Cingulate gyrus
2. Gyrus fasciolaris
3. Hippocampal formation
   a. Dentate gyrus
   b. Hippocampus
   c. Parahippocampal gyrus
4. Indusium griseum
5. Olfactory tubercle
6. Paraterminal gyrus (precommissural septum)
7. Prepyriform cortex
8. Secondary olfactory area (entorhinal area)
9. Subcallosal gyrus
10. Subiculum

13.8.2.2 Nuclei

Subcortical nuclear groups that are generally considered to be part of the limbic system nowadays include the

- Amygdala (amygdaloid nucleus)
- Anterior thalamic nucleus
- Dorsal tegmental nucleus
- Epithalamic nucleus
- Habenula
- Hypothalamic nuclei
- Mammillary bodies
- Raphe nucleus
- Septal nucleus (septal area)
- Superior central nucleus
- Ventral tegmental area

13.8.2.3 Connecting Pathways

Connecting pathways of the limbic system include the

- Anterior commissure
- Cingulum
- Dorsal longitudinal fasciculus
- Fornix
- Lateral longitudinal striae
- Mammillotegmental tract
- Mammillothalamic tract
- Medial forebrain bundle
- Medial longitudinal striae
- Stria terminalis
- Stria medullaris thalami

13.9 INTERNAL ANATOMY OF THE TEMPORAL LOBES

13.9.1 HIPPOCAMPAL FORMATION

The hippocampal formation consists of the

- Dentate gyrus
- Hippocampus
- Parahippocampal gyrus

13.9.1.1 Dentate Gyrus

This gyrus lies between the hippocampal fimbria and the parahippocampal gyrus. Anteriorly, it is continuous with the uncus. Posteriorly, it is continuous with the indusium griseum. Histologically, it is made up of the following three layers:

- Molecular layer (outer)
- Granular layer
- Polymorphic layer (inner)

13.9.1.2 Hippocampus

This grey matter structure lies mainly in the floor of the inferior horn of the lateral ventricle. Anteriorly, it forms the pes hippocampus. Posteriorly, it ends inferior to the splenium of the corpus callosum. Axons from each alveus converge medially to form the fimbria and crus of the fornix. Histologically, the hippocampus is made up of the following three layers:

- Molecular layer (outer)
- Pyramidal layer
- Polymorphic layer (inner)

Afferent connections of the hippocampus include fibres that originate from the

- Cingulate gyrus
- Dentate gyrus
- Hippocampus (the opposite one)
- Indusium griseum
- Parahippocampal gyrus
- Secondary olfactory area (entorhinal area)
- Septal nucleus (septal area)

13.9.1.3 Parahippocampal Gyrus

This gyrus is separated from the remaining cerebral cortex by the collateral sulcus. Anteriorly, it is continuous with the uncus. The subiculum of the parahippocampal gyrus allows the passage of nerve fibres from the secondary olfactory cortex (entorhinal area) to the dentate gyrus.

13.9.2 AMYGDALA

The amygdala is also known as the amygdaloid nucleus, body, or complex. It is continuous with the tail of the caudate nucleus, lying anterior and superior to the tip of the inferior horn of the lateral ventricle.

13.9.2.1 Afferent Connections

Afferent connections received by the amygdala include the

- Amygdala (the opposite one, via the anterior commissure)
- Dopaminergic brain stem nuclei
- Frontal association area
- Lateral olfactory stria
- Noradrenergic brain stem nuclei
- Septal nucleus (septal area)
- Serotonergic brain stem nuclei
- Temporal association area
- Uncus

13.9.2.2 Efferent Connections

Parts of the brain to which efferent connections pass from the amygdala include the

- Hypothalamus (via the stria terminalis)
- Septal nucleus (septal area) (via the stria terminalis)
- Corpus striatum
- Frontal association area
- Lateral olfactory stria
- Temporal association area
- Thalamus

13.10 MAJOR WHITE MATTER PATHWAYS

13.10.1 CORPUS CALLOSUM

This is the largest set of interhemispheric connecting fibres. It lies inferior to the longitudinal fissure and superior to the diencephalon. It connects homologous neocortical areas.

13.10.1.1 Divisions

The main divisions of the corpus callosum (rostral first) are the

- Rostrum
- Genu
- Body
- Splenium

These are shown in the diagrammatic sketch of the corpus callosum of Figure 13.5, which also shows some adjacent structures.

13.10.2 FORNIX

This is the major efferent subcortical white matter tract of the hippocampus. The two crura of the fornix, each formed from axons from the alveus of the hippocampus, converge inferior to the corpus callosum and form the body of the fornix. The body of the fornix is connected anteriorly with the inferior surface of the corpus callosum via the septum pellucidum. The body of the fornix then divides into the two columns of the fornix.

13.10.2.1 Destination of Fibres in the Fornix

The efferent connections of the hippocampus, via the fornix, include the

- Anterior hypothalamus
- Anterior nucleus of the thalamus
- Habenular nucleus
- Lateral preoptic area
- Mammillary body (medial nucleus)
- Septal nucleus (septal area)
- Tegmentum of the mesencephalon

13.10.3 PAPEZ CIRCUIT

This is the concept introduced by Papez, in 1937, of a supposed limbic system reverberating circuit constituting the neuronal mechanism of emotion. It consisted of the

- Hippocampus
- Hypothalamus
- Anterior nucleus of the thalamus
- Cingulate gyrus

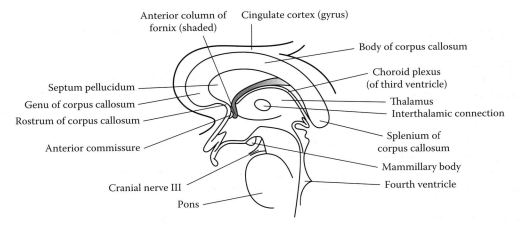

FIGURE 13.5 Sketch of the corpus callosum in a midsagittal section of the adult human brain. The adjacent cingulate cortex and septum pellucidum are also indicated. Note that the rostral direction is towards the left.

The postulated circuit was as follows:

> Hippocampus → (via the fornix)
> Mammillary bodies of the hypothalamus → (via a synaptic connection)
> Anterior nucleus of the thalamus → (the neuroimpulse then radiates up)
> Cingulate gyrus → (via the cingulum)
> Hippocampus

13.10.4 ARCUATE BUNDLE

This is a specific group of association fibres arranged in a curved shape running parallel to the cortical surface that, on the dominant (usually left) side, connects the more rostral Broca's area with Wernicke's area.

13.10.5 ANTERIOR COMMISSURE

This small nerve fibre bundle crosses the midline in the lamina terminalis and connects homologous areas of the neocortex and paleocortex. Parts of the limbic system in the two cerebral hemispheres that are connected via the anterior commissure include the

- Amygdala
- Hippocampus
- Parahippocampal gyrus

13.11 CRANIAL NERVES

13.11.1 OLFACTORY NERVE

This contains the central processes of the olfactory receptors, which pass from the olfactory mucosa, through the cribriform plate of the ethmoid, to synapse with the olfactory bulb mitral cells. Axons then pass in the olfactory tract to the primary olfactory cortex (also known as the periamygdaloid and prepyriform areas) via the lateral olfactory striae.

13.11.2 OPTIC NERVE

This contains retinal ganglion cell axons that pass to the optic chiasma. At the optic chiasma,

- Medial retinal fibres, containing temporal visual field information, pass to the contralateral optic tract
- Lateral retinal fibres, containing nasal visual field information, pass to the ipsilateral optic tract

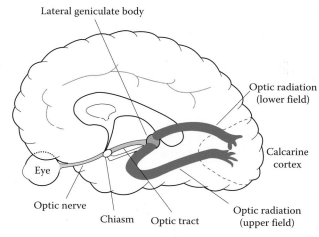

FIGURE 13.6 Medial sagittal view of the brain, showing the visual pathways that traverse the brain from the front to the back. (Reproduced from Fowler, T.J. and Scadding, J.W., *Clinical Neurology*, 3rd edn., Hodder, London, U.K., 2003. With permission.)

Most optic tract fibres synapse in the thalamic lateral geniculate body, while a minority (concerned with papillary and ocular reflexes) pass directly to the pretectal nucleus and superior colliculi, bypassing the lateral geniculate body. From the lateral geniculate body, the optic radiation passes, via the retrolenticular part of the internal capsule, to the visual cortex (see Figure 13.6).

13.11.3 OCULOMOTOR NERVE

This nerve has two motor nuclei:

- The main oculomotor nucleus (also known as the somatic efferent nucleus)—supplies all the extrinsic ocular muscles with the exception of the superior oblique and lateral rectus
- The accessory parasympathetic nucleus (also known as the Edinger–Westphal nucleus)—sends preganglionic parasympathetic fibres to the constrictor pupillae and ciliary muscles

13.11.4 TROCHLEAR NERVE

This supplies one extrinsic ocular muscle, namely, the superior oblique.

13.11.5 TRIGEMINAL NERVE

This is the largest cranial nerve.

13.11.5.1 Nuclei

The trigeminal nerve has four nuclei, the

- Main sensory nucleus
- Spinal nucleus
- Mesencephalic nucleus
- Motor nucleus

13.11.5.2 Sensory Components

The main divisions and branches of the trigeminal nerve, which together constitute the main sensory innervation of most of the head and face, are as follows:

1. Ophthalmic nerve or division
   a. Frontal nerve: innervates, via the supraorbital and supratrochlear branches, the
      i. Upper eyelid
      ii. Scalp (anterior to the lambdoid suture)
   b. Lacrimal nerve: innervates the
      i. Lacrimal gland
      ii. Lateral conjunctiva
      iii. Upper eyelid
   c. Nasociliary nerve: innervates the
      i. Eyeball
      ii. Medial lower eyelid
      iii. Nasal skin
      iv. Nasal mucosa
2. Maxillary nerve or division
   a. Infraorbital nerve: innervates the
      i. Skin of the cheek
   b. Superior alveolar nerve: innervates the
      i. Upper teeth
   c. Zygomatic nerve: innervates the
      i. Skin of the temple (via the zygomatico-temporal branch)
      ii. Skin of the cheek (via the zygomaticofacial branch)
   d. Branches from the sphenopalatine ganglion include the
      i. Greater palatine nerve
      ii. Lesser palatine nerve
      iii. Long sphenopalatine nerve
      iv. Nasal branches
      v. Pharyngeal branches
      vi. Short sphenopalatine nerve
3. Mandibular nerve or division
   a. Auriculotemporal nerve: innervates the
      i. Skin of the temple
      ii. Auricle division

   b. Buccal nerve: innervates the
      i. Skin of the cheek
      ii. Mucous membrane of the cheek
   c. Inferior alveolar nerve: innervates the
      i. Lower teeth
      ii. Lower lip
      iii. Skin of the chin
   d. Lingual nerve: innervates the
      i. Anterior two-thirds of the tongue
      ii. Mucous membrane of the mouth

13.11.5.3 Motor Component

The motor component of the trigeminal nerve supplies the

- Muscles of mastication
- Anterior belly of the digastric
- Mylohyoid
- Tensor tympani
- Tensor veli palatini

13.11.6 ABDUCENS NERVE

This supplies one extrinsic ocular muscle, namely, the lateral rectus.

13.11.7 FACIAL NERVE

13.11.7.1 Nuclei

The facial nerve has three nuclei:

- Main motor nucleus
- Parasympathetic nuclei
- Sensory nucleus (the superior part of the tractus solitarius nucleus)

13.11.7.2 Main Motor Nucleus

This supplies the

- Muscles of facial expression
- Auricular muscles
- Posterior belly of the digastric
- Stapedius
- Stylohyoid

Corticonuclear fibres from the contralateral cerebral hemisphere are received by the part of the main motor nucleus supplying the lower face muscles. Corticonuclear fibres from both cerebral hemispheres are received by the part of the main motor nucleus supplying the upper face muscles.

13.11.7.3 Parasympathetic Nuclei

These include the

- Lacrimal nucleus: supplies the
  Lacrimal gland
- Superior salivary nucleus: supplies the
  Nasal gland
  Palatine gland
  Sublingual gland
  Submandibular gland

13.11.7.4 Sensory Nucleus

This receives taste fibres, via the geniculate ganglion, from the

- Anterior two-thirds of the tongue
- Floor of the mouth
- Hard palate
- Soft palate

13.11.7.5 Chorda Tympani

This is a branch of the facial nerve given off before it passes through the stylomastoid foramen. The chorda tympani joins the lingual branch of the mandibular division of the trigeminal nerve.

13.11.8 VESTIBULOCOCHLEAR NERVE

This nerve consists of the following two parts, the

- Cochlear nerve—concerned with hearing
- Vestibular nerve—concerned with the maintenance of equilibrium

13.11.8.1 Cochlear Nerve

Its fibres are the central processes of the cochlear spiral ganglion cells, terminating in the anterior and posterior cochlear nuclei.

13.11.8.2 Vestibular Nerve

Its fibres are the central processes of vestibular ganglion neurons, terminating in the lateral, medial, superior, and inferior vestibular nuclei.

13.11.9 GLOSSOPHARYNGEAL NERVE

13.11.9.1 Nuclei

The glossopharyngeal nerve has three nuclei

- Main motor nucleus

- Parasympathetic nucleus (the inferior salivary nucleus)
- Sensory nucleus (part of the tractus solitarius nucleus)

13.11.9.2 Main Motor Nucleus

This supplies the

- Stylopharyngeus

Corticonuclear fibres from both cerebral hemispheres are received by the main motor nucleus.

13.11.9.3 Parasympathetic Nucleus

This receives inputs from the

- Hypothalamus
- Olfactory system
- Tractus solitarius nucleus
- Trigeminal sensory nucleus

Preganglionic fibres reach the otic ganglion via the tympanic plexus and the lesser petrosal nerve. Postganglionic fibres supply the parotid gland by means of the auriculo-temporal branch of the mandibular nerve.

13.11.9.4 Sensory Nucleus

This receives taste information from the posterior one-third of the tongue.

13.11.10 VAGUS NERVE

13.11.10.1 Nuclei

The vagus nerve has three nuclei, the

- Main motor nucleus
- Parasympathetic nucleus (the dorsal nucleus)
- Sensory nucleus (the inferior part of the tractus solitarius nucleus)

13.11.10.2 Main Motor Nucleus

This supplies the

- Intrinsic muscles of the larynx
- Constrictor muscles of the pharynx

Corticonuclear fibres from both cerebral hemispheres are received by the main motor nucleus.

13.11.10.3 Parasympathetic Nucleus

This receives inputs from the

- Hypothalamus
- Glossopharyngeal nerve
- Heart
- Lower respiratory tract
- Gastrointestinal tract, as far as the transverse colon

It supplies the

- Involuntary muscle of the heart
- Lower respiratory tract
- Gastrointestinal tract, as far as the distal one-third of the transverse colon

13.11.10.4 Sensory Nucleus

This receives taste information from the inferior ganglion of the vagus nerve.

13.11.11 Accessory Nerve

This nerve consists of the following two parts

- Cranial root
- Spinal root

13.11.11.1 Cranial Root

This supplies, via the vagus nerve, muscles of the

- Larynx
- Pharynx
- Soft palate

13.11.11.2 Spinal Root

This supplies the

- Sternocleidomastoid
- Trapezius

13.11.12 Hypoglossal Nerve

This supplies the

- Intrinsic muscles of the tongue
- Styloglossus
- Hyoglossus
- Genioglossus

13.12 SPINAL CORD

13.12.1 Divisions

From rostral to caudal, the spinal cord is divided into the following five parts:

- Cervical—8 pairs of spinal nerves
- Thoracic—12 pairs of spinal nerves
- Lumbar—5 pairs of spinal nerves
- Sacral—5 pairs of spinal nerves
- Coccygeal—1 pair of spinal nerves

13.12.2 Ascending White Column Tracts

The anatomy of the ascending white column tract is shown in Figure 13.7.

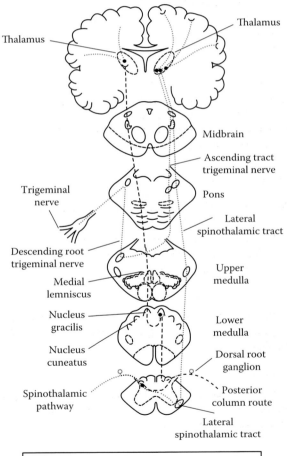

··············	Spinothalamic (pain, temperature)
- - - - - - -	Posterior columns (position, vibration)

FIGURE 13.7 Ascending sensory pathways. (Reproduced from Fowler, T.J. and Scadding, J.W., *Clinical Neurology*, 3rd edn., Hodder, London, U.K., 2003. With permission.)

13.12.2.1 Anterior

The ascending anterior white column tracts include the

- *Anterior spinothalamic tract*—carries light touch and pressure sensations

13.12.2.2 Lateral

The ascending lateral white column tracts include the

- *Anterior and posterior spinocerebellar tracts*— carry proprioceptive, pressure, and touch sensations
- *Lateral spinothalamic tract*—carries pain and temperature sensations

- *Spino-olivary tract*—carries proprioceptive and cutaneous sensations
- *Spinotectal tract*—involved with spinovisual reflexes

13.12.2.3 Posterior

The ascending posterior white column tracts include the

- *Fasciculus cuneatus*—carries discriminative touch and proprioceptive sensations
- *Fasciculus gracilis*—carries vibration sensations

13.12.3 DESCENDING WHITE COLUMN TRACTS

The anatomy of the descending white column tracts is shown in Figure 13.8.

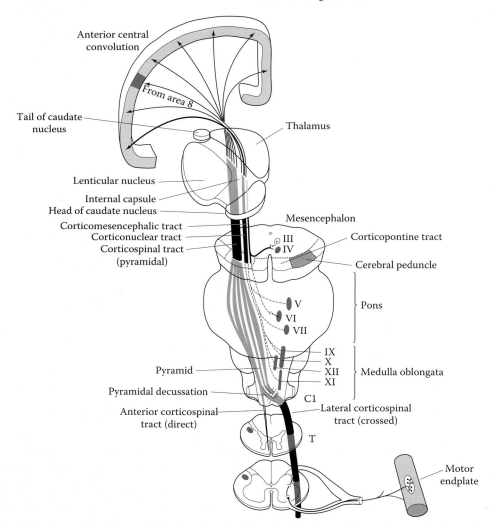

FIGURE 13.8 Course of the corticospinal tracts. (Reproduced from Fowler, T.J. and Scadding, J.W., *Clinical Neurology*, 3rd edn., Hodder, London, U.K., 2003. With permission.)

13.12.3.1 Anterior

The descending anterior white column tracts include the

- *Anterior corticospinal tract*—involved with voluntary movement
- *Reticulospinal fibres*—involved with motor function
- *Vestibulospinal tract*—involved with muscle tone control
- *Tectospinal tract*—involved with a head-turning reflex and movement of the upper limbs in response to acoustic, cutaneous, and visual stimuli

13.12.3.2 Lateral

The descending lateral white column tracts include the

- *Lateral corticospinal tract*—involved with voluntary movement
- *Rubrospinal tract*—involved with muscular activity

- *Lateral reticulospinal tract*—involved with muscular activity
- *Descending autonomic fibres*—involved with visceral function control
- *Olivospinal tract*—?involved with muscular activity

13.13 MAJOR NEUROCHEMICAL PATHWAYS

13.13.1 Nigrostriatal Dopaminergic Pathway

This is shown in Figure 13.9. The presynaptic components of this pathway are formed by

- *A8 dopaminergic neurons*—located in the reticular formation of the mesencephalon
- *A9 dopaminergic neurons*—located in the pars compacta of the substantia nigra

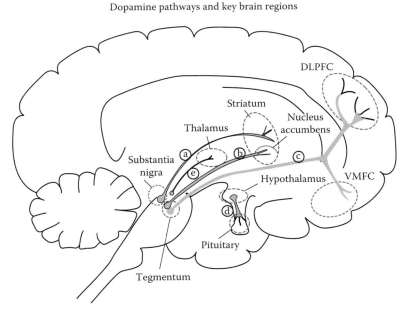

Dopamine pathways and key brain regions

FIGURE 13.9 Major dopamine pathways in the brain. (a) The nigrostriatal dopamine pathway, which projects from the substantia nigra to the corpus striatum of the basal ganglia, is part of the extrapyramidal system and controls motor function and movement. (b) The mesolimbic dopamine pathway projects from the midbrain ventral tegmental area to the nucleus accumbens, a part of the limbic system thought to be involved in many behaviours such as pleasurable sensations, the powerful euphoria of drugs of abuse, and delusions and hallucinations of psychosis. (c) The mesocortical dopamine pathway is related to the mesolimbic pathway and also projects from the ventral tegmental area but sends its axons to areas of the prefrontal cortex, where they may have a role in mediating cognitive symptomatology (DLPFC) and affective symptomatology (ventromedial prefrontal cortex) of schizophrenia. (d) The tuberoinfundibular dopamine pathway projects from the hypothalamus to the anterior pituitary gland and controls prolactin secretion. (e) A fifth dopamine pathway arises from multiple sites, including the periaqueductal grey, ventral mesencephalon, hypothalamic nuclei, and lateral parabrachial nucleus, and projects to the thalamus. Its function is not currently well known. (Reproduced from Stahl, S.M., *Stahl's Essential Psychopharmacology*, 3rd edn., Cambridge University Press, Cambridge, U.K., 2008. With permission.)

Their axons pass, via the medial forebrain bundle, to terminate mostly in the

- Caudate nucleus
- Putamen
- Amygdala

This pathway is concerned with sensorimotor coordination.

13.13.2   MESOLIMBIC–MESOCORTICAL DOPAMINERGIC PATHWAY

The two parts of this pathway are shown in Figure 13.9. This pathway originates in

- *A10 dopaminergic neurons*—located in the ventral tegmental area of the mesencephalon

Their axons pass, via the medial forebrain bundle, to terminate mostly in the

- Nucleus accumbens
- Olfactory tubercle
- Bed nucleus of the stria terminalis

- Lateral septum
- Cingulate cortex
- Entorhinal cortex
- Medial prefrontal cortex

13.13.3   ASCENDING NORADRENERGIC PATHWAY FROM THE LOCUS COERULEUS

This is shown in Figure 13.10. The main noradrenergic nucleus is the locus coeruleus, located in the dorsal pons. At least five noradrenergic tracts arise from it:

1. Three ascend, via the medial forebrain bundle, to supply mainly the
   a. Ipsilateral cerebral cortex
   b. Thalamus
   c. Hypothalamus
   d. Limbic system
   e. Olfactory bulb
2. The fourth, via the superior cerebellar peduncle, supplies the cerebellar cortex.
3. The fifth descends in the mesencephalon and spinal cord.

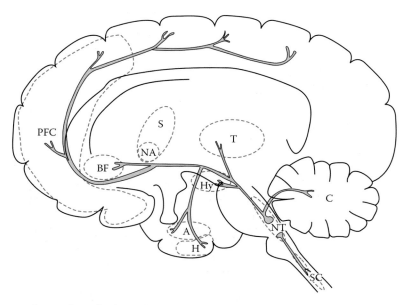

FIGURE 13.10   Major noradrenergic projections. Ascending noradrenergic projections originate mainly in the locus coeruleus of the brainstem; they extend to multiple brain regions, as shown here, and regulate mood, arousal, cognition, and other functions. Descending noradrenergic projections extend down the spinal cord and regulate pain pathways A, amygdala; BF, basal forebrain; C, cerebellum; H, hippocampus; Hy, hypothalamus; NA, nucleus accumbens; NT, brainstem neurotransmitter centres; PFC, prefrontal cortex; S, striatum; SC, spinal cord; T, thalamus. (Reproduced from Stahl, S.M., *Stahl's Essential Psychopharmacology*, 3rd edn., Cambridge University Press, Cambridge, U.K., 2008. With permission.)

13.13.4 BASAL FOREBRAIN CHOLINERGIC PATHWAY

This is shown in Figure 13.11. Cholinergic neurons of this pathway originate in the basal forebrain, including

- *Ch4 cholinergic neurons*—located in the nucleus basalis of Meynert
- *Ch2 and Ch3 cholinergic neurons*—located in the diagonal band nucleus (of Broca)
- *Ch1 cholinergic neurons*—located in the medial septal nucleus

Their main innervation is as follows:

- Ch4—cerebral cortex, amygdala, and corpus striatum
- Ch1—hippocampal formation
- Ch2—hippocampal formation
- Ch3—olfactory bulb

(Note that most of the cholinergic innervation of the corpus striatum is intrinsic and not from this pathway.)

13.13.5 BRAIN STEM CHOLINERGIC PATHWAY

This is shown in Figure 13.12. Cholinergic neurons of this pathway originate in the brainstem, including

- *Ch5 cholinergic neurons*—located in the pedunculopontine nucleus
- *Ch6 cholinergic neurons*—located in the laterodorsal tegmental nucleus

Their (Ch5 and Ch6) main innervation is to the

- Thalamus
- Cerebral cortex
- Basal forebrain
- Corpus striatum
- Globus pallidus
- Subthalamic nucleus
- Substantia nigra

Ch5 neurons are more closely interconnected with extrapyramidal structures, while Ch6 neurons send more projections to nuclei of the limbic system and to medial prefrontal cortex.

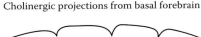

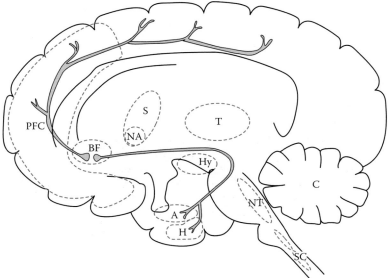

FIGURE 13.11 Basal forebrain cholinergic pathway. Cholinergic neurons originating in the basal forebrain project to the prefrontal cortex, hippocampus, and amygdala; they are believed to be involved in memory A, amygdala; BF, basal forebrain; C, cerebellum; H, hippocampus; Hy, hypothalamus; NA, nucleus accumbens; NT, brainstem neurotransmitter centres; PFC, prefrontal cortex; S, striatum; SC, spinal cord; T, thalamus. (Reproduced from Stahl, S.M., *Stahl's Essential Psychopharmacology*, 3rd edn., Cambridge University Press, Cambridge, U.K., 2008. With permission.)

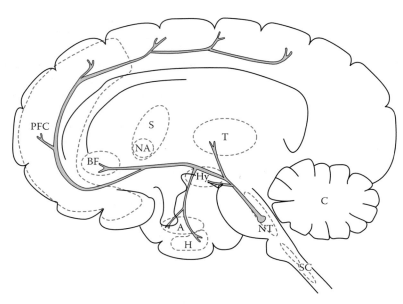

FIGURE 13.12 Brainstem cholinergic pathway. Acetylcholine projections originating in the brainstem extend to many regions, including the prefrontal cortex, basal forebrain, thalamus, hypothalamus, amygdala, and hippocampus. These projections regulate arousal, cognition, and other functions A, amygdala; BF, basal forebrain; C, cerebellum; H, hippocampus; Hy, hypothalamus; NA, nucleus accumbens; NT, brainstem neurotransmitter centres; PFC, prefrontal cortex; S, striatum; SC, spinal cord; T, thalamus. (Reproduced from Stahl, S.M., *Stahl's Essential Psychopharmacology*, 3rd edn., Cambridge University Press, Cambridge, U.K., 2008. With permission.)

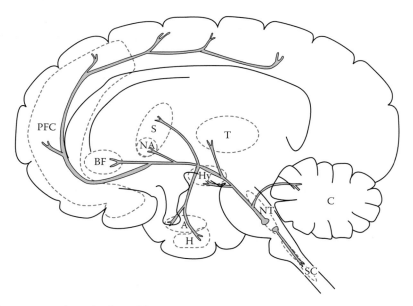

FIGURE 13.13 Major serotonergic projections. Like noradrenaline, serotonin has both ascending and descending projections. Ascending serotonergic projections originate in the brainstem and extend to many of the same regions as noradrenergic projections, with additional projections to the striatum and nucleus accumbens. These ascending projections may regulate mood, anxiety, sleep, and other functions. Descending serotonergic projections extend down the brainstem and through the spinal cord; they may regulate pain A, amygdala; BF, basal forebrain; C, cerebellum; H, hippocampus; Hy, hypothalamus; NA, nucleus accumbens; NT, brainstem neurotransmitter centres; PFC, prefrontal cortex; S, striatum; SC, spinal cord; T, thalamus. (Reproduced from Stahl, S.M., *Stahl's Essential Psychopharmacology*, 3rd edn., Cambridge University Press, Cambridge, U.K., 2008. With permission.)

13.13.6 GLUTAMATE SYSTEM

Neurons using glutamate, an excitatory neurotransmitter, include

- Cerebral cortical pyramidal cells
- Hippocampal pyramidal cells
- Primary sensory afferents
- Cerebellar granule cells
- Cerebellar climbing fibres

The cerebral cortex contains abundant N-methyl-D-aspartate (NMDA) receptors, which serve an integral role in corticocortical and corticofugal glutamatergic neurotransmission.

13.13.7 ASCENDING SEROTONIN SYSTEM

This is shown in Figure 13.13. During embryogenesis, two groups of serotonergic neurons develop:

- *A superior group*—located at the boundary between the mesencephalon and the pons
- *An inferior group*—located from the pons caudally to the cervical spinal cord

The superior group gives rise to the superior raphe nuclei and is largely responsible for the origin of ascending serotonergic fibres projecting to the forebrain. The main superior raphe nuclei are the

- Caudal linear nucleus (the most rostral)
- Dorsal raphe nucleus
- Median raphe nucleus
- Supralemniscal nucleus

Ascending fibres pass from the superior raphe nuclei, via pathways such as the dorsal raphe cortical tract (the largest pathway in primates) and the medial forebrain bundle (the largest pathway in the rat), to innervate the forebrain. Particularly important destinations include the

- Suprachiasmatic nucleus
- Substantia nigra
- Limbic system
- Periventricular regions
- Primary sensory areas of the cerebral cortex
- Association areas of the cerebral cortex

BIBLIOGRAPHY

Alexander GE, DeLong MR, and Strick PL. 1986: Parallel organization of functionally segregated circuits linking basal ganglia and cortex. *Annual Review of Neuroscience* 9:357–381.

Fitzgerald MJT, Gruener G, and Mtui E. 2012: *Clinical Neuroanatomy and Neuroscience*, 6th edn. Edinburgh, U.K.: Saunders Elsevier.

Moore DP and Puri BK. 2012: *Textbook of Clinical Neuropsychiatry and Behavioral Neuroscience*, 3rd edn. London, U.K.: Hodder Arnold.

Puri BK and Logan BM 2010: Neuroanatomy. In Puri BK and Treasaden IH (eds.) *Psychiatry: An Evidence-Based Text*. London, U.K.: Hodder Arnold.

Snell RS. 2010: *Clinical Neuroanatomy*, 7th edn. Baltimore, MD: Lippincott, Williams & Wilkins.

14 Neuropathology

14.1 DEMENTIAS

14.1.1 ALZHEIMER'S DISEASE

The neuropathology of presenile dementia (later called Alzheimer's disease by Emil Kraepelin) was first described in 1906 by Aloysius (or 'Alois') Alzheimer (1864–1915) (Berrios, 1991).

14.1.1.1 Macroscopic Neuropathology

Macroscopic changes in Alzheimer's disease include

- Global brain atrophy and low brain mass
- Ventricular enlargement (particularly of the lateral ventricular inferior horn)
- Sulcal widening

The atrophy is usually most marked in the frontal, medial temporal, and parietal lobes.

14.1.1.2 Histopathology

Histological changes in the cerebral cortex in Alzheimer's disease include

- Neuronal loss
- Shrinking of dendritic branching
- Reactive astrocytosis
- Neurofibrillary tangles—intracellular
- Neuritic plaques (senile plaques)—extracellular

There is a positive correlation between the number of neurofibrillary tangles and neuritic plaques, on the one hand, and, on the other, the degree of cognitive impairment.

Histological changes seen commonly in the hippocampus include

- Granulovacuolar degeneration
- Hirano bodies
- Neurofibrillary tangles
- Neuritic plaques (senile plaques)

14.1.1.3 Ultrastructural Pathology

Neuritic plaques contain a core made of amyloid. This consists of 8 nm extracellular filaments made up mainly of the amyloid-β peptide Aβ, which is a 39–43-amino acid peptide. Scattered deposits of amyloid-β protein in the brain in Alzheimer's disease have been found to localize to activated microglia.

Aβ is derived from the membrane-bound β-amyloid precursor protein (APP).

14.1.1.4 Neurochemical Pathology

Neurochemical changes that have been reported in Alzheimer's disease include

- ↓ Acetylcholinesterase
- ↓ Choline acetyltransferase
- ↓ GABA
- ↓ Noradrenaline

14.1.2 PICK'S DISEASE

Pick's disease is one histological type of frontotemporal dementia.

14.1.2.1 Macroscopic Neuropathology

Macroscopic changes in Pick's disease include

- Selective asymmetrical atrophy of the anterior temporal lobes and frontal lobes
- Knife-blade gyri
- Ventricular enlargement

14.1.2.2 Histopathology

Histological changes in Pick's disease include

- Pick's bodies
- Neuronal loss
- Reactive astrocytosis

These changes may be seen in the

- Cerebral cortex
- Basal ganglia
- Locus coeruleus
- Substantia nigra

14.1.2.3   Ultrastructural Pathology

Pick's bodies consist of

- Straight neurofilaments
- Paired helical filaments
- Endoplasmic reticulum

14.1.3   MULTI-INFARCT DEMENTIA

ICD-10 classes multi-infarct dementia under vascular dementia.

14.1.3.1   Macroscopic Neuropathology

Macroscopic changes in multi-infarct dementia include

- Multiple cerebral infarcts
- Local or general brain atrophy
- Ventricular enlargement
- Arteriosclerotic changes in major arteries

Clinically, the following relationships have been found usually to hold approximately for the total volume of the infarcts:

- $50\,mL < volume \leq 100\,mL$: cognitive impairment
- Volume $> 100\,mL$: dementia

14.1.3.2   Histopathology

Histological changes include those of infarction and ischaemia.

14.1.4   LEWY BODY DISEASE

The generic term 'dementia with Lewy bodies' was proposed at the first International Workshop on Lewy Body Dementia in 1995 (McKeith, 2006). It was described in 1923 by Friedrich Lewy in a large proportion of his patients suffering from paralysis agitans, which had coincident plaques and neurofibrillary tangles (Holdorff, 2002). Lewy body dementia includes the following types of dementia:

- Diffuse Lewy body disease
- Senile dementia of Lewy body type
- Lewy body variant of Alzheimer's disease

14.1.4.1   Histopathology

Histological changes in the brain in dementia caused by Lewy body disease include

- Lewy bodies
- Neuronal loss
- Neurofibrillary tangles
- Neuritis plaques (senile plaques)

Compared with Parkinson's disease, in which Lewy bodies are also found, in dementia caused by Lewy body disease, the density of Lewy bodies is much higher in the

- Cingulate gyrus
- Parahippocampal gyrus
- Temporal cortex

14.1.4.2   Ultrastructural Pathology

Lewy bodies contain

- Protein neurofilaments
- Granular material
- Dense core vesicles
- Microtubule assembly protein
- Ubiquitin
- Tau protein

14.1.5   CREUTZFELDT–JAKOB DISEASE

Creutzfeldt–Jakob disease (CJD) is transmitted by infection with a prion. In addition to the brain changes mentioned in the succeeding text, CJD is also associated with degeneration in spinal cord long descending tracts. It has an incubation period of many years. Infection may be transmitted from surgical specimens, postmortem preparations (such as corneal grafts), and human pituitary glands; the latter have been used to produce human somatotropin for clinical use. In 1995 in Britain, a new variant of CJD (nvCJD) was reported, which, it has been suggested, may be linked to transmission, possibly via the food chain, from the neuropathologically related disorder bovine spongiform encephalopathy (BSE).

14.1.5.1   Macroscopic Neuropathology

There may be little or no gross atrophy of the cerebral cortex evident in rapidly developing cases. In those surviving the longest, changes seen may include

- Selective cerebellar atrophy
- Generalized cerebral atrophy
- Ventricular enlargement

14.1.5.2   Histopathology

Histological changes in the brain in dementia caused by CJD include

- Status spongiosus
- Neuronal degeneration without inflammation
- Astrocytic proliferation

14.1.6 PUNCH-DRUNK SYNDROME

This is also known as post-traumatic dementia, dementia pugilistica, or boxing encephalopathy. In addition to occurring in boxers who have received repeated punches to the head, other contact sports involving repeated head injury, such as rugby union, may also put participants at risk.

14.1.6.1 Macroscopic Neuropathology
Typical macroscopic changes include

- Cerebral atrophy
- Ventricular enlargement
- Perforation of the cavum septum pellucidum
- Thinning of the corpus callosum

14.1.6.2 Histopathology
Histological changes in the brain in punch-drunk syndrome include

- Neuronal loss
- Neurofibrillary tangles

14.2 CEREBRAL TUMOURS

14.2.1 TYPES

The main types of cerebral tumours, listed in order of relative frequency, are

- Gliomas
- Metastases
- Meningeal tumours
- Pituitary adenomas
- Neurilemmomas
- Haemangioblastomas
- Medulloblastomas

14.2.2 GLIOMAS

These are tumours derived from glial cells and their precursors and include

- Astrocytomas—derived from astrocytes
- Oligodendrocytomas—derived from oligodendrocytes
- Ependymomas—derived from ependymal cells

14.2.3 METASTASES

Cerebral metastases derive particularly from primary neoplasia in the

- Lung
- Breast
- Kidney
- Colon
- Ovary
- Prostate
- Thyroid

14.2.4 MENINGEAL TUMOURS

These include

- Meningiomas
- Meningeal sarcomas—very rare
- Primary malignant melanomas derived from pia–arachnoid melanocytes—very rare

14.2.5 PITUITARY ADENOMAS

These include, in approximate order of relative frequency (commonest first),

- Sparsely granulated PRL (prolactin/lactotrophin/ mamotrophin) cell adenomas
- Oncocytomas
- Null cell adenomas
- Gonadotroph cell adenomas
- Corticotroph cell adenomas
- Densely granulated GH (growth hormone/ somatotropin) cell adenomas
- Sparsely granulated GH cell adenomas
- Mixed (GH cell–PRL cell) adenomas
- Silent 'corticotroph' adenomas, subtype 2
- Unclassified adenomas
- Acidophil stem cell adenomas
- Silent 'corticotroph' adenomas, subtype 1
- Silent 'corticotroph' adenomas, subtype 3
- Mammosomatotroph cell adenomas
- Thyrotroph cell adenomas
- Densely granulated GH cell adenomas

14.2.6 NEURILEMMOMAS

These are also known as schwannomas. They are derived from Schwann cells and include acoustic neuromas.

14.2.7 HAEMANGIOBLASTOMAS

These are derived from blood vessels.

14.2.8 MEDULLOBLASTOMAS

These cerebellar tumours are embryonal tumours.

14.3 SCHIZOPHRENIA

14.3.1 GROSS NEUROPATHOLOGY

14.3.1.1 Brain Mass

There is a slight but significant reduction in brain mass in schizophrenia, compared with controls, allowing for differences in height, body mass, sex, and year of birth (Brown et al., 1986; Pakkenburg, 1987; Bruton et al., 1990).

14.3.1.2 Brain Length

Bruton et al. (1990) found a significant reduction in the maximum anteroposterior length of formalin-fixed cerebral hemispheres in schizophrenia, compared with age- and sex-matched normal controls. Both hemispheres were shorter in schizophrenia compared with the controls.

14.3.1.3 Cerebral Volumes

In the postmortem brains of patients with schizophrenia, compared with age- and sex-matched controls, Pakkenburg (1987) found a significant reduction in the volumes of the

- Cerebral hemispheres
- Cerebral cortex
- Central grey matter

The volumes of the white matter did not differ significantly.

14.3.1.4 Hippocampus and Parahippocampal Gyrus

Altshuler et al. (1990) studied the area and shape of the anterior hippocampus and parahippocampal gyrus in postmortem brains from schizophrenic, nonschizophrenic suicide, and nonpsychiatric controls. No significant differences were found in hippocampal area, but the parahippocampal gyrus was significantly smaller in the schizophrenic group compared with the control group.

Bogerts et al. (1990) also studied postmortem brains of schizophrenic patients and control subjects. Compared with the controls, in the schizophrenic group, the hippocampal formation was significantly smaller in the right and left hemispheres. The reduction in hippocampal volume in the male schizophrenics was greater than in the female schizophrenics.

14.3.1.5 Ventricular Volume

Ventricular enlargement has been found in a number of postmortem studies of schizophrenic brains (e.g. Brown et al., 1986; Pakkenburg, 1987; Bruton et al., 1990).

The ventricular enlargement particularly affects the temporal horn (Crow et al., 1989), indicating temporal lobe neuropathology.

14.3.1.6 Temporal Lobe

The major of postmortem studies have found a reduction in temporal lobe volume in schizophrenia. While the grey matter is reduced in volume, particularly at the level of the amygdala and anterior hippocampus, the volume of the white matter tends not to be reduced.

14.3.2 MORPHOMETRIC STUDIES

14.3.2.1 Temporal Lobe

Pyramidal cell disorientation in the hippocampus has been reported by Kovelman and Scheibel (1984) and by Conrad et al. (1991), although this failed to be found by Altshuler et al. (1987).

Jeste and Lohr (1989) found that schizophrenic patients had a significantly lower pyramidal cell density than normal controls in the left CA4 hippocampal region.

Cytoarchitectural abnormalities have been reported in the entorhinal cortex in schizophrenia (Arnold et al., 1991). These changes, which suggest disturbed development, included

- Aberrant invaginations of the surface
- Disruption of cortical layers
- Heterotopic displacement of neurons
- Paucity of neurons in superficial layers

Arnold et al. (1995) found that schizophrenic postmortem brains had a smaller neuron size in the hippocampal regions of

- The subiculum
- CA1
- Layer II of the entorhinal cortex

It is of note that the subiculum, CA1, and the entorhinal cortex are the major subfields of the hippocampal region that maintain the afferent and efferent connections of the hippocampus with widespread cortical and subcortical targets. It was therefore concluded that the smaller size of neurons in these subfields may reflect the presence of structural or functional impairments that disrupt these connections, which in turn could have behavioural sequelae.

Reduced hippocampal mossy cell fibre staining has also been reported by Goldsmith and Joyce (1995).

Akbarian et al. (1993b) found a distorted distribution of nicotinamide-adenine dinucleotide phosphate-diaphorase (NADPH-d) neurons in the hippocampal formation and in the neocortex of the lateral temporal lobe, consistent with anomalous cortical development in the lateral temporal lobe.

14.3.2.2 Other Cortical Areas

Compared with control brains, Benes et al. (1986) found significantly lower neuronal density in the following cortical regions in schizophrenic brains:

- Prefrontal cortex—layer VI
- Anterior cingulate cortex—layer V
- Primary motor cortex—layer III

The glial density also tended to be lower throughout most layers of all three aforementioned regions. However, there were no differences in the neuron: glia ratios or neuronal size between the two groups. These results suggest the occurrence of a dysplastic process rather than degeneration in schizophrenia.

Benes et al. (1987) confirmed the presence of greater numbers of long, vertical, associative axons in the anterior cingulate cortex of schizophrenic patients relative to control subjects. On the basis of this finding, they suggested that there might be an increase of associative inputs into the anterior cingulate cortex in schizophrenia.

Akbarian et al. (1993a) found a distorted distribution of NADPH-d neurons in the dorsolateral prefrontal area of schizophrenic postmortem brains, consistent with anomalous cortical development in this region.

Akbarian et al. (1995) have also found that the prefrontal cortex of schizophrenics shows reduced expression for glutamic acid decarboxylase (GAD) in the absence of significant cell loss, suggesting an activity-dependent down-regulation of neurotransmitter gene expression.

14.3.2.3 Other Brain Regions

The results of studies of the corpus callosum and cerebellum have yielded inconsistent results.

14.3.3 SYNAPTIC PATHOLOGY

14.3.3.1 Synaptic Vesicles

Soustek (1989) found clusters of large numbers of synaptic vesicles in presynaptic knobs in the cerebral cortex of schizophrenic postmortem brains but not in brains from control subjects.

14.3.3.2 Synaptophysin

Synaptophysin is a presynaptic vesicle protein, the distribution and abundance of which provide a synaptic marker that can be reliably measured in postmortem brain.

Eastwood et al. (1995) found that in schizophrenic brains, compared with controls, synaptophysin mRNA was reduced bilaterally in

- CA4
- CA3
- The subiculum
- The parahippocampal gyrus

(The effect of antipsychotic medication was discounted as a separate rat study showed no effect of haloperidol treatment on hippocampal synaptophysin mRNA.) Furthermore, Eastwood and Harrison (1995) found decreased synaptophysin in the medial temporal lobe in schizophrenia, compared with controls, using immunoautoradiography. Significant reductions were found in the

- Dentate gyrus
- Subiculum
- Parahippocampal gyrus

14.3.4 GLIOSIS

Almost all recent quantitative studies investigating the regions of greatest structural differences in schizophrenic patients have not shown significant gliosis (e.g. Jellinger, 1985; Roberts et al., 1987; Bruton et al., 1990). This negative finding is consistent with either of the following possibilities:

- The structural change in schizophrenic brains results from an embryonic insult prior to the third trimester (since the developing brain does not show reactive gliosis until approximately the third trimester).
- A neuropathological process occurs at or after the third trimester but does not usually initiate a glial reaction.

14.3.5 ANTIPSYCHOTIC MEDICATION

It has been suggested that some of the neuropathological (and magnetic resonance imaging [MRI]) changes seen in schizophrenia may be the result of pharmacotherapy with antipsychotic medication (Puri, 2011).

14.4 AUTISM

14.4.1 HISTOLOGICAL CHANGES

Bauman and Kemper (1985) studied the brain of a 29-year-old autistic man and found, compared with the brain of an age- and sex-matched normal control, abnormalities in the

- Hippocampus
- Subiculum
- Entorhinal cortex
- Septal nuclei
- Mammillary body
- Amygdala (selected nuclei)
- Neocerebellar cortex
- Roof nuclei of the cerebellum
- Inferior olivary nucleus

Neuropathological studies suggest that the microscopic neuroanatomical abnormalities in autism begin early in gestation, probably in the second trimester (Bauman, 1991).

14.4.2 CEREBELLAR PATHOLOGY

Both neuropathological and structural neuroimaging studies have indicated that hypoplastia of the cerebellar vermis as well as hypoplasia of the cerebellar hemispheres occurs in some subjects with autism.

14.4.2.1 Reduced Purkinje Cell Count

Ritvo et al. (1986) compared the cerebellums of four autistic subjects with those of three comparison subjects without central nervous system pathology and one with phenytoin toxicity. Total Purkinje cell counts were found to be significantly lower in the cerebellar hemisphere and vermis of each autistic subject than in the comparison subjects.

14.4.2.2 Neocerebellar Abnormality

In their study of subjects with autism, Courchesne et al. (1988) measured the size of the cerebellar vermis using MRI and compared these with its size in controls. The neocerebellar vermal lobules VI and VII were found to be significantly smaller in autism. This appeared to be a result of developmental hypoplasia rather than shrinkage or deterioration after full development had been achieved. In contrast, the adjacent vermal lobules I–V, which are ontogenetically, developmentally, and anatomically distinct from lobules VI and VII, were found to be of normal size. Maldevelopment of the vermal neocerebellum had occurred in both retarded and nonretarded patients

with autism. The authors suggested that this localized maldevelopment might serve as a temporal marker to identify the events that damage the brain in autism, as well as other neural structures that might be concomitantly damaged. They concluded that the neocerebellar abnormality may

- Directly impair cognitive functions that may be attributable to the neocerebellum
- Indirectly affect, through its connections to the brain stem, hypothalamus, and thalamus, the development and functioning of one or more systems involved in cognitive, sensory, autonomic, and motor activities
- Occur concomitantly with damage to other neural sites, the dysfunction of which directly underlies the cognitive deficits in autism

14.5 MOVEMENT DISORDERS

14.5.1 PARKINSON'S DISEASE

Idiopathic Parkinson's disease is characterized by a loss of dopaminergic neurons in the substantia nigra.

14.5.1.1 Macroscopic Neuropathology

Macroscopic changes in idiopathic Parkinson's disease include

- Depigmentation of the substantia nigra—particularly the zona compacta
- Depigmentation of the locus coeruleus

Diffuse cortical atrophy may take place.

14.5.1.2 Histopathology

Histological changes in idiopathic Parkinson's disease include

1. Neuronal loss
2. Reactive astrocytosis
3. The presence of Lewy bodies in the
   a. Substantia nigra
   b. Dorsal motor nucleus of the vagus
   c. Hypothalamus
   d. Nucleus basalis of Meynert
   e. Locus coeruleus
   f. Edinger–Westphal nucleus
   g. Raphe nuclei
   h. Cerebral cortex
   i. Olfactory bulb
4. The presence of melanin-containing macrophages

14.5.1.3   Neurochemical Pathology

Neurochemical changes in idiopathic Parkinson's disease include reduced inhibitory dopaminergic action of the nigrostriatal pathway on striatal cholinergic neurons.

14.5.2   HUNTINGTON'S DISEASE (CHOREA)

Huntington's disease (or chorea) results from a mutation of the protein huntingtin and is characterized by a selective loss of discrete neuronal populations in the brain with progressive degeneration of efferent neurons of the neostriatum and sparing of dopaminergic afferents, resulting in progressive atrophy of the neostriatum.

14.5.2.1   Macroscopic Neuropathology

Macroscopic changes in Huntington's disease include

- Small brain with reduced mass
- Marked atrophy of the corpus striatum—particularly the caudate nucleus
- Marked atrophy of the cerebral cortex—particularly the frontal lobe gyri (the parietal lobe is less often affected)
- Dilatation of the lateral and third ventricles

14.5.2.2   Histopathology

Histological changes in Huntington's disease include

1. Neuronal loss in the cerebral cortex—particularly the frontal cortex
2. Neuronal loss in the corpus striatum—particularly neurons using as neurotransmitters
   a. GABA and enkephalin
   b. GABA and substance P
3. Astrocytosis in affected regions

In the affected regions, there is relative sparing of the following neuronal populations:

- Diaphorase-positive neurons containing nitric oxide synthase (NOS)
- Large cholinesterase-positive neurons

14.5.2.3   Neurochemical Pathology

Neurochemical changes that have been reported in Huntington's disease include

- ↓ GABA
- ↓ GAD
- ↓ Acetylcholine
- ↓ Substance P

- ↑ Somatostatin
- ↓ Corticotrophin-releasing factor (CRF)
- Dopamine hypersensitivity

Evidence has been put forward suggesting that phospholipid-related signal transduction in advanced Huntington's disease is impaired (Puri, 2001).

14.5.3   TARDIVE DYSKINESIA

Tardive dyskinesia is a syndrome of potentially irreversible involuntary hyperkinetic dyskinesias that may occur during long-term treatment with antipsychotic (neuroleptic) medication. The most important hypotheses concerning the neurochemical pathology of tardive dyskinesia are

- Dopamine hypersensitivity
- Free-radical-induced neurotoxicity
- GABA insufficiency
- Noradrenergic dysfunction

14.5.3.1   Dopamine Hypersensitivity Hypothesis

According to this hypothesis, the following sequence of events takes place:

Long-term treatment with antipsychotic (neuroleptic) medication

- → Chronic dopamine receptor blockade
- → Dopamine D2 receptor hypersensitivity in the nigrostriatal pathway
- → Tardive dyskinesia

Evidence in favour of this hypothesis includes

- Studies of denervation-induced hypersensitivity in muscles
- Animal experiments in which, following discontinuation of antipsychotic drugs, acute dopamine agonist challenges → ↑ oral stereotyped behaviour
- Animal experiments in which repeated antipsychotic treatment may → ↑ brain dopamine D2 receptors

Problems with the hypothesis include the following:

- Differences in the chronology of onset of symptoms between humans and animal models.
- Only limited support for dopamine hypersensitivity from post-antipsychotic dopamine turnover experiments in monkeys.

- Postmortem human brain tissue studies have not shown significant differences in D2 receptor binding between schizophrenic patients with tardive dyskinesia and schizophrenic patients without tardive dyskinesia.
- Blood biochemical assays have not shown consistent significant differences between patients with tardive dyskinesia and patients without tardive dyskinesia with respect to
  - Prolactin
  - Somatotropin
- No consistent significant differences have been shown between patients with tardive dyskinesia and patients without tardive dyskinesia with respect to
  - Plasma homovanillic acid
  - Urinary homovanillic acid
  - CSF homovanillic acid
- Dopamine agonists do not strikingly exacerbate tardive dyskinesia.
- Dopamine antagonist antipsychotics may sometimes worsen tardive dyskinesia.

A modification of this hypothesis includes a role for dopamine D1 receptors, but many of the previously mentioned problems also apply again. Moreover, postmortem human brain tissue studies have not shown significant differences in D1 receptor binding between schizophrenic patients with tardive dyskinesia and schizophrenic patients without tardive dyskinesia.

14.5.3.2   Free-Radical-Induced Neurotoxicity

According to this hypothesis, the following sequence of events takes place:

Long-term treatment with antipsychotic (neuroleptic) medication

- → ↑ Catecholamine turnover
- → Free-radical by-products
- → Membrane lipid peroxidation in the basal ganglia (the basal ganglia have a high oxidative metabolism)
- → Tardive dyskinesia

Evidence in favour of this hypothesis includes the following:

- α-Tocopherol (vitamin E) is of benefit in rodent models of antipsychotic-induced dyskinesia.
- Some studies have shown ↑ blood or CSF levels of lipid peroxidation by-products in patients with tardive dyskinesia compared with those without tardive dyskinesia.

Problems with the hypothesis include

- Vitamin E treatment of tardive dyskinesia in general does not lead to major clinical improvement.

14.5.3.3   GABA Insufficiency

According to one version of this hypothesis, the following sequence of events takes place:

Long-term treatment with antipsychotic (neuroleptic) medication

- → Destruction of GABAergic neurons in the striatum
- → ↓ Feedback inhibition
- → Tardive dyskinesia

According to another version, the sequence of events is

Long-term treatment with antipsychotic (neuroleptic) medication

- → ↓ GABAergic neuronal activity in the pars reticulata of the substantia nigra
- → ↓ Inhibition of involuntary movements
- → Tardive dyskinesia

Evidence in favour of these hypotheses includes the following:

1. It has been shown that striatonigral GABAergic neurons feed back on dopaminergic nigrostriatal neurons to reduce their activity.
2. Antipsychotic-treated dyskinetic monkeys have been found to have a decrease in GAD, compared with similarly treated monkeys without tardive dyskinesia, in the
   a. Substantia nigra
   b. Globus pallidus
   c. Subthalamic nucleus
3. Patients with tardive dyskinesia have been found on postmortem to have a significant decrease in GAD activity, compared with patients without tardive dyskinesia, in the subthalamic nucleus
4. The following GABAergic agonists have generally shown promise as potential therapeutic agents
   a. Benzodiazepines
   b. Baclofen
   c. Gamma-vinyl GABA

Problems with the hypothesis include the following:

- Rodent models of tardive dyskinesia do not show consistent GABA function changes with antipsychotic treatment.
- It has not so far proved possible effectively to treat tardive dyskinesia with GABAergic drugs.

14.5.3.4 Noradrenergic Dysfunction

According to this hypothesis, noradrenergic overactivity contributes to the pathophysiology of tardive dyskinesia. Evidence in favour of these hypotheses includes the following:

- Patients with tardive dyskinesia have been found to have significantly greater dopamine β-hydroxylase activity than those without tardive dyskinesia.
- Platelet ^{3}H-dihydroergocryptine-α2 adrenergic receptor binding and CSF noradrenaline have been found to be significantly correlated with the severity of tardive dyskinesia

Problems with the hypothesis include

- It has not so far proved possible effectively to treat tardive dyskinesia with noradrenergic drugs.

REFERENCES

Akbarian S, Bunney WE Jr, Potkin SG, Wigal SB, Hagman JO, Sandman CA, and Jones EG. 1993a: Altered distribution of nicotinamide-adenine dinucleotide phosphate-diaphorase cells in frontal lobe of schizophrenics implies disturbances of cortical development. *Archives of General Psychiatry* 50:169–177.

Akbarian S, Kim JJ, Potkin SG, Hagman JO, Tafazzoli A, Bunney WE Jr, and Jones EG. 1995: Gene expression for glutamic acid decarboxylase is reduced without loss of neurons in prefrontal cortex of schizophrenics. *Archives of General Psychiatry* 52:258–266.

Akbarian S, Vinuela A, Kim JJ, Potkin SG, Bunney WE Jr, and Jones EG. 1993b: Distorted distribution of nicotinamide-adenine dinucleotide phosphate-diaphorase neurons in temporal lobe of schizophrenics implies anomalous cortical development. *Archives of General Psychiatry* 50:178–187.

Altshuler LL, Casanova MF, Goldberg TE, and Kleinman JE. 1990: The hippocampus and parahippocampus in schizophrenia, suicide, and control brains. *Archives of General Psychiatry* 47:1029–1034.

Altshuler LL, Conrad A, Kovelman JA, and Scheibel A. 1987: Hippocampal pyramidal cell orientation in schizophrenia. A controlled neurohistologic study of the Yakovlev collection. *Archives of General Psychiatry* 44:1094–1098.

Arnold SE, Franz BR, Gur RC, Gur RE, Shapiro RM, Moberg PJ, and Trojanowski JQ. 1995: Smaller neuron size in schizophrenia in hippocampal subfields that mediate cortical–hippocampal interactions. *American Journal of Psychiatry* 152:738–748.

Arnold SE, Hyman BT, Van Hoesen GW, and Damasio AR. 1991: Some cytoarchitectural abnormalities of the entorhinal cortex in schizophrenia. *Archives of General Psychiatry* 48:625–632.

Bauman ML. 1991: Microscopic neuroanatomic abnormalities in autism. *Pediatrics* 87:791–796.

Bauman M and Kemper TL. 1985: Histoanatomic observations of brain in early infantile autism. *Neurology* 35:866–874.

Benes FM, Davidson J, and Bird ED. 1986: Quantitative cytoarchitectural studies of the cerebral cortex of schizophrenics. *Archives of General Psychiatry* 43:31–35.

Benes FM, Majocha R, Bird ED, and Marotta CA. 1987: Increased vertical axon numbers in cingulate cortex of schizophrenics. *Archives of General Psychiatry* 44:1017–1021.

Berrios GE. 1991: Alzheimer's disease: A conceptual history. *International Journal of Geriatric Psychiatry* 5:355–365.

Bogerts B, Falkai P, Haupts M, Greve B, Ernst S, Tapernon-Franz U, and Heinzmann U. 1990: Post-mortem volume measurements of limbic system and basal ganglia structures in chronic schizophrenics. Initial results from a new brain collection. *Schizophrenia Research* 3:295–301.

Brown R, Colter N, Corsellis JA, Crow TJ, Frith CD, Jagoe R, Johnstone EC, and Marsh L. 1986: Postmortem evidence of structural brain changes in schizophrenia. Differences in brain weight, temporal horn area, and parahippocampal gyrus compared with affective disorder. *Archives of General Psychiatry* 43:36–42.

Bruton CJ, Crow TJ, Frith CD, Johnstone EC, Owens DG, and Roberts GW. 1990: Schizophrenia and the brain: A prospective clinico-neuropathological study. *Psychological Medicine* 20:285–304.

Conrad AJ, Abebe T, Austin R, Forsythe S, and Scheibel AB. 1991: Hippocampal pyramidal cell disarray in schizophrenia as a bilateral phenomenon. *Archives of General Psychiatry* 48:413–417.

Courchesne E, Yeung Courchesne R, Press GA, Hesselink JR, and Jerningan TL. 1988: Hypoplasia of cerebellar vermal lobules VI and VII in autism. *New England Journal of Medicine* 318:1349–1354.

Crow TJ, Ball J, Bloom SR, Brown R, Bruton CJ, Colter N, Frith CD, Johnstone EC, Owens DG, and Roberts GW. 1989: Schizophrenia as an anomaly of development of cerebral asymmetry. A postmortem study and a proposal concerning the genetic basis of the disease. *Archives of General Psychiatry* 46:1145–1150.

Eastwood SL, Burnet PW, and Harrison PJ. 1995: Altered synaptophysin expression as a marker of synaptic pathology in schizophrenia. *Neuroscience* 66:309–319.

Eastwood SL and Harrison PJ. 1995: Decreased synaptophysin in the medial temporal lobe in schizophrenia demonstrated using immunoautoradiography. *Neuroscience* 69:339–343.

Gentleman SM. 2010: Neuropathology. In Puri BK and Treasaden IH (eds.) *Psychiatry: An Evidence-Based Text*, pp. 435–444. London, U.K.: Hodder Arnold.

Goldsmith SK and Joyce JN. 1995: Alterations in hippocampal mossy fiber pathway in schizophrenia and Alzheimer's disease. *Biological Psychiatry* 37:122–126.

Holdorff B. 2002; Friedrich Heinrich Lewy and His Work. *Journal of the History of the Neurosciences* 11(1):19–28.

Jellinger K. 1985: Neuromorphological background of patho-chemical studies in major psychoses. In Beckman H (ed.) *Pathochemical Markers in Major Psychoses*, pp. 1–23. Heidelberg, Germany: Springer Verlag.

Jeste DV and Lohr JB. 1989: Hippocampal pathologic find-ings in schizophrenia. A morphometric study. *Archives of General Psychiatry* 46:1019–1024.

Kovelman JA and Scheibel AB. 1984: A neurohistologi-cal correlate of schizophrenia. *Biological Psychiatry* 19:1601–1621.

McKeith IG. 2006: Consensus guidelines for the clinical and pathologic diagnosis of dementia with Lewy bodies (DLB): Report of the Consortium on DLB International Workshop. *Journal of Alzheimer's Disease* 9:417–423.

Pakkenberg B. 1987: Post-mortem study of chronic schizophrenic brains. *British Journal of Psychiatry* 151:744–752.

Puri BK. 2001: Impaired phospholipid-related signal transduc-tion in advanced Huntington's disease. *Experimental Physiology* 86:683–685.

Puri BK. 2011: Brain tissue changes and antipsychotic medi-cation. *Expert Review of Neurotherapeutics* 11:943–946.

Ritvo ER, Freeman BJ, Scheibel AB, Duong T, Robinson H, Guthrie D, and Ritvo A. 1986: Lower Purkinje cell counts in the cerebella of four autistic subjects: Initial findings of the UCLA-NSAC autopsy research report. *American Journal of Psychiatry* 143:862–866.

Roberts GW, Colter N, Lofthouse R, Johnstone EC, and Crow TJ. 1987: Is there gliosis in schizophrenia? Investigation of the temporal lobe. *Biological Psychiatry* 22:1459–1468.

Soustek Z. 1989: Ultrastructure of cortical synapses in the brain of schizophrenics. *Zentralblatt für Allgemeine Patholic und Pathologische Anatomie* 135:25–32.

15 Neuroimaging Techniques

15.1 X-RAY

15.1.1 BASIS

Radiography utilizes x-rays.

15.1.2 TYPE OF IMAGING

X-ray radiography is a form of structural imaging.

15.1.3 NEUROPSYCHIATRIC APPLICATIONS

The main use nowadays of skull radiography is

- Assessment of trauma

It may also be useful in the detection of intracranial expanding lesions.

15.2 CT

CT is x-ray computerized tomography or computed tomography. It was previously known as computerized axial tomography, or CAT.

15.2.1 BASIS

The basis of CT is as follows:
X-ray beams are passed through a given tissue plane in different directions:

Scintillation counters record the emerging x-rays.
Computer reconstruction of emerging x-ray data.
Radiodensity maps.

This procedure is repeated for successive adjacent planes, thereby building up an image of, for example, the whole brain.

15.2.2 TYPE OF IMAGING

CT is a form of structural imaging.

15.2.3 NEUROPSYCHIATRIC APPLICATIONS

Where available, CT and MRI have largely replaced skull radiography. Its clinical uses include the detection of

- Shifts of intracranial structures
- Intracranial expanding lesions
- Cerebral infarction
- Cerebral oedema
- Cerebral atrophy and ventricular dilatation
- Atrophy of other structures
- Demyelination changes and other causes of radiodensity change

It is also widely used in neuropsychiatric research.

15.3 PET

PET is positron emission tomography.

15.3.1 BASIS

The basis of PET neuroimaging is as follows:

A positron-emitting radioisotope or radiolabelled ligand is introduced into the cerebral circulation; routes commonly used are
- Intravenous administration (the radioactive substance is in solution)
- By inhalation (the radioactive substance is in gaseous form)

Blood flow ± cerebral tissue binding in the brain.
Emission of positrons.
Positron–electron interactions.
Dual γ-photon emissions.
Detection of γ-photons.
Computer reconstruction of emerging γ-photon data.
Slice images of the distribution of the radioisotopes in the brain.

The positron-emitting radioisotopes used can be produced in small cyclotrons.

15.3.2   Type of Imaging

PET is a form of functional imaging.

15.3.3   Neuropsychiatric Applications

PET neuroimaging can give information about

- Metabolic changes
- Regional cerebral blood flow (rCBF)
- Ligand binding

Clinical applications of PET include

- Cerebrovascular disease
- Alzheimer's disease
- Epilepsy, prior to neurosurgery
- Head injury

Some measurements made by PET, for example, the study of rCBF, are likely to be increasingly replaced by functional magnetic resonance imaging (fMRI), since the latter does not require the use of radioactive isotopes. On the other hand, fMRI is not a suitable replacement for PET for ligand-binding studies.

15.4   SPECT

SPECT is single-photon emission computerized tomography. It is also known as SPET or single-photon emission tomography.

15.4.1   Basis

The basis of SPECT neuroimaging is as follows:

A radioisotope or radiolabelled ligand is introduced into the cerebral circulation; routes commonly used are
- Intravenous administration (the radioactive substance is in solution)
- By inhalation (the radioactive substance is in gaseous form)

Blood flow ± cerebral tissue binding in the brain.
Single γ-photon emissions.
Detection of γ-photons.
Computer reconstruction of emerging γ-photon data.
Slice images of the distribution of the radioisotopes in the brain.

15.4.2   Type of Imaging

SPECT is a form of functional imaging.

15.4.3   Neuropsychiatric Applications

SPECT neuroimaging can give information about

- rCBF
- Ligand binding

It is also of use in conditions in which the onset of the symptomatology being studied (e.g. epileptic seizures, auditory hallucinations) may occur at a time when the patient is not in or near a scanner; a suitable radioligand (e.g. 99 m technetium hexamethylpropylene amine oxime [HMPAO]) can be administered at the material time and the patient scanned afterward.

Clinical applications of SPECT include

- Alzheimer's disease

The resolution of SPECT is generally poorer than that of PET, and both are likely to be increasingly replaced by fMRI. However, fMRI is not a suitable replacement for SPECT for ligand studies or for the type of study mentioned earlier in which the onset of the symptomatology being studied may occur at a time when the subject is not in or near a scanner.

15.5   MRI

MRI is magnetic resonance imaging. It was previously referred to as NMR or nuclear magnetic resonance. In vivo NMR is now taken to include arterial spin labelling (ASL), diffusion kurtosis imaging (DKI), diffusion tensor imaging (DTI), diffusion-weighted imaging (DWI), MRI, magnetic resonance angiography (MRA), magnetic resonance spectroscopy (MRS), and fMRI. In addition, it is possible to carry out in vitro NMR studies of tissues at higher magnetic field strengths (say, over 11 T) than are currently allowed for human subjects.

15.5.1   Basis

The basis of MRI is as follows:
The patient is placed in a strong static magnetic field → alignment of proton spin axes:

Pulses of radio-frequency waves at specified frequencies are administered.
This additional energy is absorbed.
Some protons jump to a higher quantum level.
Radio waves are emitted when these protons return to the lower quantum level.

The radio-frequency (rf) wave frequencies are measured.

Precession in each voxel is determined and T_1 (longitudinal relaxation time) and T_2 (transverse relaxation time) calculated.

Proton density, T_1, $T_2 \rightarrow$ pixel intensities.

Anatomical magnetic resonance images.

(The data are actually collected in the temporal domain and need to be converted into the frequency domain using Fourier transformation.)

In some circumstances, it may be useful to administer a paramagnetic contrast-enhancing agent such as gadolinium-DTPA.

fMRI can use the blood oxygen level-dependent (BOLD) effect, whereby whereas oxyhaemoglobin is diamagnetic, deoxyhaemoglobin is paramagnetic and so may be used as an endogenous contrast agent. Images from the first published human study of V1 activation during photic stimulation using BOLD fMRI, by Bruce Rosen's group at Harvard Medical School, are shown in Figure 15.1.

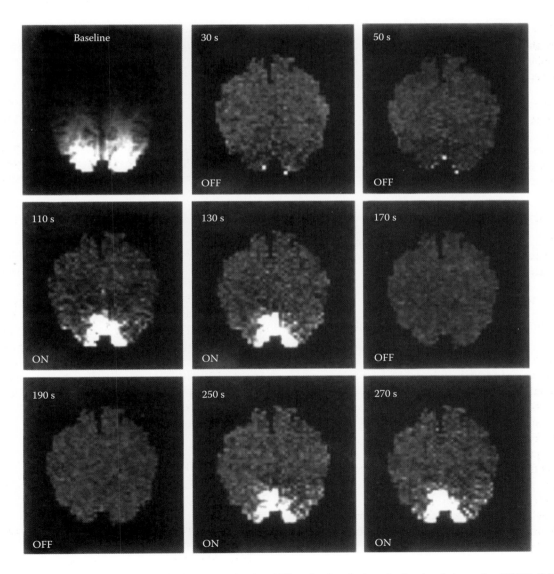

FIGURE 15.1 Images from the first published human study of V1 activation during photic stimulation using BOLD fMRI. The upper left image was acquired during darkness (baseline) and this baseline image was subtracted from subsequent images. OFF, darkness; ON, photic stimulation. (Reproduced from Kwong, K.K. et al., *Proc. Natl. Acad. Sci. USA*, 89, 5675, 1992. With permission.)

15.5.2   TYPE OF IMAGING

DKI, DTI, DWI, MRI, and MRA are forms of structural imaging. DKI and DTI are particularly useful for mapping white matter tracts in the brain.

ASL, MRS, and fMRI are types of functional imaging. ASL allows cerebral blood flow to be measured noninvasively. MRS allows the relative concentrations in the brain (and other organs) of certain substances to be measured noninvasively.

15.5.3   NEUROPSYCHIATRIC APPLICATIONS

MRI is useful in most clinical and research studies requiring high-resolution neuroanatomical imaging.

BIBLIOGRAPHY

Ketonen LM and Berg MJ. 1996: *Clinical Neuroradiology.* London, U.K.: Arnold.

Kwong KK, Belliveau JW, Chesler DA et al. 1992: Dynamic magnetic resonance imaging of human brain activity during primary sensory stimulation. *Proceedings of the National Academy of Sciences of the United States of America* 89:5675–5679.

Puri BK. 2000: MRI and MRS in neuropsychiatry. In Young IR, Grant DM, and Harris RK (eds.) *Methods in Biomedical Magnetic Resonance Imaging and Spectroscopy,* pp. 1135–1142. New York, NY: Wiley.

Puri BK. 2010: Neuroimaging. In Puri BK and Treasaden IH (eds.) *Psychiatry: An Evidence-Based Text,* pp. 445–464. London, U.K.: Hodder Arnold.

Yousem DM and Grossman RI. 2010: *Neuroradiology: The Requisites,* 3rd edn. Philadelphia, PA: Mosby Elsevier.

16 Neurophysiology

16.1 PHYSIOLOGY OF NEURONS, SYNAPSES, AND RECEPTORS

16.1.1 NEURONS

16.1.1.1 Resting Membrane Ion Permeabilities

The comparative permeabilities to different ions of the resting neuronal membrane are as follows:

- K^+ (potassium ions)—relatively permeable
- Na^+ (sodium ions)—relatively impermeable
- Cl^- (chloride ions)—freely permeable
- Organic anions—relatively impermeable

16.1.1.2 Resting Membrane Potential

There is a negative resting membrane potential of around −70 mV. It is maintained by the sodium pump, which actively transports Na^+ out of the cell and K^+ into the cell. Energy for this process is provided by ATP.

16.1.1.3 Changes in Membrane Ion Permeabilities

The neuronal membrane ion permeabilities may change in response to stimulation:

- Depolarization—the membrane potential increases, that is, it becomes less negative.
- This increases the probability of an action potential (AP) being generated.
- Hyperpolarization—the membrane potential decreases, that is, it becomes more negative.

This decreases the probability of an action potential being generated.

16.1.1.4 Action Potential

Details of the AP are shown in Figure 16.1.

Neuronal stimulation leads to local depolarization.

If (degree of depolarization) > (a critical threshold) → nerve impulse or AP

During an AP, the membrane potential rapidly becomes positive, before returning to become negative. This is caused by an increase first in Na^+ permeability, allowing the inflow of Na^+, and then in K^+ permeability (with a rapid reduction in Na^+ permeability at the same time), causing an outflow of K^+ and thereby restoring the negative membrane potential. The sodium pump then restores the original ionic concentrations.

16.1.1.5 Propagation of Action Potential

An AP is propagated by the depolarization spreading laterally to adjacent parts of the neuron.

16.1.1.6 All-or-None Phenomenon

The passage of an AP along a neuron is an all-or-none phenomenon.

16.1.1.7 Absolute Refractory Period

This is the period during which the active part of the neuronal membrane has a reversed polarity so that conduction or initiation of another AP is not possible in it.

16.1.1.8 Relative Refractory Period

This is the period of repolarization after an AP, during which hyperpolarization occurs, making it more difficult for stimulation to allow the membrane potential to reach the critical threshold.

16.1.1.9 Conduction in Unmyelinated Fibres

The greater the diameter of the fibre, the faster is the rate of transmission.

16.1.1.10 Conduction in Myelinated Fibres

The AP appears to jump from one node of Ranvier to the next, skipping the intervening myelinated parts. This rapid form of conduction is known as saltatory conduction.

16.1.2 SYNAPSES

16.1.2.1 Synaptic Cleft

This is the gap at a synapse between the membrane of a presynaptic fibre and that of the postsynaptic fibre.

16.1.2.2 Location

Synapses may be found between

- Two neurons
- Motor neurons and muscle cells
- Sensory neurons and sensory receptors

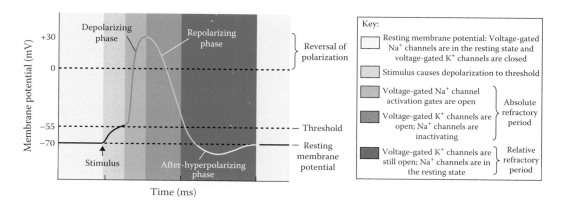

FIGURE 16.1 AP or impulse. When a stimulus depolarizes the membrane to threshold −55 mV, an AP is generated. The AP arises at the trigger zone (at the junction of the axon hillock and the initial segment) and then propagates along the axon to the axon terminals. (Redrawn from Tortora, G.J. and Derrickson, B., *Principles of Anatomy and Physiology*, 11th edn., Wiley-Blackwell, New York, 2006. With permission.)

16.1.2.3   Types

There are two types of synapse:

1. Chemical—the commoner type, in which a chemical neurotransmitter is stored in presynaptic vesicles
2. Electrical—faster than chemical synapses, with direct membrane to membrane connection via gap junctions

16.1.2.4   Synaptic Transmission

At chemical synapses, the following events take place during synaptic transmission:

Arrival of AP at presynaptic membrane.
Influx of Ca^{2+} (calcium ions).
Presynaptic vesicles fuse to the presynaptic membrane.
Release of neurotransmitter into the synaptic cleft.
Passage of neurotransmitter across the synaptic cleft.
Binding of neurotransmitter to postsynaptic receptors.
Ion permeability changes in postsynaptic membrane.
Postsynaptic depolarization or hyperpolarization (depending on the type of neurotransmitter).

16.1.2.5   Excitatory Postsynaptic Potentials

Excitatory postsynaptic potentials, or EPSPs, occur in the postsynaptic membrane (because of depolarization) following release of an excitatory neurotransmitter from the presynaptic neuron at central excitatory synapses.

16.1.2.6   Inhibitory Postsynaptic Potentials

Inhibitory postsynaptic potentials, or IPSPs, occur in the postsynaptic membrane (because of hyperpolarization) following release of an inhibitory neurotransmitter from the presynaptic neuron at central inhibitory synapses.

16.1.2.7   Summation

One EPSP on its own is not usually sufficient to initiate an AP. However, temporal and/or spatial summation may allow the degree of depolarization to reach the critical threshold, as shown in Figure 16.2. IPSPs, on summating with EPSPs, counter the effect of the latter.

16.1.3   Receptors

16.1.3.1   Sensory Receptors

The main types of sensory receptor in humans are

- Mechanoreceptors
- Thermoreceptors
- Light receptors
- Nociceptors
- Chemoreceptors

16.1.3.2   Adaptation

In response to a continuous prolonged appropriate stimulus, most sensory receptors exhibit adaptation:

- Phasic receptors—the receptor firing stops.
- Tonic receptors—the receptor firing frequency falls to a low maintained level.

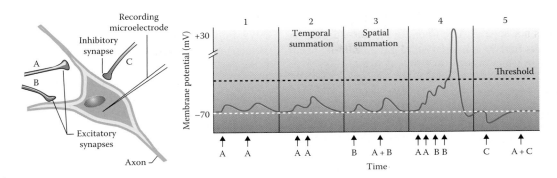

FIGURE 16.2 Interaction of excitatory postsynaptic potentials (EPSPs) and inhibitory postsynaptic potentials (IPSPs) at the postsynaptic neuron. Presynaptic neurons (A–C) were stimulated at times indicated by the arrows, and the resulting membrane potential was recorded in the postsynaptic cell by a recording microelectrode. (Redrawn from Widmaier, E.P. et al., *Vander's Human Physiology*, 11th edn., McGraw Hill, Berkshire, England, 2008. With permission.)

16.2 PITUITARY HORMONES

16.2.1 ANTERIOR PITUITARY HORMONES

The following table gives the anterior pituitary hormones and their corresponding hypothalamic-releasing factors (hormones) and release-inhibiting factors (hormones).

Anterior Pituitary Hormone	Hypothalamic-Releasing Factor (Hormone) and/or Release-Inhibiting Factor (Hormone)
Corticotropin (adrenocorticotropic hormone, ACTH)	Corticotropin-releasing factor (hormone) (CRF or CRH)
Follicle-stimulating hormone (FSH)	Gonadotropin-releasing factor (hormone) (GnRF or GnRH)
Luteinizing hormone (LH)	GnRF or GnRH
Melanocyte-stimulating hormone (MSH)	MSH release inhibitory factor (MIH)
Prolactin	Prolactin-releasing factor (PRF)
	Prolactin release inhibitory factor (PIF) (dopamine)
Somatotropin (growth hormone, GH)	Growth hormone-releasing factor (hormone) (GRF or GRH; somatocrinin)
	GH release inhibitory factor (somatostatin)
Thyrotropin (thyroid-stimulating hormone, TSH)	Thyrotropin releasing factor (hormone) (TRF or TRH)

16.2.1.1 ACTH

This is a single-chain peptide that stimulates the production by the adrenal glands of the steroid hormone cortisol.

16.2.1.2 FSH

FSH consists of two peptide chains, α and β. FSH stimulates the gonads (ovaries and testes).

In males, FSH stimulates seminiferous tubule Sertoli cells to promote the growth of spermatozoa and also stimulates the release of inhibin A (the α subunit) and inhibin B (the β subunit). (In turn, inhibin causes a negative feedback on the secretion of FSH by the anterior pituitary gland.)

In females, FSH stimulates the development of follicles. It also stimulates the activity of aromatase, which in turn stimulates the conversion of ovarian androgens into oestrogens. As in males, FSH stimulates the release of inhibin (from stromal cells of the ovary), which in turn causes a negative feedback on the secretion of FSH by the anterior pituitary gland.

16.2.1.3 LH

LH consists of two peptide chains, α and β; the α-chain of LH is the same as that of FSH. LH stimulates the gonads (ovaries and testes).

In males, LH stimulates the testicular Leydig cells to produce testosterone.

In females, LH stimulates the ovaries to produce androgens. In menstruating females, a surge of LH midcycle induces ovulation.

16.2.1.4 MSH

MSH does not appear to be found in the human anterior pituitary. Its functions in relation to pigmentation appear to have been taken over by ACTH and β-lipotropin.

16.2.1.5 Prolactin

Prolactin is a single-chain peptide hormone that acts on the mammary glands to stimulate the secretion of milk (normally during lactation). It also inhibits activity of the testes and ovaries.

16.2.1.6 GH

GH is a peptide hormone that stimulates the hepatic secretion of IGF-1 (insulin-like growth factor-1; previously termed somatomedin C). In turn, binding of IGF-1 to widespread IGF-binding proteins (IGF-BP) leads to the stimulation of anabolism (e.g. by stimulating the retention of calcium, phosphorus, and nitrogen, thereby promoting growth in bones) and stimulating the widespread biosynthesis of protein and collagen. Another important action of IGF-1 is in terms of opposing the action of insulin.

16.2.1.7 TSH

TSH consists of two peptide chains, α and β; the α-chain of TSH is the same as that of LH (and of FSH). TSH stimulates the synthesis by the thyroid gland of the thyroid hormones T_4 and T_3. TSH also stimulates the release of T_4 and T_3 from the thyroid gland. (In turn, T_3 exerts a negative feedback control on the secretion of TRH and TSH.)

16.2.2 Posterior Pituitary Hormones

The hypothalamus is responsible for the neurosecretion of the two posterior pituitary hormones:

- Arginine vasopressin (AVP) (argipressin or antidiuretic hormone [ADH])
- Oxytocin

Note that, strictly speaking, these are actually hypothalamic hormones rather than pituitary hormones, as they are synthesized in the supraoptic and paraventricular nuclei of the anterior hypothalamus and then transported to and stored in the posterior pituitary gland.

16.2.2.1 AVP or ADH

AVP or ADH is a nonapeptide that acts on the distal convoluted tubule and collecting ducts of the renal nephron to exert an antidiuretic effect.

16.2.2.2 Oxytocin

Oxytocin is a nonapeptide that stimulates contraction of the uterine myometrium during parturition (and perhaps during sexual intercourse), and postpartum, it stimulates the ejection of milk from the mammary glands during lactation. In rats, it has been found that centrally administered oxytocin has a satiety action (in both males and females). Oxytocin also has a natriuretic action in both males and females.

16.3 INTEGRATED BEHAVIOURS

16.3.1 Regulatory Behaviour

A regulatory behaviour is one that is controlled by a homeostatic mechanism. Examples include behaviours related to hunger (feeding) and thirst (drinking).

In contrast, a non-regulatory behaviour is one that is not controlled by a homeostatic mechanism. Examples include sexual behaviour and parenting behaviour.

16.3.2 Pain

The neural pathway for pain is as follows:

Pain detection by receptors (e.g. nociceptors in the skin)

- Dorsal root ganglion neurons to spinal cord
- Ventral spinothalamic tract
- Medial lemniscus
- Ventrolateral thalamus
- Primary somatosensory cortex

According to the gate theory of pain, gates in the spinal cord, involving activity in spinal cord interneurons, can modify the perception of pain. These gates may also exist in the brain stem and even the cerebral cortex. This theory may explain why shifting attention away from the source of pain to something else may help reduce the severity of the pain that the subject is conscious of.

Hormonal substances, such as endorphins, may also influence the perception of pain. For example, during times of war, a soldier at the front may hardly feel any pain initially following a traumatic bodily injury such as the loss of part of a limb. In contrast, the same injury incurred in civilian life during peace time may cause the same person to scream out in agony.

16.3.3 Motor Function

At its simplest, motor activity involves the following pathway:

Activity in the motor cortex (primary motor cortex—precentral gyrus, Brodmann area 4)

- Ipsilateral corticospinal tract
- Pyramidal decussation
- Ipsilateral (mainly) ventral corticospinal tract (moves midline muscles) and contralateral (mainly) lateral corticospinal tract (moves limb muscles)

16.3.4   Arousal

Further details regarding sleep and arousal are given in Section 16.4. Here, we consider the changes in thalamo-cortical systems that occur in sleep and arousal. Basically, the hypothalamus appears to contain neuronal circuits that mediate homeostatic sleep mechanisms.

One important subcortical circuit involved is as follows. Output from the ventrolateral preoptic area, suprachiasmatic nucleus, and tuberomammillary nucleus of the hypothalamus synchronizes the non-rapid eye movement–rapid eye movement (NREM–REM) sleep cycle mechanisms of the pontine brain stem. The parts of the latter that appear to be particularly involved are the

- Locus coeruleus
- Raphe nuclei
- Dorsolateral tegmental nucleus
- Pedunculopontine tegmental nucleus

A second subcortical system of importance involves output from the ventrolateral preoptic area, suprachiasmatic nucleus, and tuberomammillary nucleus of the hypothalamus to the thalamus and thence to the cerebral cortex.

16.3.5   Sexual Behaviour

This is a non-regulatory form of behaviour with complex control mechanisms.

Sex hormones have an important effect on the brain. In male fetuses, during development testosterone masculinizes the brain. This is the *organizing effect* of the hormone. This effect is particularly noteworthy in the hypothalamic preoptic area; this area is much larger in males following exposure to testosterone.

In the adult brain, sex hormones have an *activating effect*. In male adults, testosterone acts on the amygdala to stimulate the motivation to carry out sexual activity. Testosterone also acts on the hypothalamus to stimulate copulatory behaviour. In particular, stimulation of the medial preoptic area, in the presence of circulating testosterone, induces copulatory behaviour in primates. (Destruction of the medial preoptic area in male monkeys, in which testosterone is circulating, is associated with an abolition of mating, but masturbation in the presence of out-of-reach females has been noted.) In female adults, ovarian hormones also appear to act on the amygdala to stimulate the motivation to carry out sexual activity. In infrahuman quadrupedal mammals, the action of ovarian hormones on the ventromedial hypothalamus (VMH) stimulates lordosis (arching of the back, staying still with the back side elevated—a position that is receptive for copulatory behaviour).

Humans are aware of the importance of cognitive influences on sexual behaviour. The influence of cerebral cortex in the context is clearly important but complex. For instance, while frontal lobe patients often are associated with a loss of sexual inhibition, loss of libido may also occur in some cases.

16.3.6   Hunger

Feeding is a regulatory behaviour that particularly involves inputs from the following systems:

- Digestive system (including insulin) and satiety signals
- Hypothalamus
- Cognitive factors

16.3.6.1   Insulin

The most important hormone that affects caloric homeostasis is insulin. When hungry, first the smell and then the taste of a meal cause signals to be sent in the following way:

Smell of food ± taste of food

- Aroma and taste signals
- Cerebral cortex
- Hypothalamus
- Dorsal motor nucleus of the vagus nerve (cranial nerve X)
- Vagal cholinergic fibres
- Pancreas
- Insulin secretion from pancreatic B cells

This is known as the cephalic phase of insulin secretion.

Entry of food into the stomach and duodenum leads to a further secretion of insulin; this is the gastrointestinal phase of insulin secretion.

Breakdown products from digested food enter the bloodstream and directly act on the pancreas, further stimulating the secretion of insulin. This is known as the substrate phase of insulin secretion.

16.3.6.2 Satiety Signals

Gastric distension, for example, following the ingestion of food, gives rise to satiety signals along the following pathway:

Food ingestion

- Gastric distension
- Stimulation of gastric wall stretch receptors
- Vagal nerve transmission
- Nucleus of tractus solitarius and area postrema (in the brain stem)
- Hypothalamus
- Cerebral cortex
- Perception of gastric distension

There exist other systems that also provide feedback to the brain from the alimentary canal. For example, as the ingested (and partially digested) food reaches the intestines, many different peptides are released. Just one of these, cholecystokinin (CCK), can stimulate vagal afferents carrying pyloric gastric stretch receptor signals to the brain stem, thereby providing synergy with the satiety signal system just mentioned earlier. Moreover, infrahuman mammalian experiments have demonstrated the satiety action of CCK directly infused into the hypothalamus. Another neuropeptide that may affect hunger is oxytocin, intracerebroventricular injection of which decreases food intake in rats.

Caloric intake also has a direct satiety effect, although the precise mechanism(s) by which this occur(s) is(are) not clear at the time of writing.

Satiety signals are also given rise to by postgastric actions of ingested food. One mechanism involved is undoubtedly related to the liver.

The hormone leptin (or Ob protein), biosynthesized in adipose tissue, has a circulating plasma concentration that is positively correlated with overall adiposity. Leptin has a satiety action when experimentally directly infused into cerebral ventricles, and hypothalamic leptin receptors have been identified.

16.3.6.3 Hypothalamus

Rodent experiments from the 1950s onward have suggested that

- The ventrolateral hypothalamus (VLH) contains a hunger centre; bilateral damage to this area causes aphagia in rats.
- The VMH contains a satiety centre; damage to this area may cause hyperphagia in rats.

This is known as the dual centre hypothesis. More recent evidence has suggested that this simple hypothesis is, in fact, incorrect. The true reason why bilateral ventromedial hypothalamic damage leads to hyperphagia is related to

- An increase in parasympathetic tone
- An increase in vagal reflexes (and therefore an increased rate of gastric emptying)
- A reduction in sympathetic tone
- A resetting of a hypothetical homeostatic set point
- An increase in the accumulation of stored fat
- A reduction in satiety duration following feeding

Opposite effects occur following bilateral VLH damage.

The neuropeptide Y (NPY) appears to act on the paraventricular nucleus to increase food intake.

16.3.6.4 Ghrelin

Ghrelin is a ligand for the growth hormone secretagogue receptor (GHSR). It is an octanoylated 28-amino-acid peptide produced and secreted by gastric oxyntic gland cells. It has been proposed that ghrelin acts as an enteric signal that stimulates appetite.

16.3.6.5 Cognitive Factors

As with sexual behaviour, cognitive factors are clearly of importance in the integrated behaviour of hunger and feeding. The ability of people to fast, for example, shows that cognitive activity can override satiety signalling and any putative hypothalamic factors.

The amygdala is thought to play some role in hunger and feeding. It is known, for example, that damage to the amygdala is associated with the abolition of taste-aversion learning and also with a change in the types of food that are preferred.

Damage to the inferior prefrontal cortex often appears to be associated with reduced food intake. This may, however, be at least partly related to the fact that this part of the cerebral cortex receives olfactory signals, so that damage to the cortex may reduce the ability to respond to the aroma and taste of food.

16.3.7 Thirst

Drinking is a regulatory behaviour. There are two types of homeostatic mechanisms that are of relevance and that give rise to two different types of thirst. They are

- Osmotic homeostasis (related to osmotic thirst)
- Volume homeostasis (related to hypovolaemic thirst)

16.3.7.1 Osmotic Thirst

Osmotic thirst occurs when the concentrations of solutes in body fluids such as the plasma become too high. This may occur as a result of a rise in concentration of one or more solutes (e.g. following sodium loading after eating a meal rich in sodium salts such as sodium chloride and monosodium glutamate). It may also occur as a result of water deprivation (dehydration) or the copious loss of dilute fluids such as sweat. Under any of these circumstances, the osmotic homeostatic mechanism requires that water be drunk.

Before the behaviour associated with osmotic thirst kicks in, the body relies on its large posterior pituitary stores of AVP to try to rectify the osmolality of the extracellular and intracellular fluid compartments. The mechanism appears to involve the following pathway:

Increase in solutes/water deprivation/dehydration/loss of dilute fluid

- Raised extracellular fluid osmolality (and therefore also raised intracellular fluid osmolality via osmosis)
- Stimulation of osmoreceptor cells in the organ of the lamina terminalis, subfornical organ, median preoptic nucleus, and magnocellular neurons in the supraoptic nucleus and paraventricular nucleus
- Projections from the organ of the lamina terminalis to the median preoptic nucleus and to the magnocellular AVP-secreting cells of the supraoptic nucleus and paraventricular nucleus further stimulate these other brain regions
- Secretion of AVP from the posterior pituitary
- Stimulation of AVP V_2 renal receptors
- Increased water permeability of distal convoluted tubules and collecting ducts of nephrons
- Increased water retention, increased urinary osmolality, and reduced urinary volume
- Restoration of extracellular fluid osmolality

At the time of writing, the neural pathways in the forebrain that are related to thirst have not been clearly identified.

Another mechanism involved in osmotic homeostasis and osmotic thirst is the increased urinary excretion of sodium ions as a result of the actions of atrial natriuretic peptide (ANP) and oxytocin. ANP is released from the cardiac atria in response to increased atrial distension, in turn caused by hyperosmolality of the extracellular fluid. The release of oxytocin from the posterior pituitary has been mentioned in Section 16.2.2.

16.3.7.2 Hypovolaemic Thirst

Hypovolaemic thirst occurs when the total volume of body fluids such as the plasma becomes too low. This may occur as a result of blood loss, for example. The hypovolaemic homeostatic mechanism requires that fluids that contain solutes be drunk; if only pure water were drunk, then hyposmolality would result. In experiments, hypovolaemic rats that are given a choice of pure water or concentrated sodium chloride solution have been observed to drink enough of each in order to be imbibing isotonic levels overall.

One mechanism involved is the following:

Blood loss of greater than 10% of normal blood volume

- Detection by stretch receptors in veins that enter the cardiac right atrium; larger blood volume decreases are also detected by stretch receptors in the aortic arch and carotid sinus.
- Vagal nerve transmission.
- Nucleus of tractus solitarius (in the medulla oblongata).
- Supraoptic nucleus and paraventricular nucleus of hypothalamus (including via a noradrenergic pathway from ventrolateral medulla A_1 cells).
- Secretion of AVP from the posterior pituitary.
- Stimulation of AVP V_2 renal receptors.
- Increased water permeability of distal convoluted tubules and collecting ducts of nephrons.
- Increased water retention, increased urinary osmolality, and reduced urinary volume.
- Reverses hypovolaemia.

Another mechanism that also operates starts with the kidneys, as follows:

Hypovolaemia

- Reduced renal perfusion pressure and reduced delivery of sodium ions to the distal tubule of the nephron.
- Renal secretion of renin.
- Catalyses the conversion of hepatic angiotensinogen into angiotensin I.
- Conversion into angiotensin II (A II) (catalysed by angiotensin-converting enzyme from the lungs).
- Vasoconstriction and stimulation of adrenal secretion of aldosterone.
- Aldosterone stimulates renal conservation of sodium ions.
- Reverses hypovolaemia.

A II also acts as a neurotransmitter in the brain in the following way:

A II

- Binding to A II receptors in the subfornical organ (which does not have a blood–brain barrier)
- Supraoptic nucleus and paraventricular nucleus
- Secretion of AVP from the posterior pituitary
- Stimulation of AVP V_2 renal receptors
- Increased water permeability of distal convoluted tubules and collecting ducts of nephrons
- Increased water retention, increased urinary osmolality, and reduced urinary volume
- Reverses hypovolaemia

The central actions of A II also stimulate thirst.

16.4   AROUSAL AND SLEEP

16.4.1   SLEEP ARCHITECTURE

16.4.1.1   REM and NREM Sleep
Sleep is divided into the following two phases:

- REM sleep—during which the eyes undergo rapid movements and there is a high level of brain activity
- NREM sleep—during which there is reduced neuronal activity

16.4.1.2   Stages of Sleep
The following stages normally occur during normal NREM sleep:

- Stage 0—quiet wakefulness and shut eyes; electroencephalogram (EEG): alpha activity
- Stage 1—falling asleep; EEG: low amplitude, ↓ alpha activity, low-voltage theta activity
- Stage 2—light sleep; EEG: 2–7 Hz, occasional sleep spindles and K complexes
- Stage 3—deep sleep; ↑ delta activity (20%–50%)
- Stage 4—deep sleep; ↑↑ delta activity (>50%)

Stage 3 + stage 4 = slow-wave sleep (SWS)

16.4.2   PHYSIOLOGICAL CORRELATES OF SLEEP

16.4.2.1   REM Sleep
Features of REM sleep include

- ↑ Recall of dreaming if awoken during REM sleep
- ↑ Complexity of dreams

- ↑ Sympathetic activity
- Transient runs of conjugate ocular movements
- Maximal loss of muscle tone
- ↑ Heart rate
- ↑ Systolic blood pressure
- ↑ Respiratory rate
- ↑ Cerebral blood flow
- Occasional myoclonic jerks
- Penile erection or ↑vaginal blood flow
- ↑ Protein synthesis (rat brain)

16.4.2.2   NREM Sleep
Features of NREM sleep include

- ↓ Recall of dreaming if awoken during REM sleep
- ↓ Complexity of dreams
- ↑ Parasympathetic activity
- Upward ocular deviation with few or no movements
- Abolition of tendon reflexes
- ↓ Heart rate
- ↓ Systolic blood pressure
- ↓ Respiratory rate
- ↓ Cerebral blood flow
- Penis not usually erect

16.4.3   CAUSES OF THE SLEEPING–WAKING CYCLE

There are two main theories accounting for the sleeping–waking cycle:

- Monoaminergic (or biochemical, two-stage, Jouvet's) model
- Cellular (or Hobson's) model

16.4.3.1   Monoaminergic Model
In this model:

- NREM sleep is associated with serotonergic neuronal activity—raphe complex
- REM sleep is associated with noradrenergic neuronal activity—locus coeruleus

16.4.3.2   Cellular Model
In this model, three groups of central neurons are of importance. These groups, and their corresponding neurotransmitters, are the

- Pontine gigantocellular tegmental fields (nucleus reticularis pontis caudalis)—acetylcholine
- Dorsal raphe nuclei—serotonin
- Locus coeruleus—noradrenaline

16.5   EEG

16.5.1   RECORDING TECHNIQUES

16.5.1.1   Conventional

The conventional EEG recording involves placing electrodes on the scalp and is therefore noninvasive. The positions of the electrodes are usually according to the International 10–20 System, which entails measurements from the following scalp landmarks:

- The nasion
- The inion
- The right auricular depression
- The left auricular depression

In this system, proportions of scalp distances are 10% or 20%, and midline electrodes are denoted by the subscript z.

In ambulatory electroencephalography, the output is stored on a suitable portable recorder.

16.5.1.2   Specialized

Specialized recording techniques include the following:

- Nasopharyngeal leads—electrodes are positioned in the superior part of the nasopharynx; can be used to obtain recordings from the inferior and medial temporal lobe.
- Sphenoidal electrodes—electrodes are inserted between the mandibular coronoid notch and the zygoma; can be used to obtain recordings from the inferior temporal lobe.
- Electrocorticography—electrodes are placed directly on the surface of the brain.
- Depth electroencephalography—electrodes are placed inside the brain.

16.5.2   NORMAL EEG RHYTHMS

16.5.2.1   Classification according to Frequency Band

Normal EEG rhythms are classified according to frequency as follows:

- Delta: frequency < 4 Hz
- Theta: 4 Hz ≤ frequency < 8 Hz
- Alpha: 8 Hz ≤ frequency < 13 Hz
- Beta: frequency ≥ 13 Hz

16.5.2.2   Lambda Activity

Lambda activity occurs over the occipital region in subjects with their eyes open. It is related to ocular movements during visual attention.

16.5.2.3   Mu Activity

Mu activity occurs over the motor cortex. It is related to motor activity and is abolished by movement of the contralateral limb.

16.5.3   SPIKES AND WAVES

16.5.3.1   Spikes

Spikes are transient high peaks that last less than 80 ms.

16.5.3.2   Sharp Waves

Sharp waves are conspicuous sharply defined wave formations that rise rapidly, fall more slowly, and last more than 80 ms.

16.5.4   EFFECT OF DRUGS

16.5.4.1   Antidepressants

In general, antidepressants cause

- ↑ Delta activity

16.5.4.2   Antipsychotics

In general, antipsychotic drugs cause

- ↓ Beta activity
- ↑ Low-frequency delta activity and/or ↑ theta activity

16.5.4.3   Anxiolytics

In general, anxiolytics, including barbiturates and benzodiazepines, cause

- ↑ Beta activity
- ↓ Alpha activity (sometimes)

16.5.4.4   Lithium

Therapeutic levels of lithium lead to only small EEG effects that are likely to be missed on visual analysis of routine recordings.

BIBLIOGRAPHY

Carpenter RHS. 2012: *Neurophysiology: A Conceptual Approach*, 5th edn. London, U.K.: Hodder Arnold.

Hall JE. 2011: *Guyton and Hall Textbook of Medical Physiology*, 12th edn. Philadelphia, PA: Saunders, Elsevier.

Puri BK. 2010: Neurophysiology of integrated behaviour. In Puri BK and Treasaden IH (eds.) *Psychiatry: An Evidence-Based Text*, pp. 361–373. London, U.K.: Hodder Arnold.

Stein JF and Stoodley C. 2006: *Neuroscience: An Introduction.* Chichester, England: Wiley-Blackwell.

Strutton P. 2010: Basic concepts in neurophysiology. In Puri BK and Treasaden IH (eds.) *Psychiatry: An Evidence-Based Text*, pp. 354–360. London, U.K.: Hodder Arnold.

Tortora GJ and Derrickson B. 2006: *Principles of Anatomy and Physiology*, 11th edn. New York, NY: Wiley-Blackwell.

Widmaier EP, Raff H, and Strang KT. 2008: *Vander's Human Physiology*, 11th edn. Berkshire, England: McGraw Hill.

17 Neurochemistry

17.1 TRANSMITTER SYNTHESIS, STORAGE, AND RELEASE

17.1.1 TRANSMITTER SYNTHESIS

The synthesis of the neurotransmitters noradrenaline (NA), serotonin (5-HT), dopamine (DA), γ-aminobutyric acid (GABA), and acetylcholine (ACh) is considered later in this chapter (Sections 17.3.3.6, 17.3.4.3, 17.3.3.3, 17.3.5.1, and 17.3.2.3, respectively).

17.1.2 TRANSMITTER STORAGE

The transmitter at a synaptic cleft is stored in presynaptic vesicles. Each vesicle contains one quantum, usually corresponding to several thousand molecules, of transmitter.

17.1.3 TRANSMITTER RELEASE

Transmitter release from synaptic vesicles takes place by exocytosis in a process controlled by Ca^{2+} influx. Because the number of vesicles released is an integer, transmitter release is essentially quantal in nature. The Ca^{2+} enters via voltage-dependent ion channels. Importantly, Na^+ influx and/or K^+ efflux is not needed for transmitter release. Ca^{2+} influences or regulates

- The probability of vesicular transmitter release
- Vesicular fusion
- The transport of synaptic vesicles to the presynaptic active zone of exocytosis
- Post-tetanic potentiation
- Tonic depolarization of the presynaptic neuron

17.2 ION CHANNELS

Ion channels are now classified into families on the basis of genetic sequence homology and, usually, pore-lining α-subunit topology. The main families are as follows:

- 6-Transmembrane (TM)
- 2-TM
- 4-TM or 8-TM
- Ionotropic glutamate receptors
- Nicotinic ACh and related receptors
- Intracellular calcium ion channels
- Chloride ion channels

17.2.1 6-TRANSMEMBRANE (TM) FAMILY

These are voltage-gated ion channels that each contain six transmembrane segments (hence their name). Members of this family include the following ion channels:

- Voltage-gated sodium channels
- Voltage-gated calcium channels
- Voltage-gated potassium channels
- Calcium-activated potassium channels
- Hyperpolarization-activated cation channels involved in rhythmic activities
- Cyclic nucleotide-gated cation channels involved in sensory transduction
- Vanilloid receptors involved in sensory transduction

17.2.2 2-TM FAMILY

These ion channels each have two transmembrane segments in each pore-lining subunit. They include

- Kir (inwardly rectifying potassium ion channels)
- Amiloride-sensitive epithelial sodium ion channel
- The P_{2X} adenosine-5'-triphosphate (ATP) receptor
- The Phe-Met-Arg-Phe-amide–activated sodium ion channel

17.2.3 4-TM OR 8-TM FAMILY

These are two-pore potassium ion channels. They are leak channels that partly help bring about the resting membrane potential of cells.

17.2.4 IONOTROPIC GLUTAMATE RECEPTORS

These ligand-gated channels have a pore-lining domain that is similar to that of the Kir α-subunit, except that it is 'upside down'.

17.2.5 NICOTINIC ACH AND RELATED RECEPTORS

These receptors each contain five subunits. Members of this family include

- Nicotinic ACh receptor
- $5-HT_3$ serotonergic receptor
- Glycine receptor
- $GABA_A$ receptor

17.2.6 Intracellular Calcium Ion Channels

Members of this family include

- IP₃ (inositol triphosphate) receptors
- Ryanodine receptors

17.2.7 Chloride Ion Channels

These have a widespread distribution.

17.3 RECEPTORS

17.3.1 Structure

In general, the receptors to which neurotransmitters bind are proteins located on the external surface of cell membranes. Until the 1980s, receptors were classified and identified pharmacologically but not according to their structures. Since 1983, however, when the primary amino acid sequence of a receptor subunit of the nicotinic ACh receptor was discovered, the DNA of an increasing number of receptor proteins have been sequenced, and hence, their amino acid sequences discovered. This has led to a further clarification of receptor classification. It has also become evident that, as expected, for receptors of classical neurotransmitters, the amino acids forming the binding site are on or close to the extracellular side of the receptor.

17.3.2 Function

The main function of a receptor is the molecular recognition of a signalling molecule, which in the case of neurotransmission is a neurotransmitter, leading in turn to signal transduction. A receptor generally responds to neurotransmitter binding in one of two ways:

- Neurotransmitter binding → opening of transmembrane ion channel
- Receptor–neurotransmitter → second messenger system activation/inhibition

17.3.2.1 G Proteins

G proteins (named after their ability to bind guanosine triphosphate [GTP] and guanosine diphosphate [GDP]) are often involved in transmembrane signalling, linking receptors to intracellular effector systems. For neurotransmitter binding, the following types of G protein may be involved:

- Gs
- Gi
- Go
- Gq

17.3.2.2 Second Messengers

Two of the most important second messenger systems are as follows:

- Receptor–neurotransmitter complex → G protein binding to receptor–neurotransmitter complex → adenylate cyclase activation (or inhibition) → cyclic AMP (cAMP).
- Neurotransmitter binding → hydrolysis of phosphatidylinositol bisphosphate (a membrane phospholipid) → diacylglycerol and IP₃ (inositol triphosphate); diacylglycerol activates protein kinase C (PKC), while IP₃ causes endoplasmic reticulum calcium release, in turn activating calmodulin-dependent protein kinase.

17.3.2.3 Acetylcholine (ACh) (Figure 17.1)

1. ACh is synthesized from acetyl-coA and choline in the cytoplasm of the cholinergic nerve terminals. Choline comes from dietary sources. The availability of choline is increased by lecithin (yellow-brownish substance found in egg yolk) but decreased by hemicholinium (a drug used in research). Black widow spider venom produces a rapid release of ACh.
2. The final step in the synthesis is catalyzed by the enzyme choline acetyltransferase (ChAT). In Alzheimer's disease, ChAT is less active and leads to a reduction in the synthesis of ACh. The deficit

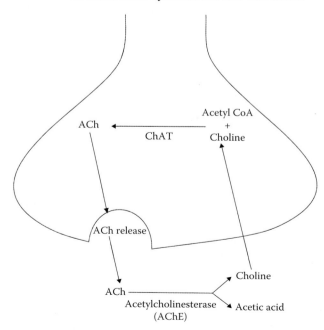

FIGURE 17.1 The synthesis and degradation of ACh.

in ACh results in reduced neurotransmission and memory deficits.

3. ACh is the primary excitatory transmitter at the neuromuscular junction and preganglionic autonomic nerves. The main cholinergic neurons are found in the basal nucleus of Meynert. Alzheimer's disease is associated with a reduction of cholinergic neurons in the subcortical areas of the brain, leading to reduced availability of ACh. Local cholinergic neurons are found in the cortex and striatum and their main function is for motor control.

4. ACh is then packaged into synaptic vesicles and transported to synapses.

5. Cholinergic nerve transmission is terminated by the enzyme acetylcholinesterase (AChE). AChE is found on the postsynaptic membrane of cholinergic synapses. ACh binds to AChE and is hydrolyzed into acetic acid and choline. The hydrolysis inactivates the ACh and the nerve impulse is stopped. Acetylcholinesterase inhibitors (AChEIs; e.g. rivastigmine) prevent the hydrolysis of ACh, which increases the concentration of ACh in the synaptic cleft. AChEIs are used in the treatment of Alzheimer's disease. Nerve gas or organophosphate, a chemical weapon, inhibits the AChEI and causes continuous muscle contraction in victims.

17.3.3 Cholinergic Receptors

Cholinergic receptors transduce signals via coupling with G proteins. At the time of writing, the following types are recognized:

17.3.3.1 Muscarinic Receptors (Figure 17.2)

Mechanisms of actions: Binding of ACh to excitatory M_1, M_3, and M_5 receptors activates the Gq/11 family of G proteins that in turn activates phospholipase C (PLC) and can lead to membrane phosphatidylinositol-4,5-bisphosphate (PIP_2) breakdown, PKC activation, and intracellular calcium mobilization. M_1, M_3, and M_5 are PLC coupled to Ca^{2+}/Na^+ channels. Activation of these ion channels leads to depolarizing currents and increased cell excitability thereby promoting the propagation of nerve impulses.

M_2 and M_4 are coupled to K+ channels. It is the activation of these K+ channels that leads to hyperpolarizing currents and reduced cell excitability thereby preventing propagation of nerve impulses.

Locations of muscarinic receptors: Parasympathetic nervous system, midbrain, medulla, pons, corpus striatum, cerebral cortex, hippocampus, thalamus, hypothalamus, and cerebellum.

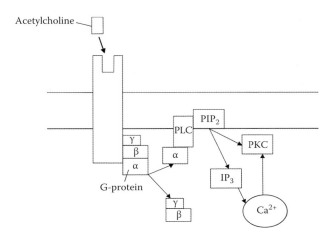

FIGURE 17.2 Muscarinic receptors (M_1, M_3, M_5).

Type of receptors: Muscarinic receptors are classified as M_1, M_2, M_3, M_4, and M_5. The M_1 receptor is the most significant receptor in the central nervous system (CNS) and is highly expressed in human brain and nerves. M_1, M_3, and M_5 receptor subtypes have a stimulatory effect on the target tissues, whereas the M_2 and M_4 subtypes are inhibitory.

Clinical relevance:

1. M_1 agonists increase ACh transmission in the brain and alleviate some of the symptoms of Alzheimer's disease.

2. M_3 agonists, such as pilocarpine, are used to treat chronic open-angle glaucoma and acute angle-closure glaucoma.

3. Antidepressants: paroxetine is the most anticholinergic selective serotonin reuptake inhibitor (SSRI).

4. Anticholinergic drugs (e.g. benzhexol) are used to block DA uptake and improve pseudoparkinsonism induced by antipsychotics. These drugs are reported to have mood-elevating effect that may lead to misuse and worsen amnesia in elderly.

5. Psychotropic drugs (e.g. chlorpromazine, tricyclic antidepressants [TCAs], and paroxetine) have high affinity at muscarinic receptors and lead to anticholinergic effects. Chlorpromazine is associated with potent anticholinergic actions and prevents extrapyramidal side effects (EPSE).

6. Atropine is an antagonist at the muscarinic ACh receptor. Scopolamine, a muscarinic antagonist, is used to treat nausea and morning sickness.

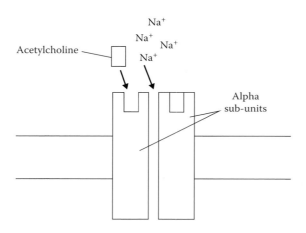

FIGURE 17.3   Nicotinic acetylcholine receptors.

17.3.3.2   Nicotinic Receptors (Figure 17.3)

Mechanisms of actions: The nicotinic receptor is activated by the binding of two ACh molecules that permits the movement of sodium ions.

Locations of the nicotinic receptors: Neuromuscular junctions, autonomic nervous system ganglia, substantia nigra, locus coeruleus, septum, corpus striatum, cerebral cortex, hippocampus, thalamus, hypothalamus, and cerebellum.

Types of receptors: There are two types: N_N and N_M.

Clinical relevance:

1. Nicotine found in tobacco is an agonist at the nicotinic receptors. Nicotine can improve cognitive performance and reduce anxiety. Its dependence potential is related to its ability to release DA in the nucleus accumbens.

   The prevalence of smoking in schizophrenia patients is two to three times higher than the general population. Patients with schizophrenia may smoke heavily as a result of antipsychotic medication, which produces marked DA receptor blockade. A very high level of smoking is necessary to overcome this blockade and produce the reward effects.
2. Antagonists at nicotinic receptors include tubocurarine (an old anaesthesia agent).

17.3.3.3   Dopamine (DA) (Figure 17.4)

1. DA is produced from tyrosine that is a dietary amino acid. A small of part of tyrosine derives from phenylalanine by hydroxylation. Phenylalanine hydroxylase is absent in phenylketonuria (PKU).
2. Tyrosine hydroxylase is the rate-limiting step in the synthesis of the catecholamines. Hence, increasing tyrosine does not influence the catecholamine levels. Carbidopa increases the availability of dopa by inhibiting DOPA decarboxylase and improve parkinsonism:
   - L-dopa: The administration of L-dopa can increase the production of DA. Amphetamine can release DA directly in the mesolimbic pathway. Electroconvulsive therapy (ECT) increases the DA function. ECT also increases oral intake and decreases psychomotor retardation.
3. DA: DA is stored in vesicles in the nerve terminals and is released by depolarization. The largest production site is the substantia nigra. Cocaine has high affinity to the DA transporter and prevents DA reuptake and increases its availability in the synapses in the mesolimbic pathway. Bupropion inhibits DA reuptake.
4. Reuptake and monoamine oxidase A (MAO-A): The DA transporter is a high-affinity uptake system that takes DA back to the nerve terminal. DA is metabolized by MAO-A. MAO-A is more effective in degrading NA, DA, and serotonin (5-HT) than monoamine oxidase B (MAO-B). MAO-B inhibitors slow the progression of Parkinson's diseases.
5. Catechol-o-methyl transferase (COMT) is responsible for extra-neuronal metabolism of DA (e.g. in liver and kidney).
6. MAO-B is the nonneuronal MAO and the end product is Homovanillic acid (HVA). HVA is an indicator of DA turnover.

There are four types of DA pathways:

1. Nigrostriatal pathway: from the substantia nigra to the striatum
2. Mesocortical pathway: from the ventral tegmental area to the cortex
3. Mesolimbic pathway: from the ventral tegmental area to the limbic system
4. Tuberoinfundibular: local network of DA in hypothalamus

Functions of DA

1. DA allows the expression of cortically initiated voluntary movements through its actions in the striatum.
2. The mesolimbic pathways promote drive and reinforcement.

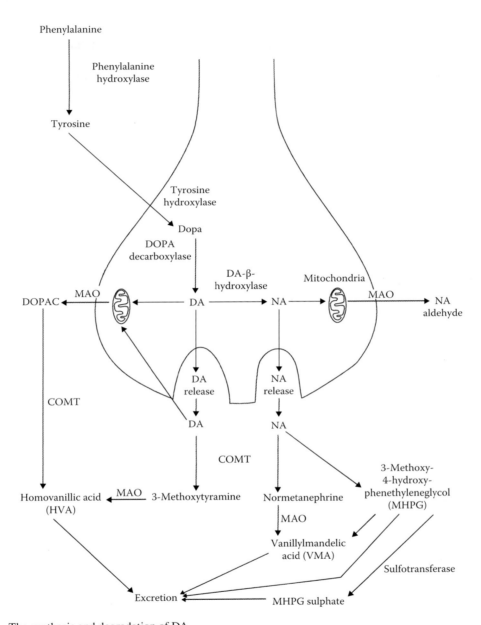

FIGURE 17.4 The synthesis and degradation of DA.

17.3.3.4 Disease Processes Involving DA

Schizophrenia

↓ DA in the mesocortical pathway: Anergy and loss of drive (negative symptoms)

↑ DA in the mesolimbic pathway

The DA hypothesis proposes that increased levels of DA or DA receptors cause schizophrenia.

Galactorrhoea is seen in antipsychotic treatment as a result of blockade of DA receptors located on the lactotroph cells in the anterior pituitary and causes excessive release of prolactin.

Depression: The mesolimbic DA system is implicated. There is low cerebrospinal fluid (CSF) HVA in depressed patients and signify low DA turnover.

Obsessive-compulsive disorder (OCD): ↑ DA in the nigrostriatal pathway (e.g. compulsive behaviour)

Bipolar disorder: ↑ DA in the nigrostriatal pathway (↑ sensory stimuli and movement), ↑ CSF HVA in manic patients

17.3.3.5 Dopamine Receptors

The dopaminergic receptors are coupled to G proteins, via which they produce their physiological effects. At the time of writing, the main dopaminergic receptors and their main effectors (via G protein α-subunits) are believed to be

- $D_1 \to \uparrow$ adenylate cyclase (via Gs)
- $D_2 \to \downarrow$ adenylate cyclase, $\uparrow K^+$, $\downarrow Ca^{2+}$ (via Gi/Go)
- $D_3 \to \downarrow$ adenylate cyclase, $\uparrow K^+$, $\downarrow Ca^{2+}$ (via Gi/Go)
- $D_4 \to \downarrow$ adenylate cyclase, $\uparrow K^+$, $\downarrow Ca^{2+}$ (via Gi/Go)
- $D_5 \to \uparrow$ adenylate cyclase (via Gs)

The D_1-like receptors comprise D_1 and D_5 receptor subtypes that are associated with stimulation of adenylate cyclase. D_1 receptors are found in the striatum, limbic system, thalamus, and hypothalamus.

The D_2-like receptors comprise D_2, D_3, and D_4 receptor subtypes that are associated with inhibition of adenylate cyclase. D_2 receptors are found in the striatum, limbic system, thalamus, hypothalamus, and pituitary gland. D_3 and D_4 receptors are found in the limbic system (see Figure 17.5).

Schizophrenia is associated with dopaminergic hyperactivity. Excessive DA activates the inhibitory G protein and inhibits the adenyl cyclase. There is an imbalance between D_1 and D_2 receptor functions in schizophrenia.

Long-term consumption of cocaine, methamphetamine, heroin, and alcohol reduces the levels of striatal D_2 receptors compared to healthy controls.

The ability of antipsychotics (e.g. chlorpromazine, haloperidol, risperidone) to reduce positive symptoms (e.g. hallucinations and delusions) by blocking the D_2 receptors in the mesolimbic and mesocortical pathways supports the DA hypothesis of schizophrenia.

For example, risperidone is an antagonist that is more D_2 selective. Risperidone has a higher affinity for the D_2 receptors than for the D_3 receptors. Seventy-five per cent of blockade of D_2 receptors is useful to achieve therapeutic response.

Antipsychotics may block the D_2 receptors in the nigrostriatal pathway and cause EPSE. EPSE emerge when 80% D_2 receptors in the nigrostriatal pathway are blocked.

The second-generation antipsychotics, which have little or no affinity for D_1 receptors, can prevent side effects associated with D_1 antagonism that are found in the older antipsychotics. DA agonists, such as apomorphine and bromocriptine, have greater potency at D_2 receptors. Bromocriptine is used to suppress prolactin secretion arising from the pituitary tumours.

Clozapine is used in treatment-resistant schizophrenia, and it has considerably higher affinity for other receptors (e.g. 5-HT$_{2A/2C}$, α_1-, α_2-, and D_4 receptors) than for D_2 receptors. Clozapine is almost 20–25 times more potent at the D_4 receptors than the D_2 receptors. Its antipsychotic effects are thought to be mediated primarily by 5-HT$_{2A/2c}$ and D_2 receptor antagonism.

Parkinson's disease is associated with dopaminergic hypoactivity as a result of degeneration of cells in the pars compacta of substantia nigra. It leads to a relative excess of cholinergic activity. DA agonists such as bromocriptine are sometimes used as adjuncts to L-dopa in treatment for Parkinson's disease.

The decrease in number of D_2 receptors in the striatum in old people inversely correlates with severity of cognitive impairment.

17.3.3.6 Noradrenaline (NA) (Figure 17.6)

1. NA is synthesized by the hydroxylation of DA by DA-β-hydroxylase. It is mainly stored in the presynaptic complexes with ATP and metallic ions. It is released from the storage vesicles by Ca^{2+}-dependent process. Its release from the storage is inhibited by antihypertensive agents such as guanethidine. Alpha-methyl-paratyrosine (AMPT) inhibits the tyrosine hydroxylase and results in depressive relapse in antidepressant-treated patients.

2. NA is mainly produced by the locus coeruleus. NA is involved in attention, learning, and emotional behaviour. In the adrenal medulla, NA is methylated to adrenaline and it is involved

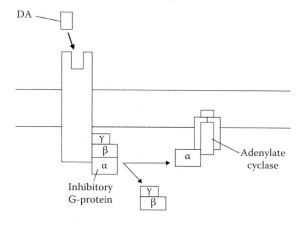

FIGURE 17.5 DA D_2 receptor.

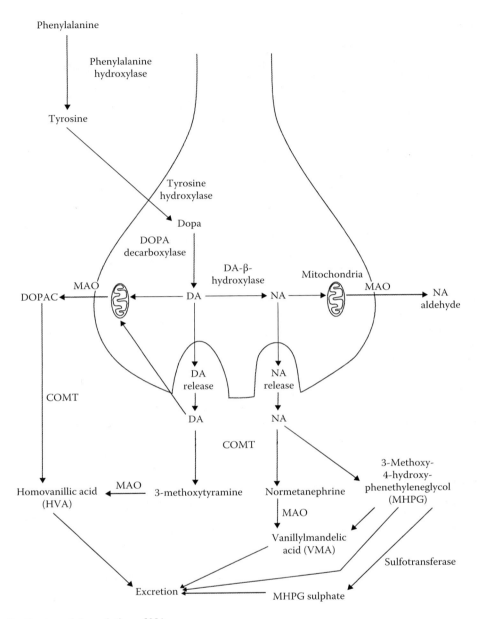

FIGURE 17.6 Synthesis and degradation of NA.

in the fight and flight response. In peripheral tissues, NA plays a role in stress responses.

3. NA metabolism: NA is metabolized by COMT to normetanephrine and then by MAO-B to vanillyl mandelic acid (VMA). It can also be metabolized to 3-methoxy-4-hydroxyphenylglycol (MHPG) by MAO and COMT in a stepwise manner. Forty per cent of plasma MHPG is derived from the brain and it indicates the NA turnover in the CNS. Reserpine and

tetrabenazine prevent vesicular accumulation of NA and leads to depression. This supports the NA theory of depressive disorder.

4. NA reuptake: NA is transported back into neurons by a high-affinity uptake system and it is energy consuming. Reuptake is more affected by secondary amines than tertiary amines. Cocaine also inhibits the presynaptic reuptake of NA. TCA and serotonin–noradrenaline reuptake inhibitors (SNRIs) are potent blockers for

NA reuptake. SNRIs (e.g. venlafaxine) restore the levels of NA in the synaptic cleft by binding at the NA reuptake transporters, preventing the reuptake and subsequent degradation. During opioid and alcohol withdrawal, high concentration of NA in the synapse is a result of attenuation of the autoinhibitory mechanisms.

5. Monoamine oxidase inhibitors (MAOIs) (irreversible MAOIs, phenelzine and tranylcypromine, or reversible MAOI, moclobemide) inhibit MAO and increase the brain levels of NA. This will help to treat depression. Tyramine-rich foods such as cheese (except cream and cottage), bean curd, offal (liver), Chianti, alcohol, smoked and pickled fish, sausage, and banana skin should be avoided as it can inhibit the peripheral metabolism of pressor amines.

Conversion to adrenaline: The conversion from NA to adrenaline involves phenylethanolamine-N-methyl transferase.

17.3.3.7 NA and Psychiatric Disorders

Generalized anxiety disorder and panic disorder: There is increased NA transmission from both the locus coeruleus and the caudal raphe nuclei. The NA projection from the ventral locus coeruleus to the hypothalamus will produce autonomic symptoms such as increased heart rate, dilated pupils, tremor, and sweating. The NA projection from the dorsal locus coeruleus to the cortex and hippocampus affects fear-related processing and fear responses.

OCD: Increased in NA transmission from the locus coeruleus to the frontal cortex, thalamus, hypothalamus, and limbic system

Depression: Reduced NA transmission from the locus coeruleus and the caudal raphe nuclei. SNRIs increase the NA level in frontal and prefrontal cortex. This will improve mood and attention in depressed patients. Chronic antidepressant treatment leads to changes in NA reuptake transporter gene expression.

Bipolar disorder: Increased NA transmission in the caudal nucleus and the locus coeruleus.

Alzheimer's disease, Korsakoff's psychosis, Parkinson's disease, and progressive supranuclear palsy: These disorders are associated with significant loss of NA neurons.

17.3.4 Adrenoceptors

The adrenergic receptors are coupled to G proteins, via which they produce their physiological effects. At the time of writing, the main adrenergic receptors and their main effectors (via G protein α-subunits) are believed to be

- $\alpha_{1A} \rightarrow \uparrow Ca^{2+}$ (via Gi/Go)
- $\alpha_{1B} \rightarrow \uparrow IP_3$ (via Gq)
- $\alpha_{1C} \rightarrow \uparrow IP_3$ (via Gq)
- $\alpha_{1D} \rightarrow \uparrow IP_3$ (via Gq)
- α_{2A} (human)/a_{2D} (probably rat homologue) $\downarrow$ adenylyl cyclase, $\uparrow K^+$, $\downarrow Ca^{2+}$ (via Gi)
- $\alpha_{2B} \rightarrow \downarrow$ adenylate cyclase (via Gi)
- $\alpha_{2C} \rightarrow \downarrow$ adenylate cyclase (via Go)
- $\beta_1 \rightarrow \uparrow$ adenylate cyclase (via Gs)
- $\beta_2 \rightarrow \uparrow$ adenylate cyclase (via Gs)

17.3.4.1 α-Adrenoceptors

α_1-Receptors act via stimulation of phosphoinositol. They are located postsynaptically. Their functions include arousal and causing vascular smooth muscles to contract. Some TCAs and antipsychotics cause sedation and postural hypotension that is a result of blocking the α_1-receptors.

The α_2-receptors act via the activation of inhibitory G proteins. They are found both pre- and postsynaptically. The α_2-adrenoceptors are widely distributed throughout the body and are found in adrenergic neurons, blood vessels, pancreas, and smooth muscle. When stimulated, these receptors reduce the blood pressure and suppress symptoms of opiate withdrawal. By coupling to the inhibitory G proteins, the α_2-adrenoceptors have an inhibitory effect on neurotransmission when bound by an agonist. The α_2-receptor densities are found to be increased on platelets of depressed patients and the brains of suicide victims. Lofexidine is an α_2-receptor agonist. These receptors are blocked by mianserin. Mirtazapine exerts α_2-autoreceptor and heteroreceptor antagonism.

The presynaptic α_2-receptors control NA release. The NA in the synapse activates the presynaptic α_2-receptors and leads to increase in potassium conductance and hyperpolarization of the cells. This autoinhibitory mechanism reduces NA release. When antidepressants such as TCAs block the NA reuptake, more NA is released in the synapses and enhances the autoinhibitory mechanism. This leads to downregulation of the presynaptic α_2-receptors. The tolerance of autoinhibitory effect takes place over a few weeks. Hence, the antidepressant can lead to therapeutic effect on depressed mood by increasing the availability of NA through reuptake inhibition and reduction of autoinhibitory mechanism after a time period of several weeks. In clinical practice, psychiatrists often remind the patients taking antidepressants for the first time to wait for several weeks before they can see the treatment response.

The autoinhibitory process can be mimicked by α_2-adrenoceptor agonists such as clonidine that reduces the NA release. In opioid withdrawal, there is an attenuation of the autoinhibitory mechanisms that leads to higher level of NA in the synapses. Clonidine can be used to reduce the NA levels and it can also stop the lactate-induced panic attacks. On the other hand, α_2-adrenoceptor antagonists such as yohimbine stop the autoinhibitory process and increase the availability of NA. Although yohimbine has antidepressant properties, it causes anxiety and increases the frequency of panic attacks.

The postsynaptic α_2-receptors are involved in growth hormone production. Administration of α_2-agonists such as clonidine to patients suffering from depressive or panic disorder shows a blunted growth hormone response. This observation resulted from the downregulation of postsynaptic α_2-receptors in depressed patients.

The adverse effects associated with first-generation antipsychotics such as tachycardia, impotence, and dizziness are caused by the nonselective binding to α-adrenoceptors.

17.3.4.2 β-Adrenoceptors

β-Receptors act via activation of stimulatory G protein. β-Receptors also stimulate melatonin production in the pineal gland. There are three types of β-receptors: β_1-receptors predominate in the cortex. Stimulation of β_1-receptors also increases the rates and force of cardiac contractions. β_2-Receptors predominate in the cerebellum. Stimulation of β_2-receptors causes bronchodilation. β_3-Receptors predominate in the brown fat. Chronic antidepressant treatments affect the G protein-coupled adenylate cyclase and induce a reduction in β_1-receptor density in the brain. The β-receptor density is increased in the brains of suicide victims and MAOIs produce β-receptor downregulation.

Phobia: There is an excess of NA in the principal noradrenergic pathways in the brain, and this results in a downregulation of postsynaptic adrenergic receptors. Transmissions of NA from the caudal raphe nuclei and the locus coeruleus are increased in phobia.

The effect of acute and chronic antidepressant treatment on β_1-receptors is summarized as follows:

There is an increase of NA and the density of postsynaptic β_1-receptors that stimulate the cAMP formation during acute antidepressant treatment (Figure 17.7).

The long-term increase in NA leads to downregulation of the postsynaptic β_1-receptors and reduce cAMP formation (Figure 17.8). Nevertheless, the amount of cAMP production is still higher than those depressed patients without treatment.

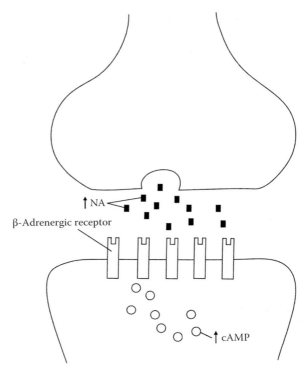

FIGURE 17.7 The effect of acute antidepressant treatment on β_1-receptors.

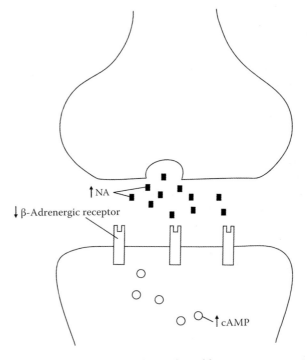

FIGURE 17.8 The effect of chronic antidepressant treatment on β_1-receptors.

17.3.4.3 Serotonin (5-HT)

5-HT is a monoamine neurotransmitter. 5-HT is produced by dorsal and median raphe nuclei. 5-HT plays a key role in appetite, sleep, mood, impulse control, suicide, and personality. 5-HT in the CNS accounts for less than 20% of the total body 5-HT. Eighty per cent of 5-HT are found in the intestine and platelets (Figure 17.9).

1. 5-HT is synthesized from dietary amino acid, L-tryptophan. Tryptophan hydroxylase does not saturate and higher level of 5-HT can be achieved by taking L-tryptophan alongside with antidepressants. On the other hand, depletion of 5-HT can be achieved by inhibiting tryptophan hydroxylase, removing L-tryptophan from the diet or adding natural amino acid such as alanine to compete for the transport process with L-tryptophan. This will lead to depression.
2. Release of 5-HT: The release of 5-HT is dependent on calcium ions.
3. 5-HT and platelets: Most of the peripheral 5-HTs are stored in the platelets. When depressed patients take the SSRI, this will lead to reduction of the 5-HT levels in the platelet but increase in the plasma 5-HT levels.
4. Degradation of 5-HT: 5-HT is taken back into the neuron and degraded by MAO-A. SSRI blocks the 5-HT reuptake. This will lead to mood improvement in depressed patients, but nausea and impaired sexual function may arise as possible side effects.
5. 5-Hydroxyindoleacetic acid (5-HIAA): 5-HIAA will be transferred out of the brain via CSF or blood. The concentration of 5-HIAA in CSF correlates with the concentration in brain tissue. CSF 5-HIAA is a useful index of central 5-HT turnover. Low CSF 5-HIAA is found in patients with violent behaviours and untreated depression.

17.3.4.4 Serotonin and Psychiatric Disorders

Anxiety and OCD: m-Chlorophenylpiperazine (mCPP) is a direct 5-HT receptor agonist and it can induce anxiety and obsessional symptoms. mCPP demonstrates the role of 5-HT dysfunction in anxiety disorders and OCD.

Depression: 5-HT transmission from the caudal raphe nuclei and rostral raphe nuclei is reduced in patients

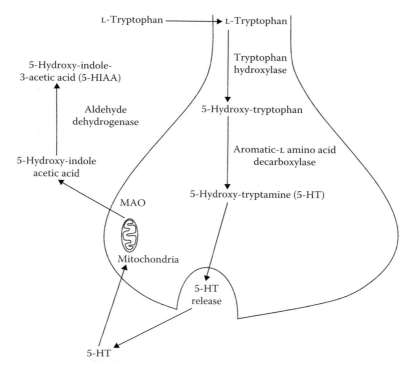

FIGURE 17.9 The synthesis and degradation of serotonin.

with depression. It leads to insomnia and suicide ideation. Presynaptic 5-HT dysfunction is a state marker in depression.

Mania: 5-HT transmission from the caudal raphe nuclei and rostral raphe nuclei is increased in patients with mania.

Schizophrenia: There is an interesting relationship between 5-HT and DA. The two 5-HT pathways that are affected in schizophrenia include (1) the projections from dorsal raphe nuclei to the substantia nigra and (2) the projections from the rostral raphe nuclei ascending into the cerebral cortex, limbic regions, and basal ganglia. 5-HT$_{2A}$ receptor agonism inhibits DA release. When there is excess 5-HT produced by these two pathways, there is a reduction of the availability of DA that can give rise to the negative symptoms of schizophrenia. Second-generation antipsychotics such as risperidone bind to the D$_2$, 5-HT$_{2A}$, and α_2-adrenergic receptors in the brain. Risperidone competes with 5-HT and its antagonism at 5-HT$_{2A}$ receptors causes an increase in DA to relieve negative symptoms. As risperidone also blocks D$_2$ receptors, the positive symptoms are reduced at the same time.

Alzheimer's disease: 5-HT transmission from the rostral raphe nuclei to the temporal lobe is reduced in patients suffering from Alzheimer's disease.

Cloninger's type 2 alcoholism: This is characterized by young men with impulsive behaviours and low 5-HT levels.

17.3.5 Serotonergic Receptors

The main serotonergic receptors, grouped according to their relative homologies, and their signalling systems, believed to exist at the time of writing, are as follows (Table 17.1):

- 5-HT$_{1A}$ → ↓ adenylate cyclase
- 5-HT$_{1B}$ → ↓ adenylate cyclase
- 5-HT$_{1Da}$ → ↓ adenylate cyclase
- 5-HT$_{1Db}$ → ↓ adenylate cyclase
- 5-HT$_{1E}$ → ↓ adenylate cyclase
- 5-HT$_{2A}$ → ↑ IP$_3$
- 5-HT$_{2B}$ → ↑ IP$_3$
- 5-HT$_{2C}$ → ↑ IP$_3$
- 5-HT$_3$—ion channel
- 5-HT$_{5A}$—signalling system not known at the time of writing
- 5-HT$_{5B}$—signalling system not known at the time of writing
- 5-HT$_6$ → ↑ adenylate cyclase
- 5-HT$_7$ → ↑ adenylate cyclase

17.3.5.1 γ-Aminobutyric Acid (GABA)

GABA is the main inhibitory neurotransmitter in the CNS. GABAergic inhibition is seen at the hypothalamus, hippocampus, cerebral cortex, and cerebellum.

Biosynthesis

GABA is derived from glutamic acid via the action of glutamic acid decarboxylase (GAD) (see Figure 17.10). GAD is a marker of GABAergic neurons. It requires pyridoxal phosphate that is a vitamin B$_6$ cofactor. Inhibitors of this enzyme may cause seizure. In schizophrenia, there is a decreased expression of the messenger RNA for this enzyme in the prefrontal cortex.

Metabolism

The metabolic breakdown of GABA to glutamic acid and succinic semialdehyde involves the action of GABA transaminase (GABA-T). GABA-T is often the target for anticonvulsants (e.g. sodium valproate). Inhibitor of this enzyme will increase GABA levels and prevent convulsion.

17.3.5.2 GABA and Disease Processes

Generalized anxiety disorder: ↓ GABA activity

  Schizophrenia: ↑ GABA activity

  Depression: GABA$_B$ agonists enhance monoaminergic neurotransmission.

17.3.5.3 GABA Receptors

The GABA receptor superfamilies may be large, with multiple types of GABA subunits having been cloned. In general, there are two main types of receptor, the main effects of which are

GABA$_A$ → ↑ Cl$^-$ (via a receptor-gated ion channel)

GABA$_A$ receptors gate a chloride ion channel and are responsible for inhibitory activity. It has at least 16 different subunits (e.g. there is a binding site for alcohol to increase sedation). For example, diazepam is a GABA-A agonist.

GABA$_B$ → ↑ K$^+$ ± Ca^{2+} effects (via G protein coupling)

GABA$_B$ receptors are positively coupled to G proteins and presynaptically modulate transmitter release. Baclofen (a medication used to treat spasticity) only binds to GABA$_B$ receptors (see Figure 17.11).

TABLE 17.1

Summary of the 5-HT Receptors

Receptor Type	Locations	Mechanisms	Clinical Relevance
5-HT$_{1A}$	1. Widely expressed throughout the brain 2. High density in the hippocampus, raphe nucleus, and medial temporal cortex 3. Lower density in the prefrontal cortex and basal ganglia	Coupled to a G protein that inhibits the intracellular messenger adenylate cyclase 5-HT$_{1A}$ acts as an accelerator of DA release	Depression: ↑ 5-HT$_{1A}$ receptor density in the hippocampus and medial temporal cortex ↓ 5-HT$_{1A}$ receptor density in the cerebellum, basal ganglia, and prefrontal cortex. Chronic antidepressant treatment leads to downregulation Buspirone exerts anxiolytic and antidepressant effects through partial agonism at the 5-HT$_{1A}$ receptor Aripiprazole is a 5-HT$_{1A}$ agonist
5-HT$_{1B}$	Autoreceptors	Coupled to a G protein that inhibits the intracellular messenger adenylate cyclase	Reduce 5-HT release Implicated in Cloninger's type II alcoholism
5-HT$_{1D}$	Autoreceptors	Coupled to a G protein that inhibits the intracellular messenger adenylate cyclase	Blunted growth hormone response to sumatriptan in depressed patients
5-HT$_2$	Cortex	Phosphoinositol turnover The secondary messenger (IP$_3$) will regulate substrate proteins (e.g. receptors, ion channels, cytoskeletal proteins, and transcription factors). This will lead to short- and long-term regulation of neuronal function 5-HT$_{2A}$ inhibits DA release upon binding of 5-HT. 5-HT$_{2A}$ receptor antagonism leads to anxiolytic effects. 5-HT$_{2A}$ receptor agonism is associated with circadian rhythm disturbance and sexual dysfunction 5-HT$_{2B}$ causes mild anxiety and hyperphagia upon stimulation 5-HT$_{2c}$ regulates DA and NA release Fluoxetine reduces binge eating and bulimia through 5-HT$_{2c}$ agonism. Weight gain and anxiolytic effects are associated with 5-HT$_{2c}$ antagonism	Depression: ↑ receptor density on platelets of depressed patents; ↓ in the 5-HT$_2$ receptor density in the frontal, temporal, parietal, and occipital cortical regions after chronic antidepressant (TCA and SSRI) treatment Slow-wave sleep regulation Implicated in anxiety disorders ↑ in 5-HT$_2$ receptor binding in suicide victims Second-generation antipsychotics: 5-HT$_{2A}$ antagonists Hallucinogens stimulate 5-HT$_{2A}$ receptors in the frontal cortex and reduce activities of GABAergic neurons Lysergic acid diethylamide (LSD) is a partial 5-HT$_2$ agonist Mianserin is a 5-HT$_2$ antagonist
5-HT$_{2C}$	Choroid plexus	Phosphoinositol turnover	Implicated in feeding Agomelatine is a 5-HT$_{2C}$ antagonist
5-HT$_3$	1. Brain stem: the putative vomiting centre and the nucleus tractus solitarius 2. Vagus nerve 3. Limbic system, hippocampus, and the cerebral cortex	Ligand-gated channel and causes depolarization 5-HT$_3$ receptors regulate inhibitory interneurons in the brain and also mediate vomiting via the vagal nerve	Controls DA release Gastrointestinal side effects and nausea associated with SSRIs (5-HT$_3$ agonism) Mirtazapine does not have nausea side effects due to its antagonism on 5-HT$_3$ receptors Anxiety disorders Alcohol acts on 5-HT$_3$ receptors

TABLE 17.1 (continued)

Summary of the 5-HT Receptors

Receptor Type	Locations	Mechanisms	Clinical Relevance
5-HT$_4$	1. Brain stem (caudate nucleus, lenticular nucleus, putamen and globus pallidus) 2. Substantia nigra 3. Low levels in hippocampus and frontal cortex 4. Heart	Coupled to a G protein that stimulates the intracellular messenger adenylate cyclase and regulates neurotransmission 5-HT$_4$ mediates DA release	This receptor mediates cortisol secretion and contraction of colon and bladder
5-HT$_6$	1. High levels: olfactory tubercle, corpus striatum, nucleus accumbens, dentate gyrus, and hippocampus 2. Low levels: cerebellum and amygdala	Coupled to a G protein that stimulates the intracellular messenger adenylate cyclase and regulates neurotransmission	5-HT$_6$ receptors may regulate release of neurotrophic factors. Antagonism may enhance cognition
5-HT$_7$	1. Thalamus	Coupled to a G protein that stimulates the intracellular messenger adenylate cyclase and regulates neurotransmission	5-HT$_7$ receptors may be involved in circadian rhythms. Antagonism may enhance cognition

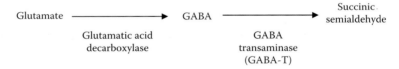

FIGURE 17.10   Synthesis and degradation of GABA.

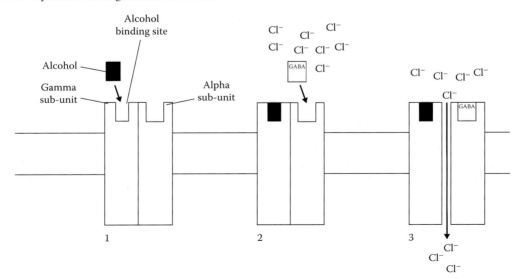

FIGURE 17.11   The GABA$_A$ receptor.

1. Benzodiazepine binds to the benzodiazepine binding site that overlaps between the γ_2- and α_1-subunits of GABA$_A$ receptors. If a patient is oversedated after an overdose of benzodiazepine, the administration of flumazenil will displace benzodiazepine from its binding sites and reverse its sedative effect. Hence, flumazenil can lead to anxiogenic effects in normal adults.

2. After the binding of benzodiazepine to its receptor, the GABA binds to the GABA receptor that overlaps between the α_1- and β_2-receptors. New benzodiazepines such as zopiclone show high affinity only to the α_1-subunits of GABA$_A$ receptors. The benzodiazepine-mediated increases in GABA neurotransmission may lead to a decrease in the restraining influence of the cortex, resulting in disinhibition observed in patients taking benzodiazepine.

3. The influx of chloride ions leads to sedative effects. Alcohol opens the Cl$^-$ ions directly and it has been misused as an anxiolytic agent.

17.3.5.4 Glutamate

Glutamate is an excitatory amino acid that is essential in learning and memory. It is also a potent neurotoxin that gives rise to excitotoxicity. The main glutamate pathways include

1. The corticocortical pathways
2. The pathways between the thalamus and the cortex
3. The extrapyramidal pathway (the projections between the cortex and striatum)

Glutamate is involved in the process of long-term potentiation that is seen as the basis of learning and memory.

17.3.5.5 Clinical Relevance of Glutamate

1. In schizophrenia patients, the glutamatergic pathways are hypoactive. Similarly, the N-methyl-D-aspartate (NMDA) antagonists produce broad-spectrum cognitive impairments, and pronounced negative symptom. NMDA receptors will be the next targets of antipsychotic treatments. In contrast, the glutamatergic pathways are hyperactive in epilepsy.

2. Lamotrigine and lithium reduce the glutamate transmission in depressed patients.

3. The NMDA glutamate receptor is blocked by phencyclidine (PCP).

17.3.6 Glutamate Receptors

The types of glutamate receptor recognized are

- NMDA receptors
- a-Amino-3-hydroxy-5-methyl-4-isoxazolepropionic acid (AMPA) receptors
- Kainic acid (KA) receptors
- Metabotropic glutamate receptors (mGluRs) (=trans-ACPD receptors)

The first three classes are ionotropic glutamate receptors that are coupled directly to cation-specific ion channels.

17.3.6.1 NMDA Receptors

The NMDA receptor is the main mediator of excitatory neurotransmission. At the time of writing, the NMDA receptor subtype is believed to include two families of subunits:

- NMDAR1 (=NR1)
- NMDAR2 (=NR2)

In turn, the following splice variants of NMDAR1 have been recognized:

- NMDAR1A (=NR1a)
- NMDAR1B (=NR1b)
- NMDAR1C (=NR1c)
- NMDAR1D (=NR1d)
- NMDAR1E (=NR1e)
- NMDAR1F (=NR1f)
- NMDAR1G (=NR1g)

Variants of NMDAR2 are modulatory subunits that form heteromeric channels but not homomeric channels.

17.3.6.2 AMPA Receptors

AMPA receptors can be formed from one or any two of the following:

- GluR1
- GluR2
- GluR3
- GluR4

17.3.6.3 KA Receptors

KA receptors include

- GluR5
- GluR6
- GluR7
- KA1
- KA2

17.3.6.4 mGluRs

The mGluRs are coupled to G proteins, unlike the other classes of glutamate receptor. At the time of writing, the following subtypes have been cloned:

- mGluR1
- mGluR2
- mGluR3
- mGluR4
- mGluR5
- mGluR6

These have been categorized into the following subgroups:

- Subgroup I = mGluR1 and mGluR5
- Subgroup II = mGluR2 and mGluR3
- Subgroup III = mGluR4 and mGluR6

The effector system for subgroup I involves stimulation of PLC, while that for both subgroup II and subgroup III involves inhibition of adenylate cyclase (Figure 17.12).

1. NMDA receptor is a ligand-gated ion channel. Its activation is dependent on the binding of both glycine and glutamate (G). Glutamate produces slow, long-lasting depolarizations by opening the calcium (Ca^{2+}) channels. NMDA receptors are usually blocked by magnesium (Mg^{2+}) ions.

This block is released by AMPA receptor-induced depolarization. This allows NMDA receptor activation and Ca^{2+} influx. Prolonged Ca^{2+} influx leads to excitotoxicity. Chronic antidepressant treatment reduces the affinity of glycine site and reduces excitotoxicity.

2. The NMDA receptor can be modulated by a number of antagonists, including competitive antagonists at the glycine and glutamate binding sites or noncompetitive NMDA receptor channel blockers such as PCP and ketamine. High concentration of alcohol antagonizes the receptor function. Memantine (M) is a low-affinity voltage-dependent uncompetitive antagonist at the NMDA receptors, and it can reduce the calcium influx and stop the excitotoxicity. Memantine is used to treat moderate to severe dementia.

3. Memantine (M) has low affinity to the NMDA receptors with rapid off-rate kinetics that allows NMDA receptors to be activated by the relatively high concentrations of glutamate released following depolarization of the presynaptic neurons.

17.3.6.5 Neuropeptides

Neuropeptides have a higher potency and affinity for their receptors and they are active in lower concentrations than classical neurotransmitters (Table 17.2).

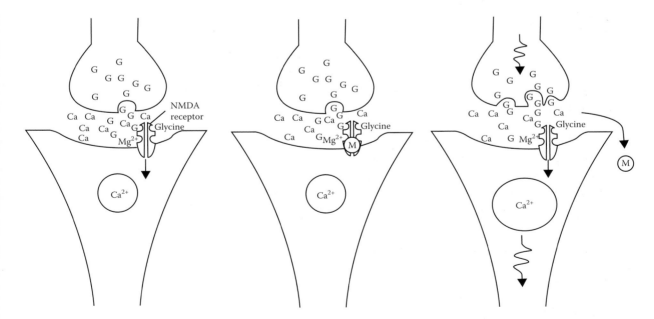

FIGURE 17.12 NMDA receptors (M stands for memantine).

TABLE 17.2
Summary of Neuropeptides and Clinical Relevance

Neuropeptides	Functions	Clinical Relevance
Corticotropin release factor (CRF)	CRF controls the release of adrenocorticotropic hormone from the anterior pituitary Injections of CRH lead to depressive symptoms such as reduced appetite and sex drives, weight loss, and altered circadian rhythms NA causes CRH release. Then CRH stimulates the locus coeruleus firing by stopping its inhibitory controls	1. ↑ CRF concentration in CSF of depressed patients 2. ↓ CRF level in CSF of depressed patients after normalization with antidepressant treatment 3. ↑ CRF mRNA in the postmortem brains of suicide victims 4. ↓ CRF receptors in the postmortem brains of suicide victims 5. Blunted ACTH release in response to CRF challenge in depressed patients 6. CRH overactivity provokes excessive NA release in panic attacks and alcohol withdrawal
Somatostatin	It has inhibitory effects on growth hormone release	1. ↓ CSF concentration in unipolar and bipolar depression 2. ↓ in Alzheimer's disease
Thyrotropin-releasing hormone (TRH)	TRH is the smallest brain peptide and has the ability to reverse sedation caused by drugs due to release of DA and ACh in the brain	1. ↑ concentration in CSF of depressed patients 2. 25%–30% of euthyroid depressives have blunted TSH response to TRH challenge or abnormal T_3/T_4 levels 3. TRH may have a role in learning and memory
Cholecystokinin (CCK)	CCK regulates the postprandial release of bile locally in the gut and control the appetite in the CNS	1. CCK_A receptors seem to be involved in appetite and feeding 2. CCK_B is involved in emotional behaviour
Vasoactive intestinal peptide (VIP)	VIP is found in the cerebral cortex, hypothalamus, amygdala, hippocampus, autonomic ganglia, intestinal, and respiratory tracts	1. VIP stimulates the release of ACTH, growth hormone, and prolactin 2. VIP inhibits the release of somatostatin

17.3.7 ENDOGENOUS OPIOIDS

Endogenous opioids isolated from the CNS are derived from peptide precursor molecules:

- POMC → corticotropin, β-lipotropin
- Proenkephalin → met-enkephalin, leu-enkephalin
- Prodynorphin → dynorphin A, dynorphin B, α-neoendorphin

The enkephalins met-enkephalin and leu-enkephalin are each pentapeptides.

ACKNOWLEDGMENTS

The authors of this book would like to acknowledge Dr. Gavin S. Dawe, BSc Neuroscience (Hons), PhD (Pharmacology), Associate Professor, Department of Pharmacology, Yong Loo Lin School of Medicine, National University of Singapore, and Dr. Ee-Peng Lim PhD, Postdoctoral Fellow, Department of Pharmacology, Yong Loo Lin School of Medicine, National University of Singapore, for their contribution to this chapter.

REFERENCES

Argyropoulos S, Campbell A, and Stein G. 2007: Anxiety disorders. In Stein G and Wilkinson G (eds.) *Seminars in General Adult Psychiatry*, pp. 315–350. London, U.K.: Gaskell.

Basu A, Pereira J, and Aitchison KJ. 2007: The pharmacological management of schizophrenia. In Stein G and Wilkinson G (eds.) *Seminars in General Adult Psychiatry*, pp. 238–294. London, U.K.: Gaskell.

Bernadt M. 2007: Drug treatment of depression. In Stein G and Wilkinson G (eds.) *Seminars in General Adult Psychiatry*, pp. 71–112. London, U.K.: Gaskell.

Carpenter RHS. 2002: *Neurophysiology*, 4th edn. London, U.K.: Arnold.

Charney DS and Bremer JD. 2004: The neurobiology of anxiety disorders. In Charney DS and Nestler EJ (eds.) *Neurobiology of Mental Illness*, 2nd edn, pp. 605–627. New York: Oxford University Press.

Cho RY, Gilbert A, and Lewis DA. 2004: The neurobiology of schizophrenia. In Charney DS and Nestler EJ (eds.) *Neurobiology of Mental Illness*, 2nd edn, pp. 299–310. New York: Oxford University Press.

Delgado PL, Price LH, Miller HL et al. 1994: Serotonin and the neurobiology of depression. Effects of tryptophan depletion in drug-free depressed patients. *Archives of General Psychiatry* 51:865–874.

Drummond LM and Finberg NA. 2007: Phobias and obsessive compulsive disorder. In Stein G and Wilkinson G (eds.) *Seminars in General Adult Psychiatry*, pp. 351–379. London, U.K.: Gaskell.

Duman RS. 2004: The neurochemistry of depressive disorders. In Charney DS and Nestler EJ (eds.) *Neurobiology of Mental Illness,* 2nd edn, pp. 421–439. New York: Oxford University Press.

Emslie-Smith D, Paterson CR, Scratcherd T, and Read NW. (eds.) 1988: *Textbook of Physiology*, 11th edn. Edinburgh, U.K.: Churchill Livingstone.

Evers MM and Martin DB. 2004: Principles of the pharmacotherapy dementia. In Charney DS and Nestler EJ (eds.) *Neurobiology of Mental Illness,* 2nd edn, pp. 863–872. New York: Oxford University Press.

Farmer A and Lange K. 2007: The causes of depression. In Stein G and Wilkinson G (eds.) *Seminars in General Adult Psychiatry*, pp. 48–70. London, U.K.: Gaskell.

Garlow SJ and Nemeroff CB. 2004: The neurochemistry of depressive disorders: Clinical studies. In Charney DS and Nestler EJ (eds.) *Neurobiology of Mental Illness,* 2nd edn, pp. 421–439. New York: Oxford University Press.

Guyton AC and Hall JE. 2000: *Textbook of Medical Physiology*, 10th edn. Philadelphia, PA: WB Saunders.

Kelly C and McCreadie R. 2000: Cigarette smoking and schizophrenia. *Advances in Psychiatric Treatment* 6:327–331.

Krystal JH, Abi-Dargham A, Laruelle M, and Moghaddam B. 2004: Pharmacological models of psychoses. In Charney DS and Nestler EJ (eds.) *Neurobiology of Mental Illness,* 2nd edn, pp. 287–298. New York: Oxford University Press.

Lawrence NS and Stein EA. 2003: Neuroimaging studies of human drug addiction. In Fu CHY, Senior C, Russell TA, Weinberger D, and Murray R (eds.) *Neuroimaging in Psychiatry*, pp. 101–130. London, U.K.: Martin Dunitz.

Nutt D. 1993: Neurochemistry and neuropharmacology. In Morgan G and Butler S (eds.) *Seminars in Basic Neurosciences*, pp. 71–112. London, U.K.: Gaskell.

Puri BK and Tyrer PJ. 2004: *Sciences Basic to Psychiatry*, 3rd edn. Edinburgh, U.K.: Churchill Livingstone.

Rogawski MA. 2000: Low affinity channel blocking (uncompetitive) NMDA receptor antagonists as therapeutic agents—Toward an understanding of their favorable tolerability. *Amino Acids* 19(1):133–149.

Sham P, Woodruff P, and Hunter M. 2007: The aetiology of schizophrenia. In Stein G and Wilkinson G (eds.) *Seminars in General Adult Psychiatry*, pp. 202–237. London, U.K.: Gaskell.

Stryer L. 1995: *Biochemistry*, 4th edn. New York: WH Freeman.

Volkow ND, Chang MO, Wang GJ et al. 2001: Low level of brain dopamine D2 receptors in methamphetamine abusers: Association with metabolism in the orbitofrontal cortex. *American Journal of Psychiatry* 158:2015–2021.

18 General Principles of Psychopharmacology

18.1 HISTORICAL OVERVIEW

18.1.1 ANTIDEPRESSANTS

18.1.1.1 Tricyclic Antidepressants and MAOIs

Tricyclic antidepressants and monoamine oxidase inhibitors (MAOIs) were introduced between 1955 and 1958:

- MAOIs—this arose from the observation of elevated mood in patients with tuberculosis being treated with the MAOI iproniazid, and less toxic MAOIs were subsequently developed; Kline was one of the first to report the value of MAOI treatment in depression.
- Tricyclic antidepressants—Kuhn observed the antidepressant action of imipramine while studying chlorpromazine-like agents.

18.1.1.2 SSRIs

The selective serotonin reuptake inhibitors (SSRIs) were introduced in the late 1980s.

18.1.1.3 RIMA, SNRI, NARI, and NaSSA

The reversible inhibitor of monoamine oxidase-A (RIMA), serotonin–noradrenaline reuptake inhibitor (SNRI), selective noradrenaline reuptake inhibitor (NARI), and noradrenergic and specific serotonergic antidepressant (NaSSA) were introduced in the 1990s.

18.1.2 LITHIUM

In 1886, Lange proposed the use of lithium for treating excited states (Schioldann, 2009). Lithium was introduced by Cade in 1949. Following his finding from animal experiments that lithium caused lethargy, Cade observed (in 1948) that it led to clinical improvement in a patient with mania (Cade, 1949).

18.1.3 ANTIPSYCHOTICS

18.1.3.1 Reserpine

Reserpine was introduced by Sen and Bose in 1931; in 1953, Kline confirmed that it was a treatment for schizophrenia.

18.1.3.2 Typical Antipsychotics

Important dates in the introduction of typical antipsychotics in psychiatric treatment in the twentieth century include the following:

- 1950—chlorpromazine synthesized by Charpentier, who was attempting to synthesize an antihistaminergic agent for anaesthetic use; Laborit then reported that chlorpromazine could induce an artificial hibernation.
- The efficacy of chlorpromazine in the treatment of psychosis was reported by Paraire and Sigwald in 1951 and by Delay and Deniker in 1952 (López-Muñoz et al., 2005).
- 1958—haloperidol was synthesized by Janssen.

18.1.3.3 Clozapine

Important dates in the introduction and, after 1988, the reintroduction of the atypical antipsychotic clozapine include the following:

- 1958—clozapine synthesized as an imipramine analogue; its actions appeared to be closer to chlorpromazine than to imipramine.
- 1961–1962—first clinical trial in schizophrenia (University Psychiatric Clinic, Bern) gave disappointing results; low doses of clozapine were used.
- 1966—Gross and Langner reported good results in chronic schizophrenia (Gross and Langner, 1966).
- 1975 and thereafter—clozapine was withdrawn from general clinical use in some countries owing to cases of fatal agranulocytosis (including eight such deaths in Finland in 1975).
- 1988—Kane and colleagues reported positive results from their multicentre double-blind study of clozapine versus chlorpromazine in treatment resistant schizophrenia; subsequent studies showed that social functioning also improved in response to clozapine (Kane et al., 1988).

18.1.4 ANXIOLYTICS

18.1.4.1 Barbiturates
The first barbiturate, barbituric acid (malonylurea), was synthesized in 1864. The barbiturates were introduced in 1903.

18.1.4.2 Benzodiazepines
The benzodiazepine chlordiazepoxide was synthesized in the late 1950s by Sternbach (working for Roche) and introduced in 1960.

18.2 CLASSIFICATION

The examples given in each class of drug are not meant to be exhaustive.

18.2.1 ANTIPSYCHOTICS (NEUROLEPTICS)

18.2.1.1 First-Generation (Typical) Antipsychotics

- Phenothiazines—aliphatic
  Chlorpromazine
  Levomepromazine (methotrimeprazine)
  Promazine
- Phenothiazines—piperazines
  Fluphenazine
  Trifluoperazine
  Perphenazine
  Prochlorperazine
- Phenothiazines—piperidines
  Pipotiazine palmitate
  Pericyazine
- Butyrophenones
  Haloperidol
  Benperidol
- Thioxanthenes
  Flupentixol
  Zuclopenthixol
- Diphenylbutylpiperidines
  Pimozide
  Fluspirilene
- Substituted benzamides
- Sulpiride (some class this as an atypical antipsychotic)
- Metoclopramide

18.2.1.2 Second-Generation (Atypical) Antipsychotics
The atypical antipsychotics include

- Clozapine
- Quetiapine
- Risperidone
- Amisulpride
- Olanzapine
- Aripiprazole
- Paliperidone

18.2.2 ANTIMUSCARINICS (ANTICHOLINERGICS)

Antimuscarinic (anticholinergic) drugs used in the treatment of parkinsonism resulting from pharmacotherapy with antipsychotics include

- Procyclidine
- Orphenadrine
- Trihexyphenidyl (benzhexol)
- Biperiden
- Benzatropine

18.2.3 PROPHYLAXIS OF BIPOLAR MOOD DISORDER

The drugs most commonly used in the prophylaxis of bipolar mood disorder are

- Lithium salts (carbonate and citrate)
- Carbamazepine

18.2.4 ANTIDEPRESSANTS

18.2.4.1 Tricyclic Antidepressants
Tricyclic antidepressants include

- Dibenzocycloheptanes
  Amitriptyline
  Nortriptyline
- Iminodibenzyls
  Clomipramine
  Imipramine
  Trimipramine
- Others
- Dosulepin (dothiepin)
  Doxepin
  Lofepramine

18.2.4.2 Tricyclic-Related Antidepressants
Tricyclic-related antidepressants include

- Trazodone

18.2.4.3 Tetracyclic Antidepressants
Tetracyclic antidepressants include

- Mianserin

18.2.4.4   MAOIs

MAOIs include

- Hydrazine compounds
  Phenelzine
  Isocarboxazid
- Non-hydrazine compounds
  Tranylcypromine

18.2.4.5   SSRIs

SSRIs include

- Fluvoxamine
- Fluoxetine
- Sertraline
- Paroxetine
- Citalopram
- Escitalopram

18.2.4.6   RIMA

There is currently one RIMA in clinical use:

- Moclobemide

18.2.4.7   SNRI

At the time of writing, there is one SNRI in clinical use:

- Venlafaxine

18.2.4.8   NARI

The NARI in clinical use is

- Reboxetine

18.2.4.9   NaSSA

The NaSSA in clinical use is

- Mirtazapine

18.2.4.10   Others

Other antidepressants include

- Duloxetine
- Agomelatine

18.2.5   NONBENZODIAZEPINE HYPNOTICS

The following short-acting hypnotics are less likely to cause dependency than benzodiazepines and may be used for the short-term relief of insomnia:

- Zaleplon—may be used for up to a fortnight
- Zolpidem—may be used for up to a month
- Zopiclone—may be used for up to a month

18.2.6   BENZODIAZEPINES

Long-acting benzodiazepines include

- Diazepam
- Chlordiazepoxide
- Nitrazepam

Short-acting benzodiazepines include

- Lorazepam
- Temazepam

18.2.7   OTHER ANXIOLYTICS

Nonbenzodiazepine anxiolytics in clinical use include

- Azaspirodecanediones—buspirone
- β-Adrenoceptor blocking drugs—for example, propranolol

18.2.8   DRUGS USED IN ALCOHOL DEPENDENCE

The following drugs are used in alcohol dependence:

- Acamprosate
- Disulfiram
- Benzodiazepines
- Clomethiazole

18.2.9   DRUGS USED IN OPIOID DEPENDENCE

The following drugs are used in opioid dependence:

- Methadone
- Lofexidine
- Naltrexone
- Buprenorphine

18.2.10   ANTIANDROGENS

At the time of writing, there is one antiandrogen used for psychiatric reasons:

- Cyproterone acetate

18.2.11   DRUGS FOR ALZHEIMER'S DISEASE

These include

- Donepezil
- Galantamine
- Rivastigmine
- Memantine

18.3 OPTIMIZING PATIENT COMPLIANCE

Factors that can help optimize patient compliance include

- Patient education
- Setting reasonable expectations
- ↓ Number of tablets to be taken
- ↓ Dosage frequency
- Labelling medicine containers clearly
- Parenteral/depot administration
- Using alternative medication if there are troublesome side effects
- Involving family members

It is particularly important to avoid polypharmacy, if possible, and to prescribe a simple, straightforward drug regime for elderly patients. Containers used by the elderly should take into account the possibility that the patient may have arthritis and may also be designed to allow the pharmacist to place the appropriate medication for each intake in clearly labelled boxes.

18.4 PLACEBO EFFECT

18.4.1 DEFINITION

A placebo refers to any therapy or component of therapy that is deliberately used for its nonspecific, psychological, or psychophysiological effect or its presumed specific effect, but that is without specific activity for the condition being treated.

18.4.2 MECHANISMS OF THE PLACEBO EFFECT

White et al. (1985) have proposed the following biopsychosocial model for the mechanisms of the placebo effect:

- Homeostatic mechanisms
  Central nervous system function
  Autonomic nervous system function
  Peripheral nervous system function
  Endocrine function
  Immune function
- Classical conditioning
- Operant conditioning
- Cognitive–affective–behavioural self-control
- Hypnosis
- The doctor's attitude
- The patient's expectations
- Transitional object phenomena

18.4.3 PILL FACTORS

The strength of the placebo effect varies with the physical form of the medication, including the size, type, colour, and number of pills (Blakwell et al., 1972; Buckalew and Coffield, 1982). For example, the relative placebo effect for the following physical forms has been found to be stronger:

- Multiple pills > single pills
- Larger pills > smaller pills
- Capsules > tablets

Again, examples of the relative potency of medication varying with pill colour include the following (Schapira et al., 1970):

- Anxiety symptoms responded better to green tablets.
- Depressive symptoms responded better to yellow tablets.

18.4.4 CONTROLLING FOR THE PLACEBO EFFECT

The previously mentioned factors can be taken into account in clinical practice. In clinical trials, it is important to control for the placebo effect, and this is achieved in the randomized double-blind placebo-controlled design (see Chapter 23).

18.5 PRESCRIBING FOR PSYCHIATRIC PATIENTS

Prescribing for psychiatric patients includes taking into consideration the following factors (Cookson et al., 2002):

- The symptoms to be targeted in the short and long term
- Age
- Physical health
- Circumstances
- Drugs already being taken, including home remedies
- The effectiveness, or otherwise, of previous drug treatments
- Personality
- Lifestyle
- Social setting
- The choice of actual drugs
  Dose size
  Dose schedule
- When to review outcome and who should help report it
- The role of the community psychiatry nurse and the GP in providing medication and monitoring progress

18.6 PHARMACOKINETICS

18.6.1 ABSORPTION

18.6.1.1 Routes of Administration

18.6.1.1.1 Enteral Administration

Enteral administration routes employ the gastrointestinal tract, from which the drug is absorbed into the circulation. They include administration via the following routes:

- Oral
- Buccal
- Sublingual
- Rectal

18.6.1.1.2 Parenteral Administration

This includes administration via the following routes:

- Intramuscular
- Intravenous
- Subcutaneous
- Inhalational
- Topical

18.6.1.2 Rate of Absorption

The rate of absorption of a drug from its site of administration depends on the following factors:

- The form of the drug
- The solubility of the drug, which is influenced by factors such as
  The pK_a of the drug
  Particle size
  The ambient pH
- The rate of blood flow through the tissue in which the drug is sited

18.6.1.3 Oral Administration

18.6.1.3.1 Mechanisms of Absorption

The main mechanisms of absorption of drugs from the gastrointestinal tract are

- Passive diffusion
- Pore filtration
- Active transport

18.6.1.3.2 Site of Absorption

The main site of absorption of most psychotropic drugs (which tend to be lipophilic at a physiological pH) from the gastrointestinal tract is the small intestine.

18.6.1.3.3 Factors Influencing Absorption

Factors influencing absorption of drugs from the gastrointestinal tract include

- Gastric emptying
- Gastric pH
- Intestinal motility
- Presence/absence of food—the presence of food delays gastric emptying
- Intestinal microflora
- Area of absorption
- Blood flow

The antimuscarinic actions of some psychotropic medication lead to delayed gastric emptying.

18.6.1.4 Rectal Administration

18.6.1.4.1 Advantages

Advantages of rectal administration over the oral route include the following:

- It can be used if the patient cannot swallow—for example, because of vomiting.
- Gastric factors are bypassed.
- It can be used for drugs that are irritant to the stomach.
- There is reduced first-pass metabolism.
- It can be useful in uncooperative patients.
- It can be used to administer diazepam during an epileptic seizure, for example, in a patient with a learning difficulty.

18.6.1.4.2 Disadvantages

Disadvantages of rectal administration include the following:

- Embarrassment.
- Presence of a variable amount of faecal matter → unpredictable rate of absorption.
- Local inflammation may occur following the frequent use of this route.

18.6.1.5 Intramuscular Administration

18.6.1.5.1 Factors Influencing Absorption

The rate of absorption of drugs administered intramuscularly is increased in the following circumstances:

- Lipid-soluble drugs
- Drugs with a low relative molecular mass
- Increased muscle blood flow—for example, after physical exercise or during emotional excitement

18.6.1.5.2 Disadvantages

Disadvantages of intramuscular administration include the following:

- Pain.
- Usually unacceptable for self-administration.
- Risk of damage to structures such as nerves.
- Some drugs, for example, paraldehyde, may cause sterile abscess formation.
- Reduced muscle blood flow (e.g. in cardiac failure) leading to reduced absorption.
- Tissue binding or precipitation from solution after intramuscular administration (e.g. for chlordiazepoxide, diazepam, phenytoin) leading to reduced absorption.
- This route should not be used if the patient is receiving anticoagulant therapy.
- Increased creatine phosphokinase occurs, which may interfere with diagnostic cardiac enzyme assays.

18.6.1.6 Intravenous Administration

18.6.1.6.1 Advantages

Advantages of intravenous administration include the following:

- Rapid intravenous administration → rapid action; useful in emergency situations.
- Drug dose can be titrated against patient response.
- Large volumes can be administered slowly.
- This route can be used for drugs that cannot be absorbed by other routes.
- First-pass metabolism is bypassed.

18.6.1.6.2 Disadvantages

Disadvantages of intravenous administration include the following:

- Adverse effects may occur rapidly.
- Dangerously high blood levels may be achieved.
- It is difficult to recall the drug once administered.
- Risk of sepsis.
- Risk of thrombosis.
- Risk of air embolism.
- Risk of injection into tissues surrounding the vein, which may lead to necrosis.
- Risk of injection into an artery, which may lead to spasm.
- Cannot be used with insoluble drugs.

18.6.2 Distribution

The rate and degree of distribution of psychotropic drugs between the lipid, protein, and water components of the body are influenced by the

- Lipid solubility of the drug
- Plasma-protein binding
- Volume of distribution
- Blood–brain barrier
- Placenta

18.6.2.1 Lipid Solubility

Increased lipid solubility is associated with increased volume of distribution. This is the case for most psychotropic drugs at physiological pH.

18.6.2.2 Plasma–Protein Binding

Drugs circulate around the body partly bound to plasma proteins and partly free in the water phase of plasma. This plasma-protein binding, which is reversible and competitive, acts as a reservoir for the drug. The main plasma-binding protein for acidic drugs is albumin, while basic drugs, including many psychotropic drugs, can also bind to other plasma proteins such as lipoprotein and α_1-acid glycoprotein. The extent of plasma-protein binding varies with a number of factors:

- Plasma drug concentration
- Plasma-protein concentration—reduced in
  Hepatic disease
  Renal disease
  Cardiac failure
  Malnutrition
  Carcinoma
  Surgery
  Burns
- Drug interactions
  Displacement
  Plasma-protein tertiary structure change
- Concentration of physiological substances—for example, urea, bilirubin, and free fatty acid
  Displacement
  Plasma-protein tertiary structure change

18.6.2.3 Volume of Distribution

This is a theoretical concept relating the mass of a drug in the body to the blood or plasma concentration:

$$\text{Volume of distribution} = \frac{\text{Mass of a drug in the body at a given time}}{\text{Concentration of the drug at that time in the blood or the plasma}}$$

A higher volume of distribution in general corresponds to a shorter duration of drug action. Factors that may influence the volume of distribution include

- Drug lipid solubility—increased lipid solubility (e.g. most psychotropic drugs) is associated with an increased volume of distribution
- Adipose tissue—for example, some psychotropic drugs → weight gain → increased adipose tissue → an increased volume of distribution
- Increasing age: proportion of lean tissue → increased volume of distribution
- Sex
- Physical disease

18.6.2.4 Blood–Brain Barrier and Brain Distribution

18.6.2.4.1 *Components*

Components of the blood–brain barrier include

- Tight junctions between adjacent cerebral capillary endothelial cells
- Cerebral capillary basement membrane
- Gliovascular membrane

18.6.2.4.2 *Drug Lipid Solubility*

A high rate of penetration of the blood–brain barrier occurs for nonpolar highly lipid-soluble drugs, since the brain is a highly lipid organ. Most psychotropic drugs, being highly lipid soluble, can therefore easily cross the blood–brain barrier.

18.6.2.4.3 *Infection*

Infection may alter the normal functioning of the blood–brain barrier.

18.6.2.4.4 *Receptors*

The existence of specific brain receptors for many psychotropic drugs leads to psychotropic drug protein binding in the brain, thereby forming a central nervous system reservoir. This does not occur in the CSF, with its very low protein concentration.

18.6.2.4.5 *Active Transport*

Active transport mechanisms are used to cross the blood–brain barrier by some physiological substances and drugs, for example, levodopa.

18.6.2.4.6 *Diffusion*

Some small molecules diffuse readily into the brain and CSF from the cerebral circulation, for example, lithium ions.

18.6.2.5 Placenta

Drugs may transfer into the fetal circulation from the maternal circulation across the placenta by means of

- Passive diffusion
- Active transport
- Pinocytosis

Since drugs may cause teratogenesis during the first trimester, they should be avoided during this time if at all possible.

18.6.3 METABOLISM

While some highly water-soluble drugs, for example, lithium, are excreted unchanged by the kidneys, others, such as most highly lipid-soluble psychotropic drugs, first undergo metabolism (biotransformation) to reduce their lipid solubility and make them more water soluble, prior to renal excretion. Metabolism sometimes results in the production of pharmacologically active metabolites, for example, amitriptyline → nortriptyline. Sites of metabolism include the following:

- Liver—this is the most important site of metabolism.
- Kidney.
- Adrenal (suprarenal) cortex.
- Gastrointestinal tract.
- Lung.
- Placenta.
- Skin.
- Lymphocytes.

18.6.3.1 Hepatic Phase I Metabolism (Biotransformation)

This leads to a change in the drug molecular structure by the following nonsynthetic reactions:

- Oxidation—the most common
- Hydrolysis
- Reduction

The most important type of oxidation reaction is that carried out by microsomal mixed-function oxidases, involving the cytochrome P450 isoenzymes.

18.6.3.2 Hepatic Phase II Metabolism (Biotransformation)

This is a synthetic reaction involving conjugation between a parent drug/drug metabolite/endogenous substance and a polar endogenous molecule/group. Examples of the latter include

- Glucuronic acid
- Sulphate
- Acetate
- Glutathione
- Glycine
- Glutamine

The resulting water-soluble conjugate can be excreted by the kidney if the relative molecular mass < approximately 300. If the relative molecular mass > approximately 300, the conjugate can be excreted in the bile.

18.6.3.3 First-Pass Effect

The first-pass effect (first-pass metabolism or presystemic elimination) is the metabolism undergone by an orally absorbed drug during its passage from the hepatic portal system through the liver before entering the systemic circulation. It varies between individuals and may be reduced by, for example, hepatic disease, food, or drugs that increase hepatic blood flow.

18.6.4 Elimination

Elimination (excretion) of drugs and drug metabolites can take place by means of the

- Kidney—the most important organ for such elimination
- Bile and faeces
- Lung
- Saliva
- Sweat
- Sebum
- Milk

With the exception of pulmonary excretion, in general, water-soluble polar drugs and drug metabolites are eliminated more readily by excretory organs than are highly lipid-soluble nonpolar ones.

18.7 PHARMACODYNAMICS

18.7.1 Antipsychotics

18.7.1.1 First-Generation Antipsychotics

Many of the actions of chlorpromazine, the archetypal antipsychotic, are believed to result from antagonist action to the following neurotransmitters:

- Dopamine
- Acetylcholine—muscarinic receptors
- Adrenaline/noradrenaline
- Histamine

Many of these actions also occur, to varying extents, with other typical antipsychotics.

18.7.1.1.1 Antidopaminergic Action

In general, typical antipsychotics are postulated to act clinically by causing postsynaptic blockade of dopamine D_2 receptors; their antagonism at these receptors is related to their clinical antipsychotic potencies. It is the antidopaminergic action on the mesolimbic–mesocortical pathway that is believed to be the effect required for this clinical action.

The antidopaminergic action on the tuberoinfundibular pathway causes hormonal side effects. Hyperprolactinaemia, resulting from the fact that dopamine is prolactin-inhibitory factor, causes

- Galactorrhoea
- Gynaecomastia
- Menstrual disturbances
- Reduced sperm count
- Reduced libido

The antidopaminergic action on the nigrostriatal pathway causes extrapyramidal symptoms:

- Parkinsonism
- Dystonias
- Akathisia
- Tardive dyskinesia

18.7.1.1.2 Antimuscarinic Action

The central antimuscarinic (anticholinergic) actions may cause

- Convulsions
- Pyrexia

Peripheral antimuscarinic symptoms include

- Dry mouth
- Blurred vision
- Urinary retention
- Constipation
- Nasal congestion

18.7.1.1.3 *Antiadrenergic Action*

Antiadrenergic actions may cause

- Postural hypotension
- Ejaculatory failure

18.7.1.1.4 *Antihistaminic Action*

Antihistaminic effects include drowsiness.

18.7.1.2 Second-Generation Antipsychotics

The second-generation or atypical antipsychotics have a greater action than do first-generation or typical antipsychotics on receptors other than dopamine D_2 receptors. For example, clozapine, the archetypal atypical antipsychotic, has a higher potency of action than do typical antipsychotics on the following receptors:

- $5\text{-}HT_2$
- D_4
- D_1
- Muscarinic
- α-Adrenergic

18.7.2 Drugs Used in the Treatment of Mood Disorder

18.7.2.1 Lithium

Lithium ions, Li^+, are monovalent cations that cause a number of effects, some of which may account for its therapeutic actions, including

- ↑ Intracellular Na^+
- ↓ Na,K-ATPase pump activity
- ↑ Intracellular Ca^{2+} in erythrocytes in mania and depression
- ↑ Erythrocyte choline
- ↑ Erythrocyte phospholipid catabolism (via phospholipase D)
- ↓ Ca^{2+} in platelets in bipolar disorder
- ↑ Serotonergic neurotransmission
- ↓ Central $5\text{-}HT_1$ and $5\text{-}HT_2$ receptor density (demonstrated in the hippocampus)

- ↑ Dopamine turnover in hypothalamic-tuberoinfundibular dopaminergic neurons
- ↓ Central dopamine synthesis (dose dependent)
- Normalization of low plasma and CSF levels of GABA in bipolar disorder
- ↑ GABAergic neurotransmission
- ↓ Low-affinity GABA receptors in the corpus striatum and hypothalamus (chronic lithium administration)
- ↑ Met-enkephalin and leu-enkephalin in the basal ganglia and nucleus accumbens
- ↑ Dynorphin in the corpus striatum

18.7.2.2 Tricyclic Antidepressants

The most important postulated modes of action in the brain of tricyclic antidepressants in achieving therapeutic effects are

- Inhibition of reuptake of noradrenaline
- Inhibition of reuptake of serotonin

For this reason, tricyclic antidepressants are also known as monoamine reuptake inhibitors, or MARIs. Peripherally, most tricyclic antidepressants also have an antimuscarinic action, which gives rise to peripheral antimuscarinic side effects such as

- Dry mouth
- Blurred vision
- Drowsiness
- Urinary retention
- Constipation

Postural hypotension occurs as a result of the antiadrenergic action.

18.7.2.3 SSRIs

The most important postulated mode of action in the brain of SSRIs in achieving therapeutic effects is

- Inhibition of reuptake of serotonin

Their relatively selective action on serotonin reuptake means that SSRIs are less likely than tricyclic antidepressants to cause antimuscarinic side effects. They are, however, more likely to cause gastrointestinal side effects such as nausea and vomiting.

18.7.2.4 MAOIs

The most important postulated mode of action in the brain of MAOIs in achieving therapeutic effects is

- Irreversible inhibition of MAO-A and MAO-B

In the central nervous system, MAO-A (monoamine oxidase type A) acts on

- Noradrenaline
- Serotonin
- Dopamine
- Tyramine

In the central nervous system, MAO-B (monoamine oxidase type B) acts on

- Dopamine
- Tyramine
- Phenylethylamine
- Benzylamine

The inhibition of peripheral pressor amines, particularly dietary tyramine, by MAOIs can lead to a hypertensive crisis when foodstuffs rich in tyramine are eaten (see Chapter 19).

18.7.2.5   RIMA

The most important postulated mode of action in the brain of the RIMA in achieving therapeutic effects is

- Reversible inhibition of MAO-A

18.7.2.6   SNRI

The most important postulated modes of action in the brain of the SNRIs in achieving therapeutic effects are

- Inhibition of reuptake of noradrenaline
- Inhibition of reuptake of serotonin

18.7.2.7   NARI

The most important postulated mode of action in the brain of the NARI in achieving therapeutic effects is

- Selective inhibition of the reuptake of noradrenaline

18.7.2.8   NaSSA

The most important postulated modes of action in the brain of the NaSSA in achieving therapeutic effects are

- Increased release of noradrenaline by antagonism of inhibitory presynaptic α_2-adrenoceptors
- Increased release of serotonin by enhancement of a facilitatory noradrenergic input to serotonergic cell bodies
- Increased release of serotonin by antagonism of inhibitory presynaptic α_2-adrenoceptors on serotonergic neuronal terminals

18.7.2.9   Asenapine

This recently introduced sublingually administered tetracyclic antipsychotic is indicated in the treatment of mania. It has high affinity for

- α_{2B}-Adrenergic receptors
- Serotonin 5-HT$_{2A}$ receptors
- Serotonin 5-HT$_{2B}$ receptors
- Serotonin 5-HT$_{2C}$ receptors
- Serotonin 5-HT$_6$ receptors
- Serotonin 5-HT$_7$ receptors
- Dopamine D$_3$ receptors

Cognitive, antianxiety, and mood stabilization beneficial actions may result from strong antagonism to 5-HT$_6$ and 5-HT$_7$ receptors. There is little binding of asenapine to muscarinic receptors, thereby leading to a low likelihood of antimuscarinic side effects.

18.7.2.10   Agomelatine

This recently introduced antidepressant has the following actions:

- Agonist at MT$_1$ melatonergic receptors
- Agonist at MT$_2$ melatonergic receptors
- Antagonist at 5-HT$_{2C}$ receptors

18.7.3   ANXIOLYTICS AND HYPNOTICS

18.7.3.1   Benzodiazepines

The most important postulated mode of action in the brain of benzodiazepines in achieving central therapeutic effects is

- Binding to GABA$_A$ receptors

18.7.3.2   Buspirone

The most important postulated mode of action in the brain of the azaspirodecanedione buspirone in achieving central therapeutic effects is

- Partial agonism at 5-HT$_{1A}$ receptors

18.7.3.3   β-Adrenoceptor Blocking Drugs

The most important postulated mode of action of the β-adrenoceptor blocking drugs in achieving anxiolytic effects is

- Antagonism at peripheral β-adrenoceptors

18.7.3.4 Zopiclone

The cyclopyrrolone zopiclone is believed to achieve a central hypnotic effect by acting on the same receptors as do benzodiazepines.

18.7.3.5 Zolpidem

The imidazopyridine zolpidem is believed to achieve a central hypnotic effect by acting on the same receptors as do benzodiazepines.

18.7.3.6 Zaleplon

The pyrazolopyrimidine zaleplon is believed to achieve a central hypnotic effect by acting on the same receptors as do benzodiazepines.

18.7.4 DRUGS FOR ALZHEIMER'S DISEASE

These have the following actions:

- Donepezil—reversible inhibitor of acetylcholinesterase
- Galantamine—reversible inhibitor of acetylcholinesterase
- Rivastigmine—reversible inhibitor of acetylcholinesterase
- Memantine—NMDA antagonist

18.7.5 ANTIEPILEPTIC AGENTS

18.7.5.1 Carbamazepine

Carbamazepine, which has a tricyclic antidepressant-like structure, may achieve its anticonvulsant effect on the basis of the following actions:

- Binding to and inactivation of voltage-dependent Na^+ channels
- Increased K^+ conductance
- Partial agonism at the adenosine A_1 subclass of P_1 purinoceptors

18.7.5.2 Sodium Valproate

Sodium valproate may achieve its anticonvulsant effect on the basis of the following actions:

- Increased GABA
  Decreased GABA breakdown
  Increased GABA release
  Decreased GABA turnover
  Increased $GABA_B$ receptor density
  Increased neuronal responsiveness to GABA
- Reduced Na^+ influx
- Increased K^+ conductance

18.7.5.3 Phenytoin

The mechanism of anticonvulsant action of phenytoin is unknown but may involve

- Membrane stabilization
  Na^+ channel binding
  Ca^{2+} channel binding
- Benzodiazepine receptor binding
- GABA receptor function modulation

18.7.5.4 Phenobarbitone

The actions of phenobarbitone may be similar to those given earlier for phenytoin.

18.7.5.5 Gabapentin

Gabapentin is believed to achieve its anticonvulsant effect by means of the following action:

- Binding to a unique cerebral receptor site

18.7.5.6 Vigabatrin

Vigabatrin is believed to achieve its anticonvulsant effect by means of the following action:

- Inhibition of GABA transaminase, leading to increased GABA release

18.7.5.7 Lamotrigine

Lamotrigine is believed to achieve its anticonvulsant effect by means of the following action:

- Inhibition of glutamate release

18.7.5.8 Levetiracetam

Levetiracetam, the S-enantiomer of etiracetam, may achieve its anticonvulsant effect by means of the following actions:

- Binding to synaptic vesicle glycoprotein 2A (SV2A)
- Inhibition of presynaptic Ca^{2+} channels

18.7.5.9 Lacosamide

Lacosamide, a functionalized amino acid, may achieve its anticonvulsant effect by means of the following action:

- ↑ slow inactivation of voltage-gated Na^+ channels

18.7.6   Neurochemical Effects of ECT

18.7.6.1   Noradrenaline

Electroconvulsive therapy (ECT) probably leads to increased noradrenergic function. In particular, ECT acutely causes

- Increased cerebral noradrenaline activity
- Increased cerebral tyrosine hydroxylase activity
- Increased plasma catecholamines, particularly adrenaline

Chronic ECS (electroconvulsive shock) leads to

- Reduced β-adrenergic receptor density

The last effect may be a result of receptor downregulation.

18.7.6.2   Serotonin

ECT probably leads to increased serotonergic function. In particular, ECT acutely causes

- Increased cerebral serotonin concentration

Chronic ECT leads to

- Increased 5-HT$_2$ receptor density

18.7.6.3   Dopamine

ECT probably leads to increased dopaminergic function. In particular, ECT acutely causes

- Increased cerebral dopamine concentration
- Increased cerebral concentration of dopamine metabolites
- Increased behavioural responsiveness to dopamine agonists

In rat substantia nigra, repeated ECSs lead to

- Increased dopamine D$_1$ receptor density
- Increased second-messenger potentiation at dopamine D$_1$ receptors

18.7.6.4   GABA

ECT may cause a functional increase in GABAergic activity.

18.7.6.5   Acetylcholine

ECT probably leads to decreased central cholinergic function. In particular, ECT acutely causes

- Reduced cerebral acetylcholine concentration
- Increased cerebral acetyltransferase activity
- Increased cerebral acetylcholinesterase activity
- Increased CSF acetylcholine concentration

Chronic ECS leads to

- Reduced muscarinic cholinergic receptor density in the cerebral cortex
- Reduced muscarinic cholinergic receptor density in the hippocampus
- Reduced second-messenger response in the hippocampus

18.7.6.6   Endogenous Opioids
Chronic ECS leads to

- Increased cerebral met-enkephalin concentration and synthesis
- Increased cerebral β-endorphin concentration and synthesis
- Changes in opioid ligand binding

18.7.6.7   Adenosine
Chronic ECS leads to

- Increased cerebral adenosine A$_1$ purinoceptor density

BIBLIOGRAPHY

Blackwell B, Bloomfield SS, and Buncher CR. 1972: Demonstration to medical students of placebo responses and nondrug factors. *Lancet* 1:1279–1282.

Buckalew LW and Coffield KE. 1982: An investigation of drug expectancy as a function of capsule color and size and preparation form. *Journal of Clinical Psychopharmacology* 2:245–248.

Cookson J, Taylor J, and Katona C. 2002: *Use of Drugs in Psychiatry: The Evidence from Psychopharmacology,* 5th edn. London, U.K.: Gaskell.

Ettinger RH. 2011: *Psychopharmacology.* London, U.K.: Pearson.

Gross H and Langner E. 1966: Effect profile of a chemically new broad spectrum neuroleptic of the dibenzodiazepine group. *Wiener Medizinische Wochenschrift* 116:814–816.

Healy D (ed.). 2008: *Psychiatric Drugs Explained,* 5th edn. Edinburgh, U.K.: Churchill Livingstone.

Kane J, Honigfeld G, Singer J, and Meltzer H. 1988: Clozapine for the treatment-resistant schizophrenic: A double-blind comparison versus chlorpromazine/benztropine. *Archives of General Psychiatry* 45(9):789–796.

King DJ (ed.). 2004: *Seminars in Clinical Psychopharmacology,* 2nd edn. London, U.K.: Gaskell.

López-Muñoz F, Alamo C, Cuenca E, Shen WW, Clervoy P, and Rubio G. 2005: History of the discovery and clinical introduction of chlorpromazine. *Annals of Clinical Psychiatry* 17(3):113–135.

Puri BK. 2013: *Drugs in Psychiatry*, 2nd edn. Oxford, U.K.: Oxford University Press.

Schapira K, McClelland HA, Griffiths NR et al. 1970: Study of the effects of tablet colour in the treatment of anxiety states. *BMJ* 2:446–449.

Schioldann J. 2009: *History of the Introduction of Lithium into Medicine and Psychiatry*, p. 390. Adelaide, Australia: Adelaide Academic Press.

Silverstone T and Turner P. 1995: *Drug Treatment in Psychiatry*, 5th edn. London, U.K.: Routledge.

White L, Tursky B, and Schwartz G (eds.). 1985: Proposed synthesis of placebo models. In *Placebo: Theory, Research, and Mechanisms*, pp. 431–447. New York: Guildford Press.

19 Psychotropic Drugs and Adverse Drug Reactions

19.1 DO PSYCHOTROPIC DRUGS WORK?

There is controversy over the issue of whether or not psychotropic drugs really do have beneficial psychotropic actions that are significantly greater than those of placebos. Based on his meta-analytic statistical reviews, Irving Kirsch has argued that antidepressant medication is not significantly better than placebo at treating depression (Kirsch, 2009a,b). Moncrieff (2007) has also published a strong critique of psychotropic drugs.

19.1.1 CATIE AND CUtLASS

These two large studies compared first-generation antipsychotics with second-generation antipsychotics.

19.1.1.1 CATIE

CATIE (Clinical Antipsychotic Trials of Intervention Effectiveness), funded by the National Institute of Mental Health (Bethesda, MD), compared olanzapine, quetiapine, risperidone, and ziprasidone (second-generation antipsychotics) and perphenazine (a first-generation antipsychotic). Almost 1500 chronic schizophrenia patients were randomly assigned to treatment with one of these antipsychotic drugs in a double-blind design, with the primary outcome measure being discontinuation of treatment for any cause (Lieberman et al., 2005). Key results were as follows:

- The efficacy of the first-generation antipsychotic was similar to that of the second-generation antipsychotics.
- Olanzapine was the most effective in terms of the rates of discontinuation.
- Olanzapine was associated with greater weight gain and increases in measures of glucose and lipid metabolism.

19.1.1.2 CUtLASS

CUtLASS (Cost Utility of the Latest Antipsychotic drugs in Schizophrenia Study), funded by the Health Technology Assessment Programme (Southampton, U.K.), compared first-generation antipsychotics and second-generation antipsychotics (apart from clozapine). Two hundred and twenty-seven patients with schizophrenia and related disorders were assessed for medication review because of inadequate response or adverse effects and randomly prescribed either first-generation antipsychotics or second-generation antipsychotics (other than clozapine), the individual medication choice in each arm being made by each patient's psychiatrist (Jones et al., 2006). Key results were as follows:

- Patients in the first-generation antipsychotic arm showed a trend towards greater improvement in Quality of Life Scale and symptom scores.
- Overall, patients reported no clear preference for either first- or second-generation antipsychotics.

19.2 TYPES OF ADVERSE DRUG REACTIONS

19.2.1 CLASSIFICATION

Adverse drug reactions may be classified as

- Intolerance
- Idiosyncratic reactions
- Allergic reactions
- Drug interactions

19.2.2 CAUSAL RELATIONSHIP

The following criteria have been suggested as making it more likely that a causal connection exists between a drug and an alleged effect (Edwards, 1995):

- There is a close temporal relationship between the effect and the taking of the drug, or toxic levels of the drug or its active metabolites in body fluids have been demonstrated.
- The effect differs from manifestations of the disorder being treated.
- No other substances are being taken or withdrawn when the effect occurs.
- The reaction disappears when treatment is stopped.
- The effect reappears with a rechallenge test.

19.2.3 INTOLERANCE

In drug intolerance, the adverse reactions are consistent with the known pharmacological actions of the drug. These adverse drug reactions may be dose related.

19.2.4 IDIOSYNCRATIC REACTIONS

Idiosyncratic adverse drug reactions are reactions that are not characteristic or predictable and that are associated with an individual human difference not present in members of the general population.

19.2.5 ALLERGIC REACTIONS

Allergic reactions to drugs involve the body's immune system, with the drug interacting with a protein to form an immunogen that causes sensitization and the induction of an immune response. Criteria suggesting an allergic reaction include the following:

- A different time course from that of the pharmacodynamic action, for example:
  Delayed onset of the adverse drug reaction.
  The adverse drug reaction manifests only following repeated drug exposure.
- There may be no dose-related effect, with sub-therapeutically small doses leading to sensitization or allergic reactions.
- A hypersensitivity reaction, unrelated to the pharmacological actions of the drug, occurs.

Types of allergic reaction to drugs include

- Anaphylactic shock—type I hypersensitivity reaction
- Haematological reactions—type II, III, or IV hypersensitivity reaction; for example:
  Haemolytic anaemia
  Agranulocytosis
  Thrombocytopenia
- Allergic liver damage—type II ± III hypersensitivity reaction
- Skin rashes—type IV hypersensitivity reaction
- Generalized autoimmune (systemic lupus erythematosus-like) disease—type IV hypersensitivity reaction

19.2.6 DRUG INTERACTIONS

Adverse drug reactions may result from interactions between different drugs. These may result from

- Pharmacokinetic interactions
- Pharmacodynamic interactions

19.2.6.1 Pharmacokinetic Interactions

Pharmacokinetic interactions between drugs include

- Precipitation or inactivation following the mixing of drugs
- Chelation
- Changes in gastrointestinal tract motility
- Changes in gastrointestinal tract pH
- Drug displacement from binding sites
- Enzyme induction
- Enzyme inhibition
- Competition for renal tubular transport
- Changes in urinary pH → changes in drug excretion

19.2.6.2 Pharmacodynamic Interactions

Pharmacodynamic interactions between drugs include

- Inhibition of drug uptake
- Inhibition of drug transport
- Interaction at receptors
- Synergism
- Changes in fluid and electrolyte balance

19.3 PSYCHOTROPIC MEDICATION

19.3.1 FIRST-GENERATION ANTIPSYCHOTICS

In Chapter 18, the major categories of adverse drug reactions are given that are believed to be caused by antagonist action to the following neurotransmitters:

- Dopamine
- Acetylcholine—muscarinic receptors
- Adrenaline/noradrenaline
- Histamine

Other important adverse drug reactions include

- Photosensitization
- Hypothermia or pyrexia
- Allergic (sensitivity) reactions
- Neuroleptic malignant syndrome

19.3.1.1 Photosensitization

Photosensitization is more common with chlorpromazine than with other typical antipsychotics.

19.3.1.2 Hypothermia or Pyrexia

Interference with temperature regulation is a dose-related side effect.

19.3.1.3 Allergic (Sensitivity) Reactions

Sensitivity reactions include

- Agranulocytosis
- Leukopenia
- Leukocytosis
- Haemolytic anaemia

19.3.1.4 Neuroleptic Malignant Syndrome

Neuroleptic malignant syndrome is characterized by

- Hyperthermia
- Fluctuating level of consciousness
- Muscular rigidity
- Autonomic dysfunction
  Tachycardia
  Labile blood pressure
  Pallor
  Sweating
  Urinary incontinence

Laboratory investigations commonly, but not invariably, demonstrate

- ↑ Creatinine phosphokinase
- ↑ White blood count
- Abnormal liver function tests

Neuroleptic malignant syndrome requires urgent medical treatment.

19.3.1.5 Chronic Pharmacotherapy

Long-term high-dose pharmacotherapy may cause ocular and skin changes, such as

- Opacity of the lens
- Opacity of the cornea
- Purplish pigmentation of the skin
- Purplish pigmentation of the conjunctiva
- Purplish pigmentation of the cornea
- Purplish pigmentation of the retina

19.3.2 SECOND-GENERATION ANTIPSYCHOTICS

19.3.2.1 Clozapine

Clozapine may cause neutropenia and potentially fatal agranulocytosis, because of which regular haematological monitoring is required. Other side effects of clozapine include hypersalivation and side effects common to chlorpromazine, including extrapyramidal symptoms.

19.3.2.2 General Side Effects

Treatment with second-generation antipsychotics may be associated with

- Weight gain
- Hyperglycaemia—for example, with clozapine and olanzapine
- Type 2 diabetes mellitus—for example, with clozapine and olanzapine
- Dizziness
- Postural hypotension
- Extrapyramidal symptoms and occasionally tardive dyskinesia
- Neuroleptic malignant syndrome (rare)

Given the risk of hyperglycaemia, metabolic syndrome, and type 2 diabetes mellitus, when treating a patient with a second-generation antipsychotic drug, the patient's body mass and plasma glucose level should be monitored regularly.

19.3.3 ANTIMUSCARINIC DRUGS

Antimuscarinic drugs used in parkinsonism may give rise to the following side effects:

- Antimuscarinic side effects (see Chapter 18)
- Worsening of tardive dyskinesia
- Gastrointestinal tract disturbances
- Hypersensitivity

19.3.4 LITHIUM

19.3.4.1 Renal Function

Since lithium ions are excreted mainly by the kidneys, renal function must be checked prior to commencing pharmacotherapy with lithium.

19.3.4.2 Plasma Levels

The therapeutic index of lithium is low and therefore regular plasma lithium level monitoring is required. (Therapeutic index = [toxic dose]/[therapeutic dose].) The dose is adjusted to achieve a lithium level of 0.4–1.0 mM for prophylactic purposes, with lower levels being used in the elderly.

19.3.4.3 Side Effects

Side effects of lithium therapy include

- Fatigue
- Drowsiness
- Dry mouth
- A metallic taste
- Polydipsia

- Polyuria
- Nausea
- Vomiting
- Weight gain
- Diarrhoea
- Fine tremor
- Muscle weakness
- Oedema

Oedema should not be treated with diuretics since thiazide and loop diuretics reduce lithium excretion and can thereby cause lithium intoxication.

19.3.4.4   Intoxication

Signs of lithium intoxication include

- Mild drowsiness and sluggishness → giddiness and ataxia
- Lack of coordination
- Blurred vision
- Tinnitus
- Anorexia
- Dysarthria
- Vomiting
- Diarrhoea
- Coarse tremor
- Muscle weakness

19.3.4.5   Severe Overdosage

At lithium plasma levels of greater than 2 mM, the following effects can occur:

- Hyperreflexia and hyperextension of the limbs
- Toxic psychoses
- Convulsions
- Syncope
- Oliguria
- Circulatory failure
- Coma
- Death

19.3.4.6   Chronic Therapy

Long-term treatment with lithium may give rise to

- Thyroid function disturbances
  Goitre
  Hypothyroidism
- Memory impairment
- Nephrotoxicity
- Cardiovascular changes
  T-wave flattening on the ECG
  Arrhythmias

Thyroid function tests are usually carried out routinely every 6 months in order to check for lithium-induced disturbances.

19.3.5   Carbamazepine

Since carbamazepine may lower the white blood count, regular monitoring of plasma carbamazepine levels should be carried out.

19.3.6   Tricyclic Antidepressants

The psychopharmacological basis of important side effects of tricyclic antidepressants is as follows:

- Blockade of ACh muscarinic receptors
- Blockade of histamine H_1 receptors
- Blockade of α_1-adrenoceptors
- Blockade of 5-HT$_{2/1c}$ serotonergic receptors
- Membrane stabilization

19.3.6.1   Blockade of Muscarinic Receptors

This leads to antimuscarinic side effects (see Chapter 18).

19.3.6.2   Blockade of Histamine H_1 Receptors

This can lead to

- Weight gain
- Drowsiness

19.3.6.3   Blockade of α_1-Adrenoceptors

This can lead to

- Drowsiness
- Postural hypotension
- Sexual dysfunction
- Cognitive impairment

19.3.6.4   Blockade of 5-HT$_{2/1c}$ Receptors

This can lead to

- Weight gain

19.3.6.5   Membrane Stabilization

Membrane stabilization can lead to

- Cardiotoxicity
- ↓ Seizure threshold

19.3.6.6 Cardiovascular Side Effects

These include

- ECG changes
- Arrhythmias
- Postural hypotension
- Tachycardia
- Syncope

19.3.6.7 Allergic and Haematological Reactions

These include

- Agranulocytosis
- Leukopenia
- Eosinophilia
- Thrombocytopenia
- Skin rash
- Photosensitization
- Facial oedema
- Allergic cholestatic jaundice

19.3.6.8 Endocrine Side Effects

These include

- Testicular enlargement
- Gynaecomastia
- Galactorrhoea

19.3.6.9 Others

Other side effects include

- Tremor
- Black tongue
- Paralytic ileus
- Sweating
- Hyponatraemia—particularly in the elderly
- Neuroleptic malignant syndrome—very rare with tricyclic antidepressants
- Abnormal liver function tests
- Movement disorders
- Pyrexia
- (Hypo)mania
- Blood glucose changes

19.3.7 SSRIs

Important side effects that may occur with SSRIs include

- Dose-related gastrointestinal side effects
  Nausea
  Vomiting
  Diarrhoea
- Headache

- Restlessness
- Sleep disturbance
- Anxiety
- Delayed orgasm

19.3.8 MAOIs

19.3.8.1 Dangerous Food Interactions

As mentioned Chapter 18, the inhibition of peripheral pressor amines, particularly dietary tyramine, by MAOIs can lead to a hypertensive crisis when foodstuffs rich in tyramine are eaten. Foods that should therefore be avoided when on treatment with MAOIs include

- Cheese—except cottage cheese and cream cheese
- Meat extracts and yeast extracts
- Alcohol—particularly chianti, fortified wines, and beer
- Non-fresh fish
- Non-fresh meat
- Non-fresh poultry
- Offal
- Avocado
- Banana skins
- Broad-bean pods
- Caviar
- Herring—pickled or smoked

19.3.8.2 Dangerous Drug Interactions

Medicines that should be avoided by patients taking MAOIs include

- Indirectly acting sympathomimetic amines, for example:
  Amphetamine
  Fenfluramine
  Ephedrine
  Phenylpropanolamine
- Cough mixtures containing sympathomimetics
- Nasal decongestants containing sympathomimetics
- L-dopa
- Pethidine
- Tricyclic antidepressants

19.3.8.3 Other Side Effects

Other side effects of MAOIs include

- Antimuscarinic actions.
- Hepatotoxicity.
- Appetite stimulation.
- Weight gain.
- Tranylcypromine may cause dependency.

19.3.9 Benzodiazepines

An important side effect of benzodiazepines is psychomotor impairment. If benzodiazepines are taken regularly for 4 weeks or more, dependence may develop, so that sudden cessation of intake may then lead to a withdrawal syndrome whose main features include

- Anxiety symptoms
  - Palpitations
  - Tremor
  - Panic
  - Dizziness
  - Nausea
  - Sweating
  - Other somatic symptoms
- Low mood
- Abnormal experiences
  - Depersonalization
  - Derealization
  - Hypersensitivity to sensations in all modalities
  - Distorted perception of space
  - Tinnitus
  - Formication
  - A strange taste
- Influenza-like symptoms
- Psychiatric/neurological symptoms
  - Epileptic seizures
  - Confusional states
  - Psychotic episodes
- Insomnia
- Loss of appetite
- Weight loss

19.3.10 Buspirone

The main side effects of buspirone are

- Dizziness
- Headache
- Excitement
- Nausea

19.3.11 Disulfiram

If alcohol is drunk while disulfiram is being taken regularly, acetaldehyde accumulates. Thus, ingesting even small amounts of alcohol then causes unpleasant systemic reactions, including

- Facial flushing
- Headache
- Palpitations
- Tachycardia
- Nausea
- Vomiting

Ingestion of large amounts of alcohol while being treated with disulfiram can lead to

- Air hunger
- Arrhythmias
- Severe hypotension

19.3.12 Cyproterone Acetate

Side effects of this antiandrogen agent in males include

- Inhibition of spermatogenesis
- Tiredness
- Gynaecomastia
- Weight gain
- Improvement of existing acne vulgaris
- ↑ Scalp hair growth
- Female pattern of pubic hair growth

Liver function tests should be carried out regularly owing to a theoretical risk to the liver. Dyspnea may result from high-dose treatment.

19.4 OFFICIAL GUIDANCE

The official guidance in Britain on the use of antipsychotic drugs and benzodiazepines is given in this section. The BNF is the abbreviation for the latest *British National Formulary*, a bi-annual publication of the British Medical Association and the Royal Pharmaceutical Society of Great Britain.

19.4.1 Antipsychotic Doses above the BNF Upper Limit

The Royal College of Psychiatrists has published advice on the use of antipsychotic doses above the BNF upper limit. This advice is reproduced in the BNF:

Unless otherwise stated, doses in the BNF are licensed doses—any higher dose is therefore *unlicensed*:

1. Consider alternative approaches including adjuvant therapy and newer or second-generation antipsychotics such as clozapine.
2. Bear in mind risk factors, including obesity; particular caution is indicated in older patients, especially those over 70.
3. Consider potential for drug interactions.

4. Carry out ECG to exclude untoward abnormalities such as prolonged QT interval; repeat ECG periodically and reduce dose if prolonged QT interval or other adverse abnormality develops.
5. Increase dose slowly and not more often than once weekly.
6. Carry out regular pulse, blood pressure, and temperature checks; ensure that patient maintains adequate fluid intake.
7. Consider high-dose therapy to be for limited period and review regularly; abandon if no improvement after 3 months (return to standard dosage).

In addition, the *British National Formulary* offers the following advice:

> *Important*: When prescribing an antipsychotic for administration on an emergency basis, the intramuscular dose should be *lower* than the corresponding oral dose (owing to absence of first-pass effect), particularly if the patient is very active (increased blood flow to muscle considerably increases the rate of absorption). The prescription should specify the dose for *each route* and should *not* imply that the same dose can be given by mouth or by intramuscular injection. The dose of antipsychotic for emergency use should be reviewed at least *daily*.

19.4.2 BENZODIAZEPINES

In Britain, the Committee on Safety of Medicines has issued the following advice with respect to the prescription of benzodiazepines:

1. Benzodiazepines are indicated for the short-term relief (2–4 weeks only) of anxiety that is severe, disabling or subjecting the individual to unacceptable distress, occurring alone or in association with insomnia or short-term psychosomatic, organic or psychotic illness.
2. The use of benzodiazepines to treat short-term 'mild' anxiety is inappropriate and unsuitable.
3. Benzodiazepines should be used to treat insomnia only when it is severe, disabling or subjecting the individual to extreme distress.

19.4.3 PREVENTION OF ADVERSE DRUG REACTIONS

The BNF gives the following advice for preventing adverse drug reactions:

1. Never use any drug unless there is a good indication. If the patient is pregnant do not use a drug unless the need for it is imperative.
2. It is very important to recognize allergy and idiosyncrasy as causes of adverse drug reactions. Ask if the patient had previous reactions.
3. Ask if the patient is already taking other drugs *including self-medication*; remember that interactions may occur.
4. Age and hepatic or renal disease may alter the metabolism or excretion of drugs, so that much smaller doses may need to be prescribed. Pharmacogenetic factors may also be responsible for variations in the rate of metabolism, notably of isoniazid and the tricyclic antidepressants.
5. Prescribe as few drugs as possible and give very clear instructions to the elderly or any patient likely to misunderstand complicated instructions.
6. When possible use a familiar drug. With a new drug be particularly alert for adverse reactions or unexpected events.
7. If serious adverse reactions are liable to occur warn the patient.

19.5 REPORTING

19.5.1 BRITAIN

In Britain, the CSM holds an information database for adverse drug reactions. Doctors practicing in Britain are asked to report adverse drug reactions to the Medicines and Healthcare products Regulatory Agency via the internet on the following web site: www.mca.gov.uk/yellowcard.

19.6 ADROIT

ADROIT (Adverse Drug Reactions On-line Information Tracking) is an online service used in Britain to monitor adverse drug reactions.

19.6.1 NEWER DRUGS

In the BNF, these are indicated by the symbol ∇. The BNF advises that doctors are asked to report all suspected reactions.

19.6.2 ESTABLISHED DRUGS

The BNF advises that doctors are asked to report all serious suspected reactions. These include those that are fatal, life threatening, disabling, incapacitating, or that result in or prolong hospitalization.

BIBLIOGRAPHY

British Medical Association and Royal Pharmaceutical Society of Great Britain. *British National Formulary.* London, U.K.: British Medical Association & Royal Pharmaceutical Society of Great Britain.

Cookson J, Taylor J, and Katona C. 2002: *Use of Drugs in Psychiatry: The Evidence from Psychopharmacology,* 5th edn. London, U.K.: Gaskell.

Edwards JG. 1995: Adverse reactions to and interactions with psychotropic drugs: Mechanisms, methods of assessment, and medicolegal considerations. In King DJ (ed.) *Seminars in Clinical Psychopharmacology,* pp. 480–513. London, U.K.: Gaskell Press.

Ettinger RH. 2011: *Psychopharmacology.* London, U.K.: Pearson.

Healy D (ed.). 2008: *Psychiatric Drugs Explained,* 5th edn. Edinburgh, Scotland: Churchill Livingstone.

Jones PB, Barnes TR, Davies L, Dunn G, Lloyd H, Hayhurst KP, Murray RM, Markwick A, and Lewis SW. 2006: Randomized controlled trial of the effect on Quality of Life of second- vs first-generation antipsychotic drugs in schizophrenia: Cost Utility of the Latest Antipsychotic Drugs in Schizophrenia Study (CUtLASS 1). *Archives of General Psychiatry* 63:1079–1087.

Kirsch I. 2009: *The Emperor's New Drugs: Exploding the Antidepressant Myth.* London, U.K.: The Bodley Head.

Kirsch I. 2009: Antidepressants and the placebo response. *Epidemiologia e Psichiatria Sociale* 18:318–322.

Lieberman JA, Stroup TS, McEvoy JP, Swartz MS, Rosenheck RA, Perkins DO, Keefe RS, Davis SM, Davis CE, Lebowitz BD, Severe J, Hsiao JK, and Clinical Antipsychotic Trials of Intervention Effectiveness (CATIE) Investigators. 2005: Effectiveness of antipsychotic drugs in patients with chronic schizophrenia. *New England Journal of Medicine* 353:1209–1223.

Moncrieff J. 2007: *The Myth of the Chemical Cure: A Critique of Psychiatric Drug Treatment.* Basingstoke, Hampshire, England: Palgrave Macmillan.

Puri BK. 2013: *Drugs in Psychiatry,* 2nd edn. Oxford, U.K.: Oxford University Press.

20 Genetics

20.1 DNA AND THE DOUBLE HELIX

A pair of complementary bases, for example, C with G, or A with T, is referred to as a base pair. The human genome is made up of approximately 3.2×10^9 base pairs organized into 23 pairs of chromosomes. Somatic cells have 44 autosomes and 2 sex chromosomes for the diploid count of 46. Gametes such as sperms and ova have the haploid count of 23 chromosomes. Somatic cells are divided by mitosis where chromosomes are duplicated during the prophase of the cell cycle. Gametes are formed by meiosis. The first meiotic division involves duplication of chromosomal material, while the second meiosis produces four gametes without chromosomal duplication.

Genes are made up of DNA that consists of two anti-parallel strands held together in a double helix by hydrogen bonds between complementary nitrogenous bases. Adenine (A) always pairs with thymine (T). Guanine (G) always pairs with cytosine (C). Approximately 30% of human genes are involved in the development and function of the central nervous system (CNS).

20.2 CHROMOSOMES

20.2.1 NUMBER

In normal humans, the genome is distributed on 46 chromosomes in each somatic cell nucleus:

- One pair of sex chromosomes (normal females: XX, normal males: XY)
- 44 autosomes = 22 pairs of chromosomes

20.2.2 KARYOTYPE

This is an arrangement of the chromosomal makeup of somatic cells that can be produced by carrying out the following procedures in turn: arrest cell division at an appropriate stage, disperse the chromosomes, fix the chromosomes, stain the chromosomes, photograph the chromosomes, identify the chromosomes, and arrange the chromosomes.

20.2.3 CENTROMERE

This is the constricted region of each chromosome that is particularly evident during mitosis and meiosis. The centromere plays a major role in chromosome assortment during cell division as it attaches itself to the spindle apparatus (Figure 20.1).

20.2.4 TELOMERE

Telomere confers stability to chromosomes by protecting ends and allowing the chromosome ends to be copied properly during replication.

Each chromatid has telomere capping at the ends with centromere in the centre.

20.2.5 METACENTRIC CHROMOSOMES

These are chromosomes with a centrally or almost centrally positioned centromere.

20.2.6 ACROCENTRIC CHROMOSOMES

These are chromosomes in which the centromere is very near to one end.

20.2.7 CHROMOSOMAL MAP

The system agreed at the International Paris Conference in 1971 is as follows:

First position—a number (1–22) or letter (X or Y) that identifies the chromosome

Second position—p (short arm of chromosome) or q (long arm of chromosome)

Third position (region)—a digit corresponding to a stretch of the chromosome lying between two relatively distinct morphological landmarks

Fourth position (band)—a digit corresponding to a band derived from the staining properties of the chromosome (Table 20.1)

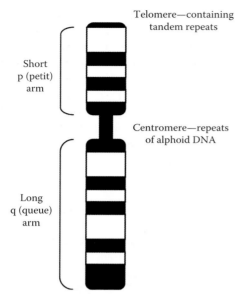

Short
p (petit)
arm

Telomere—containing
tandem repeats

Centromere—repeats
of alphoid DNA

Long
q (queue)
arm

FIGURE 20.1   Structure of chromosome.

20.3   AUTOSOMAL ABNORMALITIES

20.3.1   DOWN'S SYNDROME

The causes of Down's syndrome are

1. Approximately 95% of cases result from trisomy 21 (47, +21) following nondisjunction during meiosis.
2. Approximately 4% result from translocation involving chromosome 21; exchange of chromosomal substance may occur between chromosome 21 and
   a. Chromosome 13
   b. Chromosome 14
   c. Chromosome 15
   d. Chromosome 21
   e. Chromosome 22
3. The remaining cases are mosaics.

Note that almost all subjects with Down's syndrome who live beyond the age of 40 years show evidence of Alzheimer's disease.

TABLE 20.1

Relationship between Chromosome Number and Psychiatric Disorders

Chromosome	Gene and Psychiatric Disorder	Chromosome	Gene and Psychiatric Disorder
Chromosome 1	DISC-1: schizophrenia and bipolar disorder DISC-2: schizophrenia Presenilin 2: Alzheimer's disease	Chromosome 14	Presenilin 1: Alzheimer's disease
Chromosome 2	2q: autistic spectrum disorder	Chromosome 15	Angelman's syndrome (maternal microdeletion) Prader–Willi syndrome (paternal microdeletion)
Chromosome 4	Alcohol dehydrogenase gene Huntington's disease (CAG trinucleotide repeat) 4p: Wolf–Hirschhorn disease	Chromosome 17	Neurofibromatosis Familial frontotemporal dementia Smith–Magenis syndrome
Chromosome 5	5p: cri-du-chat syndrome	Chromosome 18	Edward's syndrome (trisomy)
Chromosome 6	6p: dysbindin gene and schizophrenia	Chromosome 19	APOE gene: Alzheimer's disease CADASIL gene: Notch 3
Chromosome 7	7q: autism Williams syndrome (microdeletion)	Chromosome 20	PrP in inherited CJD
Chromosome 8	8p: neuregulin and schizophrenia	Chromosome 21	Amyloid precursor protein gene: Alzheimer's disease Down's Syndrome (trisomy)
Chromosome 11	11p: brain-derived neurotrophic factor gene and bipolar affective disorder	Chromosome 22	DiGeorge Syndrome (velocardiofacial syndrome) COMT gene: schizophrenia and bipolar disorder
Chromosome 13	Patau's syndrome (trisomy) Wilson's disease	X or Y chromosome	Fragile X syndrome Lesch–Nyhan syndrome Klinefelter's syndrome XXY Turners (XO) syndrome

20.3.2 EDWARD'S SYNDROME

This is caused by trisomy 18 (47, +18).

20.3.3 PATAU'S SYNDROME

This is caused by trisomy 13 (47, +13).

20.3.4 CRI-DU-CHAT SYNDROME

This partial aneusomy results from the partial deletion of the short arm of chromosome 5. Its characteristic kitten-like high-pitched cry has been localized to 5p15.3. Its other clinical features have been localized to 5p15.2, known as the cri-du-chat critical region or CDCCR.

20.4 SEX CHROMOSOME ABNORMALITIES

20.4.1 KLINEFELTER'S SYNDROME

In this syndrome, phenotypic males possess more than one X chromosome per somatic cell nucleus. Genotypes include

- 47,XXY (i.e. one extra X chromosome per somatic cell nucleus); this is the most common genotype in Klinefelter's syndrome
- 48,XXXY
- 49,XXXXY
- 48,XXYY

20.4.2 XYY SYNDROME

In this syndrome, phenotypic males have the genotype 47,XYY.

20.4.3 TRIPLE-X SYNDROME

In this syndrome, phenotypic males have the genotype 47,XYY.

20.4.4 TETRA-X SYNDROME

In this syndrome, also known as super-female syndrome, phenotypic females have the genotype 48,XXXX.

20.4.5 TURNER SYNDROME

In this syndrome, phenotypic females have the genotype 45,X (=45,XO).

20.4.6 ALZHEIMER'S DISEASE

The gene for amyloid precursor protein (APP) is located on the long arm of human chromosome 21 and is a member of a gene family that includes the amyloid precursor–like proteins (APLP) 1 and 2. This may explain the link between Alzheimer's disease and Down's syndrome (see preceding text). The apolipoprotein E e4 allele is common in Alzheimer's disease, while the e2 allele is less common than would be expected by chance. It may be that the e4 allele is associated with increased accumulation of β-amyloid protein, while the reverse is true for the e2 allele.

20.5 CELL DIVISION

20.5.1 MITOSIS

This is the process of nuclear division allowing many somatic cells to undergo cell division via the following stages: interphase, prophase, metaphase, anaphase, and telophase.

20.5.2 MEIOSIS

This process involves two stages of cell division and occurs in gametogenesis via the following stages: interphase, prophase I, metaphase I, anaphase I, telophase I, prophase II, metaphase II, anaphase II, and telophase II.

Chromosomal division takes place once during meiosis, so that the resulting gametes are haploid. Recombination takes place during prophase I.

20.6 GENE STRUCTURE

Genes, the biological units of heredity, consist of codons grouped into exons with intervening nucleotide sequences known as introns. The introns do not code for amino acids. Genes also contain nucleotide sequences at their beginning and end that allow transcription to take place accurately. Thus, starting from the 5′ end (upstream), a typical eukaryotic gene contains the following:

- Upstream site–regulating transcription
- Promoter (TATA)
- Transcription initiation site
- 5′ Noncoding region
- Exons: gene contains regions that are expressed
- Introns: intervening sequences that are not expressed in the final protein and spliced out of mature mRNAs
- 3′ Noncoding region, containing a poly A addition site

20.7   DNA REPLICATION

Replication proceeds in the 5′–3′ direction with new nucleotides being added to the 3′ end. One strand, known as the leading strand, is formed continuously, moving into the direction of the fork (see Figure 20.2). The other strand, called the lagging strand (aka Okazaki fragments), is formed in 100–1000 nucleotide blocks. The process is described as semi-discontinuous because of the different ways in which the two DNA strands are synthesized.

At the end of DNA synthesis, there will be two chromatids for each chromosome. Each chromatid comprises one original parental strand and one newly synthesized complementary strand. This pattern of replication whereby one parental strand is retained in each daughter cell is known as semiconservative.

20.7.1   TRANSCRIPTION

Chromatin exists in two forms, euchromatin and heterochromatin. Euchromatin is loosely packed, whereas heterochromatin is tightly condensed. Euchromatin is transcriptionally active and heterochromatin is generally not transcriptionally active.

Transcription is the step in gene expression in which information from the DNA molecule is transcribed on to a primary RNA transcript.

Transcription is initiated in the upstream locus control region (LCR). The transcription factors with specific structural domains such as zinc fingers bind to the LCR. This process allows previously concealed strands of DNA to be unfolded and prepared for transcription (see Figure 20.3).

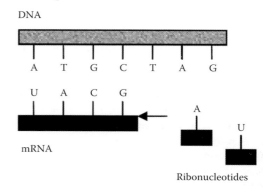

FIGURE 20.3   Transcription.

This is followed by splicing and nuclear transport, so that the information (minus that from introns) then exists in the cytoplasm of the cell on messenger RNA (mRNA). The splicing out of the introns is guided by recognition of the GT and AG dinucleotides that mark the beginning and the end of the intron. A mutation at these two sites is called a splice-site mutation and leads to serious effects on the protein structure and function. For example, clinical features of Fragile X syndrome are due to failure of FMR1 gene transcription due to hypermethylation resulting in the absence of the FMR1 gene protein.

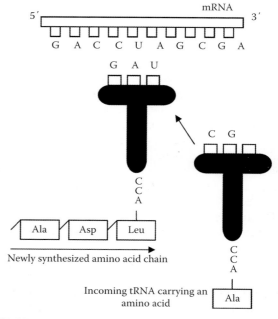

FIGURE 20.4   Translation.

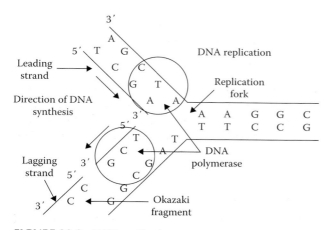

FIGURE 20.2   DNA replication process.

20.7.2 Translation

Following transcription, splicing, and nuclear transport, translation is the process in gene expression whereby mRNA acts as a template allowing the genetic code to be deciphered to allow the formation of a peptide chain. This process involves tRNA molecules.

Each tRNA contains a set of three nucleotides, referred to as an anticodon, which is complementary to a set of three bases in the mRNA known as a codon (see Figure 20.4). A codon consists of three bases that code for a specific amino acid. With four bases, there are $4 \times 4 \times 4 = 64$ possible codons. As there are only 20 amino acids, several different codons may specify the same amino acid. The translation is regulated by signal sequences known as the 'stop transfer' and the 'start transfer' sequences. The amino acid residues then form the newly synthesized polypeptide chain.

20.8 POSTTRANSLATIONAL MODIFICATION

The newly synthesized polypeptide chains can be modified by the addition of chemical groups. This process is known as posttranslational modification. Other examples include the formation of disulfide bonds, the cleavage of transport polypeptides, hydroxylation, and phosphorylation. Phosphorylation is an important event in signal transduction and plays a key role in psychiatry (e.g. aripiprazole increases the level of glycogen synthase kinase 3-beta phosphorylation and offers more neuroprotective effects than haloperidol in schizophrenia) (Sham et al., 2007).

20.9 MUTATIONS

A mutation is a change in DNA sequence that can be transmitted from the parent cell to its daughter cells. There are two types of mutations: germline mutation refers to mutation that originates from a gamete that is subsequently fused with another gamete during fertilization, leading to the conception of an individual who has the mutation in every cell. A somatic mutation occurs after fertilization and is only present in a subpopulation of somatic cells.

Deletion involves loss while insertion involves gain of genetic material. Small deletions and insertions are caused by slippage or mispairing between complementary strands due to close homology of adjacent sequences. Large deletions and insertions account for 5% of known pathogenic mutations. Most large deletions and insertions are caused by unequal crossing-over between homologous sequences.

TABLE 20.2
Classification of Mutations

Mutations	Loss-of-Function Mutations	Gain-of-Function Mutations
Impact	Reduced activity or quantity of the gene product	Presence of an abnormal gene product with toxic effects on the cell
Mode of inheritance	Usually recessive (autosomal or X-linked) inheritance. Loss-of-function mutations may not have harmful effects in the heterozygous state, as 50% of normal enzyme activity is usually sufficient for normal function	Often dominant (autosomal or X-linked) inheritance
Diseases	Inborn errors of metabolism	Huntington's disease

Substitution mutations resulting in silent, missense, or nonsense mutations can be transition (purine to purine or pyrimidine to pyrimidine) or transversion (purine to pyrimidine or pyrimidine to purine) mutations. A silent mutation does not alter the amino acid residue encoded. A missense mutation results in the change of amino acid residue encoded, while a nonsense mutation results in the creation of a stop codon, resulting in the premature termination of the protein. Most mutations have the effect of a loss of function. If the number of nucleotides deleted or inserted in an exon involves multiples of three, then the sequence of codons or the reading frame is preserved. If it does not, the reading frame will be disrupted, resulting in a frameshift mutation with a truncated protein product (Table 20.2).

20.10 TECHNIQUES IN MOLECULAR GENETICS

20.10.1 Restriction Enzymes

Restriction enzymes, also known as restriction endonucleases, cleave DNA only at locations containing specific nucleotide sequences. Different restriction enzymes target different nucleotide sequences, but a given restriction enzyme targets the same sequence.

20.10.2 Gene Library

This is a set of cloned DNA fragments representing all the genes of an organism or of a given chromosome.

20.10.3   Molecular Cloning

This technique can be used to create a gene library. It can be carried out by splicing a given stretch of (human) DNA, cleaved using a restriction enzyme, into a bacterial plasmid having at least one antibiotic resistance gene. After reintroduction of the resulting recombinant plasmid into bacteria, antibiotic selective pressure causes these bacteria to reproduce. Multiple recoverable copies of the original (human) DNA are contained in the resulting bacterial colonies.

20.10.4   Gene Probes

These are lengths of DNA that are constructed so that they have a nucleotide sequence complementary, or almost complementary, to that of a given part of the genome, with which, therefore, they can hybridize under suitable conditions.

20.10.5   Oligonucleotide Probes

These are small gene probes that can be used to detect single-base mutations.

20.11   POLYMERASE CHAIN REACTION

Polymerase chain reaction (PCR) is the most versatile technique for cloning or making copies of DNA. PCR starts with a mixture in a buffer solution comprising of (1) template (e.g. DNA to be copied); (2) Taq polymerase (an enzyme needed for DNA synthesis); (3) the four deoxyribonucleotide triphosphates; and (4) DNA primers = short sequence comprising of 15–20 nucleotides that hybridizes to the target sequence to be replicated but not to itself or copies of itself, for example, GATCCAG.

The process of PCR involves three steps as outlined in Table 20.3. Each three-step cycle is repeated 30–35 times (after 35 cycles more unwanted by-products are produced than useful DNA). PCR requires very small amounts of DNA and can detect small mutations (<1 kb). It can be completed in less than 1–2 h. Flanking DNA sequence must be known in order to design the primers.

TABLE 20.3

Steps Involved in Copying DNA

Step	Description	Temperature (°C)
1. Denaturation	DNA strands are separated	93
2. Annealing	Primers attach to the separate DNA strands	40–55
3. Extension	Nucleotides are added to make new strands: the polymerase reaction	72

Source: Lewis, G.H. et al., *Mastering Public Health: A Postgraduate Guide to Examinations and Revalidation*, London, U.K.: Hodder Arnold, 2008.

20.12   SEPARATING AND VISUALIZING DIFFERENT DNA SEQUENCES

Once DNA has been replicated, for example, by PCR, it can be sequenced to identify the order of nucleotides (A, C, G, or T); see Figure 20.5.

The most common method of sequencing uses chain termination. A primer, containing DNA with tagged or terminator nucleotides, is added to denatured DNA strands. The primer bases bind to the relevant bases on the DNA to form base pairs. However, every time a terminator sequence binds, it will block further synthesis and the strand will not be further extended, thereby creating many different lengths of sequences, all ending with the same base pair (see Figure 20.6).

20.13   RESTRICTION FRAGMENT LENGTH POLYMORPHISM

Restriction enzyme is a nuclease that recognizes a specific nucleotide sequence of 4–12 bases and cleaves the DNA within or adjacent to that sequence. A polymorphism can be defined based on whether the DNA is cleaved by a restriction enzyme. Restriction fragment length polymorphism (RFLP) can be used as DNA markers and are usually inherited in a simple

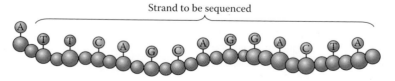

FIGURE 20.5   Strand to be sequenced. (From Lewis, G.H. et al., *Mastering Public Health: A Postgraduate Guide to Examinations and Revalidation*, CRC press, Oxford, U.K., 2008, p. 197.)

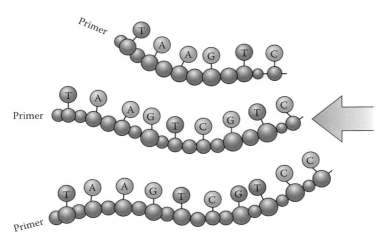

FIGURE 20.6   DNA sequences of varying lengths. (From Lewis, G.H. et al., *Mastering Public Health: A Postgraduate Guide to Examinations and Revalidation*, CRC press, Oxford, U.K., 2008, p. 197.)

Allele 1	GAATTC...	GACTTC.....	GAATTC......
Fragment cut by restriction enzymes	X ⟵	⟶ X	
Allele 2	GAATTC...	GAATTC.....	GAATTC......
Fragment cut by restriction enzymes		X ⟵	⟶ X

FIGURE 20.7   Polymorphism and restriction enzyme.

Mendelian fashion. If a nucleotide substitution changes the recognition site for a restriction enzyme, one allele will be intact (e.g. AC in allele 1) and restricted (e.g. AA in allele 2), as shown in Figure 20.7. After PCR, the reaction products can be digested with restriction enzyme, and the genotype will be determined after electrophoresis.

Polymorphisms of the serotonin transporter gene have been reported to be associated with obsessive–compulsive disorder, suicidal behaviour, autism, and intense fear. Polymorphisms of the tryptophan hydroxylase gene have been associated with suicidal behaviour, bipolar disorder, early smoking initiation, and alcohol abuse.

20.14   GEL ELECTROPHORESIS

During gel electrophoresis, DNA fragments of different sizes move at different speeds under an electric field (larger fragments migrate more slowly towards a positive electric charge). Fragments carrying different genotypes can then be identified according to their final position on the gel. The same process can also be used with RNA and protein fragments.

20.14.1   SOUTHERN BLOTTING

This is a technique that allows the transfer of DNA fragments from gel, where electrophoresis and DNA denaturation have taken place, to a nylon or nitrocellular filter. It involves overlaying the gel with the filter and in turn overlaying the filter with paper towels. A solution is then blotted through the gel to the paper towels. Autoradiography can then be used to identify the fragments of interest on the filter. The technique is named after its inventor, Edwin Southern (Figure 20.8).

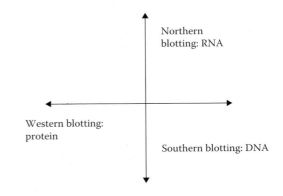

FIGURE 20.8   Classification of blotting.

20.15　GENOME-WIDE STUDIES USING MICROARRAY TECHNOLOGY

Microarrays or gene chips are based on sequence-specific hybridization. In brief, different DNA sequences of interest are applied onto glass slides. Fluorescent-labelled DNA probes from the test sample will bind to the complementary target sequences on the slides that are then scanned to quantify fluorescent signals corresponding to the specific DNA sequences. The time for analysis of gene expression or polymorphic markers is short as several thousand hybridizations can be analysed simultaneously under the same conditions.

20.15.1　RECOMBINATION

As mentioned earlier, recombination takes place during prophase I of meiosis. There is alignment and contact of homologous chromosome pairs during prophase I, allowing genetic information to cross over between adjacent chromatids. This process of crossover or recombination causes a change in the alleles carried by the chromatids at the end of the first meiotic division.

The unit to measure genetic distance or recombination frequency is centimorgan. Recombination, the random assortment of chromosomes during meiosis, and DNA mutations are the three essential processes that establish the genetic makeup of an individual.

The further apart two loci are, the more there will be recombination between the two loci and the less likely the two will be transmitted together (see Figure 20.9).

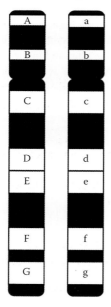

FIGURE 20.9　Probability of recombination depends upon distance.

The closer the two loci, the less there will be recombination between the two loci and the more likely the two will be transmitted together. The probability of a recombination is very low for loci D and E. It is very high for loci A and G.

Recombination rate can be used as an estimate of the distance between two points on a chromosome and this forms the theoretical basis of *linkage analysis*. The *recombination fraction* is the number of recombinants divided by the total number of offspring and it is proportional to the physical distance between two loci over short distances only. The recombination fraction is a measure of how often the alleles at two loci are separated during meiotic recombination. Its value can vary from 0 to 0.5.

20.15.2　MAXIMUM LIKELIHOOD SCORE

This is the value of the recombinant fraction that gives the highest value for the LOD score. It represents the best estimate that can be made for the recombinant fraction from the given available data.

20.16　LINKAGE ANALYSIS

20.16.1　GENETIC MARKERS

A DNA polymorphism, such as a RFLP, if linked to a given disease locus, can be used as a genetic marker in linkage analysis without its precise chromosomal location being known. Genetic markers can also be used in presymptomatic diagnosis and prenatal diagnosis.

20.16.2　LINKAGE

This is the phenomenon whereby two genes close to each other on the same chromosome are likely to be inherited together.

20.16.3　LINKAGE PHASES

For two alleles occurring at two linked loci in a double heterozygote, the following linkage phases can occur:

- Coupling: the two alleles are on the same chromosome
- Repulsion: the two alleles are on opposite chromosomes of a pair

20.16.4　LINKAGE ANALYSIS

Linkage analysis is based on the principle of co-segregation of a trait (disorder) with marker gene(s) within families. The genes tend to segregate (i.e. passed on) together from parent to offspring because the gene causing the disorder and the marker allele are physically linked to each other on the same chromosome.

Linkage analysis is based on three principles:

1. Affected members of a pedigree will have the same mutation on the marker allele.
2. Unaffected offspring within a family will tend to have the same genotype(s) on the marker.
3. Hence, affected individuals will have different genotypes from unaffected individuals for the marker.

Figure 20.10 shows the linkage of disease-causing gene (disease D) and allele of marker (colour blindness) on X chromosome. If a marker is close to a disease-causing gene, alleles of the marker will tend to co-segregate with the disorder in families or be shared between affected relatives.

The strength of linkage is expressed as logarithm of the odds (LOD) score. The LOD score for a given recombinant fraction is the logarithm to base 10 of the odds $P_1:P_2$, where P_1 is the probability of there being linkage for a given recombinant fraction and P_2 is the probability of there being no measurable linkage. Thus the LOD score gives a measure of the probability of two loci being linked. The LOD score method was devised by Morton. A cumulative LOD score exceeding 3 is regarded as strong evidence for linkage while a cumulative LOD

TABLE 20.4
Summary of Findings in Linkage Studies of Major Psychiatric Disorders

Disorders	Findings
Schizophrenia	A genome scan meta-analysis produced significant genome-wide evidence for linkage on chromosome 2q
Depressive disorder	No consistent findings
Anxiety disorders	Chromosomes 7p and 1
	Chromosomes 13 and 15q
Alcohol dependence	A1 alleles of the dopamine D2 receptor

TABLE 20.5
Compare and Contrast Linkage and Association Studies

Linkage Studies	Association Studies
To study the association between a disease and a genetic	To study the association between a specific allele and a disease
Use families	Use cases and controls or families with unaffected controls
Detectable over large distances > 10 cM	Detectable only over small distances, 1 cM
Can usually only detect large effects RR > 2 because it is systematic	Capable of detecting small effects OR < 2 but prone to false positives

score below −2 is regarded as strong evidence against linkage (Tables 20.4 through 20.6).

20.17 QUANTITATIVE GENETICS

Quantitative genetics in psychiatry is concerned with

1. The mode of inheritance
2. Genetic factors as an aetiology of a psychiatric illness
3. Relative contribution of genetic and environmental factors

20.18 BASIC CONCEPTS OF QUANTITATIVE GENETICS

20.18.1 PATTERN OF INHERITANCE

In this section, R and S are dominant alleles, and r and s the corresponding recessive alleles.

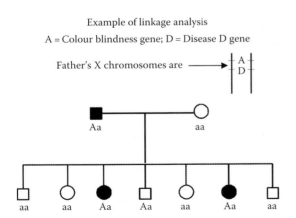

Example of linkage analysis
A = Colour blindness gene; D = Disease D gene

Offspring with marker A will have disease D.
As the genes are on the X chromosome, disease D and colour blindness only occur in female offspring but not male offspring.

FIGURE 20.10 Linkage of disease D gene and colour blindness gene.

TABLE 20.6

Summary of Findings in Association Studies of Major Psychiatric Disorders

Disorders	Findings
Schizophrenia (Crocq et al., 1992; Williams et al., 1996)	Dopamine D3 receptor gene and 5-HT2A receptor gene
	Catechol-*o*-methyl transferase (COMT) gene
	Recently discovered candidate genes, dysbindin, neuregulin, G27/D-amino acid oxidase
	Velocardiofacial syndrome on chromosome 22q
Depressive disorder	With inconsistent results
Bipolar disorder (Lange and Farmer, 2007)	Genes encoding for the tyrosine hydroxylase, serotonin transporter, and COMT
	Anticipation (the phenomenon whereby a disease has an earlier age of onset and increased severity in succeeding generations) has been described in bipolar disorder
Posttraumatic stress disorders (Lee et al., 2005)	Serotonin transporter promoter gene
Alzheimer's disease	Amyloid precursor gene on chromosome 21
	Presenilin 1 gene on chromosome 14
	Presenilin 2 gene on chromosome 14
	Apolipoprotein E (APOE) gene on chromosome 19
Autism	Chromosome 7q
Hyperkinetic disorder (Gill et al., 1997; Smalley et al., 1998)	Dopamine D4 receptor gene
	Allele of the dopamine transporter gene

20.18.1.1 Law of Uniformity

Consider two homozygous parents with genotypes RR and rr, respectively. Mating (X) results in the next (F1) generation having the genotype shown:

Parents: RR x rr
F1: Rr

20.18.1.2 Mendel's First Law

This is also known as the law of segregation:

Parents: Rr × Rr
F1: RR: Rr: rr = 1:2:1

20.18.1.3 Mendel's Second Law

This is also known as the law of independent assortment:

Parents: RRSS × rrss
F1: RrSs
F2: independent assortment of different alleles Æ
RRSS, RRSs, …, rrss

20.19 AUTOSOMAL DOMINANT INHERITANCE

Autosomal dominant disorders result from the presence of an abnormal dominant allele causing the individual to manifest the abnormal phenotypic trait. Features of autosomal dominant transmission include the following:

- The phenotypic trait is present in all individuals carrying the dominant allele.
- The phenotypic trait does not skip generations—vertical transmission takes place.
- Males and females are affected.
- Male to male transmission can take place.
- Transmission is not solely dependent on parental consanguineous matings.
- If one parent is homozygous for the abnormal dominant allele, all the members of F1 will manifest the abnormal phenotypic trait.

Variable expressivity can cause clinical features of autosomal dominant disorders to vary between affected individuals. This, together with reduced penetrance, may give the appearance that the disorder has skipped a generation. The sudden appearance of an autosomal dominant disorder may occur as a result of a new dominant mutation.

20.20 AUTOSOMAL DOMINANT DISORDERS

20.20.1 HUNTINGTON'S DISEASE

Huntington's disease (chorea) is a progressive, inherited neurodegenerative disease that is characterized by autosomal dominant transmission and the emergence of abnormal involuntary movements and cognitive deterioration, with progression to dementia and death over 10–20 years. The huntingtin gene responsible is located on the short arm of chromosome 4; this genetic mutation consists of an increased number of cytosine–adenine–guanine (CAG) repeats. (The normal number of such repeats at this locus is between 11 and about 34.) The age of onset is strongly determined by the number of repeat units, but once symptoms develop, the rate of progression is relatively uninfluenced by CAG repeat length.

20.20.2 PHACOMATOSES

The phacomatoses (or phakomatoses), which exhibit neurocutaneous signs, include

- Tuberous sclerosis
- Neurofibromatosis
- Von Hippel–Lindau syndrome
- Sturge–Weber syndrome

There are three main forms of tuberous sclerosis:

- TSC1 (tuberous sclerosis type 1), caused by a gene on chromosome 9
- TSC2 (tuberous sclerosis type 2), caused by a gene on chromosome 16
- TSC3 (tuberous sclerosis type 3), caused by a translocation that involves chromosome 12

Neurofibromatosis is caused by an abnormality in the NF-1 gene (in the region 17q11.2).

20.20.3   EARLY-ONSET ALZHEIMER'S DISEASE

A minority of cases of Alzheimer's disease are inherited as an early-onset autosomal dominant disorder. The mutations concerned tend to be found on chromosome 14 or chromosome 21.

20.20.4   OTHER AUTOSOMAL DOMINANT DISORDERS

Other disorders that can be inherited in an autosomal dominant manner include

- Acrocephalosyndactyly type I
- Acrocallosal syndrome
- Acrodysostosis
- De Barsy syndrome
- Early-onset familial Parkinson's disease
- Periodic paralyses
- Velocardiofacial syndrome
- Von Hippel–Lindau syndrome
- Treacher Collins' syndrome

20.21   AUTOSOMAL RECESSIVE INHERITANCE

Autosomal recessive disorders result from the presence of two abnormal recessive alleles causing the individual to manifest the abnormal phenotypic trait. Features of autosomal recessive transmission include the following:

- Heterozygous individuals are generally carriers who do not manifest the abnormal phenotypic trait.
- The rarer the disorder, the more likely it is that the parents are consanguineous.
- The disorder tends to miss generations but the affected individuals in a family tend to be found among siblings—horizontal transmission takes place.

- Where both parents carry one abnormal copy of the gene, there is a 25% chance of a child inheriting both mutations, hence expressing the disease.
- In addition, there is a 50% chance of the child inheriting one of the mutations and be a genetic carrier for the disease. When both parents are affected, all the children will be affected.

Examples of autosomal recessive disorder include

1. Protein metabolism: phenylketonuria
2. Fat metabolism: Niemann–Pick disease, Tay–Sachs disease, and Smith–Lemli–Opitz syndrome
3. Mucopolysaccharidoses: Hurler's syndrome
4. Obesity and learning disability: Laurence–Moon–Biedl syndrome
5. Ataxia and learning disability: ataxia-telangiectasia and Marinesco–Sjögren syndrome
6. Short stature and learning disability: Virchow–Seckel dwarf

20.22   X-LINKED RECESSIVE INHERITANCE

In X-linked recessive disorders, a recessive abnormal allele is carried on the X chromosome. All male (XY) offspring inheriting this allele manifest the abnormal phenotypic trait. In contrast, a single recessive mutation for a gene on the X chromosome in women is compensated for by the normal allele on the other X chromosome so that the disease does not occur. Other features of X-linked recessive transmission include the following:

- Male to male transmission does not take place.
- Female heterozygotes are carriers. A heterozygous 'carrier' woman passes the allele to half of her sons (who will express the disease), who express it and half of her daughters (who do not).
- Males are far more likely to be affected with X-linked recessive disorders, and females are more likely to be carriers. Hence, the incidence of disease is very much higher in males than females.

20.23   AUTOSOMAL RECESSIVE DISORDERS

20.23.1   DISORDERS OF PROTEIN METABOLISM

There are many disorders of protein metabolism that can be inherited in an autosomal recessive manner. They include the following:

- Phenylketonuria (incidence 1 in 12,000). A reduction in phenylalanine hydroxylase causes an increase in circulating phenylalanine. The Guthrie test is used to screen for this disorder.

- Hartnup disorder or disease (incidence 1 in 14,000). This is a renal-transport amino aciduria in which there is reduced absorption of neutral amino acids (including tryptophan) from the alimentary canal and renal tubules, causing reduced biosynthesis of nicotinic acid.
- Histidinaemia (incidence 1 in 18,000). This is a reduction in histidase causing an increased level of histidine in the blood and urine.
- Homocystinuria (incidence 1 in 50,000). This is a reduction in cystathionine β-synthase causing an increased level of homocysteine in the blood and urine.
- Maple-syrup urine disorder (incidence 1 in 120,000). This is a reduction in oxoacid decarboxylase causing the presence of branched-chain amino acids (valine, leucine, and isoleucine) in the blood and urine.
- Carbamoyl phosphate synthetase deficiency (or hyperammonaemia) (incidence <1 in 100,000). This is a urea cycle disorder in which hyperammonaemia occurs.
- Argininosuccinate synthetase deficiency (or citrullinaemia) (incidence <1 in 100,000). This is a urea cycle disorder in which there is increased citrulline in the blood and urine.
- Argininosuccinate lyase deficiency (or argininosuccinic aciduria) (incidence <1 in 100,000). This is a urea cycle disorder in which there is increased argininosuccinic acid in the blood and urine.
- Arginase deficiency (or argininaemia) (incidence <1 in 100,000). This is a urea cycle disorder in which there is increased arginine in the blood.
- Cystathioninuria (incidence of about 1 in 200,000). A reduction in g-cystathionase causes increased cystathionine in the blood and urine.

Further disorders are

- Cystinuria
- Hydroxyprolinaemia
- Hyperlysinaemia
- Nonketotic hyperglycinaemia
- Ornithinaemia
- Stimmler syndrome
- Type II tyrosinaemia
- Oasthouse urine syndrome

20.23.2   DISORDERS OF CARBOHYDRATE METABOLISM AND LYSOSOMAL STORAGE

These disorders can be inherited in an autosomal recessive manner. They include the following:

- Gaucher's disease (incidence of type I Gaucher's disease is between 1 in 600 and 1 in 2400 in Ashkenazi Jewish populations). This is a reduction in lysosomal cerebroside β-glucosidase causing an abnormal accumulation of glucosylceramide.
- Tay–Sachs disease (incidence 1 in 4000 in Ashkenazi Jewish populations). This is a G_{M2} gangliosidosis in which a reduction in lysosomal hexosaminidase A causes an abnormal accumulation of G_{M2} ganglioside.
- Sanfilippo syndrome (or MPS type III) (incidence 1 in 24,000). This is a mucopolysaccharidosis. Types A, B, C, and D are recognized.
- Hurler's syndrome (or MPS type I) (incidence about 1 in 100,000). This is a mucopolysaccharidosis. A reduction in lysosomal α-L-iduronidase causes abnormal accumulation of dermatan sulphate and heparin sulphate.
- Metachromatic leukodystrophy (incidence about 1 in 100,000). This is a sulfatidosis (sulphatidosis).
- Sandhoff disease (incidence about 1 in 300,000). This is a G_{M2} gangliosidosis in which there is an abnormal accumulation of G_{M2} gangliosides and oligosaccharides.
- Niemann–Pick disease (types I and II; both are rare). Type I is caused by a reduction in lysosomal sphingomyelinase causing abnormal accumulation of sphingomyelin.
- G_{M1} gangliosidoses (types I, II, and III; all are rare). Type I is the infantile type, type II is the juvenile type, and type III is the adult type. In all three types, there is a reduction in lysosomal β-galactosidase causing an abnormal accumulation of G_{M1} ganglioside.

Further disorders are

- Fucosidosis
- Galactosaemia
- Hereditary fructose intolerance
- Krabbe disease
- Mannosidosis
- Pompe disease
- Von Gierke disease

20.23.3 OTHER DISORDERS

There are many other disorders inherited in an autosomal recessive manner. Many are rare or very rare. They include

- Alexander disease
- Cerebelloparenchymal disorders
- Coat disease
- Cockayne syndrome
- Cohen syndrome
- Friedreich's ataxia
- Macrocephaly
- Oculocerebral syndrome
- Oculorenocerebellar syndrome
- Refsum disease
- Rubinstein syndrome
- Turcot syndrome
- Wilson disease (hepatolenticular degeneration)

20.24 X-LINKED DOMINANT INHERITANCE

In X-linked dominant disorders, a dominant abnormal allele is carried on the X chromosome. If an affected male mates with an unaffected female, all the daughters and none of the sons are affected. If an unaffected male mates with an affected heterozygous female, half the daughters and half the sons, on average, are affected. Again, male to male transmission does not take place.

20.24.1 X-LINKED DOMINANT DISORDERS

Disorders that can be inherited in an X-linked dominant manner include

- Ornithine transcarbamylase (incidence of about 1 in 500,000)—a urea cycle disorder in which hyperammonaemia occurs
- Aicardi syndrome (learning disability, agenesis of corpus callosum, and early death in males)
- Coffin–Lowry syndrome
- Rett syndrome

20.24.2 X-LINKED RECESSIVE DISORDERS

Disorders that can be inherited in an X-linked recessive manner include the following:

- Hunter's syndrome (MPS type II) (incidence about 1 in 100,000)—a mucopolysaccharidosis in which there is a reduction in lysosomal iduronate 2-sulphatase.

- Lesch–Nyhan syndrome (incidence about 1 in 100,000)—a reduction in hypoxanthine–guanine phosphoribosyltransferase causes increased synthesis of urate and hyperuricaemia.
- Cerebellar ataxia.
- Fragile X syndrome.
- Lowe syndrome.
- Testicular feminization syndrome.
- X-linked spastic paraplegia.
- W syndrome.

20.25 OTHER CONCEPTS OF INHERITANCE

20.25.1 ANTICIPATION

This refers to the occurrence of an autonomic dominant disorder at earlier ages of onset or with greater severity in the succeeding generations. In Huntington's disease, it has been shown to be caused by expansions of unstable triplet repeat sequences.

20.25.2 MOSAICISM

Abnormalities in mitosis can give rise to an abnormal cell line. Such mosaicism may affect somatic cells (somatic mosaicism) or germ cells (gonadal mosaicism).

20.25.3 UNIPARENTAL DISOMY

This refers to the phenomenon in which an individual inherits both homologues of a chromosome pair from the same parent.

20.25.4 GENOMIC IMPRINTING

This refers to the phenomenon in which an allele is differentially expressed depending on whether it is maternally or paternally derived.

20.25.5 MITOCHONDRIAL INHERITANCE

Since mtDNA (mitochondrial DNA) is essentially maternally inherited, mitochondrial inheritance may explain some cases of disorders that affect both males and females but that are transmitted through females only and not through males.

20.26 FAMILY STUDIES

Family studies investigate the degree of familial clustering of a disorder by comparing the frequency of a disorder in the relatives of affected index cases (i.e. probands) with the frequency in a representative sample drawn from a general population. First-degree relatives share 50% of their genes. Second-degree relatives have, on average, 25% of the genome in common with the proband. Depending on the prevalence of disorders, there are several recruitment strategies: for relatively uncommon disorders such as schizophrenia, probands are usually ascertained from a tertiary or specialist centre such as patients admitted to a university hospital or attending a specialist clinic. For relatively common disorders such as depression or anxiety, patients can be recruited from GP clinics or counselling centres.

There are two types of ascertainment bias: cohort effects and volunteer bias. Cohort effects refer to the changes in the characteristics of a disorder over time, which may be relevant if probands have a wide age range (e.g. the clinical features of first episode schizophrenia of a 20-year-old consist of more positive symptoms compared to chronic schizophrenia of a 50-year-old). Volunteer bias occur in studies where probands with less severe disorders (e.g. for studies of Alzheimer's disease, mild cases of dementia) are more likely to give consent and be recruited for the study.

20.26.1 DIFFICULTIES

Difficulties (and possible solutions) with family studies applied to psychiatric disorders include

- Psychiatric disorders need to be considered longitudinally. Lifetime expectancy rates or morbid risks can be used.

- At the time of the study, some relatives may not have reached an age range during which the disorder manifests itself. Weinberg's age-correction method can be used.
- Genetic factors are not separated well from environmental factors. Twin and adoption studies can be used.

20.27 MORBID RISK

The morbid risk (MR) (aka lifetime incidence) is used to express the rates of illness in relatives. It is calculated from the number of affected relatives divided by the total number of relatives. As not all relatives would have gone through the period of risk (e.g. schizophrenia symptoms may not manifest in a 5-year-old cousin), adjustment has to be made for the effect of age of onset. One major limitation of family studies is that it does not distinguish between genetic and shared environmental effects (Table 20.7).

20.28 TWIN STUDIES

The main purpose of twin studies is to identify the relative contribution of genetic and environmental factors to the aetiology.

TABLE 20.7
Summary of Morbid Risks of Major Psychiatric Disorders

Disorders	MR in First-Degree Relatives	MR in General Population	Other Information
Schizophrenia (Hutchinson et al., 1996)	3.5% (Caucasians) to 24.6% (second generation of Afro-Caribbean)	0.5%	Age of onset: Males = 21 years Female = 28 years
Depressive disorder (McGuffin and Katz, 1989)	9.1%	3%	Age of onset = 27 years
Bipolar disorder (Vallès et al., 2000)	5%	0.3%	Unipolar depression in first-degree relatives: 11.5% Age of onset = 21 years
Anxiety disorders (Noyes et al., 1978)	18%	3%	Age of onset = 11 years
Obsessive–compulsive disorder (Paul, 2008)	10%	1.9%	Age of onset = 20 years
Eating disorder	6%–10%	1%–2%	• Family studies support familiar transmission • Age of onset = 10–16.
Alzheimer's disease	15%–19% Three times the risk of general population	5%	Most cases are sporadic cases without family history
Autism (Rutter et al., 1990)	3%	0.06%	Autism is associated with fragile X syndrome
Attention deficit and hyperkinetic disorder	Two times of the general population	—	—

Twin studies are based on a number of assumptions:

1. Monozygotic (MZ) twins are genetically identical because they are developed from the same fertilized ovum.
2. MZ and dizygotic (DZ) twin pairs are assumed to share environmental risk factors for the disorder to the same degree.
3. The null hypothesis assumes that the risk of the disorder is the same in MZ and DZ twins.
4. The null hypothesis assumes that the risk of the disorder is the same in twins and singletons.

20.28.1 METHODOLOGY

The rates of illness in co-twins of MZ and DZ probands are compared. MZ twins share 100% of the genome, whereas DZ twins share, on average, 50% of their genome. The rate of concurrence of a disorder in the co-twin of a proband is the concordance rate:

1. Probandwise rate (as a percentage) =

$$\frac{\text{(number of co-twins of probands in whom the disorder is concurrent)}}{\text{(total number of co-twins)}} \times 100\%$$

Twin pairs are most usefully counted probandwise, that is, if both members of an affected twin pair are ascertained independently, they are counted as two pairs. This approach allows comparison between the MR of the general population to develop the disorder and the rate of the disorder in co-twins of the probands, which is a prerequisite for model fitting and calculating heritability.

2. Pairwise rate (as a percentage) =

$$\frac{\text{(number of concordant pairs of twins)}}{\text{(total number of twin pairs)}} \times 100\%$$

The alternative approach is to count pairwise, where each pair is counted once. However, this rate cannot be directly compared with the population MR.

The resemblance for the disorder in twin pairs is initially expressed as the probandwise concordance rate. Probandwise concordance is more commonly used than pairwise concordance. A higher concordance rate in MZ compared to DZ pairs suggests a genetic contribution to the disorder. In Table 20.8, bipolar disorder and

TABLE 20.8

Twin Concordance Values for Major Psychiatric Disorders

Disorders	MZ Concordance (%)	DZ Concordance (%)
Schizophrenia	46	14
Bipolar disorder	40	5
Depressive disorder	67	20
Generalized anxiety disorder	34	17
Panic disorder	42	17
OCD	87	47
Alcohol dependence	63	44
Anorexia nervosa	22	10
Alzheimer disease	31	9
Autism	96	27

schizophrenia have higher concordance rate in MZ than DZ pairs, which signify the importance of genetic contribution in aetiology compared to other disorders.

Twin data can be interpreted in the framework of a liability-threshold model to estimate heritability. Each person has an underlying liability that is determined by both genetic and environmental factors and the frequency of distribution of liability follows normal distribution. The liability distribution is set to have mean = 0 and variance = 1. Individuals below a particular threshold on this liability distribution are unaffected, while those above the threshold are affected. In Figure 20.11, the area under the curve above the threshold of schizophrenics' relatives is larger than general population.

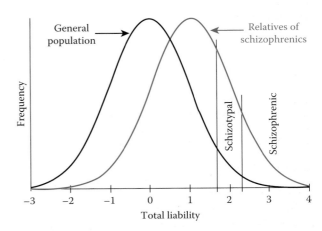

FIGURE 20.11   Liability threshold model for transmission of schizophrenia.

20.28.2 DIFFICULTIES

Difficulties (and possible solutions) with twin studies applied to psychiatric disorders include the following:

- Pairwise and probandwise concordance rates usually give different results. Take note of the method used to determine the concordance rate.
- Zygosity was determined less accurately in older twin studies. (Use modern, more accurate methods.)
- Diagnostic variability occurred in older twin studies. (Use more detailed modern diagnostic criteria.)
- Sampling bias may occur. (Use twin registers.)
- Twins are at greater risk of central nervous system abnormalities resulting from birth injury or congenital abnormalities (risk to MZ twins > risk to DZ twins), which may introduce errors if central nervous system abnormalities contribute to the disorder being studied.
- Assortative mating may lead to a relative increase in the rate of illness in DZ twins compared with MZ twins.
- Age-correction techniques may introduce errors, so do not use them.
- The environment does not necessarily affect twins equally. Use adoption studies.

20.29 ADOPTION STUDIES

20.29.1 METHODOLOGY

Individuals are studied who have been brought up by unrelated adoptive parents from an early age, instead of by their biological parents. Types of adoption studies include the following:

- Adoptee studies:
  It compares the adopted children of affected and unaffected biological parents. An improved version of this design incorporates the affection status of the adoptive parents. If the affection status of the biological parents is related to MR in the adoptee, after adjusting for the affection status of the adoptive parents, then genetic factors are implicated.
- Adoptee family studies:
  It compares MR in the biological and adoptive families of affected adoptees. An improved version of this design includes the biological

and adoptive families of unaffected adoptees. A greater MR among biological than among adoptive family members of affected but not unaffected adoptees would implicate genetic factors.
- Cross-fostering studies:
  The risk of the disorder is compared in adoptees who have affected biological parents but unaffected adopting parents and in adoptees with unaffected biological parents but affected adopting parents.
- Adoption studies involving monozygotic twins (Table 20.9).

20.29.2 DIFFICULTIES

Difficulties with adoption studies applied to psychiatric disorders include the following:

- Few cases fulfil the criteria for adoption studies.
- Adoption studies take a long time to carry out.
- Information about the biological father may not be available.

TABLE 20.9

Summary of Findings in Adoption Studies of Major Psychiatric Disorders

Disorders	Findings
Schizophrenia (Kety et al., 1994)	In family adoption studies, the rate of schizophrenia spectrum disorders is 13% among the biological relatives of affected adoptees, 3% among biological relatives of control adoptees, 1% among the adoptive relatives of affected adoptees, and 3% among the adoptive relatives of control adoptees
Depressive disorder (Wender et al., 1986)	Eightfold increase in the rate for affective disorder among the relatives of index adoptees with affective disorder and 15-fold increases in suicide rates
Alcohol dependence	Increased risk of alcohol misuse and dependence in the adopted-away sons of alcohol-dependent biological parents than in the adopted-away sons of non-alcohol-dependent biological parents
Hyperkinetic disorder (Van den Oord et al., 1994)	Adoption studies show that the biological parents of children with the attention deficit hyperactivity disorder are more likely to have the same or a related disorder than are the adoptive parents

- Adoption may cause indeterminate psychological sequelae for the adoptees.
- The process of adoption is unlikely to be random.
- In MZ twin studies, it cannot be assumed that the environmental influences on each twin are more or less equivalent following adoption.

ACKNOWLEDGMENTS

The authors of this book would like to acknowledge Professor Pak Sham, BA (Cantab), BM BCh (Oxon), MSc (Lond), PhD (Cantab), MRCPsych, Chair Professor in Psychiatric Genomics and Department Head, Department of Psychiatry, Queen Mary Hospital; the University of Hong Kong; and Dr. Ene-Choo Tan, PhD, Research Scientist in Genetics, KK Women's and Children's Hospital, Singapore, for their contribution to this chapter.

BIBLIOGRAPHY

Bertelsen A, Harvald B, and Hauge M. 1977: A Danish twin study of manic-depressive disorders. *British Journal of Psychiatry* 130:330–351.

Carey G and Gottesman I. 1981: Twin and family studies of anxiety, phobic and obsessive disorders. In Klein DF and Rabkin J (eds.) *Anxiety: New Research and Changing Concepts*, pp. 117–136. New York: Raven Press.

Crocq MA, Mant R, Asherson P et al. 1992: Association between schizophrenia and homozygosity at the Dopamine D₂ receptor gene. *Journal of Medical Genetics* 29:858–860.

Gill M, Daly G, Heron S et al. 1997: Confirmation of association between attention deficit hyperactivity disorder and a dopamine transporter polymorphism. *Molecular Psychiatry* 2:311–313.

Heath AC, Bucholz KK, Madden PA et al. 1997: Genetic and environmental contributions to alcohol dependence risk in a national twin sample: Consistency of findings in women and men. *Psychological Medicine* 27:1381–1396.

Hutchinson G, Takei N, Fahy TA, Bhugra D, Gilvarry C, Moran P, Mallett R, Sham P, Leff J, and Murray RM. 1996: Morbid risk of schizophrenia in first-degree relatives of white and African–Caribbean patients with psychosis. *The British Journal of Psychiatry* 169:776–780.

International l Molecular Generic Study of Autism Consortium. 1998: A full genome scan for autism with evidence for linkage to a region on chromosome 7q. *Human Molecular Genetics* 7:571–578.

Kendler KS, Neale MC, Hearh AC et al. 1994: A twin-family study of alcoholism in women. *American Journal of Psychiatry* 151:707–715.

Kessler RC, Berglund P, Demler O et al. 2005: Lifetime prevalence and age-of-onset distributions of DSM-IV disorders in the National Comorbidity Survey Replication. *Archives of General Psychiatry* 62:593–602.

Kety SS, Wender PH, Jacobsen B et al. 1994: Mental illness in the biological and adoptive relatives of schizophrenic adoptees. Replication of the Copenhagen Study in the rest of Denmark. *Archives of General Psychiatry* 51:442–455.

Lange K and Farmer A. 2007: The causes of depression. In Stein G and Wilkinson G (eds.) *Seminars in General Adult Psychiatry*, 2nd edn., pp. 48–70. London, U.K.: Gaskell.

Lee HJ, Lee MS, Kang RH et al. 2005: Influence of the serotonin transporter promoter gene polymorphism on susceptibility to posttraumatic stress disorder. *Depression and Anxiety* 21:135–139.

Lewis CM, Levinson DF, Wise LH et al. 2003: Genome scan meta-analysis of schizophrenia and bipolar disorder. Part II. Schizophrenia. *American Journal of Human Genetics* 73:34–48.

Lewis GH, Sheringham J, Kalim K et al. 2008: *Mastering Public Health: A Postgraduate Guide to Examinations and Revalidation*. Oxford, U.K.: CRC Press.

Maier W. 2003: Genetics of anxiety. In Kasper S, den Boer JA, and Ad Sitsen JM (eds.) *Handbook of Depression and Anxiety*, 2nd edn., revised and expanded, pp. 189–205. New York: Marcel Dekker.

McGuffin P and Katz R. 1989: The genetics of depression and manic-depressive disorder. *British Journal of Psychiatry* 155:294–304.

McGuffin P, Owen MJ, O'Donovan MC, Thapar A, and Gottesman II. 1994: *Seminars in Psychiatric Genetics*. London, U.K.: Gaskell.

Noyes R Jr, Clancy J, Crowe R et al. 1978: The familial prevalence of anxiety neurosis. *Archives of General Psychiatry* 35:1057–1074.

Ogilvie AD, Battersby S, Bubb VJ et al. 1996: Polymorphism in serotonin transporter gene associated with susceptibility to major depression. *Lancet* 347:731–733.

Paris Conference. 1971: (Supplement 1975) Standardization in human cytogenetics. *Cytogenetics and Cell Genetics* 15(4):203–238.

Pauls DL. 2008: The genetics of obsessive compulsive disorder: A review of the evidence. *American Journal of Medical Genetics* 148:133–139.

Pauls DL, Alsobrook JP, Goodman W et al. 1995: A family study of obsessive compulsive disorder. *American Journal of Psychiatry* 152:76–84.

Puri BK and Tyrer PJ. 2004: *Sciences Basic to Psychiatry*, 3rd edn. Edinburgh, U.K.: Churchill Livingstone.

Rasmussen SA and Eisen JL. 1990: The epidemiology of obsessive compulsive disorder. *Journal of Clinical Psychiatry* 51(suppl.):10–13.

Rutter ML, MacDonald H, LeCouteur A et al. 1990: Genetic factors in child psychiatric disorder. II Empirical findings. *Journal of Child Psychology and Psychiatry* 31:39–83.

Sadock BJ and Sadock VA. 2003: *Kaplan & Sadock's Synopsis of Psychiatry*. Philadelphia, PA: Lippincott Williams & Wilkins.

Sham P, Woodruff P, Hunter M, and Leff J. 2007: The aetiology of schizophrenia. In Stein G and Wilkinson G (eds.) *Seminars in General Adult Psychiatry*, 2nd edn., pp. 202–237. London, U.K.: Gaskell.

Smalley SL, Bailey JG, Cantwell DP et al. 1998: Evidence that the dopamine D4 receptor is a susceptibility gene in attention deficit hyperactivity disorder. *Molecular Psychiatry* 3:427–430.

Vallès V, Van Os J, Guillamat R, Gutiérrez B, Campillo M, Gento P, and Fañanás L. 2000: Increased morbid risk for schizophrenia in families of in-patients with bipolar illness. *Schizophrenia Research* 42:83–90.

Van den Oord EJ, Boomsma DL, and Verhulst FC 1994: A study of problem behaviors in 10–15 year old biologically related and unrelated international adoptees. *Behavior Genetics* 24:193–205.

Wender PH, Kety SS, Rosenthal D et al. 1986: Psychiatric disorders in the biological and adoptive families of adopted individuals with affective disorders. *Archives of General Psychiatry* 43:923–929.

Williams J, Spurlock G, McGuffin P et al. 1996: Association between schizophrenia and T102C polymorphism of the 5-hydroxytryptamine type 2a-receptor gene. European Multicentre Association Study of Schizophrenia (EMASS) Group. *Lancet* 347:1294–1296.

Young ID. 2005: *Medical Genetics*. Oxford, U.K.: Oxford University Press.

21 Psychiatric Epidemiology*

21.1 DISEASE FREQUENCY

21.1.1 INCIDENCE

The incidence of a disease is the rate of occurrence of new cases of the disease in a defined population over a given period of time. It is equal to the number of new cases over the given period of time divided by the total population at risk (see the succeeding text) during the same period of time.

21.1.1.1 Units

The unit of incidence is T^{-1}, that is, $(time)^{-1}$. For instance, Dunham (1965) gave the incidence of schizophrenia as

$$= 0.00022 \text{ year}^{-1}$$

$$= 0.00022 \text{ per year}$$

$$= 0.22 \text{ per } 1,000 \text{ per year}$$

$$= 22 \text{ per } 100,000 \text{ per year, etc.}$$

(see Table 21.1.)

21.1.2 PREVALENCE

The prevalence of a disease is the proportion of a defined population that has the disease at a given time:

- *Point prevalence.* This is the proportion of a defined population that has a given disease at a given point in time.
- *Period prevalence.* This is the proportion of a defined population that has a given disease during a given interval of time.
- *Lifetime prevalence.* This is the proportion of a defined population that has or has had a given disease (at any time during each individual's lifetime thus far) at a given point in time.
- *Birth defect rate.* This is the proportion of live births that has a given disease.
- *Disease rate at postmortem.* This is the proportion of bodies, on which postmortems are carried out that has a given disease.

21.1.2.1 Units

Prevalence, being a proportion or ratio of two numbers, does not have units. A given prevalence value may, however, be multiplied by 100 to express it as a percentage. For example, according to Jablensky and Sartorius (1975), the annual prevalence of schizophrenia is

$$= 0.002 - 0.004$$

$$= 2 - 4 \text{ per } 1000$$

$$= 0.2\% - 0.4\%$$

(Note that the annual prevalence is a type of period prevalence.)

21.1.3 POPULATION AT RISK

This is the population of individuals free of a given disease, who have not already had the disease by the time of the commencement of a given period of time, who are at risk of becoming new cases of the disease.

21.1.4 CHRONICITY

The chronicity of a disease is its average duration. It has the units of time.

21.1.5 STEADY-STATE RELATIONSHIP BETWEEN POINT PREVALENCE AND INCIDENCE

In the steady state, in which the incidence of a disease is constant over a given time period and the time between caseness onset and ending is constant, the following relationship holds:

$$P = ID$$

where
  P is the point prevalence
  I is the incidence
  D is chronicity

---

* This chapter may usefully be read in conjunction with Chapter 6, which deals with the principles of evaluation and psychometrics. In addition to topics that are epidemiological in nature, this chapter also includes a few related subjects that are of value in the analysis of trial data.

TABLE 21.1

Measures of Incidence

Concept	Alternative Name	Definition
Incidence	Incidence rate	Number of new events during a specified time period
Cumulative incidence	Risk	Proportion of a population who develops the disease of interest in a defined time period

Note: Incidence (unlike prevalence) is not affected by disease survival. The denominator should include those who are 'at risk'.

21.2 CASE IDENTIFICATION, CASE REGISTERS, AND MORTALITY AND MORBIDITY STATISTICS

21.2.1 CASE IDENTIFICATION

21.2.1.1 Caseness

An overall threshold is ideally defined in order to establish caseness, that is, to differentiate cases of a given psychiatric disorder from noncases. Classification systems and screening can be used to help identify cases.

21.2.1.2 Classification

Classification systems that are useful in case identification are those that provide specific operational diagnostic criteria as guides for making each psychiatric diagnosis. A widely used example in psychiatry is that of DSM-5.

21.2.1.3 Screening

Screening, by means of psychiatric assessment instruments, can be used to identify cases. The instruments used should have good sensitivity and specificity:

$$\text{Sensitivity} = \frac{\text{True} +\text{ve}}{(\text{True} +\text{ve}) + (\text{False} -\text{ve})}$$

$$\text{Specificity} = \frac{\text{True} -\text{ve}}{(\text{True} -\text{ve}) + (\text{False} +\text{ve})}$$

In terms of the generalized diagnostic and test results shown in Table 21.2, the sensitivity and specificity are given by

$$\text{Sensitivity} = \frac{a}{a + c}$$

$$\text{Specificity} = \frac{d}{b + d}$$

TABLE 21.2

Generalized Diagnostic and Test Results

Test Result	True Diagnosis Positive	Negative
Positive	a	b
Negative	c	d

Source: Puri, B.K., Epidemiology, In: Puri, B.K. and Tyrer, P.J., *Sciences Basic to Psychiatry*, 2nd edn., Churchill Livingstone, Edinburgh, U.K., 1998.

The predictive value of a positive test result (or positive predictive value) is the proportion of the positive results that is truly positive, while the predictive value of a negative test result (negative predictive value) is the proportion of the negative results that is truly negative. The efficiency of the test is the proportion of all the results that is true. In terms of the notation of Table 21.2, these are given by the following expressions:

$$\text{Positive predictive value} = \frac{a}{a + b}$$

$$\text{Negative predictive value} = \frac{d}{c + d}$$

$$\text{Efficiency} = \frac{a + d}{a + b + c + d}.$$

The sensitivity, specificity, predictive values, and efficiency of a test are often expressed in terms of percentages, simply by multiplying the earlier formulae by 100.

Three further measures (which may also be expressed as percentages by multiplication by 100) that may be derived from Table 21.2 are

$$\text{Screen prevalence} = \frac{a + b}{a + b + c + d}$$

$$\text{Disease prevalence} = \frac{a + c}{a + b + c + d}$$

$$\text{Test accuracy} = \frac{a + d}{a + b + c + d}.$$

21.2.1.4 Likelihood Ratio

This is a function of both the sensitivity and the specificity of a test and indexes how much the test result will change the odds of having a disease/disorder:

- The likelihood ratio for a *positive* result, LR+, is given by

$$LR+ = \frac{\text{Sensitivity}}{1 - \text{Specificity}}$$

- It indexes the increase in the odds of having a disease when the test result is positive.
- The likelihood ratio for a *negative* result, LR−, is given by

$$LR- = \frac{1 - \text{Sensitivity}}{\text{Specificity}}$$

- It indexes the decrease in the odds of having a disease when the test result is negative.

21.2.1.5 Pretest Odds

The pretest odds are a function of the prevalence of the disease and may be calculated as follows:

$$\text{Pretest odds} = \frac{\text{Prevalence}}{1 - \text{Prevalence}}$$

(Prevalence, in this context, is also sometimes known as the pretest probability.)

21.2.1.6 Posttest Odds

The posttest odds of a disease are the odds that a patient has a disease and incorporate information relating to

- Disease prevalence
- The patient pool
- The likelihood ratio
- Pretest odds (i.e. risk factors for the patient)

The posttest odds are calculated as follows:

$$\text{Posttest odds} = (\text{Pretest odds}) \times (\text{Likelihood ratio})$$

21.2.2 CASE REGISTERS

Examples of case registers that have proved useful in epidemiological studies and psychiatric research generally include

- Swedish and Danish twin registers
- Psychiatric case registers, containing records of those who have been treated for psychiatric disorders in certain hospitals or catchment areas

Limitations of case registers include

- The registered individuals may move out of the defined geographic area.
- The registers may not be kept up to date for other reasons.

21.2.2.1 Mortality Statistics

21.2.2.1.1 Mortality Rate

This is the number of deaths in a defined population during a given period of time divided by the population size during that time period. This measure is also sometimes referred to as the 'crude mortality ratio' or CMR. It may be expressed as a percentage by multiplying the ratio by 100:

- Standardized mortality rate. This is the mortality rate adjusted to compensate for a confounder.
- Age-standardized mortality rate. This is the mortality rate adjusted to compensate for the confounding effect of age.
- Standardized mortality ratio (SMR). The SMR is the ratio of the observed standardized mortality rate, derived from the population being studied, to the expected standardized mortality rate, derived from a comparable standard population. It may be expressed as a percentage by multiplying the ratio by 100 (Table 21.3).

21.2.2.2 Life Expectancy

This is a measure of the mean length of time that an individual can be expected to live based on the assumption that the mortality rates used remain constant. It is calculated from the ratio of the total time a hypothetical group of people is expected to live to the size of that group.

TABLE 21.3

Summary of Mortality Indices

Index (Commonly Expressed per 1,000 or per 100,000)	Typical Reference Period	Numerator	Denominator
Crude mortality rate (10.2/1000 in the United Kingdom)	1 Year	Number of deaths	Midyear population
Age-specific mortality rate Proportionate mortality as % of total deaths of respective age group	1 Year	Number of deaths aged X X = specific age	Midyear population aged X X = specific age
Case fatality rate	Within a specified time period	Mortality due to a condition	The population of people with that condition
Child mortality rate (0.2/1000 in the United Kingdom)	1 Year	Number of deaths in children aged 1–4 years	Midyear number of children aged 1–4 years
Infant mortality rate (4.9/1000 in the United Kingdom)	1 Year	Number of deaths under 1-year-old	Number of live births
Postnatal mortality rate	1 Year	Number of deaths in infants aged 4–52 weeks	Number of live births
Neonatal mortality rate (3.4/1000 in the United Kingdom)	1 Year	Number of deaths in the first 28 days	Number of live births
Stillbirth (in England and Wales, there are 3000 stillbirths per year; the stillbirth rate in England and Wales = 5/1000)	Born after 24 weeks	Number of fetus born after the 24th week of pregnancy who does not show any signs of life	Number of live births
Perinatal mortality rate (8.4/1000 in the United Kingdom)	1 Year	Number of stillbirths + deaths <7 days	Number of live births + stillbirths

21.2.2.2.1　Morbidity Rate

This is the rate of occurrence of new nonfatal cases of a given disease in a defined population at risk during a given period of time:

- *Standardized morbidity rate.* This is the morbidity rate adjusted to compensate for a confounder.
- *Age-standardized morbidity rate.* This is the morbidity rate adjusted to compensate for the confounding effect of age.
- *Standardized morbidity ratio.* The standardized morbidity ratio is the ratio of the observed standardized morbidity rate, derived from the population being studied, to the expected standardized morbidity rate, derived from a comparable standard population. It may be expressed as a percentage by multiplying the ratio by 100.

21.3　MEASUREMENTS OF RISK

The terms described in this section can usefully be related to the 2 × 2 contingency table shown in Table 21.4, as used in analytical epidemiological studies. Similarly, they also

TABLE 21.4

Generalized 2 × 2 Contingency Table Used in Analytical Epidemiological Studies

Exposure to Risk Factor	Outcome		Total
	Disease	No Disease	
Positive	a	b	a + b
Negative	c	d	c + d
Total	a + c	b + d	a + b + c + d

Source: Puri, B.K., Epidemiology, In: Puri, B.K. and Tyrer, P.J., *Sciences Basic to Psychiatry*, 2nd edn, Edinburgh, U.K., Churchill Livingstone, 1998.

apply to the critical appraisal of, for example, prospective cohort studies, such as the one shown in Table 21.5.

21.3.1　RELATIVE RISK

In terms of analytical epidemiological studies, the relative risk of a disease with respect to a given risk factor is

---

TABLE 21.5

Generalized Prospective Cohort Study Results

Group	Outcome Positive	Negative	Total
Cohort	a	b	$a + b$
Control	c	d	$c + d$
Total	$a + c$	$b + d$	$a + b + c + d$

---

the ratio of the incidence of the disease in people exposed to that risk factor to the incidence of the disease in people not exposed to that same risk factor. In Table 21.4, this equates to the ratio of $a/(a + b)$ to $c/(c + d)$.

In terms of prospective cohort studies, the relative risk is the ratio of the probability of a positive outcome in the cohort group (exposed) to the probability of a positive outcome in the control group (not exposed). In Table 21.5, this again equates to the ratio of $a/(a + b)$ to $c/(c + d)$.

Thus, in terms of both Tables 21.4 and 21.5,

$$\text{Relative risk} = \frac{a(c + d)}{c(a + b)}$$

The relative risk does not have any units, being the ratio of two numbers, and it can take on any nonnegative real value; that is, relative risk ≥ 0.

21.3.2 Attributable Risk

This is the incidence of the disease in the group exposed to the risk factor of interest minus the incidence in the group not exposed to this risk factor. The attributable risk is also known as the 'risk difference' or the 'absolute excess risk'. In terms of Table 21.4,

$$= \text{Attributable risk}$$

$$= \text{Risk difference}$$

$$= \text{Absolute excess risk}$$

$$= \text{Absolute risk increase}$$

$$= \frac{a}{(a + b)} - \frac{c}{(c + d)}$$

21.3.3 Relative Risk Increase

This is the absolute risk increase as a proportion of the risk in the unexposed group and is given by

$$\text{Relative risk increase} = \frac{a/(a + b) - c/(c + d)}{c/(c + d)}$$

21.3.4 Absolute Risk Reduction

This is another measure of the difference in the risk between the two groups being studied but this time indexing the risk reduction following exposure to the index factor. In the notation of the tables of this section, it is given by

$$\text{Absolute risk reduction} = \frac{c}{(c + d)} - \frac{a}{(a + b)}$$

21.3.5 Relative Risk Reduction

This is the absolute risk reduction as a proportion of the risk in the unexposed group and is given by

$$\text{Relative risk reduction} = \frac{c/(c + d) - a/(a + b)}{c/(c + d)}$$

21.3.6 Number Needed to Treat

The number needed to treat (NNT) expresses the benefit of an active treatment over a placebo. It can be used in summarizing the results of a trial and in individualized medical decision-making. It takes the value of the nearest integer (or whole number) equal to or higher than the following expression:

$$\frac{1}{c/(c + d) - a/(a + b)}$$

21.3.7 Odds Ratio

If Table 21.5 is taken to refer to a retrospective study, in which the variable consists of exposure or nonexposure to a given factor, while the outcome consists of being in the disease group or the control group, the odds that

TABLE 21.6

Generalized Retrospective (Case–Control) Study Results

Outcome	Variable		Total
	Exposure	No Exposure	
Disease group	a	b	$a + b$
Control	c	d	$c + d$
Total	$a + c$	$b + d$	$a + b + c + d$

subjects in the disease group were exposed to the factor are given by a/b. Similarly, the odds that subjects in the control group were exposed to the factor are given by c/d.

These results follow from the following definition:

$$\text{Odds of an event taking place } = \frac{\text{Probability of that event}}{1 - \text{Probability of that event}}$$

The odds ratio is the ratio of the odds that subjects in the disease group were exposed to the factor to the odds that subjects in the control group were exposed to the factor. In terms of Table 21.6, we have

$$\text{Odds ratio} = \frac{ad}{bc}$$

In the case of retrospective epidemiological studies (see Table 21.4), if the disease is relatively rare, we have

$$a \ll b \Leftrightarrow a+b \approx b$$

and

$$c \ll d \Leftrightarrow c+d \approx d$$

Hence, in this case,

$$\text{Relative risk} \approx \frac{ad}{bc} = \text{odds ratio}$$

21.4 STUDY DESIGN

21.4.1 HIERARCHY OF RESEARCH METHODS

Beginning with the type of research method generally considered to have the lowest credibility and in increasing order of generally accepted strength of evidence, the types of research studies that are most often used are as follows:

- Case reports
- Case series
- Cross-sectional studies
- Retrospective studies
- Prospective studies/trials
- Randomized double-blind placebo-controlled clinical trials
- Meta-analyses (or other systematic reviews) of randomized double-blind placebo-controlled clinical trials

This hierarchical order should not necessarily be taken as being set in stone. For example, case reports involving the first use of an innovative treatment can be of great value.

21.4.2 CONFOUNDING

One of the most important confounding factors in studies is age, particularly, for example, in the calculation of morbidity and mortality rates in epidemiological studies. There are various methods that may be used to compensate for confounding variables. These include

- Standardization (e.g. age can be compensated for by means of age standardization)
- Stratification
- Randomization
- Matching (in terms of the confounder[s]) of controls with patients/subjects/index cases
- Restriction (to restrict entry into the study of subjects who are not affected by the confounder[s])
- Mathematical and statistical modelling techniques

Summary of epidemiological findings in common psychiatric disorders (Table 21.7 through 21.18).

TABLE 21.7
Epidemiology of Schizophrenia and Schizoaffective Disorder

	Schizophrenia	Schizoaffective Disorder
Incidence	Approximately 15/100,000 per annum in most industrialized countries (Johnstone et al., 2004)	Incidence is not known but less common than schizophrenia
Prevalence and lifetime risk	*Adults in general population* 1-Year prevalence: 1% Lifetime prevalence: 1.4% *Lifetime risk of first-degree relatives:* 5%–16% In the United Kingdom, the risk of the siblings of Afro-Caribbean probands to develop schizophrenia is 16%. In contrast, the risk of the siblings of Caucasian to develop schizophrenia is 2% (Sugarman and Craufrud, 1994)	Prevalence is less than 1%, possibly in the range of 0.5%–0.8% in the United States (Sadock and Sadock, 2003)
Geographic pattern	Worldwide incidence is fairly similar	No specific geographic pattern
Person	*Gender*: • M = F • The mortality rate in men with schizophrenia is twice of women • Men are associated with more structural brain abnormalities • Women show a bimodal peak of incidence in their late 20s and 50s *Age*: • Onset is usually in late adolescence and young adulthood. • Mean onset age for men is between 15 and 25 years and for women is between 25 and 35 years (Semple et al., 2005) *Socioeconomic (SE) status*: • The association between schizophrenia and low social class is now seen as a consequence rather than an aetiology of schizophrenia • There is social drift in people with schizophrenia as a result of the illness, and unemployment rate can be as high as 70% • Low birth weight and urban birth are risk factors for schizophrenia • Patients in developing countries tend to have more acute onset and better outcome than patients in developed countries *Ethnicity*: • There is an increase in frequency of schizophrenia among Afro-Caribbean in the United Kingdom as a result of environmental factors (Sugarman and Craufrud, 1994) *Life events*: • Symptoms may start to appear after stressful life events • Misuse of cannabis plays a role in people who are homozygous for val/val in COMT gene *Disease*: • There is a negative association between rheumatoid arthritis and schizophrenia	*Gender*: Women > men; age of onset is later for women than men. Male patients may exhibit antisocial behaviour *Age*: The depressive type of schizoaffective disorder may be more common in older than in younger persons. The bipolar type is more common in younger adults than in older adults *Inheritance*: There is an increased risk of schizophrenia among the relatives of probands with schizoaffective disorder (Sadock, 2003)

(continued)

TABLE 21.7 (continued)
Epidemiology of Schizophrenia and Schizoaffective Disorder

	Schizophrenia	Schizoaffective Disorder
Person	*Comorbidity*: • 90% are smoker (three times increase in risk as compared to the general population) (Kelly and McCreadie, 2000) • 60% suffer from depression • 35%–50% misuse substances • 10% have obsessive–compulsive symptoms (Fabisch et al., 2001) • 10% of schizophrenia is caused by cannabis misuse *Inheritance*: • Heritability: 82%–85% (Farmer et al., 1987; Cardno et al., 1999) • 40% of the first-degree relatives have abnormal smooth pursuit eye movement *Mortality*: • At least two times higher than the general population as a result of suicide or metabolic diseases • Life expectancy is 10 years less than general population • 10% commit suicide. Risk factors include male gender, younger than 30 years, university education, paranoia, depression, and substance abuse *Forensic aspects (Swinson et al., 2007)*: • Around 50 homicides per year are committed by those in recent contact with mental health services in the United Kingdom. This figure represents 9% of all homicides • 5% of homicide perpetrators have a diagnosis of schizophrenia. This figure is much lower than the comorbidity of alcohol and drug misuse. 60% of homicide perpetrators have misused alcohol and drug in the past	

TABLE 21.8

Epidemiology of Mood Disorders

	Depressive Disorder	Bipolar Disorder	Dysthymia	Cyclothymia
Incidence	In the United Kingdom, the incidence of depressive disorder fell from 22.5 to 14.0 per 1,000 person-years at risk (PYAR) from 1996 to 2006 The incidence of depressive symptoms rose by threefold from 5.1 to 15.5 per 1,000 PYAR (Rait et al., 2009)	4.6/100,000 in the United Kingdom London: 6.2/100,000 Nottingham: 3/100,000 Liverpool: 1.7/100,000 The incidence is also increased in people of African origin and the minority ethnic groups as compared with the Caucasian (Lloyd et al., 2005)	One-year incidence in adolescents is 3.4% (Garrison et al., 1997)	Unknown
Prevalence and lifetime risk	*Prevalence in general population*: 2%–5% *Prevalence in medical outpatients*: 5%–10% *Prevalence in medical inpatients*: 10%–20% *Lifetime risk for adults in the general population* Overall: 10%–20%; 1 in 4 women and 1 in 10 men have depressive disorder in their lifetime *Lifetime risk for first-degree relatives*: 20% *Children and adolescents*: • 0.5%–2.5% among children • 2%–8% among adolescents *Seasonal pattern*: • In the United Kingdom, the lifetime prevalence of major depression with a seasonal pattern is 0.4% • The prevalence of both major and minor depression with a seasonal pattern is 1.0% • Male gender and older age are associated with seasonal pattern (Blazer et al., 1998)	*Prevalence*: In the United States, the prevalence of bipolar I disorder is 0.4%–1.6%, and the prevalence of bipolar II disorder is 0.5% (Sadock, 2003) *Lifetime risk for adults in the general population*: 1%–1.5% *Lifetime risk for first-degree relatives*: 4%–18% of relatives have bipolar disorder 9%–25% of relatives have unipolar depression *Mania in old people*: 0.1% *Rapid cycling* Rapid cycling affects 13%–30% of bipolar patients (Hajek et al., 2008)	5% of general population Dysthymia is more common than severe depressive episode in chronically medically ill	3%–6% of the general population
Geographic pattern	People living in deprived industrial areas are more likely to be treated for depression than people living in other areas Peak of admission: spring	No significant geographic pattern Peak of admission: summer	No significant geographic pattern	No significant geographic pattern

(*continued*)

TABLE 21.8 (continued)

Epidemiology of Mood Disorders

	Depressive Disorder	Bipolar Disorder	Dysthymia	Cyclothymia
Person	*Gender*: • F:M = 2:1 *Age*: • The peak age of the first onset of depression is 30 years. (>50% of depressed people have their first depressive episode before the age of 40 years) • People younger than 40 years are three times more likely to develop depression than older people (Coryell et al., 1992) • An older age of onset is not associated with a family history of depression (Brodaty et al., 1991) *Social factors*: • Unemployment (twice the risk) • Separation or divorce • Brown and Harris study: risk factors for depression in women: 3 or more children under the age of 11 years, unemployment, and lack of confiding relationship (Brown and Harris, 1978) *Life events*: • Depression occurs after stressful life events, for example, divorce, bereavement, job loss, and adverse childhood experience involving loss and abuse *Diseases*: • The first major depressive episode in old people is often associated with an undiagnosed neurological disorder (e.g. Parkinson's disease, multiple sclerosis, cerebrovascular accident, and epilepsy) or other medical disorders (postmyocardial infarction, diabetes, and cancer) (Robinson and Starkstein, 1990)	*Gender*: • F = M Rapid cycling more common in women *Age*: • The age of onset of bipolar disorder is earlier than in unipolar disorder (mean age = 30 years, range: 15–50 years) • The first onset is usually a depressive episode *SE status*: • Bipolar disorder is found in occupations that require creativity such as artists, writers, and pop stars *Comorbidity*: • Substance misuse: 50% • Attempted suicide: 25%–50% • Completed suicide: 10% *Inheritance*: • Genetic component plays a significant role in transmitting bipolar disorder (Sadock and Sadock, 2003) • Heritability: 79%–93% (Kendler et al., 1995; McGuffin et al., 2003; Kieseppa et al., 2004) *Risk factors for relapse*: • Stopping lithium: increase in risk by 28 times in 3 months after stopping lithium) • Substance misuse leads to poor response to lithium • Stressful life events *Mortality*: • ↑ Risk of violent deaths by three times *Prognosis*: • Bipolar disorder patients with only manic episodes have better outcome than patients with severe depressive episode. • Patients with mixed episodes have the worse prognosis	*Gender*: • F:M = 2:1 *Age*: • Early onset—late adolescence or 20s • Late onset—30–50 years of age, often after a depressive episode (double depression) *SE status*: • Common in people with low income *Life events*: • Common in unmarried • Early onset is associated with childhood trauma • Late onset often occurs after a major depressive episode • Chronic life difficulties and diseases (Stein and Wilkinson, 2007)	*Gender*: • F = M *Age*: • Early onset—late adolescence or 20s • Late onset—30–50 years of age, often after an affective episode *Life events*: • Misuse of psychoactive substances is a frequent precipitant *Inheritance*: • Familial aggregation in both unipolar and bipolar disorders (Stein and Wilkinson, 2007)

TABLE 21.8 (continued)

Epidemiology of Mood Disorders

	Depressive Disorder	Bipolar Disorder	Dysthymia	Cyclothymia
Person	*Comorbidity*: • 2/3 of patients have anxiety disorders, substance misuse, and personality disorders • 1/3 of patients with insomnia have a moderate depressive episode Suicide risk is increased by 20 times in patients with depression *Inheritance*: • 55% share with the personality trait neuroticism • Heritability: 33%–48% (Kendler et al., 1992; McGulffin et al. 1996; Kendler and Prescott 1999)			

TABLE 21.9

Epidemiology of Suicide and Deliberate Self-Harm

	Suicide	Deliberate Self-Harm (DSH)
Incidence	• 11/100,000 for men and contribute to 2% of all male deaths (United Kingdom) • 3/100,000 for women and contribute to 1% of all female deaths (United Kingdom) • Suicide accounts for 1% of all deaths in the United Kingdom (Power, 1997) *Findings from National Confidential Inquiry into Suicide and Homicide by People with Mental Illness (Swinson et al., 2007)*: • 4500–5000 general population suicides occur per year in England and Wales • 160–200 psychiatric inpatients die by suicide annually; most common method is by hanging • 1 suicide per GP every 5 years	140/100,000 for men in Europe 193/100,000 for women in Europe 140,000 hospital attendances per year of DSH in the United Kingdom
Prevalence and lifetime risk	*Adults*: • Epidemiological data suggest the 12-month prevalence rate for suicide attempts is between 0.4% and 0.6% (Kessler et al., 1999, 2005) • 8–25 suicide attempts result in one death (Moscicki, 2001) *Lifetime risk of suicide in people with alcohol misuse*: 3%–4%; M:F = 2:1; mean age of suicide is 47 years, One-third have history of DSH and occur when patient is intoxicated with alcohol *Suicide in children and adolescents*: • Suicidal ideation: 10% • Attempted suicide: 2%–4% of adolescents • Suicide: 7.6 per 100,000 among the 15–19-year-olds *Goth subculture in the United Kingdom (Young et al., 2006)*: • Lifetime risk of suicide attempt: 47%	*DSH among young people in the United Kingdom*: 7%–14% (Hawton and James, 2005, Skegg, 2005) *Goth subculture in the United Kingdom (Young et al., 2006)*: Lifetime self-harm: 53% 50% of people present with DSH are repeaters
Geographic and temporal pattern	• Lithuania, Estonia, and Latvia are the countries with the highest suicide rates in the world • Lithuania has the highest annual rate for men (79.3/100,000) • China has the highest for women (17.8/100,000) (Yip and Liu, 2006) • The United Kingdom has lower rate of suicide compared to other European countries such as France and Russia • There are higher suicide rates in Scotland as compared to the rate in England and Wales • In England and Wales, suicide is more common in spring and summer • The suicide rate is usually reduced during war (e.g. WWII)	• The rate of DSH ranges from 2% in Lebanon to 20% in New Zealand • In England and Wales, both suicide and DSH are common in the cities • Seasonal variation is not seen in the DSH
Person	*Gender*: • In the United Kingdom, the M:F ratio is 3:1 and the rate of women is rising • For the rest of the world, men have higher suicide rate compared to women with the exception of China (Yip and Liu, 2006). Hence, China is the only country where the M:F ratio in suicide is close to 1:1 *Age*: • Highest suicide rates in men older than 75 years and women older than 65 years in England and Wales • Advancing age is a risk factor, and 90% of old people committed suicide because of depression	*Gender*: • Women > men *Age*: • Peak age for women: 15–24 years • Peak for men: 25–34 years • The age of onset at which people first deliberately harm themselves is decreasing *SE status*: • More people from the lower social class exhibit DSH

TABLE 21.9 (continued)

Epidemiology of Suicide and Deliberate Self-Harm

	Suicide	Deliberate Self-Harm (DSH)
Person	*Methods of suicide*: • Psychiatric patients tend to use violent methods such as hanging, shooting, and jumping from heights • 2/3 of British men and 1/3 of British women committed suicide by hanging or vehicle exhaust fumes • Drowning is more frequent among old people • Jumping from height is more frequent in young people who committed suicide *SE status*: • Poverty is associated with an increased risk of suicide *Ethnicity*: • In the United Kingdom, immigrants from India, especially the women, are at high risk • Young Pakistani and Bangladeshi women have higher than expected suicide rates (Bhugra and Desai, 2002) • For ethnic minorities in the United Kingdom, the most common method of suicide is hanging • Violent methods are more common than among ethnic minorities as compared to the Caucasians • People of Afro-Caribbean origin who committed suicide have the highest rates of schizophrenia (74%), unemployment, living alone, previous violence, and drug misuse (Isabelle et al., 2003) *Social factors*: • Higher risk in the low and high social class • Low risk in the middle social class • Suicide rates in the divorced and widowed are higher than people who are married • Unemployment, low SE status, and certain occupations such bar owners, doctors, pharmacists, artists, and farmers are risk factors • Institutions, for example, prisons • Organization with easy access to firearms: army and police • Suicide attempts occur after significant life events are common among people with poor social support and living alone *Diseases*: • Previous suicide attempt • Concurrent mental disorders: severe depression, bipolar depression, postnatal depression, postpartum psychosis, and alcohol and drug abuse • Young men recovered from schizophrenia and regain insight • Chronic medical illnesses associated pain • Anhedonia, alcohol misuse, and anxiety are short-term predictors of suicide	*Ethnicity and subculture*: • In the United Kingdom, the rate of DSH is raised among Asian women • The Goth subculture in the United Kingdom is strongly associated with self-harm *Life events*: • Adverse life events (e.g. interpersonal conflicts) are frequently reported to have occurred before the act of self-harm *Diseases*: • People who deliberately harm themselves have higher than expected incidence of physical illness and recent admissions to the hospital (Stein and Wilkinson, 2007) *DSH and suicide*: • A history of DSH is a long-term predictor of suicide, and the risk of suicide is 100 times greater than that of general population • 15% of people attempting self-harm will have another episode within 1 year • 1% of patients eventually kill themselves in the year following DSH • 3%–5% of patients kill themselves in the 5–10 years following DSH *Prevention*: • A contact card scheme such as the Bristol Green Card Scheme reduces the admission rate associated with DSH

(continued)

TABLE 21.9 (continued)

Epidemiology of Suicide and Deliberate Self-Harm

	Suicide	Deliberate Self-Harm (DSH)
Person	• Two in five people who committed suicide saw their GP in the week preceding their suicide (Power, 1997) • One in four contacted the mental health service in the year before their death *Post-discharge suicide*: • In the United Kingdom, nearly a quarter of the inpatient deaths occur within the first 7 days of admission • 30% occur on the ward, and the most common method is hanging • Post-discharge suicide is most frequent in the first 2 weeks after leaving hospital, and the highest number occurred on the first day (Meehan et al., 2006) *Inheritance*: • The tendency to attempt suicide is associated with familial pattern through the inheritance of depressive disorder or modelling	

TABLE 21.10
Epidemiology of Anxiety Disorders

	Generalized Anxiety Disorder (GAD)	Panic Disorders	Social Phobia	Agoraphobia
Incidence	*GAD*: 4.3% (Beesdo et al., 2010) Other anxiety disorders: 23% (phobia or panic disorder) (Beesdo et al., 2010)	*General population*: One-year incidence: 10% For patients presenting to emergency departments with chest pain, 25% have panic disorder (Ham et al., 2005)	*General population*: One-year incidence: 6%	Large numbers of people in the community who have agoraphobia without panic disorder do not seek help In the United States, about 2/1000 PYAR (Bienvenu et al., 2006)
Prevalence and lifetime risk	*General adults*: One-year prevalence: 3%–8% *Children and adolescents*: The prevalence is 2%. Girls have higher rates of anxiety disorders than boys *Old people*: The prevalence of old people (> 65-year-old) is 5%–15%	*General adults*: Lifetime prevalence is 8.6% in the United Kingdom (Birchall et al., 2000) *First-degree relatives of panic disorder*: 8%–31% *Children and adolescents*: <1%	*Lifetime prevalence*: 6% *Children and adolescents*: Social phobia: 1% Simple phobias: 2%–9% Specific phobia: 3%	*Lifetime prevalence*: 4% (Stein and Wilkinson, 2007) 6-month prevalence: 3%–6%, 4% for women and 2% for men
Person	*Gender*: Women > Men *Age*: The mean age of onset is usually in the 20s *Life events*: Life event is an important precipitant for anxiety disorder, and it may lead to alcohol misuse *Comorbidity*: GAD is probably the most common psychiatric disorder that coexists with another psychiatric disorder (e.g. social phobia, specific phobia, panic disorder, and depressive disorder) Endocrine disorders such as hyperthyroidism are associated with anxiety symptoms	*Gender*: Women > Men *Age*: Bimodal peak: 15–24 years and 45–54 years *Life events*: Recent history of divorce or separation (Sadock, 2003) *Disease*: Mitral valve prolapse (20%), hypertension, cardiomyopathy, COPD, and irritable bowel syndrome	*Gender*: The F:M ratio may be closer to 1:1 in social phobia *Age*: First onset: 11–15 years *Life events*: being criticized or scrutinized and resulted in humiliation *Psychiatric comorbidity*: depressive disorder and alcohol misuse and an increased rate of DSH *Inheritance*: Social phobia is more common among relatives of patients with social phobia as compared to the general population (Gelder et al., 2001)	*Gender*: Women > Men *Age*: 25–35 years Agoraphobia may occur before the onset of panic disorder *SE status*: common in housewives *Life events*: Onset usually follows a traumatic event (Sadock and Sadock, 2003) *Disease*: Half of patients have panic disorder as well (Sadock and Sadock, 2003)

(continued)

TABLE 21.10 (continued)

Epidemiology of Anxiety Disorders

	Generalized Anxiety Disorder (GAD)	Panic Disorders	Social Phobia	Agoraphobia
Person	*Inheritance*: Genetic factors play a role.	*Comorbidity*: • Depressive disorder (70%) • Social phobia (50%) • Agoraphobia (40%) • Alcohol misuse (30%) *Inheritance*: • Heritability: 44% (Kendler et al., 1992) • Risk is increased by five times for developing panic disorder in the first-degree relatives of probands with panic disorder		*Comorbidity*: • Panic disorder • Depression • Other anxiety disorders

TABLE 21.11

Epidemiology of OCD Spectrum Disorders and Post-Traumatic Stress Disorder

	Obsessive–Compulsive Disorder (OCD)	Body Dysmorphic Disorder (BDD)/Dysmorphophobia	Post-Traumatic Stress Disorder
Incidence	0.55 per 1000 person-years (Nestadt et al., 1998)	Unknown	On average, about 10% of people experiencing a significant traumatic event actually go on to develop PTSD (Kessler et al., 1995)
Prevalence and lifetime risk	*Prevalence*: 1% *Lifetime prevalence*: 2%–5% *Children and adolescents* 2 in 100 children and adolescents 1%–13% of boys 1%–11% of girls	One-year prevalence: 0.77% (Phillips, 2004) Affecting 1 in 200 people in the community	Lifetime prevalence: 1 in 100 *Prevalence based on circumstances*: 1 in 5 fire fighters 1 in 3 teenager survivors of car crashes 1 in 2 female rape victims 2 in 3 prisoners of war
Person	*Gender*: F:M = 1.5:1 Women: Compulsive washing and avoidance are more common. Men checking rituals or ruminations (more common) *Age*: Mean age of onset is around 20 years (70% before 25 years, 15% after 35 years). Men have early age of onset (adolescence) One of the commonest psychiatric disorders in children, affecting 1%–5% of children and adolescents in community samples *SE status*: 50% of OCD patients are unmarried *Disease*: Pediatric autoimmune neuropsychiatric disorders associated with streptococcal infections. Postencephalitis *Comorbidity*: Avoidance, histrionic, and dependent personality traits (40%) Tic disorder (40%) Depression (60%) *Inheritance*: OCD occurs in 10% of the first-degree relatives of patients, compared with 2% in general population	*Gender*: women > men *Age*: between 15 and 30 years old. Onset is in adolescence. *SE status*: People with BDD are likely to be unmarried. *Comorbidity*: BDD may be comorbid with depression (60%), trichotillomania (26%), social phobia (11%–13%), substance misuse, OCD (8%–37%), and suicide attempt (25%) (Phillips, 2004) *Inheritance*: BDD are found in 10% of family members of the probands. *Frequencies of imagined defects* (Phillips, 2004): Skin 70% Hair 55% Nose 40% Stomach/breast/eyes/thighs/teeth: 20% Ugly face: 15%	*Gender*: F:M = 2:1 Men's trauma is due to combat experience, and women's trauma is related to assault or rape *Age*: most prevalent in young adults *SE status*: low SE status and low education; other factors: those single, divorced, widowed, and socially withdrawn *Ethnicity*: Afro-Caribbean/Hispanic *Comorbidity*: Depression Anxiety disorders Alcohol misuse *Inheritance*: First-degree biological relatives of persons with a history of depression have an increased risk for developing PTSD following a traumatic event

TABLE 21.12

Epidemiology of Somatization Disorder and Hypochondriasis

	Somatization Disorders (Briquet's Syndrome)	**Hypochondriasis**
Prevalence	*General population*: 4% *Medical patients*:10%–20% *Primary care*: 70% of patients with emotional disorder present in primary care with a somatic complaint Lifetime prevalence of somatoform pain disorder is 10% one in five surgery attenders has chronic somatic symptoms longer than 2-year duration	In medical outpatients: approximately 5% (Barsky et al., 1990) Transient hypochondriasis is common
Person	*Gender*: F:M = 2:1 *Age*: Between 20 and 30s; before the age of 30 years *Comorbidity*: • Depression in 40% of people with somatoform pain disorder • Substance misuse: Opioid or analgesic is common *Diseases*: Complicated medical history with spurious physical diagnosis *Family*: • Family history of psychopathy or alcoholism, broken home, early abuse, and school refusal • Exposure to parents who are sensitive to body discomfort	*Gender*: Men = women *Age*: Peak incidence: 40–50-year-olds. *Life events*: An adverse childhood environment (e.g. sexual abuse, domestic violence, parental upheaval) can predispose to hypochondriasis *Comorbidity*: • GAD (50%) • *Other comorbidities*: depression, OCD, and panic disorder

TABLE 21.13

Epidemiology of Eating Disorders

Anorexia Nervosa (AN)	Bulimia Nervosa (BN)
Incidence	
• 14.6/100,000 in women • 1.8/100,000 in men • 20/100,000 for women aged 10–39 within primary care	Incidence in primary care in the Netherlands: 11.4/100,000 (1985–1989) (Hoek, 1991)
Prevalence	
In adolescence: • 0.5% of 12–19-year-olds • 8–11 times more common in girls • Among 15-year-old school children • 700 per 100,000 (girls) and 90 per 100,000 (boys) *In adults*: • AN: 0.5% • Eating problems not meeting full diagnostic criteria: 5%	*In adolescence*: Increased over the past three decades. Among young women: 1% 1% of adolescent girls and young women *In adults*: BN: 1%–2%
Person	
Gender: F:M = 10:1 *Age*: • Mean age: 15/16 years • Median age: 17 years *SE status*: • Higher social class • Certain social groups: dancers and athletes *Ethnicity*: • The clinical profile of eating disorders in Hong Kong has increasingly conformed to that of Western countries (Lee et al., 2009) • AN exhibited an increasingly fat-phobic pattern • Nonfat-phobic AN patients exhibited significantly lower premorbid body weight, less body dissatisfaction, less weight control behaviour, and lower EAT-26 scores than fat-phobic AN patients *Risk factors*: • History of sexual abuse, alcohol and substance misuse, enmeshed family relationship, and IDDM *Life events*: • For fat-phobic AN patients, episode of AN is precipitated by negative remarks made by the others on their body images • In Singapore, some young, nonfat-phobic AN patients develop the first episode of AN before public examinations *Comorbidity*: • >80% of people with AN have additional psychiatric comorbidity during the course of their lives • Depression (70%) and OCD (30%) are most frequent comorbidity • Suicide rate is increased by 32 times in AN patients compared to general population	*Gender*: F:M = 10:1 *Age*: Median age = 18 years *SE status*: All social classes are affected *Ethnicity*: In Hong Kong, BN has become more common, and the pattern is similar to Western countries (Lee et al., 2009) *Life events*: • BN seems to arise as a result of exposure to premorbid dieting and other risk factors (premorbid and parental obesity, innate tendency to overeat and enjoy food, critical comments about weight, shape, and eating) *Other risk factors* include depression, alcohol and substance misuse during childhood, low parental contact and high parental expectations, abuse, and neglect *Comorbidity*: • Additional psychiatric features are common; depressive and anxiety symptoms predominate • Patients often have problems of impulse control: self-mutilation (10%), suicide attempts (30%), promiscuity (10%), and shoplifting (20%) *Genetics*: • Familial disposition • The risk for first-degree relatives is increased fourfold *Prognosis* • 20% continue to have BN after 2–5, and a further 25% still had bulimic symptoms • The use of purgative is a poor prognostic factor (Wihelm and Clarke, 1998)

(*continued*)

TABLE 21.13 (continued)

Epidemiology of Eating Disorders

	Anorexia Nervosa (AN)	Bulimia Nervosa (BN)
Person	*Genetics*: • AN is more common in monozygotic twins compared to dizygotic twins • Depression and OCD are common among first-degree relatives of AN patients (Stein and Wilkinson, 2007) *Mortality*: • The risk is increased by five times in AN patients compared to general population *Prognosis* • 50% of patients have good recovery with normalization in three outcome parameters: weight, menstrual pattern, and eating behaviour • 30% of patients have fair outcome with improvement in one to two parameters • 20% have poor outcome with no improvement and result in death • Persistent vomiting is a poor prognostic factor (Wihelm and Clarke, 1998) *Poor prognostic factors for both AN and BN*: lower initial body weight, failure to respond to treatments, disturbed family relationships, and severe personality disorder	

TABLE 21.14

Epidemiology of Personality Disorders

	Borderline Personality Disorder (BPD)	Antisocial Personality Disorder (ASPD)
Prevalence	*Community*: 0.7%–2.0% (Coid, 2003) *Elderly*: 0.8% *Psychiatric inpatients*: 15% (Widiger and Weissman, 1991)	*Community*: 0.6%–3.0% in the community (Coid, 2003)
Geographic pattern	The clinical profiles of BPD in Eastern countries have increasingly conformed to that of Western countries	• Western societies emphasize on individualization, competitiveness, and rivalry between individuals that may promote the expression of antisocial behaviours • In contrast, collectivistic culture in Eastern societies may put less emphasis on individualization but more concerns of the consequence of one's behaviour. This leads to less antisocial behaviour in Eastern countries • Higher rates are found in urban rather than rural settings
Person	*Gender*: • F:M = 3:1 • Men with BPD compared with men suffering from other personality disorders have shown more evidence of dissociation, image distortion, frequency of childhood sexual abuse, longer experiences of physical abuse, and experiences of loss at an early age • Research suggests that men with BPD are more regularly diagnosed with substance abuse problems than women with BPD *Age*: • Onset is in adolescence and early 20s • Three-quarters of people with BPD are women and usually within childbearing age *Life events*: • Childhood physical or sexual abuse (between 40% and 70% of people with BPD report having been sexually abused, often by a noncaregiver) *Comorbidity* • Substance misuse (15%) and bulimia are common comorbidity (Zimmennan and Mattia, 1999) • Rapid and reactive shifts into depression are common (60%); affective instability, impulsive behaviour, and panic attacks may occur (30%) • 10% commit suicide (Work Group on Borderline Personality Disorder, 2001) *Genetics*: • Increased prevalence of major depression and alcohol and other substance misuse disorders is reported in first-degree relatives *Poor prognosis*: Poor prognostic factors include sexual abuse in childhood and victims of incest (Paris et al., 1993; Stone, 1993) *Mortality*: 1 in 10 committed suicide	*Gender*: • M:F = 6:1 *Age*: • There is a 10-fold increase in antisocial behaviours during adolescence *Family background*: • Parental criminality, parental aggression, poor supervision from parents, harsh and erratic discipline, and being rejected as a child *SE status*: • Social adversity • Parental criminal behaviours • Maternal deprivation • Paternal alcohol misuse • Low education background and association with conduct disorder *Comorbidity*: • Alcoholism and substance misuse are common • Among women, there is an association with somatization disorder • Inpatients have higher rates of psychiatric comorbidity *Genetics*: MZ: DZ = 60%:30% (Sadock, 2003)

TABLE 21.15

Epidemiology of Substance Misuse

Alcohol misuse	• Among British adults, 75% are normal drinkers, 8% are abstainers, 8% are hazardous drinkers, 5% are harmful drinkers, and 4% are dependent on alcohol
	• If the father is dependent on alcohol, the child has 80% chance to develop alcohol misuse. Hence, the risk is around four times higher than a child whose father is not dependent on alcohol
	• The lifetime risk for alcohol dependence: 10% for men and 3%–5% for women
	• The prevalence of abuse: 20% for men and 10% for women
	• The lifetime prevalence of psychiatric comorbidity (e.g. PTSD, depression) for women with alcohol abuse is as high as 70%
	• Women are more likely to develop medical complications at a younger age as compared to men
Substance misuse	• For adolescents and young adults in the United Kingdom, 50% have taken illicit drugs at some point in time. 20% used illicit substance in the previous month. 5% used at least two substances in the past 1 month
	• The peak age of substance misuse is 20 years
	• M:F = 3:1
	• For opiate misuse, mortality is increased by 12 times, and suicide rate is increased by 10 times

Source: Mynors-Wallis, L. et al., *Shared Care in Mental Health*, Oxford University Press, Oxford, U.K., 2002.

TABLE 21.16

Epidemiology of Common Psychiatric Disorders in Childhood and Adolescence

	Attention Deficit and Hyperkinetic Disorder (ADHD)	Autism	Conduct Disorders	School Refusal and Truancy
Incidence	• <1.0% (United Kingdom) • 3.0%–7.0% of prepubertal elementary school children (United States)	5 per 10,000 (United States)	1.0%–10.0%	Not known
Prevalence	• 1.7% of primary school boys • 1 in 200 in the population suffers severe hyperkinetic disorders	2/10,000	• 6.2%–10.8% among 10-year-olds • Boys: 9% • Girls: 2% • 33%–50% among child psychiatric clinic attendees	• Data from National Centre for Health Statistics (United States) [National Centre for Health Statistics 1993]: 5 school-loss days per person (5–17-year-olds) were caused by acute and chronic conditions • 4 school-loss days per person (5–17-year-olds) were caused by acute conditions only
Person	*Gender*: M:F = 2:1–9:1 *Age*: Symptoms present by 3 years of age but not diagnosed until older than 7 years *Comorbidity*: • Conduct disorder and oppositional defiant disorder: 50%–80% • Academic difficulties • Anxiety and depressive disorders *Genetics*: • First-degree biological relatives are at high risk to develop ADHD	*Gender*: M:F = 4:1–5:1 Girls with autism are more likely to suffer from severe learning disability *Age*: Onset is before the age of 3 years *Disease*: • Association with fragile X syndrome (≈1% of autistic children) • Tuberous sclerosis (up to 2%) *Genetics*: Evidence suggests that two regions on chromosomes 2 and 7 contain genes related to autism	*Gender*: M:F = 4:1–12:1 *Age*: Certain behaviours such as truancy begin before the age of 13 years *SE status*: Low *Family environment*: Harsh, punitive parenting, family discord, lack of appropriate parental supervision, and lack of social competence *Genetics*: More common in children with parents suffering ASPD and alcohol dependence than in general population	*Gender and ethnicity for school refusal*: Caucasian girls have higher rate of absence for acute reasons and chronic reasons in comparison to boys of Afro-Caribbean origin (Berg and Nursten, 1996) *Age of onset (school refusal)*: • Between 5 and 7 • At 11 years • Especially at 14 years and older *Age of onset (truancy)*: • 5% before age of 8 • Median age is 14 years (Berg and Nursten, 1996)

(continued)

TABLE 21.16 (continued)

Epidemiology of Common Psychiatric Disorders in Childhood and Adolescence

	Attention Deficit and Hyperkinetic Disorder (ADHD)	Autism	Conduct Disorders	School Refusal and Truancy
Person	• Parents of children with ADHD show an increased incidence of hyperkinesis, sociopathy, alcohol misuse, and conversion disorder *Risk factors*: Parental exposure to alcohol, nicotine, and maternal toxaemia (Sadock, 2003)		*Prognosis*: • 40% will become delinquent young adults (Goodman and Scott, 2005) • Early onset of conduct disorder is associated with higher than to develop ASPD in adulthood	*SE status (school refusal)*: The rate of school refusal is inversely related to family income (Adams and Bensen, 1992) *Life events (school refusal)*: Illnesses and family problems (e.g. caring for a young sibling, violence, and bullying in school) *Comorbidity associated with school refusal*: Separation anxiety (younger children), school phobia, and depressive disorder (older children) *Prognosis of truancy* (Berg and Nursten, 1996): *Boys*: Drug misuse (30%), antisocial personality (25%), and phobia (20%) *Girls*: Phobia (32%), drug misuse (25%), and antisocial personality (11%)

TABLE 21.17

Epidemiology of Common Psychiatric Disorders in Postpartum Period

	Postnatal Blues	Postpartum Depression	Postpartum Psychosis
Incidence	50% of women	10%–15% in the first year of the postnatal period	• 1.5 per 1000 childbirths • Affective presentation: 70% • Schizophreniform presentation: 25% • Confusion: 5%
Geographic pattern	No geographic pattern	• Lower incidence rates in some countries (e.g. Japan) • Higher in deprived inner city areas • In India, social status of women is lower than men. The birth of a female infant often leads to disappointment	No geographic pattern
Person	*Onset*: The third to tenth day postpartum *Prognosis*: Postnatal blues usually resolve in 2–3 days	*Onset*: within 6 weeks postdelivery *SE status*: unemployment and lack of supportive relationship *Life events*: unhappy marriage, relationship problems with partner, absence of a confiding relationship, other young children at home, ambivalent feelings of becoming a mother, and delivery of a premature and unwell baby *Past history*: Patients have often experienced anxiety and depressive symptoms in the last trimester of pregnancy. Past depressive episode is also a risk factor *Prognosis*: Each episode of postnatal depression lasts 2–6 months	*Onset*: within first 2 weeks following delivery *SE status*: little evidence for psychosocial causation *Diseases*: Some cases are caused by general medical conditions associated with perinatal events (infection, drug intoxication, and blood loss) *Past psychiatric history*: schizophrenia or affective disorders (20%–50%) *Family*: About 50% of affected women have a family history of mood disorders *Prognosis*: • 70%: full recovery • 50%: risk of future psychotic episodes • 20% risk of future puerperal psychosis

TABLE 21.18

Epidemiology of Common Psychiatric Disorders in Old People

	Dementia	Depression	Suicide	Late Onset Psychosis/Late Paraphrenia
Incidence	Risk increases with age: 1% at 60 years old and doubles every 5 years (Semple et al., 2005)	8.4% (Harris et al., 2006)	40 per 100 000	10–26 per 100, 000 per year
Prevalence	• 1 in 20 people older than 65 years and 1 in 5 older than 80 years develop dementia • Alzheimer's disease: 50% • Vascular dementia: 20% • Lewy body dementia: 15%	• Prevalence of depressive symptoms: 15% • 2%–4% major depression • 12%–20% minor degree of depression • 80% of old people who committed suicide suffer from depression • 20% of elderly inpatients fulfil the diagnostic criteria for depression	Not applicable	• *Overall*: 0.1%–4% • First onset of schizophrenia after the age of 60 is very rare • Only 1.5% of all people with schizophrenia have onset older than 60 years • 60% of people with late paraphrenia resemble paranoid schizophrenia
Person	*Gender*: M = F *Age*: Risk increases with age: 2% at the age 65–70 and 20% at the age of 80 and above *Risk factors*: smoking, sedentary lifestyle, high-fat/salt diet, head injury *Disease*: high blood pressure, high cholesterol, and obesity; learning disability and Down syndrome *Family*: Genetic risk of Alzheimer's disease is associated with apolipoprotein E4 (APOE4) allele Family history of Down syndrome and Parkinson's disease also increases the risk of dementia	*Gender*: Elderly women have higher prevalence *SE status*: No instrumental social support, social isolation, financial difficulty, nursing home resident are less likely to be treated by GP for depression as compared to adults and younger people *Life events*: Widowhood and having chronic illness associated with functional limitation and poor self-rated health are precipitating factors to depression *Genetics*: Genetic factors are less important (cf depression in young people) *Comorbidity*: Depression is the most common cause of obsessional symptoms in old people. Depression is more common in mild dementia than in severe dementia	*Gender*: M:F = 3:2 *SE status*: Financial problem is a risk factor Life events: widowhood *Disease*: Physical illness (e.g. chronic pain, terminal illness) is a major risk factor. Personality factors and depression are important associated factors	*Gender*: F:M = 3:1 *SE status*: • Social isolation (80% of people with late paraphrenia are socially isolated) • Single and never married *Comorbidity*: • Sensory impairment in hearing and vision • People with late paraphrenia are four times more likely to suffer from hearing impairment • Neurological disorders are common *Family history*: Family history of schizophrenia is a risk factor for late paraphrenia Relatives of people with late paraphrenia are 3.5 times more likely to develop schizophrenia as compared to the general population

REFERENCES

Adams PF and Benson V. 1992: Current estimates from the National Health Interview Survey, National Centre for Health Statistics. *Vital and Health Statistics* 10:184.

Barsky AJ, Wyshak G, Klerman GL, and Latham KS. 1990: The prevalence of hypochondriasis in medical outpatients. *Social Psychiatry and Psychiatric Epidemiology* 25:9–94.

Beesdo K, Pine DS, Lieb R, and Wittchen HU. 2010: Incidence and risk patterns of anxiety and depressive disorders and categorization of generalized anxiety disorder. *Archives of General Psychiatry* 67(1):47–57.

Berg I and Nursten J. 1996: *Unwillingly to School*, 4th edn. London, U.K.: Gaskell.

Bhugra D and Desai M. 2002: Attempted suicide in South Asian women. *Advance in Psychiatric Treatment* 8:418–423.

Bienvenu OJ, Onyike CU, Stein MB, Chen LS, Samuels J, Nestadt G, and Eaton WW. 2006: Agoraphobia in adults: Incidence and longitudinal relationship with panic. *The British Journal of Psychiatry* May, 188:432–438.

Birchall H, Brandon S, and Taub N. 2000: Panic in a general practice population: Prevalence, psychiatric comorbidity and associated disability. *Social Psychiatry and Psychiatric Epidemiology* 35(6):235–241.

Blazer DG, Kessler RC, and Swartz MS. 1998: Epidemiology of recurrent major and minor depression with a seasonal pattern. The National Comorbidity Survey. *The British Journal of Psychiatry* 172:164–167.

Brodaty H, Peters K, Boyce P et al. 1991: Age and depression. *Journal of Affective Disorders* 23(3):137–149.

Brown GW and Harris TO. 1978: *Social Origins of Depression: A Study of Psychiatric Disorders in Women*. London, U.K.: Tavistock Publications.

Cardno AG, Marshall EJ, Coid B et al. 1999: Heritability estimates for psychotic disorders: The Maudsley twin psychosis series. *Archives of General Psychiatry* 56:162–168.

Coid J. 2003: Epidemiology, public health and the problem of personality disorder. *The British Journal of Psychiatry* 182:s3–s10.

Coryell W, Endicott J, and Keller M. 1992: Major depression in a nonclinical sample. Demographic and clinical risk factors for first onset. *Archives of General Psychiatry* 49:117–125.

Dunham HW. 1965: *Community and Schizophrenia: An Epidemiological Analysis*. Detroit, MI: Wayne State University Press.

Fabisch K, Fabisch H, Langs G, Huber HP, and Zapotoczky HG. 2001: Incidence of obsessive-compulsive phenomena in the course of acute schizophrenia and schizoaffective disorder. *European Psychiatry* 16(6):336–341.

Farmer AE, McGuffin P, and Gottesman II. 1987: Twin concordance for DSM-III schizophrenia. Scrutinizing the validity of the definition. *Archives of General Psychiatry* 44:634–641.

Garrison CZ, Waller JL, Cuffe SP, McKeown RE, Addy CL, and Jackson KL. 1997: Incidence of major depressive disorder and dysthymia in young adolescents. *Journal of the American Academy of Child and Adolescent Psychiatry* April, 36(4):458–465.

Gelder M, Mayou R, and Cowen P. 2001: *Shorter Oxford Textbook of Psychiatry*, 9th edn. Oxford, U.K.: Oxford University Press.

Goodman R and Scott S. 2005: *Child Psychiatry*, 2nd edn. Oxford, U.K.: Blackwell Publishing.

Hajek T, Hahn M, Slaney C, Garnham J, Green J, Růzicková M, Zvolský P, and Alda M. 2008: Rapid cycling bipolar disorders in primary and tertiary care treated patients. *Bipolar Disorders* 10(4):495–502.

Ham P et al. 2005: Treatment of panic disorder. *American Family Physician* 71(4):733–739.

Harris T, Cook DG, Victor C, DeWilde S, and Beighton C. 2006: Onset and persistence of depression in older people—Results from a 2-year community follow-up study. *Age Ageing* 35:25–32.

Hawton K and James A. 2005: ABC of adolescence: Suicide and deliberate self harm in young people. *BMJ* 330:891–894.

Hoek HW. 1991: The incidence and prevalence of anorexia nervosa and bulimia nervosa in primary care. *Psychological Medicine* 21:455–460.

Isabelle MH, Robinson J, Bickley H et al. 2003: Suicides in ethnic minorities within 12 months of contact with mental health services: National clinical survey. *The British Journal of Psychiatry* 183:155–160.

Jablensky A and Sartorius N. 1975: Culture and schizophrenia. *Psychological Medicine* 5:113–124.

Johnstone EC, Cunningham Owens DG, Lawrie SM, Sharpe M, and Freeman CPL. 2004: *Companion to Psychiatric Studies*, 7th edn. London, U.K.: Churchill Livingstone.

Kelly C and McCreadie R. 2000: Cigarette smoking and schizophrenia. *Advance in Psychiatric Treatment* 6:327–331.

Kendler KS, Neale MC, Kessler RE et al. 1992: A population-based twin study of major depression in women. The impact of varying definitions of illness. *Archives of General Psychiatry* 49:257–266.

Kendler KS, Pedersen NL, Neale MG, and Mathe AA. 1995: A pilot Swedish twin study of affective illness including hospital–and population-ascertained subsamples: Results of model fitting. *Behavior Genetics* 25:217–232.

Kendler KS and Prescott CA. 1999: A population-based twin study of lifetime major depression in men and women. *Archives of General Psychiatry* 56:39–44.

Kessler RC, Berglund P, Borges G, Nock M, and Wang PS. 2005: Trends in suicide ideation, plans, gestures, and attempts in the United States, 1990–1992 to 2001–2003. *JAMA* 293:2487–2495.

Kessler RC, Borges G, and Walters EE. 1999: Prevalence and risk factors for lifetime suicide attempts in the National comorbidity survey. *Archives of General Psychiatry* 56:617–626.

Kessler RC, Sonnega A, Bromet E et al. 1995: Posttraumatic stress disorder in the National comorbidity survey. *Archives of General Psychiatry* 52:1048–1060.

Kieseppa T, Partonen T, Haukka J et al. 2004: High concordance of bipolar', disorder in a nationwide sample of twins. *American Journal of Psychiatry* 161:1814–1821.

Lee S, Ng KL, Kwok K, and Fung C. 2009: The changing profile of eating disorders at a tertiary psychiatric clinic in Hong Kong (1987–2007). *International Journal of Eating Disorders* 43(4):307–314.

Lewis GH, Sheringham J, Kalim K, and Crayford JBC. 2008: *Mastering Public Health*, pp. 151–153. London, U.K.: Royal Society of Medicine Press Ltd.

Lieb R, Pfister H, Mastaler M, and Wittchen H. 2000: Somatoform syndromes and disorders I in a representative population sample of adolescents and young adults: Prevalence, co-morbidity and impairments. *Acta Psychiatrica Scandanavica* 101:194–208.

Lloyd T, Kennedy N, Kirkbride J et al. 2005: Incidence of bipolar affective disorder in three UK cities results from the ÆSOP study. *The British Journal of Psychiatry* 186:126–131.

McGuffin P, Katz R, Watkins S, and Rutherford J. 1996: A hospital-based twin register of the heritability of DSM-IV unipolar depression. *Archives of General Psychiatry* 53:129–136.

McGuffin P, Rijsdijk F, Andrew M et al. 2003: The heritability of bipolar affective disorder and the genetic relationship to unipolar depression. *Archives of General Psychiatry* 60:497–502.

Meehan J, Kapur N, and Hunt IM. 2006: Suicide in mental health in-patients and within 3 months of discharge: National clinical survey. *The British Journal of Psychiatry* 188:129–134.

Moscicki EK. 2001: Epidemiology of completed and attempted suicide: Toward a framework for prevention. *Clinical Neuroscience Research* 1:310–323.

Mynors-Wallis L, Moore M, Maguire K, and Hollingery T. 2002: *Shared Care in Mental Health*. Oxford, U.K.: Oxford University Press.

National Centre for Health Statistics. 1993: Advance report of final natality statistics. *Monthly Vital Statistics Report,* 42(3) (suppl). Hyattsville, MD: Public Health Service.

Nestadt G, Bienvenu OJ, Cai G, Samuels J, and Eaton WW. 1998: Incidence of obsessive-compulsive disorder in adults. *Journal of Nervous and Mental Disease* 186(7):401–406.

Paris J, Zweig-Frank H, and Guzder H. 1993: The role of psychological risk factors in recovery from borderline personality disorder. *Comprehensive Psychiatry* 34:410–413.

Phillips KA. 2004: Body dysmorphic disorder: Recognizing and treating imagined ugliness. *World Psychiatry* 3(1):12–17.

Power K et al. 1997: Case-control study of GP attendance rates by suicide patients with or without a psychiatric history. *The British Journal of General Practice* 417:211–217.

Puri BK and Tyrer PJ. 2004: *Sciences Basic to Psychiatry*, 3rd edn. Edinburgh, U.K.: Churchill Livingstone.

Rait G, Walters K, Griffin M, Buszewicz M, Petersen I, and Nazareth I. 2009: Recent trends in the incidence of recorded depression in primary care. *The British Journal of Psychiatry* 195(6):520–524.

Robinson R and Starkstein SE. 1990: Current research in affective disorders following stroke. *The Journal of Neuropsychiatry and Clinical Neurosciences* 2:1–14.

Sadock BJ and Sadock VA. 2003: *Kaplan and Sadock's Comprehensive Textbook of Psychiatry*, 9th edn. Philadelphia, PA: Lippincott Williams & Wilkins.

Semple D, Smyth R, Burns J, Darjee R, and McIntosh A. 2005: *Oxford Handbook of Psychiatry,* 134, p. 252. Oxford, U.K.: Oxford University Press.

Skegg K. 2005: Self-harm. *Lancet* 28:1471–1483.

Stein G and Wilkinson G. 2007: *Seminars in General Adult Psychiatry,* 2nd edn. London, U.K.: The Royal College of Psychiatrists.

Stone M. 1993: Long-term outcome in personality disorders. *The British Journal of Psychiatry* 162:299–313.

Sugarman PA and Craufurd D. 1994: Schizophrenia in the Afro-Caribbean community. *The British Journal of Psychiatry* 164:474–480.

Swinson N, Ashim B, Windfuhr K et al. 2007: National confidential inquiry into suicide and homicide by people with mental illness: New directions. *The Psychiatrist Bulletin* 31:161–163.

Trimble M. 2004: *Somatoform Disorders—A Medicolegal Guide*, pp. 41–49. Cambridge, U.K.: Cambridge University Press.

Widiger TA and Weissman MM. 1991: Epidemiology of borderline personality disorder. *Hospital and Community Psychiatry* 10:1015–1021.

Wilhelm KA and Clarke SD. 1998: Eating disorders from a primary care perspective. *Medical Journal of Australia Practice Essentials* 168:458–463.

Work Group on Borderline Personality Disorder. 2001: Practice guideline for the treatment of patients with borderline personality disorder. *The American Journal of Psychiatry* 158(suppl):1–52.

Yip PSF and Liu KY. 2006: The ecological fallacy and the gender ratio of suicide in China. *The British Journal of Psychiatry* 189:465–466.

Young R, Sweeting H, and West P. 2006: Prevalence of deliberate self harm and attempted suicide within contemporary Goth youth subculture: Longitudinal cohort study. *BMJ* 332(7549):1058–1061.

Zimmennan M and Mattia JL. 1999: Axis I diagnostic comorbidity and borderline personality disorder. *Comprehensive Psychiatry* 40:245–252.

22 Biostatistics

22.1 DESCRIPTIVE AND INFERENTIAL STATISTICS

22.1.1 DESCRIPTIVE STATISTICS

Descriptive statistics are ways of organizing and describing data. Examples include

- Diagrams
- Graphical representations
- Numerical representations
- Tables

22.1.2 INFERENTIAL STATISTICS

Inferential statistics allow conclusions to be inferred from data. An example is inferring a likely range of values for the population mean from the sample mean.

22.1.3 HYPOTHESIS TESTING: SIGNIFICANCE TESTS

A value or range of values for an unknown population parameter is hypothesized. A study/experiment is then carried out, and the value of the observed random variable is used to test whether or not the hypothesis should be rejected.

22.1.3.1 Null Hypothesis

The initial hypothesis is the null hypothesis, H_0, usually representing no change:

$$H_0: \theta = \theta_0$$

where
θ is the unknown parameter
θ_0 is its hypothesized value

22.1.3.2 Alternative Hypothesis

The alternative hypothesis, H_1, may, for example, be one of the following types:

- $H_1: \theta \neq \theta_0$
- $H_1: \theta > \theta_0$
- $H_1: \theta < \theta_0$
- $H_1: \theta = \theta_1$

22.1.3.3 Simple Hypothesis

A simple hypothesis is one involving a single value for the population parameter.

22.1.3.4 Composite Hypothesis

A composite hypothesis is one involving more than one value for the population parameter.

22.1.3.5 One-Sided Significance Test

A one-sided significance test is a hypothesis test involving a composite alternative hypothesis of the following types:

- $H_1: \theta > \theta_0$
- $H_1: \theta < \theta_0$

22.1.3.6 Two-Sided Significance Test

A two-sided significance test is a hypothesis test involving a composite alternative hypothesis of the following type:

- $H_1: \theta \neq \theta_0$

22.1.3.7 Critical Region

The critical region is the region of the range of the random variable X such that if the observed value x falls in it, the null hypothesis, H_0, is rejected.

22.1.3.8 Critical Value

The critical value(s) is (are) the value(s) of the test statistic expected from the null hypothesis, H_0, that defines the boundary (boundaries) of the critical region.

22.1.3.9 Significance Level

The significance level, α, is the size of the critical region and represents the following probability:

$$\alpha = P(\text{Type I error})$$

where a type I error is the error of wrongly rejecting H_0 when it is true.

305

22.1.3.10 Steps in Carrying Out a Significance/Hypothesis Test

Hypothesis testing is carried out as follows:

- Formulate H_0.
- Formulate H_1.
- Specify α.
- Decide on the study/experiment to be carried out.
- Calculate the test statistic.

Test statistic

$$= \frac{\text{Appropriate statistic} - \text{Hypothesized parameter}}{\text{Standard error of statistic}}$$

- From the sampling distribution of the test statistic, create the test criterion for testing H_0 versus H_1.
- Carry out the study/experiment.
- Calculate the value of the test statistic from the sample data.
- Calculate the value of the difference, d, between the value of the test statistic from the sample and that expected under H_0 (the critical value(s), defining the critical range).
- If $P(d) < \alpha$, the result is statistically significant at the level of α (the 'p value') and H_0 is rejected.
- If $P(d) \geq \alpha$, the result is not statistically significant at the level of α and H_0 cannot be rejected.
- If H_0 is composite, the hypothesis test is designed so that the critical region size is the maximum value of the probability of rejecting H_0 when it is true.

22.1.4 ESTIMATION: CONFIDENCE INTERVALS

From sample statistics, confidence statements can be made about the corresponding unknown parameters, by constructing confidence intervals. A confidence interval can be two sided or one sided; two-sided confidence intervals need not necessarily be symmetrical (central).

If a $100(1 - \alpha)\%$ confidence interval from a statistic (or statistics) is calculated, this implies that if the study were repeated with other random samples taken from the same parent population and further $100(1 - \alpha)\%$ confidence intervals similarly individually calculated, the overall proportion of these confidence intervals that included the corresponding population parameter(s) would tend to $100(1 - \alpha)\%$.

The two-sided central confidence interval for the unknown parameter θ of a distribution with confidence level $(1 - \alpha)$ can be derived from the random interval of the following type:

$$(\theta_-(X), \theta_+(X))$$

By substituting the observation x for X, the realization of the random interval

$$(\theta_-(x), \theta_+(x))$$

is the two-sided central confidence interval for θ, in which

- $\theta_-(x) =$ lower confidence limit (confidence bound) for θ.
- $\theta_+(x) =$ upper confidence limit (confidence bound) for θ.

22.1.5 ADVANTAGES OF CONFIDENCE INTERVALS OVER p VALUES

There has been a recent move away from simply quoting p values in psychiatric research to giving instead, or additionally, the corresponding confidence intervals. Advantages of estimation over hypothesis testing include the following:

- Testing the null hypothesis is often inappropriate for psychiatric research; for example, they may reverse an investigator's idea (for instance, that a new treatment will be more effective than a current one) and substitute instead the notion of no effect or no difference.
- A hypothesis test evaluates the probability of the observed study result, or a more extreme result, occurring if the null hypothesis was in fact true.
- Proper understanding of a study result is obscured in hypothesis testing by transforming it onto a remote scale constrained from zero to one.
- Obtaining a low p value, particularly $p < 0.05$, is widely interpreted as implying merit and leads to the findings being deemed important and publishable, whereas this status is often denied study results that have not achieved this arbitrary level.
- The p value on its own implies nothing about the magnitude of any difference between treatments.
- The p value on its own implies nothing even about the direction of any difference between treatments.

- This overemphasis on hypothesis testing and the use of p values to dichotomize results into significant and nonsignificant have detracted from more useful procedures for interpreting the results of psychiatric research.
- Levels of significance are often quoted alone in the abstracts and texts of published papers without mentioning actual values, proportions, and so on, or their differences.
- Confidence intervals do not carry with them the pseudoscientific hypothesis testing language of significance tests.
- Estimation and confidence intervals give a plausible range of values for the unknown parameter.
- Inadequate sample size is indicated by the relatively large width of the corresponding confidence interval.

22.2 SPECIFIC BIOSTATISTICAL TESTS

22.2.1 t-TEST

The t-test is used for testing the null hypothesis that two population means are equal when the variable being investigated has a normal distribution in each population and the population variances are equal; that is, the t-test is a parametric test.

22.2.1.1 Independent Samples t-Test

This procedure tests the null hypothesis that the data are a sample from a population in which the mean of a test variable is equal in two independent (unrelated) groups of cases.

Assuming equal population variances (which can be checked using Levene's test), the standard error of the difference between two means, $\bar{x}_1$ and $\bar{x}_2$, of two independent samples (taken from the same parent population) of respective sizes n_1 and n_2 and respective standard deviations s_1 and s_2, $(s_1 \approx s_2)$ is given by

$$\text{Standard error of difference} = s\sqrt{\frac{1}{n_1} + \frac{1}{n_2}}$$

where the pooled standard deviation s is given by

$$s = \sqrt{\frac{(n_1 - 1)s_1^2 + (n_2 - 1)s_2^2}{(n_1 + n_2 - 2)}}$$

If the population variances cannot be assumed to be equal, then the standard error is given by

$$\text{Standard error of difference} = \sqrt{\frac{s_1^2}{n_1} + \frac{s_2^2}{n_2}}$$

22.2.1.2 Paired Samples t-Test

This procedure tests the null hypothesis that two population means are equal when the observations for the two groups can be paired in some way. Pairing (a repeated measures or within-subjects design) is used to make the two groups as similar as possible, allowing differences observed between the two groups to be attributed more readily to the variable of interest.

For n pairs, the appropriate standard error is given by

$$\text{Standard error of difference of paried observation} = \frac{s_d}{\sqrt{n}}$$

where s_d is the standard deviation of the differences of the paired observations.

22.2.2 CHI-SQUARE TEST

The chi-square (χ^2) test is a nonparametric test that can be used to compare independent qualitative and discrete quantitative variables presented in the form of contingency tables containing the data frequencies.

22.2.2.1 Null Hypothesis

For a given contingency table, under H_0,

$$\text{Expected value of a cell} = \frac{(\text{Row total})(\text{Column total})}{\text{Sum of cells}}$$

22.2.2.2 Calculation of χ^2

The value of χ^2 for a contingency table is calculated from

$$\chi^2 = \sum \left[\frac{(O - E)^2}{E} \right]$$

where
O is the observed value
E is the expected value

In order to use the χ^2 distribution, the number of degrees of freedom of a contingency table, ν, is given by

$$\nu = (r-1)(k-1)$$

where

r is the number of rows
k is the number of columns

22.2.2.3 2 × 2 Contingency Table

A 2 × 2 contingency table has one degree of freedom (Table 22.1).

For a 2 × 2 contingency table, the following formula can be used to calculate χ^2:

$$\chi^2 = \frac{(az - by)^2(a+b+y+z)}{(a+b)(y+z)(a+y)(b+z)}$$

22.2.2.4 Small Expected Values

For a contingency table with more than one degree of freedom, the following criteria (Cochran, 1954) should be fulfilled for the test to be valid:

- Each expected value ≥ 1.
- In at least 80% of cases, expected value > 5.

For a 2 × 2 contingency table, all the expected values need to be at least 5 in order to use the aforementioned formula; therefore, the overall total must be at least 20. If the total is less than 20, Fisher's exact probability test can be used. If $20 \leq$ total < 100, then a better fit with the continuous χ^2 distribution is provided by using Yates' continuity correction:

$$\chi^2_{\text{corrected}} = \frac{\{|az - by| - 1/2(a+b+y+z)\}^2(a+b+y+z)}{(a+b)(y+z)(a+y)(b+z)}$$

TABLE 22.1

Observed Values in a 2 × 2 Contingency Table

	—	—	**Total**
—	a	y	$a+y$
—	b	z	$b+z$
Total	$a+b$	$y+z$	$a+b+y+z$

Source: Reproduced from Puri, B.K., *Statistics for the Health Sciences*, WB Saunders, London, U.K., 1996. With permission.

22.2.2.5 Goodness of Fit

The χ^2 test can be used to test how well an observed distribution fits a given distribution, such as the normal distribution. This can be applied to both discrete and continuous data and tests the hypothesis that a sample derives from a particular model.

22.2.3 Fisher's Exact Probability Test

This test determines exact probabilities for 2 × 2 contingency tables. With the nomenclature of Table 22.1, the formula used is

$$\text{Exact probability of table} = \frac{(a+y)!(b+z)!(a+b)!(y+z)!}{(a+b+y+z)!a!b!y!z!}$$

In order to test H_0, in addition to calculating the probability of the given table, the probabilities also have to be calculated of more extreme tables occurring by chance.

22.2.4 Mann–Whitney U Test

This is a nonparametric alternative to the independent samples t-test. The test statistic, U, is the smaller of U_1 and U_2:

$$U_1 = n_1 n_2 + \frac{1}{2}n_1(n_1 + 1) - R_1$$

$$U_2 = n_1 n_2 + \frac{1}{2}n_2(n_2 + 1) - R_2$$

where

n_1 is the number of observations in the first group
n_2 is the number of observations in the second group
R_1 is the sum of the ranks assigned to the first group
R_2 is the sum of the ranks assigned to the second group

For $n_1 \geq 8$ and $n_2 \geq 8$, $U \approx N(\mu, \sigma^2)$, where

$$\mu = \frac{n_1 n_2}{2}$$

$$\sigma^2 = \frac{n_1 n_2(n_1 + n_2 + 1)}{12}$$

22.2.5 Confidence Interval for the Difference between Two Means

The $100(1 - \alpha)\%$ confidence interval for the difference between two means is given by

Difference $- t_{1-\alpha/2}$ (Standard error of difference)

To $\rightarrow$ Difference $t_{1-\alpha/2}$ (Standard error of difference)

22.2.6 Confidence Interval for the Difference between Two Proportions

For large sample sizes and population proportions not too close to 0 or 1, the $100(1 - \alpha)\%$ confidence interval for the difference between two proportions is given by

Difference $- z_{1-\alpha/2}$(Standard error of difference)

To $\rightarrow$ Difference $+ z_{1-\alpha/2}$(Standard error of difference)

where the standard error of the difference is given by

$$\text{Standard error of difference} = \sqrt{\frac{\hat{p}_1(1-\hat{p}_1)}{n_1} + \frac{\hat{p}_2(1-\hat{p}_2)}{n_2}}$$

where
$\hat{p}_1$ is the sample estimate of first proportion
$\hat{p}_2$ is the sample estimate of second proportion
n_1 is the sample size of the first group
n_2 is the sample size of the second group

22.2.7 Confidence Interval for the Difference between Two Medians

For the following confidence intervals to be valid, the assumption is made that the two distributions whose possible difference is being estimated have the same shape but may differ in location.

22.2.7.1 Two Unpaired Samples

In order to determine the $100(1 - \alpha)\%$ confidence interval for the difference between two medians, the value of K must first be calculated from

$$K = \frac{n_1 n_2}{2} - z_{1-\alpha/2}\sqrt{\frac{n_1 n_2 (n_1 + n_2 + 1)}{12}}$$

where
n_1 and n_2 are the sample sizes
$n_1 > 25$
$n_2 > 25$
K is rounded up to the nearest integer

The total number of possible differences is equal to $n_1 n_2$.

The $100(1 - \alpha)\%$ confidence interval for the median of these differences is from the Kth smallest to the Kth largest of the $n_1 n_2$ differences ($K \in \mathbb{Z}^+$).

If n_1 and/or n_2 is less than or equal to 25, then tables based on the value of the corresponding Mann–Whitney test statistic can be used.

22.2.7.2 Two Paired Samples

In this case, the value of K is calculated from

$$K = \frac{n(n+1)}{4} - z_{1-\alpha/2}\sqrt{\frac{n(n+1)(2n+1)}{24}}$$

where
n is the number of paired cases
$n > 50$
K is rounded up to the nearest integer

The total number of possible means of two differences (including differences with themselves) is equal to $n(n + 1)/2$.

The $100(1 - \alpha)\%$ confidence interval for the median of these mean differences is from the Kth smallest to the Kth largest of the $n(n + 1)/2$ mean differences ($K \in \mathbb{Z}^+$).

If $n \leq 50$, then tables based on the value of the corresponding Mann–Whitney test statistic can be used.

22.3 MORE COMPLEX METHODS

22.3.1 Factor Analysis

Factor analysis is an attempt to express a set of multivariate data as a linear function of unobserved, underlying dimensions or (common) factors together with error terms (specific factors). The common factors associated with each observed variable have individual loadings.

22.3.2 Principal Components Analysis

Principal components analysis is used to produce uncorrelated linear combinations of the observed variables of a multivariate dataset. The first component has maximum variance. Successive components account for progressively smaller parts of the total variance. Each component is uncorrelated with preceding components.

A plot of the variance of each principal component against the principal component number is known as a scree plot.

22.3.3 CORRESPONDENCE ANALYSIS

A correspondence analysis is similar to a principal components analysis but is applied to contingency tables. It allows a 2D contingency table to be presented as a 2D graph in which one set of coordinates represents the rows of the table and the other set represents the columns. Rather than partitioning the total variance, as in principal components analysis, there is a partition of the value of χ^2 for the contingency table.

22.3.4 DISCRIMINANT ANALYSIS

This is a method of classification applied to a multivariate dataset. Independent variables used to discriminate among the groups are known as discriminating variables. The discriminant function is a linear function of discriminating variables that maximizes the distance (or separation) between groups.

22.3.5 CLUSTER ANALYSIS

This is also a method of classification applied to a multivariate dataset that derives homogeneous groups or clusters of cases based on their values for the variable set. Hierarchical methods can be applied to the clusters.

22.3.6 MULTIVARIATE REGRESSION ANALYSIS

In this method, a linear multivariate regression equation is fitted to a multivariate dataset. The multiple regression coefficient is the maximum correlation between the dependent variable and multiple non-random independent variables, using a least-squares method.

22.3.7 PATH ANALYSIS

A series of multiple regression analyses are used to allow hypotheses of causality between variables to be modelled and tested. A path diagram allows these variables and their hypothetical relationships to be represented graphically. It shows arrows between the variables, with regression coefficients (known as path coefficients) associated with these arrows. χ^2 tests are used to test the model.

22.3.8 CANONICAL CORRELATION ANALYSIS

This is an extended form of multivariate regression in which the number of dependent variables is no longer confined to one. The maximum correlation between the set of independent variables and the set of dependent variables is known as the canonical correlation and gives information about interrelationships among the variables.

22.4 META-ANALYSIS, SURVIVAL ANALYSIS, AND LOGISTIC REGRESSION

22.4.1 META-ANALYSIS

22.4.1.1 Definition
The term meta-analysis is used to describe the process of evaluating and statistically combining results from two or more existing independent randomized clinical trials addressing similar questions in order to give an overall assessment.

22.4.1.2 Difficulties
Difficulties associated with meta-analysis include the following:

- The existence of publication bias—trials showing a statistically significant difference are more likely to be published than those not finding a statistically significant result.
- Researchers finding 'nonsignificant' results may be less likely formally to write up their results for publication.
- Arriving at selection criteria to determine which studies to include and which not to include in the meta-analysis.
- The different centres in which the different clinical trials have taken place may differ with respect to important variables in such a way as seriously to question the validity of combining their data.
- If the meta-analysis is of clinical trials carried out on widely differing population groups, to whom can the results of the meta-analysis properly be applied?

22.4.2 SURVIVAL ANALYSIS

This is a collection of statistical analysis techniques that can be applied to situations in which the time to a given event, such as death, illness onset, or recovery, is measured, but not all individuals necessarily have to have reached this event during the overall time interval studied.

22.4.2.1 Survival Function

The survival function, $S(t)$, is given by

$$S(t) = P(t_s > t)$$

where

t is the time

t_s is the survival time

The survival function is also given by

$$S(t) = 1 - (\text{Cumulative distribution function of } t_s)$$

22.4.2.2 Survival Curve

This is a plot of $S(t)$ (on the ordinate) versus t (on the abscissa). Instead of being drawn as continuous curves, sometimes survival curves are drawn in a stepwise fashion, with the steps occurring between estimated cumulative survival probabilities.

22.4.2.3 Hazard Function

This measures the likelihood of an individual experiencing a given event, such as death, illness onset, or recovery, as a function of time.

22.4.3 LOGISTIC REGRESSION

This is a regression model used to predict the probability of a dichotomous variable, such as better/not better at the end of the treatment period, on the basis of a set of independent variables, x_1 to x_n:

$$P(\text{event}) = \frac{1}{1 + \exp(-(\alpha_0 + \alpha_1 x_1 + \cdots + \alpha_n x_n))}$$

where the coefficients α_0 to α_n are estimated using a maximum likelihood method.

BIBLIOGRAPHY

Altman DG. 1991: *Practical Statistics for Medical Research*. London, U.K.: Chapman & Hall.

Bryman A and Cramer D. 1994: *Quantitative Data Analysis for Social Scientists*, revised edition. London, U.K.: Routledge.

Cochran WG. 1954: Some methods for strengthening the common χ^2-test. *Biometrics* 10:417–451.

Coolican H. 2009: *Research Methods and Statistics in Psychology*, 5th edn. London, U.K.: Hodder Arnold.

Dunn G and Everitt B. 1995: *Clinical Biostatistics: An Introduction to Evidence-Based Medicine*. London, U.K.: Arnold.

Everitt B and Hay D. 1992: *Talking about Statistics: A Psychologist's Guide to Design and Analysis*. London, U.K.: Arnold.

Puri BK. 2002: *Statistics in Practice: An Illustrated Guide to SPSS*, 2nd edn. London, U.K.: Arnold.

23 Research Methodology and Critical Appraisal

23.1 RESEARCH STUDY DESIGN

23.1.1 TYPES

Research studies may be classified as being case–control studies, in which patients affected by the index disease are compared with matched control subjects, and cross-sectional, in which subjects' data are collected at the same time (or, more usually, during the same time interval), and longitudinal studies. Confounding variables that may affect case–control studies include recall bias and selection bias. Cross-sectional studies may be confounded by a cohort effect whereby subjects with different ages may have different temporally influenced characteristics (e.g. with respect to experiencing epidemics at different ages or different sociocultural attitudes). Longitudinal studies are ones in which a cohort of subjects are followed up over time; they may be prospective, retrospective (here, information bias may pose a problem), or indeed of mixed design (in which the selection process is made on the basis of a retrospective study, which is then followed by a prospective study of the selected subjects). Confounding variables that might affect longitudinal studies may include a history effect (in which an effect is incorrectly attributed to the age of the subjects), a morbidity effect (with increasing levels of certain illnesses occurring with age), a mortality effect (with the effect of death leading to fewer subjects over time in the cohort), or a practice/testing effect (because subjects will already have experienced taking part in the testing earlier in the study, leading to learning). Furthermore, a Darwinian-type survival of the fittest effect may occur in a longitudinal study whereby the fittest subjects survive over time, so that some of the characteristics of the subjects who have survived to the last part of the study may be markedly different from those of the subjects generally who were alive at the start of the study.

In a crossover design, the subjects act as their own controls. For example, in a placebo-controlled double crossover trial with two arms, at the time of crossover, the subjects who had been receiving the placebo during the first part of the study now cross over to the active treatment, while the subjects who had been receiving the active treatment now cross over to the placebo. In contrast, in a placebo-controlled single crossover trial with two arms, at the time of crossover, the subjects who had been receiving the placebo during the first part of the study now cross over to the active treatment, while the subjects who had receiving the active treatment continue to receive the active treatment for the rest of the duration of the trial. A trial is double-blind if both the subjects and the observers are blinded to group allocation.

Table 23.1 compares and contrasts the strengths and weaknesses of different designs.

23.1.2 HIERARCHY OF EVIDENCE

See Chapter 21.

23.1.3 SELECTION PROCESS

The stages in the selection process for recruitment into a randomized clinical trial are shown in Figure 23.1.

Many major medical and scientific journals now require the reporting of the results of a randomized interventional trial to follow the CONSORT guidelines. CONSORT stands for Consolidated Standards of Reporting Trials. Such a report should include a CONSORT diagram, as shown in Figure 23.2.

23.2 CLINICAL TRIALS

23.2.1 DEFINITION

Clinical trials are planned experiments carried out on humans to assess the effectiveness of different forms of treatment.

TABLE 23.1

Comparing Design Strengths and Weaknesses

Parameter	Cross-Sectional Surveys	Case–Control Studies	Prospective Cohort Studies	RCTs
Cost	Low	Low	High	High
Setup	Quick and easy	Quick and easy	Complex	Complex
Recall bias	Low	High	Low	Low
Rare diseases	Impractical	Practical	Impractical	Practical
Rare exposures	Impractical	Disadvantage	Advantage	Deliberate
Long disease course	NA	Advantage	Disadvantage	NA
Diseases with latency	NA	Advantage	Disadvantage	NA
Follow-up period	None	Short	Long	Specified
Attrition rate	NA	Low	High	Moderate
Estimate incidence	NA	Poor	Good	NA
Estimate prognosis	NA	Fair	Good	NA
Examine several possible risks	NA	Good	Impractical	Impractical
Examine several possible outcomes	NA	Impractical	Good	NA
Inference to target population	Strong	Less strong	Strong	Strong

Source: Ajetunmobi, O., *Making Sense of Critical Appraisal*, Arnold, London, U.K., 2002, p. 59, Table 2.1.
Note: RCTs, randomized clinical trials; NA, not applicable.

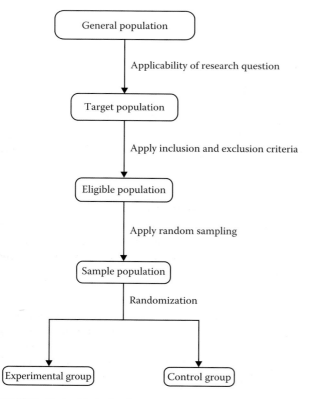

FIGURE 23.1 The selection process. (From Ajetunmobi, O., *Making Sense of Critical Appraisal*, Arnold, London, U.K., 2002, p. 61, Figure 2.2.)

23.2.2 CLASSIFICATION

The following classification of clinical trials is used by the pharmaceutical industry:

- Phase I trial—clinical pharmacology and toxicity
- Phase II trial—initial clinical investigation
- Phase III trial—full-scale treatment evaluation
- Phase IV trial—postmarketing surveillance

23.2.3 ADVANTAGES OF RANDOMIZED TRIALS

In a randomized trial, all the subjects have the same probability of receiving each of the different forms of treatment being compared. The advantages of such randomization include the following:

- The effects of concomitant variables are distributed in a random manner between the comparison groups; these variables may be unknown.
- The allocation of subjects is not carried out in a subjective manner influenced by the biases of the investigators.
- Statistical tests used to analyse the results are on a firm foundation as they are based on what is expected to occur in random samples from parent populations having specified characteristics.

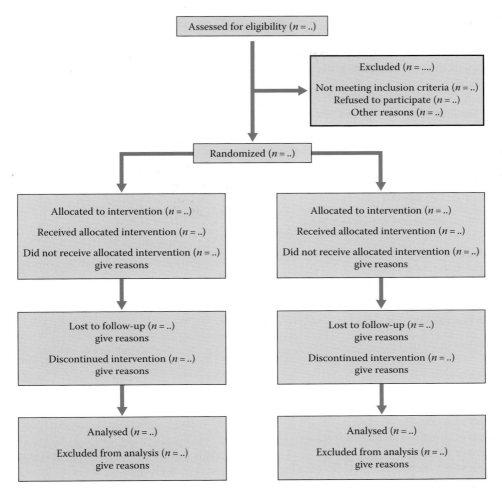

FIGURE 23.2 Example of a CONSORT diagram for an individually randomized trial. (From Stahl, D. and Leese, M., Research methods and statistics, in: *Psychiatry: An Evidence-Based* Text, Puri, B.K. and Treasaden, I.H. (eds.), Hodder Arnold, London, U.K., 2010, p. 39, Figure 4.3.)

The gold standard of clinical trials is the randomized double-blind controlled trial in which

- Allocation of treatments to subjects is randomized
- Each subject does not know which treatment has been received by him or her
- The investigator(s) does not know the treatment allocation before the end of the trial

23.2.4 DISADVANTAGES OF NON-RANDOMIZED TRIALS

Non-randomized trials may have concurrent or historical (i.e. nonconcurrent) controls. Both types of non-randomized trials have associated disadvantages in comparison with randomized trials.

23.2.4.1 Concurrent Controls

It is not usually possible to confirm that the different treatment groups are comparable. Volunteer bias may also occur, with volunteers faring better than those who refuse to participate in a trial.

23.2.4.2 Historical Controls

Here the control group consists of a group previously given an older/alternative treatment. This group is compared with suitable subjects receiving a new treatment being tested. Disadvantages of using historical controls include the following:

- It cannot be assumed that everything apart from the new treatment being tested has remained unchanged over time.

- The monitoring and care of current subjects receiving the new treatment are likely to be greater than was that of the historical controls.
- The efficacy of the new treatment is likely to be overestimated.
- The findings of such a trial may be not be widely accepted because of the lack of randomization.

23.3 PROBLEMS OF MEASUREMENT IN PSYCHIATRY

23.3.1 AIMS OF MEASUREMENT

The main aims of measurement in psychiatry are

- To help in the diagnostic process or in other forms of categorization
- To measure symptomatology ± its change

23.3.2 PROBLEMS OF MEASUREMENT

Problems in measurement in psychiatry include

- Defining caseness
- Assessment of behaviour
- Assessment of cognitive performance
- Assessment of mood
- Assessment of delusions and hallucinations
- Assessment of personality
- Assessment of psychophysiological functioning
- Assessing the degree to which an individual suffers from a psychiatric/psychological disorder

23.3.3 MEASUREMENT METHODS

A range of measurement methods can be employed in psychiatric/psychological assessments. Examples include

- Observer-rated scales—structured and semi-structured standardized psychiatric interview schedules
- Screening instruments
- Behavioural observation studies
- Self-predictions
- Self-recording—for example, diaries
- Self-rating scales for the assessment of mood
- Self-rating scales for the assessment of personality
- Psychophysiological techniques
- Naturalistic observations
- Psychometric measurements—for example, of intelligence and personality

23.3.4 LATENT TRAITS (CONSTRUCTS)

Psychological concepts such as attitude and intelligence are considered to be latent traits or hypothetical constructs that are believed to exist. Although not directly observable, constructs can be used to explain phenomena that can be observed and to make predictions. In the development and use of psychometric tests, in particular, factor analysis may be used to identify factors, corresponding to latent traits or hypothetical constructs, that may account for correlations observed between the scores on tests or subtests by a large sample of subjects.

23.3.5 RELIABILITY

23.3.5.1 Definition

The reliability of a test or measuring instrument describes the level of agreement between repeated measurements. It can be expressed as the ratio of the variance of the true scores to the variance of the observed scores:

$$\text{Reliability} = \frac{\sigma_t^2}{\sigma_t^2 + \sigma_e^2}$$

where
σ_t^2 is the true score variance
σ_e^2 is the measurement error variance

With this definition, the range of values that the reliability can take is given by

$$0 \le \text{reliability} \le 1$$

A low value, close to zero, implies low reliability, while a high value, close to one, implies high reliability.

23.3.5.2 Interrater Reliability

Interrater reliability describes the level of agreement between assessments of the same material made by two or more assessors at roughly the same time.

23.3.5.3 Intrarater Reliability

Intrarater reliability describes the level of agreement between assessments made by two or more assessors of the same material presented at two or more times.

23.3.5.4 Test–Retest Reliability

Test–retest reliability describes the level of agreement between assessments of the same material made under similar circumstances but at two different times.

23.3.5.5 Alternative Forms Reliability

Alternative forms reliability describes the level of agreement between assessments of the same material by two supposedly similar forms of the test or measuring instrument made either at the same time or immediately consecutively.

23.3.5.6 Split-Half Reliability

Split-half reliability describes the level of agreement between assessments by two-halves of a split test or measuring instrument of the same material made under similar circumstances. Since some tests or measuring instruments contain different sections measuring different aspects, in such cases, it may be appropriate to create the halves by using alternative questions, thereby maintaining the balance of each half.

23.3.6 STATISTICAL TESTS OF RELIABILITY

23.3.6.1 Percentage Agreement

Measuring the percentage agreement is the simplest but most unsatisfactory method of assessing the reliability, since it does not take into account agreement between observers owing to chance.

23.3.6.2 Product–Moment Correlation Coefficient

The product–moment correlation coefficient, r, may give spuriously high results, particularly if there is chance agreement of many values. It may even give the maximum value of one for the agreement between two raters, even if they do not agree at all, if, for example, one of the raters consistently rates scores on the test or measuring instrument at twice the values rated by the other rater.

23.3.6.3 Kappa Statistic

The kappa statistic, or kappa coefficient, κ, is a measure of agreement in which allowance is made for chance agreement. It is most appropriate when different categories of measurement are being recorded and are calculated from the following formula:

$$k = \frac{P_o - P_c}{1 - P_c}$$

where
  P_c is the chance agreement
  P_o is the observed proportion of agreement

The range of values that κ can take is

- $\kappa = 1$: complete agreement
- $0 < \kappa < 1$: observed agreement > chance agreement
- $\kappa = 0$: observed agreement = chance agreement
- $\kappa < 0$: observed agreement < chance agreement

The weighted kappa, κ_w, is a version of κ that takes into account differences in the seriousness of disagreements (represented by the weightings).

23.3.6.4 Intraclass Correlation Coefficient

The intraclass correlation coefficient, r_i, is more appropriate than κ or r if agreement is being measured for several items that can be regarded as part of a continuum or dimension. For two raters, the value of r_i is derived from the corresponding value of r:

$$r_i = \frac{\left\{\left[\sum\left(s_1^2 + s_2^2\right) - \left(s_1 - s_2\right)^2\right]r - \left(\bar{x}_1 - \bar{x}_2\right)^2 / 2\right\}}{\left\{\left(s_1^2 + s_2^2\right) + \left(\bar{x}_1 - \bar{x}_2\right)^2 / 2\right\}}$$

where
  r is the product–moment correlation coefficient between the scores of the two raters
  s_1 is the standard deviation of the scores for the first rater
  s_2 is the standard deviation of the scores for the second rater
  $\bar{x}_1$ is the mean of the scores for the first rater
  $\bar{x}_2$ is the mean of the scores for the second rater

It follows that

if $\bar{x}_1 = \bar{x}_2$ and $s_1 = s_2$
then $r_i = r$
else $r_i < r$

For more than two raters, the value of r_i is derived from the corresponding two-way ANOVA for (raters × subjects):

$$r_i = \frac{n_s\left(s_{ms} - e_{ms}\right)}{n_s s_{ms} + n_r r_{ms} + \left(n_s n_r - n_s - n_r\right)e_{ms}}$$

where
  n_r is the number of raters
  n_s is the number of subjects
  e_{ms} is the error mean square
  r_{ms} is the raters mean square
  s_{ms} is the subjects mean square

23.3.6.5 Cronbach's Alpha

Cronbach's alpha, α, gives a measure of the average correlation between all the items when assessing split-half reliability. It thereby indicates the internal consistency of the test or measuring instrument.

23.3.7 VALIDITY

23.3.7.1 Definition

The validity of a test or measuring instrument is the term used to describe whether it measures what it purports to measure.

23.3.7.2 Face Validity

Face validity is the subjective judgement as to whether a test or measuring instrument appears on the surface to measure the feature in question. In spite of its name, it is not strictly a type of validity.

23.3.7.3 Content Validity

Content validity examines whether the specific measurements aimed for by the test or measuring instrument are assessing the content of the measurement in question.

23.3.7.4 Predictive Validity

Predictive validity determines the extent of agreement between a present measurement and one in the future.

23.3.7.5 Concurrent Validity

Concurrent validity compares the measure being assessed with an external valid yardstick at the same time.

23.3.7.6 Criterion Validity

Criterion validity refers to predictive and concurrent validity together.

23.3.7.7 Incremental Validity

Incremental validity indicates whether the measurement being assessed is superior to other measurements in approaching true validity.

23.3.7.8 Cross-Validity

Cross-validation of a test or measuring instrument is used to determine whether, after having its criterion validity established for one sample, it maintains criterion validity when applied to another sample.

23.3.7.9 Convergent Validity

Convergent validity is established when measures expected to be correlated, since they measure the same phenomena, are indeed found to be associated.

23.3.7.10 Divergent Validity

Divergent validity is established when measures discriminate successfully between other measures of unrelated constructs.

23.3.7.11 Construct Validity

Construct validity is determined by establishing both convergent and divergent validity and is closely connected with the theoretical rationale underpinning the test or measuring instrument. It involves showing the power of the hypothetical construct(s) or latent traits both to explain observations and to make predictions.

23.3.8 TYPE I ERROR

A type I error is the error of wrongly rejecting H_0 when it is true. As mentioned earlier, the probability of making a type I error is denoted by α, the significance level:

$$\alpha = P(\text{type I error})$$

23.3.9 TYPE II ERROR

A type II error is the error of wrongly accepting H_0 when it is false. The probability of making a type II error is denoted by β:

$$\beta = P(\text{type II error})$$

23.3.10 POWER

The power of a test is the probability that H_0 is rejected when it is indeed false. It is related to β, the probability of making a type II error, in the following way:

$$\text{Power} = 1 - \beta$$

23.3.11 SENSITIVITY

The sensitivity of a test or measuring instrument is the proportion of positive results/cases correctly identified:

$$\text{Sensitivity} = \frac{\text{True positive}}{\text{True positive} + \text{False negative}}$$

This ratio needs to be multiplied by 100 if the sensitivity is to be given as a percentage.

23.3.12 SPECIFICITY

The specificity of a test or measuring instrument is the proportion of negative results/cases correctly identified:

$$\text{Specificity} = \frac{\text{True negative}}{\text{True negative} + \text{False positive}}$$

This ratio needs to be multiplied by 100 if the sensitivity is to be given as a percentage.

23.3.13 ROC CURVE

The receiver operating characteristic, or ROC, curve for a test is a plot of sensitivity versus $(1 - \text{specificity})$, as shown in Figure 23.3. This figure shows that the closest point on the ROC curve to the ideal state is the best compromise between sensitivity and specificity for the test. The area under the ROC curve represents how accurate the test is, that is, the probability of identifying true positives and true negatives correctly.

23.3.14 PREDICTIVE VALUES

The predictive value of a positive result from a research measure is the proportion of the positive results that is true positive:

Predictive value of a positive result

$$= \frac{\text{True positive}}{\text{True positive} + \text{False positive}}$$

The predictive value of a negative result from a research measure is the proportion of the negative results that is true negative:

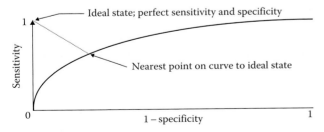

FIGURE 23.3 The ROC plot. (From Ajetunmobi, O., *Making Sense of Critical Appraisal*, Arnold, London, U.K., 2002, p. 74, Figure 3.1.)

Predictive value of a negative result

$$= \frac{\text{True negative}}{\text{True negative} + \text{False negative}}$$

23.3.15 LIKELIHOOD RATIOS

Likelihood ratios for tests are derived from their sensitivity and specificity values. For tests in which the result is binary (positive or negative), likelihood ratios are calculated as follows:

$$\text{Likelihood ratio for a positive result} = \frac{\text{Sensitivity}}{1 - \text{Specificity}}$$

$$\text{Likelihood ratio for a negative result} = \frac{1 - \text{Sensitivity}}{\text{Specificity}}$$

Note also the following relationships between the odds ratio (see Chapter 21) and the likelihood ratio:

$$\text{Posttest odds} = \text{Pretest odds} \times \text{Likelihood ratio}$$

where
  Pretest odds = (pretest probability)/(1 − pretest probability)
  Note that posttest probability = (posttest odds)/(posttest odds + 1)

23.3.16 BIAS

23.3.16.1 Selection Bias

Selection bias occurs when a characteristic associated with the variable(s) of interest leads to higher or lower participation in the research study, such as an epidemiological cross-sectional survey.

23.3.16.2 Observer Bias

In epidemiological studies, observer bias occurs when the researcher has clues about whether the subject is in the case or comparison group, leading to a biased assessment. This is particularly likely in studies involving retrospective assessments.

23.3.16.3 Recall Bias

In epidemiological studies, recall bias occurs when there is a difference in knowledge between the subjects in the case and in the comparison groups, leading to a biased recall.

For example, in case–control studies, the knowledge on the part of subjects (or, in the case of childhood disorders, their parents) as to whether or not they have a given disorder may bias their recall of exposure to putative risk factors.

23.3.16.4   Information bias

Information bias includes both observer bias and recall bias.

23.3.16.5   Confounding bias

In epidemiological studies, confounding bias occurs when the actual, but unexamined, underlying cause of the disorder being researched is associated with both the suspected risk factor and the disorder.

BIBLIOGRAPHY

Ajetunmobi O. 2002: *Making Sense of Critical Appraisal.* London, U.K.: Arnold.

Altman DG. 1991: *Practical Statistics for Medical Research.* London, U.K.: Chapman & Hall.

Bryman A and Cramer D. 1994: *Quantitative Data Analysis for Social Scientists*, revised edition. London, U.K.: Routledge.

Dunn G and Everitt B. 1995: *Clinical Biostatistics: An Introduction to Evidence-Based Medicine.* London, U.K.: Arnold.

Everitt B and Hay D. 1992: *Talking about Statistics: A Psychologist's Guide to Design and Analysis.* London, U.K.: Arnold.

Stahl D and Leese M. 2010: Research methods and statistics. In Puri BK and Treasaden IH (eds.) *Psychiatry: An Evidence-Based Text*, p. 39. London, U.K.: Hodder Arnold.

24 Physical Therapies

24.1 NEUROSTIMULATION THERAPIES

Neurostimulation therapies are physical interventions that treat psychiatric disorders through delivery of electric current or magnetic field.

The following four types of neurostimulation therapies are currently used in psychiatry:

1. Electroconvulsive therapy (ECT)
2. Repetitive transcranial magnetic stimulation (rTMS)
3. Vagus nerve stimulation (VNS)
4. Deep brain stimulation (DBS)

24.2 ELECTROCONVULSIVE THERAPY

The following are key historical points in the development of ECT:

- During the early twentieth century, it was hypothesized that schizophrenia and epilepsy are more or less mutually exclusive disorders.
- In 1934, Meduna, on the basis of this hypothesis, attempted to treat schizophrenia by inducing seizures chemically.
- In 1938, Cerletti and Bini induced seizures electrically.

24.2.1 ECT INDICATIONS AND CONTRAINDICATIONS

24.2.1.1 Indications for ECT

The National Institute for Health and Clinical Excellence (NICE) guidelines recommended that ECT be used only to achieve rapid and short-term improvement of severe symptoms after an adequate trial of other treatment options has proven ineffective and/or when the condition is considered to be potentially life-threatening in individuals with the following:

Depression

- Severe depressive illness: 60%–80% remission rate; maximum response typically attained after 2–4 weeks; relapse rate without maintenance antidepressant treatment after ECT is 50%–95%.

- Life-threatening depression: refusal to eat.
- Depression with strong suicidal ideation.
- Psychotic depression.
- Stupor.
- Puerperal depressive illness: the use of ECT during pregnancy is known to cause complications, but the risks associated with ECT need to be balanced against the risks of using pharmacological treatments.

Mania

- Prolonged manic episode
- Treatment-resistant mania with life-threatening physical exhaustion

Schizophrenia

- Catatonic schizophrenia
- Schizoaffective disorder
- Treatment-resistant schizophrenia

Other indications

- Affective symptoms in Parkinson's disease
- Neuroleptic malignant syndrome

24.2.1.2 Contraindications against ECT

Raised intracranial pressure is an absolute contraindication to ECT. Relative contraindications include

- Cerebral aneurysm
- Recent cerebrovascular accident
- Recent myocardial infarction
- Cardiac arrhythmia
- Intracerebral haemorrhage
- Acute/impending retinal detachment
- Phaeochromocytoma
- Raised anaesthetic risk
- Sickle cell disease
- Unstable vascular aneurysm or malformation

24.2.1.3   Medications to Avoid before ECT

- Benzodiazepines have anticonvulsant activity. If there is a need for benzodiazepine before ECT, choose a short-acting benzodiazepine such as alprazolam and lorazepam.
- Lithium may result in postictal delirium and confusion.

24.3   PREPARATION FOR ECT

According to the NICE guidelines, the decision as to whether ECT is clinically indicated should be based on a documented assessment of the risks and potential benefits to the patient, including

- The risks associated with the anaesthesia
- Current comorbidities
- Anticipated adverse events, particularly cognitive impairment
- The risk of not having ECT

Pre-ECT assessment and investigations

- Review psychiatric history, medical history, drug history, and previous ECT record (to check the previous electric stimulus and response).
- Perform a physical examination with special focus on cardiovascular, respiratory, and neurological systems.
- Baseline MMSE is required for old people.
- Assess the patient's dentition, especially for old people or people who have poor dental care.
- Order full blood count (FBC), urea and electrolytes (U&E), and liver function tests (LFT).
- Order ECG and chest x-ray (CXR) for patients who are older than 45 years.
- Consult an anaesthetist for preanaesthesia assessment.
- Consult a cardiologist if there is cardiovascular risk.
- Order an x-ray for spine if there is evidence of a spinal cord disorder.
- Perform CT or MRI if neurological sign is present.
- A patient receiving ECT in the morning should remain 'nil by mouth' from the previous midnight.

Consent

The NICE guidelines recommend the following:

- *Autonomy*: Valid consent should be obtained in all cases in which the individual has the ability to grant or refuse consent. Consent should be obtained without pressure or coercion, which may occur as a result of the circumstances and clinical setting.
- *Nonmaleficence*: Prior to obtaining consent for ECT, the psychiatrist must ensure that ECT is indeed indicated, and the patient has the capacity to give consent.
- *Partnership*: The decision to use ECT should be made jointly by the individual and the clinician(s) responsible for treatment, on the basis of an informed discussion. The involvement of patient advocates and/or carers to facilitate informed discussion is strongly encouraged.
- *Education*: This discussion should be enabled by the provision of full and appropriate information about the general risks associated with ECT and about the risks and potential benefits specific to that individual. The psychiatrist must ensure the patient understands the information provided and address any question that the patient may have.
- *Right to withdrawal*: The individual should be reminded of his or her right to withdraw consent at any point during the course of ECT.
- *Second opinion*: The psychiatrist should be prepared to offer the patient access to a second opinion, should the patient request it.
- *Advance directives:* In all situations in which informed discussion and consent is not possible, advance directives should be taken fully into account, and the individual's advocate and/or carer should be consulted.

24.4   ADMINISTRATION OF ECT

Bilateral and unilateral ECT

Electrode placement

- In unilateral ECT, the electrodes are placed on the nondominant cerebral hemisphere. The nondominant cerebral hemisphere should be on the right side of the head for all right-handed people and most left-handed people. Stimulating the nondominant hemisphere reduces the risk of cognitive side effects as compared to stimulation of dominant hemisphere (Figure 24.1).
- In bilateral ECT, both cerebral hemispheres are stimulated.

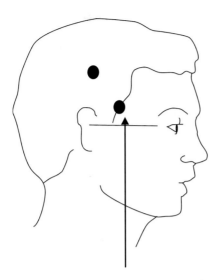 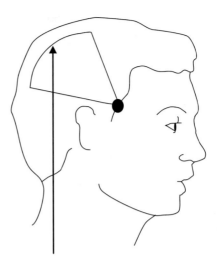

First electrode: 4 cm above the
midpoint of lateral angle of eye and
external auditory meatus

Second electrode or d'Elia
positioning: second electrode is
placed in the midpoint of the arc.
The radius of arc is around 18 cm.

FIGURE 24.1   Positioning of electrodes in unilateral ECT.

Dosing/electric stimulus

- Seizure threshold increases with age (Table 24.1). To determine seizure threshold, the psychiatrist can use age-based dosing method. The formula is as follows: Dose in energy = Age divided by 2.
- For example, a 40-year-old woman requires ECT. The initial dose is 40/2 = 20 J based in the age-based dosing method. The patient has no seizure at 20 J but has a seizure at 30 J. The psychiatrist knows that the seizure threshold is between 20 and 30 J. Then the psychiatrist takes an average by (20 + 30 J)/2 = 25 J. For unilateral ECT, the psychiatrist multiplies by 1.5 (i.e. increase by 50%) to get 37.5 J. For bilateral ECT, the psychiatrist can add 5 J to the average value (i.e. 25 J) and starts at 30 J. If the seizure duration reduces in the subsequent ECT, the psychiatrist can increase by 5 J during each session.
- Unilateral ECT requires suprathreshold stimulus. The electric stimulus has to exceed the seizure threshold by 25%–100%.
- Bilateral ECT requires a barely suprathreshold doses. The electric stimulus is just exceeding the seizure threshold.

Other stimulus parameters

The assessment report (NICE guidelines) provides data that the stimulus parameters have an important influence on efficacy (Figure 24.2).

The energy is determined by four stimulus parameters (current, stimulus duration, frequency of the pulse, and pulse width). In order to increase effectiveness, the psychiatrist can consider changing the stimulus parameters in the following order:

1. Increase stimulus duration
2. Increase the frequency
3. Increase pulse width

The current usually remains the same.

TABLE 24.1

Factors Associated with Increase or Decrease of Seizure Threshold

Increase in Seizure Threshold/ Decrease in Duration of Seizure	Decrease in Seizure Threshold/ Increase in Duration of Seizure
- Male gender	- Caffeine
- Baldness	- Low carbon dioxide saturation of blood
- Paget's disease	- Hyperventilation
- Dehydration	- Theophylline
- Previous ECT	
- Benzodiazepine	

```
% Energy Set.................. 20 %
Charge Delivered.............. 102.2 mC
Current....................... 0.91 A
Stimulus Duration............. 1.9 Sec
Frequency..................... 30 Hz
Pulse Width................... 1.00 mSec
Static Impedance.............. 2740 Ohm
Dynamic Impedance............. 300 Ohm
EEG Endpoint.................. 46 Sec
EMG Endpoint.................. N/A
Base Heart Rate............... N/A
Peak Heart Rate............... N/A
Average Seizure Energy Index.. 8334.4 µV2
Postictal Suppression Index... 68.1 %
Maximum Sustained Power....... 15554.3 µV2
Time to Peak Power............ 23 Sec
Maximum Sustained Coherence... 85.5 %
Time to Peak Coherence........ 37 Sec
```

FIGURE 24.2   Other stimulus parameters and usual values.

Frequency of session and total number of treatment

1. The usual frequency is twice a week for a total of 6–12 ECT sessions.
2. There is no difference in efficacy between twice a week and three times a week.
3. Maintenance ECT: The frequency ranges from once per week to once per month. Indications of maintenance ECT include
   a. Frequent relapse and recurrence of depressive episodes
   b. History of responsiveness to maintenance ECT
   c. Patient preference
   d. Resistance to or intolerance of antidepressants

Bilateral ECT versus unilateral ECT

- When deciding bilateral or unilateral ECT, there are two issues to consider: memory impairment and effectiveness.

Memory impairment

- Bilateral ECT is associated with greater memory impairment as compared to unilateral ECT.
- Bilateral ECT has better efficacy. As a result, bilateral ECT is preferred when there is a treatment urgency (e.g. patients with high suicide risk) or when unilateral ECT fails.

TABLE 24.2

Classification of Duration of Seizure

Duration of Seizure	Type of Seizure
0 s	Missed seizure: There is no seizure activity following delivery of electric stimulus. The psychiatrist is advised to ensure there are good electrode contacts and the ECT machine demonstrates normal operation. The psychiatrist can restimulate at 25% of higher dose after 10 s
<15 s	Short seizure: The psychiatrist is advised to increase the energy level by 25% in the next ECT session and not to restimulate to prevent prolonged seizure
25–75 s	Normal seizure: satisfactory response
>120 s	Prolonged seizure: The anaesthetist may need to abort the prolonged seizure

Effectiveness (Table 24.2)

- The effectiveness of ECT is determined by the electrode placement and stimulus intensity. Bilateral ECT was reported to be more effective than unilateral ECT.
- A barely suprathreshold unilateral ECT is ineffective. Raising the electric stimulus above the individual's seizure threshold was found to increase the effectiveness of unilateral ECT at the expense of increased cognitive impairment.
- For bilateral ECT, barely suprathreshold stimuli are effective and reduce the risk of memory impairment. The speed of clinical response can be achieved by increasing the stimulus intensity.

Monitoring during ECT

- Pulse oximetry monitors blood oxygen saturation.
- ECG monitors heart rhythm.
- EEG measures electric brain activity.
- EMG measures motor seizure activity.

Anaesthesia

1. A muscle relaxant (succinylcholine) is administered in order to prevent violent movements during the convulsion.
2. Fasciculation goes from head to toes when succinylcholine takes effect. Fasciculation usually occurs 60–120 s after injection.

3. Atropine is administered in order to reduce secretions and prevent the muscarinic actions of the muscle relaxant. Anticholinergic agent also prevents bradycardia after the seizure.

4. If there is any possibility that the patient may have low or atypical plasma pseudocholinesterase enzymes, the anaesthetist must be informed as this could lead to prolonged muscle paralysis with the muscle relaxant.

5. Bilateral or unilateral (to the nondominant cerebral hemisphere) ECT is administered under a short-acting general anaesthetic.

   a. Thiopentone increases seizure threshold and causes cardiovascular depression and apnoea. Thiopentone is commonly used.

   b. Propofol may shorten seizure.

   c. Ketamine is associated with the risk of hallucinations, tachycardia, hypertension, and decreases seizure threshold. It is not commonly used.

6. A mouthpiece is placed in the patient's mouth in order to prevent damage from biting during the convulsion.

7. Vagal tone is increased during and immediately after administration of the electric stimulus. The patient may develop bradycardia.

8. The sympathetic nervous system is activated during the seizure, and there is a significant increase in heart rate, blood pressure, and cardiac output.

9. Shortly after the seizure, there may be another period of increased vagal tone. The patient may develop bradycardia and bradyarrhythmias.

10. There may be another period of increased sympathetic tone when the patient awakens from the anaesthesia.

Interpretation of EEG strip (Figures 24.3 and 24.4)

The NICE guidelines recommend that clinical status should be assessed following each ECT session and treatment should be stopped when a response has been achieved or sooner if there is evidence of adverse effects. Cognitive function should be monitored on an ongoing basis and at a minimum at the end of each course of treatment.

The NICE guidelines also recommend that a repeat course of ECT should be considered only for individuals who have severe depressive illness, catatonia, or mania and who have previously responded well to ECT. In patients who are experiencing an acute episode but have not previously responded, a repeat trial of ECT should be undertaken only after all other options have been considered and following discussion of the risks and benefits with the individual and/or where appropriate the carer/advocate.

24.4.1 SIDE EFFECTS OF ECT

The rate of adverse events after ECT is 0.4%.
The main early side effects include

- Headache
- Myalgia
- Nausea
- Dental damage or oral lacerations
- Musculoskeletal injuries
- Temporary confusion after ECT

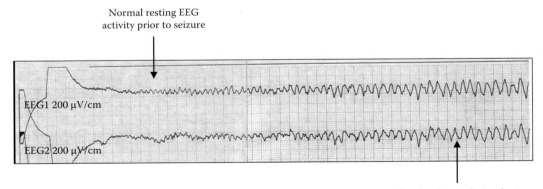

Normal resting EEG activity prior to seizure

EEG1 200 µV/cm

EEG2 200 µV/cm

After the electrical stimulus is given, a seizure is initiated. The EEG shows low voltage, fast activity, and polyspike rhythms

FIGURE 24.3   EEG—at the initiation of seizure.

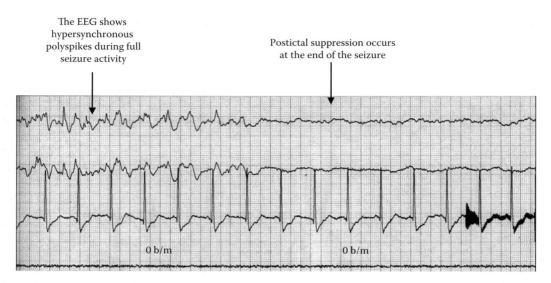

The EEG shows hypersynchronous polyspikes during full seizure activity

Postictal suppression occurs at the end of the seizure

0 b/m   0 b/m

FIGURE 24.4   EEG—at the termination of seizure.

Risk factors for post-ECT confusion

1. Bilateral ECT
2. Coadministration of anticholinergics and lithium
3. Old age
4. Underlying cognitive impairment

Strategies to prevent post-ECT confusion

1. Avoid anticholinergics and lithium before ECT.
2. Reduce pulse width.
3. Reduce the dose of electric stimulus.
4. Reduce the frequency of ECT sessions.
5. Use unilateral ECT instead bilateral ECT.

Memory impairment

- Anterograde (forgetting of events after the seizure) and retrograde amnesia (forgetting of events prior to the seizure) may occur after ECT.
- Retrograde amnesia of events immediately preceding ECT treatments may be permanent. Risk factors for retrograde amnesia include bilateral ECT, high dose of electric stimulus, and post-ECT confusion.
- Anterograde amnesia is usually transient. It usually manifests as forgetfulness regarding events that happened after the ECT treatment or misplacing belongings after ECT. Anterograde amnesia usually resolves in 6 months.

- A small number of patients experience long-lasting subjective memory impairment, which is not detected objectively by cognitive assessment.

Outcome of memory loss

- Some specific memories of events immediately before and after ECT are lost permanently.
- There is some limited evidence from RCTs to suggest that the effects on memory may not last beyond 6 months, but this has been inadequately researched.

ECT may cause depressed patients with bipolar mood disorder to become manic.

24.5   COMPLICATIONS OF ECT

A complication rate of 1 per 1400 treatments and most complications resolve without intervention.
    Complications include

- Cardiac arrhythmia
- Circulatory insufficiency
- Laryngospasm
- Prolonged apnoea
- Prolonged seizures
- Tooth damage

According to assessment report (NICE guidelines), the six reviewed studies that used brain-scanning techniques did not provide any evidence that ECT causes brain damage.

24.6 MORTALITY

- The mortality rate of ECT is 2.0–4.5 deaths per 100,000 ECT.
- There was no evidence to suggest that the mortality associated with ECT is greater than that associated with minor procedures involving general anaesthesia. The majority of deaths are related to cardiorespiratory complications. The mortality rate is higher in patients with impaired cardiac functions.
- Pre-ECT oxygenation, brief anaesthesia, muscular relaxation, and physiological monitoring reduce morbidity and mortality associated with ECT.

24.7 REPETITIVE TRANSCRANIAL MAGNETIC STIMULATION

The use of repetitive transcranial magnetic stimulation (rTMS) is gaining support among psychiatrists as evidence emerges suggesting that it may provide an alternative to ECT in treating depression and other psychiatric disorders.

The following are key historical points in the development of transcranial magnetic stimulation (TMS) and rTMS:

- In 1896, d'Arsonval observed the occurrence of phosphenes and vertigo when a subject's head is put into a coil (driven at 42 Hz) (d'Arsonval et al., 1896).
- In 1959, Kolin and colleagues stimulated the exposed frog sciatic nerve looped around the pole piece of an electromagnet and caused the gastrocnemius to contract (driven at 60 Hz and 1 kHz) (Kolin et al., 1959).
- In 1965, Bickford and Freeming successfully demonstrated noninvasive stimulation of human peripheral nerves (Bickford and Fremming 1965).
- In 1985, Barker (in Sheffield, England) reported the first magnetic stimulation of the human motor cortex (Barker et al., 1985).

24.7.1 INDICATIONS FOR rTMS

At the time of writing, there is evidence that the administration of rTMS to humans may be able to treat:

- Depression
- Poststroke rehabilitation for motor function

In addition, rTMS with appropriate stimulation parameters may result in long-term effects on synaptic efficacy.

24.7.2 MECHANISMS OF rTMS

1. TMS stimulates regions of the cerebral cortex by using a magnetic field generated by an electromagnet placed over the skull to induce electric currents.
2. rTMS delivers rhythmic pulses of electromagnetism. The intensity of rTMS is usually set as a percentage of the patient's motor threshold defined as the minimum stimulus strength required to evoke involuntary muscle movements in the hand.

24.7.3 EFFICACY OF rTMS

- Active rTMS shows modest superiority in comparison to sham rTMS in treatment-resistant depression. (Response rate for active rTMS = 25% vs. sham rTSM = 9%; remission rate for active rTMS = 17% vs. sham rTMS = 6%) (Rossini et al., 2005; Rumi et al., 2005; Fitzgerald et al., 2008).
- The combination of rTMS and antidepressant may accelerate treatment response.
- MRI can provide neuronavigation technique that is used to guide specific site on the dorsolateral prefrontal cortex (DLPFC), and this will enhance response to rTMS.

24.8 SIDE EFFECTS

Side effects of rTMS include local discomfort, headache, and the risk of developing hypomania and seizure.

24.8.1 ECT VERSUS rTMS/MST

ECT is compared with rTMS in Table 24.3.

TABLE 24.3

A Comparison of ECT with rTMS

	ECT	rTMS
Anaesthesia	Required	Not required
Seizure	Required	Not required
Treatment frequency	2–3 per week	Every day
Occurrence of amnesia	Yes	No
Focality	Relatively non-focal	More focal
Tissue impedance	Shunting occurs	No shunting
Pulse width	0.5–2 ms	0.2 ms

24.9   VAGAL NERVE STIMULATION

Vagal nerve stimulation (VNS) is generally carried out by surgically implanting a vagus nerve stimulator (a pulse generator) into the subcutaneous tissues of the upper left chest in order to deliver pulsed electric stimulation to the cervical vagal trunk. VNS is of particular use in the treatment of epilepsy.

The first use of VNS in humans was by Penry and Dean (published in 1990) for the prevention of partial seizures. Later, a neurocybernetic prosthesis implant was used in a patient with depression at the Medical University of South Carolina (Charleston, the United States).

24.9.1   INDICATIONS FOR VNS

There are two major indications for VNS:

- Epilepsy
- Treatment-resistant depression

The rationale for using VNS in treatment-resistant depression is based partly on the following findings:

- VNS has been found to reduce depressive symptoms in epileptic patients.
- Limbic blood flow is altered by VNS.
- CSF monoamine concentrations are altered by VNS.
- Antiepileptic drugs may affect mood.

Preliminary results with VNS appear to support its efficacy in treatment-resistant depression (Rush et al., 2000).

Patient selection and management should be offered jointly by a psychiatrist and a neurosurgeon.

The NICE guidelines recommend that VNS can only be used after informing the clinical governance leads in the respective trusts in the United Kingdom.

24.9.2   MECHANISMS OF ACTIONS

VNS is carried out under general anaesthesia. An incision is made of the left side of the neck, and a stimulator electrode is cuffed around the left vagus nerve.

The vagus nerve is stimulated periodically followed by a period of no stimulus. The stimulation frequency and intensity are programmed in an external electronic control.

24.9.3   EFFICACY OF VNS

VNS may deliver a delayed antidepressant effect with clinical improvement over several weeks.

In a 10-week randomized controlled trial, the response rate of active VNS was 15% as compared to 10% of sham treatment (Rush et al., 2005b).

In 10-week trial with antidepressant and VNS, the response rate was 30% and remission rate was 15% (Sackeim et al., 2001).

In trails with 1–2 years of VNS treatment, the response rate was between 27% and 46%, and remission rate was between 16% and 29% (Maranegil et al., 2002; Nahas et al., 2005; Nierenberg et al., 2008).

24.9.4   SIDE EFFECTS

Side effects of VNS include dyspnoea, pain, cough, and voice alteration (50%).

24.10   DEEP BRAIN STIMULATION

Deep brain stimulation (DBS) involves stereotactic neurosurgical implantation of electrodes under the MRI guidance. The stimulator is implanted under the chest wall. Three neuroanatomical areas are stimulated:

1. Subgenual cingulated gyrus (Brodmann area 25): Patients who respond early to stimulation of this area are more likely to maintain their response.
2. Nucleus accumbens.
3. Ventral caudate and ventral striatum.

DBS is at an investigational stage, and it may be useful for patients suffering from treatment-resistant depression. Six months after DBS, the response rate is 60% and remission rate is 35% for depression. Twelve months after DBS, the response rate is 55% and remission rate is 33% for depression (Lozano et al., 2008).

24.11   OTHER PHYSICAL THERAPIES

24.11.1   LIGHT THERAPY/PHOTOTHERAPY

This is treatment with high-intensity artificial light and may be used to treat patients suffering from seasonal affective disorder (SAD).

The light boxes used typically emit light of a strength of around 10,000 lux. By comparison, on a sunny day, the level of illumination may reach 100,000 lux, while the home environment may typically be illuminated at around 250 lux. The light spectrum used tends to be balanced but usually with potentially harmful ultraviolet B (UVB) frequencies filtered out.

24.11.1.1 Administration
- For the strength of 2500 lux, the patient is advised to receive light therapy for 2 h every morning.
- The light exposure to eyes is important because the light can alter circadian rhythm. Light therapy reduces melatonin levels.
- Therapeutic effects are seen within a few days, and it usually takes 2 weeks for full therapeutic effect.
- For relapse prevention, the patient is recommended to receive light therapy half an hour a day starting in autumn and continue throughout winter.

24.11.1.2 Efficacy
- Fifty per cent of patients with SAD show clinically significant response to light therapy.

24.11.1.3 Side Effects
- Side effects of light therapy include jumpiness, headache, and nausea (15% of patients).

24.11.2 SLEEP DEPRIVATION

24.11.2.1 Indications
The clinical indications for sleep deprivation in mood disorders include

- As an antidepressant in treatment-resistant patients
- To augment the response to antidepressants
- To hasten the onset of action of antidepressant medication or of lithium
- As a prophylaxis in recurrent mood cycles
- As an aid to diagnosis
- To predict the response to antidepressants or ECT

24.11.2.2 Administration
In total sleep deprivation, the patient is kept awake for 36 h. One variation is late partial sleep deprivation, in which the patient is kept awake from 2 a.m. until 10 p.m. Another variation entails depriving the patient only of rapid-eye-movement (REM) sleep.

24.11.3 PSYCHOSURGERY

The following are key points in the history of psychosurgery:

- From 3000 to 2000 BCE, there is evidence of trepanation.
- In the nineteenth century, Burckhardt removed postcentral, temporal, and frontal cortices from patients.
- In 1910, Pusepp resected fibres between the frontal and parietal lobes in patients with bipolar mood disorder.
- In 1936, Ody resected the right prefrontal lobe of a patient with the so-called childhood-onset schizophrenia.
- In 1935, after learning of the work of Fulton and Jacobsen involving bilateral ablation of the prefrontal cortex in chimpanzees, Moniz carried out human frontal leucotomy (work published in 1936).

24.11.3.1 Indications for Psychosurgery
Psychosurgery is seldom performed in the United Kingdom and is a last-resort treatment in other countries for

- Chronic severe intractable depression
- Chronic severe intractable obsessive–compulsive disorder
- Chronic severe intractable anxiety states

24.11.3.2 Psychosurgery Practise
Current methods for making stereotaxic lesions include

- Electrocautery
- Radioactive yttrium implantation
- Thermocoagulation
- Gamma knife

Some of the specific operations that may be used currently include

- Frontal lobe lesioning
- Cingulotomy
- Capsulotomy
- Subcaudate tractotomy
- Limbic leucotomy

REFERENCES

d'Arsonval A. 1896: Dispositifs pour la mesure des courants alternatifs de toutes fréquences. *C. R. Soc. Biol.(Paris)* 3:450–457.

Barker AT, Jalinous R, and Freeston IL. 1985: Non-invasive magnetic stimulation of human motor cortex. *The Lancet* 325(8437):1106–1107.

Bickford RG and Fremming BD. 1965: Neural stimulation by pulsed magnetic fields in animals and men. *Digest of the Sixth International Conference of Medical Electronics and Biological Engineering*, Abstract 7–6. Tokyo, Japan.

Carney S. and Geddes J. 2003: Electroconvulsive therapy: Recent recommendations are likely to improve standards and uniformity of use. *British Medical Journal* 326:1343–1344.

Cole C and Tobiansky R. 2003: Electroconvulsive therapy: NICE guidance may deny many patients treatment that they might benefit from. *British Medical Journal* 327:621.

Fitzgerald PB, Hoy K, Daskalakis ZJ, and Kulkarni J. 2009: A randomized trial of the anti-depressant effects of low- and high-frequency transcranial magnetic stimulation in treatment-resistant depression. *Depress Anxiety* 26(3):229–234.

Kennedy SH, Milev R, Giacobbe P, Ramasubbu R, Lam RW, Parikh SV, Patten SB, and Ravindran AV, Canadian Network for Mood and Anxiety Treatments (CANMAT). 2009: Canadian Network for Mood and Anxiety Treatments (CANMAT): Clinical guidelines for the management of major depressive disorder in adults. IV. Neurostimulation therapies. *Journal of Affective Disorders* 117(Suppl 1):S44–S53.

Kolin A, Brill NQ, and Broberg PJ. 1959: Stimulation of irritable tissues by means of an alternating magnetic field. *Proceedings of the Society for Experimental Biology and Medicine* 102:251–253.

Lisanby SH and Sackeim HA. 2002: Transcranial magnetic stimulation and electroconvulsive therapy: Similarities and differences. In Pascual-Leone A, Davey, NJ, Rothwell J, Wassermann EM, and Puri BK (eds.) *Handbook of Transcranial Magnetic Stimulation*, pp. 376–395. London, U.K.: Arnold.

Lock T. 1994: Advances in the practice of electroconvulsive therapy. *Advances in Psychiatric Treatment* 1:47–56.

Lozano AM, Mayberg HS, Giacobbe P, Hamani C, Craddock RC, and Kennedy SH. Sep. 15, 2008: Subcallosal cingulate gyrus deep brain stimulation for treatment-resistant depression. *Biological Psychiatry* 64(6):461–467.

Marangell LB, Rush AJ, George MS, Sackeim HA, Johnson CR, Husain MM, Nahas Z, and Lisanby SH. 2002: Vagus nerve stimulation (VNS) for major depressive episodes: One year outcomes. *Biological Psychiatry* 51(4):280–287.

Nahas Z, Marangell LB, Husain MM, Rush AJ, Sackeim HA, Lisanby SH, Martinez JM, and George MS. Sep. 2005: Two-year outcome of vagus nerve stimulation (VNS) for treatment of major depressive episodes. *Journal of Clinical Psychiatry* 66(9):1097–1104.

NICE. *Guidelines on Transcranial Magnetic Stimulation for Severe Depression*. http://guidance.nice.org.uk/IPG242 (accessed 26 July 2012).

NICE. *Guidelines on Vagus Nerve Stimulation for Treatment Resistant Depression*. http://guidance.nice.org.uk/IPG330 (accessed 26 July 2012).

Nierenberg AA, Alpert JE, Gardner-Schuster EE, Seay S, and Mischoulon D. Sep 15 2008: Vagus nerve stimulation: 2-Year outcomes for bipolar versus unipolar treatment-resistant depression. *Biological Psychiatry* 64(6):455–460.

O'Keane V, Dinan TG, Scott L, and Corcoran C. 2005: Changes in hypothalamic-pituitary-adrenal axis measures after vagus nerve stimulation therapy in chronic depression. *Biological Psychiatry* 58(12):963–968. [Epub 7 July 2005].

Pascual-Leone A, Davey NJ, Rothwell J, Wassermann EM, and Puri BK. (eds.) 2002: *Handbook of Transcranial Magnetic Stimulation*. London, U.K.: Arnold.

Penry JK and Dean JC. 1990: Prevention of intractable partial seizures by intermittent vagal stimulation in humans: Preliminary results. *Epilepsia* 31(Suppl 2):S40–S43.

Puri BK, Laking PJ, and Treasaden IH. 2002: *Textbook of Psychiatry*, 2nd edn. Edinburgh, Scotland: Churchill Livingstone.

Rossini D, Lucca A, Zanardi R, Magri L, and Smeraldi E. 2005: Transcranial magnetic stimulation in treatment-resistant depressed patients: A double-blind, placebo-controlled trial. *Journal of Psychiatric Research* 137(1–2):1–10.

Rumi DO, Gattaz WF, Rigonatti SP, Rosa MA, Fregni F, Rosa MO, Mansur C et al. 2005: Transcranial magnetic stimulation accelerates the antidepressant effect of amitriptyline in severe depression: A double-blind placebo-controlled study. *Biological Psychiatry* 57(2):162–166.

Rush AJ, George MS, Sackeim HA et al. 2000: Vagus nerve stimulation (VNS) for treatment-resistant depressions: A multicenter study. *Biological Psychiatry* 47:276–286.

Rush AJ, Marangell LB, Sackeim HA, George MS, Brannan SK, Davis SM, Howland R et al. 2005b: Vagus nerve stimulation for treatment-resistant depression: A randomized, controlled acute phase trial. *Biological Psychiatry* 58(5):347–354.

Rush AJ, Sackeim HA, Marangell LB, George MS, Brannan SK, Davis SM, Lavori P et al. 2005a: Effects of 12 months of vagus nerve stimulation in treatment-resistant depression: A naturalistic study. *Biological Psychiatry* 58(5):355–363.

Sackeim HA, Rush AJ, George MS, Marangell LB, Husain MM, Nahas Z, Johnson CR et al. 2001: Vagus nerve stimulation (VNS) for treatment-resistant depression: Efficacy, side effects, and predictors of outcome. *Neuropsychopharmacology* 25(5):713–728.

Schachter S and Schmidt D. (eds.) 2001: *Vagus Nerve Stimulation*. London, U.K.: Martin Dunitz.

Schlaepfer TE, Frick C, Zobel A, Maier W, Heuser I, Bajbouj M, O'Keane V et al. 2008: Vagus nerve stimulation for depression: Efficacy and safety in a European study. *Psychological Medicine* 38(5):651–661.

Scott AIF. 2005: College guidelines on electroconvulsive therapy: An update for prescribers. *Advances in Psychiatric Treatment* 11:150–156.

Trimble MR. 1996: *Neuropsychiatry*, 2nd edn. Chichester, U.K.: John Wiley.

U.K. ECT Review Group. 2003: Efficacy and safety of electroconvulsive therapy in depressive disorders: A systematic review and meta-analysis. *Lancet* 361(9360): 799–808.

25 Advanced Psychological Process and Treatment

25.1 SUPPORTIVE PSYCHOTHERAPY

25.1.1 OBJECTIVES

1. Maintain and improve self-esteem of the client
2. Improve symptoms
3. Prevent relapse
4. Develop adaptive and reasonable behaviour
5. Set goals and positive thinking
6. Strengthen defences and enhance adaptive capacity

25.1.2 HISTORICAL DEVELOPMENT

1. Supportive psychotherapy is based on psychodynamic therapy because it supports patient's defence mechanisms and explores conscious problems and conflicts.

25.1.3 CHARACTERISTICS

1. Supportive psychotherapy focuses on conscious conflicts but not unconscious conflicts.
2. There is no explicit interpretation of transference in supportive psychotherapy.

25.1.4 INDICATIONS

1. Crisis or common life problems.
2. Acute stress reaction.
3. Adjustment disorder.
4. Client is not ready for more sophisticated form of psychotherapy.
5. Patients with chronic medical illnesses.

25.1.5 CONTRAINDICATIONS

The following are contraindications for supportive psychotherapy. These contraindications also apply to other types of psychotherapy in general:

1. Patient has no motivation for psychotherapy, even the simplest form.
2. Acute or severe organic condition affects the client's ability to communicate (e.g. severe head injury, massive stroke, severe dementia, acute confusional state).
3. Pathological liars, malingerers, and people with psychopathy.
4. Other forms of psychotherapies are more appropriate (e.g. sensate focus therapy for sexual dysfunction, couple therapy for motivated couples who have marital problems).

25.1.6 TECHNIQUES

Open-ended question

- This allows the client to respond in more than one word (e.g. yes or no).
- This also allows the client to take an active role in therapy.
- For example, a therapist can ask, 'What concerns you today?', in the beginning of a session.

Observation

1. Pay attention to nonverbal behaviour, emotions, and other patterns of communication exhibited by the client.

Expression of interest

1. Offer acknowledging statements, 'I am glad that you make an effort to come and share with me about your hardship'.
2. Validate feelings (e.g. 'I can imagine that you have gone through a lot of hardship and people would feel sad in such situation').

Set goals

1. Goals are the desired outcomes of psychotherapy.
2. Goals have to be specific, measurable, realistic, and achievable in a preset time frame.
3. Agree on tasks to reach therapeutic goals.

Establish therapeutic alliance

1. Develop trust and respect between the therapist and the client.
2. Demonstrate empathy.

Affirmation

1. Confirm the validity of a prior judgement or behaviour (e.g. 'I must say, if I were in your position, I might have a hard time dealing with those difficult people in your company').
2. Elicit affirmative response:
   a. For example, the client has a BMI of 40. The therapist is interested to find out his exercise level.
   b. ☑ 'Do you find it difficult to do exercise?'
   c. ☒ 'Your BMI is a concern to me. How often do you exercise?'
   d. ☑ ' = recommended approach'; ☒ ' = not recommended'.

Praise

1. Compliments, statements of appreciation, and understanding:
   a. ☑ 'Thanks for coming on time today'.
   b. ☑ 'This is a very good suggestion'.
2. Praise the client for sincere and genuine input.
3. Reinforce positive behaviour.
4. Seek feedback from the client to ensure acceptance of praise.

Reflective listening

1. Repeat patient's own accounts by paraphrasing or using words that add meaning to what the client has said.
2. For example, a client complains that she does not like the way her partner comments on how she handles her children. The therapist can say, 'It seems that you are a bit annoyed by your partner's comment'.

Summary

1. Summarizing, paraphrasing, and organizing of the client's account of issues.
2. This indicates that the therapist is listening and interested in the issues.

3. Summary often links issues together and allows transition from topic to topic.
4. Summary may enhance client's awareness of potential bias of their view.

Reassurance and encouragement

1. Reassure the patient within limits of the therapist's expertise.
2. Encourage the client by instilling hope and identify 'small steps' for improvement.

Rationalization and reframing

1. Rationalization involves providing a logical explanation for an event, situation, or outcome.
2. Reframing involves providing an alternative way to look at a situation.

Avoid common pitfalls in supportive psychotherapy

1. Avoid attacks and criticism:
   a. For example, the client submitted his resignation the next day without following the therapist's advice.
   b. ☑ 'Resignation is usually the last resort. Perhaps we can explore other options which we can find satisfaction in the company'.
   c. ☒ 'It really does not make any sense to me to resign after three months just because you are not happy with your boss. I cannot agree with you and you never listen to my advice'.
2. Avoid overpowering statements:
   a. ☑ 'I hope that I have made myself clear. There are other options which you can consider'.
   b. ☒ 'As your therapist, I am trying to get you to understand that resignation at this stage is not a wise decision. Please withdraw your resignation letter'.
3. Avoid denigration:
   a. For example, the client wants to explain to the therapist why he submitted the resignation letter suddenly. The therapist does not understand his explanation:
   b. ☑ 'Sorry, I do not understand. Would you mind to explain to me again the reason for your sudden resignation?'
   c. ☒ 'What are you trying to say? I do not understand at all'.

4. Avoid dismissive response:
   a. For example, the client complains that supportive psychotherapy is not working. The therapist does not feel good about his remark:
   b. ☑ 'I am sorry to hear that you find the psychotherapy not working. May I know in which aspects of the therapy you find not working?'
   c. ☒ 'It has not been a problem for most of my clients. Most of them find the therapy useful. May I know in which aspects of the therapy you find unhelpful?'

Duration of supportive psychotherapy: several months to 1 year

25.2 BRIEF DYNAMIC PSYCHOTHERAPY

25.2.1 HISTORICAL DEVELOPMENT

Psychoanalytic theories are considered in Chapter 9.

25.2.2 OBJECTIVES

1. Improve self-understanding by developing capacity for self-reflection.
2. Increase awareness of maladaptive defences and modify such defences.
3. Understand the relationship between the past and present.

25.2.3 INDICATIONS

1. Depressive disorder
2. Anxiety disorders
3. Childhood abuse and trauma
4. Relationship problem
5. Personality disorder
6. Client's factors
   a. Strong motivation to understand about the influence of the past
   b. Adequate ego strength
   c. Tolerance to frustration
   d. Capacity to form and sustain relationship
   e. Psychological mindedness
   f. Good response to trial interpretation

25.2.4 CONTRAINDICATIONS

1. Schizophrenia
2. Delusional disorder
3. High tendency for serious self-harm
4. Severe dependence on substances
5. Very poor insight
6. General contraindications for psychotherapy apply (see supportive psychotherapy Section 25.1).

25.2.5 GENERAL TECHNIQUES

1. Establish a therapeutic alliance.
2. Set goal: the client and therapist agree to work on an emotional or psychological problem.
3. Free association by the client.
4. Focus on internal conflicts since childhood.
5. Interpret transference.
6. Confrontation: an attempt to make the client face issues that are close to consciousness but being repressed or denied by the client.
7. Working through: draw previous maladaptive patterns or defences to conscious awareness.
8. Enactment: play out the psychological phenomenon such as regression in the therapy to facilitate understanding.
9. Containment of anxiety.
10. Resolution of conflicts.
11. Modify and avoid maladaptive defences.
12. Link the past, the present, and the transference.
13. Address termination issues.

25.2.6 SUBTYPES OF BRIEF DYNAMIC PSYCHOTHERAPY

1. Brief focal psychotherapy (Malan)
   • Clarify the nature of defences and its relationship to anxiety and impulse.
2. Time-limited psychotherapy (Mann)
   • Focus on the present and chronically endured pain and negative self-image.
3. Short-term dynamic psychotherapy (Davanloo)
   • Focus on oedipal (triangular) conflict.

25.2.7 NEGATIVE REACTIONS DURING BRIEF DYNAMIC PSYCHOTHERAPY

1. Resistance: the client is ambivalent about getting help and may oppose attempts from the therapist who offers help. Resistance may manifest in the form of silence, avoidance, or absences. These can reveal a great deal about significant relationship(s) in the past.

2. Acting out: the poor containment of strong feelings triggered by the therapy (e.g. anger towards the therapist).
3. Acting in: the exploration of therapist's personal and private information by the client or presenting a symbolic gift to a therapist.
4. Negative therapeutic reaction: the sudden and unexpected deterioration or regression in apparent progression during therapy (e.g. premature termination of therapy by the client without any explanation despite a period of engagement).

25.2.8 Structure

25.2.8.1 Initial Phase

1. Identify problem and clarification.
2. Explore the nature and origin of the problem.
3. Perform a psychodynamic formulation.
4. Establish a therapeutic alliance.
5. Establish a treatment contract.

25.2.8.2 Middle Phase

1. Identify defences.
2. Challenge and modify primitive, neurotic, and immature defences.
3. Interpret unconscious motives and transference.
4. Analyse enactment and repetition of pattern.
5. Facilitate the working through of attachment and loss within the psychotherapy setting.
6. Link the past and present.

25.2.8.3 Terminal Phase

1. Termination occurs when therapeutic endeavour comes to a predefined end date set by the treatment contract.
2. Termination can be a complex and powerful event in brief dynamic psychotherapy.
3. Summarize the progress of therapy.
4. Encourage the client to look forward into the future.
5. Address transference and countertransference issues.
6. Discuss possible follow-up plan and access to external resources and other therapies.
7. Possible negative reactions from the client: grief and mourning, anger and perceptions of abandonment, enactment of negative experience of earlier separations and regression, devaluation of therapist as a result of narcissistic injury, return of symptoms, denial and resistance, avoidance of termination, acting out, and acting in.

8. Possible positive reactions from the client: gratitude, acceptance of frustration, and demonstration of capacity to handle grief and separation.

Duration of treatment: 6 months to several years

25.2.9 Case Vignette

A 30-year-old man presents with mixed anxiety and depression after he contracted STD from his ex-female partner. He was recently admitted to the ward after harming himself with self-laceration. He feels that he is symbolically castrated by his ex-partner because all ladies would avoid him. This episode reminds him of the remarks made by his mother who threatened to castrate him when he was a child. She probably ridiculed him and tried to undermine his sense of masculinity, but the client took her remarks very seriously. His father left the family when he was young. The client described his father as passive and irresponsible. He wishes to see a male psychotherapist and wants to understand the relationship between the past and the present.

25.2.10 Psychodynamic Formulation

A psychodynamic formulation is an account of the client's problems in the context of developmental history that enables the therapist to consider the psychiatric diagnosis in the context of the client's inner world, personal relationship, and past experiences. A psychodynamic formulation of the previous case is summarized in two triangles (Figures 25.1 and 25.2).

25.2.11 CASC Preparation: Explain Brief Dynamic Psychotherapy to a Client

1. Brief dynamic psychotherapy is useful for a client who wants to understand how his or her current difficulties may relate to past experiences based on the concepts developed by Sigmund Freud. Freud developed the model of the mind through psychoanalysis. Freud described that forces and processes in an unconscious mind may affect how a person behaves. The content of dreams also helps us to understand how the unconscious mind works.
2. In contrast to traditional psychoanalysis that involves frequent meetings (typically five times a week), the brief dynamic psychotherapy aims to reduce distress reported by the client through

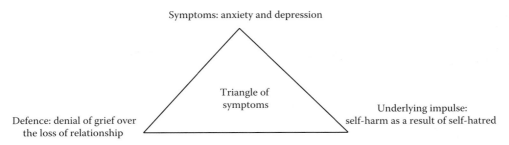

FIGURE 25.1   Triangle of symptoms.

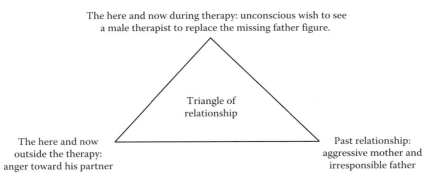

FIGURE 25.2   Triangle of relationship.

less frequent sessions over a time-limited period (e.g. weekly session over a period of 6 months–1 year).

3. The therapist works with the client to identify recurrent patterns. The therapist helps the client to draw upon feelings evoked during psychotherapy. The therapist promotes reflective thoughts and helps the client to make links with past experiences. The goals of therapy are to resolve conflict, to effect changes to improve quality of life, and to enhance the client's capacity to handle frustration.

4. This process of attempting to explore the unconscious mind may generate anxiety. Client often complains of deep-seated discomfort. Clients who are interested in brief dynamic psychotherapy must demonstrate sufficient ego strength. It is because they have to be strong enough to face the process of working through and the feelings associated with conflicts. Clients have to be in touch with painful memories and emotions during the therapy. They are also subjected to the therapist's interpretation and gentle confrontation.

5. In general, clients who are more articulate, psychologically inclined, and able to tolerate stress are more likely to benefit from brief dynamic psychotherapy. The therapist is mostly nondirective and follows the thoughts and feelings of the client.

25.2.12   RESEARCH AND BRIEF PSYCHODYNAMIC THERAPY

Research in brief dynamic psychotherapy faces the following challenges:

25.2.12.1   Structural Aspects

1. Psychodynamic psychotherapy is relatively unstructured in nature. It has less clear aims, goals, or end points compared to cognitive behaviour therapy (CBT).

2. Psychodynamic psychotherapy cannot be manualized and there is no agreement on a standard approach. The therapy cannot be reduced to treatment algorithms but depends on the therapeutic alliance and analysis of transference and countertransference.

3. There are less psychodynamic psychotherapists compared to cognitive behaviour therapists.

4. There are funding barriers to brief dynamic psychotherapy research because it is often conducted in private clinics.

25.2.12.2   Methodological Aspects

1. There is selection bias because clients presenting for brief dynamic psychotherapy are more motivated, educated, and psychologically inclined.
2. Psychotherapists cannot be blinded to the interventions, but outcome can be measured by a trained research personnel blinded to the nature of the psychotherapeutic intervention.
3. Issues of informed consent required for research and administering standardized questionnaires may affect the transference and countertransference. On the other hand, issues of transference may contaminate the client's satisfaction on therapy if this is an outcome measure.

25.2.12.3   Measurement of Outcomes

1. There is disagreement on the universal outcomes in brief dynamic psychotherapy. Possible outcomes include measures of symptom severity, 'ego strength', coping style, self-report in quality of life improvement, or client satisfaction.
2. Clients may not have a clear psychiatric diagnosis and there is often spontaneous remission of symptoms.
3. Statistically significant improvement in outcome may not equal to clinical improvement.

25.3   CBT

25.3.1   Historical Development of CBT

25.3.1.1   Cognitive Therapy

Beck proposed that negative thinking in depression originates from earlier assumptions that play a central role in the maintenance of depressive symptoms.

Beck's cognitive model of depression includes the effect of early experiences, core beliefs, underlying assumptions, cognitive distortions, automatic thoughts, and the negative cognitive triad. Depression can be treated by modifying one of the components based on Beck's cognitive model.

25.3.1.2   Behaviour Therapy

Mowrer's two-factor model states that fear of a specific stimulus is acquired through classical conditioning and the client tries to reduce fear by avoiding the conditioned stimulus through operant conditioning.

Ayllon and Azrin's token economy model is a controlled environment where reinforcers were applied to systematically change a client's behaviour.

25.3.2   Objectives

1. Alleviate symptoms such as anxiety or depression by helping the client to identify and challenge negative cognitions.
2. Develop alternative and flexible schemas.
3. Rehearse new cognitive and behavioural responses in difficult situations.

25.3.3   Characteristics

1. Collaborative empiricism: engagement and collaboration between the therapist and the client.
2. Focus on specific issues.
3. Homework is assigned.
4. Time-limited.
5. Focus on here and now.
6. Outcome can be measured by direct observation, physiological measures, standardized instruments, and self-report measures such as the Beck Depression Inventory, the Beck Anxiety Inventory, and the Fear Questionnaire.

25.3.4   Indications

1. Mood disorders: depressive disorder and bipolar disorder
2. Generalized anxiety disorder, panic disorder, and obsessive compulsive disorder
3. Phobia: social phobia, agoraphobia, and simple phobia
4. Eating disorders: anorexia nervosa and bulimia nervosa
5. Impulse control disorders
6. Schizophrenia (target at delusions and hallucinations, coping enhancement, enhance adherence to treatment, and relapse prevention)
7. Personality disorders (refer to dialectical behavioural therapy)
8. Substance abuse
9. Liaison psychiatry (chronic pain, chronic fatigue, physical illnesses)
10. Paraphilia

25.3.5   Contraindications

1. Severe dementia
2. Profound learning disability
3. Delirium
4. No evidence of cognitive errors
5. No motivation or no interest for CBT
6. General contraindications for psychotherapy apply (see Section 25.1)

25.3.6 TECHNIQUES

25.3.6.1 Cognitive Techniques

Cognitive restructuring helps the client to identify negative thoughts, dysfunctional assumptions, and maladaptive core beliefs relating to their underlying problems. It also tests the validity of those thoughts, assumptions, and beliefs. The goal is to produce more adaptive and positive alternatives:

1. Identify negative automatic thought (NAT) (e.g. I am going to receive the bad news when I step into by office).
2. Identify dysfunctional or faulty assumption (e.g. at my workplace, people do not like me because I expressed my negative feelings last week).
3. Identify maladaptive core belief and rate its strength (e.g. I am an unpopular person).
4. Restructure the maladaptive core belief.
5. Formulate alternative positive belief.
6. Rate the impact of maladaptive belief on emotion.
7. Rate the impact of new core belief on emotion.

25.3.6.2 Behavioural Techniques

RAT PAD (think of the rat in the Skinner's box)

R—rehearsal: help the client to anticipate challenges and develop strategies to overcome such difficulties.

A—assignment: graded assignment on exposure.

T—training to be self-reliant.

P—pleasure and mastery.

A—activity scheduling: to increase contact with positive activities and decrease avoidance and withdrawal.

D—diversion or distraction techniques.

25.3.7 SOCRATIC QUESTIONING

1. What is your view of the event?
2. What is the evidence of your belief?
3. Is there any alternative explanation?
4. What would you tell a close friend if he or she is in the same situation as you?
5. Are you condemning yourself based on a single event?
6. Do you think that you have bias?
7. Have you overestimated the risk?

25.3.8 DURING EACH SESSION

1. Weekly update.
2. Bridge from the previous session.
3. Review homework assignment.
4. Set agenda for this session.
5. Work on the agenda.
6. Provide brief summaries.
7. Assign homework assignment.
8. Summarize the session and offer feedback.

25.3.9 STRUCTURE

25.3.9.1 Early Phase (Session 1–4)

1. Establish therapeutic relationship.
2. Educate the client about the model of CBT and the influence of thoughts on behaviour and emotion.
3. Set goals for psychotherapy.
4. Identify NATs.
5. Assessment by Socratic questioning: the use of questions to reveal the self-defeating nature of the client's NATs and identify cognitive triads (automatic thoughts, cognitive distortion, and faulty assumptions).
6. Case formulation.
7. Baseline measure of symptom severity by a standard instrument.

25.3.9.2 Middle Phase (Session 5–12)

1. Keep a dysfunctional thought diary (see Figure 25.3).
2. Identify cognitive errors and core beliefs through homework assignment.
3. Practice skills for reattribution by reviewing evidence and challenging cognitive errors.
4. Behaviour therapy involves identifying safety behaviours, entering feared situation without safety manoeuvres, applying relaxation techniques, activity scheduling, and assertiveness training.
5. Review progress and offer feedbacks.

25.3.9.3 Termination (Session 13–16)

1. Prepare for termination.
2. Identify early symptoms of relapse and predict high-risk situations leading to a relapse.
3. Relapse prevention: develop coping strategies to overcome negative emotions, interpersonal conflicts, and pressure.
4. Formulate a plan for early intervention if relapse takes place.

Situation / Date / Time	Automatic Thoughts	Emotion (Mood score: 1–10; 1 = very depressed; 10 = very happy)	Behaviour	Alternative Thoughts
26 July 2012. Thursday night 8 pm My boyfriend criticised me	'I can never do the things right. I have no say in this relationship. I fail everything in my life'	Said and angry with myself (rated 2 out of 10)	Said nothing, shut myself in a room	'I am too negative. This is not a catastrophe. Our relationship will get better'

FIGURE 25.3   Dysfunctional thought diary.

5. Consolidate skills and knowledge learned in therapy.
6. Measure severity of symptoms by a standard instrument at the end of therapy.

25.4   DBT

25.4.1   HISTORICAL BACKGROUND

- Dialectical behaviour therapy (DBT) was developed by Marsha Linehan who is a clinical psychologist from Seattle, the United States.

25.4.2   OBJECTIVES

- Borderline personality disorder (BPD) is an interaction between an emotionally vulnerable person and an invalidating environment. As a result, the client has chronic feeling of emptiness and does not find his or her life worth living, which results in multiple self-harm. The overall objective of DBT is to help the client build a life that is worth living.
- Reduces self-harm or suicidal behaviour (e.g. self-laceration).
- Reduces and stops therapy-interfering behaviour (e.g. missing session or acting out in therapy).
- Reduces or stops serious quality of life-interfering behaviour (e.g. frequent argument with family members, resulting in rejection and homelessness).
- Develop life skills.

25.4.3   INDICATIONS

1. BPD: reduce self-harm behaviour, anger, number of visits of accident and emergency department, and hospitalization.
2. Young people with repetitive self-harm.

25.4.4   CONTRAINDICATIONS

General contraindications for psychotherapy apply (see Section 25.1). In addition, there is a set of skill training rules that the client must comply:

1. Client cannot miss therapy for more than 4 weeks in a row.
2. Client cannot misuse drugs or alcohol during the course of therapy.
3. Client is not allowed to discuss past suicidal behaviour with other clients outside therapy.
4. Client must keep information obtained from group session confidential.
5. Client must not develop private relationship with other clients outside therapy.
6. Client must not attend the same skill training group with his or her sexual partner.

25.4.5   COMPONENTS OF DBT

1. Individual sessions: 45–60 min on a weekly basis, to review diary cards in the past 1 week and discuss life-threatening behaviours.
2. Skill training group by a trainer: weekly group session for 2 h
   a. First hour: mindfulness meditation practice and sharing of each member
   b. Second hour: life-skill training (mindfulness, interpersonal effectiveness, emotional regulation, and distress tolerance)
3. Brief out-of-hours telephone contact as part of the treatment contract
4. Weekly consultation group between the individual therapist and the skills trainer

25.4.6   TECHNIQUES

1. Dialectical thinking: advise the client not to think linearly. Truth is an evolving process of opposing views rather than extremes.

2. Behavioural therapy with homework assignment.
3. Mindfulness 'how' skills: observing and describing events and participating without self-consciousness.
4. Mindfulness 'what' skills: adopting nonjudgement stance, focusing on one thing at a time, and enhancing self-effectiveness.
5. Life-skill training: Zen Buddhism: emphasize on wholeness, consider alternatives, and engulf alternatives.
6. Use of metaphors: enhancing effectiveness of communication, discovering one's own wisdom, and strengthening therapeutic alliance.

Duration of treatment: 1 year.

25.5 MENTALIZATION-BASED TREATMENT

25.5.1 HISTORICAL DEVELOPMENT

1. Mentalization-based treatment (MBT) was developed by Anthony Bateman and Peter Fonagy.

25.5.2 OBJECTIVES

1. Mentalization refers to psychological mindedness and empathy. Mentalization is developed in people who have responsive parents providing secure attachment in childhood. Patients with BPD have impaired mentalization. As a result, they are not able to interpret their actions or others' actions based on the intentional mental states such as beliefs, feelings, and preferences. Impaired mentalization is associated with affect dysregulation and incoherent self.
2. MBT helps clients with BPD to develop the capacity to realize that a person has an agentive mind and to recognize the importance of mental states in other people.

25.5.3 INDICATIONS

1. BPD

25.5.4 TECHNIQUES

1. Ask the client to observe his or her state of mind.
2. Generate alternative perspective of the experience of oneself and other people.

3. Develop appropriate affect expression to handle impulse control, reduction of self-harm, passive aggression, idealization, hate, and love.
4. Establish a stable representational system.
5. Form a coherent sense of self.
6. Develop a capacity to form secure relationships.

Duration: 18 months; DBT is conducted in a day hospital.

25.6 COGNITIVE ANALYTIC THERAPY

25.6.1 HISTORICAL BACKGROUND

Cognitive analytic therapy (CAT) is developed by Anthony Ryle. CAT is a combination of cognitive and analytic therapy.

25.6.2 OBJECTIVES

1. CAT aims at changing maladaptive procedural sequences.
2. CAT focuses on specific patterns of thinking and less on interpersonal behaviour.
3. CAT focuses less on transference interpretation.

25.6.3 INDICATIONS

1. Neurotic disorders
2. Personality disorders (e.g. BPD)
3. Depression
4. Deliberate self-harm
5. Abnormal illness behaviour

25.6.4 TECHNIQUES

1. Use open questioning and descriptive reframing during the assessment.
2. Formulate a procedural sequence model. The model tries to understand the aim-directed action (e.g. formulate an aim, evaluate environmental plans, plan actions, and evaluate results of actions).
3. Identify faculty procedures:
   a. Traps: repetitive cycles of behaviour and their consequences become perpetuation.
   b. Dilemma: false choices or unduly narrowed options.
   c. Snag: extreme pessimism about the future and halt a plan before it even starts.

4. Write a reformulation letter that begins with a narrative account of the client's life story and identify repetitive maladaptive patterns. The letter also contains a diagram that illustrates the reciprocal roles between the client and procedural sequence model.
5. Change maladaptive procedural sequences and predict the likely transference and countertransference feelings. Enactments become active during sessions.
6. Towards termination, the therapist will issue a goodbye letter to the client that summarizes the progress and achievement of the therapy. The client may also issue a goodbye letter to the therapist.

Duration: 16–24 sessions.

**CASC STATION: EXPLAIN
CAT TO A CLIENT**

Client P is a 30-year-old man. He is currently unemployed and he worked as a graphic designer in the past. He feels hopeless after he was retrenched. His girlfriend has recently terminated their relationship but they are still in contact. He spends his time with his band and he is the band leader. He realizes that his members have betrayed him and he has decided to leave the band. His psychiatrist diagnosed him with moderate depressive episode and refers him for psychotherapy. During the assessment session, he wants to know what has gone wrong in his work and in the band. He hopes that the failure will not occur in his future career. He has history of hyperthyroidism.

Task: Explain CAT to this client.

---

1. CAT is a short-term focused treatment. CAT involves a combination of cognitive therapy and analysis. For cognitive therapy, the therapist will examine your behaviours and associated feelings. For example, if a specific situation makes you feel depressed, an analysis of feeling may help to identify the origin of depression.
2. The analytical component deals with conflict through explanation. The therapist will try to understand your negative feelings and resolve problematic behaviour. The client will gain more understanding through analysis and reduce the stress levels.
3. In the beginning phase, the therapist will try to understand you and formulate a model. The in-depth assessment will help the therapist to identify any faulty pattern. You need to write a letter to describe your life story. The therapist will look for repetitive faulty patterns in your life. The most important part of CAT is to change maladaptive and faulty patterns.
4. Prior to termination, the therapist will give you a letter that will summarize the progress and achievement during the therapy. You can also write a letter to the therapist to express your feelings (Figure 25.4).

25.7 INTERPERSONAL THERAPY

25.7.1 HISTORICAL BACKGROUND

Interpersonal therapy (IPT) was developed by Gerald Klerman. IPT is based on attachment theory.

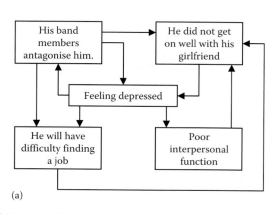

(a)

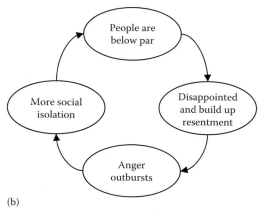

(b)

FIGURE 25.4   (a) Trap in Client P's case. (b) Dilemma faced by Client P.

25.7.2 Objectives

1. To create a therapeutic environment with meaningful therapeutic relationship and recognize the client's underlying attachment needs
2. To develop an understanding of the client's communication difficulties and attachment style both inside and outside the therapy
3. To identify the client's maladaptive patterns of communication and establishment of insight
4. To assist the client in building a better social support network and mobilize resources

25.7.3 Indications

- Depressive disorder: IPT is equally effective as CBT.
- Eating disorder: bulimia nervosa.
- Dysthymia.
- Other issues: interpersonal disputes, role transition, grief, and loss.

25.7.4 Techniques

25.7.4.1 Structure

25.7.4.1.1 *Initial Phase*

1. Define depression and explain diagnosis.
2. Offer an interpersonal formation (see Figure 25.5).
3. Explain rationales of IPT and logistics of treatment such as treatment contract.
4. Identify target interpersonal problem areas such as grief, role transition, role dispute, and interpersonal deficits.
5. Assign sick role.

25.7.4.1.2 *Middle Phase*

1. Identify 1–2 interpersonal problem areas:
   a. Assess the impact of an interpersonal event on mood.
   b. Explore patient's expectations and options in the event.
   c. Assess the relationship between the interpersonal problem and underlying attachment pattern.
   d. Fill up an interpersonal inventory card (see Figure 25.6).
   e. Perform communication analysis to identify maladaptive patterns of communication.
   f. The therapist can adopt three stances: neutral stance, passive stance, and client advocate stance on correcting communication patterns.
   g. Role-play and develop strategies to handle similar situations in the future.
2. For grief
   a. Explore grief feelings for loss of relationship or loss of status.
   b. Facilitate mourning of loss.
   c. Develop interest and relationships to substitute for the loss.
3. For interpersonal disputes
   a. Identify current stage of interpersonal disputes (e.g. renegotiation, impasse, or dissolution).
   b. Understand role expectations.
   c. Modify nonreciprocal role expectations.
   d. Examine other interpersonal relationships.
   e. Examine assumptions behind patient's behaviour and modify faulty assumptions.
4. For role transitions
   a. Accept the loss of previous roles.
   b. Develop positive attitude towards the new roles.
   c. Develop a sense of mastery in the new roles.

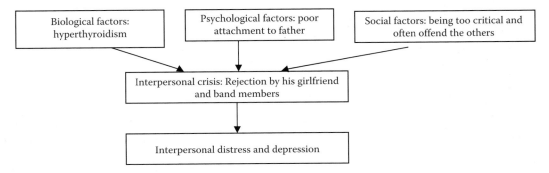

FIGURE 25.5 Interpersonal formulation (using Client P under CAT as an example).

Client Name: Client P   **Date of Birth:** 4 February 1976   **Psychiatrist-in-charge:** Dr. McFadzean
Date of first consultation: 26 July 2012

Name of significant person: Miss L   **Relationship:** Ex-girlfriend

Client's account of problems:

1. Miss L is too sensitive with unrealistic expectation.
2. Always end up in quarrel, relationship is not going anywhere.
3. Client P cannot hold his criticism and openly criticises Miss L.
4. Miss L also looks down on Client P because he is out of job.

Areas requiring further clarification:

1. Communication with band members
2. Attachment in childhood
3. Anger control

Agreed problem area:

1. Grief and loss of relationship
2. Develop more gentle way to communicate his disappointment

FIGURE 25.6   Interpersonal inventory (using Client P under CAT as an example).

5. For interpersonal role deficits
   a. Reduce social isolation.
   b. Encourage formation of new relationships.
   c. Explore repetitive patters in relationships.

25.7.4.1.3 Termination Phase

1. Discuss the impact of termination.
2. Acknowledge that termination may trigger grief feelings.
3. Assist patient to establish competency to handle interpersonal problems independently after termination.
4. Identify social support resources.

Number of sessions: 16–20 sessions.

25.7.5 CASC Preparation: Explain IPT to a Client

1. *What is IPT?* IPT is a time-limited psychotherapy. The aim of IPT is to reduce your suffering and improve interpersonal functioning. IPT focuses on interpersonal relationships as a means of bringing about change. The goal is to help you to improve your interpersonal relationships or change your expectations on interpersonal relationship.
2. *What does the therapist do?* The therapist will help you to improve the social support network so that you can manage the interpersonal distress. In order to help you to understand this concept better, I would like to give you an analogy. Some people like to climb to high places as they are adventurous and enjoy the excitement. For some people, climbing is frightening and they have no confidence to do it. They are able to climb with assistance from a trusted and significant person. This significant person also provides interpersonal reassurance. The psychotherapy itself is like climbing the mountain, and IPT is designed to help the client to recognize their interpersonal needs and to seek attachment and reassurance in the process of improving interpersonal relationship. More importantly, you will be able to express those needs to other people and promote positive responses after the therapy.
3. *How many stages does IPT have?* The therapy has three stages. In the first stage, the therapist will try his or her very best to develop a good therapeutic relationship with you and understand your problem. In the second stage, the therapist will seek your views to work on an agreed problem area. The information will be summarized in a card. The therapist will analyse the way you communicate with other people. The therapist will give you useful advice and help you to develop new skills by using role-play. The therapist will help you to work on issues related to loss and develop a new role. In the final stage, the

therapist will strengthen the skills you learned in therapy. The therapist will help to identify resources for you to handle interpersonal problems in the future. The whole IPT takes 16–20 sessions.

25.8 FAMILY THERAPY

25.8.1 HISTORICAL PERSPECTIVES

Minuchin developed *structural family therapy*. He is interested in how families are organized in the subsystems and in the boundaries between these components. A good family has clear hierarchy and boundary between the subsystems.

Milan developed *systemic family therapy* that emphasizes that family system is more than the sum of its components and the system as a whole is the focus of therapy. Symptoms of individual family members are a manifestation of the way the family system is functioning.

25.8.2 INDICATIONS

25.8.2.1 External Indicators for Family Therapy

1. Addition of members to the family (e.g. unplanned pregnancy and birth of a young sibling).
2. A family member is recently diagnosed with an illness that can be terminal or causes significant change in role (e.g. cancer in one parent).
3. Change in financial status: for example, bankruptcy in family.
4. Children leaving home: for example, empty nest syndrome.
5. Change in marital status: for example, divorced parent remarries again, affecting the children.
6. Suprasystem problems: for example, when there is a high crime rate in the neighbuorhood that affects the family, family therapy can strengthen the boundary between the family and the suprasystem by working with external agencies such as police or MP.

25.8.2.2 Internal Indicators for Family Therapy

1. Behaviour control problems (e.g. conduct disorder in a child): engage family to deliver behaviour therapy in home environment.
2. Boundary issues between family members (e.g. enmeshment): to promote communication and emotional interchange in disengaged

relationship; to create necessary separation and independence in case of enmeshment.
3. Communication problems and triangulation: introduction of humour, demonstration of warmth and empathy, role-play, and modifying both verbal and nonverbal communication.
4. Role problems (e.g. family scapegoat, parental child): identify problems and redefine roles. The same-sex parent functions as primary disciplinarian and promotes maximum ego development by setting limits and higher-level goals. The opposite-sex parent functions as the facilitator or mediator within the triangular relationship to correct inappropriate parenting from the same-sex parent.
5. Task accomplishment problems (e.g. developmental tasks): identifying the task, exploring alternative approaches, taking action, evaluating, and adjusting.

25.8.3 ASSESSMENT TECHNIQUES

1. Ask each family member to describe his or her sense of the problem.
2. Ask each individual the same question that has been asked of other family members.
3. Ask each family member to propose a solution to the problem.
4. Ask each individual's reaction to what other family members have said.
5. Assign homework or task that aims to solve problems in the family.
6. Identify nonverbal communication in the family.
7. Identify common themes in the family.
8. Individuals are requested to speak with 'I' phrases but not the 'you' phrases during assessment.

25.8.4 TYPES OF FAMILY THERAPY

25.8.4.1 Structural Family Therapy (Minuchin)

- Minuchin believed that families are systems that operate through subsystems. Each subsystem requires adequate boundary and permeability.
- Family problems arise when boundaries are too loose, resulting in enmeshment. When family members are too rigid, this will result in disengagement.
- Structural family therapy identifies the set of unspoken rules governing the hierarchy, sharing of responsibilities, and boundaries.
- The therapist presents these rules to the family in a paradoxical way to bring about changes. The therapist is active in control of the proceedings.

25.8.4.2 Systemic Family Therapy

1. *Milan associates* often involve more than two therapists working in a team to maintain the systemic perspective. One therapist is always with the family while the team observes through a one-way screen or video camera. The team offers input to the therapist via telephone or during intersession breaks to discuss the family system. There are pre- and post-session discussions.
2. *Reframing* an individual's problem as family problem (e.g. the borderline personality of a daughter is reframed as the parental problem in providing care to their child). An internal problem can be reframed as an external problem if there are unproductive conflicts in the family that exhausted everyone (e.g. the family is under the influence of anger rather than labelling a family member as an angry person).
3. Explore the coherence and understand the family as an organized coherent system.
4. *Circular questioning* is used to examine perspective of each family member on interfamily member relationship. It aims at discovering and clarifying conflicting views. Hypothesis can be formed from the conflicting views and the therapist can propose further changes.

25.8.4.3 Strategic Family Therapy

Strategic family therapy uses a complex plan rather than a simple directive to produce changes in the family. The general techniques are listed as follows:

1. *Positive connotation*: It is a form of reframing by ascribing positive motives to the symptomatic behaviour.
2. *Metaphors* allow indirect communication of ideas (e.g. a relationship metaphor describes the relationship between the therapist and a family member, and this metaphor can apply on other relationships). Metaphorical object refers to the use of a concrete object to represent abstract ideas (e.g. a blank sheet of paper in an envelope representing the family secrets).
3. Paradoxical interventions
   a. This method is used when direct methods fail or encounter strong resistance in some family members. The therapist will reverse the vector (i.e. rather than a top-down approach that always starts from the parents, a bottom-up approach from children to

their parents is allowed). This therapist will also disqualify anyone who is an authority on the problems including the parents (e.g. the children are allowed to challenge their parents and undesired behaviour is encouraged. Paradoxically, change and improvement will take place as family members cannot tolerate the paradoxical pattern).
   b. Another technique is symptom prescription when symptoms are allowed to take place in specific time and place. Paradoxically, symptom will disappear.
   c. Declaration of impotence by therapist is used when family members gang up and attack the therapist. Such declaration will put an end to the battle and this often leads to complementary relationship between the therapist and the family. It is paradoxical because the therapist declares impotence on the one hand but collects professional fee and planning treatment on the other hand.
   d. The therapist can pass pessimistic views on the family and hope that they change quickly after hearing the negative remarks.
4. *Prescribing family rituals*: Rituals refer to membership, brief expression, and celebration. (e.g. the therapist passes a metaphor object to the family and any family member can use this object to call for a meeting at home). Ritual prescription refers to setting up a timetable that assigns one parent to take charge on an odd day and a child to take charge on an even day. Ritual prescription is useful for a family with parental child.
5. Other strategies include humour, getting help from a consultation group that observes through the one-way mirror to offer advice, and debate among family members.

There are two types of strategic family therapy:

1. Strategic approach (Haley and Madanes)
   a. Clear generational boundaries are emphasized in normal family development.
   b. Concerns with the family dysfunction are manifested by a symptom (e.g. anorexia nervosa in a daughter).
   c. Family rules usually follow a hierarchical model. Improving the hierarchical and boundary problems would prevent dysfunctional

feedback loops (e.g. the therapist focuses on the hierarchy between the parents and their daughter with anorexia nervosa. This will change the anorexia nervosa of daughter).

d. Four types of family problems usually result from
   i. Desire to be loved
   ii. Desire to control and dominate
   iii. Desire to love and protect other family members
   iv. Desire to repent and forgive

2. Mental Research Institute (MRI) strategic family therapy
   a. Define problem in behavioural term.
   b. The family members attempt to solve their problems by setting up a feedback loop that worsens the problems.
   c. For example, if the daughter suffers from anorexia nervosa, the family has made the problems worse by giving harsh feedbacks.
   d. In MRI strategic family therapy, the family therapist focuses on correcting the daughter's diet and eating habits.
   e. Then the therapist identifies the feedback loop that prevents the daughter from eating and sets behavioural goals.
   f. The family therapist helps the family by
      i. Identifying the feedback loop
      ii. Finding the rules that govern it
      iii. Changing the loop and the rules

25.8.4.4 Eclectic Family Therapy

- It concentrates on the present situation of the family and examines how family members communicate with one another.
- It is flexible and allows time for the family to work together on problems raised in the treatment.
- It is commonly used in adolescents and their family.

25.9 GROUP THERAPY

25.9.1 Historical Development

1. In 1907, Joseph Pratt started an education group for tuberculosis patients. The study of veterans of World War I and II had great influence on the development of group therapy (Pratt, 1907).
2. In the second Northfield experiments, Michael Foulkes used the whole veteran ward as a therapeutic community to increase discipline and morale while decreasing delinquency (Foulkes, 1946). He developed group analysis when the patient was considered as a nodal point of social interactions and offered deeper interpretation of hidden communication and problems in a group. He also introduced group matrix that is a total network of communications that evolves in group therapy.

3. In the United States, Kurt Lewin developed the field theory that states that individual dynamics are shaped by the surrounding social forces. This concept evolves into the encounter group that emphasizes on self-awareness and personal growth (Lewin, 1943).

4. In 1961, Bion introduced two concepts of group (Bion, 1961):
   a. The basic assumption group refers to the primitive state of mind and members gather together, which poses a threat to the group.
   b. The work group is rational, purposeful, and cooperative.

25.9.2 Indications

Group members require careful selection. The general inclusion criteria include

1. High motivation
2. Interest to explore the past issues
3. Ability to empathize and sympathize
4. Positive group experience
5. Compatible problems: long-standing psychological problems

25.9.3 Contraindications

Medical or psychiatric factors

1. Severe head injury or other organic condition that affects the ability to communicate
2. Paranoid schizophrenia or paranoid personality disorder
3. Severe narcissistic personality disorder
4. Severe hypochondriasis
5. Severe antisocial personality disorder or people with psychopathy

Personal factors

1. Poor motivation
2. Strong denial
3. Inability to self-disclose
4. Lack of empathy
5. Negative group experience

6. Problems incompatible with group therapy (e.g. marital problem)
7. Frequent acting-out behaviour
8. Hidden agenda (e.g. aim to develop a romantic relationship with one of the group members)

25.9.4 TYPES OF GROUP THERAPY

25.9.4.1 Classification Based on Service Administration

1. Open group therapy: allows replacement of group members.
2. Closed group therapy: no replacement of group members is allowed.
3. Heterogeneous group: allows a mixture of clients with different backgrounds and conditions.
4. Homogeneous group: only allows group members of the same gender, similar background, or same condition (e.g. anger problem).
5. Continuous group therapy: there is no definite end date of group therapy. The therapy may last for years. Old members leave and new members join.
6. Brief group therapy: there is a definite end date and members are expected to join and complete group therapy at the same time.
7. Leadership: active or passive leadership; co-leadership (i.e. two group leaders).

25.9.4.2 Classification Based on Technique

1. *Milieu group therapy:* Mainly developed for therapeutic community, and the whole community (e.g. the ward) is viewed as a large group. Rappaport described four characteristics in milieu group therapy:
   a. Democratization (equal sharing of power)
   b. Permissiveness (tolerance of others' behaviour outside the setting)
   c. Reality confrontation (confront with the views from others)
   d. Communalism (sharing of amenities)
      Further details on therapeutic community are considered in Norton and Warren (2009).

2. *Supportive group therapy:*
   a. For clients with chronic psychiatric disorders such as schizophrenia attending a day hospital, which offers supportive group therapy.

   b. Supportive group therapy involves empathy, encouragement, and explanation (e.g. Schizophrenia Fellowship).
3. *Analytic group therapy:*
   a. Analyse cyclical relational patterns.
   b. Interpret transference and countertransference in interpersonal terms.
   c. Interpret conflicts in a group and relate with experience outside the group.
   d. Dream analysis in a group.
4. *Outpatient group therapy*
   a. It may involve a self-help group targeting at homogenous group of clients focusing on one disorder (e.g. for anxiety disorders or Alcoholics Anonymous, AA).
   b. Outpatient group therapy is for short term and involves direct didactic instruction.
5. *Psychodrama*
   a. The group enacts the life of one member as a role-play. The other members exchange roles in the role-play and all group members express their views after the role-play.
   b. Psychodrama leads to better understanding and development of strategies to handle similar situations in the future.

25.10 THERAPEUTIC PROCESS

25.10.1 PREGROUP THERAPY ASSESSMENT

1. Assess the client's suitability for group therapy.
2. Socialize with the client.
3. Assess his or her ability to communicate and empathize.
4. Set personal and interpersonal goals.
5. Inform the rules of group therapy.
6. Discuss the common pitfalls in group therapy.
7. Discuss strategies to reduce anxiety in group participation and dropouts from group therapy.
8. Establish a treatment contract.

25.10.2 YALOM'S 11 THERAPEUTIC FACTORS

25.10.2.1 Early Stages

1. Instillation of hope: sense of optimism about progress and improvement.
2. Universality: one member's problems also occur in other members. Hence, the member is not alone.
3. Information giving: members will receive information on their illness and associated problems.

25.10.2.2   Middle Stage

1. Altruism: one member feels better by helping other members and sharing their solutions.
2. Corrective recapitulation of the primary family: the group mirrors one's own family and provides a chance for self-exploration of past family conflicts.
3. Improved social skills by social learning.
4. Imitative behaviour is established by vicarious learning or observation of the others.
5. Interpersonal learning is established by corrective experience in social microcosm.

25.10.2.3   End Stage

1. Group cohesiveness occurs after intermember acceptance and understanding. The cohesiveness leads to the sense of safety and containment of negative feelings.
2. Catharsis: group members feel encouraged and supported by expressing emotionally laden materials.
3. Existential factors: after group therapy, group members have more self-understanding and insight in responsibility and capriciousness of existence.

25.10.3   ROLE OF THE THERAPIST

1. The therapist can draw heavily upon a group setting to exercise the full range of therapeutic skills. Group therapy reduces the chance of intense transference reactions from group members.
2. The therapist may have particular inclinations and motivations (e.g. past experience of alcohol misuse in AA groups).
3. The therapist can encourage a combination of individual and group therapy. This will positively integrate these two forms of therapy for maximal benefit.

25.10.4   ADVANTAGES OF GROUP THERAPY

1. Reduction of cost.
2. The context of the group may give members value and a sense of group identity to assist them to cope with current problems in life.

25.10.5   COUNTERTHERAPEUTIC PROCESS

1. The countertherapeutic process may lead to individual disappointment, pessimism, and antagonism of therapist.

2. Bion's basic assumption group
   a. Dependence
   b. Fight–flight
   c. Pairing
3. Resistance is an attempt to break the framework of the group (e.g. scapegoating: subclassifying a group of people and attacking them and/or monopolizing the group).

Other problems of group therapy include repetitive stress injury, enhancing abnormal illness behaviour, danger of charismatic leadership, and dissemination of false information.

25.11   COUPLE THERAPY

25.11.1   OBJECTIVES

1. Couple therapy involves the therapist (or sometimes two therapists) seeing two clients who are in a relationship, not necessarily in a marriage.

25.11.2   INDICATIONS

1. Interpersonal problems in a relationship
2. Issues or difficulties related to a marriage or partnership
3. Grief in a couple (e.g. loss of a child)
4. Sexual problems

25.11.3   CONTRAINDICATIONS

1. Ongoing violent behaviour that is not under control
2. Clear evidence that one partner is using the couple therapy to terminate a relationship

25.11.4   ISSUES TO BE CONSIDERED BEFORE ARRANGING COUPLE THERAPY

1. Therapist-related issues
   a. Age and life experiences of the therapist are essential because couples may look for therapists who are married or who have been married.
   b. The gender of the therapist plays a key role as the therapist may identify with the same-sex client.
   c. Culture and religious background of the therapist in relation to the background of the couple should be considered.

d. The therapist needs to monitor his or her own countertransference (e.g. rescue fantasies or overidentification with the client).
2. Therapy-related issues
    a. The relationship between couple therapy and other ongoing therapies such as individual psychotherapy
    b. Confidentiality, neutrality, and triangulation between the couple and the therapist
3. Couple-related issues
    a. It requires motivation from the couple to attend the session and it is a challenge to establish therapeutic alliance with both partners.
    b. During the course of couple therapy, there will be decompensation from one or both clients.
    c. The therapist may face resistance and acting out that result in early termination.

25.11.5 TYPES OF COUPLE THERAPY

Couple therapy follows one of the following psychotherapeutic models:

1. The CBT model: identify reinforcement of undesirable behaviour in the couple.
2. The psychodynamic model: understand the client's emotional needs and the relationship to the needs of the partner.
3. The emotionally focused model (Greenberg and Johnson, 1988): rigid interaction patterns are systemic in nature and result in negative emotional states. In this model, emotion is the target and the agent of change. The therapist is a process consultant.
4. The transactional model: behaviours are analysed in terms of the 'child, adult, and parent' within a client and how the client reacts with the partner.

25.11.6 TECHNIQUES OF COUPLE THERAPY

1. Reciprocity negotiation: The couples develop an ability to express their offers and understand their partner's request. This allows an exchange of positive behaviours and reactions.
2. Communication training: This encourages mutual exchange of emotional messages.
3. System approaches: This approach focuses on hidden rules and identifies underlying disagreement to resolve enmeshment. It also involves a behavioural technique called paradoxical

injunction. Provocative statements are used to stir up counterresponse. This response is a double-end sword because it also offers benefits by bringing changes. An example is that the therapist prescribes the symptom and advises one partner to continue the problem behaviour. This will stir up counterresponse from the couple because they are uncomfortable to continue. The discomfort will lead to changes. System task involves making a timetable to allocate specific time for interaction.
4. Structural move: Experiment of disagreement focuses on a topic when one partner always dominates and the other habitually gives in to avoid disagreement. This exercise helps the passive partner to express an opinion forcefully and the other needs to value the expression. Role reversal helps one partner to understand the viewpoints and experiences of the other partner. Sculpting involves one partner taking up the position in silence and expresses his or her own feelings without words while the other partner has to guess the feelings.

25.12 MOTIVATIONAL INTERVIEWING

25.12.1 INDICATIONS

1. Substance misuse
2. Noncompliance to psychotropic medications

25.12.2 TECHNIQUES

Main techniques include

1. Express empathy and establish understanding from the client's perspectives.
2. Develop discrepancy in their behaviour and their personal goals/values.
3. Identify advantages and disadvantages of change.
4. Roll with client's resistance by understanding the client's hesitancy to change.
5. Support self-efficacy to reach personal goals and allow client to realize optimism about change.
6. Provide a menu of options for change.

25.12.3 EYE MOVEMENT AND DESENSITIZATION REPROCESSING

Eye movement and desensitization reprocessing (EMDR) focuses on traumatic experiences, negative cognitions, and affective responses. The aim is to desensitize the individual to the affective responses. This is accompanied by bilateral stimulation and rapid eye movement when the client is asked to follow the regular movement of the therapist's forefinger.

The procedural phases of EMDR include the following:

1. Assessment of target memory of image.
2. Desensitization by holding the target image together with the negative cognition in mind.
3. Bilateral stimulation continues until the memory has been processed with the chains of association.
4. Installation of positive images.
5. Scanning of body to identify any sensations.
6. Closure and debriefing on the experience of the session.

25.12.4 GRIEF COUNSELLING

Grief counselling allows the client to talk about the loss; to express feelings of sadness, guilt, or anger; and to understand the course of the grieving process. This therapy also allows the client to accept the loss, working through the grief process and adjust one's life without the deceased.

CASC STATION FOR GRIEF COUNSELLING

You are the consultant psychiatrist in charge of a psychotherapy service. A 35-year-old housewife with agoraphobia was referred to you urgently by her GP to continue psychotherapy as her previous therapist has passed away.

Task: Assess this client's suitability to continue psychotherapy.

25.12.5 APPROACH TO THIS CASC STATION

25.12.5.1 Issues the Candidate Needs to Explore

Issues related to the previous therapist

1. The cause of death of the previous therapist and how the client was informed
2. The type and quality of the therapeutic relationship between the deceased therapist and client
3. The type of treatment offered (e.., CBT)
4. The stage and progress of previous therapy

Issues relating to the client

1. Does the client feel responsible for the previous therapist's death (for real or imagined reasons)?
2. Comorbidity of the client (e.g. depression, panic disorder, or substance abuse).
3. Premorbid personality of the client and coping styles.
4. Previous experience of separations and grief process.
5. Look for acting-out behaviour that caused the GP to refer the case to you urgently.

Issues relating to the future therapy

1. Address new issues that are raised in the beginning of new therapy.
2. Explore expectations of the client to either continue the previous form of therapy or receive grief counselling.
3. Explore idealization of the previous therapist and potential devaluation of the current therapist.

25.13 BRIEF INSIGHT-ORIENTED THERAPY

Brief insight-oriented psychotherapy is based on psychoanalytic theory with different techniques and time frames. Insight refers to a person's understanding of his or her psychological function and personality. Treatment framework involves the therapist assisting the client to gain new and better insight into possible explanations for his or her feelings, responses, behaviours, and interpersonal relationships. It also expects that the client develops insight into his or her responses to the therapist and other significant relationship in the past.

25.14 ART THERAPIES

Objective: Art therapist provides a psychotherapeutic intervention that enables the client to effect change and growth by using the art materials to gain insight and promote the resolution of difficulties.

25.14.1 TYPES OF ART THERAPY

Art therapy is based on pictures and drawings. Therapeutic relationship progresses as art process progresses. The art therapist acts as a facilitator and the therapist is invited in the multidisciplinary team meeting to share his or her interpretation of a client's drawings.

Drama therapy encourages the clients to experience their physicality, to develop an ability to express a whole range of emotions, and to increase their insight and knowledge of themselves and other people.

Music therapy facilitates interaction and development of insight into a client's behaviour and emotional difficulties through listening to music.

Details of the scientific background of music therapy are considered in Puri (2009).

REFERENCES

Anna Freud Centre. http://www.annafreudcentre.org/shortcourses.php (accessed on 26 July 2012).

Aveline M and Dryden W. 1988: *Group Therapy in Britain*. Milton Keynes, England: Open University Press.

Barker P. 1998: *Basic Family Therapy*. Oxford, U.K.: Blackwell Science.

Barnes B, Ernst S, and Hyde K. 1999: *An Introduction to Group Work. A Group-Analytic Perspective*. Hampshire, England: Palgrave Macmillan.

Bateman A and Fonagy P. 2004: *Psychotherapy for Borderline Personality Disorder: Mentalization Based Treatment*. New York: Oxford University Press.

Bion WR. 1961: *Experiences in Groups*. London, U.K.: Tavistock.

Coetzee RH and Regel S. 2005: Eye movement desensitisation and reprocessing: An update. *Advances in Psychiatric Treatment* 11:347–354.

Council Report CR 95. 2001: *Curriculum for Basic Specialist Training and the MRCPsych Examination*. London, U.K.: Royal College of Psychiatrists.

Cowen P, Harrison P, and Burns T. 2012: *Shorter Oxford Textbook of Psychiatry*, pp. 571–600. Oxford, U.K.: Oxford University Press.

Crowe M and Ridley J. 2000: *Therapy with Couples*, 2nd edn. London, U.K.: Blackwell Science.

Denman C. 2001: Cognitive-analytical therapy. *Advances in Psychiatric Treatment* 7:243–256.

Foulkes SH. 1946: Group analysis in a military neurosis centre. *Lancet* 1:303–310.

Gabbard GO. 2000: *Psychodynamic Psychotherapy*, 3rd edn. Washington, DC: American Psychiatric Press.

Gabbard GO. 2005: Major modalities in psychoanalytic/psychodynamic. In Gabbard GO, Beck JS, and Holmes J (eds.) *Oxford Textbook of Psychotherapy*, pp. 3–14. Oxford, U.K.: Oxford University Press.

Greenberg LS and Johnson SM. 1988: *Emotionally Focused Therapy for Couples*. New York, NY: Guilford Press.

Hallstrom C and McClure N. 2005: *Your Questions Answered: Depression*. London, U.K.: Churchill Livingstone.

Hawton K, Salkovskis PM, Kirk J, and Clarl DM. 2001: *Cognitive Behaviour Therapy for Psychiatric Problems: A Practical Guide*. New York: Oxford University Press.

Hook J. 2007: Group psychotherapy. In Naismith J and Grant S. (eds.) *Seminars in the Psychotherapies*. London, U.K.: Gaskell.

Johnstone EC, Cunningham ODG, Lawrie SM, Sharpe M, and Freeman CPL. 2004: *Companion to Psychiatric Studies*. 7th edn. London, U.K.: Churchill Livingstone.

Lackwood K. 1999: Psychodynamic psychotherapy. In Stein S, Hiagh R, and Stein J (eds.) *Essentials of Psychotherapy*, pp. 134–154. Oxford, U.K.: Butterworth Heinemann.

Lewin K. 1943: Defining the "Field at a Given Time." *Psychological Review* 50:292–310.

Norton K and Warren F. 2009: Therapeutic communities. In Puri BK and Treasaden IH (eds.) *Psychiatry: An Evidence-Based Text*, pp. 1003–1008. London, U.K.: Hodder Arnold.

Palmer RL. 2002: Dialectical behaviour therapy for borderline personality disorder. *Advances in Psychiatric Treatment* 8:10–16.

Pratt JH. 1907: The organization of tuberculosis classes. *Medical Communications of the Massachusetts Medical Society* 20:475–492.

Puri BK. 2009: Other Individual Psychotherapies. In Puri BK and Treasaden IH (eds.) *Psychiatry: An Evidence-Based Text*, pp. 994–1002. London, U.K.: Hodder Arnold.

Puri BK and Treasaden IH. 2009: *Psychiatry: An Evidence-Based Text*. London, U.K.: Hodder Arnold.

Sadock BJ and Sadock VA. 2003: *Kaplan and Sadock's Comprehensive Textbook of Psychiatry*, 9th edn. Philadelphia, PA: Lippincott Williams and Wilkins.

Schaverien J and Odell-Miller H. 2005: The art therapies. In Gabbard GO, Beck JS, and Holmes J (eds.) *Oxford Textbook of Psychotherapy*, pp. 87–94. Oxford, U.K.: Oxford University Press.

Shemilt J and Naismith J. 2007: Psychodynamic theories II. In Naismith J and Grant S (eds.) *Seminars in the Psychotherapies*, pp. 63–99. London, U.K.: Gaskell.

Stuart S and Robertson M. 2003: *Interpersonal Psychotherapy: A Clinician's Guide*. London, U.K.: Arnold.

Turner T. 2003: *Your Questions Answered: Depression*. London, U.K.: Churchill Livingstone.

University of Ottawa. http://www.uottawapsychiatry.ca/en/uottawaresidents/Psychotherapy_Center_p3513.html (accessed on 28 July 2012)

Ursano RJ and Silberman EK. 1988: Individual psychotherapies. In Talbott JA, Hales RE, and Yudofsky SC (eds.) *The American Psychiatric Textbook of Psychiatry*. Washington, DC: American Psychiatric Press.

26 Schizophrenia and Delusional Disorders

26.1 SCHIZOPHRENIA

26.1.1 HISTORY

- In 1860, Morel used the term démence précoce for a disorder of deteriorating adolescent psychosis (Noll, 2011).
- In 1863, Kahlbaum described katatonie (Starkstein et al., 1995).
- In 1871, Hecker described hebephrenie (Hecker and Kraam, 2009).
- In 1894, Sommer included deteriorating paranoid syndromes in the concept of primary dementia.
- In 1868, Griesinger believed that insanity could develop in the absence of mood disturbance, primary insanity (primäre Verücktheit), and that all functional psychoses were expressions of single disease entity (Einheitspsychoses) (Dollfus and Petit, 1993).
- In 1896, Emil Kraepelin grouped together catatonia, hebephrenia, and the deteriorating paranoid psychoses under the name dementia praecox. He differentiated dementia praecox with its poor prognosis from the manic–depressive psychoses with their relatively better prognoses. He considered dementia praecox to be a disease of the brain (Kraepelin, 1987).
- In 1911, Bleuler introduced the term schizophrenia, applied it to Kraepelin's cases of dementia praecox, and expanded the concept to include what today may be considered schizophrenic spectrum disorders. He considered symptoms of ambivalence, autism, affective incongruity, and disturbance of association of thought to be fundamental (the 'four A's'), with delusions and hallucinations assuming secondary status. Bleuler was influenced by the writings of Sigmund Freud. He added schizophrenia simplex to Kraepelin's list (Berrios, 2011).
- In 1931, Hughlings Jackson considered positive symptoms as 'release phenomena' occurring in healthy tissue; negative symptoms were attributed to neuronal loss (Jackson, 1931).
- In 1959, Kurt Schneider emphasized the importance of delusions and hallucinations in defining his first-rank symptoms (Schneider, 1959).
- In 1960, Langfeldt sought to distinguish between schizophrenia and the better-prognosis schizophreniform psychoses and process versus nonprocess schizophrenia (Langfeldt, 1969).
- In 1972, Cooper compared patients admitted to psychiatric hospitals in New York and London. He found identical symptomatology, but schizophrenia diagnosed nearly twice as often in New York compared to London (Gurland, 1972).
- In 1973, the WHO conducted the International Pilot Study of Schizophrenia. This study found, using narrow criteria, a 1-year incidence of schizophrenia of 0.7–1.4 per 10,000 population aged 15–54, across all countries. It was confirmed that psychiatrists in the United States and the former USSR diagnosed schizophrenia twice as often as those in seven other countries (Columbia, Czechoslovakia, Denmark, Nigeria, India, Taiwan, and the United Kingdom). This led to a realization that psychiatric diagnoses had to be defined operationally (Sartorius et al., 1972).

26.2 CLASSIFICATION OF SCHIZOPHRENIA

26.2.1 SCHNEIDERIAN FIRST-RANK SYMPTOMS

In defining his first-rank symptoms, Schneider stated that in the absence of organic brain disease, the following are highly suggestive of schizophrenia:

- Auditory hallucinations
  - Repeat the thoughts out loud (e.g. Gedankenlautwerden, écho de la pensée)
  - In the third person
  - In the form of a running commentary
- Delusions of passivity
  - Thought insertion, withdrawal, and broadcasting
  - Made feelings, impulses, and actions
- Somatic passivity
- Delusional perception

Second-rank symptoms include perplexity, emotional blunting, hallucinations, and other delusions.

First-rank symptoms can occur in other psychoses and, although highly suggestive of schizophrenia, are not pathognomonic.

26.2.2 ST. LOUIS CRITERIA (FEIGHNER ET AL., 1972)

The sufferer is continuously ill for at least 6 months, with no prominent affective symptoms, presence of delusions, hallucinations, or thought disorder. Personal and family histories are taken into account (e.g. marital status, age under 40, premorbid social adjustment).

26.2.3 CATEGO (WING ET AL., 1974)

This uses the Present State Examination to generate diagnoses by means of a computer program. It is based on the Schneiderian concept of schizophrenia. No account is taken of symptom duration.

26.2.4 RESEARCH DIAGNOSTIC CRITERIA (SPITZER ET AL., 1975)

These are a 2-week duration, lack of affective symptoms, and presence of thought disorder, hallucinations, or delusions similar to Schneider's first-rank symptoms.

26.2.5 INTERNATIONAL CLASSIFICATION OF DISEASES, TENTH REVISION: ICD-10 (WHO, 1992)

There are fundamental, characteristic distortions of thinking and perception and inappropriate or blunted affect. There is clear consciousness. Intellectual capacity is usually maintained, but some cognitive deficits can evolve over time (see Table 26.1).

Symptoms are divided into groups:

1. Thought echo and thought alienation
2. Delusions of passivity; delusional perception
3. Auditory hallucinations in the form of a running commentary, or discussing the patient, or hallucinatory voices coming from some part of the body
4. Persistent delusions, culturally inappropriate and impossible
5. Persistent hallucinations in any modality, accompanied by fleeting delusions without affective content, or by persistent over-valued ideas, or occurring every day for weeks

6. Formal thought disorder comprising interruptions in the train of thought, incoherence, irrelevant speech, or neologisms
7. Catatonic behaviour (e.g. excitement, stupor, posturing, waxy flexibility, negativism and mutism)
8. Negative symptoms (e.g. apathy, paucity of speech, and blunted or incongruous affect)
9. A significant and consistent change in the overall quality of some aspects of personal behaviour (e.g. loss of interest, aimlessness, idleness, self-absorbed attitude, and social withdrawal)

Diagnostic guidelines require a minimum of one clear symptom (two if less clear-cut) belonging to groups (1) to (4), or symptoms from at least two of the groups (5) to (8) should have been present for most of the time during a period of one month or more.

Symptom (9) applies only to a diagnosis of simple schizophrenia, and a duration of at least one year is required.

Schizophrenia is not diagnosed if extensive affective symptoms are present, unless they postdate the schizophrenic syndrome. If both schizophrenic and affective symptoms develop together and are evenly balanced, the diagnosis of schizoaffective disorder is made.

Schizophrenia is not diagnosed in the presence of overt brain disease, or during drug intoxication or withdrawal.

The pattern of course is classified as (1) continuous; (2) episodic, progressive deficit; (3) episodic, stable deficit; (4) episodic, remittent; (5) incomplete remission; and (6) complete remission.

26.2.5.1 Subtypes

In ICD-10, the following subtypes of schizophrenia are distinguished:

- *Paranoid schizophrenia.* This is the commonest subtype. Hallucinations and/or delusions are prominent. Disturbances of affect, volition, speech, and catatonic symptoms are relatively inconspicuous. Auditory, olfactory, gustatory and somatic hallucinations, and visual hallucinations may occur. Commonly, there are delusions of control, influence, passivity, and persecution.
- *Hebephrenic schizophrenia.* The age of onset is usually between 15 and 25 years. There is a poor prognosis. Affective changes are prominent. Fleeting and fragmentary delusions and

TABLE 26.1

Compare and Contrast ICD-10 and Proposed DSM-5 Diagnostic Criteria for Schizophrenia

	ICD-10 (F20.) (WHO, 1992)	DSM-5 (APA, 2013)
F20 Schizophrenia Number of symptoms	At least one of: Thought disturbances, passivity, hallucinatory voices, and persistent delusional beliefs Or two or more of: Other persistent hallucinations, formal thought disorder, catatonic behaviour, and negative symptoms	295.90 Schizophrenia At least two of the following: delusions, hallucinations, disorganized speech, grossly disorganized or catatonic behaviour, and negative symptoms. Out of the two symptoms, at least one should be delusions, hallucinations, or disorganized speech At least two items of less specific symptoms Absence of substance abuse or general medical condition Specify if catatonic features are present Specify the number of episodes and remission status (partial or full)
Deterioration in occupational and social function	It is not a compulsory criterion	It is a compulsory criterion
Duration of symptoms	The symptoms have to be present for at least 1 month for schizophrenia The symptoms have to be present for at least 1 year for simple schizophrenia	The minimum duration of disturbance is at least 6 months. The minimum duration of symptoms is at least 1 month
Inclusion of simple schizophrenia and schizophreniform disorder	F20.6 simple schizophrenia: 1-year of negative symptoms and deterioration in personal behaviour as a result of loss of drive or interest and social withdrawal No mention of schizophreniform disorder	No mention of simple schizophrenia 295.40 Schizophreniform disorder: Duration is between 1 and 6 months; specifier includes with or without good prognostic factors (e.g. acute onset, absence of negative symptoms, confusion, good premorbid functioning)
Other types of schizophrenia	F20.0 Paranoid schizophrenia F20.1 Hebephrenic schizophrenia: flatten and incongruity of affect, stereotypies, incoherent speech, with minimal positive symptoms F20.2 Catatonic schizophrenia: duration for 2 weeks, similar to the DSM-5 criteria with additional symptom such as command automatism F20.3 Undifferentiated schizophrenia F20.5 Residual schizophrenia: reduction in activity, blunting of affect, lack of initiative, and poor communication and self-care	Catatonic disorder associated with another medical condition: motoric immobility (catalepsy/waxy flexibility/stupor), excessive motor activity, extreme negativism or mutism, peculiarities of voluntary movement (stereotypies, mannerisms), echolalia, or echopraxia The DSM-5 does not propose subtype of schizophrenia
Delusional disorder	F22. Delusion disorder: 3 months in duration, no hallucinations F22.8 Other persistent delusional disorders: delusional dysmorphobia, involutional paranoid state, and paranoia querulans F22.9 Persistent delusional disorder, unspecified	F297.1 Delusional disorder Duration: at least 1 month Not meeting the diagnostic criteria for schizophrenia, but tactile or olfactory hallucinations may be present Mood disturbance only lasts for a brief period of time No significant impairment of functioning Subtypes include • Erotomanic type • Grandiose type • Jealous type • Persecutory type • Somatic type • Mixed type • Unspecified type

(continued)

TABLE 26.1 (continued)

Compare and Contrast ICD-10 and Proposed DSM-5 Diagnostic Criteria for Schizophrenia

	ICD-10 (F20.)	Proposed DSM-5
Brief psychosis	F23 Acute and transient psychotic disorder: symptoms not exceeding 2 weeks, with or without associated acute stress. This disorder accounts for around 10% of all psychotic disorder. 30% of patients can remain in remission without medication (Philmann and Marneros, 2005) F23.0 Acute polymorphic psychotic disorder without symptoms of schizophrenia: duration < 3 months F23.1 Acute polymorphic psychotic disorder with symptoms of schizophrenia: duration < 1 month F23.2 Acute schizophrenia-like psychotic disorder: duration < 1 month F23.3 Other acute predominantly delusional psychotic disorders: duration < 3 months F23.8 Other acute and transient psychotic disorders F23.9 Acute and transient psychotic disorder, unspecified	298.8 Brief psychotic disorder: presence of one (or more) of the following: delusions, hallucinations, disorganized speech (e.g. frequent derailment or incoherence), and grossly disorganized or catatonic behaviour. Duration is between 1 day and 1 month Specifier includes with stressful event, without stressful event, and with postpartum onset Substance-induced psychotic disorder: Psychotic symptoms develop within 1 month of substance intoxication or withdrawal Psychotic disorder associated with another medical condition: hallucination subtype, delusion subtype, and disorganized speech subtype The number of subtypes of brief psychotic disorder proposed by DSM-5 is less than ICD-10
Schizoaffective disorder	F20.0 Schizoaffective disorder—manic type: duration at least 2 weeks F25.1 Schizoaffective disorder—depressive type: duration at least 2 weeks F25.2 Schizoaffective disorder—mixed type: Schizophrenia and affective symptoms are prominent F25.8 Other schizoaffective disorders F25.9 Schizoaffective disorder, unspecified	295.70 Schizoaffective disorder—bipolar type and depressive type The psychosis is present for at least 2 weeks in the absence of mood symptoms The mood symptoms account for at least 50% in the course of illness Specify the number of episodes and remission status (e.g. partial or full)
Post-schizophrenic depression	F20.4 Post-schizophrenic depression Prolonged depressive symptoms when psychotic symptoms subside and depression occurs within 12 months of schizophrenia	Not mentioned
Schizotypal disorder	This disorder is listed under schizophrenia. Clinical features include quasipsychotic experience, odd belief, speech, behaviour, idea of reference, excess social anxiety, paranoia, and absence of close friends	This disorder is considered to be a personality disorder, but DSM-5 also lists this disorder under schizophrenia. It must fulfil two core criteria for personality disorder: impairment in self and interpersonal functioning. Further details are found in Chapter 29

hallucinations; irresponsible behaviour; fatuous, disorganized thought; rambling speech; and mannerisms are common. Negative symptoms, particularly flattening of affect and loss of volition, are prominent. Drive and determination are lost, goals abandoned, and behaviour becomes aimless and empty. The premorbid personality is characteristically shy and solitary.

• *Catatonic schizophrenia.* One or more of the following behaviours dominate: stupor, excitement, posturing, negativism, rigidity, waxy flexibility, command automatism, and perseveration of words or phrases. Catatonic symptoms alone are not diagnostic of schizophrenia; they may be provoked by brain disease, metabolic disturbance, alcohol and drugs, and mood disorders. Psychomotor disturbances may alternate between extremes; violent excitement may occur. It may be combined with a dreamlike state with vivid scenic hallucinations.

- *Simple schizophrenia.* There is an insidious onset of decline in functioning. Negative symptoms develop without preceding positive symptoms. Diagnosis requires changes in behaviour over at least a year, with marked loss of interest, idleness, and social withdrawal.
- *Residual or chronic schizophrenia.* This is characterized by negative symptoms. There is past evidence of at least one schizophrenic episode and a period of at least 1 year in which frequency of positive symptoms has been minimal and negative schizophrenic syndrome has been present. There is absence of depression, institutionalization, or dementia or other brain disorders.
- *Undifferentiated schizophrenia.* General criteria for schizophrenia are satisfied but not conforming to the earlier syndromes.
- *Post-schizophrenic depression.* This is a depressive episode arising after a schizophrenic illness. Schizophrenic illness must have occurred within the last 12 months, some symptoms still being present. Depressive symptoms fulfil at least the criteria for a depressive episode and are present for at least 2 weeks. There is an increased risk of suicide.

26.2.6   Type 1 and Type 2 Schizophrenia (Crow, 1980)

Crow described a two-syndrome hypothesis of schizophrenia—a categorical approach:

- *Type 1 schizophrenia.* This type is characterized by prominent positive symptoms, acute onset, good premorbid adjustment, good treatment response, intact cognition, intact brain structure, and a reversible neurochemical disturbance.
- *Type 2 schizophrenia.* This type is characterized by prominent negative symptoms, insidious onset, poor premorbid adjustment, poor treatment response, impaired cognition, structural brain abnormalities (ventricular enlargement), and an underlying pathology based on neuronal loss, therefore irreversible.

26.2.7   SAPS and SANS

In 1984, Andreasen developed structured scales for the assessment of positive and negative symptoms: the Scale for the Assessment of Positive Symptoms (SAPS) and the Scale for the Assessment of Negative Symptoms (SANS).

26.2.8   Liddle's Syndromes (Liddle, 1987)

Liddle found that the pattern of symptoms in schizophrenia segregated into three distinguishable syndromes—a dimensional approach:

- *Psychomotor poverty syndrome.* There is poverty of speech, flatness of affect, and decreased spontaneous movement.
- *Disorganization syndrome.* There are disorders of the form of thought and inappropriate affect.
- *Reality distortion syndrome.* There are delusions and hallucinations.

A subsequent PET study of regional cerebral blood flow (Liddle et al., 1992) showed that each of these three syndromes is associated with a specific pattern of perfusion.

26.2.8.1   Psychomotor Poverty Syndrome

Hypoperfusion of the left dorsal prefrontal cortex extends to medial prefrontal cortex and anterior cingulate cortex. There is hyperperfusion in the head of the caudate nucleus, which receives substantial projections from the dorsolateral prefrontal cortex. Some changes are also found on the right (laterality only a matter of degree). Hypofrontality in schizophrenia is more often seen in chronic patients and is associated with inactivity and catatonic symptoms. In normal subjects, prefrontal activity increases when involved in internal generation of action.

26.2.8.2   Disorganization Syndrome

There is hypoperfusion of the right ventral prefrontal cortex and increased activity in anterior cingulate and dorsomedial thalamic nuclei that project to the prefrontal cortex. There is relative hypoperfusion of Broca's area and bilateral hypoperfusion of parietal association cortex. Evidence suggests that in primates the ventral prefrontal cortex plays a role in suppression of interference from irrelevant mental activity. The anterior cingulate plays a role in attentional mechanisms. The suggestion is that these patients are engaged in an ineffective struggle to suppress inappropriate mental activity.

26.2.8.3   Reality Distortion Syndrome

There is increased activity in the left parahippocampal region and left striatum. This is consistent with the proposal that delusions and hallucinations arise from a disorder of internal monitoring resulting in failure to recognize internally generated mental acts. Abnormalities of function underlying schizophrenic symptoms are not confined to single loci but involve distributed neuronal networks.

26.2.9 Neurodevelopmental Classification (Murray et al., 1992)

On the basis of genetic, epidemiological, neuropathological, neuroimaging, and gender difference studies, schizophrenia has been subdivided into the following three groups:

- *Congenital schizophrenia.* The abnormality is present at birth and may be caused by genetic predisposition and/or environmental insult (e.g. maternal influenza, obstetric complication, early brain injury, or infection). The person is more likely to have minor physical abnormalities, abnormal personality, or social impairment in childhood; to present early; to exhibit negative symptoms; and to show morphological brain changes and cognitive impairment. The person is more likely to be male and to have a poor outcome.
- *Adult-onset schizophrenia.* The person is more likely to exhibit positive and affective symptoms. The person may have a genetic predisposition to manifest symptomatology anywhere along a continuum from bipolar mood disorder to schizoaffective disorder to schizophrenia.
- *Late-onset schizophrenia.* This presents after age 60 years, with good premorbid functioning. It is most common in females. It is often associated with auditory and visual sensory deprivation. It is sometimes related to paranoid personality or to mood disorder. Organic brain dysfunction is often present.

CASC STATION ON THE SYMPTOMS OF SCHIZOPHRENIA

A 17-year-old female is admitted to the psychiatric ward with a weeklong history of complaining of 'increasing interference to her mind'. She suffers from schizophrenia, and she has been adherent to medication. She seems to be irritable and anxious.

Task: Take a history to establish the causes of her stress.

Approach to this station: In this station, the candidate is expected to determine whether the patient is suffering from schizophrenia and to rule out differential diagnoses such as substance misuse, organic disorder, or affective disorder with psychotic features. Candidates who perform poorly focused only on schizophrenia and did not consider other differential diagnoses that may lead to the patient's described symptoms. The simulated patient in the exam appears to be calm and denies other first-rank symptoms. However, by careful history taking, it is possible to determine that the symptoms and presentation are most likely related to psychotic illness.

CASC Grid

Opening statement: 'Hello, my name is Dr Ford. I would like to ask you a few questions. Would that be okay? Can you tell me how you've been feeling? I understand from the nurse that you've been experiencing some stress. Can you tell me more about this?'

(A) Schizophrenia Symptoms	(A1) Thought	(A2) Passivity Experiences	(A3) Delusions	(A4) Hallucination
	'I can imagine that it is quite stressful if your thoughts are being interfered with. Can you tell me more about this?' 'Are you able to think clearly?' 'Does your mind go blank suddenly?'	'Do you feel that the thoughts are being put into/taken out of your head?' 'Do you feel that everyone knows what's on in your mind? Do you feel that people can read your mind?' 'Do you feel that your thoughts are being broadcasted out so that everyone can receive your thoughts?'	'Do you feel that people are talking about you or laughing at your expense? Do you think that people are following you/out to get you?' 'Do you realize that things happening to you have a special meaning to you?' (delusional perception) 'Do you feel that someone wants to harm you at this moment? If so, who is behind it? Could it be a misunderstanding?'	'Do you hear voices when there's no one around? If yes, how do the voices address you?' 'Do the voices give you instructions? If yes, what kinds of instructions do they give?' 'Do you see things that other people cannot see?' 'Do you experience funny sensations in your body or as if something strange is going to happen to you?'

(B) Other Psychiatric Comorbidities	(B1) Anxiety State	(B2) Affective Disorder	(B3) Substance Abuse	(B4) Insight, Side Effects, and Risk Assessment
	'Do you feel anxious most of the time? Are there specific things/ situations that make you feel anxious? Do you experience shaking/ sweating/heart racing/ choking/fainting/ dizziness?' 'How do you cope with anxiety? Do you take drug to control it?'	'How is your mood today? Do you feel sad? Do you feel high, like the top of the world?' 'What is the reason behind your low mood? Is it because of the voices?'	'Do you use recreational drugs or alcohol? If so, what do you use? How often do you use it? When was the last intake?' 'Do you feel shaky without those drugs?'	'How do you feel about your illness?' 'Do you receive any treatment at this moment? Do you experience any side effect?' 'Do you have the feeling that life is not worth living? Do you have thoughts of hurting yourself or other people?'

(C) Issues Related to Young People	(C1) Academic Performance	(C2) Recent Life Event	(C3) Relationship with Parents	(C4) Relationship Problems and Peers
	'Are you in school at this moment? Do you experience any academic difficulty?' 'How did you do in your study in the past?' 'Do you feel that those voices are affecting your concentration?'	'Did you experience any unhappy events prior to admission?' 'Is there a change in your environment recently?' 'Do you have any financial problem at this moment?'	'Can you tell me more about your parents? How do they treat you? Are they overprotective?' 'Do you feel that your parents are critical or overinvolved?' (assess expressed emotion [EE]) 'What's the family's view of your admission? Are they concerned about you?' 'Do you have any family member suffering from similar illness?'	'Are you in a relationship at this moment? If yes, can you tell me more about your relationship?' 'How about your friends? Do they know that you are here? Do they know about your illness? Are they supportive?'

(D) Past Medical History and Background History	(D1) Recent Illness	(D2) Chronic Medical Illness	(D3) Previous Traumatic Events	(D4) Explain your Preliminary Formulation to the Patient
	'Have you fallen sick recently?' 'Have you received any treatment such as antibiotics?' 'Did you travel to other countries recently?'	'Do you suffer from chronic disease that requires frequent treatment?' Explore history of epilepsy, head injury, asthma, etc. If chronic illness is present, explore the effect on his or her development, relationship with her family, and possible developmental lag.	Explore history of psychological, physical, and sexual abuse. 'Do you have traumatic experience in the past? If yes, can you tell me more?'	If you have identified a stressor, check with the patient and see whether he or she agrees that this is the source of his or her stress.

26.3   EPIDEMIOLOGY OF SCHIZOPHRENIA

26.3.1   Statistics

- The incidence of schizophrenia is between 15 and 30 new cases per 100,000 of the population per year:
- The point prevalence is approximately 1%.
- The lifetime risk is approximately 1%.
- The age of onset is usually between 15 and 45 years, earlier in men than in women.
- It is equally common in males and females. There is a higher incidence in those not married.
- It is most common in social classes IV and V.
- Prevalence varies geographically. Rates from urban areas are generally higher than in rural areas, with marked exceptions—the highest prevalence measured (17.4 per 1000 population) was from a sparsely populated rural area in the west of Ireland.

Further details on epidemiology of schizophrenia are found in Chapter 21.

26.3.2   Theories

The following are theories accounting for geographical variance in the prevalence of schizophrenia:

- *Social drift.* Goldberg and Morrison (1963) studied fathers' birth certificates and found schizophrenic males had lower social class distribution than their fathers. They attributed these findings to social drift, that is, migration of those affected to areas where social demands may be less. Men were more likely to drift into inner city areas.
- *Social residue.* Healthy people migrate away from undesirable areas, leaving schizophrenics behind.
- *Breeder or social causation.* This theory assumes that environmental factors either are causative or have to be present for the predisposed individual to develop schizophrenia. Castle et al. (1993) found that schizophrenic patients in Camberwell were more likely to have been born in a socially deprived area and to have fathers with manual jobs. Those developing schizophrenia were more likely than controls to have been born into socially deprived households. This suggested that some environmental factor of aetiological importance in schizophrenia is more likely to affect those born into households of lower socio-economic status and in the inner city.

Theories emphasizing environmental influences need not exclude the importance of biological factors, such as exposure to toxins, increased incidence of obstetric complications, and a higher rate of infectious disease in cities. Social factors more common in cities include stressful life events, social isolation, and social overstimulation.

26.4   AETIOLOGY OF SCHIZOPHRENIA

26.4.1   Genetics in Schizophrenia

The heritability of schizophrenia is between 82% and 85% (Farmer et al., 1987: Cardno et al., 1999). Twin, family, and adoption studies have consistently demonstrated familial aggregation of schizophrenia, largely attributable to genetic factors.

26.4.1.1   Family Studies
Table 26.2 shows the approximate lifetime risks for the development of schizophrenia in the relatives of patients with schizophrenia.

26.4.1.2   Twin Studies
The concordance rate for monozygotic (MZ) twins is approximately 45%, that for dizygotic (DZ) twins approximately 10% (Gottesman and Shields, 1972).

Studying adult offspring of 21 MZ and 41 DZ twin pairs discordant for schizophrenia, Gottesman and Bertelsen found the risk of developing schizophrenia was 17% among the adult children of the MZ and DZ probands, 17% among the offspring of phenotypically normal MZ co-twins, and only 2% among the offspring of phenotypically normal DZ co-twins. This suggests that

TABLE 26.2

Approximate Lifetime Risks for the Development of Schizophrenia in the Relatives of Patients with Schizophrenia

Relationship	Lifetime Expectancy Rate to the Nearest Percentage Point
Parents	6
All siblings	10
Siblings (when one parent has schizophrenia)	17
Children	13
Children (when both parents have schizophrenia)	46
Grandchildren	4
Uncles, aunts, nephews, and nieces	3

the normal MZ co-twins carried and transmitted the relevant genotype without expressing it themselves.

26.4.1.3 Adoption Studies

When children of schizophrenic mothers have been adopted soon after birth by nonschizophrenic families, they have a similar likelihood of developing schizophrenia (approximately 13%) as the rates suggested by family studies. There appears to be no such increased risk of developing schizophrenia in the children of nonschizophrenic parents who are similarly adopted (Kety et al., 1971).

The following are possible modes of inheritance:

- *Single major locus.* Some forms possibly exist but would account for a very small proportion of observed cases. To date, no single genetic focus responsible for the development of schizophrenia has been reliably demonstrated.
- *Polygenic.* There might be a threshold of gene numbers required for expression of schizophrenia.
- *Multifactorial.* There may be aetiological heterogeneity with various genetic and environmental subtypes. There is probably a spectrum of causes ranging from wholly genetic, through those with mixed aetiology, to the totally environmental.

26.4.1.4 Linkage Studies

Bassett and associates reported a man who presented with schizophrenia plus minor physical abnormalities both shared by his maternal uncle. Cytogenetic analysis revealed translocation of part of chromosome 5; this led the writers to postulate that this segment of chromosome 5 may be site of a putative schizophrenia gene.

Sherrington and associates collected seven extended schizophrenic families from Iceland and England, probed chromosome 5, and found evidence highly suggestive of linkage between markers on chromosome 5 and schizophrenia. However, this finding has never been replicated, and the study has subsequently been criticized on methodological grounds.

The following candidate genes and chromosomes are implicated in the aetiology of schizophrenia:

- Chromosome 1q22: CArboxyl-terminal Pdz ligand of neuronal Nitric Oxide synthas (CAPON)
- Chromosom 1q23: RGS4 I (regulator of G-protein signalling 4)
- Chromosom 1q42.1: DISC1 (disrupted in schizophrenia 1)
- Chromosom 5q33: EPN4
- Chromosome 5q34: GABA(A) receptors

- Chromosome 6p22: DTNBP1 (dystrobrevin-binding protein 1)
- Chromosome 6q23: TAAR6 (trace amine associate receptor 6)
- Chromosome 8p12: NRG1 (neuregulin)
- Chromosome 8p21: PPP3CC (protein phosphatase 3 calcineurin gamma catalytic gene)
- Chromosome 13q34: G72
- Chromosome 22q11: PRODH (proline dehydrogenase (oxidase) 1), ZDHHC8, catechol-*o*-methyltransferase (COMT)

There are problems in applying linkage methodology to schizophrenia:

- Schizophrenia is probably genetically heterogeneous.
- Linkage analysis is usually applied to conditions transmitted by simpler Mendelian inheritance.
- Diagnostic and penetrance problems probably require a much higher lod score than the usual +3 before linkage for psychiatric diagnoses can be regarded as proved.

26.4.2 PRENATAL FACTORS IN SCHIZOPHRENIA

People developing schizophrenia as adults are born disproportionately more often during late winter and early spring. A similar but less marked seasonal effect is reported for bipolar affective disorders but not for neurotic or personality disorders. Seasonally varying environmental causes have been sought, and prenatal infection is currently the most favoured explanation.

An excess of minor physical abnormalities is reported in schizophrenics; examples are low-set ears, greater distance between the eyes, and a single transverse palmar crease. Dermatoglyphics are determined by genes, and deleterious events in the second trimester of pregnancy can alter their form. Schizophrenics have deviations from normal in ridge patterns of fingers, palms, and soles. Schizophrenic probands of MZ twin pairs discordant for schizophrenia have significantly more finger and palm epidermal ridge anomalies than their healthy co-twins (Bracha et al., 1991).

Structural abnormalities in the brains of many schizophrenics suggest a neurodevelopmental rather than degenerative process. Most studies investigating brain morphology in schizophrenia report nonprogressive ventricular and cortical sulcal enlargement and structural abnormalities in the limbic areas. Structural changes reflect an early acquired hypoplasia, not degeneration. Cytoarchitectural changes in limbic and prefrontal areas are strong indicators of early disordered brain development. Altered distribution of cortical layers of NADPH-d neurons is consistent with a disturbance of development, in which the normal pattern of programmed cell death is compromised, resulting in defective migration of neurons.

Murray suggests that neural dysplasia results in premorbid cognitive deficits, abnormal personality, negative symptoms, and abnormal CT scans in schizophrenia. Maturational brain changes in adolescence, possibly myelination or synaptic pruning, reveal immature neuronal circuitry with consequent onset of hallucinations and delusions.

The neurodevelopmental model of schizophrenia accounts for the following findings:

- Individuals who were in their second trimester of fetal life during the influenza epidemic in Finland in 1957 had an increased risk of later schizophrenia (Mednick et al., 1988).
- The winter excess of births in schizophrenics is due to a seasonal prevalence of a viral infection or other perinatal hazard.
- Males have an earlier onset of schizophrenia than females, possibly due to increased vulnerability to neurodevelopmental damage (generally commoner in males).
- The smaller proportion of male schizophrenics is genetically determined; there is evidence that concordance rates for schizophrenia are lower in male than in female identical twins.

Obstetric complications (premature rupture of membrane, premature birth (<37 weeks), and use of resuscitator or incubation) are more frequent in schizophrenics than in normal controls. This is noted particularly in schizophrenics without a positive family history for psychosis, implying that obstetric factors may augment or substitute for a genetic cause.

26.4.3 PERSONALITY IN SCHIZOPHRENIA

Only schizotypal personality disorder is aetiologically related to schizophrenia. Among the schizotypal criteria, eccentricity, affect constriction, and excessive social anxiety are linked to schizophrenia. There may be a milder phenotype along the schizophrenia spectrum.

26.4.4 SOCIAL FACTORS IN SCHIZOPHRENIA

26.4.4.1 Rural or Urban Setting

The higher prevalence of schizophrenia in urban areas is a result of interaction of genetic factors, migration, higher rates of social deprivation, and social problems in the inner city.

26.4.4.2 Ethnicity

Afro-Caribbean immigrants to the United Kingdom have higher risk of schizophrenia. This phenomenon is seen in the second generation.

26.4.4.3 Expressed Emotion

In 1968, Brown and Birley found that schizophrenics had experienced significantly more independent life events in the 3 weeks prior to onset of relapse than had controls. In 1976, Vaughn and Leff found an increased relapse rate of schizophrenia in those who lived with families in which the relatives displayed high EE (critical comments, overinvolvement) (see Figure 26.1). Changes in physiological arousal may account for this effect.

There was a poverty of the social milieu of patients with chronic schizophrenia, associated with increased negative symptoms, particularly social withdrawal, affective blunting, and poverty of speech (Wing and Brown, 1961).

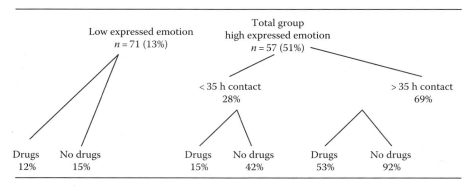

FIGURE 26.1   Relapse rates of 128 schizophrenics over a 9-month period. (From Vaughn, C.E. and Leff, J.P., *Br. J. Psychiatry,* 129, 125, 1976.)

26.4.5   CASC STATION ON SCHIZOPHRENIA AND CANNABIS

A 19-year-old man is admitted because he experiences a psychotic episode. He smokes cannabis regularly. His mother has browsed through the Internet and has some questions for you. She wants to know the relationship between cannabis use and schizophrenia.

Task
Explain to her the relationship between schizophrenia and cannabis. Address her views, concerns, and expectations.

How to fail this station: Candidates who perform well in this station address the controversy surrounding the role of cannabis in the aetiology of schizophrenia and the complicating effects of cannabis on the course of illness. Candidates may fail if they do not broadly describe their experience in clinical practice and the research evidence relating to the association between cannabis and psychosis.

26.4.5.1   Approach to This Station

26.4.5.1.1   Background Information

Cannabis leads to a twofold increase in risk of schizophrenia and a fourfold increase in risk of psychosis (Arseneault et al., 2004).

26.4.5.1.2   Role of Genetic Factors

Explain to his mother that not all cannabis users develop schizophrenia. It depends on the COMT genotype. People who have homozygous VAL/VAL alleles in the COMT genotype have relatively higher risk. People who are homozygous for MET/MET alleles in the COMT genotype have no increase in risk.

26.4.5.1.3   Explain Effects of Cannabis

1. Amotivational syndrome
2. Flashback phenomena
3. Changes in affect
4. Change in heart rate, red eyes, motor incoordination, poor concentration, and memory problems

26.4.5.1.4   Obtain More Information About Her Son's Usage of Cannabis

1. Duration and frequency of use
2. Peer influence
3. Other substance use, for example, alcohol
4. Economic impact
5. Predisposing factors: personality and peer pressure

26.4.5.1.5   Explain the Roles of Cannabis after Development of Schizophrenia

1. Self-medication
2. Worsening of psychotic symptoms (e.g. idea of reference, paranoia)
3. Worsening of other symptoms (e.g. agitation, confusion)
4. Worsening of negative symptoms

26.4.5.1.6   Explain the Challenges in Dual Diagnosis

1. The difficulties of assessment: emphasize on the need to be clear of the chronological sequence of cannabis misuse and development of psychosis.
2. Other substance use such as alcohol may affect efficacy of antipsychotics.
3. Amotivational syndrome, reluctance to quit cannabis (require motivational interviewing), and its effects on the therapeutic alliance.
4. Potential involvement of substance abuse service.
5. Importance of psychoeducation to prevent further substance use.

26.4.6   NEUROTRANSMITTERS IN SCHIZOPHRENIA

26.4.6.1   Dopamine

The mesolimbic–mesocortical system is a dopaminergic system originating in the ventral tegmental area of the brain. The mesolimbic system projects to the limbic system, while the mesocortical system innervates the cingulate, entorhinal, and medial prefrontal cortices.

The dopamine hypothesis of schizophrenia asserts that the clinical features are the result of central dopaminergic hyperactivity in the mesolimbic–mesocortical system. The following is put as evidence in favour of the dopamine hypothesis:

- All clinically effective antipsychotic drugs occupy a substantial proportion of D_2 receptors in the brain (70%–80% D_2 receptor occupancy in the striatum at normal doses).
- Amphetamine, a dopamine agonist, can cause a state similar to that of acute schizophrenia.
- Dopamine agonists exacerbate psychotic symptoms.
- Comparing actions of a and b isomers of flupenthixol in patients with acute schizophrenia, only those receiving the dopamine antagonist improved (Johnstone et al., 1978).
- Postmortem studies have found increased D_2 receptors in the basal ganglia and limbic regions of schizophrenic brains.

- In animals, administration of dopamine agonists produces a behavioural picture said to be similar to human psychosis. This is reversed by giving dopamine antagonists.
- In drug-naive schizophrenics, the number of D_2 receptors in the striatum was two to three times that of controls as measured by PET (Wong et al., 1986).

Evidence against the dopamine hypothesis includes

- The concentration of dopamine metabolite homovanillic acid (HVA) in the cerebrospinal fluid in schizophrenics has generally not been found to be higher than in control subjects.
- D_2 receptor blockade caused by antipsychotics is an acute effect, but the therapeutic effect is observed 3–4 weeks later.
- 15%–30% of schizophrenics fail to respond to dopamine antagonists.
- Antipsychotics have a better effect on positive than on negative symptoms.
- Clozapine, an effective antipsychotic, has less D_2 blocking activity than conventional antipsychotics.
- Some studies have failed to replicate Wong's findings of increased D_2 receptors in striatum of brains of living schizophrenics.

Explanations that may account for contradictory results

- Schizophrenia is clinically complex, and the aetiology is heterogeneous.
- Schizophrenia may involve reduced dopaminergic activity in the prefrontal cortical area and compensatory overactivity in subcortical or limbic areas.
- There are potential problems in patient selection and study methodology.
- Identification of D_1, D_3, D_4, and D_5 receptors has suggested that they alone or in addition to D_2 receptors may be the appropriate target for antipsychotic drug therapy.
- Clozapine acts in part by antagonism of D_1, D_2, and particularly D_4 receptors; it is effective during long-term use in up to 60% of neuroleptic-resistant patients.
- D_1 antagonist alone failed to show antipsychotic efficacy. Specific D_3 and D_4 antagonists have not yet been studied.

- During treatment with haloperidol, the ratio of dopamine metabolite (HVA) to serotonin and noradrenaline metabolites in CSF of schizophrenics increased significantly and correlated with reduction of symptoms. This supports the hypothesis that interactions between different monoamine neurotransmitters are involved in expression of schizophrenic symptoms.

26.4.6.2 Serotonin (5-HT)

There is some evidence that serotonergic dysfunction may be associated with schizophrenia:

- The hallucinogen LSD (see Chapter 32) acts at serotonin receptors.
- Antipsychotic risperidone is a potent $5-HT_2$ receptor antagonist (it also blocks D_2 receptors, however).
- Ritanserin, a selective $5-HT_2$ antagonist, reduced negative symptoms when given as adjunctive therapy in neuroleptic-treated schizophrenics.

26.4.6.3 Glutamate

Glutamate stimulates the NMDA receptor. Phencyclidine ('angel dust'—see Chapter 32) causes schizophrenic-like effects by blocking NMDA receptors. A balance exists between excitatory glutamatergic and inhibitory dopaminergic terminals in the corpus striatum, regulating GABAergic neurons. These function in the 'thalamic filter', which seems to be hypoactive in schizophrenia. According to this theory, hypoactivity of GABA neurons is corrected by either reducing dopaminergic activity or increasing glutamatergic activity.

26.4.7 Structural Cerebral Abnormalities in Schizophrenia

Johnstone et al. (1976) conducted a CT scan study, finding that chronically hospitalized schizophrenic patients had larger lateral ventricles than controls. This has been confirmed by numerous neuroimaging studies.

In 1990, Andreasen et al. conducted a large study in people matched for age, sex, height, weight, and level of education. The ventricle/brain ratio was greater in schizophrenics than in controls. The differences were small, and there was overlap with the normal population; it was more marked in males.

MRI has shown a diffuse reduction in the volume of cortical grey matter in schizophrenic patients, this being associated with poor premorbid function. These findings are consistent with neurodevelopmental changes having taken place in such patients.

The following are further structural changes in schizophrenia found in some studies:

- Reduced size of frontal lobes or some division thereof
- Reduced size of temporal lobe, particularly on the left
- Reduced size of hippocampus and amygdala, particularly on the left
- Reduced size of parahippocampal gyrus

26.4.8 Neuropathological Abnormalities in Schizophrenia

26.4.8.1 Postmortem Studies

Compared with control subjects, the brains of schizophrenic patients have shown the following in some studies:

- Lower fixed brain weight
- Reduced brain length
- Reduced size of the parahippocampal gyrus

26.4.8.2 Histological Studies

Compared to controls, the brains of schizophrenics have shown the following in some studies:

- Hippocampal pyramidal cell disarray
- Reduced hippocampal cell numbers
- Reduced cell numbers in the entorhinal cortex
- Reduced hippocampal cell size
- Disturbed cytoarchitecture in the entorhinal cortex

26.4.9 Functional Brain Abnormalities in Schizophrenia

Hypofrontality is associated with the presence of negative symptoms and autism.

Combining functional imaging with task activation, Weinberger et al. (1986) measured regional cerebral blood flow at rest and during the Wisconsin Card Sorting Test (activates frontal lobes normally). Impaired performance by schizophrenics was mirrored by a smaller increase in blood flow to prefrontal cortex.

26.4.10 Deficits in Cognition in Schizophrenia

Cognitive impairment is common among patients suffering from schizophrenia. The cognitive deficits of schizophrenia are summarized in Figure 26.2.

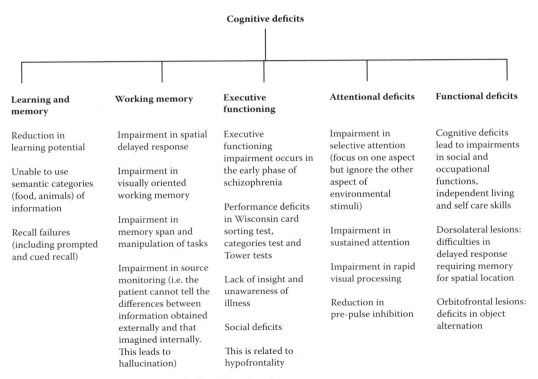

FIGURE 26.2 A summary of cognitive deficits in schizophrenia.

26.5 MANAGEMENT OF SCHIZOPHRENIA

26.5.1 PHYSICAL EXAMINATION

1. Vital signs: heart rate and temperature.
2. Measure BMI.
3. Neurological examination looking for side effects associated with antipsychotics such as extrapyramidal side effects (EPSE).

26.5.2 INVESTIGATIONS

1. Full blood count (FBC)
2. Liver function tests (LFTs)
3. Renal function tests (RFTs)
4. Electrolytes
5. Thyroid function tests
6. Fasting lipids and glucose
7. Pregnancy test β-HCG (for females)
8. Toxicology screen
9. Electrocardiogram
10. CT brain scan or MRI brain scan
11. Prolactin level if patient complains of galactorrhoea

26.5.3 GENERAL MANAGEMENT STRATEGIES (SCOTTISH SCHIZOPHRENIA GUIDELINES AND NICE GUIDELINES)

1. Assess symptoms and establish a diagnosis based on the ICD-10 or DSM-V criteria.
2. Establish therapeutic alliance and formulate and implement a treatment plan.
3. Phase-specific management:
   A. *Acute phase*:
      a. Community mental health teams are an acceptable way of organizing community care.
      b. Crisis resolution and home treatment teams should be used to manage crises of patients and should augment services provided by early intervention and assertive outreach teams.
      c. Alternatives to acute inpatient care should be developed.
      d. Antipsychotic therapy should be initiated as part of a comprehensive package of care.
      e. Atypical antipsychotic should be introduced at the earliest convenience. Atypical drugs at the lower end of the dose range should be used in the first episode of schizophrenia.
      f. Massive loading doses (rapid neuroleptization) should be avoided.
      g. The choice of medication depends on the risk–benefit ratio and the potential side effect on a patient.
      h. Where a potential to cause weight gain or diabetes has been identified for the atypical antipsychotic prescribed, there should be routine monitoring for these potential risks.
      i. Use of adjunctive medication to prevent harm and reduce symptoms.
   B. *Stabilization phase*:
      a. In the early post-acute period, patients should be helped to understand their illness and should be encouraged to write an account of their illness in their notes.
      b. The assessment of needs for health and social care for people with schizophrenia should be comprehensive and address medical, social, psychological, occupational, economic, physical, and cultural issues.
      c. Minimize the likelihood of relapse.
      d. Enhance adaptation.
      e. Facilitate continued reduction in symptoms and promote the process of recovery.
   C. *Maintenance phase*:
      a. Ensure symptom remission or control.
      b. Maintain/improve level of functioning and quality of life.
      c. Continuation of antipsychotic drugs for 1 or 2 years after a relapse is recommended.
      d. Monitor adverse effects related to treatment.
      e. Withdrawal of antipsychotic medication should be gradual and monitored.
      f. Following the withdrawal of drugs, patients should continue to be monitored for signs of relapse for at least 2 years after the last acute episode.
4. Review the use of alcohol and illicit drugs and provision of access to specialist addiction services.
5. Psychosocial rehabilitation.
6. Assessment for the need of life and social skills training and a person and their carer's need for psychotherapy. Cognitive behavioural therapy (CBT) and family intervention should be available. Cognitive remediation therapy aims to improve cognitive dysfunction in poor memory, executive dysfunction, and attentional deficits.

26.5.4   PROMOTING RECOVERY

26.5.4.1   Primary Care

1. General practitioners (GPs) should develop case registers for people with schizophrenia.
2. GPs should regularly monitor the physical health of patients with schizophrenia. Particular attention should be paid to endocrine disorders, for example, diabetes, hyperprolactinaemia, blood pressure, lipids, side effects of medication, and lifestyle risk factors, for example, smoking.
3. GPs should re-refer patients to secondary care particularly if
   a. Treatment adherence is problematic.
   b. There is poor response to treatment.
   c. Comorbid substance misuse is suspected.
   d. Level of risk to self or others is raised.
   e. When patient first joins the practice.

26.5.4.2   Secondary Care

- A full assessment of health and social care needs should be made regularly.
- Carers should have their needs assessed.

26.5.5   SERVICE INTERVENTIONS

- Assertive outreach teams should be developed for patients who engage poorly with services, are high users of inpatient care, or are homeless.
- Crisis resolution and home treatment teams should be available for those in acute crisis.
- The Care Programme Approach (CPA) ensures services are managed and integrated.

26.5.6   HOSPITALIZATION

Those with acute schizophrenia often require admission to hospital, if necessarily compulsorily, for assessment, investigations, and treatment. Before discharge, Section 117 of the Mental Health Act 1983 for detained patients, and the CPA for all patients, requires that an 'assessment of needs' be made. A key worker should be assigned to monitor a patient's progress and to administer depot medication.

Attendance at a day hospital or centre may be considered, and there should be appropriate communication with the patient's GP.

Electroconvulsive therapy is used in the treatment of catatonic stupor.

26.5.7   DRUG TREATMENTS FOR SCHIZOPHRENIA

The efficacy of neuroleptics for acute symptoms has been demonstrated beyond doubt. 'Positive' symptoms respond better than 'negative' symptoms. Bear in mind the following:

1. 5%–25% of schizophrenics are unresponsive to conventional neuroleptics.
2. 5%–10% are intolerant owing to adverse neurological effects (parkinsonism, akathisia, dyskinesia).
3. 40%–60% of schizophrenics are noncompliant with oral medication. Possible reasons are
   a. Limited insight into the disease
   b. Limited beneficial effect
   c. Unpleasant side effects
   d. Pressure from family and friends
   e. Poor communication with the medical team
      Depot neuroleptics increase compliance and reduce relapse rates
4. Continuous therapy is superior to intermittent treatment. It results in fewer relapses and a lower overall dose of neuroleptics.
5. Of patients who stop medication, 60%–70% relapse within a year, and 85% within 2 years, compared to 10%–30% of those who continue on active medication (Table 26.3).

TABLE 26.3
Properties of the Typical Antipsychotics

Typical Antipsychotics	Properties
Typical antipsychotics in general	1. The most common EPSE is acute dystonia (90%)
	2. In acute dystonia, young men are at the highest risk
	3. In tardive dyskinesia, elderly women are at the highest risk
Haloperidol	1. High risk for EPSE
	2. High risk for galactorrhoea
	3. Low risk for weigh gain, postural hypotension, or sedation
Trifluoperazine	1. Low risk for weight gain or postural hypotension
Sulpiride or amisulpride	1. Sulpiride carries low risk of weight gain
	2. Amisulpride carries low risk of dyslipidaemia, weight gain, and glucose intolerance
	3. Sulpiride and amisulpride carry low risk of postural hypotension
	4. Sulpiride and amisulpride carry low risk of sedation

Source: Taylor, D. et al., *The Maudsley Prescribing Guideline*, Informa Healthcare, London, U.K., 2009.

26.5.8   Use of Atypical Neuroleptics

Atypical neuroleptics are distinguished from conventional neuroleptics by not producing catalepsy in animals and not elevating prolactin levels in humans. There is a considerably lower potential for EPSE and tardive dyskinesia. EPSE occur in up to 90% of patients taking neuroleptic medication.

26.5.8.1   NICE Guidelines on Atypical Antipsychotics

In the United Kingdom, the NICE issued guidelines in June 2002 with respect to the prescription of atypical antipsychotics for patients with schizophrenia. They are as follows:

- The atypical antipsychotics (amisulpride, olanzapine, quetiapine, risperidone, and zotepine) should be considered when deciding on the first-line treatment of newly diagnosed schizophrenia.
- An atypical antipsychotic is considered the treatment of choice for managing an acute schizophrenic episode when discussion with the individual is not possible.
- An atypical antipsychotic should be considered for an individual who is suffering from unacceptable side effects with a conventional antipsychotic.
- An atypical antipsychotic should be considered for an individual in relapse whose symptoms were previously inadequately controlled.
- Changing to an atypical antipsychotic is not necessary if a conventional antipsychotic controls symptoms adequately and the individual does not suffer unacceptable side effects.
- Clozapine should be introduced if schizophrenia is inadequately controlled despite the sequential use of two or more antipsychotics (one of which should be an atypical antipsychotic) each for at least 6–8 weeks (Table 26.4).

26.5.9   Treatment-Resistant Schizophrenia

Kane's Criteria for Treatment-Resistant Schizophrenia

26.5.9.1   Past Psychiatric History

1. In the past 5 years, the patient has no good functioning.
2. In the past 5 years, two different antipsychotics have been tried for 6 weeks with at least 1000 mg chlorpromazine equivalent but unsatisfactory response.

26.5.9.2   Cross Sectional Measures

1. The score of Brief Psychiatric Rating Scale (BPRS) is larger than 45.
2. The score of Clinical Global Index (CGI) is larger than 4.

26.5.9.3   Prospective Trials

1. Trial of 4 weeks of haloperidol at 15 mg–60 mg per day (if not tried before).
2. The BPRS score is larger than 35 (after the trial of haloperidol).

If a patient has failed to respond to a trial of three neuroleptics of different classes, using an adequate dose for an adequate duration, an atypical agent such as clozapine can be tried. Clozapine can cause agranulocytosis, so regular blood counts are necessary. The incidence of agranulocytosis is 0.8% at 12 months and 0.9% at 18 months, with a peak risk in the third month; it is higher in women and older patients.

Kane et al. (1988) showed that clozapine was significantly better than chlorpromazine in the treatment of schizophrenics previously resistant to haloperidol. Improvement was observed in both positive and negative symptoms.

26.5.9.4   Clozapine Patient Management System

In the United Kingdom, patients receiving clozapine are required to have their full blood counts monitored at regular intervals. The CPMS is summarized in Table 26.5.

26.6   MEDICATION ADHERENCE

Schizophrenia patients are often nonadherent to antipsychotics. The NICE guidelines recommend the following interventions to enhance adherence:

1. Improve communication: Adapt the communication style to suit the patient's needs.
2. Increase patient's involvement: The analysis of risks and benefits will help the patient to make the decision.
3. Understand the patient's perspectives: Explore about general or specific concerns (e.g. adverse effects or worries about dependence).
4. Determine the type of nonadherence: Intentional (due to beliefs and concerns) or unintentional nonadherence (practical difficulties and cost).
5. Provide information: Provide further information in the form of leaflet.
6. Monitor adherence in a nonjudgemental way: The psychiatrist should explain why he or she is interested in patient's adherence and let patient understand the good intention.

TABLE 26.4

Properties of the Atypical Antipsychotics

Atypical Antipsychotics	Properties
Clozapine	1. Agranulocytosis is the most common in Ashkenazi Jews
	2. The most common side effect is sedation till the next morning
	3. The second most common side effect is hypersalivation
	4. Clozapine (like olanzapine) carries the highest risk of weight gain
	5. Clozapine is least likely to cause tardive dyskinesia
Risperidone	1. Higher risk for EPSE and galactorrhoea as compared to other second-generation antipsychotics
	2. Risperidone carries low risk of sedation
Paliperidone	1. Side effects include EPSE, corrected QT (QTc) prolongation, hyperprolactinaemia, metabolic syndrome, and increase in risk of seizure
	2. Renal impairment is a contraindication because paliperidone is mainly excreted by kidney
Olanzapine	1. Olanzapine carries the highest risk of weight gain among all antipsychotics
	2. Olanzapine carries low risk of EPSE
	3. Olanzapine carries low risk of hyperprolactinaemia
	4. Olanzapine carries the lowest risk of QTc prolongation
Quetiapine	1. Quetiapine has high affinity for muscarinic receptors
	2. Quetiapine carries the lowest risk for EPSE
	3. Quetiapine carries the lowest risk of sexual dysfunction
	4. Quetiapine carries low risk of hyperprolactinaemia
Ziprasidone	1. Ziprasidone carries low risk of dyslipidaemia, weight gain, and glucose intolerance
Aripiprazole	1. Aripiprazole carries the lowest risk of QTc prolongation
	2 Aripiprazole carries low risk of sexual dysfunction
	3. Aripiprazole carries low risk for EPSE
	4. Aripiprazole carries low risk of dyslipidaemia, weight gain, and glucose intolerance
	5. Aripiprazole carries low risk of hyperprolactinaemia
	6. Aripiprazole carries low risk of postural hypotension
	7. Aripiprazole carries low risk of sedation
Asenapine	1. Asenapine has less potential to raise prolactin than risperidone
	2. Asenapine is associated with lower risk of weight gain

Source: Taylor, D. et al., *The Maudsley Prescribing Guideline*, Informa Healthcare, London, U.K., 2009.

7. Further intervention to increase adherence: If nonadherence continues to be an issue, the psychiatrist can suggest the patient to record his or her medicine taking by multicompartment medicine system. The patient can monitor the relationship between severity of symptoms and level of adherence. The psychiatrist can simplify the dosing regimen and offer advice to help the patient to cope with the side effects.

26.6.1 PSYCHOSOCIAL TREATMENTS FOR SCHIZOPHRENIA

26.6.1.1 General Principles

1. Establishing, maintaining, and developing a therapeutic alliance. Engagement, rapport, and building basic trust in a patient who may have difficulty trusting.

2. Understanding and respecting patient's views and decisions about treatment options and lifestyle.

3. Psychological interventions should be supportive in nature, focus on here and now, and reality based. To be flexible and eclectic, tailored to the patient's needs as they emerge (e.g. addressing developmental issues and losses).

4. To foster and encourage independence and optimal social and occupational functioning and promote self-management of the illness.

26.6.1.2 Psychoeducation

1. The main objective is to provide the patient with information about the illness, the range of treatments available, and the effect of using recreational drugs such as amphetamines. The patients are informed of the choices.

TABLE 26.5

Clozapine Patient Management System (CPMS)

Time	Actions
0	1. Perform assessment and discuss with patient and carers
	2. Information and advice regarding swapping to clozapine from another antipsychotic should be sought from the pharmacy
	3. Decide whether it is an inpatient or outpatient initiation. Inpatient initiation is indicated for elderly and adolescents 16–18-year-olds, concurrent medical problems, and medication
	4. Register patient with the Clozaril Patient Management System (CPMS) and obtain an initial FBC
	5. Start clozapine at 12.5 mg once a green blood result is issued by the CPMS
	6. For inpatient treatment, physical monitoring is required every hour for 6 h, and patient needs to be accompanied by a carer
	7. For outpatient treatment, patient and carer must be provided with emergency contact details for the first 24 h
	8. Inform his or her GP on the start date
	9. Baseline physical examination: weight, temperature, pulse, and BP (both lying and standing)
	10. For patients with diabetes: HbA1c at baseline; for patients without diabetes: fasting blood glucose
	11. Other baselines: LFTs, RFTs, lipids, and ECG
0–18 weeks	1. FBC: at least weekly for the first 18 weeks of clozapine treatment
	2. Fasting plasma glucose at 1 month, then 4–6 monthly
	3. LFTs, RFTs, lipids: every 6 months for the first year
	4. Follow standardized clozapine initiation charts
	5. A slower dose titration in the inpatient setting is required for older adults (>65's)
	6. The usual dose is 200–450 mg daily with a maximum dose of 900 mg daily. Older adults may need a lower daily dose
	7. For outpatient treatment, increments should not be done over weekend or holidays
18–52 weeks	1. FBC: at least two weekly from week 18 to week 52 of clozapine treatment
	2. Fasting plasma glucose at 1 month, then 4–6 monthly
	3. LFTs, RFTs, lipids: every 6 months for the first year
First to second year	1. FBC: at least four weekly after 1 year of clozapine treatment with stable blood results and the CPMS agreement
	2. LFTs, RFTs, lipids, fasting glucose every year
Second year	1. FBC: for at least 4 weeks
	2. LFTs, RFTs, lipids, fasting glucose every year

Sources: Taylor, D. et al., *The Maudsley Prescribing Guideline*, Informa Healthcare, London, U.K., 2009; NICE, *NICE Guidelines for Schizophrenia*, http://guidance.nice.org.uk/CG82 (accessed on August 1, 2012).

2. Psychoeducation for individuals with first episode of psychosis or schizophrenia should encourage blame-free acceptance of illness.
3. Develop strategies to promote control of illness by recognizing and responding to early warning signs and seek professional advice.

26.6.1.3 Social Milieu

Wing and Brown (1970) found that negative symptoms varied in intensity with social stimulation within psychiatric institutions.

The Team for the Assessment of Psychiatric Services (TAPS) study (Leff et al., 1994) reported on long-stay patients discharged into the community. It found that, provided reprovision was well resourced with staffed homes for the more disabled, there was no increase in death rate, suicides, crime, or vagrancy at 1- and 5-year follow-up, compared to matched controls. Between discharge and 5 years, negative symptoms reduced significantly in response to a more stimulating environment. Positive symptomatology remained stable.

26.6.1.4 Grief Work on Losses

To work through both losses from prior to the illness onset and also losses arising from the disruption, disorganization, and disability associated with schizophrenia.

26.6.1.5 Supportive Psychotherapy

Refinements of individual supportive psychological treatments, that is, targeted psychological treatments for specific components of illness or symptoms, developed for affected individual, for example, coping techniques to deal with psychotic symptoms.

26.6.1.6 Cognitive Behavioural Therapy

Components of CBT should involve

1. Advising the patients to keep a record to monitor their own thoughts, feelings, or behaviours with respect to their symptoms or recurrence of symptoms
2. Promoting alternative ways of coping with the target symptoms
3. Reducing stress
4. Improving functioning
5. Reducing negative symptoms by activity scheduling

Specific techniques targeting at auditory hallucination

1. Distraction method: Wearing headphones to focus attention away and the hallucinations are extinguished with decreased reactivity.
2. Desensitization: Describe, record, and recognize the connection between stressors and hallucinations and explore what the voices mean to them.

The NICE guidelines also recommend the therapist to deliver CBT on a one-to-one basis over at least 16 planned sessions. The therapist should follow a treatment manual to help the patient to establish links between their thoughts, feelings, or actions and their current or past symptoms. This will help them to reevaluate their perceptions, beliefs, and reasoning behind the target symptoms.

26.6.1.7 Expressed Emotion

Psychoeducational family programmes to increase medication compliance and coping with stressors are successful in reducing the risk of relapse. Families with high EE were identified using the Camberwell Family Interview. Education and family sessions in the home run in parallel with a relatives group. The programme is aimed at teaching problem-solving skills, lowering criticism and overinvolvement, and reducing contact between patients and relatives while expanding social networks.

26.6.1.8 Family Intervention

The NICE guidelines recommend the following:

1. The therapist should include the service user if possible and offer at least 10 planned sessions over a period of 3 months to 1 year.
2. Single-family intervention focusing on 'here and now' and the family system (boundaries, coalitions, triangulation) is recommended.
3. Family intervention should take into account the relationship between the main carer and the service user.
4. Therapist should establish a working relationship with family and provide structure and stability.
5. Cognitive techniques can be used to challenge unhelpful attributions such as guilt.
6. Behavioural approaches include goal setting and problem-solving.

26.6.1.9 Art Therapy

The NICE guidelines recommend art therapies conducted by art therapists registered by the Health and Care Professional Council. The objectives of art therapy include

1. Helping people with schizophrenia to experience themselves differently and develop new ways of relating to others
2. Expressing themselves and organizing their experience into a satisfying aesthetic form
3. Accepting and understanding feeling that may have emerged during the creative process when doing the artwork

26.6.1.10 Rehabilitation

1. Objectives
   a. Achieve the highest possible levels of social and vocational functioning and well-being for individuals with severe and persistent mental disorders
   b. Reduce interference from symptoms and neurocognitive impairments
2. Cognitive restructuring
   a. Attention (using various computer software): to increase attention span and to improve the efficiency of information processing
   b. Memory: memory notebook, mnemonics, rehearsal
   c. Executive function: to attempt remediation

3. Social skill and assertive community training
   a. Promote independent living and enhance social relations
   b. Focus on food preparation, money management, personal self-care, and interpersonal relationship
   c. Reduce disabilities and enhance abilities
   d. Reduce unacceptable community behaviours such as violence or substance abuse
   e. Crisis intervention in community and reduced hospitalization
4. Supported employment and vocational rehabilitation
   a. Enhance occupational potential
   b. Increase income and improve socioeconomic status

26.6.2 PROGNOSIS FOR SCHIZOPHRENIA

Schizophrenia is a heterogeneous disorder, and there are no reliable predictors of outcome. Approximately 25% of cases of schizophrenia show good clinical and social recovery, while most studies show that fewer than a half of patients have a poor long-term outcome. Factors associated with a good prognosis include

26.6.2.1 Sociodemographics
- Being female
- Being married

26.6.2.2 Past History
- Good premorbid social adjustment
- Family history of affective disorder
- Short duration of illness prior to treatment

26.6.2.3 Pathology
- No ventricular enlargement

26.6.2.4 Course of Illness
- An abrupt onset of the illness
- Later onset of the illness

26.6.2.5 Symptoms
- An affective component to the illness
- Paranoid, compared with nonparanoid
- Lack of negative symptoms
- Lack of cognitive impairment

26.6.2.6 Treatment
- Good initial response to treatment

26.6.2.7 Suicide

Ten per cent of schizophrenics commit suicide, and for most sufferers, it happens early in their illness. Roy (1982) reported that suicide was more likely in the following cases:

- Being male
- Being young
- Being unemployed
- Having chronic illness, relapses, and remissions
- Having a high educational attainment prior to onset
- Akathisia
- Abrupt stoppage of drugs
- Recent discharge from inpatient care

Finally, paranoid schizophrenics are three times more likely than nonparanoid patients to commit suicide.

26.6.2.8 Violence (Bobes et al., 2009)

Violence in people with schizophrenia is uncommon, but they do have a higher risk than general population. Prevalence of recent aggressive behaviour among outpatients with schizophrenia is 5%. The types of violence and aggression are classified as follows: verbal aggression (45%), physical violence towards objects (30%), violence towards others (20%), and self-directed violence (10%). Family members are involved in 50% of the assaults with strangers being attacked in 20%. Psychiatrists need to be competent in identifying patients at risk and protecting both patients and others.

26.6.3 PRODROME OF SCHIZOPHRENIA

Prodrome refers to a range of subjective experiences before the onset of schizophrenia (Yung and McGorry, 1996).

26.6.3.1 Attenuated Positive Symptoms
1. Unusual perception.
2. Odd beliefs.
3. Vague and circumstantial speech.
4. Preoccupation with religion, occult, and philosophy.
5. Suspiciousness.
6. Prepsychotic anxiety.
7. Praecox feeling refers to a subjective sense by the clinician that the patient is odd. The patient is usually concrete, woolly, exhibiting mild formal thought disorder, or socially blamed or reporting perceptual disturbance.

26.6.3.2 Negative Symptoms

1. Blunted affect
2. Amotivation
3. Isolation and social withdrawal

26.6.3.3 Cognitive Symptoms

1. Deterioration in academic, work, social functioning, and self-care
2. Reduced attention and concentration

26.6.3.4 General Symptoms

1. Sleep disturbance: usually initial insomnia
2. Irritability
3. Depressed mood
4. Poor hygiene

26.6.3.5 Interventions for Prodrome

1. Careful observation.
2. Consider differential diagnoses including organic diagnoses.
3. Consider comorbidity such as substance abuse.
4. Strive to minimize risk of relapse.
5. Aim to eliminate exposure to cannabis and psychostimulants by psychoeducation, enhance stress management, and employ maintenance antipsychotic treatment.
6. Discuss prudent treatment options such as starting antipsychotics and CBT.

26.6.3.6 Prognosis

The conversion to schizophrenia is 35%.
70% achieve full remission within 3–4 months.
80% achieve stable remission within 1 year.

26.6.3.7 Predictors for Further Progression to Psychosis or Schizophrenia (Cannon et al., 2008)

1. Genetic risk with recent deterioration in function
2. Higher levels of unusual thought content
3. Higher levels of suspicion/paranoia
4. Greater social impairment
5. History of substance abuse

26.7 CATATONIA

26.7.1 AETIOLOGY

1. Schizophrenia
2. Depression or mania (more common than schizophrenia)
3. Organic disorders, for example, CNS infection
4. Epilepsy
5. Medications (ciprofloxacin)
6. Recreational drugs (cocaine)
7. Psychogenic catatonia
8. Lethal catatonia (extreme psychotic excitement that differs from neuroleptic malignant syndrome [NMS])

26.7.2 CLINICAL FEATURES

1. Ambitendency.
2. Automatic obedience.
3. Mitgehen.
4. Mitmachen.
5. Mannerism.
6. Negativism.
7. Echolalia.
8. Echopraxia.
9. Logorrhoea.
10. Stereotypy.
11. Waxy flexibility/catalepsy.
12. Gegenhalten (negativism): Patient resists the attempts of examiner to move part of body in equal strength to applied force.
13. Verbigeration: morbid repetition of words.

26.7.3 MANAGEMENT

26.7.3.1 Investigations

- Haematology: FBC
- Biochemistry: RFTs, LFTs, creatinine kinase, and blood glucose
- Endocrine: thyroid function tests
- Urine drug screen
- Heavy metal screening
- Imaging: CT scan or MRI scan of the brain
- Microbiology: urine and blood culture, syphilis, and HIV
- Heavy metal screening
- Autoantibody screen
- Lumbar puncture
- Electrophysiology: ECG and EEG

26.7.4 MEDICATIONS

1. Benzodiazepines (e.g. intramuscular lorazepam up to 4 mg per day)
2. Electroconvulsive therapy

26.7.5 Prognosis

Two-thirds of patients improve with treatment.

26.8 DELUSIONAL (PARANOID) DISORDERS

26.8.1 ICD-10 Issues (WHO, 1992)

According to ICD-10, a delusional disorder is an ill-defined condition, manifesting as a single delusion or a set of related delusions, being persistent, sometimes lifelong, and not having an identifiable organic basis. There are occasional or transitory auditory hallucinations, particularly in the elderly.

Delusions are the most conspicuous or only symptom and are present for at least 3 months. For the diagnosis, there must be no evidence of schizophrenic symptoms or brain disease.

ICD-10 includes the previously used term late paraphrenia, although there is some evidence that there are differences between persistent delusional disorder and late paraphrenia. Howard et al. (1994) showed, using MRI scans in a group of late-onset schizophrenics and late-onset delusional disorders, that lateral ventricle volumes in the delusional disorder patients were much greater than those of schizophrenics and almost twice those of controls.

Monodelusional disorders feature a stable, encapsulated delusional system, which takes over much of a person's life. The personality is preserved.

26.8.2 Epidemiology of Delusional Disorders

There is a point prevalence of 0.03% and a lifetime risk of 0.05%–0.1%.

Munro (1991) reports from his series of patients with monodelusional disorder:

- A mean age of onset of 35 years for males and 45 years for females
- Onset gradual and unremitting in 62%
- Equal sex ratio of sufferers
- Sufferers often unmarried, with high marital breakdown and low fecundity
- Introverted, long-standing interpersonal difficulties
- Family history of psychiatric disorder but not of delusional disorder or schizophrenia
- Evidence of minimal brain disorder in 16%

26.8.3 Specific Delusional (Paranoid) Disorders

26.8.3.1 Pathological (Delusional) Jealousy

This is also called the Othello syndrome, morbid jealousy, erotic jealousy, sexual jealousy, psychotic jealousy, or conjugal paranoia. The person holds the delusional belief that his or her sexual partner is being unfaithful and will go to great lengths to find evidence of infidelity. Underclothing may be examined for semen stains, belongings may be searched, and the partner may be interrogated and followed. It is more common in men.

Pathological jealousy may be associated with the following conditions:

- Organic disorders and psychoactive substance use disorders (e.g. alcohol dependence, cerebral tumour, endocrinopathy, dementia, cerebral infection, use of amphetamines or cocaine)
- Paranoid schizophrenia
- Depression
- Neurosis or personality disorder

Treatment should be directed at the underlying disorder. If no primary cause is identified, pharmacotherapy with a neuroleptic and/or psychotherapy may be helpful. There may be a risk of violence to the partner, and it may be best to recommend that the couple separate.

26.8.3.2 Erotomania (De Clérambault's Syndrome)

The person holds the delusional belief that someone, usually of a higher social or professional status or a famous personality or in some other way 'unattainable', is in love with him or her. The patient may make repeated attempts to contact that other person. Eventually, rejections may lead to animosity and bitterness on the part of the patient towards the object of attention.

In hospital and outpatient clinical psychiatry, patients are more likely to be female than male, whereas in forensic psychiatry, male patients are commoner. Overall, females outnumber males.

26.8.3.3 Cotard's Syndrome

This condition, also called délire de négation, is a nihilistic delusional disorder in which the patient believes that, for example, all his or her wealth has gone or that relatives or friends do not exist. It may take a somatic form with the patient believing that parts of his or her body do not exist. It can be secondary to very severe depression or to an organic disorder.

26.8.3.4 Capgras Syndrome

Although Capgras syndrome is also called illusion des sosies, or illusion of doubles, it is not an illusion but a delusional disorder. The essential feature of this rare condition is that a person who is familiar to the patient is believed to have been replaced by a double. It is more common in females. Common primary causes are schizophrenia, mood disorder, and organic disorder. Derealization often occurs.

26.8.3.5 Fregoli Syndrome

In this very rare delusional disorder, the patient believes that a familiar person, who is often believed to be the patient's persecutor, has taken on different appearances. Primary causes include schizophrenia and organic disorder.

26.8.3.6 Induced Psychosis (Folie À Deux)

This rare delusional disorder is shared by two, or rarely more than two, people who are closely linked emotionally. One of the people has a genuine psychotic disorder; his or her delusional system is induced in the other person, who may be dependent or less intelligent than the first person. Geographical separation leads to recovery of the well person.

26.9   SCHIZOAFFECTIVE DISORDERS

26.9.1   TYPES OF DISORDER

The term 'schizoaffective psychosis' was introduced by Kasanin in 1933 to describe a condition with both affective and schizophrenic symptoms, with sudden acute onset after good premorbid functioning, and usually with complete recovery.

ICD-10 describes these as disorders in which both affective and schizophrenic symptoms are prominent within the same episode of illness, either simultaneously or within a few days of each other. It distinguishes various types:

- *Manic type*—the person usually makes a full recovery.
- *Depressive type*—prognosis not as good as that of the manic subtype, with a greater chance of developing 'negative' symptoms.
- *Mixed type*.

26.9.2   RELATIONSHIP BETWEEN AFFECTIVE AND SCHIZOPHRENIC COMPONENTS

There is no consensus concerning the nosological status of schizoaffective disorder. Opposing views include the Kraepelinian binary system and continuum theories:

- *Binary theorists* (e.g. Winokur, Kendler) hold the traditional notion that there are two separate illnesses, schizophrenia and manic–depressive psychosis, having different aetiologies and requiring different treatments.
- *Continuum theorists* (e.g. Crow, Kendall) doubt that there are distinct illnesses but rather that features of psychosis vary quantitatively along a continuum, with schizophrenia and manic depression at opposing poles and schizoaffective disorder somewhere in between.

In 1991, Tsuang studied a subgroup of patients with strictly defined schizoaffective disorder. It was found that the morbid risk of schizophrenia in relatives of schizoaffectives was similar to that of a schizophrenic group and fell between schizophrenia and affective disorder for the risk of affective disorder in relatives. It was concluded that this condition was different from schizophrenia or manic depression.

In 1993, Goldstein et al. found that, among probands with schizoaffective disorder, relatives had higher rates of schizophrenia and unipolar depression than relatives of males. Among relatives, males were at higher risk for schizophrenia spectrum disorders than females. This points to a stronger relationship between schizoaffective disorder and schizophrenia.

In 1994, DeLisi et al. reported the following in relationship to schizophrenia and affective disorder:

- At least one-third of schizophrenics have depressive symptoms.
- Affective disorder is more frequent in the families of schizophrenics than in controls.
- Unipolar depression is more common in families of schizoaffectives than schizophrenia-only probands. Bipolar disorder is as frequent in families of both.
- Affective disorder is frequently inherited from the same parental line as schizophrenia.
- Bipolar disorder is more frequent in male relatives, and unipolar disorder more frequent in female relatives.

It was concluded that the same genes contribute to schizophrenia and affective disorder, and sex and phenotypic expression are related.

26.9.3   PROGNOSIS FOR SCHIZOAFFECTIVE DISORDERS

The prognosis of schizoaffective disorders lies between that of mood disorders and schizophrenia.

REFERENCES

American Psychiatric Association. 2013: *Desk Reference to the Diagnostic Criteria from DSM-5.* Washington, DC: American Psychiatric Association Press.

Andreasen NC. 1983: *Scale for the Assessment of Negative Symptoms (SANS).* Iowa City, IA: University of Iowa.

Andreasen NC. 1984: *Scale for the Assessment of Positive Symptoms (SAPS).* Iowa City, IA: University of Iowa.

Andreasen NC, Swayze VW, Flaum M et al. 1990: Ventricular enlargement in schizophrenia evaluated with computed tomographic scanning. *Archives of General Psychiatry* 47:1008–1015.

Arseneault L, Cannon M, Witton J, and Murray RM. 2004: Causal association between cannabis and psychosis: Examination of the evidence. *The British Journal of Psychiatry* 184:110–117.

Bassett A, McGillivray B, Jones B, and Pantzar J. 1985: Partial trisomy chromosome 5 cosegregating with schizophrenia. *Lancet* i:1023–1026.

Berrios GE. 2011: Eugene Bleuler's place in the history of psychiatry. *Schizophrenia Bulletin* 37(6):1095–1098.

Bobes J, Fillat O, and Arango C. 2009: Violence among schizophrenia out-patients compliant with medication: Prevalence and associated factors. *Acta Psychiatrica Scandinavica* 119:218–225.

Bracha HS, Torrey EF, Bigelow LB et al. 1991: Subtle signs of prenatal maldevelopment of the hand ectoderm in schizophrenia: A preliminary monozygotic twin study. *Biological Psychiatry* 30:719–725.

Brown GW and Birley JLT. 1968: Crises and life changes and the onset of schizophrenia. *Journal of Health and Social Behaviour* 9:203.

Cannon TD, Cadenhead K, Cornblatt B et al. 2008: Prediction of psychosis in youth at high clinical risk: A multi site longitudinal study in North America. *Archives of General Psychiatry* January, 65(1):28–37.

Cardno AG, Marshall EJ, Coid S et al. 1999: Heritability estimates for psychotic disorders: The Maudsley twin psychosis series. *Archives of General Psychiatry* 56:162–168.

Castle DJ, Scott K, Wessely S, and Murray RM. 1993: Does social deprivation during gestation and early life predispose to later schizophrenia? *Social Psychiatry and Psychiatric Epidemiology* 28:1–4.

Chua SE and McKenna PJ. 1995: Schizophrenia—A brain disease? A critical review of structural and functional cerebral abnormality in the disorder. *British Journal of Psychiatry* 166:563–582.

DeLisi LE, Henn S, Bass N et al. 1994: Depression in schizophrenia: Is the Kraepelinian binary system dead? *Proceedings of the 9th World Congress of Psychiatry 1993.* Macclesfield, U.K.: Gardiner–Caldwell Communications.

Dollfus S and Petit M. 1993: Current aspects and pertinence of the concept in schizophrenic states. *Encephale* 19(2):109–115.

Duinkerke SJ, Botter PA, Jansen AA et al. 1993: Ritanserin, a selective 5-HT2/1c antagonist, and negative symptoms in schizophrenia: A placebo-controlled double-blind trial. *British Journal of Psychiatry* 163:451–455.

Farmer AE, McGuffin P, and Gottesman II. 1987: Twin concordance for DSM-III schizophrenia. Scrutinizing the validity of the definition. *Archives of General Psychiatry* 44:634–641.

Feighner JP, Robins E, Guze SB et al. 1972: Diagnostic criteria for use in psychiatric research. *Archives of General Psychiatry* 26:57–63.

Fleming M. 2006: Implementing the Scottish schizophrenia guidelines through the use of integrated care pathways. In Hall J and Howard D (eds.) *Integrated Care Pathways in Mental Health,* pp. 157–174. London, U.K.: Churchill Livingstone.

Goldberg EM and Morrison SL. 1963: Schizophrenia and social class. *British Journal of Psychiatry* 109:785–802.

Goldstein JM, Faraone SV, Chen WJ, and Tsuang MT. 1993: The role of gender in understanding the familial transmission of schizoaffective disorder. *British Journal of Psychiatry* 163:763–768.

Gottesman II and Shields J. 1972: *Schizophrenia and Genetics: A Twin Study Vantage Point.* New York: Academic Press.

Gurland B, Fleiss JL, Sharpe L, Simon R, Barrett JE Jr, Copeland J, Cooper JE, and Kendell RE. 1972: The mislabeling of depressed patients in New York state hospitals. *Proceedings of the Annual Meeting of the American Psychopathological Association* 60:17–31.

Hecker E and Kraam A. 2009: Hebephrenia. A contribution to clinical psychiatry' by Dr. Ewald Hecker in Gorlitz (1871). *History of Psychiatry* 20(77):87–106.

Howard RJ, Almeida O, Levy R et al. 1994: Quantitative magnetic resonance imaging volumetry distinguishes delusional disorder from late onset schizophrenia. *British Journal of Psychiatry* 165:474–480.

Jackson JH. 1931: *Selected Writings.* London, U.K.: Hodder and Stoughton.

Johnstone EC, Crow TJ, Frith CD, Husband J, and Kreel L. 1976: Cerebral ventricular size and cognitive impairment in chronic schizophrenia. *Lancet* ii:924–926.

Johnstone EC, Crow TJ, Frith CD et al. 1978: Mechanism of the antipsychotic effect in the treatment of acute schizophrenia. *Lancet* ii:848–851.

Kahn RS, Davidson M, Knott P et al. 1993: Effect of neuroleptic medication on cerebrospinal fluid monoamine metabolite concentrations in schizophrenia. *Archives of General Psychiatry* 50:599–605.

Kane JM and Freeman HL. 1994: Towards more effective antipsychotic treatment. *British Journal of Psychiatry* 165(Suppl 25):22–31.

Kane JM, Honigfield G, Singer J et al. 1988: Clozapine for the treatment-resistant schizophrenic: A double-blind comparison with chlorpromazine. *Archives of General Psychiatry* 45:789–796.

Kety SS, Rosenthal D, Wender PH et al. 1971: Mental illness in the biological and adoptive families of adopted schizophrenics. *American Journal of Psychiatry* 128:302.

Kraepelin E. 1987: *Memoirs.* Berlin, Germany: Springer-Verlag.

Langfeldt G. 1969: Schizophrenia: diagnosis and prognosis. *Behavioral Science* 14(3):173–182.

Leff J, Thornicroft G, Coxhead N et al. 1994: The TAPS project: 22. A five-year follow-up of long-stay psychiatric patients discharged to the community. *British Journal of Psychiatry* 165(Suppl 25):13–17.

Lewis SW and Murray RM. 1988: Obstetric complications, neurodevelopmental deviance and risk of schizophrenia. *Journal of Psychiatric Research* 21:473.

Liddle PF, Friston KJ, Frith CD et al. 1992: Patterns of cerebral blood flow in schizophrenia. *British Journal of Psychiatry* 160:179–186.

Lieberman JA and Sobel SN. 1993: Predictors of treatment response and course of schizophrenia. *Current Opinion in Psychiatry* 6:63–69.

Mednick SA, Machon RA, Huttunen MO, and Bonnet D. 1988: Adult schizophrenia following prenatal exposure to an influenza epidemic. *Archives of General Psychiatry* 45:189–192.

Meltzer HY, Myung AL, and Ranjan R. 1994: Recent advances in the pharmacotherapy of schizophrenia. *Acta Psychiatrica Scandinavica* 90(Suppl 384):95–101.

Murray RM, Lewis SW, Owen MJ, and Foester A. 1988: Neurodevelopmental origins of dementia praecox. In Bebbington P and McGuffin P (eds.) *Schizophrenia: The Major Issue*, pp. 90–103. London, U.K.: Heinemann.

Murray RM, O'Callaghan E, Castle DJ, and Lewis SW. 1992: A neurodevelopmental approach to the classification of schizophrenia. *Schizophrenia Bulletin* 18:319–332.

NICE. *NICE Guidelines for Medication Adherence*. http://guidance.nice.org.uk/CG76 (accessed on 1 August 2012).

NICE. *NICE Guidelines for Schizophrenia*. http://guidance.nice.org.uk/CG82 (accessed on 1 August 2012).

Noll R. 2011: *American Madness: The Rise and Fall of Dementia Praecox*. Cambridge, MA: Harvard University Press.

Pillmann F and Marneros A. 2005: Longitudinal follow-up in acute and transient psychotic disorders and schizophrenia. *British Journal of Psychiatry* 187:286–287.

Rajagopal S. 2007: Catatonia. *Advances in Psychiatric Treatment* 13:51–59.

Roy A. 1982: Suicide in chronic schizophrenia. *British Journal of Psychiatry* 141:171–177.

Sartorius N, Shapiro R, Kimura M, and Barrett K. 1972: WHO international pilot study of schizophrenia. *Psychological Medicine* 2(4):422–425.

Schneider K. 1959: *Clinical Psychopathology*. New York: Grune & Stratton.

Sherrington R, Brynjjolfsson J, Petursson H et al. 1988: Localisation of a susceptibility locus for schizophrenia on chromosome 5. *Nature* 336:164–167.

Spitzer RL, Endicott J, and Robins E. 1975: *Research Diagnostic Criteria (RDC) for a Selected Group of Functional Disorders*. New York: New York State Psychiatric Institute.

Starkstein SE, Goldar JC, and Hodgkiss A. 1995: Karl Ludwig Kahlbaum's concept of catatonia. *History of Psychiatry* 6(22):201–207.

Syvälahti EKG. 1994: Biological factors in schizophrenia: Structural and functional aspects. *British Journal of Psychiatry* 164(Suppl 23):9–14.

Taylor D, Paton C, and Kapur S. 2009: *The Maudsley Prescribing Guideline*. London, U.K.: Informa Healthcare.

Torgersen S. 1994: Personality deviations within the schizophrenia spectrum. *Acta Psychiatrica Scandinavica* (Suppl 384):40–44.

Tsuang MT. 1991: Morbidity risks of schizophrenia and affective disorders among first-degree relatives of patients with schizoaffective disorders. *British Journal of Psychiatry* 158:165–170.

Vaughn CE and Leff JP. 1976: Influence of family and social factors on the course of psychiatric illness. *British Journal of Psychiatry* 129:125–137.

Watt RJ. 2001: Diagnosing schizophrenia. In Lieberman JA and Murray RM (eds.) *Comprehensive Care of Schizophrenia. A Textbook of Clinical Management*, pp. 1–26. London, U.K.: Martin Dunitz.

Weinberger DR, Berman KF, and Zec RF. 1986: Physiological dysfunction of dorsolateral prefrontal cortex in schizophrenia: I. Regional cerebral blood flow evidence. *Archives of General Psychiatry* 43:114–124.

Wilson IC, Garbutt JC, Lanier CF et al. 1983: Is there a tardive dysmentia? *Schizophrenia Bulletin* 9(2):187–192.

Wing J, Cooper JE, and Sartorius N. 1974: *The Description of Psychiatric Symptoms: An Introduction Manual for the PSE and CATEGO System*. Cambridge U.K.: Cambridge University Press.

Wing JK and Brown GW. 1961: Social treatment of chronic schizophrenia: A comparative survey of three mental hospitals. *Journal of Mental Science* 107:847.

Wing JK and Brown GW. 1970: *Institutionalism and Schizophrenia*. Cambridge, U.K.: Cambridge University Press.

Wong DF, Wagner HN, Tune LE et al. 1986: Positron emission tomography reveals elevated D2 dopamine receptors in drug naive schizophrenics. *Science* 234:1558–1563.

World Health Organization. 1973: *Report of the International Pilot Study of Schizophrenia*. Geneva, Switzerland: WHO.

World Health Organization. 1992: *The ICD-10 Classification of Mental and Behavioural Disorders*. Geneva, Switzerland: WHO.

Yung AR and McGorry PD. 1996: The prodromal phase of first-episode psychosis: Past and current conceptualizations. *Schizophrenia Bulletin* 22(2):353–370.

27 Mood Disorders, Suicide, and Parasuicide

27.1 HISTORY

- In 1921, Kraepelin divided the functional psychoses into two broad categories: dementia praecox and manic–depressive insanity. He thought of the latter as a disorder in which discrete episodes of illness alternated with clearly defined well periods during which patients returned to their previous state of health.
- In 1949, Cade first initiated the use of lithium, but it was not widely used until the 1960s.
- In the 1950s, tricyclic and monoamine oxidase inhibitor (MAOI) antidepressants were introduced.
- In the 1970s, anticonvulsants were first used for bipolar disorders. Specific psychological treatments (e.g. cognitive therapy) were introduced.
- In the 1980s, selective serotonin reuptake inhibitors (SSRIs) were introduced.

27.2 CLASSIFICATIONS OF MOOD DISORDERS

27.2.1 ICD-10 Classifications (WHO, 1992)

27.2.1.1 F30 Manic Episode

The fundamental disturbance is an elevation of mood to elation, with concomitant increase in activity level. Three degrees of manic episode are specified by ICD-10, all used for a single manic episode only:

- Hypomania. There is persistent elevated mood, increased energy and activity, feelings of well-being, and reduced need for sleep. Irritability may replace elation. Work is considerably disrupted. There are no hallucinations or delusions.
- Mania without psychotic symptoms. Mood is elevated, with almost uncontrollable excitement. There is overactivity; pressured speech; reduced sleep; distractible, inflated self-esteem; and grandiose thoughts. Perceptual heightening may occur. The person may spend excessively and become aggressive, amorous, or facetious.
- Mania with psychotic symptoms. The symptoms are as mentioned earlier but with delusions and hallucinations, usually grandiose. There may be sustained physical activity, aggression, and self-neglect (Table 27.1).

27.2.1.2 F31 Bipolar Affective Disorder

There are repeated episodes of mood disturbance, sometimes elevated, sometimes depressed.

Repeated episodes of mania are classified as bipolar (sufferers resemble those who also have depressive episodes in their family history, premorbid personality, age of onset and prognosis). It includes the following:

1. Bipolar affective disorder with
   a. Current episode hypomanic
   b. Current episode manic without psychotic symptoms
   c. Current episode manic with psychotic symptoms
2. Bipolar affective disorder with
   a. Current episode having mild/moderate depression
   b. Current episode having severe depression without psychotic symptoms
   c. Current episode having severe depression with psychotic symptoms
3. Bipolar affective disorder with
   a. Current episode mixed

27.2.2 DSM-5 (APA, 2013)

296 Bipolar I disorder

1. Duration: at least 1 week
2. Number of episode: at least one manic episode
3. Manic episode: at least three or more of the following symptoms or four or more if only irritability is present
   a. Inflated self-esteem or grandiosity
   b. Decreased need for sleep

TABLE 27.1

Compare and Contrast ICD-10 and DSM-5 Criteria on Bipolar Disorder

ICD-10 (WHO, 1992)	DSM-5 (APA, 2013)
F30 Manic episode (hypomania, mania with and without psychotic symptoms)	296 Bipolar I disorder
	296.89 Bipolar II disorder
	301.13 Cyclothymic disorder
F31 Bipolar affective disorder (current episode hypomanic, manic with and without psychotic features, moderate depression with and without somatic symptoms, severe depression with and without psychotic features)	Substance-induced bipolar disorder
	293.83 Bipolar disorder associated with another medical condition
	296.80 Bipolar disorder not elsewhere classified

TABLE 27.2

Comparison between the ICD-10 and Proposed DSM-5 Criteria for Depressive Disorder

ICD-10 (WHO, 1992)	DSM-5 (APA, 2013)
F32 Depressive episode (mild/moderate/severe)	296.99 Disruptive mood dysregulation disorder
F33 Recurrent depressive episode (mild/moderate/severe)	296.2 Major depressive disorder, single episode
F34 Persistent mood disorder (cyclothymia, dysthymia, and other persistent mood disorders)	296.3 Major depressive disorder, recurrent
	300.4 Dysthymia (persistent depressive disorder)
F38 Other mood disorders (mixed affective episode, recurrent brief depressive episode)	625.4 Premenstrual dysphoric disorder
	Substance-induced depressive disorder
	293.83 Depressive disorder associated with another medical condition
	311 Depressive disorder not elsewhere classified

   c. More talkative than usual or pressure of speech

   d. Flight of ideas or racing thoughts

   e. Distractibility

   f. Increase in goal-directed activity or psycho-motor agitation

   g. Excessive involvement in activities that have a high potential for painful and negative consequences (e.g. overspending, sexual indiscretions, or foolhardy investments)

4. Functional impairment and exclusion of other causes

5. Specifiers: current or most recent episode manic, hypomanic, depressed, mixed features, psychotic features, catatonic features, atypical features, melancholic features, rapid cycling, with suicide risk severity, with anxiety, with seasonal pattern, and with postpartum onset

296.89 Bipolar II disorder

1. Duration: at least 4 days.

2. Number of episode: one major depressive episode and at least one hypomanic episode.

3. Hypomanic episode has the same requirement of the number of symptoms as manic episode.

4. The only difference is that patients should have no impairment in functioning.

5. Specifiers are the same as manic episode.

301.13 Cyclothymia

1. Duration is for at least 2 years (at least 1 year in children and adolescents).

2. There have been numerous episodes with hypomanic symptoms that do not meet criteria for a hypomanic episode and numerous episodes with depressive symptoms that do not meet criteria for a major depressive episode.

3. The symptoms have been present for 2 years for adults and 1 year for children and adolescents.

4. Symptom-free period should be less than 2 months at a time.

Substance-induced bipolar disorder

1. Manic episode develops soon after misusing a substance which is able to cause manic symptoms

2. Following ingestion of substances (e.g. amphetamine, cannabis, and cocaine) or withdrawal of substances (Table 27.2)

27.2.2.1 ICD-10 Criteria for Depressive Episode (F32)

There is depression of mood, reduced energy, and fatiguability. Mood is pervasively depressed. Other features are reduced attention and concentration, lowered self-esteem, ideas of guilt and worthlessness, pessimistic thoughts, thoughts of self-harm or suicide, and disturbed sleep.

Somatic changes include reduced appetite leading to weight loss (at least 5% of body weight in a month), constipation, early-morning awakening (more than 2 h before usual), diurnal variation of mood, anhedonia, loss of normal reactivity of mood, reduced libido, amenorrhoea, and psychomotor retardation or agitation.

A duration of 2 weeks is required for the diagnosis. This applies to the first episode only. Severity is graded:

- Mild depressive episode
- Moderate depressive episode
- Severe depressive episode without psychotic symptoms
- Severe depressive episode with psychotic symptoms

296.2 Major depressive episode, single episode

1. At least five symptoms for 2-week duration
2. At least one of the following: low mood and loss of interest or pleasure
3. Other symptoms include
   a. Significant weight loss or weight gain
   b. Insomnia or hypersomnia on a daily basis
   c. Psychomotor agitation or retardation
   d. Low energy level
   e. Feelings of worthlessness or guilt
   f. Poor concentration
   g. Recurrent suicidal thoughts
4. Other criteria: functional impairment, no history of manic or hypomanic episode, and exclusion of other psychiatric diagnosis
5. Subtype: mixed feature

27.2.2.2 ICD-10 Criteria for Recurrent Depressive Disorder (F33)

There are repeated episodes of depression, without episodes of mania. Recovery between episodes is usually complete, but a minority becomes chronic, especially in the elderly. It includes

1. Recurrent depressive disorder with
   a. Current episode mild
   b. Current episode moderate
   c. Current episode severe without psychotic symptoms
   d. Current episode severe with psychotic symptoms
2. Recurrent depressive disorder, currently in remission

296.3 Major depressive episode, recurrent episode

1. The presence of at least two or major depressive episodes.
2. To be considered separate episodes, there must be an interval of at least 2 consecutive months in which criteria are not met for a major depressive episode.
3. Specifiers: mild, moderate, and severe without psychotic features/with psychotic features, chronic, mixed features.

27.2.2.3 ICD-10 Criteria for Dysthymia (F34)

This is a chronic, less severe depression, usually with an insidious onset. Symptoms include excessive guilt, difficulty in concentrating, loss of interest, pessimism, low self-esteem, low energy, irritability, and reduced productivity. For the diagnosis it must be present for at least 2 years.

300.4 Dysthymia (persistent depressive disorder)

1. Similar to the ICD-10, the depressed mood should last for 2 years for adults and 1 year for children and adolescents.
2. Depressive symptoms include change in appetite, change in sleep pattern, low energy, low self-esteem, poor concentration and hopelessness.
3. Symptom free period should be less than 2 months.
4. No psychosis disorder or substance-abuse.
5. Significant impairment in functioning.
6. Specifier: early onset (<21 years), late onset (>21 years), atypical features.

625.4 Premenstrual dysmorphic disorder

During the final week before the onset of menses, the patient experiences affective lability, irritability, marked anxiety and other DSM-5 depressive symptoms. The above symptoms improve shortly after menses.

Substance-induced depressive disorder

Depressive episode develops soon after misusing a substance which is able to cause depressive symptoms

296.99 Disruptive mood dysregulation disorder

1. Recurrent severe temper outbursts.
2. Frequency: three or more times per week.
3. Irritability in between temper outbursts.
4. Duration at least 12 months and symptom free period should be less than 3 months.
5. At least two different settings.
6. Age of onset: between 6 to 10 years.

27.2.3 Other Classifications of Depression

Depression is variously classified, and the usefulness of differing categories is still under debate.

27.2.3.1 Endogenous versus Reactive Depression

This is a distinction drawn by Roth and the Newcastle School in the 1950s (Richmond, 2006):

1. The endogenous form (melancholia) is thought to be of biological origin, with the following symptoms (*mnemonics: MAD GRADS*):
   a. Motor retardation or agitation.
   b. Anorexia and weight loss.
   c. Diurnal variation.
   d. Guilt is excessive.
   e. Reactivity of mood is absent.
   f. Anhedonia.
   g. Distinct quality of mood.
   h. Sleep is characterized by terminal insomnia.
2. The reactive form is thought to be of psychological origin. Depression is moderate; anxiety, irritability, initial insomnia, and mood remain reactive.

However, triggering events are present in both types.

Kendall (1965) failed to find a point of rarity in symptomatology between neurotic and psychotic depression, so concluded that there are no essential differences between them.

27.2.3.2 Unipolar versus Bipolar Depression

This is a distinction due to Leonhard, Angst, and Perris in the 1950s (Angst and Sellaro, 2000):

- Unipolar depression is more common in females. Episodes are longer, with somatic symptoms, anxiety, agitation, suicidal ideas, weight loss, and initial insomnia.
- In bipolar depression a seasonal pattern and hypersomnia tend to be more commonly present. There are more male sufferers, more family

history of mania, an earlier and more acute onset (15 years earlier than 'unipolars' on average), and more episodes.

No difference is observed in sleep EEGs of these two groups.

27.2.3.3 Rapid-Cycling Bipolar Disorder

This refers to those patients who experience four or more affective episodes in 12 months. It is more common in women, predicts poorer prognosis with more lifetime affective episodes and a poorer response to lithium and other treatments. Twenty per cent are induced by antidepressant drugs.

27.2.3.4 Other Classes

27.2.3.4.1 Double Depression

This is a major depression superimposed upon dysthymia.

27.2.3.4.2 Depressive Stupor

The person is unresponsive, akinetic, mute, and fully conscious. Following an episode, the patient can recall the events that took place at the time. Episodes of excitement may occur between episodes of stupor.

27.2.3.4.3 Recurrent Brief Depression

In 1990, Angst proposed diagnostic criteria for this condition—dysphoric mood or loss of interest for a duration of less than 2 weeks, with at least four of the following: poor appetite, sleep problems, agitation, loss of interest, fatigue, feelings of worthlessness, difficulty concentrating, and suicidality. One or two episodes per month for at least a year are characteristic.

27.2.3.4.4 Masked Depression

In masked depression, depressed mood is not always complained of, rather somatic or other complaints. It is more common in the undeveloped world and in those unable to articulate their emotions (e.g. those with learning disability or dementia). The presence of biological symptoms is helpful in making the diagnosis. Diurnal variation in abnormal behaviour may mirror diurnal variation in mood.

27.2.3.4.5 Seasonal Affective Disorder (Lee, 2007)

Definition: Seasonal Affective Disorder (SAD) is a form of recurrent depressive disorder which the sufferers consistently experience low mood in winter months. Symptoms include increase appetite, craving for sugar or rice, low energy, increased sleep, and weight gain.

Epidemiology: 3% in Europe

Aetiology

1. Melatonin/pineal gland abnormalities, replaced by theories on disordered brain serotonin regulation and phase-advanced circadian rhythms.
2. Biologically vulnerable individuals are affected by the actual effect of the changes in the seasons and specific anniversary or environmental factors in winter.

Clinical features: The clinical features of SAD are similar to those of atypical depression. These include hypersomnia, hyperphagia, tiredness, and low mood in winter.

ICD-10 criteria (WHO, 1992):

1. Three or more episodes of mood disorder must occur with onset within the same 90-day period of the year for 3 or more consecutive days.
2. Remission also occurs within a particular 90-day period of the year.
3. Seasonal episodes substantially outnumber any nonseasonal episodes that may occur.

In SAD there is a regular temporal relationship between the onset of depressive episodes and a particular time of year. Depressive episodes commence in autumn or winter months and end in the spring or summer months as the hours of daylight increase.

Note that the onset of bipolar disorders may be seasonal. Hyperphagia, hypersomnia, and weight gain are more frequent than in matched nonseasonal patients.

Atypical depression: Atypical depression is more common in younger individuals and in women. It is more likely to have chronic course with poor inter-episode recovery. Atypical depression responds better to MAOIs. The symptoms are summarized in *mnemonics RAILS*:

- Reactive mood
- Appetite increased
- Interpersonal rejection sensitivity
- Leaden (heavy) paralysis
- Sleep increased

Mixed affective states: Kraepelin maintained that mood, cognition, and behaviour may vary independently, producing mixed affective states which are usually transitional but are sometimes persistent.

Bereavement reactions: Grief usually has three phases. The *stunned* phase lasts from a few hours to a few weeks. This gives way to the *mourning* phase, with intense yearning and autonomic symptoms. After several weeks the phase of *acceptance and adjustment* takes over. Grief typically lasts about 6 months.

Atypical grief is divided by Parkes (1985) into

- Inhibited grief: absence of expected grief symptoms at any stage
- Delayed grief: avoidance of painful symptoms within 2 weeks of loss
- Chronic grief: continued significant grief related symptoms 6 months

It is important to understand the differences between depression and bereavement. The following features are more common in depression, but not in bereavement:

- Active suicidal ideation
- Depressive symptoms which are out of proportion with loss
- Feelings of guilt not related to the deceased
- Marked functional impairment for longer than 2 months
- Marked psychomotor changes lasting more than a few days
- Preoccupation with worthlessness

Management

1. Grief is usually managed in the outpatient setting but inpatient setting in indicated for patients at high suicide risk.
2. Psychiatrist needs to assess and distinguish normal grief from the abnormal grief.
3. Grief work is a supportive psychotherapy while allows expression of the loss and its meaning and work through the issues. It also provides a secure base, identifies factors which block natural grief and addressees social isolation and spiritual issues.
4. Family involvement and psychoeducation.
5. If psychotropic drug is indicated, careful dosing is required to avoid side effects. Maintenance treatment is required for severe prolonged grief.
6. Rehabilitative efforts emphasize on stage-appropriate tasks such as developing vocational and social skills.

CASC STATION ON GRIEF AND BEREAVEMENT

A 50-year-old woman is referred by her GP. The referral states that she has been depressed since the sudden death of her husband 18 months ago. She has no previous psychiatric history. She herself identifies her problem as 'loneliness'. She states that since her husband's death, she has cried daily while looking at his photograph and that the distress she felt after his death has persisted since.

Task: Take a history to assess her grief.

(A) Identify Details of Death and Immediate Reaction	(A1) Identify the Nature and Circumstances of Death	(A2) Further Information Based on the Cause of Death	(A3) Assess Her Reactions	(A4) Assess Current Situation	(A5) Assess Her Current Feelings (Depending on Patient's Response)
	'How did your husband pass away? Was his death sudden or unexpected? Was it caused by a medical misadventure? Did he commit suicide?'	• Medical misadventure: medicolegal issues • Murder: progress of police investigation • AIDS: her concern about HIV status • Civil disaster: 'Was his body found?' • Chronic illness: 'Did you look after him for long time before he passed away?'	'How did you react at the time of his death?' (e.g. tearful, depression, disbelief, acting out, atypical pain, or physical symptoms) 'Do you also experience symptoms which are similar to those experienced by your husband before he died?'	• Assess current level of perceived social support • Identify the source of social support such as friends and relatives 'Have you picked up his work or interests?'	'I can imagine how difficult it is to look after him for long time before he left. How do you feel at this moment? Do you feel relieved?' 'Do you feel guilty that you survive after the accident?' 'Did you have intense reaction at certain period such as one year after his death?'
(B) Bereavement	(B1) Funeral Arrangement 'Were you involved in organizing his funeral? Did you attend his funeral? Did you have a chance to say goodbye to him?'	(B2) Mood 'How is your mood at this moment?' 'How is your sleep and appetite at this moment?' 'Have you lost weight?' 'How do you find your concentration?'	(B3) Identify Stage of: DABDA 'People usually go through the following stages after their loved ones passed away. May I know which stage are you in?' Denial, Angry, Bargaining, Depression, Acceptance	(B4) Assess Coping and Support 'How are you coping so far?' 'Do you turn into alcohol or tranquilizers?' 'Can you look after yourself?' 'Do you have children? Do they see you often?'	(B5) Functioning 'Are you able to resume what you normally did before his death?'

(C) Identify Features Suggestive of Abnormal Grief	(C1) Prolonged Grief	(C2) Inhibited Grief	(C3) Handling of Possessions	(C4) Psychotic Experiences	(C5) Risk Assessment
	'Is your feeling as intense as 6 months ago?' 'Is your feeling easily triggered?'	'Have you tried to avoid morning and grieving?' 'Do you allow yourself to express feeling towards his death?'	'After our loved ones passed away, some people keep their rooms and possessions as if they were still alive. How about yourself?'	'Do you hear voices when no one is around? Are the voices belonging to your husband?'	'Do you have any intention to end your life? If yes, why? Do you want to join him in the afterworld?'

(D) Identify Factors Impeding Grief Resolution	(D1) Explore Past Relationship with Deceased	(D2) Explore Past Experience	(D3) Personality	(D4) Past Psychiatric and Medical History	(D5) Seek Her Views on Treatment
	'How was your relationship with him? Were you dependent on him? Was there any unhappy experience?' Identify anger, violence, conflict, ambivalence, dependency, or passive aggression	Explore childhood loss and previous traumatic bereavement *Look for early disturbances in attachment:* • Affectional bonds • Security • Reciprocity • Response to separations 'Do you feel that history is repeating itself?'	'Can you describe your character?' 'How would the others describe you a person?' Look for dependency, narcissism, excessive denial, or projection	Explore past history of depression, low self-esteem, psychosis, and chronic physical illness	'Are you keen to go for counselling to talk about your experience after your husband's departure?'

27.3 EPIDEMIOLOGY OF MOOD DISORDERS

27.3.1 DEPRESSIVE EPISODES

Problems are encountered in epidemiological studies of mood disorders because of the differing use of diagnostic categories, screening instruments, and definitions of caseness.

Broadly, depressive episodes are more common in females: the annual incidence in men in the population is between 80 and 200 per 100,000, the corresponding figure for women being between 250 and 7,800 per 100,000. There is a raised incidence in those who are not married. The point prevalence in Western countries is 1.8%–3.2% for men and 2.0%–9.3% for women.

The point prevalence of depressive symptoms is 10%–30% (women 18%–34%, men 10%–19%). In the general population of Western countries, the lifetime risk of suffering from depressive episodes is 5%–12% for men and 9%–26% for women.

The average age of onset of depressive episodes is around the late thirties; however, they can start at any age.

Brown and Harris (1978) found that 15% of urban women had severe depressive symptoms, and there was a higher prevalence in working-class than in middle-class women.

Bt 2030, unipolar depressive disorder is predicted to be ranked as the number one cause of global burden of diseases in terms of disability-adjusted life years (DALYs).

27.3.2 BIPOLAR MOOD DISORDER

The sex ratio is equal, and it is more common in the upper social classes. The point prevalence in Western countries is 0.4%–1.2% in the adult population. In the general population of Western countries, the lifetime risk of suffering from a bipolar disorder is 0.6%–1.1%. The average age of onset is around the mid-twenties. Being unmarried is associated with higher rates of bipolar disorder. Common comorbidities include anxiety disorder (92%), substance misuse disorder (71%), and antisocial personality disorder (29%) (Kessler et al., 1997).

Further details on the epidemiology of mood disorder are considered in Chapter 21.

27.4 AETIOLOGY OF MOOD DISORDERS

27.4.1 GENETIC FACTORS

27.4.1.1 Family Studies

Family studies compare the rate of affective illness in relatives of index cases versus relatives of controls. There are differences in morbid risk noted for unipolar (9.1%) versus bipolar disorder (11.5%) (McGuffin and Katz, 1989). In unipolar probands there is an increased risk of unipolar depression in first-degree relatives, but the amount of bipolar illness is virtually the same as in the general population (combined risk = 7%–8%). In bipolar probands there is an increased risk of both bipolar and unipolar disorder in first-degree relatives (combined risk = 18%–20%). Family studies have demonstrated that children of parents suffering from bipolar disorder

have a ninefold increase in lifetime bipolar disorder risk compared to the general population. The heritability for bipolar disorder is 85% and depression is 60%. There are gender differences. Men are at risk of depression if there is family history of alcoholism and antisocial behaviour. Women are at risk if there is family history of anxiety disorder.

27.4.1.2 Twin Studies

Twin studies compare concordance rates in monozygotic (MZ) to dizygotic (DZ) twins and need twins reared apart to separate genetic from environmental influences. In a large Danish twin study of affective disorder (Bertelson et al., 1977), the concordance rate for MZ twins was 67%, compared with 20% for DZ twins. The MZ to DZ concordance ratio for bipolar disorder of 79:19 compared with 54:24 for unipolar disorder.

27.4.1.3 Adoption Studies

Adoptee studies compare the rates of illness in biological versus adoptive relatives of affectively ill patients which separates genetic and environmental influences. In adoptees with bipolar disorder, 28% of biological parents suffer from a mood disorder compared with 12% of adoptive parents. By comparison, 26% of the biological parents of bipolar non-adoptees were found to suffer from a mood disorder.

27.4.1.4 Molecular Genetics (Berrettini, 2004)

Linkage studies using classical autosomal markers such as red cell types, histocompatibility antigens (HLA types) to identify linkage with genes of disease. Early studies showed that bipolar disorder has been cross-linked to colour blindness and glucose-6-phosphate deficiency. Recent studies have demonstrated that bipolar disorder complex genetic heterogeneity. Multiple partially overlapping sets of susceptibility genes which interact with the environment can predispose bipolar disorder. Confirmed linkages in bipolar disorder include 4p15, 12q24, 18p11, 18q22, 22q11–13, and 21q22. The serotonin transporter (5HTT) gene has been studied, and the 5HTT promoter short allele is found to have a significant association with bipolar disorder.

Egeland et al. (1987) found linkage to chromosome 11 in an old-order Amish pedigree. This finding is now thought to have been a statistical artefact and has not been replicated. In linkage studies of complex diseases such as manic–depressive disorder, spurious linkage may be produced because of phenotypic misclassification and misspecification of the disease model.

Segregation analysis uses statistical method to examine pedigrees and hypothesized modes of inheritance. There are no consistent findings in affective disorder due to complex genetic mechanisms.

Recombinant DNA techniques resulting in development of new generation of markers. For example, the restriction fragment length polymorphisms (RFLPs) allow candidate gene approach. In bipolar disorder, candidate genes include genes encoding for tyrosine hydroxylase, serotonin transporter, catechol-*o*-methyltransferase (COMT), and brain-derived neurotropic factor (BDNF). In unipolar depressive disorder, there is lack of consistent results.

27.4.2 PERSONALITY FACTORS IN MOOD DISORDER

27.4.2.1 Cyclothymic Personality Disorder

This is characterized by persistent instability of mood with numerous periods of mild depression and mild elation. It may predispose to bipolar disorder.

27.4.2.2 Depressive Personality Disorder

This is related to the mood disorders, overlapping substantially with them, but not congruent with them. It often coexists with mood disorders. Core phenomena are excessive negative, pessimistic beliefs about oneself and others. Symptoms include unhappy, gloomy mood; low self-esteem; being self-critical, brooding, negativistic, and judgemental towards others; pessimism; and prone to feelings of guilt.

27.4.3 PSYCHOSOCIAL STRESSORS IN MOOD DISORDER

27.4.3.1 Childhood Factors

1. Childhood sexual abuse
2. Maternal loss and disruption of bonding
3. Poor care and overprotection in parenting
4. Poor relationship with adults and low intelligence

27.4.3.2 Adulthood Factors

Vaughn and Leff (1976) showed that high expressed emotion (EE) increased the risks of relapse in depressed patients. Compared to schizophrenics, depressives were more sensitive to critical remarks. However, hostility and over-involvement did not add to the significant association. The effect of critical comments (criticism index) was not mitigated by reducing the number of hours depressed people spent in contact with their relatives (unlike schizophrenia, in which it was).

Women

Brown and Harris (1978), in a community survey in Camberwell, South London, identified vulnerability factors which increase the risk of depression in women if a provoking agent is present. Four vulnerability factors are

- Having three or more children at home under the age of 14 years
- Not working outside the home
- Lack of a confiding relationship
- Loss of the mother before the age of 11 years

Men (Bebbington, 2003)

1. Marital breakdown is an important cause of depression for men.

27.4.3.3 Recent Life Events

Excess life events occur in the 6 months before a depressive episode starts:

- Loss of a child
- Death of a spouse
- Divorce
- Marital separation
- Gaol term
- Death of a close family member
- Recent unemployment (three times increase in risk)
- Suicide in relatives

The first manic episodes are often precipitated by life events such as bereavement, personal separation, work-related problems, or loss of role (Ambelas, 1987). High expressed emotion and sleep deprivation are important precipitating factors.

Social support: Buffer of social support reduces depression. The main effect hypothesis suggests that lack of social support leads to depression.

Vulnerability factors may operate by reducing self-esteem.

Kendler et al. (1995) compared stressful life events in twins with and without depression. He found that, in those with the lowest risk (MZ co-twin unaffected), the probabilities of onset of major depression were 0.5% and 6.2%, respectively, for those unexposed and exposed to the life event. In those at highest genetic risk (MZ co-twin affected), these probabilities were 1.1% and 14.6%, respectively. He concluded that genetic factors influence the risk of the onset of major depression in part by altering the sensitivity of individuals to the depression-inducing effect of stressful life events.

27.4.4 PHYSICAL ILLNESS IN MOOD DISORDER

Viral infection, particularly influenza, hepatitis A, and brucellosis are sometimes accompanied or followed by depressed mood. More recently, a significant association has been found between the occurrence of anti-Borna Disease Virus (BDV) antibodies and mood disorder (unipolar and bipolar) (Terayama et al., 2003).

Endocrine disorders commonly predispose to depression. Eighty-three per cent of people with Cushing's syndrome develop affective disorder (e.g. mood changes 50%, depression 30%, and mania) during the course of their disorder. Depression is a frequent (50%) and early presentation of people with Addison's disease. It is also seen in hypothyroidism and hypo- and hyperparathyroidism. Physical illnesses associated with depression include Parkinson's disease (50%), epilepsy (25%), congestive heart disease (27%), and hypothyroidism. Physical illnesses associated with mania include cerebral tumour, epilepsy, AIDS, and multiple sclerosis (Lange and Farmer, 2007).

Cerebrovascular accident (CVA) is associated with depression and mania. If CVA occurs in the right cerebral hemisphere, depression will develop especially in people with past or family history of depression. If CVA occurs in the left frontal part of the brain, depression will develop regardless of past history or family history. One in four people will develop a major depression after CVA. Mania is associated with right-sided CVA, and it is commonly associated with lesions in the frontal and temporal lobes, especially in patients with family history of mania.

Mania is associated with right-sided hemispheric damage. Head injury victims are more irritable than euphoric.

Medications associated with depression include clonidine, metoclopramide, theophylline, indomethacin, and nifedipine. Medications associated with mania include anticholinergic drugs, dopamine agonists (e.g. bromocriptine

and levodopa), corticosteroids, anabolic steroids, and thyroxine. Withdrawal from baclofen, clonidine, and fenfluramine is associated with mania.

27.4.5 PSYCHOLOGICAL FACTORS IN MOOD DISORDER

Seligman gave naive dogs unavoidable electric shocks and found that, after learning that there was nothing that could be done to influence the outcome of events, the dogs finally developed a condition which he thought resembled depression in humans, with reduced appetite, reduced sex drive, and disturbed sleep. He called this condition learned helplessness.

It has been suggested that in humans depression is more likely to occur if the helplessness is perceived to be attributable to a personal source, thus leading to lowered self-esteem. Global stable attributions are likely to be the longest lasting.

Beck et al. (1979) proposed a cognitive model of depression from which cognitive therapy has developed. Three concepts seek to explain the psychological substrate of depression:

1. Cognitive triad. The depressed person has:
   a. A negative personal view
   b. A tendency to interpret his or her ongoing experiences in a negative way
   c. A negative view of the future
2. Schemas. These are stable cognitive patterns forming the basis for the interpretation of situations.
3. Cognitive errors. These are systematic errors in thinking that maintain depressed people's beliefs in negative concepts.

Cognitive distortions include
Beck's negative triad: self, environment, and future
Common cognitive errors in depression: *CBT SLOPS out MDE*

C—Catastrophic thinking
B—Black and white thing (dichotomous thinking)
T—Tunnel vision
S—Selective abstraction
L—Labelling
O—Overgeneralization
P—Personalization
S—Should statement
M—Magnification and minimization
D—Discarding evidence or arbitrary inference
E—Emotional reasoning

CASC STATION ON ASSESSING COGNITIVE DISTORTIONS

A 20-year-old cricket player presents with depressive disorder. His coach comments that he has been absent for all the practices in the past 3 months. He missed hitting one ball which was easily thrown and believed this single act led to the loss of the match and will eventually lead to the loss of the entire season. The coach has read something on cognitive–behavioural therapy and hopes you can refer him for psychotherapy.

Task: Assess his cognitive distortions.

APPROACH TO THIS CASC STATION

Opening: I wonder if you would be able to tell me how things have been for you. It sounds like you are having a rough time in the cricket club, but tell me how you feel about yourself.

Cognitive Biases in Beck's Theory of Depression	Questions
Minimization	Did you play a part in any success or winning of cricket games?
	How do you see your role in the club?
	Do you feel that you have underestimated your contribution?
	Have you won any awards before? (e.g. player of the year)
	Have you hit any difficult balls before? Would you say those were remarkable?
	How many matches have you won?
	How many points have you scored this season? Over how many games?
	That sounds like a good average, what do you think?
Magnification	How did you play in the match before that miss? Aren't those successes important as well?
	Will one miss lead to the loss of an entire match? What about the whole season?
	Aren't there many turns to bat in each match and many more matches for the season?
Overgeneralization	How have things been outside cricket? We all have various roles outside work, as a husband, father, son, and friend, how do you see yourself in these different roles?
Selective abstraction	Based on what you've told me, you've contributed a lot to the team (points, trophies, etc.), how do you feel about these successes?
Personalization	I am sorry to hear that the team lost the game. Who do you think is responsible for the loss? (patient may say it's him)
	Are you the only batter on the team? Cricket is a team sport. What about the other players, aren't they responsible as well?
	It seems that you attribute failure of the team solely on yourself. Are there other factors contributing to the loss of the game?
Arbitrary inference	What do your coach and teammates think about you now? (mind-reading error)
	How does this single miss affect the outcome of the season? (fortune-telling error)
Dichotomous thinking	It seems that you're either a complete success if you had hit that ball or a complete failure if you don't. Are there any shades in between?
Catastrophic thinking	It sounds like you consider your situation to be rather depressing. Is a disaster going to happen? Will you lose control?
Labelling	What does missing this ball say about you? (patient will then label himself)
	You're calling yourself a loser. Would you call a teammate who merely missed one ball a loser?

(continued)

Schemata	Questions
Underlying beliefs	Did you have any unhappy experience when you were young?
	In order to be happy, what must happen first?
Negative automatic	Cognitive triad: How do you see yourself, the world, and your future?
thoughts	How are these thoughts being triggered? Are they related to recent unhappy events in the cricket club?
Vicious cycle	How do you see the relationship between your mood and negative thoughts?
	Do you feel that things may change and get better? Do you think that you can be helped in anyway?

Summarizing: You have told me that things have been pretty awful for you and you feel pretty dreadful about yourself. It seems that you have attributed failure to yourself and minimize your success. It might take some time for us to help you, but hopefully we can figure out the best way of getting things back on track.

Acknowledgement: Dr. Terence Leong, Consultant Psychiatrist, Department of Psychological Medicine, National University Hospital, Singapore.

27.4.6   NEUROTRANSMITTERS IN MOOD DISORDER

According to Schildkraut in 1965 the monoamine hypothesis of mood disorders stated that depression was associated with a depletion, and mania with an excess, of central monoamine. Evidence favouring this hypothesis includes the following findings:

- Tricyclic antidepressants inhibit the reuptake of noradrenaline and serotonin by presynaptic neurons, leading to an increase in the availability of these monoamines in the synaptic cleft.
- Monoamine oxidase inhibitors increase the availability of monoamines, by inhibiting their metabolic degradation by monoamine oxidase.
- SSRIs increase the availability of serotonin by inhibiting the reuptake of serotonin.
- Use of antidepressants in bipolar disorder can precipitate mania.
- Amphetamine releases catecholamines from the neurons; it is a central nervous system stimulant that lifts mood.
- Reserpine, an antihypertensive drug derived from the Indian plant Rauwolfia, depletes central monoaminergic neuronal stores of catecholamines and serotonin. Its use can lead to severe depression and suicide.
- The cerebrospinal fluid level of the serotonin metabolite 5-hydroxyindoleacetic acid (5-HIAA) is often reported as being reduced in depressed patients.
- Impaired repression at a 5-hydroxytryptamine 1A receptor gene polymorphism is associated with major depression and suicide (Lemonde et al., 2003).
- The antidepressant effects of light therapy combined with sleep deprivation are influenced by a functional polymorphism within the promoter of the serotonin transporter gene (Benedetti et al., 2003).

Evidence against the monoamine hypothesis includes the following:

- Antidepressant pharmacotherapy takes at least a fortnight to effect a clinical improvement. This time interval is much greater than the relatively rapid onset of biochemical action.
- Not all drugs that act as monoamine reuptake inhibitors have a therapeutic antidepressant action (e.g. cocaine).

27.4.6.1   Serotonin (5-HT)

Additional evidence for abnormal serotonergic function in mood disorders includes the following:

- In subgroups of depressed patients, low levels of 5-HIAA have been reported in cerebrospinal fluid.
- In depressed patients, a low density of brain and platelet serotonin transporter sites has been found, as well as a high density of brain and platelet serotonin binding sites.
- Dietary tryptophan depletion induced a prompt relapse in depressed patients who had responded to SSRIs.
- There is a low plasma tryptophan in depressed patients.

- Blood platelet studies: reduced 5-HT uptake and changes in 5-HT2 receptors have been studied in platelets in depression in normal subjects. The uptake of 5-HT into platelets is reduced in depression (Lange and Farmer, 2007).

The connection of 5-HT metabolism between 5-methoxy-indole metabolism in the pineal and overlaps and impacts on sleep, pain mechanisms and depression

- There is a decreased 5-HT transporter binding density in depression.
- Serotonin function is reduced in depression and may be normalized with active treatment.

27.4.6.2 Adaptive Changes in Receptors

Depression is associated with an increase in the density of $\alpha2$ adrenergic presynaptic receptors in the locus coeruleus and increased density of β-adrenergic receptors in the cerebral cortex.

During antidepressant treatment, changes take place in cerebral α- and β-adrenergic and serotonin receptors, showing only after 2 weeks of treatment, at the same time as the therapeutic effect. A decrease in the sensitivity (downregulation) of β-adrenergic receptors is particularly evident.

27.4.6.3 Brain-Derived Neurotropic Factor

The BDNF is associated with production of new neurons and important for mood regulation and memory. Both serotonin and noradrenaline play roles in modulation of BDNF (Dunman et al., 1997). The levels of BDNF are reduced in depression and causes hippocampal atrophy in depressed patients (Sheline et al., 1996). Antidepressant restores BDNF function.

27.4.7 NEUROENDOCRINE FACTORS IN MOOD DISORDER

27.4.7.1 Brain–Steroid Axis

Disturbances of the hypothalamic–pituitary–adrenal axis are reported in depression. In normal humans, cortisol secretion is episodic and follows a circadian rhythm. Peak cortisol secretion is in the morning; between noon and 4 a.m., secretion remains low, being lowest just after the onset of sleep.

In biological depression, there is disruption in the normal circadian rhythm of cortisol secretion, the morning peak being increased and longer lasting. A phase shift with the morning peak occurring earlier has been reported.

In depressed patients, increased secretion has been reported in corticotropin (ACTH), cortisol, β-endorphin, and prolactin.

In the dexamethasone suppression test (DST), plasma cortisol levels are measured following the administration of the long-acting potent synthetic steroid dexamethasone the previous evening. In normal subjects, dexamethasone leads to a suppression in the level of cortisol over the next 24 h through negative feedback. In depressed patients with biological symptoms, non-suppression of cortisol has been reported in over 60%. The DST has not proved to be a useful laboratory test for depression because a relatively high level of cortisol non-suppression has been found in other psychiatric disorders. The DST can be affected by factors such as age, bodyweight, drugs, ECT, and endocrinopathies. The DST is usually state-dependent and in most subjects normalizes as the patient recovers.

Corticotropin-releasing factor (CRH or CRF) is an important hypothalamic peptide in the regulation of appetite and eating. In the CRH stimulation test, the administration of CRH to normal humans leads to the release of corticotropin. In depression there is a consistent reduction of corticotropin response.

The noradrenergic neurons of the locus coeruleus express glucocorticoid receptors, through which corticosteroids can regulate its functioning. It is hypothesized that steroids may be important in causing and perpetuating depression.

27.4.7.2 Brain–Thyroid Axis

Thyroid-releasing hormone (TRH) causes the release of thyroid-stimulating hormone (TSH) from the adenohypophysis. In normal subjects there is a circadian pattern of TSH secretion, with a nocturnal rise which is blunted in depression and returns with sleep deprivation. In the TRH stimulation test, the TSH response to intravenous TRH is measured. About 25% of depressed patients show a blunted TSH response to TRH stimulation. This does not often normalize as the subject recovers from depression. Blunting is also found in panic disorder. TRH stimulation studies in depression have also shown that approximately 15% of patients have a raised TSH response; many of these patients have been found to have antimicrosomal thyroid and antithyroglobulin antibodies, indicating that depression can be associated with symptomless autoimmune thyroiditis.

27.4.7.3 Melatonin

Patients with depression have disordered biological rhythms—short REM latency (time from falling asleep to onset of REM sleep), early-morning awakening, and diurnal mood variation. The suprachiasmatic nucleus (SCN) of the hypothalamus plays a major role in regulating diurnal rhythms. Information about light conditions from the retina, via the retinohypothalamic pathway, controls the SCN. This influences the pineal which excretes melatonin.

The biosynthesis of melatonin from its precursor, serotonin, occurs via *N*-acetylation followed by *O*-methylation. The step involving serotonin *N*-acetyltransferase is probably rate-limiting and is stimulated at night. Melatonin receptors are numerous in the SCN, and parts of the hypothalamus where releasing and inhibiting hormones end. Darkness stimulates melatonin release and light blocks its synthesis. When compared with normal subjects, patients with SAD have been found to have an increased sensitivity of melatonin biosynthesis to inhibition by phototherapy. Furthermore, sleep deprivation and flying overnight from west to east may trigger relapse of mania.

27.4.7.4   Water and Electrolyte Changes

There are increases in the body's residual sodium (which is an index of intracellular sodium ion concentration) in both depression and mania. Erythrocyte sodium ion concentrations decrease following recovery from depression or mania as a result of increased Na^+–K^+-ATPase activity.

27.4.8   Neuroanatomy and Imaging

The following neuroanatomical areas are implicated in depression (Charney and Nestler, 2004):

1. Amygdala: associated with memory of emotional reactions
2. Anterior cingulate cortex: associated with negative anticipation or poor judgement
3. Cerebellum: psychomotor retardation
4. Hippocampus: memories
5. Insular cortex: process information in an emotionally relevant context and associated with negative interpretation of events
6. Nucleus accumbens: lack of motivation
7. Prefrontal cortex: associated with impairment in executive functions

27.4.8.1   Structural Imaging

Depression

1. Ventricular enlargement
2. Sulcal widening
3. Hippocampus atrophy (Sheline, 2003)
4. Reduction in size in the frontal lobe, cerebellum, and basal ganglia

27.4.8.2   Bipolar Disorder

1. Asymmetry in temporal lobe (Swayze et al., 1992)
2. Smaller dorsolateral prefrontal cortex (Lyoo et al., 2004)
3. Increased white matter intensities (Woods et al., 1995)

27.4.8.3   Functional Imaging

Depression

1. Increased blood flow in the amygdala and ventrolateral prefrontal cortex in depression, and antidepressant may normalize amygdala activity (Sheline, 2001; Drevets, 2003).
2. Reduced glucose metabolism and blood flow in frontal regions.

27.4.8.4   Bipolar Disorder

1. Increase in amygdala activation
2. Increased cerebello-posterior cortical metabolism

27.5   MANAGEMENT OF DEPRESSIVE DISORDER

27.5.1   Investigations

1. FBC, LFT, RFT, TFT, and ECG are required in the assessment of the first depressive episode.
2. CT or MRI is indicated if there are neurological signs or symptoms.

27.5.2   Pharmacotherapy: NICE Guidelines (Table 27.3)

27.5.2.1   Unipolar Depression

Categories
Frank et al. (1991) have categorized outcomes of treatment according to the '5 Rs':

- Response.
- Remission. This is a return to the patient's premorbid self.
- Relapse. This is a return of depressive symptoms in the time between initial response and recovery. Risk is particularly high (40%–60%) following the withdrawal of antidepressants within the first 4 months of achieving a response. The risk of relapse is reduced to 10%–30% by continuation of pharmacotherapy.
- Recovery. A patient who has achieved a stable remission for at least 4–6 months is assumed to have recovered from the index episode.
- Recurrence. This is a return of depression after recovery from the index episode. Risk factors for recurrent depression include frequent and/or multiple prior episodes, seasonal pattern, and a family history of mood disorder.

TABLE 27.3

Pharmacological Treatment of Depressive Disorder

Stages	Recommendations from the NICE Guidelines

Starting antidepressant treatment	1. Explain the following to the patient:
	   a. The gradual development of the full antidepressant effect
	   b. The importance of taking medication as prescribed and the need to continue beyond remission
	   c. The risk and nature of discontinuation symptoms (particularly with drugs with a shorter half-life, such as paroxetine and venlafaxine, usually mild with duration of less than 1 week)
	   d. Addiction does not occur with antidepressants
	 2. If a person experiences side effects early in treatment, consider stopping or changing to a different antidepressant
	 3. If anxiety, agitation, or insomnia is problematic, consider short-term benzodiazepine (<2 weeks)

Frequency of monitoring	1. For patients who are not considered to be at increased risk of suicide, normally see them after 2 weeks 2. For patients who are considered to be at increased risk of suicide or are younger than 30 years, normally see them after 1 week and then frequently until suicide risk has subsided
Clinical response	1. If improvement is not occurring on the first antidepressant after 2–4 weeks, check that the drug has been taken as prescribed 2. If antidepressant is taken as prescribed, increase the dose based on the summary of product characteristics 3. If there is improvement by 4 weeks, continue treatment for another 2–4 weeks 4. Consider switching antidepressants if the response is inadequate, there is presence of side effects, or the patient requests to change drug
Switching antidepressants	1. Consider a different SSRI or better tolerated new generation antidepressant 2. Normally switch within 1 week for drugs with short half-life 3. Consider at least 2-week washing period when switching: from fluoxetine to other antidepressants, from paroxetine to TCA (because of anticholinergic side effects), from other antidepressants to new serotonergic antidepressants or MAOI and from a nonreversible MOAI to other antidepressants
Augmentation	1. Mood stabilizers: lithium 2. Antipsychotics: aripiprazole, olanzapine, quetiapine, or risperidone 3. Another antidepressant: mianserin (be aware of blood dyscrasia) or mirtazapine
Discontinuation of antidepressants	1. Gradually reduce the dose over 4 weeks 2. Longer period is required for drugs with shorter half-life (e.g. paroxetine and venlafaxine) 3. Shorter period is required for drugs with long half-life (e.g. fluoxetine) 4. If patient experiences significant discontinuation symptoms, consider reintroducing the original antidepressant at the dose that was effective

Acute treatment: This is initial treatment which aims to achieve a response.

Continuation treatment: This begins when a patient has achieved a significant response to treatment. The aim is to prevent relapse and consolidate response into remission.

Maintenance treatment: This follows continuation treatment for those patients with a history of recurrent depression. A recurrence rate of 85% is seen in those patients with recurrent depression within 3 years following the discontinuation of pharmacotherapy. After 6 months, continuation becomes maintenance treatment by arbitrary definition.

In an MRC trial in 1965, 269 patients with operationally defined depression were randomly assigned to treatment groups, with the following results at 4 weeks:

- A tricyclic antidepressant (imipramine) response rate of 53%
- A MAOI (phenelzine) response rate of 30%
- A placebo response rate of 39%
- An ECT response rate of 71%

Drugs: The first-line treatment of depression is with antidepressants. It is important that patients receive an adequate dose for an adequate duration, conventionally 6 weeks. Antidepressants should be continued for 4–6 months after the amelioration of symptoms of the acute episode. Maintenance therapy usually with the same agent is used to treat the acute and continuation phases.

Lithium is efficacious in preventing recurrent depressive episodes but less so than tricyclic antidepressants.

Patients maintained on the full effective treatment dose of antidepressants have proportionately fewer relapses than those whose dose is cut down to a lower maintenance level.

27.5.2.2 Sequenced Treatment Alternatives to Relieve Depression (STAR*D) Trial (Trivedi et al., 2006)

*Objective of the STAR*D trial*: The purpose of this trial is to determine the effectiveness of different treatments for people with major depressive disorder (MDD) who have not responded to initial treatment with an antidepressant.

*Methodology of the STAR*D trial*: The STAR*D project enrolled 4000 outpatients (ages 18–75) diagnosed with nonpsychotic MDD in the United States. Participants will be initially treated (open label) with citalopram, the Level 1 treatment, for a minimum of 8 weeks. Patients who experienced minimal benefit were strongly encouraged to complete 12 weeks of treatment in order to maximize the chances of symptom remission (unless no benefit at all is seen after 8 weeks). All participants received a brief depression educational programme. There were four levels and participants who either did not have an adequate response to or could not tolerate one level were eligible to move to higher level. At each level change, participants were asked to indicate the unacceptability of the potential treatment strategies (e.g. to augment or to switch medications). Participants would then be eligible for random assignment to one of the treatment options.

The Level 2 treatment strategies include (i) switching to other antidepressants (sertraline, venlafaxine, bupropion) and cognitive therapy, (ii) medication and psychotherapy augmentation, (iii) antidepressant only switch, (iv) antidepressant only augmentation, (v) psychotherapy only switch, and (vi) psychotherapy only augmentation.

The Level 3 treatment strategies include switching to (i) mirtazapine or nortriptyline or (ii) lithium or thyroid hormone (T_3) augmentation.

The Level 4 treatment strategies include two switch options: (i) to tranylcypromine or (ii) to mirtazapine plus venlafaxine.

Summary of results

1. One-third of participants reached a remission or virtual absence of symptoms during the initial phase of the study, with an additional 10%–15% experiencing some improvement.
2. There were consistent findings across both standard and patient-rated depression rating scales.

3. The remission rate was 30% (higher than expected) because of the systematic and comprehensive approach to care.
4. One in three depressed patients who previously did not achieve remission using an antidepressant became symptom-free with the help of augmenting with another antidepressant. One in four achieved remission after switching to a different antidepressant.
5. At Level 3, 20% of participants became symptom-free after 9 weeks. Patients taking T_3 complained of fewer side effects than those taking lithium. The discontinuation rate for T_3 was 10% and the rate for lithium was 23%.
6. The Level 4 findings suggested that the venlafaxine or mirtazapine treatment may be a better choice than the MAOI.

Switching to or adding cognitive therapy after a first unsuccessful attempt at treating depression with an antidepressant medication is generally as effective as switching to or adding another medication. Participants on cognitive therapy took longer to achieve remission.

27.5.2.3 Atypical Depression

This responds better to monoamine oxidase inhibitors than to tricyclic antidepressants.

27.5.2.4 Psychotic Depression

Spiker et al. (1985) found a superior response when an antidepressant and an antipsychotic were used in combination, in delusional depression:

1. 41% responded to amitriptyline alone.
2. 19% responded to perphenazine alone.
3. 78% responded to a combination of amitriptyline and perphenazine.

27.5.2.5 Resistant Major Depression

Up to 20% of patients may be resistant to first-line treatment with antidepressant medication, and another 20%–30% may have only a partial response. Patients with a partial response have a significantly higher rate of relapse during the first 6 months following response.

Those patients not showing a response to adequate first-line drug treatment may respond to augmentation with various agents including lithium, T_3, or tryptophan. ECT should be tried if these measures fail.

CASC STATION ON TREATMENT-RESISTANT DEPRESSION

A 40-year-old male executive suffers from depression and has failed to make a clinically significant response after an adequate dose of amitriptyline and fluoxetine given for an adequate period of time. He has prepared a list of antidepressants which he tried before with dosage and duration.

Task:

1. Explore the underlying reasons for poor response and explain possible management options.
2. Patient will seek your view on lithium augmentation and address his concerns.

CASC Grid

(A) Causes of Poor Response	(A1) Wrong Diagnosis	(A2) Substance-Abuse	(A3) Compliance and Tolerability of Previous Medication	(A4) Perpetuating Psychosocial Factors and Predisposing Factors	(A5) Side Effects with Previous Medication?
	Explore the following: • Other psychiatric diagnosis: PTSD • Grief reaction • Other medical diagnosis: hypothyroidism, multiple sclerosis • Medication: corticosteroid, cardiac drugs	Explore history of drug and alcohol misuse	'Are you taking the antidepressant on a daily basis?' 'Do you experience any side effect?'	Explore marital problems, work-related problems, financial problems Ask about family history of depression, severity, completed suicide, and family members' responses to treatment	Explore common side effects such as nausea, headache, sexual dysfunction, and sedation

(B) Explain Management of Possible Treatment-Resistant Depression	(B1) Explore the Dose and Duration of the Current Drugs	(B2) Inform the Possibility of Substitution by an Antidepressant from Different Class	(B3) Offer Other Treatments	(B4) Discuss Augmentation with Another Antidepressant	(B5) Augmentation with Other Agents
	'Can you tell me which antidepressant have you tried? Can you tell me the duration and dosage? Can you tell me which one works and which one doesn't' Explore the possibility to increase the dose and duration of current medication	For example, SNRI venlafaxine	ECT Psychotherapy such as CBT or IPT with medication	Examples: SSRI + bupropion SSRI + buspirone SSRI + venlafaxine/ mirtazapine	*First-line agents:* • Add lithium (effective in 50% of cases) • Add triiodothyronine (T_3 is better tolerated than T_4 and be aware of the side effects) **Second-line agents:** • Add lamotrigine • Combine olanzapine and fluoxetine • Combine MAOI and TCA • Add tryptophan (*continued*)

(C) Seek Patient's View on Lithium Augmentation	(C1) Explain Lithium	(C2) Assess His Background Knowledge	(C3) Inform Frequency of Blood Tests	(C4) Inform Duration of Treatment and Explain Side Effects	(C5) Risk Assessment
	The best established augmentation strategy is the addition of lithium to a given antidepressant Lithium augmentation with TCA has been extensively studied, and lithium augmentation reduces the risk of remaining depressed	'How much information would you like to know about lithium? Would it be alright with you if I explain how it works?'	'You need baseline investigation result and lab test on a weekly basis for 1 month. Then I will check lithium level every 3–6 months. Renal, thyroid functions and ECT will be checked every 6 months The dose is 400 mg per day and we aim at the serum level between 0.4 and 0.6 mmol/L'	'You need regular follow-up and should carry a lithium card. You need to maintain lithium for 2–3 years' Common side effects include nausea, metallic taste, diarrhoea, frequent urination, feeling thirsty, tremor, and muscle weakness Long-term side effects include weight gain and impaired kidney and thyroid functions 'How do you feel about lithium?'	'Did you have any thyroid or kidney problem in the past?' 'Are you suicidal? Will you take an overdose of lithium? If yes, please ask your partner to keep lithium for you' 'Do you take the following medications which may interact with lithium? (e.g. diuretics, NSAIDs, ACEI, carbamazepine, and alcohol)'

27.5.3 Electroconvulsive Therapy and Physical Therapies in Mood Disorder

Double-blind placebo-controlled trials have shown electro-convulsive therapy (ECT) to be superior to placebo, especially in delusional depression. It is considered the gold standard of antidepressant therapy and is often given to patients who have not responded to antidepressants. ECT is also used in the treatment of resistant mania or manic stupor.

ECT, repetitive transcranial magnetic stimulation (rTMS), vagus nerve stimulation (VNS), and deep brain stimulation (DBS) are mentioned in Chapter 24.

27.5.4 Psychosocial Treatments

27.5.4.1 Psychotherapies

Indications to administer CBT alone without antidepressant in depression include

1. Better response to psychotherapies in the past as compared to antidepressant response to antidepressants
2. Reactive depression to life events

3. Depressed mood with strong correlation with negative cognitions (Figure 27.1)
4. Mild somatoform disorders
5. Adequate reality testing and absence of psychotic feature
6. Inability to tolerate side effects of antidepressants

27.5.4.2 CASC Preparation: Explain CBT to a Depressed Person

CBT is a structured psychotherapy with two components: cognitive and behaviour therapy. Depression can be explained by cognitive and behavioural models. According to the cognitive model, unhelpful thoughts lead to depression and unhelpful behaviours. According to the behavioural model, people with depression are often withdrawn because they have no mood to socialize and do things. CBT aims at changing unhelpful thoughts. As a result, behaviour and mood will be improved. CBT begins with assessment of the client's problems. The client is encouraged to keep a diary of life events and their thoughts, behaviours, and mood.

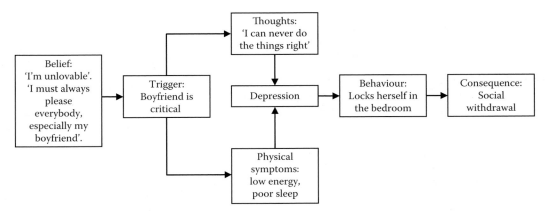

FIGURE 27.1   Cognitive model of a 20-year-old woman suffering from depressive disorder.

For cognitive therapy, the therapist helps the client to identify the pattern, namely, what happens before a mood change (i.e. the antecedents) and after the mood change (i.e. the consequences). The therapist also helps the client to identify the negative thoughts about client, his or her views about the future and the world. The client needs to challenge the negative thoughts and develop new strategies of thinking.

For behaviour therapy, the therapist helps the client to draw a list of mood-enhancing activities. The client usually starts with simple activities and move on to more sophisticated activities. The duration of activity will be increased in a gradual manner.

Nowadays, CBT can be administered by computer. This new treatment is called computerized CBT or CCBT. CCBT is commonly used in people with mild depression or young people. New form of CBT called mindfulness-based CBT involves combination of meditation techniques and CBT. The mindfulness-based CCBT aims at detaching the client's thinking process and emotions. CBT can also be offered in a group. Both CBT and antidepressants are of proven benefit in the treatment of depression. CBT does not work very well for people who are very depressed. These patients require antidepressant first.

27.5.4.3   NICE Guidelines Recommendations on CBT and Depressive Disorder

1. Adult depression
   a. For people with persistent subthreshold depressive symptoms or mild to moderate depression, individual-guided self-help based on the principles of CBT and CCBT can be offered.
   b. For people with moderate or severe depression, combination of individual CBT or group-based CBT with antidepressant is recommended.

c. For relapse prevention, CBT is recommended for clients who have received antidepressant treatment and mentalization-based CBT is recommended for stable clients with three or more previous episodes of depression.
2. Depression in children and adolescents: CBT is used as first-line treatment in moderate to severe depression for 2–3 months. If depression is unresponsive to combined treatment, individual child psychotherapy will be offered for 30 sessions.
3. Depression in clients with chronic physical health problems: individual CBT or group-based CBT are offered to clients with persistent subthreshold or mild symptoms, moderate depression, and combined with antidepressants in severe depression (Table 27.4).

27.5.5   MANAGEMENT OF BIPOLAR DISORDER (NICE GUIDELINES RECOMMENDATIONS)

27.5.5.1   Investigations

- Evaluation of physical status. FBC, LFT, U&Es, TFT, fasting glucose, lipid profile, and ECG should be considered.
- Urine pregnancy test is a must for female patients with bipolar disorder. STD screen should be ordered if history suggests.
- Urine drug screen will be useful to rule out the possibility of illicit drugs causing manic-like symptoms.
- The patient may need neurological investigations such as lumbar puncture, EEG, and MRI brain scan if there were neurological signs or symptoms which suggest an underlying neurological disorder.

TABLE 27.4

Treatment of Depressive Disorder Based on the Severity of Depression (NICE Guidelines)

Persistent subthreshold depressive symptoms (mild to depressive episode)	Persistent subthreshold depressive symptoms or mild to moderate depression with inadequate response to initial interventions (moderate and severe depressive episode)	Depression and chronic physical health problem
Individual-guided self-help based on CBT principles: written materials, for 6–8 sessions, duration over 9–12 weeks *CCBT*: explain CBT model, encourage tasks between sessions, use of thought-challenging, active monitoring of behaviour and thought patterns and duration over 9–12 weeks *Structured group physical activity programme*: 3 sessions per week, lasting 45 min to 1 h over 10–14 weeks *Group-based CBT*: by 2 trained practitioners with 10–12 meetings of 8–10 participants and duration is between 12–16 weeks	*Antidepressant* *High intensity—psychological interventions* • *Individual CBT*: 16–20 sessions over 3–4 months, 3–4 follow-up sessions subsequently over the next 3–6 months. Consider 2 sessions per week for the first 2–3 weeks • *Interpersonal therapy*: 16–20 sessions over 3–4 months and 2 sessions per week for the first 2–3 weeks • *Behavioural activation*: 16–20 sessions over 3–4 months. Consider 3–4 follow-up sessions over next 3–6 months. For moderate of severe depression, consider 2 sessions per week for the first 3–4 weeks • For complex cases, it will involve crisis intervention with the home treatment team, multidisciplinary care plan, or ECT in addition to antidepressant and high intensity psychological interventions	*Group-based CBT*: in a group of 6–8 people with a common physical health problem over 6–8 weeks *Individual CBT*: 6–8 weeks for moderate depression and 16–18 weeks for severe depression *Behavioural activation*: 16–20 sessions over 3–4 months *Behavioural couples therapy*: 15–20 sessions over 5–6 months

27.5.5.2 Pharmacotherapy

If the patient is lacking insight towards bipolar disorder, the imposition of compulsory treatment should be addressed. The treatment of acute mania is with antipsychotics (e.g. risperidone, quetiapine, or olanzapine). Lithium carbonate is used in the prophylaxis of bipolar disorder. They can also be used in the treatment of acute mania, but neuroleptics are preferred in the first instance. It is important to ensure that antidepressant is stopped because it may be the main precipitant of mania. Short-term benzodiazepine (such as lorazepam) can be used to control behavioural disturbance or agitation. If patient is admitted to the ward, the nurses should avoid excessive stimulation and engage the patient in structured routine.

A maintenance strategy consisting of lithium carbonate monotherapy in bipolar disorder is likely to result in sustained remission in approximately 50% of cases. The NICE guidelines recommend pharmacological treatment for at least 2 years after an episode of bipolar disorder.

The premature withdrawal of lithium in bipolar patients results in more than 80% of recurrences within 36 months, a 28-fold increase compared to those left on lithium. Low-dose maintenance strategies (less than the usual acute antimanic range of [0.8–1.2 mmol/L]) lead to an increased risk of relapse.

In cases of bipolar disorder which are resistant to or intolerant of lithium, alternative prophylactic treatment with carbamazepine or sodium valproate are effective, both as acute antimanic treatment and as prophylaxis.

27.5.5.3 Psychotherapy

The NICE guidelines recommend offering psychotherapy of at least 16 sessions over 6–9 months. It includes psychoeducation, general coping strategies, and CBT.

27.5.5.4 Relapse Prevention

Besides medication and psychotherapy, advice (including written information) on the importance of good sleep hygiene and regular lifestyle should be given.

For those patients who work, risks of shift work in triggering mania should be discussed. For those patients who travel, the risk of flying across various time zones should be informed. Families and careers often play an important role in relapse prevention. Joining a support group can be useful. The GP needs to encourage the patient to continue treatment. The patient is taught on identifying the triggers and early warning signs of relapse. The GP helps to monitor the early signs of relapse. Treatment plan should include risk management addressing risk of suicide, exploitation, self-neglect, or unprotected sex.

27.5.6 MANAGEMENT OF RAPID CYCLING

- The NICE guidelines recommend increasing the dose of antimanic drug or adding lamotrigine.
- For long-term management, the NICE guidelines recommend a combination of lithium and valproate as first-line treatment.
- Lithium monotherapy is the second-line treatment.
- Antidepressants should be avoided and check thyroid function tests every 6 months.

27.5.6.1 Prognosis for Mood Disorders

Depression is a chronic and recurrent condition. It has become increasingly clear that a significant proportion of patients followed in the long term after suffering from depression remain chronically ill, despite the previously held belief that patients tended to recover fully between depressive episodes. Factors predicting a prolonged time to recovery are the longer duration and the increased severity of the index episode, a history of non-affective psychiatric disorder, lower family income, and married status during the index episode.

It has been found that 15%–20% of depressed patients develop a chronic course of illness and 75%–80% suffer multiple episodes. The risk of relapse decreases the longer the patient remains well. For a first episode of depression, an older age and a history of previous non-affective psychiatric illness predict a shorter time to relapse. Continuing high levels of medication in the first few months is associated with a higher chance of remaining well. Overall, there is a suicide rate of around 15%.

The time to recovery from the index episode of major depression in patients suffering from double depression is shorter than in patients suffering major depression alone, but they tend to relapse more frequently and rapidly.

27.6 PERSISTENT MOOD DISORDERS

ICD-10 describes persistent and usually fluctuating disorders of mood in which individual episodes are rarely sufficiently severe to warrant being described as hypomanic or mild depressive episodes. They may last for years at a time, sometimes for the greater part of adult life and involve considerable subjective distress and disability.

In ICD-10, the persistent mood disorders are classed with the mood disorders rather than with the personality disorders because of evidence from family studies which suggests that the persistent mood disorders are genetically related to other mood disorders.

The two most important persistent mood disorders are cyclothymia and dysthymia.

27.6.1 CYCLOTHYMIA

Cyclothymia is defined in ICD-10 as

> A persistent instability of mood, involving numerous periods of mild depression and mild elation. This instability usually develops early in adult life and pursues a chronic course, although at times the mood may be normal and stable for months at a time. The lifetime risk of cyclothymia is between 0.4 and 3.5%, sex ratio equal. First-degree relatives of patients with cyclothymia are more likely than the general population to suffer from depressive episodes and bipolar disorder.

Some are treated successfully with lithium and/or with individual or group psychotherapy.

27.6.2 DYSTHYMIA

Dysthymia, also called depressive neurosis, is defined in ICD-10 as

> A chronic depression of mood which does not fulfil the criteria for recurrent depressive disorder.... The balance between individual phases of mild depression and intervening periods of comparative normality is very variable. Sufferers usually have periods of days or weeks when they describe themselves as well, but most of the time... they feel tired and depressed; everything is an effort and nothing is enjoyed. They brood and complain, sleep badly and feel inadequate, but are usually able to cope with the basic demands of everyday life.

Dysthymia is probably more common in women than in men. It is more common in first-degree relatives of patients with a history of depressive episodes than in the general population.

Treatment with antidepressants, individual psychotherapy, or cognitive therapy may be helpful.

27.7 SUICIDE AND PARASUICIDE (DELIBERATE SELF-HARM)

27.7.1 SUICIDE

27.7.1.1 Epidemiology

The annual incidence of suicide in England and Wales is approximately 1 in 10,000 of the population. It is more common in men than women and also more common in those aged over 45 years. The highest rates are in those who are divorced, single, or widowed. The highest rates are in social classes I and V.

Suicide is associated with unemployment and retirement. Suicide rates fell in England and Wales during the First and Second World Wars.

There is a seasonal variation in suicide rates. In the northern hemisphere, suicide rates are highest during the months of spring and early summer. In the southern hemisphere, rates are highest in the months corresponding to spring and early summer.

There is evidence that the availability of method affects gross suicide rates as well as the choice of method. Suicide rates by hanging were constant until the 1960s when there was a rise after the abolition of capital punishment. A massive reduction in the number of deaths caused by gassing followed the switch from coal gas to the safer North Sea gas in the 1960s. A marked rise in poisoning in the early 1960s was because of the increased availability of medicines such as barbiturates.

27.7.1.2 Aetiology of Suicide

27.7.1.2.1 Statistics

Ninety per cent of people who commit suicide suffer from a psychiatric disorder. Of these, approximately 50% suffer depression, 25% alcoholism, 5% schizophrenia, and 20% other (e.g. personality disorder, chronic neuroses, and psychoactive substance-abuse disorders). The rate of suicide is increased by 50 times the population rate among psychiatric inpatients. There is also an association with physical illnesses, particularly chronic painful illnesses, epilepsy (especially temporal lobe epilepsy), cancer, peptic ulcer, and gastric ulcer disease.

Following an act of deliberate self-harm, the risk of completing suicide in the subsequent year is approximately 100 times that in the general population and remains high in subsequent years.

27.7.1.2.2 Associations

Positive associations with suicide in the general population include

- Being male
- Being elderly
- Having suffered loss or bereavement
- Being unemployed
- Being retired
- Childlessness
- Living alone in a big, densely populated town
- A broken home in childhood
- Mental or physical illness
- Loss of role
- Social disorganization, including overcrowding, criminality, and drug and alcohol misuse

Negative associations include

- Religious devoutness
- Lots of children
- Times of war

27.7.1.2.3 Risk Factors

Risk factors by psychiatric diagnosis are as follows:

- Schizophrenia. There is a 10% mortality from suicide. Roy (1982) characterized schizophrenics who commit suicide as young, male, and unemployed, with chronic relapsing illness. Fewer schizophrenic patients give warning of their intention to commit suicide than patients in other diagnostic groups (23% vs. 50%). The suicide is usually after recent discharge, with good insight.
- Affective psychosis. There is a 15% mortality from suicide. Men are older, separated, widowed or divorced, living alone, and not working. Women are middle aged, middle class, with a history of parasuicide, and threats made in the last month. Those with obsessive–compulsive symptoms are about six times less likely to commit suicide than those without.
- Neuroses. Nearly 90% have a history of parasuicide, and a high proportion have threatened suicide in the preceding month. There is a tendency after a failed attempt to resort to more violent means. There is a high risk in depressive neurosis and panic disorder, but a lower risk in obsessive–compulsive disorder.

- Alcoholism. There is a 15% mortality from suicide. It tends to occur later in the course of the illness, and those affected are often also depressed. Associated with completed suicide are poor physical health, a poor work record, previous parasuicide, and a recent loss of a close relationship.
- Personality disorder. High-risk factors are lability of mood, aggressiveness, impulsivity, alienation from peers, and associated alcohol and substance misuse.

27.7.1.2.4   Life Events and Suicide

The risk of suicide increases, more among males than females, during the 5 years following the bereavement of a parent or a spouse.

Compared with psychiatric patient controls, suicides have experienced interpersonal losses more frequently, although schizophrenic suicides have experienced fewer losses than nonschizophrenic controls.

Age-related variations of stressors have been described, with conflict–separation–rejection more common in younger age groups, economic problems in middle-aged groups, and medical illness among the older age groups.

27.7.1.2.5   Biochemical Disturbances

Low 5-HIAA concentration in cerebral spinal fluid is associated with increased suicidal behaviour and aggression. Irrespective of the clinical diagnosis, the group in which CSF concentration of 5-HIAA is low often includes persons who have attempted a violent method of suicide. Serotonin may play an important role in the biology of aggression and the control of impulsive behaviour.

Postmortem ligand binding studies have found increased numbers of $5HT_2$ receptors in the prefrontal cortex of suicide victims, particularly those who used violent means. Low concentrations of serum cholesterol have been found to be prospectively associated with an increase in the risk of violent death or suicide. Biological mechanisms linking low serum cholesterol concentration and suicide have been hypothesized.

27.7.1.2.6   Sociological Theory

Durkheim in 1897 used the phenomenon of suicide to describe society (see also Chapter 7). He described four types of suicide:

- Altruistic. The individual sets no value on life and renounces his or her personal being in order

to be engulfed into something wider (e.g. religious or terrorist suicides).
- Egoistic. Suicide springs from excessive individuation of the individual from society.
- Anomic. This relates to how society regulates the individual. Suicide results from the fact that a human's activities lack regulation.
- Fatalistic. This is a rare type of suicide, the opposite of anomic, deriving from excessive regulation by oppressive regimes.

27.7.1.3   Assessment of the Individual for Suicide

Suicidal ideation should be explored in every patient and forms a part of the routine mental state examination. There is no evidence that asking patients about suicidal thoughts increases the risk of suicide.

The majority of people who commit suicide have told somebody beforehand of their thoughts. Two-thirds have seen their GP in the previous month. One-quarter have been psychiatric outpatients at the time of death; half of them will have seen a psychiatrist in the previous week.

27.7.1.4   Management of Suicidal Ideation

Once the need for treatment has been identified, it should be provided quickly. The interval between GP referral to psychiatric services and consultation has been identified as a danger period and should be minimized.

If there is a serious risk of suicide, the patient should be admitted to hospital. Any psychiatric disorder from which the patient suffers should be treated appropriately. If the patient is suffering from severe depression, electroconvulsive therapy may be required. Patients with manic depression have a mortality up to three times that of the general population, with suicide and cardiovascular disease being primarily responsible. In patients treated with lithium prophylaxis, cumulative mortality does not differ from that of the general population. A minimum of 2 years of lithium treatment is needed to reduce the high mortality resulting from manic depression. It is proposed that lithium exerts its anti-suicide effect as a result of improved serotonergic transmission.

27.7.2   PARASUICIDE

27.7.2.1   Epidemiology

There is an annual incidence of about 3 in 1000, but this is probably an underestimate. It is most common in females and in those aged below 35 years. The highest rates are in those who are divorced or single, among the lower social classes, unemployed, and living in overcrowded urban areas in which there are high rates of juvenile delinquency.

Ninety per cent of cases involve deliberate self-poisoning with drugs. Forty per cent use minor tranquilizers and a further 30% use salicylates and paracetamol.

27.7.2.2 Aetiology of Parasuicide

Compared with the general population, life events are more common in the 6 months before an act of parasuicide. These include the breakup of a relationship, trouble with the law, physical illness, and the illness of a loved one.

Predisposing factors include

- Marital difficulties
- Unemployment
- Physical illness, particularly epilepsy
- Mental retardation
- Parental neglect or abuse

Motives include interruption, attention, communication, or a true wish to die.

27.7.2.3 Assessment of the Individual for Suicide

A high degree of suicidal intent is indicated by the following:

- The act was planned and prepared.
- Precautions were taken to avoid discovery.
- The person did not seek help after the act.
- The act involved a dangerous method.
- There were final acts such as making a will or leaving a suicide note.

In interviewing the parasuicidal

- Establish rapport.
- Try to understand the attempt.
- Inquire about current problems.

TABLE 27.5

Prevention of Depressive Disorders and Suicide

Prevention	Depressive Disorders	Suicide
Primary prevention: aim to reduce incidence of the disorder	Family planning: Advise people with strong family history of depression to space out pregnancies to avoid poor parenting of child	Close monitoring during the post-discharge period: young men with schizophrenia and high education background who have regained insight, depressed elderly with somatic complaints
	Interventions in parent–child relationships with special focus on depressed mothers to improve parenting	Limiting supply of medication to prevent toxic overdose
	Events centred interventions: targeting at life events	Control methods of suicide: install suicide barriers to prevent people jumping from high places and restricting gun ownership
		Reduce unemployment and poverty
		Enhance social support and preventing marital breakdown
		Media report: straightforward and undramatic factual reporting of suicide cases
Secondary prevention: early detection and treatment of hidden morbidity and prevent progress of the disease	Early detection of depressive disorder by GPs or through public education and use of screening instruments such as general health questionnaires (GHQ), psychiatric outreach service	Early detection and treatment of psychiatric disorders
	Early intervention through CCBT in mild stage	
Tertiary prevention: aim to reduce disabilities arising as a consequence of the disorder	Community-based support project: help vulnerable families	Better community support and psychiatric outreach team to identify individuals with strong suicidal ideation and patients who are discharged from the hospital after suicide attempts
	Prevention of relapse and recurrence: continue pharmacotherapy (avoid premature termination), psychotherapy such as CBT and IPT	
	Rehabilitation: restore confidence, self-esteem, and impairment	
	Providing employment to depressed people who face social adversity	

Source: Paykel, E.S. and Jenkins, R., *Prevention in Psychiatry*, Gaskell, London, U.K., 1994.

- Elicit background information.
- Implement a mental state examination.

The presence of psychiatric disorders should be looked for, and any previous history of suicide attempts should be asked about. Social and financial support should also be detailed. Do not avoid asking about suicidal intent.

27.7.2.4 Assessment of Risk Factors for Subsequent Completion of Suicide

Tuckman and Youngman (1968) devised the following checklist. One point is awarded for each of the following:

Age > 45 years	Recent Medical Treatment
Male	Psychiatric disorder
Unemployed	Violent attempt
Not married	Suicide note
Living alone	Previous attempt
Poor physical health	

Score—2–5: subsequent suicide rate 7 per 1000 >10: subsequent suicide rate 60 per 1000

27.7.2.5 Management of Parasuicide

The individual should be treated medically as appropriate. Assess fully. Identify the risk factors. Reduce the immediate risk and treat the causes. If the patient suffers from a psychiatric disorder, this should be treated appropriately.

Management of suicidal feelings involves the following:

- Allow ventilation. Talking out avoids acting out.
- Strike a bargain on medication. Ask whether the person can cope with the responsibility of a bottle of tablets. If 'no', then admit to hospital.
- Agree a list of problem areas.
- Establish possible practical help.
- Allow for an underestimate of the true risk.

Prevention involves

- Recognizing high-risk cases and taking them seriously
- Asking patients about their suicidal ideas
- Not removing hope
- Prescribing the safest drugs
- Treating underlying illness adequately (Table 27.5)

REFERENCES

Ahrens B, Måller-Oerlinghausen B, and Grof P. 1993: Length of lithium treatment needed to eliminate the high mortality of affective disorders. *British Journal of Psychiatry* 163(Suppl 21):27–29.

Altshuler L, Bookheimer S, Proenza MA, Townsend J, Sabb F, Firestine A, Bartzokis G et al. 2005: Increased amygdala activation during mania: A functional magnetic resonance imaging study. *American Journal of Psychiatry.* 162(6):1211–1213.

Ambelas A. 1987: Life events and mania: A special relationship? *British Journal of Psychiatry* 150:235–240.

American Psychiatric Association. 2013: *Desk Reference to the Diagnostic Criteria from DSM-5.* Washington, DC: American Psychiatric Association Press.

Angst J and Sellaro R. 2000: Historical perspectives and natural history of bipolar disorder. *Biological Psychiatry* 48(6):445–457.

Beyer JL and Krishnan KR. 2002: Volumetric brain imaging findings in mood disorders. *Bipolar Disorder* 4:89–104.

Bebbington PE. 2003: The origins of sex differences in depressive disorder: Bridging the gap. *International Review of Psychiatry* 8:295–332.

Beck AT, Rush AJ, Shaw BF, and Emery G. 1979: *Cognitive Therapy of Depression.* New York: Guilford Press.

Benedetti F, Colombo C, Serretti A et al. 2003: Antidepressant effects of light therapy combined with sleep deprivation are influenced by a functional polymorphism within the promoter of the serotonin transporter gene. *Biological Psychiatry* 54:687–692.

Berrettini W. 2004: Linkage and association studies of bipolar disorder. In Charney DS and Nestler EJ (eds.): *Neurobiology of Mental Illness.*, 2nd edn. New York: Oxford University Press.

Bertelson A, Harvald B, and Hauge M. 1977: A Danish twin study of manic–depressive disorders. *British Journal of Psychiatry* 130:330.

Brown GW and Harris T. 1978: *Social Origins of Depression.* London, U.K.: Tavistock.

Cassano GB, Tundo A, and Micheli C. 1994: Bipolar and psychotic depressions. *Current Opinion in Psychiatry* 7:5–8.

Clark A. 2004: Working with grieving adults. *Advances in Psychiatric Treatment* 10:164–170.

Charney DS and Nestler EJ. 2004: *Neurobiology of Mental Illness,* 2nd edn. New York: Oxford University Press.

Castrén E, Võikar V, and Rantamäki T. 2007: Role of neurotrophic factors in depression. *Curr Opin Pharmacol* 7(1):18–21.

Drevets WC. 2003: Neuro imaging abnormalities in the amygdala in mood disorders. *Annals of the New York Academy of Sciences* 985:420–444. Review.

Duman RS and Monteggia LM. 2006: A neurotrophic model for stress-related mood disorders. *Biological Psychiatry* 59(12):1116–1127.

Duman RS, Heninger GR, and Nestler EJ. 1997: A molecular and cellular theory of depression. *Archives of General Psychiatry* 54(7):597–606.

Egeland JA, Gerhard DS, Paus DL et al. 1987: Bipolar affective disorders linked to markers on chromosome 11. *Nature* 325:783–787.

Frank E, Prien RF, Jarrett DB et al. 1991: Conceptualization and rationale for consensus definitions of terms in major depressive disorder: Response, remission, recovery, relapse, and recurrence. *Archives of General Psychiatry* 48:851–855.

Gallerani M, Manfredini R, Caracciolo S et al. 1995: Serum cholesterol concentrations in parasuicide. *British Medical Journal* 310:1632–1636.

Heikkinen M, Aro H, and Lînnqvist J. 1994: Recent life events, social support and suicide. *Acta Psychiatrica Scandinavica* 89(Suppl. 377):65–72.

Hirschfield RMA. 1994: Major depression, dysthymia and depressive personality disorder. *British Journal of Psychiatry* 165(Suppl. 26):23–30.

Johnstone EC, Freeman CPL, and Zealley AK (eds.) 1998: *Companion to Psychiatric Studies*, 6th edn. London, U.K.: Churchill Livingstone.

Keller MB. 1994: Depression: A long-term illness. *British Journal of Psychiatry* 165(Suppl. 26):9–15.

Kendler KS, Kessler R, Walters EE et al. 1995: Stressful life events, genetic liability and onset of an episode of major depression in women. *American Journal of Psychiatry* 152:833–842.

Kessler RC, Rubinow DR, Holmes C, Abelson JM, and Zhao S. 1997: The epidemiology of DSM-III-R bipolar I disorder in a general population survey. *Psychological Medicine* 27(5):1079–1089.

Ketter TA, Kimbrell TA, George MS, Dunn RT, Speer AM, Benson BE, Willis MW et al. 2001: Effects of mood and subtype on cerebral glucose metabolism in treatment-resistant bipolar disorder. *Biological Psychiatry* 49(2):97–109.

Kimbrell TA, Ketter TA, George MS et al. 2002: Regional cerebral glucose utilization in patients with a range of severities of unipolar depression. *Biological Psychiatry* 51:237–252.

King E. 1994: Suicide in the mentally ill: An epidemiological sample and implications for clinicians. *British Journal of Psychiatry* 165:658–663.

Kraepelin E. 1921: In Robertson GM (ed.) *Manic Depressive Insanity and Paranoia* (trans. Barclay RM), pp. 255–265. Edinburgh, Scotland: Churchill Livingstone.

Lange K and Farmer A. 2007: The causes of depression. In Stein G and Wilkinson G (eds.) *Seminars in General Adult Psychiatry*, pp. 48–70. London, U.K.: Gaskell.

Lee A. 2007: Clinical features of depressive disorder. In Stein G and Wilkinson G (eds.) *Seminars in General Adult Psychiatry*, pp. 1–21. London: Gaskell.

Lemonde S, Turecki G, Bakish D. et al. 2003: Impaired repression at a 5-hydroxytryptamine 1A receptor gene polymorphism associated with major depression and suicide. *Journal of Neuroscience* 23:8788–8799.

Medical Research Council. 1965: Clinical trial of the treatment of depressive illness. *British Medical Journal* i:881.

Lyoo IK, Kim MJ, Stoll AL, Demopulos CM, Parow AM, Dager SR, Friedman SD, Dunner DL, and Renshaw PF. 2004: Front all obey gray matter density decreases in bipolar I disorder. *Biological Psychiatry* 55(6):648–651.

McGuffin P and Katz R. 1989: The genetics of depression and manic-depressive disorder. *British Journal of Psychiatry*, 155, 294–304.

Nemeroff CB, Knight DL, Franks J et al. 1994: Further studies on platelet binding in depression. *American Journal of Psychiatry* 151:1623–1625.

NICE. *NICE Guidelines on Depression in Adults*. http://guidance.nice.org.uk/CG90 (accessed on 9 August 2012.)

Oakley-Browne, M. A., Joyce, P. R., Wells, J. E., et al (1995) Adverse parenting and other childhood experience as risk factors for depression in women aged 18–44 years. *Journal of Affective Disorders*, 34, 13–23.

Paykel ES, Jenkins R (1994) *Prevention in Psychiatry*. London, U.K.: Gaskell.

Parkes C.M. 1985: Bereavement. *British Journal of Psychiatry* 146:11–17.

Richmond C. 2006: Sir Martin Roth. *British Medical Journal* 333(7579):1175.

Roy, A. 1982: Suicide in chronic schizophrenia. *British Journal of Psychiatry* 141:171–177.

Sheline YI, Barch DM, Donnelly JM, Ollinger JM, Snyder AZ, and Mintun MA. 2001: Increased amygdala response to masked emotional faces in depressed subjects resolves with antidepressant treatment: An fMRI study. *Biological Psychiatry* 50(9):651–658.

Sheline YI, Gado MH, and Kraemer HC. 2003: Untreated depression and hippocampal volume loss. *American Journal of Psychiatry* 160(8):1516–1518.

Sheline YI, Wang PW, Gado MH, Csernansky JG, and Vannier MW. 1996: Hippocampal atrophy in recurrent major depression. *Proceedings of the National Academy of Sciences* 93(9):3908–3913.

Spiker, DG, Cofskyweiss J, Dealy RS et al. 1985: The pharmacological treatment of delusional depression. *American Journal of Psychiatry* 142:430–436.

Swayze VW 2nd, Andreasen NC, Alliger RJ, Yuh WT, and Ehrhardt JC. 1992: Subcortical and temporal structures in affective disorder and schizophrenia: A magnetic resonance imaging study. *Biological Psychiatry* 31(3):221–240.

Symonds RL. 1991: Books reconsidered. *Suicide: A study in sociology* by Emile Durkheim. *British Journal of Psychiatry* 159:739–741.

Syvälahti, EKG. 1994: Biological aspects of depression. *Acta Psychiatrica Scandinavica* (Suppl 377):11–15.

Taylor D, Paton C, and Kapur S. 2009: *The Maudsley Prescribing Guideline*. London, U.K.: Informa Healthcare.

Terayama, H., Nishino, Y., Kishi, M. et al. 2003: Detection of anti-Borna Disease Virus (BDV) antibodies from patients with schizophrenia and mood disorders in Japan. *Psychiatry Research* 120:201–206.

Thase, M.E. 1993: Maintenance treatments of recurrent affective disorder. *Current Opinion in Psychiatry* 6:16–21.

Trivedi MH, Rush AJ, Wisniewski SR et al. 2006: Evaluation of outcomes with citalopram for depression using measurement-based care in STAR*D: Implications for clinical practice. *American Journal of Psychiatry.* 163(1):28–40.

Tuckman J and Youngman WF. 1968: A scale for assessing risk of attempted suicides. *Journal of Clinical Psychology* 24:17–19.

Vaughn CE and Leff JP. 1976: The influence of family and social factors on the course of psychiatric illness: A comparison of schizophrenic and depressed neurotic patients. *British Journal of Psychiatry* 129:125–137.

Wender P, Kety SS, Rosenthal D et al. 1986: Psychiatric disorders in the biological and adoptive families of adopted individuals with affective disorders. *Archives of General Psychiatry* 43:923–929.

Woods BT, Yurgelun-Todd D, Mikulis D, and Pillay SS. 1995: Age-related MRI abnormalities in bipolar illness: A clinical study. *Biological Psychiatry* 38(12):846–847.

World Health Organisation. 1992: *ICD-10: The ICD-10 Classification of Mental and Behavioural Disorders: Clinical Descriptions and Diagnostic Guidelines.* Geneva, Switzerland: World Health Organisation.

28 Neurotic and Stress-Related Disorders

28.1 HISTORY

- In 1869, Beard introduced neurasthenia, comprising almost all current anxiety disorders.
- In 1893, Hecker subdivided neurasthenia into different syndromes.
- In 1900, Sigmund Freud (see Ref. Freud, 1953) distinguished between
  - Actual neuroses: somatic causation, comprising neurasthenia, anxiety neurosis (generalized anxiety, panic disorder, and agoraphobia), and hypochondriasis
  - Psychoneuroses: psychological causation, comprising hysteria and obsessions (simple phobia, social phobia, and obsessive–compulsive disorder [OCD])
- Libidinous impulses reaching the ego generate anxiety; repression and symptom formation follow.
- Fright neurosis, not related to repressed libido, was also described, similar to current post-traumatic stress disorder (PTSD).

28.2 CLASSIFICATIONS OF NEUROSIS (TABLE 28.1)

28.3 GENERAL ISSUES

28.3.1 EFFECT OF CHILDHOOD NEUROSIS

Robins (1966) found that most children with neurotic disorders do not suffer neurosis in adulthood. Adult neurotics develop neurosis in adult life.

In childhood, there is excess neurosis in males. After puberty, there is excess in females.

28.3.2 EFFECT OF PERSONALITY DISORDER

The prevalence of personality disorder in neurosis is 12% in primary care and 40% in psychiatric outpatients. Psychological treatment, particularly self-help, is more effective in neurotic patients without personality disorder. Neurotic patients with personality disorder respond better to antidepressant drug treatment.

28.3.3 MORTALITY

There is increased mortality in severe neurotic disorder. The relative risk of death in the decade following treatment for neurosis is 1.7. The biggest cause of increased risk is accidental death, particularly suicide (relative risk = 6.1). There is also a major excess of deaths from nervous, circulatory, and respiratory disease. Suicide is most likely in the first year after discharge.

28.4 PHOBIC ANXIETY DISORDERS

The Greek word *phobos* means panic or terror. In phobic anxiety disorders, anxiety is evoked predominantly by certain well-defined situations, characteristically avoided. Contemplation of a feared situation generates anticipatory anxiety.

In defining fear as phobic, the following are considered:

- It is out of proportion to objective risks.
- It cannot be reasoned or explained away.
- It is beyond voluntary control.
- It leads to avoidance.

Marks et al. (1993) classify adult fears as normal or abnormal fears. The latter are grouped as follows:

- Phobias of *external stimuli*
  - Agoraphobia
  - Social phobia
  - Animal phobia
  - Miscellaneous specific phobias
- Phobias of *internal stimuli*
  - Illness phobia
  - Obsessive phobias

28.4.1 EPIDEMIOLOGY OF PHOBIC ANXIETY DISORDER

The Epidemiologic Catchment Areas (ECA) study found

- A lifetime prevalence for all phobias from 7.8% to 23.3% between sites
- A 6 month prevalence for agoraphobia of 2.8%–5.8%

TABLE 28.1

Comparison between ICD-10 and Proposed DSM-5 Criteria

ICD-10 (WHO, 1992)

DSM-5 (APA, 2013)

Phobic anxiety disorders

F40.0 Agoraphobia

F40.1 Social phobia

F40.2 Specific phobia

- Acrophobia
- Animal phobia
- Claustrophobia
- Simple phobia

300.22 Agoraphobia

300.23 Social anxiety disorder

300.29 Specific phobia

- Animal (e.g. spiders, insects, dogs)
- Blood–injection–injury (e.g. needles, invasive medical procedures)
- Natural environment (e.g. heights, storms, water)
- Situational (e.g. airplanes, elevators, enclosed places)
- Other (e.g. situations that may lead to choking or vomiting; in children, loud sounds or costumed characters)

Other anxiety disorders

F41.0 Panic disorder

F41.1 GAD

F41.2 Mixed anxiety and depressive disorder

300.01 Panic disorder

300.02 GAD

There is no mention of mixed anxiety and depressive disorder

Other anxiety disorders

Substance-induced anxiety disorder

293.84 Anxiety disorder attributable to another medical condition

300.00 Anxiety disorder not elsewhere classified

F42 OCD

There is no mention of OCD-spectrum disorders

300.3 OCD

OCD-spectrum disorders:

300.7 BDD

300.3 Hoarding disorder

312.29 Hair-pulling disorder (trichotillomania)

698.4 Skin picking disorder

Substance-induced OCD or related disorders

294.8 OCD or related disorder attributable to another medical condition

300.3 OCD or related disorder not elsewhere classified

F43.0 Acute stress reaction

308.3 Acute stress disorder

The DSM-5 proposed 313.89 reactive attachment disorder and 313.89 disinhibited social engagement disorder

F43.1 PTSD

F43.2 Adjustment disorder

F44.0 Dissociative (conversion) disorders

- F44.0 Dissociative amnesia
- F44.1 Dissociative fugue
- F44.2 Dissociative stupor
- F44.3 Trance and possession disorder
- F44.4–7 Dissociative disorders of movement and sensation
- F44.4 Dissociative motor disorders
- F44.5 Dissociative convulsion
- F44.6 Dissociative anaesthesia and sensory loss
- F44.7 Mixed dissociative (conversion) disorders
- F44.81 MPD

309.81 PTSD

Adjustment disorder

Dissociative disorders

300.6 Depersonalization–derealization disorder

300.12 Dissociative amnesia (localized or generalized)

300.14 Dissociative identity disorder

- A 6 month prevalence for simple phobia of 4.5%–11.8%
- A 6 month prevalence for social phobia of 1.2%–2.2%

The Edmonton Study (Dick et al., 1994b) found

- A lifetime prevalence for all phobias of 8.9% (females 11.7%, males 6.1%)
- Age of first symptoms—6 years in females, 12 years in males
- High rates of comorbidity with depression, alcohol abuse, drug abuse, and OCD in all types of phobia

Phobic anxiety disorders affect females more than males (agoraphobia 75%, simple phobia 95%), except social phobia where the sex ratio is equal.

28.4.2 Aetiology of Phobic Anxiety Disorder

28.4.2.1 Genetic Factors

Phobic disorders or other psychiatric illnesses (neurosis, alcoholism, depressive illness) are more prevalent in families of phobic probands.

Kendler et al. (1993a), using the twin registry, demonstrated that familial aggregation of phobia resulted from genetic liability, not from shared environmental factors.

28.4.2.2 Psychological Factors

- *Pavlovian classical conditioning.* Watson, in the 'Little Albert' experiment on an 18-month-old child, produced fear of a toy white rat by presenting it repeatedly with a loud noise. Fear is later generalized to all furry objects (see Chapter 3).
- *Operant conditioning.* Avoidance of a phobic situation is rewarded by a reduction in anxiety that reinforces avoidance.
- *Seligman's preparedness theory.* Anxiety is easily conditioned to certain stimuli (e.g. heights, snakes, spiders) and is resistant to extinction. Prepared stimuli were dangerous to primitive man and may have been acquired by natural selection.

Phobias represent a conflict leading to avoidance of situations symbolic of that conflict. 'Little Hans' developed a phobia of horses after seeing a male horse urinate. Freud believed that fear of castration by his father was displaced on to horses after this viewing.

28.4.2.3 Comorbidity

There is overlap between anxiety disorders. For example, 55% of agoraphobics have social phobia and 30% of social phobics also have agoraphobia.

Persons with major depression have 15 times the risk of having agoraphobia and 9 times the risk of simple phobia as controls.

Twenty-five per cent of phobics report alcohol abuse/dependence; there are higher rates in agoraphobics and social phobics than in simple phobias.

28.4.3 Management of Phobic Anxiety Disorder

28.4.3.1 Psychological Approaches

Behaviour therapy is the treatment of choice. *Exposure techniques* are most widely used. Wolpe's systematic desensitization combines relaxation with graded exposure. *Reciprocal inhibition* prevents anxiety from being maintained when exposed to the phobic stimulus while relaxed.

Flooding entails maximal exposure to the feared stimulus until anxiety reduction occurs. This is not more effective than other exposure techniques.

Modelling requires the patient to observe the therapist engaging in non-avoidant behaviour when exposed to a feared stimulus.

Psychoanalytic psychotherapy has proved to be ineffective.

28.4.3.2 Pharmacological Approaches

Selective serotonin reuptake inhibitors (SSRIs) such as escitalopram, fluvoxamine, paroxetine, and sertraline are first-line treatments of phobic anxiety disorder.

Monoamine oxidase inhibitors (MAOIs) are effective in agoraphobics and social phobics: 80%–90% of pure social phobics are almost asymptomatic at week 16, but patients withdrawn from the active drug relapse (Versiani et al., 1992).

Benzodiazepines may help prevent the reinforcement of fear through avoidance.

28.4.4 Specific Phobic Disorders

28.4.4.1 Agoraphobia

In 1871, Westphal first used the term to describe patients who experienced intense anxiety when walking across open spaces.

28.4.4.1.1 *ICD-10 (WHO, 1992)*

- Symptoms are manifestations of anxiety and are not secondary to other symptoms such as delusions or obsessional thoughts.

408   Revision Notes in Psychiatry

- Anxiety is restricted to at least two of the following: crowds, public places, travelling away from home, and travelling alone.
- At least two symptoms from automatic arousal symptoms, symptoms involving the chest and abdomen, and symptoms involving mental state.
- Avoidance of the phobic situation is prominent.
- Two subtypes: agoraphobia without panic disorder or agoraphobia with panic disorder.

28.4.4.1.2   DSM-5 (APA, 2013)

- The agoraphobic situations are similar to ICD-10.
- The fear, anxiety, or avoidance lasts for at least 6 months.
- The fear is associated with difficulty to escape and help being unavailable.
- Avoidance of agoraphobic situations.
- The fear is out of proportion to the danger.

28.4.4.1.3   Course

Symptoms fluctuate, but the course is prolonged. Eighty per cent of agoraphobics are not free of symptoms after 5 years.

28.4.4.2   Social Phobias
Genetics:

1. MZ/DZ = 24%:15% (Kendler et al., 1992).
2. The relatives of socially phobic probands have a threefold elevated risk of social phobia.

Imaging: Positron emission tomography (PET) scan shows an increased blood flow in the right dorsolateral prefrontal cortex (Gelder et al., 2006).

Social phobias are characterized by a fear of scrutiny by others in small groups. This may progress to panic attacks. Avoidance is often marked (Figure 28.1).

28.4.4.2.1   ICD-10 (WHO 1992)

- Symptoms are manifestations of anxiety and not secondary to other symptoms.
- Anxiety is restricted to or predominates in particular social situations.
- The phobic situation is avoided whenever possible.
- Marked fear of being the focus of attention and marked avoidance of being the focus of attention.
- At least two symptoms: blushing or shaking, fear of vomiting, and urgency or fear of micturition or defecation.

28.4.4.2.2   DSM-5 (APA 2013)

It is characterized by marked fear or anxiety about one or more social situations in which the individual is exposed to possible scrutiny or be negatively evaluated by others. The fear is out of proportion and lasts for 6 months or longer.

28.4.4.2.3   Treatment

The treatment for social phobia is similar to panic disorder (see succeeding text). In addition, β-blockers can be used to reduce autonomic arousal, which can be particularly helpful for performance anxiety.

28.4.4.2.4   Course

The course is continuous but it may improve gradually. Alcohol and drug abuse are common.

28.4.4.3   Isolated Phobias

Isolated phobias are restricted to highly specific situations. The seriousness of the handicap depends on how easily a feared situation can be avoided.

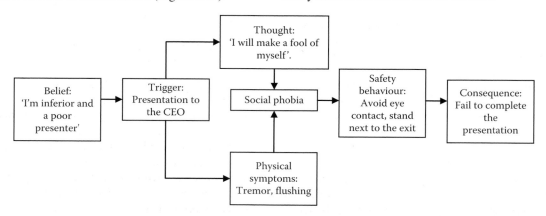

FIGURE 28.1   Cognitive model of a 35-year-old marketing manager suffering from social phobia.

- Symptoms are manifestations of anxiety and not secondary to other symptoms.
- Anxiety is restricted to the particular phobic situation.
- The phobic situation is avoided whenever possible.

Childhood phobias are always improved after 5 years. In adult phobias, 20% are unchanged, 40% are better, and 40% are worse after 5 years.

28.5 GENERALIZED ANXIETY DISORDER

The diagnostic reliability of generalized anxiety disorder (GAD) is lower than that of other anxiety disorders. Patients report uncontrollable worry. A negative response to the question 'Do you worry excessively over minor matters?' virtually rules out GAD as a diagnosis (negative predictive power 0.94). Symptoms of muscle and psychic tension are the most frequently reported by people with GAD.

GAD is associated with the highest rates of comorbidity of all anxiety disorders.

28.5.1 EPIDEMIOLOGY OF GENERALIZED ANXIETY DISORDER

The ECA study found

- A 6 month prevalence of GAD of 2.5%–6.4%
- An earlier age of onset (majority before age 20) and more gradual than other anxiety disorders

Early-onset GAD is more likely to be in a female and in a person having a history of childhood fears and/or having marital or sexual disturbance. Later onset is more likely to develop after a stressful life event.

28.5.2 AETIOLOGY OF GENERALIZED ANXIETY DISORDER

28.5.2.1 Genetic Factors

Some studies show familial aggregation of GAD, while others do not. Kendler et al. (1993a) concluded that GAD is a moderately familial disorder with a heritability of 30%.

28.5.2.2 Neurochemistry

- Noradrenaline (NA)
  - Downregulation of α_2-receptors and increase in autonomic arousal.
  - Electrical stimulation of the locus coeruleus releases NA and generates anxiety.
- Serotonin: dysregulation of the 5-HT system
- GABA: reduced GABA activity

28.5.2.3 Endocrinology

Thirty per cent of patients with GAD show reduced suppression of dexamethasone suppression test (DST).

28.5.2.4 Imaging

Structural magnetic resonance imaging (MRI) shows decreased hippocampal and medical prefrontal cortex volumes.

Proton MR spectroscopy shows decreased GABA in anterior cingulate cortex and posterior occipital cortex.

28.5.2.5 Cognitive Theories

Patients with GAD often have selective attention to negative details, distortions in information processing, and negative views on coping.

28.5.2.6 Psychoanalytic Theories

GAD represents symptoms of unresolved unconscious conflicts, early loss of parents, overprotective parenting, or parenting lacking warmth and responsiveness.

28.5.2.7 Environmental Factors

Torgersen (1983) reported that probands with GAD had lost their parents by death far more often than probands with panic disorder, suggesting that environmental factors contribute to a higher vulnerability for the development of GAD.

28.5.3 DIAGNOSTIC CRITERIA

ICD-10 criteria (F41.1): 6 month durations; at least four symptoms from the following category must be present:

- Core symptoms: persistent tension, worry, and feelings of apprehension
- Autonomic arousal symptoms: palpitation, sweating, trembling, dry mouth
- Symptoms involving the chest and abdomen: choking sensation, nausea, difficulty in breathing
- Symptoms involving mental state: giddiness, fear of losing control, derealization
- Hot flushes or cold chills
- Poor concentration, startled responses

DSM-5 (300.02) (APA, 2013)—minimum duration: 6 months

- Excessive anxiety and worry (apprehensive expectation) about two (or more) domains of activities or events (e.g. family, health, finances, and school/work difficulties)
- Core symptoms
  - Muscle tension
  - Fatigue
  - Irritability
  - Poor concentration
  - Poor sleep
  - Restlessness
- Four associated behaviours
  - Marked avoidance of activities or events with possible negative outcomes
  - Marked time and effort preparing for activities
  - Events with possible negative outcomes
  - Marked procrastination in behaviour or decision making as a result of worries
  - Repeatedly seeking reassurance

28.5.4 MEDICAL DIFFERENTIAL DIAGNOSIS

1. Cardiovascular disorders: arrhythmia, ischaemic heart disease, mitral valve prolapse, congestive heart failure
2. Thyroid disorder
3. Medication such as thyroxine, antihypertensives, antiarrhythmics, bronchodilators, anticholinergics, anticonvulsants, and NSAIDS

28.5.5 MANAGEMENT OF GENERALIZED ANXIETY DISORDER

Investigations: Full blood count, renal function tests, liver function tests, thyroid function tests, fasting glucose and lipids, urinalysis, urine toxicology, and electrocardiography (ECG)

Recommendations from the NICE guidelines:

1. Benzodiazepines should not be used beyond 2–4 weeks.
2. For longer-term treatment, the following treatment should be considered:
   a. Option A: psychological therapy (e.g. cognitive–behavioural therapy [CBT]).
   b. Option B: pharmacological therapy (e.g. an SSRI licensed for GAD).
   c. Option C: self-help (bibliotherapy based on the CBT principles).
   d. For the duration of effect, option A is longer than option B; option B is longer than option C.

3. For CBT, it should be offered in weekly sessions of 1–2 h and be completed within 4 months. The optimal range is 16–21 h in total. If the psychologist decides to offer briefer CBT, it should be about 8–10 h with integration of structured self-help material. Components of CBT include education, problem-solving, exposure-based approaches, cognitive approaches, emotion-regulation approaches, and relapse prevention. CBT is more effective than relaxation training.
4. For pharmacological therapy, the psychiatrist should consider the patient's age, previous treatment response, risk of DSH, cost, and patient's preference. Inform the patient on the potential side effects, possible discontinuation withdrawal, and the time course of treatment. An SSRI should be offered. Examples include paroxetine, escitalopram, and sertraline. If one SSRI is not suitable, consider another SSRI. The psychiatrist should review the patient within 2 weeks of starting treatment and again at 4, 6, and 12 weeks. Then the psychiatrist can review the patient at 8–12-week intervals.
5. For GAD not responding to at least two types of intervention, consider venlafaxine. Before prescribing, the psychiatrist should consider the presence of preexisting hypertension and the possibility of overdose because venlafaxine is more dangerous than other SSRIs. The psychiatrist should order an ECG to rule out cardiac arrhythmias and recent myocardial infarction. The dose should not be higher than 75 mg per day and the psychiatrist should monitor the blood pressure regularly during follow-up.
6. During reassessment, the psychiatrist should evaluate treatment response, potential substance abuse, emergence of comorbidities, day-to-day functioning, social networks, chronic stressors, and the role of agoraphobia and other avoidant symptoms.

28.5.5.1 Psychological Therapies (Figure 28.2)

Recommendations from the NICE Guidelines: For GAD, the recommendation is similar for panic disorder except the optimal range is 16–20 h in total. Briefer CBT is 8–10 h with integration of appropriate focused information and self-help materials.

28.5.5.1.1 Comorbidity and Prognosis

Comorbidity: Concurrent panic disorder (25%) and depression (80%)

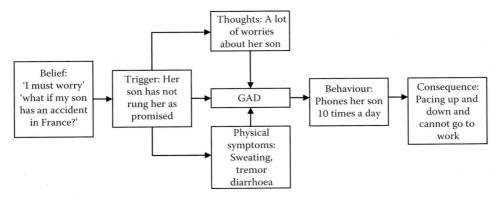

FIGURE 28.2   Example of a cognitive model of a 40-year-old mother with GAD.

28.5.5.1.2   Course

Follow-up after 6 years reveals stability of diagnosis; the most common change of diagnosis is to alcoholism. Sixty-eight per cent have mild or no residual impairment; 9% have severe impairment.

28.5.5.1.3   Prognosis (Argyropoulos et al., 2007)

Seventy per cent of patients have mild or no impairment and 9% have severe impairment. Poor prognostic factors include severe anxiety symptoms, syncope, agitation, derealization, and suicide.

CASC STATION

Dr. Sobieski, a 50-year-old female medical doctor from your hospital, has self-referred to you. She complains of being on the edge most of the time with palpitations and dizziness in the past 1 year. She migrated from Poland 15 years ago and describes herself as a lifelong worrier.

Task:

1. Take a history of her anxiety symptoms and explore the causes of her anxiety.
2. Inform Dr. Sobieski on your treatment plan.

CASC Grid

Approach to this station: Candidates have to differentiate the main causes of anxiety with her occupational background.

(A) Anxiety Symptoms Based on the ICD-10 Criteria (WHO, 1992)	(A1) Assess Autonomic Arousal Symptoms	(A2) Assess Symptoms Involving the Chest/Abdomen	(A3) Assess Mental State Symptoms	(A4) General Symptoms	(A5) Other Nonspecific Symptoms
	Palpitation	Difficulty breathing	Giddiness	Hot flushes	Exaggerated responses to minor surprises/ being startled
	Sweating	Choking sensation	Fainting	Cold chills	
	Trembling/ shaking	Chest pain	Derealization or depersonalization	Numbness	
	Dry mouth	Nausea or stomach churning	Not being able to stop worrying	Tingling/ aches—muscle tension	Persistent irritability
			Being annoyed or irritable	Restlessness	Poor sleep
			Fear of losing control	Keyed up, on the edge	Poor concentration
			Fear of dying or 'going crazy'	Trouble relaxing	Mind goes blank
			Feeling afraid as if something awful may happen	Lump in the throat	

(continued)

(B) Comorbidity and Risk Assessment	(B1) Brief Screening for Other Neurotic Disorders	(B2) Assess Possible PTSD and OCD Symptoms	(B3) Assess Depression	(B4) Assess Substance/Alcohol Abuse	(B5) Assess Fitness to Practice
	'Do you have any panic attack or difficulty in breathing?' 'Do you have any fear? (e.g. fear of going to crowded areas or presenting a case during the ward round?'	'Do you have nightmare, flashbacks related to previous trauma?' 'Do you have any excessive checking or washing behaviour?'	Assess mood and cognitive symptoms. If symptoms of GAD and depression are present, a diagnosis of mixed anxiety and depressive disorder is justified	Usage of alcohol and benzodiazepine to overcome insomnia or other recreational drugs for self-medication 'Is your anxiety worsening after stop drinking or taking tranquillizer?'	Explore cognitive symptoms that may affect her work (e.g. poor concentration, anxiety during medical procedures)

(C) Issues Related to the Patient as a Migrant Doctor from Eastern Europe	(C1) Explore the Issue of Self-Referral	(C2) The Issue of Self-Diagnosis and Self-Treatment	(C3) Factors that Delay Help-Seeking	(C4) Work-Related Problems	(C5) Culture Issues
	'I can imagine that it is hard for you as a doctor to disclose your own illness. Do you have a GP? Did you consult him for your anxiety problems? If not, why?'	'Do you recognize that you suffer from anxiety disorder? If yes, when?' 'Have you started any treatment on your own?'	Explore the following factors: e.g. low motivation, fear of damage to her reputation, discrimination, and her cultural views of mental illness	Explore relationship with peers and supervisors, bullying, complaints from patients, medicolegal issues because of negligence, medical errors, and multiple failures in the MRCP exam	Explore language problems in clinical practice, adaptation to the U.K. culture, cultural clashes with patients or colleagues

(D) Other Background History	(D1) Explore Her Reasons for Migrating to the United Kingdom	(D2) Family	(D3) Personal History	(D4) Developmental Issues	(D5) Past Medical History
	'Were you a refugee doctor?' Explore other factors such as better salary, well-recognized training, and better job prospects	Explore her marital status, the effect of migration on her marriage, any children left behind in Poland, the financial status of her family, and past family history of anxiety disorders	Explore past experience of persecution under the previous communist regime. Explore history of personal trauma and subsequent re-traumatization	Explore middle-age crisis and stagnation in career development	'Do you have any chronic medical disease like heart or lung disease?' 'Do you take medication on a long term basis?'

(E) Management Plan	(E1) Set Boundaries for Treatment and Investigations	(E2) Ethical Issues, e.g. Confidentiality	(E3) Address Medical Practice Issues	(E4) Deliver Psychotherapy in a Culturally Aware Manner	(E5) Issue of Prescribing Medication
	'Would you prefer to see a psychiatrist in this hospital or elsewhere?' Address management of the future professional interactions Investigations include FBC, TFT, calcium, phosphate, glucose, and ECG	Reassure Dr. Sobieski that you are trying your very best to help her The candidate should only mention the issues of reporting to the GMC if there is evidence of impairment in her clinical practice	Suggest to take time off, offer CBT to address distorted negative thought processes, and reduce her anxiety symptoms by relaxation training	Explore her preferences based on the cultural background of psychotherapists, e.g. gender, cultural backgrounds	Explain the possibility of taking antidepressants and provide education on the proper usage of benzodiazepine because it can cause dependence. Discuss common side effects

28.6 PANIC DISORDER

This involves recurrent unpredictable attacks of severe anxiety lasting usually for a few minutes only. There can be a sudden onset of palpitations, chest pain, choking, dizziness, depersonalization, and derealization, together with a secondary fear of dying, losing control, or going mad. It often results in a hurried exit and a subsequent avoidance of similar situations; it may be followed by persistent fear of another attack.

28.6.1 EPIDEMIOLOGY OF PANIC DISORDER

The ECA study found that 3% of the population had experienced a panic attack in the previous 6 months. All socioeconomic groups were affected, and there was no relationship with race or education. Women aged 25–44 years, with a family history of panic disorder, divorced, or separated were at highest risk. Other findings were

- Maximum period of onset from mid-teens to mid-thirties, rarely after the age of 40
- More common in females than males (2:1)
- A prevalence of strictly defined panic disorder of 0.1%–0.4%
- A 1-year prevalence of 0.2%–1.2%
- A lifetime prevalence of 1.4%–1.5%

- Discrete episode of intense fear or discomfort, abrupt onset, reaches a maximum within a few minute autonomic arousal symptoms with freedom from anxiety symptoms between attacks.
- Symptoms involving the chest and abdomen.
- Symptoms involving mental state (see A1–A3 of CASC on page 407).
- Hot flushes and chills.

28.6.3.1.2 300.01 Panic Disorder (DSM-5, APA 2013)
- Recurrent unexpected panic attacks with symptoms similar to the ICD-10 criteria.
- At least one of the attacks has been followed by at least 1 month of persistent concern or worry about additional panic attack and maladaptive change in behaviour related to the attacks.

28.6.2 AETIOLOGY OF PANIC DISORDER

28.6.2.1 Genetic Factors

The morbid risk for panic disorder in relatives of probands is 15%–30%, much higher than in the general population (2%). Female relatives are at higher risk than male relatives. There is an increased risk of alcoholism in the relatives of probands.

Kendler et al. (1993b) estimated that the heritability for panic disorder with or without phobic avoidance is 35%–40%.

28.6.2.2 Cognitive Theories
- Classical conditioning
- Negative catastrophic thoughts during panic attacks

28.6.2.3 Psychoanalytic Theories
- Panic attacks arise from unsuccessful attempts to defend against anxiety provoking impulses.

28.6.2.4 Neurochemistry (Argyropoulos et al., 2007)

28.6.2.4.1 Noradrenaline
- Hypersensitivity of presynaptic α_2-receptor and increase in adrenergic activity.
- Panic disorder is induced by yohimbine.

thyrotoxicosis, hypoparathyroidism, phaeochromocytoma, and anaemia

28.6.5 MANAGEMENT OF PANIC DISORDER

Recommendations from the NICE Guidelines:
The recommendations are similar to management on GAD.

28.6.5.1 Pharmacotherapy

The NICE guidelines recommend SSRI as the first-line treatment of panic disorder. Examples include citalopram, escitalopram, fluoxetine, fluvoxamine, paroxetine, or sertraline. If an SSRI is unsuitable and there is no improvement, consider imipramine or clomipramine but not venlafaxine.

The tricyclic antidepressants (TCAs) imipramine and clomipramine, MAOIs, and SSRIs are efficacious

TABLE 28.2
Compare and Contrast Panic Disorder and Hyperventilation Syndrome

	Panic Disorder	HVS
ICD-10 and proposed DSM-5 criteria Overlap between the two disorders	A codable disorder. 50%–60% of patients with panic disorder or agoraphobia have HVS symptoms.	Not a codable disorder. 25% of HVS patients have symptoms of panic disorder.
Aetiology	Biological and psychological causes are well defined.	Less well defined. Lactate, CCK, caffeine, and psychological stressors also play a role.
Salient clinical features	Panic disorder has more mental symptoms.	High thoracic breathing or excessive use of accessory muscles to breathe result in hyperinflated lungs.
Metabolic disturbances	The role of metabolic disturbances is less well established.	• Acute hypocalcaemia: positive Chvostek and Trousseau signs and prolonged QTc interval • Hypokalaemia with generalized weakness • Respiratory alkalosis • Acute hypophosphataemia leading to paraesthesias and generalized weakness
Management	Acute management involves reassuring patients, establish normal breathing pattern, and reduce anxiety with anxiolytics. Long-term management includes relaxation exercise and CBT.	Investigation may include d-dimer and possible *V/Q* scan to rule out pulmonary embolism. Acute and long-term management are similar to panic disorder. De-arousal strategy is useful.

Sources: Johnstone, E.C. et al., *Companion to Psychiatric Studies*, 7th edn, London, U.K.: Churchill Livingstone, 2004; Semple, D. et al., *Oxford Handbook of Psychiatry*, Oxford, U.K.: Oxford University Press, 2005.

28.6.2.4.2 Serotonin
- Subsensitivity of 5-HT$_{1A}$ receptors and exaggerated postsynaptic receptor response.
- Panic disorder is induced by d-fenfluramine.

28.6.2.4.3 GABA
- Reduction in GABA receptor sensitivity; panic attack is induced by flumazenil.

28.6.2.4.4 Others
- Cholecystokinin (CCK) and sodium lactate induce panic attack.

28.6.2.5 Neuroimaging
Structural MRI shows decreased medial temporal lobe volume.

Functional MRI shows increased haemodynamic responses in the amygdala, hippocampus, and insula.

28.6.2.6 Comorbidity
One-third develop secondary depression following the onset of panic disorder. If depression does occur, the course is poorer. Agoraphobia usually occurs with panic disorder but can occur separately.

There is an increased lifetime prevalence of alcohol abuse/dependence (54%) and drug abuse/dependence (43%) in persons with panic disorder. Some use substances as a complication of panic disorder; others develop panic disorder as a result of withdrawal from substances.

Major controversy surrounds the relationship between anxiety disorders and depression. There is evidence supporting the unitary position that anxiety and depression lie along the same continuum:

- High overlap of symptoms (65% of anxious patients have depressive symptoms) (Roth et al., 1972)
- Difficulty separating primary disorder in patients experiencing both panic attacks and depression

- Children of probands with major depression and panic disorder have higher rates of major depression and anxiety disorders.
- There is an increased rate of panic disorder but not major depression or other anxiety disorders in the relatives of panic-disorder probands.

28.6.2.7 Life Events
There is an excess of stressful life events in the year prior to the onset of panic disorder, especially illness or death of a cohabitant or relative.

28.6.2.8 Physiological Factors
Pitts and McClure (1967) provoked panic attacks in patients with anxiety neurosis but not controls, by the intravenous infusion of sodium lactate. There were higher levels of autonomic arousal in preinfusion panickers compared to non-panickers.

No single biochemical or neuroendocrine finding explains lactate-induced panic. Yohimbine, a presynaptic a$_2$-adrenergic autoreceptor blocker, induced panic attacks in a subgroup of individuals. This group showed increased noradrenergic activity and blunted growth hormone response to clonidine, supporting the hypothesis of a dysregulation of the noradrenergic system and possibly the hypothalamus–pituitary–adrenal axis in a subgroup of panic-disorder patients. There were very low rates of non-suppression during a DST in panic disorder.

Panic attacks are associated with a reduced blood flow in the frontal lobes. Panic-disorder patients not having a panic attack have reduced perfusion of the hippocampus bilaterally and an increase in blood flow to the right inferior frontal cortex.

Mitral valve prolapse occurs in 40% of panic-disorder patients compared to 9% of controls. Patients suffering from mitral valve prolapse do not suffer more panic disorder than controls. An aetiological role for mitral valve prolapse in panic disorder is unlikely.

Panic-disorder patients have abnormal sleep breath-

in the treatment of panic disorder. The downregulation of 5-HT$_2$ receptors may be responsible for therapeutic effects, which take up to 4 weeks to appear. Increased anxiety or panic may occur in the first week of treatment.

Benzodiazepines (e.g. alprazolam in high dosage) reduce the frequency of panic attacks in the short term. There is the need to maintain treatment in the long term, with the risk of dependency.

28.6.5.2 Psychological Treatment (Figure 28.3)

28.6.5.2.1 NICE Guidelines: CBT and Anxiety Disorders

1. CBT should be offered to GAD and panic disorder in primary care.
2. For panic disorder, CBT should be delivered by trained and supervised therapists, closely adhering to the treatment protocols. CBT should be offered weekly with duration of 1–2 h and be completed within 4 months. The optimal range is 7 (brief CBT) to 14 h in total.

CBT involving the cognitive restructuring of catastrophic interpretations of bodily experience is efficacious in panic disorder, as are exposure techniques that generate bodily sensations of fear during therapy with the aim of habituating the subject to them. Agoraphobic avoidance is treated by situational exposure and relaxation techniques.

Marks et al. (1993), comparing alprazolam and exposure therapy in patients suffering from panic disorder and agoraphobia, found the effect size of exposure was twice that of alprazolam; during follow-up, gains from alprazolam disappeared, but exposure gains were maintained. Treatment with a combination of exposure and alprazolam impaired improvement seen in the exposure-alone group.

28.6.5.2.2 Course and Prognosis
The course is highly variable. Sixty per cent suffer mild impairment. Ten per cent suffer severe disability. Poor outcome is predicted by lower social class and long duration of illness.

Recurrence is common when new stressors emerge in panic disorder. If a patient with panic disorder stops the SSRI, there is more than 50% chance of recurrence (Taylor et al., 2009).

28.7 OCD

28.7.1 Epidemiology of OCD

The ECA study found that OCD is very rare in children. Rutter found no cases among 2000 10- and 11-year-olds on the Isle of Wight. Other findings were

- A 6-month prevalence of OCD of 1.3%–2.0%
- A lifetime prevalence of 1.9%–3.0%
- Sex ratio equal
- Bimodal age of onset with peaks occurring at 12–14 and 20–22 years of age (decline in onset after the age of 35)

The ECA study prevalence findings were consistently higher than earlier accepted estimates.

28.7.2 Aetiology of OCD

28.7.2.1 Genetic Factors
First-degree relatives of OCD patients have a higher than normal incidence of psychiatric disorders, most commonly anxiety, phobias, depression, and schizophrenia.

First-degree relatives of OCD patients have higher than normal obsessional traits; the risk of OCD among relatives is higher in early-onset OCD probands, suggesting aetiological heterogeneity.

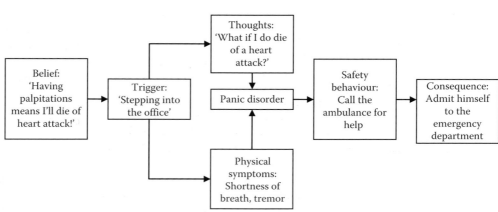

FIGURE 28.3 Cognitive model of a 45-year-old office worker suffering from panic disorder.

Twin studies suggest that monozygotic twins are more likely to be concordant than dizygotic twins for OCD (MZ/DZ = 50%–80%:25%).

Gilles de la Tourette's syndrome is a familial condition with a substantial genetic basis. Twin and family studies find high rates of OCD and obsessive–compulsive symptoms among families of patients with Tourette. This suggests that some forms of OCD may be related to Tourette's syndrome.

OCD is equally frequent in families of Tourette's probands regardless of whether the proband has OCD. The rate of OCD alone is higher in female relatives and the rate of Tourette's and tics is higher in male relatives of a Tourette patient's proband. These findings suggest that some forms of OCD are familial.

Probands with no relatives affected by OCD may represent a sporadic form of OCD that is aetiologically distinct from the familial form.

28.7.2.2 Neuroimaging

Diffusion-tensor imaging shows decreased cortico-striato-thalamo-striato-cortical circuitry.

Functional MRI shows increased orbitofrontal cortex, anterior cingulate cortex, and striatum.

28.7.2.3 Neurological Factors

The reported numbers of OCD cases increased following the 1915 and 1926 outbreaks of encephalitis lethargica (Foley, 2009).

OCD patients have more abnormal births than expected and more neurological disorders including Sydenham's chorea and encephalitis, suggestive of basal ganglia dysfunction. Childhood streptococcus infection leads to Paediatric Autoimmune Neuropsychiatric Disorders Associated with Streptococcus (PANDAS) that is associated with childhood-onset OCD. Flor-Henry observed neuropsychological deficits implicating left frontal lobe dysfunction.

Brain-imaging techniques show morphological changes of basal ganglia structures in OCD. Frontostriatal abnormality is present. Functional neuroimaging studies show increased blood flow in the basal ganglia and orbital, prefrontal, and anterior cingulate cortex. Caudate metabolic rate is reduced after treatment with drugs or behaviour therapy in those patients responsive to treatment, with the percentage change in symptom ratings correlating significantly with right caudate change.

28.7.2.4 Psychological Factors

In learning theory, obsessions are thoughts with which anxiety has become associated. Rituals or neutralizing thoughts terminate exposure to the stimulus; thus, anxiety is reduced and the rituals are negatively reinforced. The use of rituals prevents the natural reduction in anxiety that would occur if exposure to the stimulus was not cut short by the ritual or neutralizing thought.

In a cognitive model, obsessional distortion concerns exaggerated the responsibility for thoughts, with a tendency to neutralize thoughts with rituals.

In psychoanalysis, OCD symptoms are seen as defensive responses to unconscious impulses. Obsessional symptoms arise from intrapsychic anxiety because of the conflicts being expressed by the defence mechanisms of displacement, undoing, and reaction formation. The origin of obsessional personality is located at the anal-training stage of development; OCD is thought to represent regression to this stage.

Neuropsychological tests suggest the presence of amnestic deficits with respect to nonverbal memory and memory for actions. OCD patients also perform poorly on tests of frontal lobe function, particularly tests of shifting set.

28.7.3 Diagnostic Criteria

28.7.3.1 ICD-10 (F42) (WHO, 1992)

Obsessional symptoms or compulsive acts are present most days for at least two successive weeks causing distress or interfering with activities. Obsessional symptoms have the following characteristics:

- The minimum duration is at least 2 weeks.
- Recognized as the individual's own.
- At least one thought or act is resisted unsuccessfully.
- The thought of carrying out the act must not in itself be pleasurable.
- Thoughts, images, or impulses are unpleasantly repetitive.
- Interference with functioning by waste of time.
- F42.0 predominantly obsessional thoughts or ruminations.
- F42.1 predominantly compulsive acts.

28.7.3.2 DSM-5 (APA, 2013)

28.7.3.2.1   300.3 OCD

Obsessions are defined by

1. Recurrent and intrusive thoughts, urges, or images causing marked anxiety or distress
2. Attempts to suppress such thoughts, urges, or images, or to neutralize them with compulsion.

TABLE 28.3

The Most Common Obsessions and Compulsions

The Most Common Obsessions (in Descending Order)	The Most Common Compulsions (in Descending Order)
1. Fear of contamination (45%)	1. Checking (63%)
2. Doubting (42%)	2. Washing (50%)
3. Fear of illness, germs, or bodily fear (36%)	3. Counting (36%)
4. Symmetry (31%)	
5. Sexual or aggressive thoughts (28%)	

Compulsions are defined by

1. Repetitive behaviours (e.g. hand washing, ordering, checking) or mental acts (e.g. praying, counting, repeating words silently) in response to an obsession.
2. The behaviours or mental acts are aimed at preventing or reducing anxiety or distress.

Obsessions or compulsions are time-consuming (Table 28.3).

Specifier: Good or fair insight, poor insight, and absent insight

28.7.4 Management of OCD

28.7.4.1 Pharmacotherapy

Antidepressants are effective in the short-term treatment of OCD. SSRIs such as fluvoxamine, fluoxetine, paroxetine, and sertraline are commonly used. Clomipramine and SSRIs have greater efficacy than antidepressants with no selective serotonergic properties. Concomitant depression is not necessary for serotonergic antidepressants to improve symptoms. There are success rates of 50%–79%. Relapse often follows discontinuation of treatment.

For treatment-resistant OCD, there is some evidence that adding quetiapine or risperidone to antidepressants increases efficacy, but this must be weighed against less tolerability and limited data (Komossa et al., 2010).

28.7.4.2 Psychological Treatments

NICE guidelines: Evoked response prevention (ERP) and CBT for OCD and body dysmorphic disorder (BDD)

1. For initial treatment of OCD, ERP (up to 10 therapist hours per client), brief individual CBT using self-help materials and by telephone, and group CBT should be offered.
2. For adults with OCD with mild to moderate functional impairment, more intensive CBT (including ERP) (more than 10 therapist hours per client) is recommended.
3. For children and young people with OCD with moderate to severe functional impairment, CBT (including ERP) is the first-line treatment.

28.7.4.3 Physical Treatments

Psychosurgery may be indicated in the chronic unremitting OCD of at least 2 years' duration with severe life disruption, unresponsive to all recognized forms of therapy. Open, uncontrolled studies show that 65% of patients with OCD are improved or greatly improved with cingulotomy plus bifrontal operations. Deep brain stimulation at the anterior limb of internal capsule may be an option for treatment-resistant OCD.

28.7.5 Course

Favourable prognostic factors include

- Mild symptoms
- Predominance of phobic ruminative ideas, absence of compulsions
- Short duration of symptoms
- No childhood symptoms or abnormal personality traits

Poor prognostic factors include

- Males with early onset
- Symptoms involving the need for symmetry and exactness
- The presence of hopelessness, hallucinations, or delusions
- A family history of OCD
- A continuous, episodic, or deteriorating course

CASC STATION ON OCD

Station 1

A 26-year-old housewife is referred by her GP for psychiatric assessment. She complains of distressing obsessional ruminations that she may harm her 3-year-old son. According to her GP, she is evasive about the nature of harm and becomes tearful when asked about it. She expresses shame at her thoughts. She also has grossly time-consuming cleaning rituals in the morning after her husband has gone to work. These are associated with thoughts about the possibility of contamination of herself or her family with the *H1N1* influenza viruses. Her illness began following the death of her father who died of colon cancer when she was 16 years old. Subsequently, her mother died of breast cancer when she was 20. She has been married to her husband for 5 years. She had tried very hard to conceal her worries from her husband until 2 weeks ago when she could not tolerate him coming back without taking a bath and they ended up in a quarrel. She saw the GP at her husband's insistence and she has never consulted a doctor for her problems. Furthermore, her GP reports that she seems to be depressed.

Task: Take a history to establish the diagnosis of OCD.

You will speak to her husband in the next station.

CASC Grid

(A) Assess Obsessions and Compulsions	(A1) Explore the Origin of Thoughts	(A2) Elicit the Recurrent and Unpleasant Nature	(A3) Explore Other Obsessions	(A4) Elicit the Unpleasant Nature	(A5) Explore Other Compulsions
	'I am sorry to hear that you are very concerned about the *H1N1* infection'. 'Do those thoughts about contamination come from your mind? Are those thoughts imposed by outside persons or influences?'	'Do you feel that those thoughts are repetitive, unpleasant, excessive and unreasonable?' 'What do you think the chance of getting *H1N1*? Have you overestimated the risk? Do you know anyone who has contracted the disease? What precaution have you taken so far? What did you worry prior to the emergence of *H1N1*?' 'Are those thoughts keep bothering you that you'd like to get rid of but can't?'	'Are you concerned about putting things in a special order? Are you very upset by mess?' 'Do you have images or doubts keep coming to your mind?' 'Do you like to repeat things in a particular number of time? Is this number bringing you good luck?'	'How do you feel about your time consuming cleaning rituals?' 'Do you feel that your rituals are unpleasurable?'	'Do you check things very often?' 'Do you perform a regular ritual or ceremony to prevent something bad from happening?' Explore other compulsive behaviours such as checking, counting, and hoarding.

(continued)

(B) Assess Risk, Precipitants, and Impact	(B1) Risk Assessment to Her Son	(B2) Assess Risk to Herself	(B3) Precipitants	(B4) Parenting Ability	(B5) Impact of Her Illness
	Inquire her thought of harming her son in an empathetic manner. 'I am sorry to hear that you have gone through tremendous stress. Have you ever thought of harming your son? Can you tell me more about this?'	'How about harming yourself?' 'Do you feel that life is not worth living?'	Explore recent life events that may lead to exacerbation of OCD symptoms.	Ask her to take you through how she looks after her son on a typical day. Explore the impact of compulsions on her parenting ability. 'Is there other person helping her?'	'Do you take a long time to finish your daily activities?' Explore the cost incurred by her illness, e.g. high water bills, loss of occupational function due to her obsessional slowness.

(C) Explore Comorbidity and Differential Diagnosis	(C1) Assess Depressive Symptoms	(C2) Establish the Temporal Relationship Between OCD and Depressive Disorder	(C3) Exclude Postpartum Psychiatric Illnesses	(C4) Assess Personality	(C5) Other Psychiatric or Medical Conditions
	Explore her current mood, cognitive, and biological symptoms related to depression. Pay attention to psychotic symptoms such as nihilistic, guilt-ridden delusions and mood-congruent hallucinations.	If depression is present, ask the patient 'Does the low mood start before or after your recurrent thoughts of contamination?'	'Did you suffer from a period of low mood after delivery? How about low mood and confusion? Did you hear voices asking you to harm your baby? Did you follow the command?'	'Are you a perfectionistic person?' 'Are you preoccupied with details?' 'Are you rigid with rules?' 'Are you a careful and thrifty person?'	'Did you have tics before?' 'Did you have any head injury before?'

(D) Salient Features of this Case	(D1) Explore the Meaning of 'Never Consulted a Doctor for Her Problems'	(D2) Explore Concealment of Her Symptoms	(D3) Assess Her Current Marriage	(D4) Developmental Issues and Family History	(D5) Assess Her Insight and Expectations
	'Would you mind to tell me why you have not seen a doctor for your problems? Are you worried that the doctor may not understand your problem?' 'Did you seek help from other sources such as self-help book?' 'Why did you consult the GP this time? Were you prompted by your husband?'	'May I know why you tried to hide your illness from your husband in the beginning?' 'Is it because of your fear of losing your husband?' 'Are you ashamed of having psychiatric symptoms? How about potential stigma?'	'Is your husband supportive and understanding?' 'Does he offer assistance when you fall sick?' 'How is the communication at home? Is the communication open and honest?'	Brief assessment of developmental crises, e.g. separation, break-up of a relationship, and death of parents. 'How did you cope with multiple losses?' 'Are those losses and your fear of contamination related?' 'Do your family members also exhibit similar concerns of contamination and cleaning behaviour?'	'Do you think that you have a psychiatric illness? If not, what are your views and explanations?' 'Have you read any information about OCD?' 'What is your expectation on treatment?' 'What type of treatment would you prefer?' (e.g. medication, psychotherapy, or both).

Station 2

You have performed a detailed psychiatric assessment on the patient and concluded that she suffers from severe OCD with secondary depression and significant functional impairment. She has tried reading self-help book but it does not work. She has been bathing her son excessively, and as a consequence, she suffers from dermatological problems. She has history of tics. The marital relationship is poor and the couple has thought of divorce. The patient is keen to receive treatment. You have obtained permission from the patient to speak to her husband.

Task: Discuss your approach to management.

Explain management of OCD based on the recommendations from the NICE guidelines:

1. *This is a potentially complex case*: The fact that this is the first time the patient presents her problems to her GP may indicate a poor prognosis. Other indicators of poor prognosis include a strong conviction about rationality of her obsession, prominent depression, and comorbid tic disorder. The candidate needs to be honest to her husband but provides hope that her symptoms may improve with treatment.

2. *Provide accurate information on OCD*:

   I am sorry to inform you that your wife suffers from a condition called obsessive compulsive disorder or OCD. Have you heard about it? Can I tell you more about her condition? OCD is characterized by the presence of either obsessions or compulsions, but commonly both. Symptoms can cause significant distress. An obsession is an unwanted intrusive thought, image, or urge that repeatedly enters the person's mind. Compulsions are repetitive behaviours or mental acts that the person feels driven to perform. These can be observable by others, such as her cleaning behaviour, or a mental act that cannot be observed, such as her worries of getting *H1N1* in her mind. It is thought that 1 in 100 of the population have OCD.

   The candidate should address any concern raised by her husband to allay his fears and to assist him in adjusting to his wife's diagnosis.

3. *Inpatient service*: Hospitalization is indicated if (1) the patient poses a severe risk to her son and herself; (2) severe self-neglect; (3) extreme distress or functional impairment; (4) complicated comorbidity such as OCD with severe depression, anorexia nervosa, and psychosis; (5) severe reversal of day and night patterns; or (6) very severe avoidance behaviour.

4. *Investigations*: Further laboratory investigations, psychological testing, or brain imaging may be necessary if the psychiatrist needs further information to rule out certain differential diagnoses. You will administer a scale such as Yale–Brown Obsessive–Compulsive Scale (Y-BOCS) to assess the baseline severity of her OCD symptoms.

5. *Use of antidepressants (SSRI)*: This patient has severe OCD symptoms. She should be offered combined treatment with SSRI and CBT, including ERP. The candidate should emphasize the common pharmacodynamic profiles of antidepressant on depression and OCD. The dose to treat OCD is two to three times higher than the dose for antidepressants (e.g. fluoxetine 40–80 mg or fluvoxamine 150–300 mg). There may be a delay up to 12 weeks in the onset of actions. Inform the husband about the potential side effects such as worsening anxiety and nausea that will be monitored closely in the first few weeks of treatment. Her response will be reviewed at 12 weeks. If the SSRI is effective, the patient is advised to continue the medication for at least 12 months to prevent relapse. If her response is very poor or inadequate, you will offer a different SSRI or suggest clomipramine. Please note that the following drugs are not normally recommended for OCD: other TCAs, SNRIs, MAOIs, and long-term anxiolytics.

6. *Use of clomipramine and management of treatment-resistant OCD*: Clomipramine can be used when (1) there is an adequate trial of at least one SSRI that is found to be ineffective, (2) an SSRI is poorly tolerated, (3) the patient prefers clomipramine, and (4) there has been a previous good response to clomipramine. The candidate needs to carry out an ECG and a blood pressure measurement before

prescribing clomipramine. Clomipramine is a TCA (derivative of imipramine). The candidate should prescribe a small amount of tablets to prevent toxicity in overdose. If the standard daily dose (100–225 mg) is inadequate for the patient and there are no significant side effects, consider a gradual dose increase in line with prescription information provided by the manufacturers. If it is still ineffective, clomipramine can be augmented with citalopram or adding an antipsychotic to clomipramine or SSRI. Continue clomipramine for at least 12 months if it appears to be effective and reduce the dose gradually to prevent withdrawals prior to discontinuation.

7. *Psychotherapy*: The patient has severe functional impairment, and self-help method has been ineffective. She should be offered CBT (including ERP) that also involves her husband as a co-therapist. If the patient refuses to come to the clinic, you will offer home-based treatment. If her symptoms prevent home-based treatment, you will offer CBT by telephone. Briefly explain to her husband that CBT will begin with anxiety management and asking the patient to keep a diary. Then it will move onto response prevention in excessive washing with cognitive coping and composure strategies. Social and occupational rehabilitation will include training on housekeeping, childcare, and promotion on independent living. The psychologist will focus on her residual depressive symptoms once her OCD symptoms have improved. For mild OCD, the NICE guidelines recommend CBT to be given for less than 10 therapist hours. For moderate CBT, a course of an SSRI alone or more intensive CBT alone (ERP and CBT for longer than 10 therapist hours) is recommended.

8. *Assess social issues*: Seek her husband's view on the home situation and how this may affect her compliance to treatment. Explore from him the ongoing difficulties in forming relationships and the future difficulties in providing care to her son given the nature of her OCD symptoms.

9. *Improving marital relationship*: Inform her husband that the patient needs encouragement and assistance on her way to recovery. You may offer to see both patient and her husband together and the advantage of a joint interview is to inform and educate the couple more about OCD and its management. This can only be done at the patient's agreement and there may be issues that the patient does not want to be discussed. If the couple is agreeable, couple therapy will involve role-playing and coaching once her OCD symptoms have improved.

10. *Continuity of care*: 'Many OCD patients will need ongoing follow-up over years and your wife is not an exception. The follow-up will enable monitoring of treatment response, side-effects, and achievement of rehabilitative and social reintegration goals'.

28.8   OCD-SPECTRUM DISORDERS

28.8.1   Body Dysmorphic Disorder

28.8.1.1   Historical Development

The old term for this condition is dysmorphophobia, which is coined by Morselli in 1886 (Morselli, 1891).

28.8.1.2   Epidemiology (Conrado, 2009)

1. The prevalence of this disorder among the general population ranges from 1% to 2%.
2. In dermatological and cosmetic surgery patients, the prevalence is from 2.9% to 16%.

28.8.1.3   Aetiology

1. Genetics: family history of BDD, OCD, and mood disorder.
2. Neurochemistry: low serotonin levels.
3. Psychodynamic theory: displacement of conflict onto body component.
4. Development: rejection in childhood as a result of body image problem, disharmony in family.
5. Culture influence: beauty equals to perfect body.

28.8.1.4   Clinical Features

DSM-5 criteria (APA, 2013):

- Preoccupation with perceived defects or flaws in physical appearance that are not observable to others.

- The person performs repetitive behaviours or mental acts (e.g. comparing their appearance with that of others) in response to the appearance concerns.
- Specifiers include muscle dysmorphia, good or fair insight, poor insight, and absent insight.

Common behavioural problems:

- Self-harm: 70%–80%
- Social avoidance: 30%
- Suicide: 20%

Rituals:

- Camouflage: 90%
- Minor check: 90%
- Compulsion: 90%
- Skin pick: 30%

Most common body sites concerned:

- Hair: 63%
- Nose: 50%
- Skin: 50%
- Eye: 30%
- Face: 20%
- Breast: <10%
- Neck, forehead, and facial muscle: <5%

28.8.1.5 Differential Diagnosis
OCD (Table 28.4)

TABLE 28.4

Differences and Similarities between OCD and BDD

Differences	Similarities
Patients with OCD are	
1. Less likely to suffer from social phobia	1. Gender ratio (M/F = 1:1)
2. Less likely to attempt suicide	2. Both conditions show obsessions and compulsions
3. Less likely to be involved in substance abuse	3. SSRI is the main treatment
4. Having better insight	4. Both conditions cause significant distress
5. Have better relationship	

28.8.1.6 Comorbidity
1. Social phobia: 38%
2. Substance: 36%
3. Suicide: 30%
4. OCD: 30%
5. Depression: 20%

28.8.1.7 Management
1. Antidepressants: SSRIs; 50% of patients respond to SSRIs.
2. Antipsychotics: if patient does not respond to SSRIs, the psychiatrist can augment with second-generation antipsychotics.
3. Other pharmacological agents: clomipramine, buspirone, and lithium.
4. For people with BDD with moderate functional impairment, more intensive CBT (including ERP) is recommended based on the NICE guidelines.

CASC STATION ON BDD

A 23-year-old woman is referred by her GP. She is single and works as a disc jockey at a local radio station. She has been worried that her nose is too large and crooked since the age of 14. She has become increasingly worried about her nose.

Task: Take a history to establish the diagnosis of BDD.

(continued)

CASC Grid

(A) Inquire More About Her Concerns About the Nose	(A1) Onset and Extent of the Problem	(A2) Repeated Checking and Reassurance Seeking	(A3) Course of the Illness	(A4) Impact of Her Illness	(A5) Explore Coping Strategy
	'When did you start to become unhappy with how you look? *If yes*: what is your concern?' 'Does this concern preoccupy you? How much time do you spend thinking about your nose?' 'Were you under scrutiny or being bullied as a result your nose problems?' 'Was there any injury to your nose causing deformation?'	'Are you very worried about your appearance? Do you need to look into the mirror very often?' 'Do you do other things to monitor your nose? e.g. repeated measurements of its size'. 'Have you tried to hide your defect?' 'Do you pick at your nose or skin?'	'Is there any fluctuation in the intensity of your concern? Is there time when you are less preoccupied with your nose?' 'Is your concern about your nose is related to your stress level?'	'Is there any change in smell? Do you think the defect affects the function of your nose?' 'Why did you choose this job? Are you comfortable with your job arrangement?' 'Does your nose affect your social life?' 'Were you rejected in a romantic relationship because of your nose?'	'How did you cope in the past 10 years? Can you distract yourself from the nose issue?' 'Do you share your concerns with your friends and family? What do they say about your nose?'

(B) Explore BDD and Comorbidity	(B1) Other Parts of the Body	(B2) Gentle Challenge	(B3) Assess Psychosis and Mood	(B4) Assess Anxiety	(B5) Substance Abuse
	'Do you worry about the following areas such as your skin, hair, body weight, breast, eyes, teeth, legs and your face in general?' If she is concerned about her body weight, explore anorexic behaviour such as restricting dieting, excessive exercise, and purging.	'I am very sorry to hear your worries. So far, I cannot find any major defect in your nose. I have seen patients who are also very concerned about a single part of their bodies. Do you think you are over concerned?'	'Do you have other unusual experiences such as hearing voices or seeing things or strange feelings?' 'Can you tell me more about your mood? Do you feel sad at this moment?'	Look for generalized anxiety symptoms, panic attack, social phobia, and agoraphobia. Look for other compulsive behaviours such as repetitive checking and excessive washing.	'Do you turn into alcohol or tranquillizer to reduce your stress associated with your concern about your nose?' 'Do you take medication to reduce the size of the nose?'

(C) Past Cosmetic Treatment and Risk Assessment	(C1) Previous Investigations	(C2) Previous Treatment	(C3) Financial Problems	(C4) Risk to Her Nose	(C5) Suicide and Self-harm
	'Did you seek medical help for the nose problems? Have you seen a plastic surgeon? If yes, how many surgeons have you seen'	'Did you go for cosmetic surgery?' 'If yes, for how many times?' 'What was the outcome?'	'How much money have you spent on fixing your nose?' 'Do you need to borrow money for treatment?'	'If the doctors say that they cannot offer further treatment to your nose, what would you do next?'	'It seems that you are desperate to get your nose fixed. Do you feel hopeless?'

(D) Background History and Explain Diagnosis	(D1) Childhood History	(D2) Personality and Family Background	(D3) Past Medical History	(D4) Past Psychiatric History	(D5) Explain Diagnosis and Seeks Her Views
	'What kind of investigations did you go through?' 'Did you consult traditional healers or alternative therapy?'	'What is your current plan for the nose problem?'	'Do you plan to go aboard for further treatment? If yes, which countries?'	'Do you have plan to perform the operation on your own?'	'Do you have thought of harming yourself? Have you thought of ending your life?'
	Look for bullying in school and home environment. Assess temperament: 'Were you a shy child?' 'Did you have confident in yourself?'	'How do you describe yourself as a person? Are you perfectionistic?' 'How was your relationship with your parents?' 'Did they criticize your nose before?'	Look for chronic medical problems or metabolic syndrome that affects her body image.	'Did you see a psychologist or psychiatrist before? If yes, what was the reason?'	on treatment Emphasize that this disorder is an excessive preoccupation with an imagined defect in appearance that results in time-consuming checking. Seek her views on treatment issues such as SSRI or CBT.

28.9 HOARDING

28.9.1 Historical Development

Diogenes syndrome refers to hoarding behaviour in old people.

28.9.1.1 Epidemiology (Saxena et al., 2004; Samuels, 2007)

1. Hoarding is most commonly found in people with OCD.
2. 18%–42% of people with OCD report hoarding and saving compulsions.
3. 10%–15% of people with OCD have compulsive hoarding as their most prominent symptom.

28.9.1.2 Aetiology (Gaston et al., 2009)

28.9.1.2.1 Genetics

1. The hoarding symptom shows an autosomal recessive inheritance pattern and has been associated with genetic markers on chromosomes 4, 5, and 17 (Zhang, 2002).
2. 84% of hoarders reported a family history of hoarding behaviour in first-degree relatives.
3. 37% of hoarders reported a family history of OCD (Winsberg et al., 1999).

28.9.1.2.2 Functional Imaging

1. People with OCD and hoarding behaviour did not have the characteristic hypermetabolism in the orbitofrontal cortex, caudate nuclei, and thalamus.
2. People with OCD and hoarding behaviour showed significantly lower activity in the dorsal anterior cingulate gyrus and occipital cortex.
3. Diminished activity in the cingulate cortex is associated with poor treatment response and compulsive hoarding behaviour.

28.9.1.2.3 Cognitive Theory

1. Cognitive appraisals about possessions, triggering emotional responses that lead to hoarding behaviours.

2. Hoarding behaviour is maintained through reinforcements related to indecisiveness, concerns over mistakes, judgements about need, and emotional attachment to possessions.
3. Positive reinforcement is related to the pleasure gained from acquiring and saving.
4. Negative reinforcement involves avoidance of grief, anxiety, and guilt.

28.9.1.3 Clinical Features
ICD-10 does not mention about this disorder.
DSM-5 criteria (300.3) (APA 2013):

1. Persistent difficulty discarding or parting with possessions, regardless of their actual value.
2. This difficulty is caused by a perceived need to save the items and distress associated with discarding them.
3. The symptoms result in the accumulation of possessions that congest and clutter active living areas and substantially compromise their intended use.
4. Specifiers include excessive acquisition, good or fair insight, poor insight, and absent insight.

There are two types of hoarding:

1. Compulsive buying
2. Acquiring free and discarded items

28.9.1.4 Questionnaires
1. The Hoarding Scale (Frost, 1993) is a 21-item questionnaire designed to measure various aspects of hoarding behaviour.
2. The Clutter Image Rating Scale (Tolin, 2007) is a pictorial scale that contains nine photographs of severity of clutter representing each of three main rooms of most people's homes.

28.9.1.5 Differential Diagnosis
Normal hoarding: The items collected are usually organized, interesting, and valuable (Melamed, 1998).

28.9.1.6 Psychiatric Comorbidity
1. Schizophrenia
2. Learning disability
3. Neurodegenerative disorders (in particular frontal lobe dysfunction)
4. Autism-spectrum disorders
5. Eating disorders
6. Impulse-control disorders

28.10 TREATMENT

28.10.1 Psychological Treatment

28.10.1.1 Cognitive Behaviour Therapy (Saxena et al., 2004)
1. Introduce alternative behaviours.
2. Get the client organized.
3. Prevent incoming clutter.
4. Encourage discarding of objects.

28.10.2 Pharmacological Treatment
1. SSRI
2. SNRI: venlafaxine
3. Acetylcholinesterase inhibitors: donepezil or galantamine

28.10.3 Trichotillomania

28.10.3.1 ICD-10 Criteria
1. Trichotillomania is an impulse-control disorder.
2. There is persistent and recurrent failure to resist the impulse to pull out one's hair, resulting in noticeable hair loss.
3. The individual describes an intense urge to pull out hair, with mounting tension before the act and subsequent relief.
4. There is no preexisting inflammation of the skin and the hair pulling is not in response to any psychotic feature.

28.10.3.2 DSM-5 Criteria (312.39) (APA 2013)
1. Recurrent pulling out of one's hair resulting in hair loss
2. Repeated attempts to decrease or stop hair pulling

28.10.4 Skin Picking Disorder
DSM-5 criteria (698.4) (APA 2013) include

1. Recurrent skin picking resulting in skin lesions
2. Repeated attempts to decrease or stop skin picking

28.11 ACUTE STRESS REACTION

This is a transient disorder developing in an individual without other mental disorder in response to exceptional stress. It usually subsides within hours or days. The risk is increased if physical exhaustion or organic factors are present.

28.11.1 ICD-10 (WHO, 1992)

- There is an immediate temporal connection between the impact of an exceptional stressor and onset of symptoms, which is within minutes.
- In addition, symptoms
  - Show a mixed and changing picture—initial state of daze, depression, anxiety, anger, despair, overactivity, and withdrawal may all be seen, with no one symptom predominating for long.
  - Resolve rapidly, within a few hours if removal from the stressful environment is possible.

  If stress continues, symptoms diminish after 24–48 h.
- Acute stress reaction is classified as mild, moderate, or severe.

28.11.2 DSM-5 (308.3)

- The duration is between 3 days and 1 month.
- Exposure to actual or threatened death, serious injury, and sexual violation.
- Intrusion symptoms: recurrent distressing dreams, dissociative reactions, and prolonged stress.
- Dissociative symptoms: inability to experience positive emotions, altered sense of reality, and inability to remember.
- Avoidance of distressing memories and external reminders.
- Arousal symptoms including sleep disturbance, irritability, hypervigilance, problems with concentration, and exaggerated startle response.

28.11.3 MANAGEMENT

Pharmacological treatment

1. Beta blockers (e.g. propranolol).
2. α_2-Receptor antagonist clonidine reduces nightmares and emotional reactivity.

28.12 PTSD

28.12.1 AETIOLOGY OF PTSD

28.12.1.1 General Factors

About 25% of people exposed to a potentially traumatic event develop PTSD. Low education and social class, preexisting psychiatric problems, and female gender are vulnerability factors. Viewing the dead body of a relative after a disaster is predictive of lower PTSD. Psychopathic traits are protective.

Sufferers of PTSD report childhood physical sexual abuse more often than expected.

28.12.1.2 Biological Factors

People with PTSD have exaggerated physiological responses (heart rate, skin conductance, electromyographic response) to traumatic imagery. They have a heightened physiological state specific to PTSD that is difficult to simulate. This may be mediated by noradrenergic and dopaminergic neurotransmitter systems and the HPA axis. PTSD patients have low cortisol levels after trauma. There is an increase in glucocorticoid receptors in the hypothalamus and a reduction in peripheral cortisol (Saddock, 2003).

Initial mobilization and the subsequent depletion of NA following inescapable shock in animals indicate a possible catecholaminergic mediation of PTSD symptoms. Drugs effective in PTSD (MAOIs, tricyclics, benzodiazepines, and clonidine) are also effective in preventing the development of learned helplessness in animals when infused into the locus coeruleus.

There are similarities between PTSD symptoms and opioid withdrawal, leading to speculation that opioid function is disturbed in PTSD. Stress-induced analgesia is reversible by naloxone in PTSD veterans exposed to traumatic stimulus.

28.12.1.3 Psychosocial Factors (Koenen and Widom, 2009)

1. Gender: female gender
2. Intelligence: low intelligence quotient (IQ) at age 5
3. Previous trauma history
4. Previous psychiatric history: hyperactivity, antisocial behaviour
5. Severity of trauma
6. Perceived life threat
7. Peri-traumatic dissociation
8. Impaired social support
9. Low socioeconomic status

28.12.2 DIAGNOSTIC CRITERIA

28.12.2.1 ICD-10 (F43.1) (WHO, 1992)

- PTSD arises within 6 months as a delayed and/or protracted response to a stressful event of an exceptionally threatening nature.
- Symptoms include repeated reliving of the trauma. Repetitive, intrusive memories (flashbacks), daytime imagery, or dreams of the event must be present.
- Emotional detachment, persisting background numbness, and avoidance of stimuli reminiscent of original event are often present, but are not essential.
- Autonomic disturbances (hyperarousal with hypervigilance, enhanced startle reaction, and insomnia) and mood disorder contribute to the diagnosis but

are not essential. Anxiety, depression, and suicidal ideation are not uncommon. The excessive use of alcohol or drugs may complicate matters.

28.12.2.2 DSM-5 (309.81)

- Exposure to actual or threatened death, serious injury, and sexual violation.
- Intrusion symptoms: recurrent distressing dreams, dissociative reactions, and prolonged stress.
- Avoidance of distressing memories and external reminders.
- Negative alternations in cognitions and mood associated with traumatic events.
- Arousal symptoms including sleep disturbance, irritability, hypervigilance, problems with concentration, and exaggerated startle response.
- Duration of disturbance is longer than 1 month.
- Subtypes include delayed expression, PTSD in preschool children, and predominant dissociative symptoms.

28.12.3 MANAGEMENT OF PTSD

A flexible, staged approach using several techniques is advocated.

28.12.3.1 Psychological Therapy

28.12.3.1.1 Cognitive Behavioural Therapy

Cognitive techniques include challenging underlying automatic thought that accidents or disasters will occur again and cognitive distortions. Cognitive restructuring, distraction thought replacement, and thought stopping are useful. Assessment should include behaviour analysis through diary keeping. Psychoeducation should offer explanation of PTSD symptoms. Behavioural techniques include relaxation training, in vivo and in vitro exposure, and desensitization to disaster or accident scenes, rehearsal, as well as assertiveness and social skill training.

The NICE guidelines recommend that

1. Trauma-focused CBT (tf-CBT) should be offered to people with severe PTSD within 3 months of the trauma with fewer sessions in the first month after the trauma.
2. The duration of tf-CBT is 8–12 sessions with 1 session per week. When trauma is discussed in the session, it requires a longer session (90 min).

28.12.3.2 Pharmacotherapy

Fluoxetine, paroxetine, sertraline, venlafaxine, and escitalopram are beneficial in PTSD. The drugs require at least 8 weeks' duration before the effects are evident.

Carbamazepine, propranolol, and clonidine reduce hyperarousal and intrusive symptoms; fluoxetine and lithium reduce explosiveness and improve mood. Buspirone may lessen fear-induced startle; it may play an adjunctive role.

Alprazolam is no more effective than placebo, but there have been some positive reports with clonazepam.

There is an almost total lack of response to placebo in chronic PTSD.

28.12.3.3 Eye Movement Desensitization Reprocessing

Involuntary multi-saccadic eye movements occur during disturbing thoughts. It is claimed that inducing these eye movements while experiencing intrusive thoughts stops symptoms of PTSD. More information on eye movement desensitization reprocessing (EMDR) are found in Chapter 25.

28.12.4 COURSE

Half of patients still have PTSD decades later. A dose–response relationship exists between the severity of the stressor and the degree of consequent psychological distress.

Most PTSD patients also have depression, anxiety disorders, substance abuse, and/or sexual dysfunction.

CASC STATION ON PTSD

Station 1

A 33-year-old British army officer (Engineer Regiment) suffered a number of traumatic combat experiences in Afghanistan. Six months ago, he was very seriously wounded by an explosive device during an operation. He lost the eyesight of his left eye and hearing ability of his left ear. He was first treated at the deployed hospital facilities and later sent back to the United Kingdom. Currently, he cannot work and he is disturbed by recurrent nightmares and vivid intrusive recollections of his traumatic experiences. He avoids the news and TV programmes that remind him of Afghanistan and he has abused alcohol since his return. He has been married for 2 years. He presents in the company of his wife seeking treatment following his first episode of domestic violence that occurred in the setting of alcohol intoxication and argument.

Task: Take a history to establish the diagnosis of PTSD.
You will speak to his wife in the next station.

CASC Grid

Approach to the patient: Candidates are advised to consult the patient on the volume of your voice as he has hearing impairment.

(A) Explore His Trauma	(A1) Describe the Incident in Afghanistan	(A2) Immediate Outcome of the Incident	(A3) Extent of Injury and Suffering	(A4) Outcome of Other Soldiers in the Operation	(A5) Psychodynamic Issues Associated with the Incident
	Explore his role during the operation. 'Were you the commander during the operation? Were you assigned the duty to detect the bomb and ensure the safety of others?' 'What was the level of threat to your life during the bomb blast?'	'How long did you wait for the rescue to come?' 'How did you feel after the accident?' Look for the symptoms of acute stress reactions on the first few days after the incident.	Especially head injury and any organic sequelae such as intracerebral haemorrhage, loss of consciousness, and epilepsy Explore other disabling or disfiguring injuries. 'Did you suffer from any chronic pain such as low back pain or pain related to other sites of injury?'	'Were the fellow soldiers killed or injured? If yes, how many were involved? What was your relationship with them?' 'How did you know about their death?' 'Was there any debriefing? If yes, what is your view on the debriefing? Did you join them?' 'Do you have guilt of staying alive or guilt of missing the bomb?'	'I am sorry to hear that you cannot see and hear well nowadays. How do you feel about it?' 'Was it the first time you faced your own mortality?' 'Do you feel remorseful of going to Afghanistan?'
(B) PTSD Symptoms	(B1) Reexperiencing	(B2) Avoidance	(B3) Hyperarousal	(B4) Emotional Detachment	(B5) Previous Trauma and Personality
	Identify the latency period between the incident and onset of his PTSD symptoms. 'How do those memories relive themselves? How vivid are they?' 'How often do you see the images of the incident?'	'How do you spend your time?' Assess the extent and degree of avoidance of people, places, and circumstances (e.g. other army officers, army facilities, and previously enjoyed activities).	'Are you always on the edge?' Look for anxiety symptoms such as excessive sweating, palpitation, panic attacks, sleep problems, irritability, and poor concentration. Check exaggerated startle response.	Look for emotional withdrawal. 'Are you able to describe your emotion?' Look for dissociative symptoms. 'Do you feel that yourself or the environment is unreal?'	Explore other traumatic events in Afghanistan. 'Do you feel blunted or numb?' Explore previous trauma (e.g. childhood trauma, road traffic accident, army operation). 'Was this incident similar to previous unresolved trauma?'

(continued)

	'Do you have nightmare? How often do you have nightmare? Can you tell me more about the content of nightmare?'	'Do you have difficulty to recall the details leading to the incident in Afghanistan?'	'Are you in shock if someone suddenly call your name?'		'How did the previous trauma affect your character development?'
(C) Risk Assessment and Comorbidity	*(C1) Suicide*	*(C2) Dangerousness to Others*	*(C3) Substance Abuse*	*(C4) Depression*	*(C5) Other Common Comorbidities*
	Assess suicidal ideation and the level of dangerousness if he has a suicidal plan. Look for extreme pessimism because he lost his occupational ability at this age.	Assess the level and quality of dangerousness to his wife and the others. 'Would you perform dangerous act when you are angry? If yes, what would you do?'	Assess his alcohol intake before, during, and after the deployment. Explore the type of alcohol and the amount he drinks every day. Explore the purpose of alcohol usage (e.g. to reduce the anxiety level). Explore misuse of benzodiazepines, analgesics, or cannabis.	Assess his current mood, biological, and cognitive symptoms of depression.	Look for symptoms of adjustment disorder, OCD, and psychosis.
(D) Background History and Compensation Issues	*(D1) Vulnerability to PTSD*	*(D2) Marital Relationship*	*(D3) Compensation and Entitlements*	*(D4) Support and Treatment from the Army*	*(D5) Background History*
	Candidate needs to explore what made him vulnerable to PTSD, e.g. low education, maladaptive coping style, personality, low resilience, and childhood trauma	'Can you tell me more about the relationship with your wife?' 'Does the relationship change before, during, and after your deployment to Afghanistan?'	'Have you discussed with the Ministry of Defence on the arrangement of compensation and veterans allowance?' 'What is your expectation? Are you satisfied with the amount being offered?'	'Did they refer you to see other specialists for your visual and hearing problems?' 'Did they refer you to counselling?' Assess his insight to his blindness, hearing impairment, and PTSD. 'Do you cooperate with treatment?'	'Why did you join the army in the first place?' 'How does this incident affect your original intention of being an army officer?'

Station 2

After assessment of the patient, it is concluded that he suffers from PTSD with severe depression and anxiety. The onset of PTSD symptoms was 4 months after the trauma. He is not keen to receive psychiatric help from the army psychiatric service and prefers to be treated in the civilian setting. The patient is deemed to have high risk for future violence and suicide as he cannot guarantee safety and he still wants to drink. He has given you the permission to talk to his wife.

Task: Inform his wife about your management plan and address her concerns.

Explain management of PTSD based on the NICE guidelines recommendations.

When symptoms are mild and have been present less than 4 weeks after the trauma, the NICE guidelines recommend watchful waiting but this is not appropriate for this patient who has symptoms for 2 months.

The NICE guidelines classify two intervention strategies when symptoms have been present for more than 3 months or less than 3 months after a trauma. As this patient developed PTSD symptoms 4 months after the trauma, the psychotherapy arrangement will follow the recommendations stated on the right side of Table 28.5:

1. *Address the referral process*: Explore the difficulty encountered by his wife to bring the patient in to see a doctor.
2. *Assess the impact of the violent episode on his wife*: Demonstrate empathy to her sufferings.

Explore her views on patient's intention to serve the army, his deployment to Afghanistan, and the bomb blast incident.

3. *Emergency issues in regard to his high risk of violence and suicide*: You should propose to admit patient to the hospital for safety reasons and for further assessment of his physical and psychiatric status. You may advise further laboratory investigations such as liver function tests.
4. *Detoxification*: You will try to enhance the motivation of the patient to quit alcohol and initiate a detoxification programme when he stays in the hospital.
5. During the hospitalization, you may commence short-term hypnotic medication to reduce his anxiety and ease his alcohol withdrawal. After stabilization, you will offer the psychological management of PTSD. The psychologist can take this

---

TABLE 28.5
Psychological Treatment for PTSD

	Less Than 3 Months after a Trauma	More Than 3 Months after a Trauma
Types of psychotherapy	Offer trauma-focused psychological treatment, tf-CBT (tf-CBT).	Offer trauma-focused psychological treatment (tf-CBT or EMDR) on an individual outpatient basis. Do not routinely offer non-trauma-focused interventions (such as relaxation or nondirective therapy) that do not address traumatic memories.
Time frame between the traumatic event and therapy	With severe PTSD within 1 month after the event or who present with PTSD within 3 months of the event	It should be offered regardless of the time elapsed since the trauma.
Length of the session	Usually 60 min. When the trauma is discussed, longer treatment sessions (90 min) are usually necessary.	Usually 60 min. When the trauma is discussed, longer treatment sessions (90 min) are usually necessary.
Duration of therapy	Consider offering 8–12 sessions of tf-CBT (or fewer sessions about 5—if the treatment starts in the first month after the event).	Consider offering 8–12 sessions of tf-CBT psychological treatment when the PTSD results from a single event. Consider extending trauma-focused psychological treatment beyond 12 sessions if there are multiple traumatic events, traumatic bereavement, chronic disability results from the trauma, significant comorbid disorders, or social problems.
Frequency of therapy	Regular and continuous (usually at least once a week).	Regular and continuous (usually at least once a week).
Therapist requirements	Delivered by the same person.	Delivered by the same person.
No improvement after psychotherapy	Consider the following drug treatment for sleep disturbance: 1. Hypnotic medication for short-term use 2. A suitable antidepressant for longer-term use	Consider an alternative form of trauma-focused psychological treatment or pharmacological treatment in addition to trauma-focused psychological treatment.

opportunity to establish contact and therapeutic alliance to prepare for long-term psychotherapy.

6. *Explain psychotherapy*: The patient may need more than 12 sessions as he experienced multiple traumatic events in Afghanistan. If his wife requests for other forms of psychological treatment (e.g. supportive therapy, nondirective therapy, hypnotherapy, psychodynamic, or systemic psychotherapy), inform her that there is no convincing evidence for a clinically important effect.

7. *Drug treatment for PTSD*: Candidate should not offer drugs as routine first-line treatment for PTSD patients. The patient may need antidepressant as he is severely depressed. You would recommend paroxetine or mirtazapine. Antidepressant is used before psychotherapy if the patient prefers not to engage in a tf-CBT or he cannot start psychological treatment because of serious threat of further trauma. Antidepressant is indicated for PTSD patients who have gained little or no benefit from a course of tf-CBT. Antidepressant can be used as an adjunct to tf-CBT. After initiation of the antidepressant, monitor potential side effect such as akathisia, increased anxiety, and suicidal ideation. If the patient responds to the antidepressant treatment, continue the medication for 12 months. Discontinuation of antidepressant would require gradual reduction over a 4-week period.

8. *Addiction service*: Candidate should consider referring the patient to the local addiction service and encourage him to attend Alcoholics Anonymous or other appropriate support groups. It is important to liaise with his GP.

9. *Medicolegal aspects*: The candidate should offer help (e.g. writing a medical report) to the patient because he may need to put his case forward to the Ministry of Defence or other related bodies for compensation or entitlement application.

10. *Couple therapy*: Counselling of his wife and/or couple therapy will be offered after discharge if both patient and his wife are interested in couple therapy.

11. *Long-term management*: The patient is advised to participate in a rehabilitation programme with the aim to resume or maintain employment, recreational activities, and social interaction, with the support of the British Veterans Association.

28.13 ADJUSTMENT DISORDERS

States of distress and emotional disturbance arise in the period after a stressful life event. Individual predisposition plays a greater role than in other stress-induced conditions, but this condition would not have arisen without a stressor.

Manifestations vary. They include depressed mood, anxiety, worry, an inability to cope, and some inability to manage the daily routine. Conduct disorders may be associated, especially in adolescents. Regressive phenomena in children are frequently seen.

Onset is within 1 month of the stressor. The duration is usually less than 6 months, except for prolonged depressive reaction.

Grief reactions considered abnormal because of their form or content are included in this category.

28.13.1 ICD-10 (F43.2) (WHO, 1992)

The following adjustment disorders are outlined in ICD-10:

- Symptoms must occur within 1 month of exposure to an identifiable psychosocial stressor.
- F43.2 brief depressive reaction—less than 1 month.
- F43.21 prolonged depressive reaction—less than 2 years.
- F43.22 mixed anxiety and depressive reaction.
- F43.23 predominant disturbance of emotions and/or conduct.

28.13.2 DSM-5 (APA 2013)

- The development of emotional or behavioural symptoms in response to an identifiable stressor occurring within 3 months of the onset of the stressor
- Do not represent normal bereavement

Other subtypes:

- With depressed mood
- With anxiety
- With mixed anxiety and depressed mood
- With disturbance of conduct
- With mixed disturbance of emotions and conduct

28.14 DISSOCIATIVE (CONVERSION) DISORDERS

28.14.1 ICD-10 (WHO, 1992)

Dissociative (conversion) disorders are presumed to be psychogenic in origin. They are associated with traumatic events, insoluble problems, or disturbed relationships. The unpleasant affect associated with these conflicts is transformed (converted) into symptoms.

Diagnostic guidelines are as follows:

- No evidence of physical disorder that may explain symptoms
- Evidence for psychological causation—a clear association in time with stressful events

28.14.2 SPECIFIC DISSOCIATIVE CONDITIONS

28.14.2.1 Dissociative Amnesia

- Loss of memory of an important event is not due to organic disorder, fatigue, or ordinary forgetfulness.
- Partial and selective amnesia is usually centred on traumatic events.
- The extent varies from day to day. A persistent core cannot be recalled while awake.
- Perplexity, distress, or calm acceptance may accompany the amnesia.
- It begins and ends suddenly, following stress. It rarely lasts more than a couple of days, and recurrence is unusual.
- It is more common in young adults but rare in the elderly.
- Recovery is complete.

28.14.2.1.1 DSM-5 (300.12) (APA, 2013)

An inability to recall important autobiographical information, usually of a traumatic nature, that is inconsistent with normal forgetting and memory function.

There are two primary forms of dissociative amnesia:

1. Localized or selective amnesia for a specific event
2. Generalized amnesia for personal identity and life history

28.14.2.2 Dissociative Fugue

- There are all the features of dissociative amnesia (see preceding text), plus an apparently purposeful journey away from home. A new identity may be assumed.
- It is precipitated by severe stress.
- There is amnesia for the duration of the fugue, but self-care and social interaction are maintained.
- It lasts for hours to days, but recovery is abrupt and complete.

28.14.2.3 Dissociative Stupor

- The sufferer is stuporose, with no evidence of a physical or other psychiatric cause.
- Onset is sudden and stress related.
- The person sits motionless for long periods, speech and movement absent. Muscle tone, posture, breathing, and eye movements indicate that the individual is neither asleep nor unconscious.

28.14.2.4 Trance and Possession Disorders

- There is a temporary loss of personal identity and awareness of surroundings.
- Attention and awareness are limited to one or two aspects of the immediate environment.
- There are repeated movements, postures, or utterances.

This includes only an involuntary or unwanted trance, occurring outside the culturally accepted situation.

28.14.2.5 Dissociative Disorders of Movement and Sensation

- There is loss of movement or sensations, usually cutaneous, with no physical cause.
- Symptoms often reflect the person's concept of disorder, which may be at variance with physiological or anatomical principles (e.g. glove and stocking anaesthesia).
- The resulting disability helps the person to escape conflict or express dependency or resentment indirectly.
- There is calm acceptance (la belle indifférence), not common and not diagnostic. This is also seen in normal people facing serious illness.
- Premorbid personality and relationships are often abnormal.

28.14.2.6 Dissociative Convulsions

- Pseudoseizures mimic epileptic seizures, but tongue biting, serious bruising, and incontinence of urine are uncommon.
- Loss of consciousness is absent or replaced by stupor or trance.

28.14.2.7   Dissociative Anaesthesia and Sensory Loss

- There are patches of sensory loss that do not correspond to anatomical dermatomes.
- Visual loss is rarely total.
- General mobility is well preserved.
- Dissociative deafness and anosmia are uncommon.

28.14.2.8   Other Dissociative Disorders

28.14.2.8.1   Ganser Syndrome

This is a complex disorder described by Ganser, characterized by approximate answers and usually accompanied by several dissociative symptoms, often in circumstances that suggest psychogenic aetiology.

The five main features of Ganser syndrome are the following:

- Approximate answers (*vorbeireden*)
- Clouding of consciousness
- Somatic conversion
- Pseudohallucinations (often)
- Subsequent amnesia

28.14.2.8.2   Multiple Personality Disorder

Controversy exists about whether multiple personality disorder (MPD) is iatrogenic or culture specific. There is an apparent existence of two or more distinct personalities within an individual, of which only one is evident at any time. Each personality is complete, with its own memories, behaviour, and preferences.

One personality is dominant. It does not have access to memories of the other and is unaware of the existence of others. The change from one personality to another is sudden and associated with stress.

Psychoanalysis views MPD as a complex, chronic developmental dissociative disorder related to severe, repetitive childhood abuse or trauma, usually beginning before the age of 5 years. Dissociative defences are used to handle subsequent traumatic experiences.

Additionally, *mass hysteria* presents with abnormal illness behaviour transmitted in close communities spreading from individuals of high status down the hierarchy. Affected individuals are suggestible. *Couvade syndrome* presents in males whose partners are pregnant, with symptoms of morning sickness, abdominal pain, and anxiety.

28.14.3   Epidemiology of Dissociative Disorder

Relatively high frequencies of dissociative experiences are reported in patients with PTSD, women with chronic pelvic pain, substance abusers (40%), patients with eating disorders, and those with a history of childhood abuse. IQ is negatively correlated.

28.14.4   Aetiology of Dissociative Disorder

Sigmund Freud introduced the term conversion to describe the unconscious rendering of innocuous of threatening ideas by conversion into physical symptoms, which have symbolic significance. This results in the relief of emotional conflict (primary gain) and the direct advantages of assuming a sick role (secondary gain).

The spectrum of dissociation (MPD is most extreme) with increasingly complex and symptomatic forms is related to increasingly severe childhood trauma.

Levels of psychological distress are highly correlated with dissociative experiences.

Of 100 substance-dependent subjects, 39 had dissociative disorder and 43 reported childhood abuse. Patients with dissociative disorder may use substances to block out more severe abuse memories and suppress dissociative symptoms.

28.14.5   Management of Dissociative Disorder

Do not confront the individual. Complete physical investigations and emphasize that serious illness is excluded. Minimize the advantages of a sick role, and praise healthy behaviour. Allow the patient to discard symptoms without losing face.

The main treatment of MPD is long-term psychoanalytic psychotherapy aimed at the unification of divided mental processes.

28.14.6   Course

Dissociative states tend to remit after a few weeks or months. Chronic states of more than 1 or 2 years are often resistant to therapy. Those with acute, recent onset, a good premorbid personality, and resolvable conflict have a better prognosis.

In a classic paper, Slater (1965) reported on a 9-year follow-up of 85 patients who were diagnosed as hysterics by senior psychiatrists and neurologists. He found that 33% developed definite organic illness, 15% had a major mental illness, and 12 patients died, 4 from suicide of whom 2 had demyelinating neurological conditions and 8 from natural causes that could have accounted for their original presentations. Of the original sample of 85, he was left with 7 young patients who had experienced acute psychogenic reactions in the form of a conversion syndrome and 14 who were suffering from lasting personality disorders. Slater concluded that the diagnosis of hysteria should not be made.

28.15 DEPERSONALIZATION–DEREALIZATION

28.15.1 DSM-5 (300.6) (APA 2013)

The presence of persistent or recurrent depersonalization, derealization, or both:

Depersonalization: Experiences of unreality, detachment, or being an outside observer with respect to one's thoughts, feelings, sensations, or actions (e.g. unreal self, perceptual alterations, emotional and/or physical numbing, distorted sense of time)

Derealization: Experiences of unreality or detachment with respect to surroundings (e.g. other people or objects are experienced as unreal, or lifeless)

During the depersonalization and/or derealization experiences, reality testing remains intact.

REFERENCES

Agarwal N, Port JD, Bazzocchi M, and Renshaw PF. 2010: Update on the use of MR for assessment and diagnosis of psychiatric diseases. *Radiology* April; 255(1):23–41.

American Psychiatric Association. 2013: *Desk Reference to the Diagnostic Criteria from DSM-5*. Washington, DC: American Psychiatric Association Press.

Andrews G, Stewart G, Morris-Yates A et al. 1990: Evidence for a general neurotic syndrome. *British Journal of Psychiatry* 157:6–12.

Argyropoulos S, Campbell A, and Stein G. 2007: Anxiety disorders. In Stein G and Wilkinson G (eds.) *Seminars in General Adult Psychiatry,* pp. 315–350. London, U.K.: Gaskell.

Beard G. 1869: Neurasthenia, or nervous exhaustion. *The Boston Medical and Surgical Journal* 217–221.

Boer JA. den. 1988: Serotonergic mechanisms in anxiety disorders. An enquiry into serotonin function in panic disorder, PhD thesis. Utrecht, the Netherlands: University of Utrecht.

Brown TA, Barlow DH, and Liebowitz MR. 1994: The empirical basis of generalized anxiety disorder. *American Journal of Psychiatry* 151:1272–1280.

Conrado LA. 2009: Body dysmorphic disorder in dermatology: Diagnosis, epidemiology and clinical aspects. *Anais brasileiros de dermatologia* 84(6):569–581.

Craig TKJ, Boardman AP, Mills K et al. 1993: The South London somatization study: I. Longitudinal course and the influence of early life experiences. *British Journal of Psychiatry* 163:579–588.

Davidson J. 1992: Drug therapy of post-traumatic stress disorder. *British Journal of Psychiatry* 160:309–314.

Dick CL, Bland RC, and Newman SC. 1994a: Panic disorder. *Acta Psychiatrica Scandinavica* (Suppl. 376):45–53.

Dick CL, Sowa B, Bland RC, and Newman SC. 1994b: Phobic disorders. *Acta Psychiatrica Scandinavica* (Suppl. 376):36–44.

Foley PB. 2009: Encephalitis lethargica and the influenza virus. II. The influenza pandemic of 1918/19 and encephalitis lethargica: Epidemiology and symptoms. *Journal of Neural Transmission* 116(10):1295–1308.

Freud S. 1953: *The Standard Edition of the Complete Psychological Works of Sigmund Freud*. London, U.K.: Hogarth.

Frost RO and Shows DL. 1993: The nature and measurement of compulsive indecisiveness. *Behaviour Research and Therapy* 31(7):683–692.

Gaston RL, Kiran-Imran F, Hassiem F, and Vaughan J. 2009: Hoarding behaviour: Building up the 'R factor'. *Advances in Psychiatric Treatment* 15:344–353.

Gelder M, Mayou R, and Cowen P. 2006: *Shorter Oxford Textbook of Psychiatry*, 5th edn. Oxford, U.K.: Oxford University Press.

Hecker E. 1893: Über larvirte und abortive Angstzustände bei Neurasthenie. *Centralblatt für Nervenheilkunde* 4:565–569.

James IA and Blackburn I-M. 1995: Cognitive therapy with obsessive–compulsive disorder. *British Journal of Psychiatry* 166:444–450.

Johnstone EC, Cunningham ODG, Lawrie SM, Sharpe M, and Freeman CPL. 2004: *Companion to Psychiatric Studies*, 7th edn. London, U.K.: Churchill Livingstone.

Kendler KS, Neale NC, Kessler RC et al. 1992: The genetic epidemiology of phobias in women: The interrelationship of agoraphobia, social phobia, situational phobia and simple phobia. *Archives of General Psychiatry* 49:273–281.

Kendler K, Neale M, Kessler R et al. 1993a: Major depression and phobias: The genetic and environmental sources of comorbidity. *Psychological Medicine* 23:361–371.

Kendler K, Neale M, Kessler R et al. 1993b: Panic disorder in women: A population based twin study. *Psychological Medicine* 23:397–406.

Kendler KS, Karkowski LM, and Prescott CA. 1999: Fears and phobias: Reliability and heritability. *Psychological Medicine* 29:539–553.

Klerman GL. 1986: The National Institute of Mental Health's Epidemiologic Catchment Areas (NIMH-ECA) program: Background, preliminary findings and implications. *Social Psychiatry* 21:159–166.

Koenen KC and Widom CS. 2009: A prospective study of sex differences in the lifetime risk of posttraumatic stress disorder among abused and neglected children grown up. *Journal of Traumatic Stress* 22(6):566–574.

Kolada JL, Bland RC, and Newman SC. 1994: Obsessive–compulsive disorder. *Acta Psychiatrica Scandinavica* (Suppl. 376):24–35.

Komossa K, Depping AM, Meyer M, Kissling W, and Leucht S. 2010: Second-generation antipsychotics for obsessive compulsive disorder. *Cochrane Database of Systematic Reviews* December; (12):CD008141.

Leckman JF, Weissman MM, Merikangas KR et al. 1985: Major depression and panic disorder: A family study perspective. *Psychopharmacological Bulletin* 21:543–545.

Loewenstein RJ and Ross DR. 1992: Multiple personality and psychoanalysis: An introduction. *Psychoanalytic Inquiry* 12:3–48.

Marks IM and Gelder MG. 1966: Different ages of onset in varieties of phobia. *American Journal of Psychiatry* 123:218–221.

Marks IM, Swinson RP, Basoglu M et al. 1993: Alprazolam and exposure alone and combined in panic disorder with agoraphobia. *British Journal of Psychiatry* 162:776–787.

McIvor RJ and Turner SW. 1995: Assessment and treatment approaches for survivors of torture. *British Journal of Psychiatry* 166:705–711.

Melamed Y, Szor H, Barak Y, and Elizur A. 1998: Hoarding—what does it mean? *Comprehensive Psychiatry* 39(6):400–402.

NICE. *NICE Guidelines for Anxiety*. http://guidance.nice.org. uk/CG22 (accessed on 6 August 2012).

NICE. *NICE Guidelines for OCD and BDD*. http://guidance. nice.org.uk/CG31 (accessed on 6 August 2012).

NICE. *NICE Guidelines for PTSD*. http://guidance.nice.org.uk/ CG26 (accessed on 6 August 2012).

Pauls DL, Alsobrook JP, Goodman W et al. 1995: A family study of obsessive–compulsive disorder. *American Journal of Psychiatry* 152:76–84.

Piccinelli M, Pini S, Bellantuono C et al. 1995: Efficacy of drug treatment in obsessive–compulsive disorder: A meta-analytic review. *British Journal of Psychiatry* 166:424–443.

Pitts FN and McClure JN. 1967: Lactate metabolism in anxiety neurosis. *New England Journal of Medicine* 13:29–36.

Robins LN. 1966: *Deviant Children Grown Up*. Baltimore, MD: Williams & Wilkins.

Roth M, Gurney C, Garside RF et al. 1972: Studies in the classification of affective disorders: The relationship between anxiety states and depressive illnesses: I. *British Journal of Psychiatry* 121:147–161.

Sadock BJ and Sadock VA. 2003: *Kaplan and Sadock's Comprehensive Textbook of Psychiatry*, 9th edn. Philadelphia, PA: Lippincott Williams & Wilkins.

Samuels J. 2007: Compulsive hoarding and OCD: Two distinct disorders? *American Journal of Psychiatry* 164:1436.

Saxena S, Brody A, Maidment K et al. 2004: Cerebral glucose metabolism in obsessive compulsive hoarding. *American Journal of Psychiatry* 161:1038–1048.

Semple D, Smyth R, Burns J, Darjee R, and McIntosh A. 2005: *Oxford Handbook of Psychiatry*. Oxford, U.K.: Oxford University Press.

Sims A and Prior P. 1978: The pattern of mortality in severe neuroses. *British Journal of Psychiatry* 133:299–305.

Slater E. 1965: Diagnosis of hysteria. *British Medical Journal* i:1395–1399.

Spector J and Huthwaite M. 1993: Eye-movement desensitisation to overcome post-traumatic stress disorder. *British Journal of Psychiatry* 163:106–108.

Stein MB, Millar TW, Larsen DK et al. 1995: Irregular breathing during sleep in patients with panic disorder. *American Journal of Psychiatry* 152:1168–1173.

Tallis F. 1995: Reading about obsessive–compulsive disorder. *British Journal of Psychiatry* 166:546–550.

Taylor D, Paton C, and Kapur S. 2009: *The Maudsley Prescribing Guideline*, 10th edn. London, U.K.: Informa Healthcare.

Tolin DF, Frost RO, and Steketee G. 2007: An open trial of cognitive-behavioral therapy for compulsive hoarding. *Behaviour Research and Therapy* 7:1461–1470.

Torgersen S. 1983: Genetic factors in anxiety disorders. *Archives of General Psychiatry* 40:1085–1089.

Torgersen S. 1985: Hereditary differentiation of anxiety and affective neuroses. *British Journal of Psychiatry* 146:530–534.

Torgersen S. 1986: Genetics of somatoform disorders. *Archives of General Psychiatry* 43:502–505.

Tyrer P, Seivewright N, Ferguson B et al. 1993: The Nottingham study of neurotic disorder: Effect of personality status on response to drug treatment, cognitive therapy and self-help over two years. *British Journal of Psychiatry* 162:219–226.

Tyrer P, Seivewright N, Murphy S et al. 1988: The Nottingham study of neurotic disorder: Comparison of drug and psychological treatments. *Lancet* ii:235–240.

Versiani M, Nardi AE, Mundim FD. et al. 1992: Pharmacotherapy of social phobia: A controlled study with moclobemide and phenelzine. *British Journal of Psychiatry* 161:353–360.

Winsberg ME, Cassic KS, and Koran LM. 1999: Hoarding in obsessive compulsive disorder: A report of 20 cases. *Journal of Clinical Psychiatry* 60:591–597.

World Health Organization. 1992: *ICD-10: The ICD-10 Classification of Mental and Behavioural Disorders: Clinical Descriptions and Diagnostic Guidelines*. Geneva, Switzerland: World Health Organization.

Zhang H, Leckman JF, Pauls DL, Tsai CP, Kidd KK, Campos MR; Tourette Syndrome Association International Consortium for Genetics. 2002: Genomewide scan of hoarding in sib pairs in which both sibs have Gilles de la Tourette syndrome. *American Journal of Human Genetics* 70(4):896–904.

29 Personality Disorders

29.1 HISTORY

- Hippocrates described four temperaments: melancholic, sanguine, phlegmatic, and choleric.
- In 1801, Pinel described manie sans délire (Campbell, 1996).
- In 1835, Prichard described moral insanity (Kaplan, 1952).
- In 1906, Kraepelin described psychopathic personality: excitable, unstable, eccentric, liars, swindlers, antisocial, and quarrelsome subtypes (Koizumi et al., 1964).
- Schneider (1958) subsequently extended the concept of psychopathic personality to include suffering to the self as well as to society.
- In 1938, Stern coined the term 'borderline', which signified a new disorder that is at the border between schizophrenia and neurosis (Stern, 1938).
- In 1939, Henderson's psychopathic states included three subtypes: aggressive, inadequate, and creative psychopaths (Henderson, 1939).
- In 1955, Cleckley described sociopathy: unreliable, untruthful, lacking remorse, poor motivation, and antisocial behaviour (Hare and Neumann, 2008).
- In 1967, Kernberg introduced the concept of borderline personality organization and use of primitive defences (Kernberg, 1975).
- In 1978, Eysenck called for a dimensional rather than a categorical approach to the description of personality (Eysenck and Eysenck, 1975).

Details of personality development are considered in Chapter 5.

29.2 CLASSIFICATION AND MEASUREMENT

29.2.1 DIMENSIONAL APPROACH

Personality disorder differs from normal variation only in terms of degree. It assumes that universal traits are present in all people in differing degrees. Personality traits of some individuals are sufficiently maladaptive and abnormal as to constitute personality disorder.

29.2.1.1 Cattell's Trait Theory

Cattell identified 20,000 words describing personality. Using factor analysis, he derived 16 first-order personality factors (PFs). Cattell's 16-PF test was devised on the basis of this work. Second-order factor analysis resulted in three broad dimensions similar to Eysenck's dimensions:

- Sociability (extra/intra)
- Anxiety
- Intelligence

29.2.1.2 Eysenck's Theory

Factor analysis of rating scale data yields orthogonal dimensions, assumed to be normally distributed:

- Neuroticism/stability
- Extroversion/introversion
- Psychoticism/stability
- Intelligence

Personality inventories have been used to measure these traits. The Maudsley Personality Inventory (MPI) was superseded by the Eysenck Personality Inventory (EPI), which in turn was superseded by the Eysenck Personality Questionnaire (EPQ)—measuring psychoticism and containing a lie scale.

29.2.1.3 Minnesota Multiphasic Personality Inventory

In this lengthy inventory, the subject answers 'true', 'false', or 'cannot say'. It is empirically constructed and measures traits. It is widely used.

29.2.1.4 Rorschach Inkblot Test

This is a projective test analysing fantasy material.

29.2.1.5 Rotter's Internal–External Locus of Control

Individuals vary along a continuum in their perception of the locus of control of events. Those attributing events to an internal source are more confident about changing their life and environment.

29.2.2 CATEGORICAL APPROACH

This approach groups people into discrete categories. It is simple and widely used, but most individuals do not conform to categories:

- Kretschmer linked body-build with personality:
  - Pyknic—sociable and relaxed
  - Asthenic—self-conscious and solitary
  - Athletic—robust and outgoing
- Sheldon also linked build with personality:
  - Endomorphic—viscerotonic personality
  - Ectomorphic—cerebrotonic personality
  - Mesomorphic—somatotonic personality

29.3 ICD-10 AND PROPOSED DSM-5 CLASSIFICATIONS

These are primarily categorical classifications, but they incorporate a dimensional approach, allowing the recording of personality traits subthreshold for a diagnosis of personality disorder (Table 29.1).

The DSM-5 proposes criterion A for all personality disorder, which includes the following (Table 29.2):

1. Impairments in self-functioning (a or b)
   a. Identity: confused boundaries between self and others; distorted self-concept; emotional expression often not congruent with context or internal experience
   b. Self-direction: unrealistic or incoherent goals: no clear set of internal standards
2. Impairments in interpersonal functioning (a or b)
   a. Empathy: pronounced difficulty understanding impact of own behaviours on others; frequent misinterpretations of others' motivations and behaviours
   b. Intimacy: marked impairments in developing close relationships, associated with mistrust and anxiety

The DSM-5 continues to classify personality disorders under cluster A, cluster B and cluster C personality disorders as in DSM-IV-TR. The cluster system is a good way to classify personality disorder.

29.4 STATISTICS

A gradient exists in the prevalence of personality disorders from community to inpatient setting (see Table 29.3).

TABLE 29.1

Comparison between the ICD-10 and Proposed DSM-5 Criteria

	ICD-10 (WHO, 1992)	DSM-5 (APA, 2013)
General criteria	• Individual's characteristic and experience and behaviour as a whole deviate markedly from the culturally expected and accepted range in cognition, affectivity, control over impulses, and manners of relating to other people. • No emphasis on personality trait	• Impairments in cognition, affectivity, interpersonal function and impulse control • Inflexible and enduring pattern for long duration • The impairments in personality functioning and personality trait expression are not better understood as normative for the individual's developmental stage or sociocultural environment
Criteria on stability	• The behaviour must be inflexible and maladaptive • Dysfunctional across a broad range of personal and social situations • The deviation is stable and of long duration, having its onset in late childhood and adolescence	• The impairments in personality functioning and the personality trait expression are stable across time and consistent across situations
Exclusion criteria	• Other adult mental disorders • Organic brain disease, injury, and dysfunction	• Direct physiological effects of a substance (e.g. a drug of abuse, medication) • General medical condition (e.g. severe head trauma)
Criteria on functioning	• Not emphasize on functioning	• Significant impairments in self (identity or self-direction) and interpersonal (empathy or intimacy) functioning

TABLE 29.2

Comparison and Contrast between the Types of Personality Disorders Listed in ICD-10 and DSM-5

ICD-10 (WHO, 1992)	DSM-5 (APA, 2013)
F60.0 Paranoid personality disorder	Cluster A Personality disorders
F60.1 Schizoid personality disorder	301.0 Paranoid personality disorder
F60.2 Dissocial personality disorder	301.2 Schizoid personality disorder
	301.22 Schizotypal personality disorder
F60.3 Emotionally unstable personality disorder (.30 impulsive type; .31 borderline type)	Cluster B Personality disorders
	301.7 Antisocial personality disorder
	301.83 Borderline personality disorder
	301.5 Histrionic personality disorder
	301.81 Narcissistic personality disorder
F60.4 Histrionic personality disorder	Cluster C Personality disorders
F60.5 Anankastic personality disorder	301.82 Avoidant personality disorder
F60.6 Anxious (avoidant) personality disorder	301.6 Dependent personality disorder
	301.4 Obsessive-compulsive personality disorder
F60.7 Dependent personality disorder	Other Personality disorders
F60.8 Other specific personality disorders (eccentric, haltlose, immature, narcissistic, passive-aggressive, and psychoneurotic)	310.1 Personality change due to another medical condition
F60.9 Personality disorder unspecified	301.89 Other personality disorder

The following are the approximate prevalences of personality disorder:

- Community 10%
- General practice 20%
- Psychiatric outpatients 30%
- Psychiatric inpatients 40%

TABLE 29.3

Prevalence of Personality Disorders in Different Settings

Personality Disorder	Prevalence		
	Community	Outpatients	Inpatients
Paranoid	0.5%–2.5%	2%–10%	10%–30%
Schizoid	0.5%–1.5%	Uncommon	
Schizotypal	3%		
Antisocial	3% in males 1% in females	3%–30%	
Borderline	1%–2%	10%	20%
Histrionic	2%–3%		10%–15%
Narcissistic	0.4%–0.8%		2%–16%
Avoidant	0.5%–1.0%	10%	
Dependent	1%–1.7%		
Obsessive–compulsive	1.7%–2.2%	3%–10%	

The American Epidemiologic Catchment Area (ECA) study found, using a diagnostic interview schedule, a prevalence of personality disorder in the community of 6%.

29.5   CLUSTER A PERSONALITY DISORDERS

- Cluster A: paranoid, schizoid, and schizotypal personality disorders—odd or eccentric

Common defence mechanisms: projection, fantasy, and denial

29.5.1   SCHIZOID PERSONALITY DISORDER

29.5.1.1   Epidemiology

- Prevalence: 0.5%–1.5%
- Gender ratio: M/F = 2:1

29.5.1.2   Aetiology

- Genetics: Schizoid personality disorder is more common among the first-degree relatives of schizophrenia patients. The heritability of schizoid personality disorder is 0.55.
- Development: Parents are experienced as cold and neglectful, leading to the belief that relationships are not worth pursuing.

TABLE 29.4

ICD-10 Criteria and Mnemonics for Schizoid Personality Disorder

ICD-10 Criteria	Mnemonics (Robinson, 2001)
Met general criteria for personality disorder and ≥4 symptoms	*SIR SAFE*
Affect	Solitary lifestyle
1. Emotional coldness, detachment, or flattened affectivity	Indifferent to praise and criticism
2. Limited capacity to express either warm, tender feelings, or anger towards others	Relationships: no interest
3. Appear to be indifferent to either praise or criticism	Sexual experience: no interest
Behaviour	Activities: solitary
1. Few, if any, activities provide pleasure	Friendships: few friends
2. Little interest in having sexual experiences with another person (taking into account age)	Emotions: cold and detached
3. Consistent choice of solitary activities	
4. No desire for or possession of any close friends or confiding relationships (or only one)	
Cognition	
1. Excessive preoccupation with fantasy and introspection	
2. Marked insensitivity to prevailing social norms and conventions (which is unintentional)	

29.5.1.3 Diagnostic Criteria

(See Table 29.4.)

29.5.1.4 Elicit Schizoid Personality in CASC

- Do you care about what other people say about you? How do you feel if other people criticize you?
- Are you in touch with your emotion?
- Do you tend to enjoy being around with people or do you prefer to be alone?
- How many friends do you have in your whole life?
- What kind of activity do you prefer? Do you have intimacy with other people?

29.5.1.5 Differential Diagnosis

1. Other personality disorders
   - People with paranoid personality disorder are easier to be engaged, and they are more resentful than people with schizoid personality disorder.
2. Pervasive developmental disorders
   - People with schizoid personality disorder have better communication and fewer

stereotypical behaviours in comparison to people with autism and Asperger's syndrome.
3. Schizophrenia
   - People with schizoid personality disorder do not exhibit first-rank symptoms.
   - People with schizotypal disorder are more eccentric with disturbed perception and thought form.

29.5.1.6 Management

1. Most individuals rarely seek treatment because of poor insight into associated problems. They have low capacity for relationship and motivation.
2. Supportive psychotherapy is useful to establish therapeutic alliance. As trust increases, the therapist may be able to access fantasies.
3. Medications: Low-dose antipsychotics and antidepressants have been used with varied outcomes.

29.5.1.7 Course

Schizoid personality disorder has an early onset with stable course.

29.5.2 SCHIZOTYPAL DISORDER

29.5.2.1 Epidemiology

Prevalence: 3%
Gender ratio: male > female

29.5.2.2 Aetiology

- Kety et al. (1971) in an adoption study demonstrated that abnormalities were more common in the biological relatives of schizophrenics than in adoptive relatives or controls ('schizophrenia spectrum disorders'). From this derived the operational criteria for schizotypal personality disorder. Almost all studies of the families of schizophrenic probands have found an excess of both schizophrenia and schizotypal personality disorder among relatives (22% in the biological relatives of schizophrenics vs. 2% of adoptive relatives and controls).
- The heritability is 0.72.
- Common biological abnormalities shared by schizophrenia and schizotypal disorder:
  1. Dopamine dysregulation: raised CSF HVA concentrations
  2. Reduction in temporal lobe volumes
  3. Impaired smooth pursuit eye movements
  4. Impaired tests of executive functioning

TABLE 29.5

ICD-10 Criteria, Proposed DSM-5 Criteria, and Mnemonics for Schizotypal Disorder

ICD-10 Criteria	DSM-5 Criteria	Mnemonics
ICD-10 considers schizotypal disorder under schizophrenia, schizotypal, and delusional disorder rather than personality disorder.	Psychoticism a. Eccentricity: odd, unusual, or bizarre behaviour or appearance b. Cognitive and perceptual dysregulation Odd or unusual thought processes; odd sensations c. Unusual beliefs and experiences: unusual experiences of reality	*UFO IDEA* Unusual perception Friendless except first-degree family Odd beliefs and speech Ideas of reference Doubt about motives of other people Eccentric appearance and behaviour Affect: inappropriate or constricted
Duration: 2 years Appearance a. Eccentric appearance b. Odd behaviour		
Cognitive a. Odd beliefs or magical thinking that influences behaviour and inconsistent with subcultural norms b. Rumination without inner resistance c. Vague, circumstantial, metaphorical, overelaborate, or stereotyped thinking	Detachment a. Restricted affectivity: constricted emotional experience and indifference b. Withdrawal: avoidance of social contacts and activity	
Affect or emotion a. Inappropriate or constricted affect	Negative affectivity a. Suspiciousness: expectations of and heightened sensitivity to signs of interpersonal ill-intent or harm; doubts about loyalty and fidelity of others; feelings of persecution	
Perception a. Unusual perceptions and experiences b. Occasional transient quasipsychotic episodes with intense illusions, auditory or other hallucinations, and delusion-like ideas		
Relationship a. Socially withdrawn b. Suspicious or paranoid		

29.5.2.3 Clinical Features

(See Table 29.5.)

29.5.2.4 Elicit Schizotypal Disorder in CASC

- Can you share me some of your ideas at this moment?
- Do you feel that you have some special powers? How about magical power?
- Do you have any unusual experience? How do you experience it (e.g. by seeing or hearing)?
- Do you have friends? Can you trust people?
- How do other people find you? Do they find you odd?

29.5.2.5 Differential Diagnosis

1. Delusional disorder, schizophrenia, and severe depressive disorder with psychotic features
2. Other personality disorders

a. Paranoid and schizoid personality disorder: People with paranoid and schizoid personality disorder do not have perceptual or cognitive disturbances.
b. Borderline personality disorder: People with borderline personality disorder may have brief psychotic experiences, which are closely related to their affective states.
c. Avoidant personality disorder: People with avoidant personality disorder may seek closeness with other people.
3. Pervasive development disorder: autism and Asperger's syndrome

29.5.2.6 Management

1. Supportive therapy and social skill training.
2. Antipsychotic drugs (e.g. risperidone or olanzapine) may lead to mild to moderate improvement in psychotic symptoms.

TABLE 29.6

ICD-10 Criteria and Mnemonics for Paranoid Personality Disorder

ICD-10 Criteria	Mnemonics (Robinson, 2001)
At least four of the following	GET FACT
Behaviour	Grudges are held without justification
1. Tendency to bear grudges (feeling resentful about something) persistently	Excessive sensitivity to setbacks
Cognition:	Threats and hidden meanings are read into benign remarks
1. Excessive sensitivity to setbacks and rebuffs	Fidelity of spouse is unjustifiably doubted
2. Suspiciousness and a pervasive tendency to distort experience by misconstruing the neutral or friendly actions of others as hostile or contemptuous	Attacks on character or reputation are perceived
3. Combative and tenacious sense of personal rights out of keeping with the actual situation	Confides reluctantly because of fears of betrayal
4. Recurrent suspicions, without justification regarding sexual fidelity of spouse/sexual partner	Trustworthiness of others is doubted without due cause
5. Persistent self-referential attitude, associated particularly with excessive self-importance	
6. Preoccupation with unsubstantiated 'conspiratorial' explanations of events immediate either to the person or in the world at large	

29.5.2.7 Course and Prognosis

1. Schizotypal disorder has a relatively stable course, with only a small proportion (10%) of individuals going on to develop schizophrenia.
2. Clinical features such as magical thinking, paranoid ideation, and social isolation are associated with an increased risk to develop schizophrenia.

29.5.3 PARANOID PERSONALITY DISORDER

29.5.3.1 Epidemiology

- Prevalence: 0.5%–2.5%
- Gender ratio: male > female

29.5.3.2 Aetiology

1. The heritability is 0.69.
2. Paranoid personality disorder is more common among the first-degree relatives of schizophrenia patients.
3. There is a lack of protective care and support in childhood. Excessive parental rage and humiliation cause feelings of inadequacy resulted in projection onto others of hostility and rage.
4. Temperament is characterized by nonadaptability and tendency to hyperactivity and intense emotions.
5. Sensory impairments: impaired vision and hearing and victims of traumatic brain injury.
6. Social factors: new immigrants and ethnic minority.

29.5.3.3 Clinical Features

(See Table 29.6.)

29.5.3.4 Elicit Paranoid Personality Disorder in CASC

1. How do you find other people in general? Can you trust them?
2. Have you encountered any setback recently? What is the reason behind it? Do you think that there is a conspiracy that purposely screws you up?
3. How do you feel about your spouse or partner? Is he or she loyal to you?
4. How do you feel about your neighbours? Are they doing something behind you?
5. Why do you think all these people are against you? Is it because you are an important person and they screw you up on purpose?

29.5.3.5 Differential Diagnosis

- Delusional disorder: People with delusional disorder have their delusions well encapsulated and systematized, but people with paranoid personality disorder do not have well-formed delusions.
- Schizophrenia: People with schizophrenia exhibit first-rank and negative symptoms.
- Severe depressive episode with psychotic features: mood congruent delusions such as delusions of guilt or nihilistic delusions.
- Substance misuse: for example, amphetamine or cannabis.

- Other personality disorders
  - Borderline personality disorder: Transient paranoia is common but not as persistent as in paranoid personality disorder.
  - Schizoid personality disorder: appears to be more indifferent.
  - Narcissistic personality disorder: Paranoia may occur as a result to the threat of an imagined success.
  - Avoidant personality disorder: They tend to avoid other people as a result of lack of self-confidence or fear of embarrassment.

29.5.3.6 Management

1. Supportive psychotherapy or problem-solving therapy.
2. Cognitive–behavioural therapy (CBT)
   a. Cognitive therapy targets at the core beliefs such as others are malicious and deceptive. Patient needs to realize that there is a need to reduce suspiciousness.
   b. In behaviour therapy, patient is involved in role play to handle hostility and personal attacks in daily life. Patient is advised to record their ideas in the dysfunction thought diary.
3. Psychotropic medications: Antidepressants and antipsychotics are indicated to treat mood and psychotic symptoms.

29.5.3.7 Course and Prognosis

1. The hypersensitivity results in poor peer relationships and eccentricity.
2. Paranoid ideas may intensify when patient is under stress.
3. Some patients with paranoid personality disorder may develop agoraphobia.

29.6 CLUSTER B PERSONALITY DISORDERS

- Cluster B: antisocial, borderline, histrionic, and narcissistic personality disorders—dramatic, emotional, or erratic

Common defence mechanisms: splitting, dissociation, denial, acting out, and projective identification

29.6.1 BORDERLINE PERSONALITY DISORDER

29.6.1.1 Epidemiology

- Prevalence: 1%–2%
- Gender ratio: M/F = 1:2
- Age of onset: adolescence or early adulthood
- Suicide rate: 9%

29.6.1.2 Aetiology

29.6.1.2.1 Biological Factors

- Family studies show the risk of relatives of borderline personality disorder to develop the same disorder is five times higher as compared to the general population.
- Concordance rate of monozygotic (MZ) versus dizygotic (DZ) twins: 35% versus 10%.
- Borderline personality disorder is more common in first-degree relatives of patients with depression.
- Some studies demonstrate abnormal dexamethasone suppression test result, decreased REM latency, decreased thyrotropin response, and abnormal sensitivity to amphetamine in patients with borderline personality disorder.
- Specific marker for impulsivity: decreased CSF 5HIAA, which is a metabolite of serotonin.
- Chronic trauma leads to decreased hippocampal volume, decreased hemispheric integration, and hyperactive hypothalamic–pituitary–gonadal (HPA) axis.
- Goyer et al. (1994) in a PET scanning study of personality-disordered subjects found a significant inverse correlation between a history of aggressive impulse difficulties and regional cerebral metabolic rates in the frontal cortex. Those subjects with borderline personality disorders had significantly reduced frontal cortex metabolism.
- Increased bilateral activity in amygdala after exposure to emotionally aversive stimuli.
- Orbitofrontal cortex abnormalities lead to reduction in cortical modulation of amygdala. Such abnormalities are associated with impulsivity, affect dysregulation, chronic feeling of emptiness, and decreased mentalization.

29.6.1.2.2 Early Development

- Borderline personality is the result of a lack of stable involved attachment during development. This leads to an inability to maintain a stable sense of self or others without ongoing contact. The child will have limited capacity to depict feelings and thoughts in self and other people. This capacity is known as mentalization.
- Family environment is characterized high conflict and unpredictability. The caregiver is not emotionally available.

- Emotionally vulnerable temperament interacts with an invalidating environment.
- Early separation or loss.
- History of parental substance misuse or forensic history in parents.

29.6.1.2.3   Past Trauma and Abuse

- Childhood trauma: Borderline personality results from early traumatic experiences occurring within a context of sustained neglect resulting in enduring rage and self-hatred.
- Physical or sexual abuse.

29.6.1.2.4   Defence Mechanisms

- Splitting—adopting a polarized or extreme view of the world where people are either all good or all bad and fail to see that each person has good and bad aspects. For example, a patient with borderline personality disorder tries to classify the doctors of the ward into two groups, good doctors and bad doctors. The patient fails to see the strengths and weaknesses of each doctor.
- Projective identification—the patient unconsciously projects a figure onto the other people. For example, a man does not like his father and projects a bad father figure onto the male doctor (projection) and accuses the doctor as a noncaring individual. As a result of countertransference, the male doctor tries to avoid the patient as if he does not care about the patient (identification).

29.6.1.3   Clinical Features

The ICD-10 classifies emotionally unstable personality disorder into impulsive and borderline type. The DSM-5 does not propose the concept of emotionally unstable personality disorder and only has borderline personality disorder.

29.6.1.3.1   Emotionally Unstable Personality Disorder: Impulsive Type (ICD-10)

The patient met the general criteria for personality disorder and at least three of the following symptoms of impulsive type:

Affect

1. Tendency to outbursts of anger or violence, with inability to control the resulting behavioural explosions
2. Unstable and capricious mood

Behaviour

1. Marked tendency to act unexpectedly and without consideration of consequences
2. Marked tendency of quarrelsome behaviour and conflicts with others, especially when impulsive acts are thwarted or criticized
3. Difficulty in maintaining any course of action that offers no immediate reward (Table 29.7).

29.6.1.4   Elicit Borderline Personality Disorder in CASC

1. Do you have problem with your anger control? How often do you get into quarrels?
2. How often do you feel empty inside yourself? What would you do when you feel empty?
3. How is your relationship with other people?
4. How do you feel if your friend or partner left you? Do you have a strong feeling of abandonment?
5. Do you think that your friends would view you as a moody person?
6. How often do you hurt yourself (e.g. cutting or burning)? Why do you cut yourself? Do you want to reexperience the pain in the past?

29.6.1.5   Differential Diagnosis

1. Depressive disorder: People with borderline personality disorder may present with depression, but people with depressive disorder do not demonstrate primitive defence mechanisms such as splitting or projective identification.
2. Bipolar disorder: Both borderline personality disorder and bipolar disorder may present with mood swings. People with borderline personality disorder refer mood swings as fluctuations in mood from normal to irritability without hypomania or mania.
3. Post-traumatic stress disorder (PTSD): People with PTSD usually present with flashbacks, hypervigilance, and nightmares of the traumatic event but do not exhibit primitive defence mechanisms.
4. Schizophrenia: Both borderline personality disorder and schizophrenia may present with psychotic symptoms. People with borderline personality disorder present with transient psychosis or visual illusions. Negative symptoms and first-rank symptoms are uncommon in borderline personality disorder.

TABLE 29.7

Comparison of the ICD-10 Criteria, the Proposed DSM-5 Criteria, and Mnemonics for Borderline Personality Disorder

ICD-10 Criteria	DSM-5 Criteria	Mnemonics (Robinson, 2001)

Borderline type (ICD-10)
 	
The borderline type requires the person to meet the diagnostic criteria of impulsive type and an additional two symptoms in the following:
 	
Affect
1. Chronic feelings of emptiness
 	
Behaviour
1. Liability to become involved in intense and unstable relationships, often leading to emotional crises
2. Excessive efforts to avoid abandonment
3. Recurrent threats or acts of self-harm
 	
Cognition
1. Disturbances in and uncertainty about self-image, aims, and internal preferences (including sexual)
	1. Negative affectivity
	  a. Emotional lability: unstable emotional experiences and frequent mood changes
	  b. Anxiousness: intense feelings of nervousness or panic in reaction to interpersonal stresses and fears of losing control
	  c. Separation insecurity: fears of rejection by or separation from significant others and associated with fears of excessive dependency and complete loss of autonomy
	  d. Depression: frequent feelings of being down, miserable, or hopelessness
	2. Disinhibition
	  a. Impulsivity: acting on the spur of the moment in response to immediate stimuli; acting on a momentary basis without a plan or consideration of outcomes; difficulty establishing or following plans; a sense of urgency and self-harming behaviour under emotional distress
	  b. Risk taking: engagement in dangerous, risky, and potentially self-damaging activities
	3. Antagonism
	  a. Hostility: persistent or frequent angry feelings; anger or irritability
		I RAISED A PAIN
		Identity disturbance
		Relationships: unstable
		Abandonment: fear of impulsivity
		Self-harm
		Emptiness
		Dissociative symptoms
		Affective instability
		Paranoid ideation
		Anger
		Idealization and devaluation
		Negativistic – undermine the efforts of self and others

5. Other personality disorders
   a. Dependent personality disorder: People with dependent personality disorder are less chaotic in affect regulation and less impulsive.
   b. Antisocial personality disorder: People with antisocial personality disorder have history of forensic problems and do not concern about the safety of other people.
   c. Histrionic personality disorder: People with histrionic personality disorder want to be the centre of attention but usually demonstrate less self-harm, emptiness, and affective instability.
   d. Narcissistic personality disorder: People with narcissistic personality disorder see rejection as humiliating. People with borderline personality disorder see rejection as abandonment. People with borderline personality disorder feel that they are entitled to special treatment because they suffered in the past. People with narcissistic personality disorder feel that they are entitled to special treatment because of their special status.
   e. Identity confusion in normal adolescence development.

Comorbidity: depression, PTSD, substance misuse, and bulimia nervosa

29.6.2 MANAGEMENT

29.6.2.1 Inpatient Treatment and Therapeutic Communities

This is controversial. Currently, there is a trend away from long-term admissions for borderline patients, probably driven by cost containment. There is evidence to support the value of therapeutic communities such as the Henderson or the Cassel Hospital. The therapeutic community approach is a multicomponent treatment programme, incorporating individual therapy, ward groups, and patient participation in the maintenance of the community.

Indications for admission include (Paris, 2004)

1. Life-threatening suicide attempt
2. Imminent danger to other people
3. Psychosis
4. Severe symptoms interfering with functioning that are unresponsive to outpatient treatment

The risks of hospitalization to the patient include

- Stigma
- Disruption of social and occupational roles
- Loss of freedom
- Hospital-induced behavioural regression

Some consider the drawing up of a contract between the patient and doctor essential to the success of inpatient care. Miller (1989) considers a good treatment contract to incorporate the following:

- Mutual agreement by all involved parties.
- Specific, focused, achievable goals with strategies to achieve them.
- Specific responsibilities of patient and staff.
- Provision of the minimum degree of structure necessary.
- Patient foregoing his or her usual means of managing intolerable feelings; alternative strategies are provided.
- Positive reinforcement of desirable behaviour.
- Not being drawn up when staff have unresolved punitive wishes towards the patient.
- Strictly enforced, but room for negotiated modification.

The alternative approach of brief admissions at the time of crisis is increasingly popular.

The NICE guidelines recommend the following:

29.6.2.2 Psychotherapy

1. Long-term outpatient psychotherapy is recommended because patients can handle challenges in daily life with the support from psychotherapists.
2. Dialectical behaviour therapy (DBT) and mentalization-based therapy are recommended treatment for people with borderline personality disorder. Details of DBT and mentalization-based treatment are considered in Chapter 25.
3. The NICE guidelines recommend that therapists should use an explicit and integrated theoretical approach and share this with their clients.
4. The guidelines also recommend that the therapists should set therapy at twice per week and should not offer brief psychological interventions (less than 3 months duration).
5. Other psychotherapies
   a. Supportive psychotherapy: diminish suicidal behaviour and impulsive acts while awaiting a remission since the long-term prognosis of this disorder is good.
   b. CBT: Cognitive therapy focuses on maladaptive cognitions about oneself and other people. Behaviour therapy improves social and emotional functioning.
   c. Schema-focused therapy: aims at modifying schemas (e.g. fear of abandonment), reducing self-harm behaviour, and improving interpersonal relationship.
   d. Transference-focused therapy: aims at correcting distorted perceptions of significant others and decreasing symptoms and self-destructive behaviour.
   e. Family therapy is frequently offered to borderline adolescent patients and is regarded by many as the treatment of choice for these patients.
   f. Social skill training.

29.6.2.3 Pharmacotherapy

1. The psychiatrist can prescribe an SSRI (e.g. fluoxetine) to treat mood lability, rejection sensitivity, and anger.
2. If the second SSRI is not effective, the psychiatrist can consider adding a low-dose antipsychotic (e.g. quetiapine) for anger control or an anxiolytic (e.g. clonazepam) for anxiety control.
3. Mood stabilizers such as sodium valproate and carbamazepine can be added if the aforementioned medications are not effective.
4. It is recommended not to use psychotropic medications that have narrow therapeutic index such as lithium or tricyclic antidepressants, which are toxic during overdose.

29.6.2.4 Course and Prognosis

1. Impulsivity improves significantly over time. Affective symptoms have the least improvement.
2. A 15-year follow-up of 100 borderline personality-disordered patients found that 75% were no longer diagnosed as borderline. All scales showed a reduction of symptomatic behaviour, with a clear functional improvement. However, there is a high risk of suicide, with 8.5% completing suicide in the 15-year follow-up period. Those patients with chronic depression, good motivation, a psychological attitude, low impulsiveness, and a stable environment are most responsive to treatment.
3. Poor prognosis is associated with early childhood sexual abuse, early first psychiatric contact, chronicity of symptoms, high affective instability, aggression, and substance use disorder.

29.6.3 DISSOCIAL PERSONALITY DISORDER

29.6.3.1 Epidemiology

- There is a lifetime prevalence of 2.3%–3.6%.
- The male-to-female sex ratio is 7:1.
- It is twice as prevalent in inner cities compared to rural areas.
- Antisocial behaviours usually start at age 8–10 years. They do not develop after age 18.
- The highest lifetime prevalence is in the 25–44-year-old group, followed by the 18–24-year-old group.
- Subjects are less likely to be married and less well educated.

29.6.3.2 Aetiology

29.6.3.2.1 Biological Causes

Genetic causes: Most twin and adoption studies suggest that antisocial personality disorder has a partial genetic aetiology (see Table 33.2). The heritable form of criminality is associated with petty recidivism and property offences rather than violent crime (Table 29.8).

Mednick et al. (1984) studied 14,427 adoptees and their biological and adoptive parents. The effect was stronger when the biological mother was convicted than if the biological father was convicted. Association was for property offences only, playing a significant role in repeat offences; it did not apply to violent offences.

Robins (1966) found that the father's criminal behaviour was the single best predictor of antisocial behaviour in a child.

TABLE 29.8

Percentages of Convictions in Male Adoptees and the Biological and Adoptive Parents

	Conviction Rate
Neither biological nor adoptive parent convicted	13.5%
Adoptive parents convicted. Biological parents not convicted	14.7%
Adoptive parents not convicted Biological parents convicted	20.0%
Adoptive and biological parents convicted	24.5%

MZ to DZ concordance rates for adult criminality are 52%:22%. This suggests a definite genetic contribution. However, concordance rates of 87%:72% for juvenile delinquency are suggestive of a familial but not a genetic component to aetiology.

Within a family that has a member with antisocial personality disorder, males more often have antisocial personality disorder and substance-related disorders, whereas females more often have somatization disorder. However, in such families, there is an increase in the prevalence of all of these disorders in both males and females compared with the general population.

It is suggested that family background plays a part in subsequent criminality but only when there is already a genetic predisposition. The risk of criminality is increased in those with prolonged institutional care and multiple temporary placements and those where the socioeconomic status of their adoptive home is low:

- Dysfunctional serotonin: low 5HIAA in CSF and associated with hostile and aggressive behaviour.
- Imaging findings
  - Structural MRI shows reduction in volume of temporal lobes but not frontal lobes. The reduction of temporal lobe volumes is associated with violent and sexually aggressive behaviour.
  - Functional MRI shows reduction in cerebral blood flow (CBF) in the prefrontal cortex, orbitofrontal cortex, and amygdala. The reduction in CBF in amygdala is associated with callous and unemotional trait.
- EEG studies in antisocial personality disorders demonstrate abnormalities that have led to speculation that psychopathic behaviour reflects cortical immaturity. Abnormalities found in this group more often than in normal include

- Generalized widespread slow (⊖) wave activity
- 'Positive spike' abnormality over temporal lobes
- Localized temporal slow-wave activity

These abnormalities are more likely to occur in highly impulsive and aggressive psychopaths.

29.6.3.2.2 *Developmental Causes*

- Parental deprivation and antisocial behaviour. For example, witnessed abuse when the patient was young.
- Inconsistent or harsh parenting.
- Frequent moves or migration, large family size, and poverty.
- Childhood risk factors include cruelty to animals, enuresis, innate aggression, and fire setting.

29.6.3.2.3 *Psychological Causes*

- Temperament: high novelty seeking, low harm avoidance, low reward dependence, and uncooperativeness

29.6.3.3 Clinical Features

(See Table 29.9.)

29.6.3.4 Elicit Dissocial Personality Disorder in CASC

1. How do you see the authority? Are you upset if people give you order? What would you do to the authority if you are upset with them?
2. How do you see other people? Are you often involved in fights with others? Are you concerned about safety of other people?
3. How do you see about commitment or obligation? Are you able to keep your promise?

TABLE 29.9

Comparison of the ICD-10 Criteria, the Proposed DSM-5 Criteria, and Mnemonics for Dissocial Personality Disorder

ICD-10 Criteria	DSM-5 Criteria	Mnemonics
ICD-10 criteria	Antagonism	*CALL ASPD*
Affect	a. Manipulativeness: frequent use of subterfuge to influence or control others	Conduct disorder before age 15
1. Very low tolerance to frustration and a low threshold for discharge of aggression, including violence	b. Deceitfulness: dishonesty and fraudulence or misrepresentation of self	Antisocial activities
2. Incapacity to experience guilt or to profit from adverse experience, particularly punishment	c. Callousness: lack of concern for feelings or problems of others; lack of guilt or remorse	Lies frequently
Behaviour	d. Hostility: persistent or frequent angry feelings; anger or irritability in response to minor insults	Lack of superego
3. Incapacity to maintain enduring relationships, though no difficulty in establishing them		Aggression
4. Marked proneness to blame the others or to offer plausible rationalizations for the behaviour that has brought the individual into conflict with society	Disinhibition	Safety of others being ignored
Cognition	a. Irresponsibility: failure to honour obligations or commitments and lack of follow-through on agreements and promises	Planning failure
5. Callous unconcern for the feelings of others Gross and persistent attitude of irresponsibility and disregard for social norms, rules, and obligations	b. Impulsivity: acting on the spur of the moment in response to immediate stimuli; acting on a momentary basis without a plan or consideration of outcomes; difficulty establishing and following plans	Denial of obligation
	c. Risk taking: engagement in dangerous, risky, and potentially self-damaging activities, unnecessarily and without regard for consequences; boredom proneness and thoughtless initiation of activities to counter boredom; lack of concern for one's limitations and denial of the reality of personal danger	

4. Do you tell lies if there is a chance?
5. Have you ever been arrested or pulled over by the police?

29.6.3.5 Differential Diagnosis

1. Temporary antisocial behaviour (e.g. vandalism or riot), focal behaviour, not exploitive, and with conscience preserved.
2. Psychopathy is different from dissocial personality disorder in the following:
   a. People with psychopathy encounter more difficulty for inhibiting antisocial and violent behaviour (e.g. empathy, guilt, and close emotional bonds).
   b. Psychopathy is associated with higher risk of recidivism and violence. The presence of deviant sexual behaviour in psychopaths is associated with violent behaviour.
   c. EEG: Psychopaths have lower cortical arousal, measured by slower cortical evoked potentials. Autonomic arousal is also lower, leading to speculation that sensation-seeking behaviour may be an attempt to increase cortical arousal.
3. Substance misuse, for example, stimulants, PCP, and ketamine.
4. Mania/hypomania—antisocial behaviour (e.g. reckless driving or violence) as a result of impaired judgement and irritability.

29.6.3.6 Comorbidity

There is a highly significant correlation between antisocial personality disorder and drug and alcohol dependence.

A high proportion (90%) have at least one lifetime psychiatric diagnosis (e.g. somatization disorder, depression, and substance misuse).

29.6.3.7 Management

Recommendations from the NICE guidelines

1. Consider offering cognitive and behavioural interventions in order to address problems such as impulsivity, interpersonal difficulties, and antisocial behaviour. For people with forensic history, the CBT should focus on reducing offending and other antisocial behaviours.
2. When providing CBT to people with dissocial personality disorder, it is important to assess risk regularly and adjust the duration and intensity of the programme accordingly. Cognitive therapy targets at cognitive bias such as minimization of

impact of antisocial behaviour. Behaviour therapy targets at reduction of antisocial behaviour.
3. Pharmacological interventions should not be routinely used for the treatment of dissocial personality disorder.
4. Pharmacological interventions may be considered in the treatment of comorbid disorders such as depression and anxiety (e.g. SSRIs) and aggression (e.g. low-dose antipsychotics or mood stabilizers).

29.6.3.7.1 Lithium

In male convicts with a pattern of recurring easily triggered violence, a marked reduction in infractions resulted from treatment with lithium. The reduction in aggressive episodes requires lithium levels above 0.6 mmol/L. Major infractions such as assault or threatening behaviour are responsive to lithium in about 60%; minor infractions are unresponsive.

Lithium is helpful in a small number of patients with diverse personality disorders. Affective features, a family history of affective disorder, or alcoholism may help selected subjects. A 2 month trial of lithium may be necessary to establish responders.

29.6.3.7.2 Carbamazepine

Impulsive aggression is the most serious symptom of personality disorder. In patients with behavioural dyscontrol, aggressive acts are reduced by about two-thirds, and the severity of the outburst is improved. It is helpful even in the absence of epileptic, affective, or organic features.

Not all patients with dissocial personality disorder are suitable for psychotherapy. Contraindications to psychotherapy include

1. History of violence causing injury
2. Absence of remorse over violent act
3. Obvious secondary gain through therapy (e.g. avoidance of responsibility)
4. Superior intelligence with poor insight or very low intelligence
5. Lack of significant relationship in the past and historical incapacity to develop attachments
6. Offering threats to therapist
7. Intense countertransference experienced by multiple therapists

29.6.3.8 Course and Prognosis

- Early onset of childhood conduct disorder (<10 years) is the most predictive of dissocial personality disorder.

- In those with antisocial personality disorders, there is a significant association between the ability to form a relationship with the therapist and treatment outcome. In confined settings such as prison or in the military, confrontation by peers may bring changes in social behaviour.
- Prevalence seems to decrease with increasing age. Spontaneous remission may occur in middle age. There is a correlation between increasing age and remission rate.
- In general, people with dissocial personality disorder have reduction in impulsivity and increase in awareness of the consequences of reckless behaviour over time. They continue to be difficult people, resulting in interpersonal problems.
- 5% of people with dissocial personality disorder commit suicide, and suicide risk is increased by four times compared to the general population.
- There is increase in mortality as a result of accidents, drug overdose, and victims of homicide.

Positive prognostic factors include

- Show more concerns and guilt of antisocial behaviour
- Ability to form therapeutic alliance
- Positive occupational and relationship record

29.6.4   NARCISSISTIC PERSONALITY DISORDER

29.6.4.1   Epidemiology
The prevalence is between 0.4% and 0.8%.
Gender ratio: men = women

29.6.4.2   Aetiology
29.6.4.2.1   Psychological Causes
- Parenting: parental deprivation, pampering, and spoiling by parents.
- Most theories state that people with narcissistic personality disorder develop narcissism in response to their low self-esteem. People with narcissistic personality disorder have inflated self-esteem and seek information that confirms their illusory bias.
- Psychodynamic theories
  - Kohut proposed that narcissistic personality disorder is different from borderline personality disorder; idealization is a normal development for missing psychic structure; self is nondefensive and normally arrested.

- Kernberg proposed that narcissistic personality disorder is part of borderline personality disorder; idealization is a defence against envy and self is highly pathological.
- Temperament: high novelty seeking and reward dependence.

29.6.4.3   Clinical Features
(See Table 29.10.)

Types of Narcissist (Gabbard, 2000)

1. The oblivious narcissist: arrogant, self-absorbed, centre of attention, sender in a social network (e.g. Facebook), not sensitive to reaction to others, and not affected by criticisms from others
2. The hypervigilant narcissist: shy, seeking attention from others, avoiding to be centre of attention, receiver tends to detect criticism in messages, sensitive to reaction to others, and easily humiliated by others
3. Mixed oblivious and hypervigilant narcissist

29.6.4.4   Elicit Narcissistic Personality Disorder in CASC
1. How do you see other people? Do you feel that they are not up to your standard? What would you do to them? Do you feel sorry for them?
2. How do you compare yourself with others? Do you feel superior? If yes, in which aspect? Do you feel people are jealous of you?
3. Do you have fantasy? If yes, would you mind to tell me the content of your fantasy? Do you like to dream about success or power?
4. What would happen if other people criticize you? Do you see this as a blow to your ego? Do you feel angry about that?

TABLE 29.10

Comparison of the DSM-5 Criteria and Mnemonics for Narcissistic Personality Disorder

DSM-5 Criteria	Mnemonics
Antagonism, characterized by	*GAME*
a. Grandiosity: Feelings of entitlement, either overt or covert; self-centredness; firmly holding to the belief that one is better than others; condescending towards others	Grandiose fantasy of self-importance Arrogant Manipulative Envious of others
b. Attention seeking: Excessive attempts to attract and be the focus of the attention of others; admiration seeking	

5. How do you find your physical appearance? Do you think that you are physically attractive? Do you like to look at yourself in the mirror or pictures repeatedly? Do you admire your own self?

29.6.4.5 Differential Diagnosis

1. Other cluster B personality disorders, for example, histrionic personality disorder
2. Adjustment disorder with depressive features or depressive disorder with narcissistic defences
3. Hypomanic episodes
4. Substance misuse

29.6.4.6 Comorbidity

1. Anorexia nervosa
2. Depression or dysthymia
3. Hypomania
4. Substance misuse

29.6.4.7 Treatment

1. People with narcissistic personality disorder are often ambivalent about treatment, and they tend to feel that it is the others who need to change.
2. People with narcissistic personality disorder may come to seek help when they are depressed after narcissistic injury.
3. Psychotherapies such as dynamic psychotherapy and CBT are useful.

29.6.4.8 Course and Prognosis

1. Depression is perpetuated by continuing frustration and disappointment and reduced boosters for narcissism.
2. Patients may encounter difficulty with ageing as a result of high value placed on self-image and unrealistic strength. They may not be able to satisfy with life achievements.

29.6.5 HISTRIONIC PERSONALITY DISORDER

29.6.5.1 Epidemiology

Prevalence: 2%–3%
Gender ratio: M = F

29.6.5.2 Aetiology

29.6.5.2.1 Psychological Causes

- Emotional, hypersensitive, extraversion, and reward dependence
- Tendency towards attention seeking

29.6.5.2.2 Developmental Causes

- Freud: Histrionic personality results from difficulties in the Oedipal phase of psychosexual development.
- Significant separations in the first 4 years of life.
- Association with authoritarian or seductive paternal attitudes during childhood.
- Low cohesion but high control in family.
- Favouritism towards boys or male gender in a family (if patient is a woman), which leads to power imbalance in family.
- Traumatic childhood.
- Chronic physical illness in childhood and attention seeking by physical complaints.
- Absence of meaningful relationships in life.

29.6.5.2.3 Defence Mechanisms

- Dissociation
- Denial

29.6.5.3 Clinical Features

(See Table 29.11.)

29.6.5.4 Elicit Histrionic Personality Disorder in CASC

1. How do you interact with other people? Do you frequently find yourself being the centre of attention?

TABLE 29.11

Comparison of the ICD-10 Criteria and Mnemonics for Histrionic Personality Disorder

ICD-10 Criteria	Mnemonics (Robinson, 2001)
Affect	*CRAVE SIN*
1. Self-dramatization, theatricality, or exaggerated expression of emotions	Centre of attention
	Relationship: viewed to be closer to others than actually is
2. Shallow and labile affectivity	
Behaviour	Appearance: very important
3. Suggestibility (he or she is easily influenced by others or circumstances)	Vulnerable to suggestions from other people
4. Continual seeking for excitement and activities in which the individual is the centre of attention	Exaggerate expression of emotion
5. Inappropriate seductiveness in appearance or behaviour	Seductive
	Impressionistic speech but no substance in the speech
Cognition	Novelty seeking
6. Overconcern with physical attractiveness	

2. How do you find your physical appearance? Do you feel that people from the opposite gender often find you attractive?

3. Do you find yourself good in acting or pretending?

4. How do you find your emotion? Does your emotion fluctuate much?

5. Do you tend to seek excitement from time to time?

29.6.5.5 Differential Diagnosis

- Hypomania/mania: characterized by episodic mood disturbances with grandiosity and elated mood, which should not be found in histrionic personality disorder.
- Somatization/conversion disorder: people with histrionic personality disorder are more dramatic and attention seeking.
- Substance misuse.
- Other personality disorders
  - Borderline personality disorder: more self-harm, chaotic relations, and identity diffusion.
  - Dependent personality disorder: more impairment in the decision-making process.
  - Narcissistic personality disorder: people with narcissistic personality disorder need attention for being praised, and they are very sensitive to humiliation.

29.6.5.6 Comorbidity

- Somatization disorder
- Alcohol misuse

29.6.5.7 Treatment

1. Dynamic psychotherapy may be useful for people with histrionic personality disorder. Patients may see power and strength as a male attribute based on their childhood experience and feel inferior about one's own gender. As a result, they need to seek attention. Dynamic therapy can help the patients to analyse their deep-seated views and understand how their childhood experiences affect perception and personality development. The therapists should help the patients to develop their self-esteem.

2. CBT can challenge cognitive distortions and reduce emotional reasoning.

3. Psychotropic medications: SSRIs target at depressive symptoms.

29.6.5.8 Course and Prognosis

1. In general, people with histrionic personality disorder have less functional impairments compared to other personality disorders.

2. Some people with histrionic personality disorder improve with age as a result of maturity.

3. Sensation seeking may lead to substance misuse.

29.7 CLUSTER C PERSONALITY DISORDERS

- Cluster C: avoidant, dependent, and obsessive–compulsive personality disorders—anxious or fearful

Common defence mechanisms: isolation, passive aggression, hypochondriasis, and undoing

29.7.1 ANANKASTIC PERSONALITY DISORDER

29.7.1.1 Epidemiology

29.7.1.1.1 Prevalence

Prevalence in the community: 1.7%–2.2%. Anankastic personality disorder is the most common personality disorder in the community in the United Kingdom.

More common in eldest children, Caucasians, and high socioeconomic status

Gender ratio: M > F

29.7.1.2 Aetiology

29.7.1.2.1 Biological Causes

1. More common in the first-degree relatives of patients of obsessive–compulsive personality disorder.

2. The heritability is 0.78.

29.7.1.2.2 Psychological Causes

1. Early development: Excessive parental control and criticism cause insecurity. This insecurity is defended by perfectionism, orderliness, and control.

2. Psychodynamic theories
   a. Freud: fixation at the anal stage of psychosexual development
   b. Erikson's development: autonomy versus shame

29.7.1.3 Clinical Features

(See Table 29.12.)

TABLE 29.12

Comparison of the ICD-10 Criteria, DSM-5 Criteria, and Mnemonics for Anankastic Personality Disorder

ICD-10 Criteria	DSM-5 Criteria	Mnemonics (Robinson, 2001)
Affect	Compulsivity	*PERFECTION*
1. Feelings of excessive doubt and caution	Rigid perfectionism on everything being flawless, perfect, and without errors or faults, including one's own and others' performance; sacrificing of timeliness to ensure correctness in every detail; believing that there is only one right way to do things; difficulty changing ideas; preoccupation with details, organization, and order	Preoccupation with details, rules, and plans
Behaviour		Emotionally constricted
1. Perfectionism that interferes with task completion		Reluctant to delegate tasks
2. Excessive conscientiousness and scrupulousness (extremely careful)		Frugal
3. Excessive pedantry (adherence to rules and forms) and adherence to social conventions		Excessively devoted to work
		Controlling of other people
	Miserly spending style and failure to discard old items	Task completion hampered by perfectionism
		Inflexible
Cognition	Rigidity at tasks long after the behaviour has ceased to be functional or effective; continuance of the same behaviour despite repeated failures	Overconscientious in morals, ethics, and values
1. Rigidity and stubbornness		
2. Undue preoccupation with productivity to the exclusion of pleasure and interpersonal relationships		Not able to discard old items and hoards objects

29.7.1.4 Elicit Anankastic Personality Disorder in CASC

1. How do you describe yourself? Are you a perfectionistic person? Does it slow you down?
2. What is your view on rules and morals? Are you strict with moral principles?
3. Are you a careful person? Do you pay a lot of attention to details?
4. Do you like to spend money?
5. Are you able to throw away old items? If not, where do you keep them?

29.7.1.5 Differential Diagnosis

Obsessive–compulsive disorder (OCD): People with OCD present with clearly defined obsessions and compulsions. People with anankastic personality disorder are more ego-syntonic with their behaviour, and hence, they are less anxious.

Generalized anxiety disorder (GAD): People with GAD present with excessive worries related to common life events.

Schizoid personality disorder: People with anankastic personality disorder may present with constricted affect because they want to maintain control. People with schizoid personality appear to be emotionally cold because there is a fundamental lack of capacity to express emotion.

29.7.1.6 Comorbidity

1. Depressive disorder.
2. Anxiety disorders.

3. Somatoform disorders.
4. Hypochondriasis.
5. 30% of people with anankastic personality disorder suffer from OCD but not vice versa.

29.7.1.7 Management

1. Psychodynamic psychotherapy is useful. It involves an active therapist who challenges isolation of the affect and helps the patient to increase emotional awareness. The therapist also helps to modify harsh superego. Patient needs to develop the capacity to accept that he or she is a human being and cannot be perfectionistic in all areas.
2. CBT is useful to enhance tolerance of imperfection and errors. Patients should label the tasks as completed once the result is good enough.

29.7.1.8 Course and Prognosis

Adolescents with anankastic personality traits may grow out of the diagnosis.

29.7.2 ANXIOUS (AVOIDANT) PERSONALITY DISORDER

29.7.2.1 Epidemiology

Prevalence in the community is 0.5%–1.0%.
Gender: male = female

29.7.2.2   Aetiology

29.7.2.2.1   Biological Causes

1. The heritability found in anxious personalities is probably related to trait anxiety, in obsessional personalities to a more general neurotic tendency as measured by the EPI, and in hysterical personalities to extroversion.
2. The heritability is 0.28.
3. Anxious personality disorder and social phobia may be genetically related.

29.7.2.2.2   Psychological Causes

1. Temperament: neuroticism and introversion.
2. Parenting: Parents tend to be inconsistent, absent, and less in demonstrating parental love. Parents are discouraging and rarely show pride in their children. Rejection and isolation often occur. As a result, maladaptive avoidance develops as a defence against shame, embarrassment, and failure.
3. Anxious attachment: The patient wants to have close relationship, but he or she is fearful of rejection.

29.7.2.3   Clinical Features

(See Table 29.13.)

29.7.2.4   Elicit Anxious (Avoidant) Personality Disorder in CASC

1. How do you see yourself? Do you often see yourself inadequate?
2. Are you an anxious person?
3. Do you mix around with other people? Do you worry that other people may not like you?
4. Do you try to avoid social interaction? Are you concerned about criticism?
5. Do you participate in any activity that you find pleasurable?

29.7.2.5   Differential Diagnosis

1. Social phobia: People with social phobia show more impairment and distress in social situations. Their low self-esteem is lower compared to people with avoidant personality disorder.
2. Agoraphobia: People with agoraphobia have frequent panic attacks.
3. Depressive disorder: Negative self-evaluation is a result of low mood.
4. Other personality disorders
   a. Dependent personality disorder: People with avoidant personality disorder avoid contact, while people with dependent personality disorder focus on being cared for.
   b. Schizoid personality disorder: isolated but emotionally cold.
   c. Paranoid personality disorder: People with paranoid personality disorder are isolated because of lack of trust in other people.

29.7.2.6   Comorbidity

1. Social phobia

TABLE 29.13

Comparison of the ICD-10 Criteria, DSM-5 Criteria, and Mnemonics for Anxious Personality Disorder

ICD-10 Criteria	DSM-5	Mnemonics
Affect	Detachment	*AVOID*
1. Persistent, pervasive tension, and apprehension	a. Withdrawal: reticence in social situations; avoidance of social contacts and activity	Avoid involvement
		Very anxious
Behaviour	b. Intimacy avoidance: avoidance of close or romantic relationships and interpersonal attachments	Overconcern about criticism
2. Unwilling to be involved with people unless certain of being liked		Inhibited in interpersonal situations
3. Restricted lifestyle due to need for physical security		Disapproval expected at work
4. Avoidance of social or occupational activities involving significant interpersonal contact because of fear of criticism, disapproval, or rejection	c. Unwilling to get involved unless being liked	
	Negative affectivity	
Cognition	a. Worry about criticism and view oneself as socially inept	
5. Belief that one is socially inept, personally unappealing, or inferior to others		
6. Excessive preoccupation with being criticized or rejected in social situations		

29.7.2.7   Treatment

1. CBT is more useful and effective as compared to brief dynamic psychotherapy to help patients to overcome avoidance.
2. Assertiveness and social skill training is useful to help patients to make and refuse request.
3. Distress tolerance skill is important to help patients to handle anticipatory anxiety in social situations.

29.7.2.8   Course and Prognosis

1. People with avoidant personality disorder may do well in familiar environment with known people.
2. Shyness tends to decrease when the patients get older.
3. People with avoidant personality disorder and comorbid depressive disorder may have high dropout rate in treatment.

29.7.3   DEPENDENT PERSONALITY DISORDER

29.7.3.1   Epidemiology

The prevalence in the community is between 1% and 1.7%.

29.7.3.2   Aetiology

29.7.3.2.1   Biological Causes

- Twin studies suggest a biological component to submissiveness.
- The heritability is 0.57.

29.7.3.2.2   Psychological Causes

- Dependent personality traits are thought to result from parental deprivation and indulgent parents who prohibit independent activity.
- Dependent personality results from fixation at the oral stage of psychosexual development.
- Hostile dependency: dependency as a way to manage anger and aggression.
- Insecure attachment.

29.7.3.3   Clinical Features

(See Table 29.14.)

29.7.3.4   Elicit Dependent Personality Disorder in CASC

1. Can you describe your character? Are you a dependent person?
2. How do you feel about making a decision?

TABLE 29.14

Comparison of the ICD-10 Criteria and Mnemonics for Dependent Personality Disorder

ICD-10 Criteria	Mnemonics
Affect	*FEARS*
1. Uncomfortable or helpless when alone due to exaggerated fears of inability to self-care	Fear of being left alone
	Expression of disagreement is limited
Behaviour	Avoid decision-making and responsibility
2. Encourages or allows others to make most of one's important life decisions	Relationship is sought urgently with other relationship ends
3. Subordination of one's own needs to those of others on whom one is dependent, undue compliance with their wishes	Self-confidence is lacking
4. Unwilling to make even reasonable demands on the people one depends on	
Cognition	
5. Preoccupation with fears of being left to care for oneself	
6. Limited capacity to take everyday decisions without an excessive amount of advice and reassurance from others	

3. In situations when you do not agree with other people, are you able to express yourself?
4. What would happen if you are left alone? Would you be fearful?

29.7.3.5   Differential Diagnosis

1. Depressive disorder
2. Agoraphobia
3. Social phobia
4. Other personality disorders
   a. Borderline personality disorder: Both borderline personality disorder and dependent personality disorder share fear of rejection and abandonment. People with borderline personality disorder show more anger, emptiness, and dramatic responses. People with dependent personality disorder are more submissive and clinging. People with dependent personality disorder want to be controlled, but people with borderline personality disorder react strongly to the efforts to be controlled. People with borderline personality disorder show more rage and chaotic relationship.

b. Avoidant personality disorder: People with avoidant personality disorder show low self-esteem, need for reassurance, and high sensitivity for rejection. People with avoidant personality disorder react by avoiding, while people with dependent personality disorder seek out for relationship.

c. Histrionic personality disorder: People with histrionic personality disorder are more seductive, flamboyant, and manipulative to get attention.

29.7.3.6 Treatment

1. CBT and social skill training.
2. Therapy targets at increasing self-esteem, self-confidence, sense of efficacy, and assertiveness.
3. Explores fear of autonomy.
4. Family or couple therapy.

CASC STATION ON BORDERLINE PERSONALITY DISORDER

A 28-year-old woman is referred by an obstetrician for assessment of postnatal depression. She delivered a baby boy 6 weeks ago, and she claims that she does not want to look after her baby. She has a past history of borderline personality disorder. The obstetrician has made a note stating that she behaves like a child.

Take a history to assess the reasons of distress and the impact of borderline personality disorder on her mood and parenting ability.

Approach to This CASC Station

1. Explore her reasons for distress by empathic open questioning including validating statements to identify the onset and the course of the current problems. The patient may have gone through a lot of difficulties during the antenatal period. It is important to hear from her views of childbirth and explore her thoughts and feelings during pregnancy. The candidate should assess the impact of her borderline personality disorder on motherhood (e.g. was this pregnancy unplanned and based on a short intense relationship with a man? Assess her current relationship with the father of the baby.) The candidate should explore the presence of any other children and her views towards motherhood. Finally, the candidate should explore the reason why she does not want to look after her baby (e.g. complications or illness in the infant, extreme social adversity, unstable emotion). The candidate should inquire the mode of feeding (e.g. breastfeeding) and the care of the baby (e.g. the availability of friends or others who are looking after the baby). The candidate should explore her coping mechanisms and substance misuse during the antenatal and postnatal periods.

2. Candidates need to explore how the borderline personality affecting the way a depressive episode would present in this patient. For example, the effect of chronic emptiness and feeling of abandonment may affect quality of low mood. Patients with borderline personality disorder may have transient psychosis, and candidates should explore possible delusions or hallucinations, which may pose harm to the baby. Has patient used 'acting out' (e.g. severe self-injury) as a means of presentation to the obstetrician? Explore the biological (e.g. insomnia) and cognitive symptoms of depression.

3. Risk assessment includes assessment on suicidality, frequency of self-mutilation, and infanticide risk.

4. Candidates are advised to take a background history to assess the degree of impairment (e.g. duration of unemployment) and severity of the borderline personality disorder (e.g. number of hospitalizations). Look for common comorbidity such as PTSD and eating disorders. Assess her development and its relationship to her current regression. An understanding of interpersonal issues and relevant crises including coping responses is important.

5. The candidate should also hear from the patient about her unmet needs and preference for treatment. The candidate should also explore treatment (e.g. psychotherapy) received in the past and the outcomes of various treatment interventions. If the

patient requires for admission, consider mother–baby unit. In general, the NICE guidelines recommend the exploration of other options before considering admission of a person with borderline personality disorder. As a result of potential risk to the infant, inpatient treatment may be more suitable in this case. It is important to agree on the length and purpose of inpatient treatment prior to admission.

According to the NICE guidelines, the management of the patient is as follows:

6. A crisis plan needs to be developed to identify potential triggers that lead to a crisis. The plan should specify self-management strategies that are likely to be effective. The patient should be informed about access services (including a list of support numbers for out-of-hour teams and crisis teams) when self-management strategy is inadequate.

7. If the patient is admitted to the ward, the psychiatrist needs to address the issues of staff countertransference, potential splitting, and regression from time to time. During hospitalization, consideration needs to be given to teach patient on parenting skills and explore the psychological meanings of the infant to her.

8. The short-term goals include helping the patient to develop parenting skills to take care of the infant and reduce recurrent self-harm.

9. In this patient, issues of breast-feeding and its potential impact on the infant are important before considering psychotropic medication. Once she has stopped breast-feeding, antipsychotic (as monotherapy) is suitable for medium- and long-term management. Polypharmacy should be avoided.

10. If insomnia is a major problem, provide general advice on sleep hygiene and consider sedative antihistamines to avoid potential misuse of benzodiazepines.

11. For psychological treatment, she may need twice-weekly psychotherapy sessions and require longer term of psychological interventions (duration of > 3 months).

12. A formal care programme approach review should be held regularly.

BIBLIOGRAPHY

American Psychiatric Association. 2013: *Desk Reference to the Diagnostic Criteria from DSM-5*. Washington, DC: American Psychiatric Association Press.

Brennan PA and Mednick SA. 1993: Genetic perspectives on crime. *Acta Psychiatrica Scandinavica* 370(Suppl.): 19–26.

Campbell RJ. 1996: *Psychiatric Dictionary*, p. 421. Oxford, U.K.: Oxford University Press.

Coccaro EF, Bergeman CS, and McClearn GE. 1993: Heritability of irritable impulsiveness: A study of twins reared together and apart. *Psychiatry Research* 48:229–242.

Dasgupta P and Barber J. 2004: Admission patterns of patients with personality disorder. *Psychiatric Bulletin* 28:321–323.

DeBattista C and Glick ID. 1995: Pharmacotherapy of the personality disorders. *Current Opinion in Psychiatry* 8:102–105.

Eysenck HJ and Eysenck SB. 1975: *Manual of the Eysenck Personality* Questionnaire. London, U.K.: Hodder and Stoughton.

Freeman CPL. 1995: Personality disorders. In Kendell RE and Zealley AK (eds.) *Companion to Psychiatric Studies*, 5th edn. Edinburgh, Scotland: Churchill Livingstone.

Gabbard GO. 2000: *Psychodynamic Psychotherapy*, 3rd edn. Washington, DC: American Psychiatric Press.

Gelder M, Gath D, and Mayou R. 1985: *Oxford Textbook of Psychiatry*. Oxford, U.K.: Oxford University Press.

Goyer PF, Andreason PJ, Semple WE et al. 1994: Positron emission tomography and personality disorders. *Neuropsychopharmacology* 10:21–28.

Hare RD and Neumann CS. 2008: Psychopathy as a clinical and empirical construct. Annual *Review of Clinical Psychology* 4:217–246.

Harris GT and Rice ME. 1997: Risk appraisal and management of violent behavior. *Psychiatric Services* 48(9):1168–1176.

Henderson DK. 1939: *Psychopathic States*. New York: W.W. Norton & Company.

Higgitt A and Fonagy P. 1992: Psychotherapy in borderline and narcissistic personality disorder. *British Journal of Psychiatry* 161:23–43.

Kaplan H. 1952: The schizophrenic reaction with psychopathic features: clinical characteristics and response to therapy: A comprehensive study of seven cases. *American Medical Association Archives of Neurology and Psychiatry* 68(2):258–265.

Kernberg OF. 1975: *Borderline Conditions and Pathological Narcissism*. New York: Aronson.

Kety SS, Rosenthal D, Wender PH et al. 1971: Mental illness in the biological and adoptive families of adopted schizophrenics. *American Journal of Psychiatry* 128:302–306.

Koizumi K, Sukegawa H, and Takakuma E. 1964: Studies on the function of concentration maintenance (TAF): Comparison of TAF with IQ and Kraepelin character types. *Nihon Eiseigaku Zasshi* 19:8–11.

Lenzenweger MF, Lane MC, Loranger AW, and Kessler RC. 2007: DSM-IV personality disorders in the National Comorbidity Survey Replication. *Biological Psychiatry* 62(6):553–564.

Linehan MM, Armstrong HE, Svarez A et al. 1991: Cognitive–behavioural treatment of chronically parasuicidal borderline patients. *Archives of General Psychiatry* 48:1060–1064.

McGuffin P and Thapar A. 1992: The genetics of personality disorder. *British Journal of Psychiatry* 160:12–23.

Mednick SA, Gabrielli WF, and Hutchings B. 1984: Genetic influences on criminal convictions: Evidence from an adoption cohort. *Science* 224:891–894.

Miller LJ. 1989: Inpatient management of borderline personality disorder: A review and update. *Journal of Personality Disorders* 3:122–134.

Mischel W. 1983: Alterations on the pursuit of predictability and consistency of persons: Stable data that yield unstable interpretations. *Journal of Personality* 51:578–604.

NICE. *NICE Guidelines for Antisocial Personality Disorder.* http://guidance.nice.org.uk/CG77 (accessed on 1 August 2012).

NICE. *NICE Guidelines for Borderline Personality Disorder.* http://guidance.nice.org.uk/CG78 (accessed on 1 August 2012).

Paris J. 2004: Is hospitalization useful for suicidal patients with borderline personality disorder? *Journal of Personality Disorders* 18(3):240–247.

Paris J, Brown R, and Nowis D. 1987: Long-term follow-up of borderline patients in a general hospital. *Comprehensive Psychiatry* 28:530–535.

Robins LN. 1966: *Deviant Children Grown Up.* Baltimore, MD: Williams & Wilkins.

Robinson DJ. 2001: *Psychiatric Mnemonics & Clinical Guides.* Port Huron, MI: Rapid Psychler Press.

Sadock BJ and Sadock VA. 2003: *Kaplan and Sadock's Comprehensive Textbook of Psychiatry,* 9th edn. Philadelphia, PA: Lippincott Williams & Wilkins.

Schneider K. 1958: *Psychopathic Personalities.* London, U.K.: Cassell.

Shea SC. 1998: *Psychiatric Interviewing: The Art of Understanding,* 2nd edn. Philadelphia, PA: Saunders.

Stein G. 1992: Drug treatment of the personality disorders. *British Journal of Psychiatry* 161:167–184.

Stern A. 1938: Psychoanalytic investigation of and therapy in the borderline group of neuroses. *Psychoanalytic Quarterly* 7:467–489.

Swanson MCJ, Bland RC, and Newman SC. 1994: Antisocial personality disorders. *Acta Psychiatrica Scandinavica* 376(Suppl.):63–70.

Tyrer P and Ferguson B. 1987: Problems in the classification of personality disorder. *Psychological Medicine* 17:15–20.

World Health Organization. 1992: *Tenth Revision of the International Classification of Diseases.* Geneva, Switzerland: WHO.

30 Cross-Cultural Psychiatry

30.1 BASIC CONCEPTS

Culture is defined as the learned way of life of a group of people bound together by a common social heritage. People of the same cultural group behave, think, and give meaning to their life in a similar way and share a set of values and beliefs.

Ethnicity is defined as the specific patterns of a group of people by a common genetic background, country of origin, and language. Ethnicity is one of the aspects of culture.

Race is defined as the biological features of a group of people by similar skin colour and other physical characteristics.

Cultural consciousness is defined as the personal consciousness of his or her own cultural identity. Cultural consciousness is developed in the following stages: It starts with naivety and the individual has no awareness of his or her own cultural identity. Then the person comes into acceptance of his or her own cultural identity and becomes resistance to other cultures. As the patient matures, he or she redefines and reflects on his or her own cultural consciousness and leads to multiperspective internalization.

Acculturation is defined as the decision made by an individual to adopt cultural values from a dominant culture and undergo changes. For example, a Chinese immigrant to the United Kingdom finds his or her children adopt the British culture and not interested in the Chinese culture after migration to the United Kingdom. Acculturation has four components: assimilation, integration, marginalization, and separation.

Alienation is defined as the sense of powerlessness, social isolation, and entrapment because the person is not belonging to a culture and not feeling welcome. This may occur in immigrants that have newly arrived in a foreign country.

Assimilation is defined as the process of adjustment when two different cultures come into contact with each other over a long period of time. For example, the colonial Hong Kong demonstrates assimilation of British and Chinese culture.

30.1.1 CULTURAL ASSESSMENT

The DSM-5 (APA, 2013) has a section on cultural formulation interview. Selected and modified questions are listed as follows:

1. *Cultural definition of the problem*: Patients often understand their problems in their own way based on their cultural background. The understanding may be similar or different from Western medicine. How would you describe your problem?
2. *Culture perceptions of cause*: What do you think are the causes of your problems based on your own cultural belief? Could it be related to bad things in life, interpersonal problems, or spiritual issues?
3. *Cultural identity*: Do you see your cultural background causing the current problems? Do members from your cultural group offer help to cope with the current situations?
4. *Help seeking from own culture*: Do you seek help from traditional healers or therapists? In comparison to Western medicine, which type of treatment was most helpful or most unhelpful?
5. *Doctor–patient relationship*: Based on our cultural background, do you find it difficult for the doctor to understand you? Do you feel discriminated as a result of your cultural background? Do you feel psychiatric services in the trust suit people sharing the same culture with you?

30.2 INTERNATIONAL COMPARISONS

30.2.1 SCHIZOPHRENIA

Kraepelin delineated dementia praecox and manic depression. In 1904, he visited the asylum of Buitenzorg in Java to examine the similarities and differences between European patients and those from another culture. He was satisfied that he could recognize cases of dementia praecox in Java, giving credence to his diagnostic distinction. This represents one of the first investigations in transcultural psychiatry.

30.2.1.1 *International Pilot Study of Schizophrenia*

This study (WHO, 1973) was devised to determine whether schizophrenia could be recognized as the same condition in a wide variety of cultural settings. Nine centres (Columbia, Czechoslovakia, Denmark, India, Nigeria, Russia, Taiwan, the United Kingdom, and the United States) participated. The Present State Examination was translated into seven languages, and psychiatrists trained in its use interviewed 1200 patients. Diagnoses were then generated using the computer program CATEGO. The main findings were

- When narrow criteria of Schneider's first-rank symptoms were applied, an incidence of schizophrenia was found, which did not differ significantly across cultural settings. Therefore, schizophrenia is recognizable as the same condition across a wide variety of cultures.
- Broadly defined, schizophrenia has an incidence that differs significantly from one country to another.
- The outcome of schizophrenia was found to vary inversely with the social development of the society. Those from developing countries had a better prognosis than those from the developed world.

30.2.1.2 *Determinants of Outcome Study*

This study (Sartorius et al., 1986) extended its case-finding techniques to include rural primary health-care centres, traditional healers, police stations, and prisons as well as the more conventional psychiatric settings. More than 1300 cases were interviewed in 12 centres across 10 countries. The main findings were

- The incidence of narrowly defined schizophrenia was stable across a wide range of cultures, climates, and ethnic groups, confirming findings of the International Pilot Study of Schizophrenia (IPSS). The form of presentation of schizophrenia varied across cultures.
- Catatonic schizophrenia was a common form of presentation in the underdeveloped world but has become much rarer in the West. Catatonia presented in 10% of cases in developing countries but in only a handful of those in developed countries.
- Hebephrenic schizophrenia was diagnosed in 13% of cases from developed countries but in only 4% of cases from developing countries.
- In developing countries, acute schizophrenia was diagnosed more often than in developed countries.

To identify the cause of the good prognosis for schizophrenia in the less-developed world, Leff et al. (1990) determined the levels of expressed emotion (EE) in a subsample of the Chandigarh cohort of first-contact schizophrenic patients from the WHO determinants of the outcome study. At 1-year follow-up, a dramatic reduction had occurred in each of the EE components. No rural relative was rated as high EE at follow-up. It was concluded that the better outcome of this cohort of schizophrenic patients is partly attributable to tolerance and acceptance by family members.

30.2.2 NEUROSIS

Using standardized interviewing and case-finding techniques, the prevalence rates for neurosis in developing countries are comparable with or higher than those found in the West, contrary to what was previously believed.

In many Third World countries, hysteria represents a high proportion of psychiatric practice. In the West, there has been a substantial decrease in the numbers of patients with hysteria and a compensatory rise in the incidence of anxiety and depression. It is suggested that this can be seen as a shift from a somatic to a psychological mode of communication of emotional distress. The tendency to express distress in a psychological form is associated with higher social class and education. Catatonia could similarly be viewed as a nonverbal manifestation of schizophrenia.

Orley and Wing (1979) investigated the rates of psychiatric illness in two villages in East and West Africa. The rates of depression and anxiety showed large differences (22% and 10%, respectively). Compared to rates in Western countries (10%–12%), these rates are high. Communities in the developed and undeveloped world are heterogeneous, a point emphasized by the 'new cross-cultural psychiatry' (see succeeding text).

In comparing the psychopathology of Jewish and gentile East London depressives, hypochondriasis and tension are much more common in the Jewish group, whereas guilt is more common in the gentiles. Guilt is culturally determined and more common in Christians.

Somatic symptoms of depression appear to be universal, but the concept of depression of mood is not recognized in all cultures; many cultures do not have the language to express the feeling of depression as described in the West. Instead, such terms as 'sinking heart' or 'soul loss' are found. In China, 87% of people suffering from neurasthenia fulfil the criteria for major depression and respond to treatment with antidepressants.

30.2.2.1 New Cross-Cultural Psychiatry

Kleinman (1977) described the 'new cross-cultural psychiatry'. He criticized as a category fallacy the assumption that Western diagnostic categories were themselves culture-free entities.

Anthropologists have criticized the older transcultural epidemiological research for imposing Western concepts of psychopathology on non-Western people. These studies have also been criticized on the grounds of translation difficulties, the poor quality of questionnaire-generated diagnosis, a disregard for various understandings of the self, and for ignoring the cultural variation for broadly defined illness.

Beliefs about the mechanisms of illness among people in the underdeveloped world have been divided into three main ideas:

- *Object intrusion.* This is illness caused by a physical object being intruded into the person's body.
- *Spirit intrusion.* A spirit is believed to take possession of the person's body.
- *Soul loss.* The soul of the person is believed to have been stolen by spirits.

30.2.2.2 Translation and Validity of Rating Scales

In the translation of rating scales, five types of problem in validity arise:

- *Content validity.* The content of instruments must be relevant in the culture into which the instrument is translated. For example, coca paste abuse is common in Peru, so the substance abuse schedule should reflect this.
- *Semantic validity.* Words used in the original and new instruments must have the same meanings.
- *Technical validity.* Where languages are not written or illiteracy rates are high, answering a questionnaire may elicit answers that represent a misunderstanding of the intention.
- *Criterion validity.* Do responses to similar items measure the same concept in two cultures? For example, in American Indians, hallucinations normally occur during the course of bereavement, but this is not the case in North Americans generally; this must thus be accommodated.
- *Conceptual validity.* This requires that responses relate to a theoretical construct within the culture.

30.2.2.3 Classificatory Systems

Europe and North America have greatly influenced the models of mental illness and the classification of mental illness over the last century. ICD-10 has been criticized in cross-cultural terms. The international group of psychiatrists involved in drawing up the first draft consisted of 47, only 2 of whom were from Africa. Thus, conditions encountered in many other cultures that do not resemble Western categories have been assigned the title 'culture-bound' conditions or 'masked' representations of 'real' illness.

30.2.2.4 Culture-Bound Syndromes

Debate exists about what constitutes a culture-bound syndrome. The term is used to describe disorders that are considered unique to a given culture (cultural determinist view). However, the question of whether the classically described 'culture-bound syndromes' are actually unique to the given culture, or are in fact universal phenomena merely influenced by culture (universalist view), has not been settled. The following syndromes are frequently cited.

30.3 CULTURE-BOUND SYNDROMES IN ASIA

30.3.1 Amok

Occurring in Malays, amok consists of a period of withdrawal, followed by a sudden outburst of homicidal aggression in which the sufferer will attack anyone within reach. The attack typically lasts for several hours until the sufferer is overwhelmed or killed. If alive, the person typically passes into a deep sleep or stupor for several days, followed by amnesia for the event. It almost always occurs in men.

It was first described in Malays in the mid-sixteenth century. It is believed to have originated in the cultural training for warfare among Malay warriors. Later it became a personal act by an isolated individual, apparently motiveless, but the motive could be understood as the restoration of self-esteem or 'face'.

It was very common in Malaya at the beginning of the nineteenth century, but the incidence was reduced when the British took over the administration of Malaya. Today it has virtually disappeared.

It is most common in Malays, but reports of amok from other countries exist, questioning its position as a culture-bound syndrome; it is clear, however, that there is a strong cultural element.

Among Malay cases in mental hospitals, the most common diagnosis is schizophrenia. Depression, acute brain syndrome, and hysterical dissociation have also been found in some cases. The majority do not have a mental illness. Attacks are often preceded by interpersonal discord, insults or personal loss, and social drinking.

30.3.2 Latah

This usually begins after a sudden frightening experience in Malay women. It is characterized by a response to minimal stimuli with exaggerated startles, coprolalia, echolalia, echopraxia, and automatic obedience. It has been suggested that this is merely one form of what is known to psychologists as the 'hyperstartle reaction' and is universally found.

30.3.3 Koro

This is common in Southeast Asia and China; it may occur in epidemic form. It involves the belief of genital retraction with disappearance into the abdomen, accompanied by intense anxiety and the fear of impending death.

Cases of a similar condition have been described in non-Chinese subjects. In these cases, the syndrome is often only partial, such as the belief of genital shrinkage, not necessarily with retraction into the abdomen; it usually occurs within the context of another psychiatric disorder and resolves once the underlying illness has been treated.

Debate about the cultural specificity of this disorder continues. Some argue that the culturally determined syndrome is clearly different from the symptom of genital retraction occurring in some non-Chinese psychotic subjects.

The development of koro has been associated with psychosexual conflicts, personality factors, and cultural beliefs in the context of psychological stress.

30.3.4 Dhat

This is commonly recognized in Indian culture and is also widespread in Nepal, Sri Lanka, Bangladesh, and Pakistan. Dhat was prevalent in Europe in the nineteenth century because masturbation was prohibited by religion and emission was a sin. It includes vague somatic symptoms (fatigue, weakness, anxiety, loss of appetite, guilt, etc.) and sometimes sexual dysfunction (impotence or premature ejaculation), which the subject attributes to the passing of semen in urine as a consequence of excessive indulgence in masturbation or intercourse.

Patients are typically from a rural area, from a family with conservative attitudes towards sex and of average or low socioeconomic status. Literacy and religion are unimportant.

Bhatia and Malik (1991) studied male patients attending a sexual problems clinic in New Delhi. They found that 65% arrived with a primary complaint of dhat syndrome. Twenty-three per cent of these also complained of impotence or premature ejaculation. The age of presentation is early twenties, with about 50% unmarried. Most are literate. Although some suffered from depression and anxiety, those with dhat syndrome differed from the others only in the relative absence of depression and anxiety. Treatment with anxiolytics or antidepressant drugs resulted in significant improvement, however.

Dhat syndrome is considered by many to be a true culture-bound condition. The belief in the precious properties of semen is ingrained in Indian culture.

30.3.5 Frigophobia

Frigophobia is common in China and Southeast Asia. Patients believe that excessive cold results in illness and they compulsively dress in heavy or excessive clothing.

30.3.6 Taijinkyofusho

Taijinkyofusho is common in Japan. The patient fears that he or she offends the other people or makes them uncomfortable through inappropriate behaviour or self-presentation (e.g. offensive odour or physical blemish). Differential diagnosis such as social phobia should be considered.

30.4 CULTURE-BOUND SYNDROMES IN AMERICA

30.4.1 Piblokto

This dissociative state is seen among Eskimo women. The patient tears off her clothing, screams, cries, and runs about wildly, endangering her life by exposure to the cold. It may result in suicidal or homicidal behaviour.

30.4.2 Susto

Susto literally means the loss of soul. This syndrome is common in Mexico and Central and South America. The aetiology of susto includes organic causes, stress, and social inadequacy. Patients usually present with both psychiatric and physical symptoms. Psychiatric symptoms include depression, anxiety, and paranoia. Organic symptoms include indigestion and anaemia.

30.4.3 WINDIGO

This is described in North American Indians and ascribed to depression, schizophrenia, hysteria, or anxiety. It is a disorder in which the subject believes he or she has undergone a transformation and become a monster who practises cannibalism. However, it has been suggested that windigo is in fact a local myth rather than an actual pattern of behaviour.

30.4.4 UQAMAIRINEQ

Uqamairineq is common in Inuits living within the Arctic Circle. Prodromal symptoms include transient auditory or olfactory hallucinations. Patients with uqamairineq present with sudden paralysis in semi-sleeping states, anxiety, agitation, and hallucinations.

30.5 CULTURE-BOUND SYNDROMES IN AFRICA

30.5.1 BOUFFEE DELIRANTE

Bouffee delirante is common in West Africa and Haiti. Patient presents with sudden outburst of agitation, aggression, and auditory and visual hallucinations. Bouffee delirante resembles acute and transient psychosis.

30.5.2 BRAIN FAG SYNDROME

This is a widespread low-grade stress syndrome described in many parts of Africa and also in New Guinea. It is commonly encountered among students, probably because of the high priority accorded to education in African society, and is particularly prevalent at examination times.

Five symptom types have been described as comprising brain fag syndrome:

- Head symptoms—aching, burning, crawling sensations
- Eye symptoms—blurring, watering, aching
- Difficulty in grasping the meaning of spoken or written words
- Poor retentivity
- Sleepiness on studying

Guinness (1992) found the rates to be highest in rural areas serving peasant populations (34% of students), compared to peri-urban schools (22%) and schools for the professional élite (6%).

Sufferers of brain fag syndrome are resistant to psychological interpretation of their condition. It is suggested that brain fag syndrome is a form of depression in which depressive features are not articulated in Western psychological terms.

30.5.3 UFUFUYANE

Ufufuyane is common in South Africa. Clinical features include anxiety, convulsions, repeated neologisms, paralysis shouting, sobbing, trance-like stupor, and loss of consciousness. Patients may complain of nightmares with sexual themes and temporary blindness.

30.5.4 NERFIZA

Nerfiza is common in Egypt, Northern Europe, Greece, Mexico, and Central and South America. Clinical features include depression, anxiety, and fearfulness. Patients present with somatic complaints such as headache and muscle pain, appetite loss, agitation, nausea, giddiness, insomnia, fatigue, and tingling sensation.

30.6 PSYCHIATRY AND BLACK AND ETHNIC MINORITIES IN BRITAIN

Britain is a multiracial society. In some large cities, ethnic minorities represent 30% or more of the total population. Ethnic minority groups are of two types:

- Immigrants
- Second- or third-generation residents

The stresses incurred by these two groups are different. Ethnic minority groups are heterogeneous in terms of religion and cultural background.

30.6.1 IMMIGRANTS

People migrate for various reasons, and so adjustment will depend on many factors including those operating before migration, the reasons for migration, and factors operating in the host society.

30.6.1.1 Types of Migrants
- Settlers are likely to be prepared for a new way of life.
- Exiles have been forced to migrate. This may result in grief reaction for their old way of life. They may have suffered torture or other atrocities before migration.

- Migrant workers are less likely to put down roots in the host country. They may be supporting their family financially at home.
- Others: students, business people, etc.

30.6.1.2 Stresses Involved in Migration

There are various social stresses:

- Culture shock and readjustment to the host society
- Downward social mobility, poor housing, unemployment or job dissatisfaction, unfulfilled aspirations, and lack of opportunities
- Racial prejudice and discrimination in the host society
- Loss of extended family support
- Intergenerational difficulties as children integrate, bringing cultural conflict into the home

In a 3-year follow-up study of Vietnamese boat people given asylum in Norway, Hauff and Vaglum (1995) found there was no decline in psychological distress over time. One in four suffered psychiatric disorder and the prevalence of depression at 3 years was 18%. Female gender, extreme traumatic stress in Vietnam, negative life events in Norway, and chronic family separation were the predictors of psychopathology. Thus, the effects of war and persecution were long lasting and compounded by adversity in exile.

Some studies have found that the mental health of refugees improves over time, and it is possible that adverse factors in the host environment have significant effects on the readjustment and mental health of refugees.

30.6.2 Mental Illness among Ethnic Minorities

30.6.2.1 Schizophrenia

The higher than expected rates of schizophrenia among Afro-Caribbean people born in Britain have been noted since the 1960s. Studies of hospital admissions have demonstrated high rates of schizophrenia in this group compared to British whites and Asians.

The highest rates of schizophrenia in the Afro-Caribbean group occur in U.K.-born second-generation subjects (up to nine times that among Europeans). Differences persist even when age and socioeconomic status are taken into account.

These results have caused controversy, with criticisms of misdiagnosis due to unfamiliar culturally determined patterns of behaviour, acute psychotic reactions being mistaken for schizophrenia, or racism accounting for the observed differences. However, well-designed studies dealing with methodological problems fail to substantiate

these criticisms. Harvey et al. (1990) studied consecutive Afro-Caribbean and white British psychotic inpatients prospectively and found no differences in the course of illness or the pattern of symptoms. This caused them to reject the hypothesis that misdiagnosis accounts for the higher rates of schizophrenia in this group.

Schizophrenia as defined by operational research criteria is more common in people of Afro-Caribbean origin living in the United Kingdom.

Sugarman and Craufurd (1994) found a lifetime morbid risk of schizophrenia in the parents of Afro-Caribbean subjects to be the same as the risks to parents of British white schizophrenic subjects (8.9% and 8.4%, respectively). However, for the siblings of Afro-Caribbean probands, the risk was 15% compared to 1.8% for white siblings. Among the siblings of U.K.-born Afro-Caribbean probands, the risk was even higher at 27.3%. These observations suggest that schizophrenia in Afro-Caribbean patients is no less familial than the rest of the population (as evidenced by the similar risks to parents) but that the increased risk is caused by environmental factors capable of precipitating schizophrenia in those who are genetically predisposed to it.

The environmental factor postulated has not been identified to date. There is no evidence of increased rates of schizophrenia in the West Indies and therefore no evidence that Afro-Caribbeans carry a greater genetic loading for schizophrenia.

Admission rates for Asians are similar to Europeans, except for the 16–29-year age group, who tend to have lower psychiatric admission rates than Europeans. This gives rise to concerns that services are not reaching this particular group.

30.6.2.2 Suicide

30.6.2.2.1 The United Kingdom

Raleigh and Balarajan (1992) reported suicide rates among British ethnic minority groups compared to the indigenous British white population:

- Suicide rates were high among young Indian women (age-specific standardized mortality rates (SMRs) of 273 and 160 at ages 15–24 and 25–34, respectively) but low among Indian men (SMR 73).
- Suicide rates were low in Caribbeans (SMRs 81 and 62 in men and women, respectively).
- Suicide rates were high in East Africans (SMRs 128 and 148 in men and women, respectively) and were largely confined to the younger age groups.

- Immigrant groups had a higher rate of suicide by burning, with a ninefold excess among Indian women.
- Goth youth culture in the United Kingdom (Young et al., 2006): Goth refers to subgenre of punk with a dark and sinister aesthetic, distinctive clothing, and taste in music. The prevalence of self-harm in Goth youth culture is 53% (cf. 7%–14% of self-harm among young people in the United Kingdom). The prevalence of attempted suicide is 47%.

30.6.2.3 Other Countries

Aboriginal people in Australia: The gender ratio is 7:1. Hanging is the most common method. Causes include marginalization, purposeless in life, poor social support, poor education, and alcohol abuse.

China: Half of all female suicides in the world come from China. Rural women attempt suicide by pesticide ingestion.

Hong Kong: Dramatic increase of suicide by charcoal burning in airtight space (age: 25–54 years). Common causes include debts and financial difficulty.

India: High suicide rates among young Indian women are reported within India and in countries where Indian immigrants have settled. High expectations of academic and economic success, the stigma of failure, the authority of their elders, and the expected unquestioning compliance of younger family members are thought to predispose to suicide in this culture. Among Indian women, these pressures are accentuated by expected submission and deference to males and elders. Rates of suicide and attempted suicide in this group are not greatly different from those in the country of origin, suggesting that the increased rates are not particularly related to issues of migration. In India, dowry-related self-burning is well known. The common causes of suicide by burns in young women include marital problems and interpersonal difficulties with other family members. In contrast, suicide rates among older Indian women are low, which is thought to accord with the greater respect given to them by virtue of their age.

Japan: Responsibility-driven suicide is often committed by middle-aged men. Elderly accounts for 24% of suicide and associates with depression and somatic complaints.

Māori (indigenous peoples) in New Zealand: There has been recent increase of suicide among young Māori men. Depression and suicidal ideation are common among Māori adolescents.

30.6.2.4 Child and Adolescent Psychiatric Presentations

Second-generation Afro-Caribbean children presenting to child and adolescent psychiatric services differ in their patterns of presentation when compared to British white children of comparable age and socioeconomic status.

Psychotic and autistic disorders are overrepresented in Afro-Caribbean children compared to whites, with psychotic disorders present in 3.4% and 0.8%, respectively, and autistic disorders present in 3.4% and 0.6%, respectively. Studies also find that the autistic children of immigrant parents are more likely than their white counterparts to be severely or profoundly mentally handicapped. Mental handicap is also overrepresented in Afro-Caribbean children (19% vs. 11%).

Afro-Caribbean children present with a significantly higher rate of conduct disorder (35% vs. 25%) and a significantly lower rate of emotional disorder (18% vs. 27%) when compared to white counterparts.

30.6.3 Use of Psychiatric Services by Ethnic Minorities

Young, male, black, schizophrenic Afro-Caribbeans have high psychiatric admission rates compared to white British and a higher rate of compulsory admissions. In inner-city London, the ratio of black Afro-Caribbeans to whites among admissions is higher than the equivalent proportion in the population (three times higher in Hammersmith and Fulham).

Part of the explanation for this is the higher rates of schizophrenia in black Afro-Caribbeans. Bebbington et al. (1994) concluded that ethnicity was not of major importance in decisions to use the Mental Health Act in two regions in London. The use of compulsion was strongly linked with challenging behaviour and diagnosis of schizophrenia but not with ethnicity per se.

Dunn and Fahy (1990), studying police admissions under Section 136 of the Mental Health Act 1983 to a South London psychiatric hospital, found an excess of admissions of blacks. However, clinicians judged that more than 90% of detained black and white subjects were suffering from a psychiatric disorder and were therefore appropriately detained. The judgement of the police in this study was not biased towards apprehending black people as a result of unconscious racist attitudes, as previously suggested by some.

Cole et al. (1995) found that for first-episode patients, the route to psychiatric care in Haringey (North London) was different from those for chronic patients. While compulsory admission was more likely for black patients, the excess was less striking than in other studies. Black patients were no more likely to have police involvement than other patients. The most important factors in avoiding adverse pathways to care were having a supportive family or friend and the presence of a general practitioner (GP). Having a GP or close person avoided the need for compulsory detention, an effect seen in both black and white subjects.

Suggestions to account for the overrepresentation of compulsory admissions among Afro-Caribbeans include the possibility that the stigma of mental illness is greater in this community, thus resulting in delays before cases come to the attention of the services. Afro-Caribbean patients with previous psychotic episodes are more likely than their white counterparts to deny they had a problem at all; these patients are more likely to be noncompliant with antipsychotic medication and to require compulsory readmission.

30.6.3.1 Approaches to Management

30.6.3.1.1 Communication

In areas with large numbers of ethnic minorities, the service should provide for interpreters to be available for translation. It is preferable that these people have training in psychiatric and sociological terms and concepts, as well as competence in both languages. Cultural competence is required as well as a knowledge of the language. Relatives may need to be used, but caution must be taken to ensure that the patient's best interests are being represented.

30.6.3.1.2 Family

Involve the family and mobilize the community for support. They may assist in the process of assessment in helping to understand the context of experience and circumstances.

30.6.3.1.3 Psychotherapy

Religious leaders and healers can provide important alternative sources of support. Psychotherapy with ethnic minority groups needs to recognize a different philosophical framework and personal development. Thus, the Western concern with personal autonomy and independence may not be relevant in those cultures that emphasize the interdependence of the family and the community. Culturally consonant therapy should be offered.

REFERENCES

American Psychiatric Association. 2013: *Desk Reference to the Diagnostic Criteria from DSM-5.* Washington, DC: American Psychiatric Association Press.

Ball RA and Clare AW. 1990: Symptoms and social adjustment in Jewish depressives. *British Journal of Psychiatry* 156:379–383.

Bebbington PE, Feeney ST, Flannigan CB et al. 1994: Inner London collaborative audit of admissions in two health districts: II. Ethnicity and the use of the Mental Health Act. *British Journal of Psychiatry* 165:743–749.

Bhatia MS and Malik SC. 1991: Dhat syndrome: A useful diagnostic entity in Indian culture. *British Journal of Psychiatry* 159:691–695.

Bhugra D and Bhui K. 2001: *Cross-Cultural Psychiatry: A Practical Guide.* London, U.K.: Arnold.

Bhugra D, Sumathipala A, and Siribaddana S. 2007: Culture-bound syndromes: A re-evaluation. In Bhugra D and Bhui K (eds.) *Textbook of Cultural Psychiatry,* pp. 141–156. Cambridge, U.K.: Cambridge University Press.

Chaturvedi SK and Desai G. 2007: Neurosis. In Bhugra D and Bhui K (eds.) *Textbook of Cultural Psychiatry,* pp. 193–206. Cambridge, U.K.: Cambridge University Press.

Cole E, Leavey G, King M et al. 1995: Pathways to care for patients with a first episode of psychosis: A comparison of ethnic groups. *British Journal of Psychiatry* 167:770–776.

Dunn J and Fahy TA. 1990: Police admissions to a psychiatric hospital: Demographic and clinical differences between ethnic groups. *British Journal of Psychiatry* 156:373–378.

Fortune SA and Hawton K. 2007: Culture and mental disorders: Suicidal behaviour. In Bhugra D and Bhui K (eds.) *Textbook of Cultural Psychiatry,* pp. 445–458. Cambridge, U.K.: Cambridge University Press.

Goodman R and Richards H. 1995: Child and adolescent psychiatric presentations of second-generation Afro-Caribbeans in Britain. *British Journal of Psychiatry* 167:362–369.

Guinness EA. 1992: Profile and prevalence of the brain fag syndrome: Psychiatric morbidity in school populations in Africa. *British Journal of Psychiatry* 160(Suppl. 16):42–52.

Harvey I, Williams M, McGuffin P et al. 1990: The functional psychoses in Afro-Caribbean. *British Journal of Psychiatry* 157:515–522.

Hauff E and Vaglum P. 1995: Organised violence and the stress of exile: Predictors of mental health in a community cohort of Vietnamese refugees three years after resettlement. *British Journal of Psychiatry* 166:360–367.

Hotopf M and Mullen R. 1992: Koro and Capgras syndrome in a non-Chinese subject. *British Journal of Psychiatry* 161:577.

Kleinman A. 1977: Depression, somatisation and the new 'cross-cultural psychiatry'. *Social Science and Medicine* 11:3–10.

Kleinman A. 1987: Anthropology and psychiatry: The role of culture in cross-cultural research on illness. *British Journal of Psychiatry* 151:447–454.

Kon Y. 1994: Amok. *British Journal of Psychiatry* 165:685–689.

Leff J, Wig NN, Bedi H et al. 1990: Relatives' expressed emotion and the course of schizophrenia in Chandigarh: A two-year follow-up of a first-contact sample. *British Journal of Psychiatry* 156:351–356.

Littlewood R. 1990: From categories to contexts: A decade of the 'new cross-cultural psychiatry'. *British Journal of Psychiatry* 156:308–327.

Murphy JM. 1994: Anthropology and psychiatric epidemiology. *Acta Psychiatrica Scandinavica* 385(Suppl.):48–57.

Orley J and Wing JK. 1979: Psychiatric disorders in two African villages. *Archives of General Psychiatry* 36:513–521.

Patel V and Winston M. 1994: 'Universality of mental illness' revisited: Assumptions, artefacts and new directions. *British Journal of Psychiatry* 165:437–440.

Raleigh VS and Balarajan R. 1992: Suicide and self-burning among Indians and West Indians in England and Wales. *British Journal of Psychiatry* 161:365–368.

Sartorius N, Jablensky A, Korten A et al. 1986: Early manifestations and first contact incidence of schizophrenia in different cultures. *Psychological Medicine* 16:909–928.

Shepherd M. 1995: Two faces of Emil Kraepelin. *British Journal of Psychiatry* 167:174–183.

Smyth MG and Dean C. 1992: Capgras and koro. *British Journal of Psychiatry* 161:121–123.

Sugarman PPA and Craufurd D. 1994: Schizophrenia in the Afro-Caribbean community. *British Journal of Psychiatry* 164:474–480.

Thomas CS, Stone K, Osborn M et al. 1993: Psychiatric morbidity and compulsory admission among UK-born Europeans, Afro-Caribbeans and Asians in central Manchester. *British Journal of Psychiatry* 163:91–99.

Tseng WS. 2007: Culture and psychopathology. In Bhugra D and Bhui K (eds.) *Textbook of Cultural Psychiatry*, pp. 95–112. Cambridge, U.K.: Cambridge University Press.

World Health Organization. 1973: *Report of the International Pilot Study of Schizophrenia*. Geneva, Switzerland: WHO.

Young R, Sweeting H, and West P. 2006: Prevalence of deliberate self harm and attempted suicide within contemporary Goth youth subculture: Longitudinal cohort study. *British Medical Journal* 332:1058–1061.

31 Liaison, Organic, and Neuropsychiatry

31.1 LIAISON PSYCHIATRY

31.1.1 SOMATIZATION DISORDER

There are multiple, recurrent, frequently changing physical symptoms. Most patients have multiple contacts with primary and specialist medical services; there are many negative investigations. Gastrointestinal and skin symptoms are most common. Sexual and menstrual complaints are also common. Onset after the age of 40 may indicate the onset of affective disorder.

31.1.1.1 Epidemiology

There is a 0.2%–0.5% prevalence in the United Kingdom:

1. Three per cent of repeated gut clinic attenders have somatization disorder.
2. Using abridged criteria (four unexplained symptoms in males, six in females), the prevalence is:
   a. Community—4.4%
   b. Patients with medically unexplained symptoms—32%
3. It is far more common in women than men (F:M = 5:1).
4. It is more common in people with lower education and from lower socioeconomic class.
5. It usually starts in early adult life except somatoform pain disorder that starts later in life.

31.1.1.2 Aetiology

Genetic factors: Torgersen (1986) reported an MZ to DZ concordance in somatoform disorder of 29:10. This suggests that somatoform disorder has a familial transmission. There is an increased rate of dissocial personality disorder among first-degree relatives.

Environmental factors: The South London somatization study reported by Craig et al. in 1993 was a longitudinal study in primary care; it compared somatizers with those with pure emotional disorder and those with pure physical disorder. The physical symptoms of somatizers were less likely to improve; one-third went on to develop chronic somatoform disorders. Changes in physical symptoms mirrored changes in emotional arousal.

Social learning: Somatizers were more likely to report parental physical illness and to have had more physical illness themselves in childhood. Emotionally disordered subjects reported more parental lack of care. It was hypothesized that physical illness in childhood lessened the distress of lack of care, resulting in somatic rather than emotional responses as a means of attracting care or lessening hostility, which endures into adult life. Somatic symptoms represent a way of communicating emotions.

31.1.1.3 Clinical Features

ICD-10 requires the presence of all the following:

- Two years of multiple and variable physical symptoms, with no physical explanation found
- Persistent refusal to accept the advice of several doctors
- Impairment of functioning attributable to symptoms and resulting behaviour

The possibility of developing an independent physical disorder should be considered.

The emphasis on symptoms and their effects distinguishes this from hypochondriacal disorder (see following text) where the emphasis of concern is on possible underlying disease.

Briquet's syndrome or St. Louis hysteria is a multiple somatization disorder.

Somatization disorder is renamed as somatic symptom disorder in the DSM-5 (APA, 2013). Patients suffer from somatic symptoms that cause distress and result in significant disruption in life. Patients also have disproportionate and persistent thoughts about the seriousness of somatic symptoms. The symptoms lead to high level of anxiety. As a result, excessive time and energy are devoted to the symptoms concerned. The duration is at least 6 months. Specific feature includes predominant pain.

31.1.1.3.1 Comorbidities

Comorbidities include depressive disorder, anxiety disorders (e.g. generalized anxiety disorder, panic disorder, and social phobia), adjustment disorder, psychotic disorder, histrionic personality disorder, dissocial personality disorder, substance misuse, and other somatoform disorder.

31.1.1.3.2 Management

Engage the patient and spouse. Conduct no more investigations but listen empathically. Elicit childhood experience of illness and parental disability. Link physical symptoms to relevant life events (the reattribution model of Goldberg). Reduce all medication apart from antidepressants for the depressed. Limit the expectations of cure.

Psychotherapies are useful in the treatment of somatization disorder:

1. *Cognitive therapy*: Cognitive therapy is useful in the treatment of somatization disorder by helping the patient to establish the connection between emotions and somatic symptoms. Dysfunction thought diary records somatic symptoms and emotionally significant life events causing the somatic symptoms. Psychologist can help the patient to review thoughts and beliefs focusing on somatic complaints and advise the patient to consider alternatives. The goal of cognitive therapy is to help the patient to reattribute physical symptoms to underlying psychological state (e.g. stress, depression).
2. *Behaviour therapy*: Enhance activity level, encourage positive coping behaviours, and develop alternative ways to express emotions and not to focus on somatic symptoms in communications.
3. *Family support*: Educate the partner or other family members on how to respond to patient's somatic complaints.

Alexithymia (limited ability to describe emotions verbally) is common in somatoform disorder. Traditional psychotherapy with alexithymic individuals is difficult. A more reality-based educational and supportive approach is better.

31.1.1.3.3 Course and Prognosis

The course is chronic and fluctuating. Treatments use disproportionate health resources. If engaged as mentioned earlier, this significantly reduces the use of resources. However, depression and anxiety are often present and may require treatment. Prognosis is poor and 80% of patients continue to suffer from somatization disorder after 5 years.

31.1.2 SOMATOFORM AUTONOMIC DYSFUNCTION

Symptoms are presented as if caused by a disorder of a system or organ largely under autonomic control (e.g. cardiac neurosis, psychogenic hyperventilation, gastric neurosis, nervous diarrhoea).

ICD-10 (WHO, 1992)

- There are persistent and troublesome symptoms of autonomic arousal.
- Symptoms are referred to a specific organ system, with no evidence of organ pathology.
- There is distress about the possibility of disorder of the organ system, not responsive to repeated reassurance.

31.1.3 PERSISTENT SOMATOFORM PAIN DISORDER

This presents with persistent, severe, distressing pain, not explained by physical disorder. Pain occurs in association with emotional conflict and results in increased support and attention.

The prevalence of persistent pain is 3%. The onset of somatoform pain disorder is usually between 40 and 50 years. The female to male ratio is 2:1. Acute pain (<6 months) is associated with anxiety disorder. Chronic pain (≥6 months) is associated with depressive disorder. The onset of somatoform pain is usually abrupt. Treatment involves antidepressants (e.g. duloxetine, nortriptyline), gradual withdrawal of analgesics, cognitive–behavioural therapy (CBT) (challenges cognitive and behaviour activation) and relaxation techniques. In general, acute pain carries a better prognosis than chronic pain.

31.1.4 HYPOCHONDRIACAL DISORDER

31.1.4.1 Epidemiology

The prevalence of hypochondriacal disorder in the general population is 1%. The prevalence among medical patients is 5%. The onset was between 20 and 30 years. It occurs in both men and women, with no familial characteristics. Hypochondriacal disorder is associated with lower economic status and history of medical illnesses.

31.1.4.2 Aetiology

The aetiology of hypochondriacal disorder includes social learning theory and patients may adopt a sick role to avoid obligations. From the psychodynamic perspectives, aggression is transformed into hypochondriacal ideas.

ICD-10 (WHO, 1992)

- There is a persistent belief in the presence of at least one serious physical illness, despite repeated investigations revealing no physical explanation of presenting symptoms, or persistent preoccupation with presumed deformity.
- There is a persistent refusal to accept the advice of several different doctors that there is no physical illness underlying the symptoms.

Attention is usually focused on one or two organ systems only. Anxiety disorders (e.g. generalized anxiety disorder, obsessive–compulsive disorder [OCD]) and depressive disorder are common comorbidity. If depressive symptoms are prominent and precede the onset of hypochondriacal ideas, then depressive disorder may be primary.

31.1.4.3 DSM-5

The DSM-5 proposed to rename hypochondriasis as illness anxiety disorder (APA, 2013). In order to fulfil the diagnostic criteria, the patient is preoccupied with having a serious illness that is clearly excessive or disproportionate. Somatic symptoms are usually not present and only be present mild in intensity. The person also exhibits high level of anxiety and easily be alarmed about health and performs excessive health-related behaviours (e.g. repetitive checking). The duration of illness is at least 6 months. There are two types of illness anxiety disorder, the care-seeking subtype that is associated with increased rate of medical consultation and the care-avoidant subtype that is associated with avoidance of medical consultation and treatment.

31.1.4.4 Management

Psychiatrists should advise medical colleagues or general practitioners to gradually reduce the frequency of visits and unnecessary investigations by increasing the duration between appointments.

Antidepressant such as SSRI is useful.

Psychotherapies are useful to treat hypochondriacal disorder:

1. *Cognitive therapy*: Reattribution and develop alternative explanations of symptoms and concerns of serious illness. Cognitive restructuring can modify dysfunctional assumptions.

2. *Behaviour therapy*: Self-monitoring of worries, negative thoughts, and illness-related behaviours. It also involves exposure and response prevention and reducing repeated reassurance-seeking behaviours.

3. Relaxation techniques.

31.1.4.5 Course and Prognosis

The course of hypochondriacal disorder is usually episodic and patients may present with different hypochondriacal idea each time. Around 30%–50% of patients have good prognosis. Good prognostic factors include good past health, high socioeconomic status, and sudden onset of hypochondriacal ideas.

31.1.4.6 Conversion Disorder and Body Dysmorphic Disorder

Conversion disorder and body dysmorphic disorder are considered in Chapter 28.

31.2 FACTITIOUS DISORDER AND MALINGERING

31.2.1 FACTITIOUS DISORDER

In factitious disorder, the patient intentionally produces physical or psychological symptoms but the patient is unconscious about his or her underlying motives. The patient may have working experience in the healthcare setting and equip with basic medical knowledge. Common presenting signs and symptoms include bleeding, diarrhoea, hypoglycaemia, infection, impaired wound healing, vomiting, rashes, and seizures. The patient often has poor prognosis and refuse to receive psychotherapy.

31.2.2 FACTITIOUS DISORDER BY PROXY

In factitious disorder by proxy, the patient intentionally produces physical signs or symptoms in another person (usually an infant or a child) who is under the patient's care.

31.2.3 MALINGERING

In malingering, the patient intentionally produces physical or psychological symptoms and the patient is fully aware of his or her underlying motives. As a result, the patient does not want to cooperate for further assessment and evaluation because the marked discrepancy between the severity of symptoms reported and the objective physical findings will be revealed. The patient may suffer from antisocial personality disorder (Table 31.1).

TABLE 31.1

Compare and Contrast Factitious Disorder, Malingering, and Somatization Disorder

	Factitious Disorder	Malingering	Somatization Disorder
Motivation	Assume the sick role	External gain (e.g. false claim from an insurance company, avoid legal responsibility)	Internal psychological motivation
Signs or symptoms	Intentional production or feigning signs or symptoms	Intentionally produced	Unintentional and involuntary
Attitude towards medical professionals	Provide a vague and confusion history	Poor cooperation in evaluation and treatment	Frequent medical consultation to seek relief of symptoms
	Patient may go from hospital to hospital seeking hospitalization		

31.3 CARDIOLOGY AND PSYCHIATRY

The relationship between stress and the cardiovascular system (Wise and Rundell, 2002):

1. Stressful life events lead to appraisal of the current situation. Primary appraisal assesses the threatening nature of a life event. Secondary appraisal assesses the adequacy of coping strategies.
2. There will be three phases of responses. Phase 1 is an alarm reaction, phase 2 is the resistance stage, and phase 3 is the exhaustion stage.
3. The sympathetic system is activated by stressful life events. Patient will experience dilation of pupils, dry mouth, palpitations, and sweating.
4. Chronic mental stress–associated ordinary life events are the most common precipitant of myocardial ischaemia in patients with coronary artery disease. Type A behaviour (e.g. aggressiveness, impatience, and hostility) is associated with the incidence of recurrent myocardial infarction and cardiac death in patients with previous myocardial infarction. Twenty per cent of people with acute myocardial infarction suffer from depressive disorder (Friedman et al., 1987).
5. Psychosocial stress increases the levels of adrenaline and noradrenaline, which causes an increase in peripheral vascular resistance, resulting in hypertension and hypertrophy of the heart.
6. An acute emotional trigger such as provoking anger is the immediate precipitant of arrhythmias in patients who are in a chronic state of helplessness. Helplessness is an underlying sense of entrapment without possible escape. Arrhythmias can lead to sudden cardiac death.

The relationship between depression and ischaemic heart disease (IHD):

1. Twenty per cent of patients with IHD have comorbid depression.
2. Major depression as an independent risk factor for IHD.
3. After an acute myocardial infarction, major depression predicts mortality in the first 6 months. The impact of a depressive episode is equivalent to the impact of a previous infarct.

The impact of depression on heart diseases:

1. Poor compliance to cardiac treatment.
2. Autonomic disturbances in depression may lead to heart rate changes and arrhythmias.
3. Serotonin dysfunction in depression: platelet activation and thrombosis.

31.3.1 ANTIDEPRESSANT TRIALS IN PATIENTS SUFFERING FROM IHD

1. Sertraline Antidepressant Heart Attack Randomized Trial (SADHART)
   This study found sertraline to be a safe treatment for depression after myocardial infarction, but there was little difference in depression status between groups receiving sertraline and placebo after 24 weeks of treatment. However, the effect of sertraline was greater in the patients with severe and recurrent depression. This study was not designed to assess the effects of treatment on cardiovascular prognosis, but severe

TABLE 31.2
Use of Psychotropic Drugs for Patients Suffering from Atrial Fibrillation

	Antipsychotics	Antidepressants	Mood Stabilizers	Hypnotics	Dementia
Recommended	Aripiprazole	Mirtazapine (patients with AF often take NSAIDs and warfarin)	Lithium Valproate	Benzodiazepines	Rivastigmine seems to be the best
Not recommended	Clozapine Olanzapine Paliperidone	Tricyclic antidepressants	Nil	Nil	Avoid other acetylcholinesterase inhibitors in paroxysmal AF

Source: Taylor, D. et al., *The Maudsley Prescribing Guideline*, Informa Healthcare, London, U.K., 2009.

cardiovascular events during the 6-month treatment tended to be less frequent in the sertraline group. The effect of sertraline on chronic depression was not evaluated.

2. ENhancing Recovery in Coronary Heart Disease (ENRICHD) Study (Berkman et al., 2003)
   In this trial, the effects of CBT on depression and cardiac outcomes were evaluated. No significant difference in the cardiac outcomes was found between the intervention and the care as usual arms. Although substantial improvement in the severity of depression was observed 6 months after initiation of CBT, the difference between both arms diminished over time and was no longer present after 30 months.

3. Myocardial INfarction and Depression— Intervention Trial (MIND–IT) (Van Melle et al., 2007)
   Antidepressant treatment did not alter the course of chronic depression after myocardial infarction status or improve the cardiac outcomes (Table 31.2).

31.4 NEPHROLOGY AND PSYCHIATRY

31.4.1 PSYCHIATRIC ASPECTS OF CHRONIC RENAL FAILURE

Chronic renal failure is a result of irreversible loss of glomerular filtration rate (GFR). Progressive loss of GFR leads to end-stage renal failure.

The most common causes of CRF in the United Kingdom include autosomal dominant polycystic kidney disease, diabetes mellitus (DM), chronic pyelonephritis, glomerulonephritides (IgA nephropathy), hypertension, obstructive uropathy, and vascular disease.

Advanced uraemia causes lethargy, asterixis, myoclonus, deterioration in total intelligence, and impairment in working memory.

The differential diagnosis of neuropsychiatric symptoms in CRF patients includes hypercalcaemia, hypophosphataemia, hypo- or hyperglycaemia, hypo- or hypernatraemia, drug intoxication, and central nervous system (CNS) pathologies such as meningitis, encephalitis, subdural haematoma (SDH), and hypertensive encephalopathy.

Uraemic encephalopathy is associated with nonspecific EEG changes.

31.4.2 PSYCHIATRIC ASPECTS OF DIALYSIS

Psychiatrists are often asked to assess patients with chronic renal failure refusing dialysis.

Assessment should include

1. Capacity to make decisions: capacity is reduced as a result of uraemia; previous views or advanced directives should be sought and dialysis should continue to optimize the patient's condition to make decisions
2. Presence of depression, hopelessness, and suicidal plan
3. Misconception and misunderstanding of dialysis

Dialysis improves uraemic encephalopathy but sexual dysfunctions and impaired quality of life continue throughout the course of dialysis. Dialysis dementia is characterized by progressive encephalopathy, stuttering, dysarthria, dysphasia, impaired memory, depression, paranoia, myoclonic jerk, triphasic EEG abnormality, and seizures (Tables 31.3 and 31.4).

TABLE 31.3

Use of Psychotropic Drugs for Patients Suffering from Renal Impairment

Types	Antipsychotics	Antidepressants	Mood Stabilizers	Hypnotics
Recommended	*First-generation antipsychotic drug*: haloperidol 2–6 mg/day *Second-generation antipsychotic drug*: olanzapine 5 mg/day	Citalopram Sertraline	Valproate Carbamazepine Lamotrigine	Lorazepam Zopiclone
Not recommended	Sulpiride Amisulpride Avoid highly anticholinergic agent.	Tricyclic antidepressant (because of anticholinergics effects)	Lithium	Diazepam (long half-life)

Source: Taylor, D. et al., *The Maudsley Prescribing Guideline*, Informa Healthcare, London, U.K., 2009.

TABLE 31.4

Summary of Electrolyte Disturbances and Psychiatric Manifestations

	Low Levels	High Levels
Sodium	*Causes*: antidepressants, lithium, carbamazepine, diuretics, SIADH, and compulsive water drinking *Neuropsychiatric features*: anorexia, fatigue, headache confusion, and convulsion (if Na < 115)	*Causes*: dehydration, diarrhoea, CNS lesions, and severe burns *Neuropsychiatric features*: reduced consciousness (Na > 160), confusion, stupor, and coma if sodium is very high
Potassium	*Causes*: vomiting, nausea (in bulimia nervosa), laxative addiction, diuretics, hypomagnesaemia, renal tubular acidosis, and Cushing's disease *Neuropsychiatric features*: muscular weakness, lethargy, and drowsiness.	*Causes*: excessive consumption of NSAIDS, potassium supplements, acute and chronic renal impairment, tumour lysis syndrome *Neuropsychiatric features*: weakness, sensory perception deficits, and delirium
Calcium	*Causes*: hypoparathyroidism, phenytoin, secondary hyperparathyroidism *Neuropsychiatric features*: weakness, depression, delirium, and seizure	*Common causes*: hyperparathyroidism, malignancy, chronic renal failure, dehydration *Less common causes*: milk-alkali syndrome, sarcoidosis, thiazide diuretics, and vitamin D *Neuropsychiatric features*: anorexia, vomiting, nausea; late stage: drowsiness, depression, delirium, and seizure
Magnesium	*Causes*: starvation, chronic alcoholism, and acute intermittent porphyria *Neuropsychiatric features*: weakness, depression, delirium, seizure, and hallucination	*Causes*: renal failure, magnesium-containing oral medication *Neuropsychiatric features*: drowsiness, weakness, and coma
Acid–base balance	Metabolic acidosis *Causes*: starvation, alcohol, diabetic ketoacidosis, renal failure, and severe sepsis *Psychiatric features*: fatigue, anorexia, hyperventilation, laboured breathing (Kussmaul respiration), coma, and convulsions	Metabolic alkalosis *Causes*: vomiting and chloride depletion *Psychiatric features*: irritability, hypoventilation, lethargy, and confusion when pH > 7.55

Source: Maxwell, P. H., *Medical Masterclass—Nephrology*, Blackwell Science, London, U.K., 2001.

31.5 HEPATOLOGY AND PSYCHIATRY

31.5.1 HEPATIC ENCEPHALOPATHY

Hepatic encephalopathy is caused by hyperammonaemia and an increase in GABA neurotransmission.

The stage of hepatic encephalopathy is summarized as follows:

Stage 0—Subclinical, psychomotor test abnormalities
Stage 1—Lethargy, confusion, excitation, sleep disturbance, and decreased attention
Stage 2—Somnolence, inappropriate behaviour
Stage 3—Stupor but arousable, speech incomprehensible
Stage 4—Coma

The first step in management of hepatic encephalopathy is to identify the underlying cause. Daily dietary protein intake is reduced to 40 g or less, preferably restricted to high biological value protein. Patients will be given laxatives, enemas, lactulose, and antibiotics (e.g. neomycin).

31.5.2 WILSON'S DISEASE (LISHMAN, 1997)

Wilson's disease is an autosomal recessive disorder of hepatic copper metabolism. The incidence is 1 in 200,000. The gene responsible for this disorder has been located on chromosome 13 and encodes a copper-binding, membrane-spanning protein with ATPase that regulates metal transport proteins.

Patients usually present with liver disease during adolescence; however, clinical onset may be detected as early as 3 years of age. Features include hepatic dysfunction (40%); psychiatric symptoms such as depression, cognitive impairment, abnormal behaviour, and personality change (35%); and renal, haematological, and endocrine symptoms. Cirrhosis and fulminant hepatic failure are well-described complications. Ocular saccades are slowed in Wilson's disease (ocular saccades are also slow in Huntington's disease and supranuclear palsy). Other neurological features include dysphagia, drooling, slowness, flexed postures, a gaping mouth, dysarthria, coarse tremor, dystonia, rigidity, and chorea. The characteristic Kayser–Fleischer rings nearly present in all patients with neuropsychiatric symptoms and slit lamp examination can be performed to verify the diagnosis. Cirrhosis usually takes two or three decades to develop.

The diagnosis is established by low serum ceruloplasmin, an increased level of copper in the urine (>100 μg/24 h), and an elevated hepatic copper level (>250 μg of copper/1 g of liver by dry weight). The CSF urate levels parallel serum levels and these levels are low in Wilson's disease.

Pharmacological treatment includes D-penicillamine and oral zinc. Liver transplantation is indicated for patients with fulminant hepatitis or advanced cirrhosis.

31.5.3 USE OF PSYCHOTROPIC DRUGS FOR PATIENTS SUFFERING FROM LIVER DISEASES

The general principle includes fewer drugs, lower dose, and monitoring of side effects. Avoid drugs that are hepatotoxic, sedative, and cause constipation that increases the risk of hepatic encephalopathy (Table 31.5).

TABLE 31.5
Use of Psychotropic Drugs for Patients with Liver Impairment

Types	Antipsychotics	Antidepressants	Mood Stabilizers	Hypnotics
Recommended	Low dose of haloperidol Sulpiride or amisulpride: no dosage reduction is required if renal function is normal	Paroxetine Citalopram	Lithium	Lorazepam Oxazepam Temazepam Zopiclone
Not recommended	Avoid antipsychotic drugs that have extensive hepatic metabolism such as chlorpromazine that is associated with anticholinergic side effects	Avoid tricyclic antidepressant that is associated with constipation Avoid fluoxetine because of long half-life and the risk of accumulation of metabolites	Avoid carbamazepine because it induces hepatic metabolism Avoid valproate because it is highly protein bound and metabolized by liver	Avoid diazepam that has long half-life

Source: Taylor, D. et al., *The Maudsley Prescribing Guideline*, Informa Healthcare, London, U.K., 2009.

31.6 ENDOCRINOLOGY AND PSYCHIATRY (GURNELL, 2001)

31.6.1 HYPERTHYROIDISM

Clinical example: A 30-year-old woman is referred to your clinic. She is quite edgy and complains that any overindulgence has resulted in severe facial flushing. She has also been troubled by watery diarrhoea. She has lost a significant amount of weight despite good appetite and her periods have stopped. Thyroid function test shows $T_4 = 250$ mmol/L and $TSH = 0.2$ mU/L.

Epidemiology: Hyperthyroidism affects 2%–5% of all women mostly between the age of 20 and 45 years, with a F:M ratio of 5:1.

Aetiology: Common causes include Grave's disease (presence of thyroid antibodies), toxic multinodular goitre, solitary adenoma, thyrotoxicosis factitia, and drugs such as amiodarone and exogenous iodine.

Rarer causes include thyroid carcinoma, pituitary tumour, ovarian teratomas, and acute thyroiditis (viral or postirradiation). Stress can precipitate Grave's disease.

Neuropsychiatric aspects: 50% present with psychiatric symptoms. Anxiety and depression are common. Depressive symptoms are not linearly related to thyroxine levels. In the thyroid crisis, delirium will occur (3%–4%). Psychosis is rare in hyperthyroidism (1%).

Treatment: Antithyroid medication, radioactive thyroxine, or thyroid surgery is able to reverse psychiatric symptoms. If there is no response by 1 month, psychotropic medication such as antidepressant is required.

31.6.2 HYPOTHYROIDISM

Clinical example: A 45-year-old woman is no longer able to meet the demands of her job, complaining of excessive tiredness, lethargy, and constipation. The only past medical history is the history of palpitations that are now well controlled on amiodarone.

Epidemiology: Hypothyroidism is one of the most common endocrinopathies in the United Kingdom with a prevalence of 1.4% in females but rarer in men (0.1%).

31.6.2.1 Aetiology

Common causes include autoimmune hypothyroidism, Hashimoto's thyroiditis, postsurgical and postirradiation hypothyroidism, antithyroid, and other drugs such as lithium and amiodarone and in mountainous area, iodine deficiency.

Rare causes include congenital agenesis, dyshormonogenesis, tumour infiltration, and secondary hypothyroidism with TSH deficiency.

31.6.2.2 Neuropsychiatric Symptoms

Twenty per cent of patients present with psychiatric symptoms. Fatigue accompanied by mental and physical slowing is a central psychiatric feature. Depression and anxiety are very common. Cognitive assessment is important.

Myxedema causes psychotic symptoms (paranoid delusions, auditory or visual hallucinations) and delirium.

31.6.2.3 Investigations

Electroencephalogram: One-third of patients show slowing of the dominant rhythm and a reduction of the background activity.

31.6.2.4 Treatment

Lithium-induced goitre has been found in 4%–35% of patients and the goitre is reversible after stopping lithium for 1–2 months.

Thyroxine replacement therapy may reverse psychiatric symptoms. If there is no response by 1 month, psychotropic medication such as antidepressant is required.

31.6.3 CUSHING'S SYNDROME

Clinical example: A 25-year-old woman with long-standing irregular menses presents with gradually worsening hirsutism and weight gain. She has acnes on her faces and she feels depressed. Her supervisor complains that the customers do not like her physical appearance because she works in a boutique.

Aetiology: Cushing syndrome is most commonly caused by exogenous administration of corticosteroids. Other causes include ACTH-dependent causes (e.g. Cushing's disease, ectopic ACTH-producing tumours, and ACTH administration), non-ACTH-dependent causes (e.g. adrenal adenomas or carcinomas), and alcohol-dependent pseudo-Cushing's syndrome.

Neuropsychiatric symptoms: 50%–80% suffer from depression with moderate to severe symptoms. Depression will resolve with the control of hypercortisolism. Suicide has been reported in between 3% and 10% of patients. Cognitive impairment such as amnesia and attentional deficits are common.

Investigation: In dexamethasone suppression test, the cortisol level is expected to be less than 50% of the baseline value in Cushing's disease but not other causes of Cushing's syndrome.

Psychiatric side effects associated with steroid: emotional lability (e.g. euphoria, anxiety, depression, hypomania), distractibility, insomnia, auditory and visual hallucinations, delusions, intermittent memory impairment, and mutism. Higher risk if the dose of prednisolone is higher than 40 mg per day and more prone in women.

31.6.4 Addison's Disease

Clinical example: A 30-year-old woman presents with weakness, dizziness, anorexia, weight loss, and gastrointestinal disturbance. On physical examination, there is generalized hyperpigmentation of the skin and mucous membrane. She also has postural hypotension and loss of pubic hairs.

Epidemiology: 75% of adrenocortical insufficiency is caused by Addison's disease. Female to male ratio is 2:1.

Neuropsychiatric Symptoms

1. Fatigue, weakness, and apathy are common in early stage.
2. Ninety per cent of patients with adrenal disorders present with psychiatric symptoms.
3. Memory impairment is common.
4. Depression, anxiety, and paranoia tend to have a fluctuating course with symptom free intervals.
5. Psychosis occurs in 20% of patients.
6. Adrenal crisis may lead to delirium.

31.6.5 Syndrome of Inappropriate Antidiuretic Hormone Hypersecretion

Clinical example: A 20-year-old man is referred from the GP for nausea, confusion, and mild irritability. A routine electrolyte check shows that the serum Na is 120 mmol/L (normal range: 135–145 mmol/L). Physical examination reveals no evidence of dehydration and fluid overload. Subsequent investigation reveals urine Na excretion of 40 mmol/L (normal range <20 mmol/L), plasma osmolality of 250 mOsmol/kg, and urine osmolality of 800 mOsmol/kg.

Aetiology: Causes include various tumours (e.g. small cell carcinoma of the lung), chest infections, CNS causes (e.g. tumours, brain abscess, head injury, meningitis), porphyria, alcohol withdrawal, and a number of drugs such as carbamazepine, chlorpropamide, and vincristine.

Investigations: Syndrome of inappropriate antidiuretic hormone hypersecretion (SIADH) leads to water retention and low serum sodium level. To make the diagnosis, other causes of dilutional hyponatraemia such as diuretic use and excess water intake should be excluded.

31.6.6 Psychogenic Polydipsia

Psychogenic polydipsia causes dilutional hyponatraemia and reduction in serum osmolality. Unlike SIADH, patients with hysterical polydipsia produce diluted urine. Water deprivation test under careful monitoring of fluid status is diagnostic and helps to distinguish psychogenic polydipsia from SIADH. Psychogenic polydipsia is controlled by limiting fluid intake. Management involves offering reassurance to patients and relatives and fluid restriction.

31.6.7 Diabetes Mellitus

Clinical Examples

1. A 60-year-old woman suffers from depression. She has informed you that she has become thirsty and having to pass urine very often. Routine urinalysis shows glycosuria and ketones.
2. A 50-year-old man with history of schizophrenia and DM is prescribed with clozapine. He complains of sudden abdominal pain. Mental state examination reveals that he appears to be agitated and confused. This is an example of clozapine-induced hyperglycaemia and diabetic ketoacidosis.

Introduction: DM refers to a group of metabolic disorders characterized by hyperglycaemia, resulting from inadequate production and/or impaired action of insulin.

Type I DM is caused by autoimmunity governed by the HLA class II genes. Environmental factors such as viruses (Coxsackie, rubella, mumps, cytomegalovirus, Epstein–Barr virus [EBV]), infants fed on bovine serum albumin in cow's milk, and stress.

Type II DM is strongly associated with obesity. The risk to develop type II DM is 40 times higher in people with BMI> 35 as compared to those with BMI < 23. Type II DM is caused by insulin resistance and defects of insulin secretion. Type II DM has high identical twin concordance rate.

Chronic hypoglycaemia may cause psychotic symptoms.

Investigations: Glycosuria may suggest the presence of DM but requires blood test to confirm. The diagnosis of DM is made on the basis of fasting plasma glucose level of ≥7.0 mmol/L that should be confirmed on a second occasion.

31.6.8 Diabetes Insipidus

Clinical example: A 60-year-old woman has informed you that she has become thirsty and passes urine very often. She has low urine osmolality and high plasma osmolality.

Cranial diabetes insipidus (DI) is caused by post head injury, cranial surgery, radiotherapy, craniopharyngioma, and CNS infection.

Treatment of cranial DI includes symptomatic relief by the synthetic vasopressin analogue desmopressin. Desmopressin is administered orally or more conveniently via a nasal spray.

Nephrogenic DI is caused by renal disorders, hypercalcaemia, hypokalaemia, and lithium.

Treatment of nephrogenic DI: Thiazide diuretic (e.g. hydrochlorothiazide) and sodium restriction are often effective.

31.6.9 HYPERPARATHYROIDISM

Clinical example: A 57-year-old woman presents with thirst, polyuria, constipation, anorexia, malaise, and depression. She has history of renal calculus.

Hypercalcaemia is caused by primary hyperparathyroidism and contributes to psychiatric morbidity.

Neuropsychiatric symptoms include the following:

1. Disturbance of mood and drive is prevalent. Depression may progress to psychosis and suicide.
2. Delirium is caused by high calcium levels or parathyroid crisis.
3. Cognitive impairment: impaired attention, mental slowing, and impaired memory.
4. Psychosis (5%–20%): mainly persecutory delusions and hallucinations.

Treatment: Correction of serum calcium usually results in reversal of psychiatric symptoms.

31.6.10 HYPOPARATHYROIDISM

Clinical example: A 35-year-old woman is referred to the liaison team because of acute confusion. She also complains of muscle cramps and loss of sensation in her extremities. Her partner reports that the muscle cramps are caused by exercise. She had a thyroid surgery 1 month ago. On physical examination, a latent tetany is provoked by inflating a sphygmomanometer cuff to 10–20 mmHg greater than her systolic blood pressure. In addition, tapping her facial nerve in front of the ear induce a brief contraction of her facial muscles.

Epidemiology: More common in women.

Types of hypoparathyroidism.

Primary hypoparathyroidism is rare and associated with insidious onset. Psychiatric features include emotional lability, inattention, intellectual deterioration, and dementia. Prognosis for dementia is unpredictable. Skull x-ray may show symmetrical calcification in the basal ganglia.

Secondary hypoparathyroidism is more common than primary hypoparathyroidism. It is often caused by thyroid surgery and associated with acute delirium. Other psychiatric features include depression, psychosis, mania, anxiety, and irritability. The prognosis for psychiatric symptoms is favourable.

Pseudohypoparathyroidism is caused by end-organ unresponsiveness to circulating parathyroid hormone as a result of familial calcification of basal ganglia. It is associated with learning disability with poor response to treatment.

Physical features: Tetany, cramps, cataracts, and generalized seizures. In the aforementioned clinical example, the latent tetany is known as *Trousseau's sign*. The contraction of the facial muscles is known as *Chvostek's sign*.

31.7 ONCOLOGY AND PSYCHIATRY

Tumours induce release of a number of pro-inflammatory markers from macrophages and inflammatory cells such as the TNF-α that causes weight loss, fatigue, and constitutional symptoms.
Symptoms include

1. Pain
2. Nausea (25% of patients receiving chemotherapy)
3. Fatigue
4. Cognitive impairment
5. Depression and anxiety (25% of people with cancer suffer from depressive disorder)

Metastatic brain tumours occur in patients suffering from primary renal, pancreatic, gynaecological, prostate, and bladder cancer. Leptomeningeal disease is caused by non-Hodgkin's lymphoma and adenocarcinoma of lung. Effects of direct neurological insults of metastatic brain tumours include

1. Complex partial seizures
2. Delirium
3. Dementia
4. Mania

Common causes of delirium in cancer patients include

1. Hypercalcaemia
2. Hypomagnesaemia
3. Hyperviscosity syndromes

31.7.1 SIDE EFFECTS OF CHEMOTHERAPEUTIC AGENTS

Neuropsychiatric Side Effects of Chemotherapeutic Agents

1. Cognitive impairment/dementia as a result of leukoencephalopathy (e.g. cytosine arabinoside, methotrexate)
2. Acute confusion (associated with most chemotherapeutic agents)
3. Manic and depressive symptoms (e.g. steroid, interferon)
4. Psychosis (e.g. procarbazine)
5. Personality change (e.g. cytosine arabinoside)
6. Fatigue (e.g. fluorouracil, interleukin, interferon)
7. Seizures (e.g. vincristine, vinblastine, alkylating agents)
8. Anorexia (associated with most chemotherapeutic agents)
9. Neuropathies and sexual dysfunction
10. Cataracts (e.g. steroids)
11. Anticholinergic side effects (e.g. antiemetic agents)

31.7.2 CHRONIC FATIGUE SYNDROME (WESSELY ET AL., 2003)

31.7.2.1 Epidemiology

In the United Kingdom, prevalence of chronic fatigue syndrome (CFS) ranges from 0.8% to 2.6% and only 0.1% fulfil the Centres for Disease Control (CDC) (1988) criteria. The female to male ratio is 3:1. The age of onset is between 29 and 35 years. People with CFS may have lower occupational status and educational background.

31.7.2.2 Aetiology

1. *Persistent viral infection*: EBV. EBV is the most common viral cause and attributes to 9%–22% of CFS. Enteroviruses (e.g. *Coxsackie B)* also cause CFS.
2. *Immune dysfunction*: abnormal immune responses with reduced or enhanced responses after acute infection.
3. *Electrolyte imbalance*: low intracellular magnesium.
4. *Chronic candidiasis*: chronic intestinal overgrowth of *Candida albicans* produces fatigue via toxins or allergic response.

31.7.2.3 Pathology

31.7.2.3.1 Immunological Changes

1. Increase in expression of activation markers on the surface of T lymphocytes
2. Increase in number of CD 8+ cytotoxic T cells
3. Decrease in number of natural killer cell function

31.7.2.3.2 Endocrine Changes

1. Abnormality in hypothalamic–pituitary–adrenal axis
2. Hypocortisolism

31.7.2.4 Diagnostic Criteria

The American use of the CDC criteria emphasizes the presence of at least four symptoms (e.g. muscle pain, sore throat, headache, shortness of breath, chronic cough, visual problems, and difficulties in maintaining upright position) from a list of eight symptoms. In contrast, the British emphasize less on the somatic symptoms but put more emphasis on physical and mental fatigue instead.

Neurasthenia (ICD-10 F48.0): CFS is the functional medical syndrome that is the approximate equivalent of neurasthenia in psychiatry.

1. Either of the following must be present:
   a. Persistent and distressing complaints of feelings of exhaustion after minor mental effort.
   b. Persistent and distressing complaints of feelings of fatigue and bodily weakness after minor physical effort.
2. At least one of the following symptoms must be present:
   a. Feelings of muscular aches and pains.
   b. The patient is unable to recover from the symptoms in criterion 1 or 2 by means of rest, relaxation, or entertainment.
   c. The duration of the disorder is at least 3 months.
   d. Exclusion: organic emotionally labile disorder, postencephalitic syndrome, postconcussional syndrome, mood disorders, panic disorder, or generalized anxiety disorder.

Fibromyalgia is characterized by tenderness at trigger points affecting mainly the cervical and thoracic areas. Other features include fatigue, poor sleep, joint stiffness, numbness, and cognitive dysfunction. It is commonly associated with depression and anxiety.

31.7.2.5 Investigations

For all patients: FBC, ESR, CRP, U & Es, LFTs, TFTs, urine protein, and glucose.

For selected patients: EBV serology, toxoplasmosis serology, cytomegalovirus serology, human immunodeficiency virus (HIV) serology, CXR, creatinine phosphokinase, rheumatoid factor, and cerebral MRI (look for demyelination).

31.7.2.6 Management

1. Pharmacological treatment: a nonsedative SSRI such as fluoxetine may be helpful for patients with CFS and depression. Essential fatty acids may be beneficial. Avoid benzodiazepine.
2. Psychological treatment: CBT with graded activity programme, anxiety management, and interpersonal therapy.
3. Rehabilitation: exercise programme.

31.7.2.7 Prognosis

1. Between 20% and 50% of CFS patients seen in specialist care improve in the medium term, but fewer than 10% return to premorbid functioning.
2. The prognosis is better in children and in patients in primary care.
3. The principal predictors of poor outcome or treatment response include intensity of focus on symptoms of CFS, psychiatric morbidity, poor sense of control, being passive with treatment, underlying secondary gain (e.g. disability benefits), and old age.
4. There is no increase in mortality (with the exception of suicide).

CASC STATION ON CHRONIC FATIGUE SYNDROME

Name: Mr. D
Age: 33 years old
Occupation: Accountant
Marital status: Married with two children

Mr. D complains of tiredness, lethargy, and intermittent, vague, generalized muscle pains, which he dates from when he had glandular fever (infectious mononucleosis) 1 year ago. Mr. D is referred to you by his GP, who has conducted the following investigations: FBC, U & Es, LFTs, TFTs and urine analysis, all of which are within normal limits. He has been avoiding contact with his usually extensive social network. Mr. D now does not entertain any possibility of returning to his previous level of occupational functioning. His wife also says that she is not coping. The marital relationship is under significant strain.

Task: Take a history to establish the diagnosis.

CASC Grid

(A) Diagnostic Criteria of CFS	(A1) Explore about Fatigue	(A2) Onset, Course and the Nature of Fatigue	(A3) Biological Symptoms	(A4) Cognitive Symptoms	(A5) Functional Impairment and Understanding of Symptoms
	'Can you tell me more about the fatigue?' 'When did the fatigue start?' 'How long have you been fatigue?' (expected to be longer than 6 months) 'Do you know your body weight prior to the onset of fatigue?' (exclude premorbid obesity) 'Do you have any other chronic medical illnesses prior to the onset of fatigue, e.g. diabetes?' (exclusion criteria for diagnosis)	'Besides glandular fever, was there any psychosocial stressor?' 'Is the fatigue persistent or fluctuating?'	Explore the following: 1. Sore throat 2. Muscle and joint pains but no joint swelling 3. Presence of lymph nodes 4. Unrefreshing sleep 5. Post-exertional malaise (more tired after exercise and not relieved by rest)	Explore the following: 1. Mental fatigue 2. Impaired memory and concentration 3. To prompt the patient to describe other symptoms, 'Are there any other symptoms you have not told me about?'	Besides his work, assess the impact of fatigue on him as a husband and father. 'What do you think the underlying causes of the fatigue? How do you cope?'

(B) Exclude other Causes of Fatigue	(B1) Infections	(B2) General Conditions	(B3) Neuromuscular Disorders	(B4) Psychiatric Causes	(B5) Drugs and Substances
	1. Infectious mononucleosis is caused by Epstein–Barr virus (EBV) 2. Other viral infections include Q fever, toxoplasmosis, and CMV; influenza and enteroviruses; chronic active hepatitis B and C; HIV 3. Lyme disease 4. Cryptococcal meningitis	1. Autoimmune disease 2. Endocrine disorders (Addison's disease, hypothyroidism) 3. Cardiac, respiratory disease, and renal failure 4. Asthma	1. Myositis 2. Multiple sclerosis 3. Myasthenia gravis 4. Fibromyalgia: muscle pain in bilateral occiput, lower cervical, trapezius, supraspinatus, second rib, greater trochanter, and knees	1. Depression (explore suicidal thoughts) 2. Adjustment disorder 3. Anxiety and hyperventilation 4. Somatoform disorders 5. Hypochondriasis 6. Neurasthenia 7. Psychosis 8. Eating disorder 9. Narcolepsy and sleep apnoea	1. Alcohol 2. Solvents 3. Side effects of medications 4. Exposure to heavy metals (e.g. mercury) and irradiation
(C) Background History	(C1) Family History	(C2) Personal History and Personality	(C3) Current Social Situation	(C4) Sick Role and Employment	(C5) Social History
	'Do your family members or relatives have strong ideas about illness and what should be done?' 'Do they have difficulty expressing emotions (i.e. alexithymia)? Do they express their emotions through body symptoms?'	Explore childhood trauma, unhelpful parenting, long absence from school, repeated episodes of glandular fever. Explore personality: 'How do you describe yourself as a person?'	Explore current marital relationship (why the marital relationship is strained and what kinds of treatment (if any) have the couple received?), difficulties in previous relationships, and social supports	'Are you on sick leave at this moment? If so, granted by which doctor?' 'Is your company keeping your job?' 'Are you keen to return to the current company?'	Explore: 1. Social support 2. Social networks 3. Financial problems

31.8 ORGANIC PSYCHIATRY

In ICD-10, organic mental disorders are grouped on the basis of a common demonstrable aetiology being present in the form of cerebral disorder, injury to the brain, or other insult leading to cerebral dysfunction, which may be

- Primary—disorders, injuries, and insults affecting the brain directly or with predilection, such as Alzheimer's disease
- Secondary—systemic disorders affecting the brain only in so far as it is one of the multiple organs or body systems involved (e.g. hypothyroidism) (Table 31.6)

By convention, the following disorders are excluded from the category of organic mental disorders and considered separately:

- Psychoactive substance use disorders (including brain disorder resulting from alcohol and other psychoactive drugs)
- The causes of learning disability (mental retardation)

31.8.1 ORGANIC MENTAL DISORDERS

The treatment, course, and prognosis for the following disorders are essentially those of the underlying pathology.

TABLE 31.6

Summary of the Organic Causes of Dementia

Degenerative Diseases of the Central Nervous System	Intoxication	Intracranial Causes	Endocrine Disorders	Metabolic Disorders	Vascular Causes
Alzheimer's disease	Alcohol	Space-occupying lesions such as	Addison's disease	Hepatic failure	Multi-infarct (vascular)
Pick's disease	Heavy metals such as lead, arsenic,	tumours, chronic	Cushing's syndrome	Renal failure	dementia
Huntington's disease	thallium, and	subdural	Hyperinsulinism	Respiratory failure	Cerebral artery
Creutzfeldt–	mercury	haematomas,	Hypothyroidism	Hypoxia	occlusion
Jakob disease	Carbon monoxide	aneurysms, and	Hypopituitarism	Renal dialysis	Cranial arteritis
Normal-pressure	Withdrawal from	chronic abscesses	Hypoparathyroidism	Chronic uraemia	Arteriovenous
hydrocephalus	drugs	Infections	Hyperparathyroidism	Chronic electrolyte imbalance	malformation
Multiple	Withdrawal from	Head injury		($\uparrow Ca^{2+}$, $\downarrow Ca^{2+}$, $\downarrow K^+$, $\uparrow Na^+$,	Binswanger's
sclerosis	alcohol	punch-drunk		$\downarrow Na^+$)	disease
Lewy body		syndrome		Porphyria	
disease				Paget's disease	
				Remote effects of carcinoma or lymphoma	
				Hepatolenticular degeneration (Wilson's disease)	
				Vitamin deficiency (thiamine, nicotinic acid, folate, B_{12})	
				Vitamin intoxication (A, D)	

31.8.1.1 Organic Hallucinosis

Organic hallucinosis is defined as being a disorder of persistent or recurrent hallucinations, in any modality but usually visual or auditory, that occur in clear consciousness without any significant intellectual decline and that may or may not be recognized by the subject as such; delusional elaboration of the hallucinations may occur, but often insight is preserved. The causes of organic hallucinosis are shown in Table 31.7.

31.8.1.2 Organic Mood Disorder

Organic mood disorder is a disorder characterized by a change in mood, usually accompanied by a change in the overall level of activity, caused by organic pathology. Table 31.8 gives the main causes of organic mood disorder.

31.8.1.3 Organic Anxiety Disorder

Organic anxiety disorder is characterized by the occurrence of the features of generalized anxiety disorder and/or panic disorder caused by organic pathology. Some of the symptoms of anxiety, which include tremor, paraesthesia, choking, palpitations, chest pain, dry mouth, nausea, abdominal pain, loose motions and increased

TABLE 31.7

Causes of Organic Hallucinosis

Psychoactive substance use	Alcohol abuse (alcoholic hallucinosis)
	Amphetamine and related sympathomimetics
	Cocaine
	Hallucinogens, e.g. LSD
	Flashback phenomena following the use of hallucinogens
Intoxication	Drugs—amantadine, bromocriptine, ephedrine, levodopa, lisuride
Intracranial causes	Brain tumour
	Head injury
	Migraine
	Infections, e.g. neurosyphilis
	Epilepsy, particularly temporal lobe epilepsy
Sensory deprivation	Deafness
	Poor vision, e.g. cataract
	Torture, e.g. in prisoners of war
Endocrine	Hypothyroidism—'myxedematous madness'
Huntington's disease	

Source: Reproduced from Puri, B.K. et al., *Textbook of Psychiatry*, 2nd edn., Churchill Livingstone, Edinburgh, U.K., 2002. With permission.

TABLE 31.8

Causes of Organic Mood Disorder

Psychoactive substance use	Amphetamine and related sympathomimetics
	Hallucinogens, e.g. LSD
Medication	Corticosteroids
	Levodopa
	Centrally acting antihypertensives— clonidine, methyldopa, reserpine, and rauwolfia
	Alkaloids
	Cycloserine
	Oestrogens—hormone replacement therapy, oral contraceptives
	Clomiphene
Endocrine disorders	Hypothyroidism, hyperthyroidism
	Addison's disease
	Cushing's syndrome
	Hypoglycaemia, diabetes mellitus
	Hyperparathyroidism
	Hypopituitarism
Other systemic disorders	Pernicious anaemia
	Hepatic failure
	Renal failure
	Rheumatoid arthritis
	Systemic lupus erythematosus
	Neoplasia, particularly carcinoma of the pancreas, Carcinoid syndrome
	Viral infection, e.g. influenza, pneumonia, infectious mononucleosis (glandular fever), hepatitis
Intracranial causes	Brain tumour
	Head injury
	Parkinson's disease
	Infections, e.g. neurosyphilis

Source: Reproduced from Puri, B.K. et al., *Textbook of Psychiatry,* 2nd edn., Churchill Livingstone, Edinburgh, U.K., 2002. With permission.

frequency of micturition, are secondary to hyperventilation. Secondary cognitive impairment may occur. Table 31.4 shows the main causes of organic anxiety disorder; of these, it is particularly important to exclude hyperthyroidism, phaeochromocytoma, and hypoglycaemia in clinical practice.

31.8.1.4 Organic Catatonic Disorder

Organic catatonic disorder is defined as being a disorder of diminished (stupor) or increased (excitement) psychomotor activity associated with catatonic symptoms; the extremes of psychomotor disturbance may alternate.

The stuporose symptoms may include complete mutism, negativism, and rigid posturing, while excitement manifests as gross hypermotility. Other catatonic symptoms include stereotypies and waxy flexibility. Important causes of organic catatonic disorder include encephalitis and carbon monoxide poisoning.

31.8.1.5 Organic Delusional or Schizophrenia-Like Disorder

Organic delusional or schizophrenia-like disorder is defined as a disorder in which the clinical picture is dominated by persistent or recurrent delusions, with or without hallucinations. The delusions are most often persecutory, but grandiose delusions or delusions of bodily change, jealousy, disease, or death may occur. Memory and consciousness are unaffected. Causes are listed in Table 31.9.

31.8.1.6 Organic Personality Disorder

In ICD-10, organic personality disorder is defined as being characterized by a significant alteration of the habitual patterns of behaviour displayed by the subject premorbidly. Such alteration always involves more profoundly the expression of emotions, needs, and impulses. Cognition may be defective mostly or exclusively in the areas of planning one's own actions and anticipating their likely personal and social consequences. The causes of organic personality disorder are summarized in Table 31.9.

TABLE 31.9

Causes of Organic Delusional/Schizophrenia Disorder and Organic Personality Disorder

Causes of Organic Delusional/ Schizophrenia Disorder	Causes of Organic Personality Disorder
Psychoactive substance use	Intracranial (particularly affecting the frontal or temporal lobes)
• Amphetamine and related substances	• Head injury
• Cocaine	• Tumours
• Hallucinogens	• Abscesses
Intracranial causes affecting the temporal lobe (e.g. tumours, epilepsy)	• Subarachnoid haemorrhage
	• Neurosyphilis
Huntington's disease	• Epilepsy
	Huntington's disease
	Hepatolenticular degeneration (Wilson's disease)
	Medication (e.g. corticosteroids)
	Psychoactive substance use
	Endocrinopathies

31.9 NEUROPSYCHIATRIC ASPECTS OF HUMAN IMMUNODEFICIENCY VIRUS INFECTION AND ACQUIRED IMMUNODEFICIENCY SYNDROME (CITRON ET AL., 2005)

31.9.1 INTRODUCTION

31.9.1.1 Epidemiology of HIV/AIDS in the United Kingdom

- Approximately 33.5 million people worldwide are living with HIV/AIDS and 95% of them are living in developing countries.
- In the United Kingdom, around 92,636 people were infected by HIV by the end of 2010 and one-quarter of them are unaware of their infection.
- The introduction of combination antiretroviral treatment has resulted in a rapid decline in the number of acquired immunodeficiency syndrome (AIDS) cases and deaths reported each year since the mid-1990s. By the end of 2010, there have been 26,791 diagnoses of AIDS in the United Kingdom. The number of deaths among people living with HIV/AIDS has remained constant, averaging around 400–500 deaths per year in the United Kingdom.
- Heterosexual sex represented 42% of all HIV diagnoses in 2010. Most new cases contracted HIV by heterosexual sex outside of the United Kingdom, particularly in Africa.
- The number of new HIV infections among the male homosexual group has increased in the United Kingdom steadily (Dougan et al., 2007).

- Intravenous drug use and mother-to-child HIV infections have made relatively smaller contribution to the HIV epidemic in the United Kingdom when compared to other developed countries.

31.9.2 HUMAN IMMUNODEFICIENCY VIRUS

The HIV is a lentivirus and a type of retrovirus. The HIV is composed of an outer envelope and an inner core. The outer envelope is made up of knoblike glycoproteins (gp 120s) that bind to the CD4 molecules of susceptible host cells. The HIV is detected in the CNS within 14 days of infection.

31.9.3 DIAGNOSIS OF HIV INFECTION AND COUNSELING

HIV infection is confirmed by the presence of anti-HIV antibodies in the serum. Acute infection is detected by the appearance of immunoglobulin G (IgG) and immunoglobulin M (IgM) within 3 months of infection, P24 antigen, or HIV RNA by PCR. As immunodeficiency becomes more severe, the IgG titer to the core protein begins to fall and P24 antigenaemia starts to surge. The cluster of differentiation 4 (CD4) is a glycoprotein expressed on the surface of T-helper cells. The CD4 to CD8 ratio is a marker of disease progression.

After the confirmation of diagnosis, the patients may undergo tremendous psychological stress because they may need to reveal information related to the HIV status and mode of transmission (e.g. history of unprotected sex with commercial sex workers, homosexuality, or intravenous drug misuse) to their sexual partners and spouses (Table 31.10).

TABLE 31.10
Pretest and Posttest Counseling

Pretest Counseling	Posttest Counseling
1. Help the person to analyse the reasons for testing and to evaluate the likelihood that he or she is infected.	1. Ensure privacy and confidentiality.
2. Explain to the person that the test is not expected to provide a diagnosis of AIDS, any information concerning the severity of the infection, the infectiousness, and prognosis.	2. Explore the feelings of the patient while waiting for the test result.
3. Explain to the person that false positive or negative results may occur.	3. Presenting the results in a sensitive but honest manner.
4. Inform the person about the possible consequences of a positive result, individual psychological reactions, interpersonal problems, possible stigma, and difficulties in purchasing medical insurance.	4. If a patient is confirmed to be infected with HIV, then inform the person about HIV and AIDS, avoiding any unwarranted estimate of survival and definite prognosis.
5. Provide education about mode of transmission and prevention strategies.	5. Prompt the person to talk about their concerns and worries.
	6. Encourage the person to fight against the infection and seek help from infectious disease specialist.
	7. Inform the person about the resources available in the community.
	8. Provide education on safe sex techniques.

TABLE 31.11

Summary of Clinical Progression and CD4 Count

200 Cells/mL < CD4 Count < 500 Cells/mL	50 Cells/mL < CD4 Count < 200 Cells/mL	CD4 + Counts < 50 Cells/mL
Patients are at risk for developing symptomatic but non-AIDS-defining conditions associated with decreased immunological functions. HIV infection affects the brain within the first few months of infection and leads to minor cognitive impairment. Weight loss, fatigue, and thrush (oral candidiasis) may occur in the early stage of the illness.	AIDS-defining conditions including opportunistic infections, neoplasm (primary non-Hodgkin's lymphoma), and AIDS-related dementia occur. *Toxoplasma gondii* cause changes in cognition and affect.	Patients are at increased risk for fatal HIV-related illness.

The most common opportunistic infections in the CNS are *Cryptococcus neoformans* and *Toxoplasma gondii* (Table 31.11).

31.9.4 Antiretroviral Treatment

The highly active antiretroviral therapy (HAART) is composed of the following:

- Nucleoside analogue reverse transcriptase inhibitors (NARTIs): zidovudine (AZT), didanosine (ddI), zalcitabine (ddC), and lamivudine (3TC)
- Pharmacodynamics: phosphorylation to triphosphate and incorporated into growing DNA chain and blocks further DNA chain expansion
- Nonnucleoside analogue reverse transcriptase inhibitors (NNARTIs): nevirapine and efavirenz
- Protease inhibitors (PIs): indinavir, ritonavir, and saquinavir

In general, the common neuropsychiatric side effects of antiretroviral drugs include depression, mania, psychosis, vivid dreams, and suicidal ideations.

Specific neuropsychiatric side effects of each medication are listed as follows:

- *Efavirenz*: decreased concentration, depression, nervousness, and nightmares
- *Interferon*: fatigue and depression
- *Interleukin-2*: depression, disorientation, confusion, and coma
- *Steroids*: mania or depression
- *AZT*: mania and depression
- *Vinblastine*: depression and cognitive impairment

31.9.5 Psychiatric Disorders and HIV Infection

31.9.5.1 Acute Stress Reaction

Acute stress reaction is common immediately after the diagnosis of HIV infection. The patient may present in a state of shock with depersonalization and derealization. Other psychological reactions include anger, withdrawal, guilt, denial, fear of death, and despair. Counselling with infectious disease nurse is often useful.

31.9.5.2 Adjustment Disorder

Adjustment disorder may present with depression, anxiety, somatic complaints, obsessions, and compulsions. Adjustment disorder is common in patients who face family estrangement, overconcern of loved ones, unemployment, and financial difficulties. Supportive psychotherapy by infectious disease nurse or CBT by psychologist is often useful.

31.9.5.3 Depressive Disorder

31.9.5.3.1 Epidemiology of Depression in HIV-Infected Patients

- The prevalence of depression in people living with HIV is around 30%.
- Depressive disorder is more frequent in the period following the identification of seropositive; HIV infection or in the initial stages of HIV dementia.

31.9.5.3.2 Aetiology

31.9.5.3.2.1 Biological Causes

1. Association with chemotherapy for malignant lymphoma
2. Endocrine and metabolic disturbances
3. Occurrence of opportunistic infections or neoplasm

TABLE 31.12

Application of Antidepressants in HIV-Infected Patients

Selective Serotonin Reuptake Inhibitors (SSRIs)	Novel Antidepressants	Tricyclic Antidepressants (TCAs)	Electroconvulsive Therapy (ECT)
SSRIs are suitable for patients infective with HIV because SSRIs do not affect the CD4 count. Most SSRIs are equally effective. SSRIs demonstrate 70%–90% response rate and placebos only demonstrate 50% response rate	*Bupropion* (75–150 mg bid) Avoid in patients with advanced HIV, epilepsy, and AIDS-related dementia	TCAs are indicated for the following purposes: Anti-diarrhoea Sedation	ECT is used successfully in HIV-infected patients ECT is useful for patients who are too ill to tolerate
Fluoxetine (10–60 mg/day)	*Venlafaxine* (75–150 mg bid) Low protein binding, low affinity for cytochrome P450 mixed-function oxidase system	Anti-nausea Anti-anxiety Analgesics for neuropathic pain	antidepressants, severely suicidal, psychotic, and exhibit treatment resistance
Highly protein bound, long half-life and inhibition of CYP 2D6			ECT is associated with an increase in risk of confusion
Paroxetine (10–40 mg/day) Highly protein bound, anticholinergic side effects and most potent inhibitor of CYP 2D6	*Mirtazapine* (7.5–45 mg/day) Low affinity for cytochrome P450 mixed-function oxidase system and associated with sedation and weight gain		
Sertraline (25–200 mg/day) Highly protein bound and shortest half-life			
Citalopram (20–40 mg/day) Least protein bound and least interaction of cytochrome P450 mixed-function oxidase system, associated with prolonged QTc			

Source: American Psychiatric Association (APA), *Desk Reference to the Diagnostic Criteria from DSM-5*, American Psychiatric Association Press, Washington, DC, 2013.

31.9.5.3.2.2 Psychosocial Causes

1. Low level of education.
2. Multiple and frequent bereavements.
3. History of mood disorders.
4. History of substance abuse appears to be the most important predictor for depression in patients infected with HIV.
5. Unemployment.
6. Unresolved grief and multiple losses.

31.9.5.3.2.3 Clinical Characteristics

1. Biological depressive symptoms (e.g. fatigue, anorexia, weight loss, sleep disorders, and loss of libido) are similar to somatic manifestations of AIDS.
2. Cognitive depressive symptoms (e.g. memory disturbance, poor concentration, slowing of mental processes) are similar to AIDS-related dementia.
3. Psychiatrists should focus on the following symptoms such as low mood, guilt, suicidal ideation, hopelessness, and loss of interest when assessing severity of depression.

31.9.5.3.3 Management

The following investigations are required before initiation of antidepressant treatment: FBC, RFT, LFT, TFT, and ECG (Table 31.12).

31.9.5.4 Mania

31.9.5.4.1 Epidemiology

The prevalence of mania in HIV-infected patients is around 1.5%. The prevalence increases as the disease progresses.

31.9.5.4.2 Aetiology

If mania presents early in the course of HIV infection, it is usually associated with social problems. If mania presents late in the course of HIV infection, it is usually associated with HIV dementia. Other causes of mania include

1. Side effects of antiretroviral agents such as AZT and lamivudine
2. Direct effect of the HIV infection on the CNS
3. Metabolic disturbance
4. CNS opportunistic infection (e.g. *toxoplasmosis* cerebritis, *cryptococcal* meningitis)
5. CNS opportunistic tumours from non-Hodgkin's lymphoma

31.9.5.4.3 Treatment (See Tables 31.13 and 31.14)

31.9.5.4.4 Prognosis

Mania in patients infected with HIV indicates poor prognosis and affects adherence to antiretroviral drugs as a result of unrealistic optimism in the disease condition.

31.9.5.5 Cognitive Impairment and Dementia

31.9.5.5.1 Epidemiology

- Early cognitive impairment occurs in 20% of patients infected with HIV. It can be classified into cognitive, behavioural, and motor symptoms.
- Cognitive symptoms include poor memory, concentration impairment, and mental slowing. The patient may need a written reminder to help them to recall.
- Behavioural symptoms include apathy, reduced spontaneity, and social withdrawal. Depression, irritability or emotional lability, agitation, and psychotic symptoms may occur.

- Motor symptoms include loss of balance, poor coordination, clumsiness, and leg weakness.
- Later stage: Global deterioration of cognitive functions is manifested by word finding difficulties. Patients may exhibit psychomotor retardation and mutism. Speech becomes slow and monotonous. Neurological examination may reveal that the patient has difficulty in walking as a result of paraparesis. Patients may lie in bed and appear indifferent to the illness and surroundings. Bladder and bowel incontinence are common at this stage. Myoclonus and seizures may occur.
- The prevalence of dementia in patients suffering from AIDS is around 25%.
- The onset of AIDS-associated dementia is insidious and occurs later in the course of illness when there is significant immunosuppression (Table 31.15).

TABLE 31.13

Application of Mood Stabilizers in HIV-Infected Patients

Lithium Carbonate	Sodium Valproate	Carbamazepine
1. Poorly tolerated, especially in HIV nephropathy.	1. Effective in treating mania in patients infected with HIV.	1. Elevated risk of pancytopenia in HIV-infected patients.
2. Monitor closely for neurotoxicity and gastrointestinal side effects.	2. Require regular monitoring of liver functions.	2. Monitor FBC on a weekly basis when given concomitantly with zidovudine.
3. Serum levels can easily be altered due to diarrhoea or poor fluid intake.	3. Coadministration with zidovudine may increase the serum levels of zidovudine.	3. Carbamazepine induces its own metabolism and decreases its own levels as well as the levels of other drugs.

Source: American Psychiatric Association (APA), *Desk Reference to the Diagnostic Criteria from DSM-5*, American Psychiatric Association Press, Washington, DC, 2013.

TABLE 31.14

Summary of Pharmacokinetic Interactions among Antidepressants, Mood Stabilizers, and Antiretroviral Drugs

	CYP 2B6	CYP 2D6	CYP 3A4	Glucuronidation
Psychotropic drugs	Bupropion	TCA SSRI Mirtazapine	Benzodiazepine Buspirone Mirtazapine	Sodium valproate Lamotrigine Opiate analgesics
Antiretroviral drugs	PIs (e.g. ritonavir) inhibit CYP 2B6	PIs (e.g. ritonavir) inhibit CYP 2D6	NNRTIs (e.g. nevirapine) induce CYP 3A4	PIs (e.g. nelfinavir) induce glucuronidation

Abbreviations: NNRTI, nonnucleotide reverse transcriptase inhibitor; PI, protease inhibitor.

TABLE 31.15

Diagnostic Criteria of HIV-Associated Cognitive Impairment and AIDS-Associated Dementia

HIV-Associated Cognitive Impairment	AIDS-Associated Dementia
Two or more of the following for at least 1 month: • Impaired attention or concentration • Mental slowing/cognitive inefficiencies • Impaired memory • Slowed movements • Poor coordination • Personality change, irritability • Must be accompanied by mild functional impairment (e.g. work or activities of daily living). Emotional lability	Acquired abnormality in at least two of the following cognitive abilities for at least 1 month: • Attention/concentration • Speed of information processing • Abstraction/reasoning • Visuospatial skill • Memory/learning • Speech/language At least one of the following: • Presence of neurological sign, e.g. abnormality in motor function • Decline in motivation or emotional control or change in behaviour • Moderate to severe functional impairment Absence of clouding of consciousness or delirium No evidence of other etiological factor of dementia

Source: American Psychiatric Association (APA), *Desk Reference to the Diagnostic Criteria from DSM-5*, American Psychiatric Association Press, Washington, DC, 2013.

31.9.6 DIFFERENTIAL DIAGNOSIS

The differential diagnoses include

1. Opportunistic infections: *cryptococcal* meningitis, *CMV* encephalitis, *herpes simplex* encephalitis, and cerebral *toxoplasmosis.*
2. Neoplasm and cerebral lymphoma.
3. Metabolic encephalopathy.
4. HIV encephalitis or leukoencephalopathy.

The presentations of the aforementioned differential diagnoses are more acute as compared to AIDS dementia complex.

31.9.7 MANAGEMENT

31.9.7.1 Investigations

In patients suffering from AIDS-associated dementia, MRI and CT scans usually show the cerebral atrophy and white matter abnormalities. The CSF β_2-microglobulin is a sensitive marker that indicates severity of dementia.

31.9.7.2 Treatment

There is no specific medication but antiretroviral treatment may be useful.

31.10 NEUROPSYCHIATRIC ASPECTS OF PARKINSON'S DISEASE

31.10.1 INTRODUCTION

31.10.1.1 Pathophysiology of Parkinson's Disease

Parkinson's disease (PKD) is characterized by the loss of dopaminergic neurons in the substantia nigra. The loss of the dopaminergic neurons and subsequent reduction in dopamine neurotransmission in the globus pallidus and subthalamic nuclei results in classical signs of PKD such as tremor, rigidity, bradykinesia, and postural changes. In 18 F-dopa PET scanning in patients with PKD, decreased uptake of 18 F-dopa has been observed. Intraneuronal α-synuclein inclusions cause neuronal death and gliosis. An interaction between tubulin and α-synuclein accelerates α-synuclein aggregation in diseased brains, leading to the formation of Lewy bodies that are eosinophilic intracytoplasmic inclusions in neurons. In general, tubulin mutation affects microtubule function and may play an important pathological role in dementia or neurodegenerative process.

31.10.1.2 Clinical Features of PKD

The clinical features of PKD are summarized by a mnemonic TRAPPED (Bentley, 2008).

*T*remor: PKD is characterized by a unilateral, resting, and pill-rolling tremor of 4–6 Hz. The tremor is worsened by stress and reduced by relaxation.

*R*igidity: PKD is characterized by lead-pipe and cogwheel rigidity.

*A*kinesia: PKD is characterized by reduction in frequency and speed of movement.

*P*erservation: Patient continues to blink after glabellar tap.

*P*ostural instability: PKD is characterized by stopped posture with festination and shuffling gait.

*E*xpression: PKD is characterized by masklike face and reduction in blinking.

*D*epression or dementia.

31.10.1.3   Treatment of PKD

31.10.1.3.1   Pro-Dopaminergic Drugs

1. *Levodopa* (L-dopa): Examples include carbidopa and benserazide. Neuropsychiatric side effect includes dyskinesia, on and off phenomenon, insomnia, and psychosis.
2. *Dopamine agonists*: Examples include ergoline (e.g. cabergoline) and nonergoline (e.g. ropinirole). Dopamine agonists delay the time to require L-dopa and not as effective as L-dopa. It may cause confusion in old people.
3. *MAO-B inhibitors*: Examples include selegiline and rasagiline. MAO-B inhibitors delay the time to require L-dopa.
4. *COMT inhibitors*: Examples include entacapone and tolcapone. COMT inhibitors are given with L-dopa to increase its bioavailability.

31.10.1.3.2   Other Treatments

5. *Anticholinergic agent*: Example includes benzhexol. Anticholinergic agent is indicated for tremor. Confusion is a common neuropsychiatric side effect.
6. *Indirect dopamine agonist and anticholinergics agent*: Example includes amantadine. Amantadine is indicated for dyskinesia. Confusion is a common neuropsychiatric side effect.
7. *Neurosurgery*: Examples include thalamotomy, subthalamotomy, pallidotomy, implantation of subthalamic nuclei stimulators and fetal cell grafts. Stimulation of subthalamic nuclei may increase suicide risk and sexual drive.

31.10.2   Psychiatric Disorders and PKD

31.10.2.1   Depression

31.10.2.1.1   Epidemiology

- Prevalence of major depressive disorder is 20%.
- Prevalence increases to 40% if dysthymia and minor depression are included.
- Two-thirds of depressed PKD patients have comorbid anxiety.

31.10.2.1.2   Aetiology

31.10.2.1.2.1   Biological Factors

- Family history of depression
- History of left brain injury and right hemi-parkinsonism
- Hypometabolism in striatal–thalamic–frontal circuits
- Low dopamine levels in the mesolimbic system and reduction in motivation and drive

31.10.2.1.2.2   Psychosocial Factors

- Past psychiatric history of depression
- Presence of cognitive impairment
- Loss of functional independence

31.10.2.1.2.3   Clinical Features

- Depression in PKD has bimodal onset. Patients may become depressed at the time of diagnosis. Depression occurs late in the course and associated with severe bradykinesia and gait disturbance.
- Depressive symptoms precede motor symptoms in 30% of cases.
- Psychiatrists should focus more on low mood, irritability, pessimism, and suicidal thoughts when assessing depression in patients suffering from PKD.
- Comorbidity with anxiety occurs in two-thirds of cases.

31.10.2.1.2.4   Treatment

- Exclude underlying organic causes such as hypothyroidism.
- Optimize treatment of motor symptoms.
- SSRI is the first-line treatment for depression in PKD.
- Bupropion is an alternative antidepressant.
- Avoid tricyclic antidepressants that may cause confusion and cognitive impairment.
- If SSRI and bupropion fail, psychiatrist can consider ECT. ECT causes transient improvement in motor symptoms. Side effects include post-ECT confusion.

- Augmentation with direct and indirect dopamine agonists (e.g. amantadine). Dopamine agonists have antidepressant properties.
- Pallidotomy and deep brain stimulation may reduce depression.

31.10.2.2   Mania
31.10.2.2.1   Epidemiology
- The prevalence of mania is 1%.
- The prevalence of euphoria is 10%.

31.10.2.2.2   Aetiology
31.10.2.2.2.1   Biological Factors
- Dopamine agonists and anticholinergic agents can cause euphoria and mania.
- Stimulation of subthalamic nuclei may cause high sexual drive and disinhibition.

31.10.2.2.2.2   Clinical Features
- Mania usually occurs during the 'on' period (e.g. predominantly motor symptoms) of PKD.

31.10.2.2.2.3   Treatment
- Exclude other organic causes of mania.
- Reduce the dose of dopamine agonists and anticholinergic agents.
- Optimize the environment to reduce stimulation.
- Low-dose quetiapine is the best tolerated antipsychotic to treat mania.

31.10.2.3   Anxiety
31.10.2.3.1   Epidemiology
- The prevalence of anxiety disorders (e.g. generalized anxiety disorder, panic disorder, social phobia, and simple phobias) is between 25% and 50% of patients suffering from PKD.
- Around 90% of PKD patients suffering from anxiety disorder have comorbid depression.

31.10.2.3.2   Aetiology
31.10.2.3.2.1   Biological Factors
- Altered locus coeruleus activity.
- Low dopamine levels causes release of noradrenaline and anxiety symptoms.
- Reduction of cortical GABA.

31.10.2.3.2.2   Psychosocial Factors
- Past psychiatric history of anxiety disorder
- Loss of functional independence

31.10.2.3.2.3   Clinical Features
- Anxiety symptoms are more common during the 'off' periods (predominantly nonmotor symptoms such as breathing difficulties).

31.10.2.3.2.4   Treatment
- Optimize treatment of PKD.
- Consider SSRI, SNRI, or mirtazapine.
- Acetylcholinesterase inhibitors (e.g. rivastigmine) may reduce anxiety.
- Benzodiazepine may worsen motor symptoms because GABA further reduces dopamine levels in the striatum.
- Pallidotomy and deep brain stimulation may reduce anxiety.

31.10.2.4   Psychosis
31.10.2.4.1   Epidemiology
- The prevalence of psychosis is between 20% and 30% in PKD patients receiving treatment.
- A small percentage of patients have hallucinations before initiation of L-dopa or dopamine agonists.

31.10.2.4.2   Aetiology
31.10.2.4.2.1   Biological Risk Factors
- Stimulation of subthalamic nuclei
- Severe PKD
- Presence of REM sleep disturbance
- Associated with sensory deficits
- High doses of L-dopa and dopamine agonists
- Combination of medications (e.g. augmentation of dopamine agonist with amantadine)

31.10.2.4.2.2   Psychosocial Risk Factors
- Presence of depression
- Associated with cognitive impairment and dementia
- Staying in a nursing home

31.10.2.4.2.3   Clinical Features
- Visual hallucination is common and occurs in 20%–40% of PKD patients receiving anti-PKD medications.
- 10% of PKD patients who receive treatment experience both auditory and visual hallucinations.
- 5% of PKD patients who receive treatment experience delusions. Delusions are often complex and persecutory in nature.
- Loss of insight occurs when the course of PKD and cognitive impairment progresses.
- Psychotic symptom is a significant contributor to caregiver stress.

31.10.2.4.2.4 Treatment
- Exclude other organic causes of psychosis.
- Reduce the dose of dopamine agonists.
- It is not necessary to treat infrequent hallucinations or delusions.
- Low-dose quetiapine is the best tolerated antipsychotic.
- If comorbid dementia exists, consider adding an acetylcholinesterase inhibitor.
- ECT is indicated for psychomotor symptoms.
- For treatment-resistant psychosis, low-dose clozapine (e.g. 25 mg/day) is often effective. Side effects of clozapine include blood dyscrasia.

31.10.2.5 Sleep Disturbances
31.10.2.5.1 Epidemiology
- 60%–90% of PKD patients suffer from sleep disturbances.

31.10.2.5.2 Clinical Features
- REM behaviour disorder (e.g. periodic limb movement, restless leg syndrome)
- Nightmares
- Obstructive sleep apnoea

31.10.2.6 Cognitive Impairment and Dementia
31.10.2.6.1 Epidemiology
- 20%–40% of patients suffering from PKD suffer from dementia.
- 65% of patients suffering from PKD develop dementia by age of 85 years.

31.11 NEUROPSYCHIATRIC ASPECTS OF CEREBROVASCULAR ACCIDENT

31.11.1 INTRODUCTION

31.11.1.1 Types of Cerebrovascular Accident
Ischaemic stroke: 88%

- Lacunar infarct: 25%
- Atherosclerotic cerebrovascular disease: 20%
- Cardiogenic embolism: 20%
- Cryptogenic type: 30%
- Other causes: 5%

Haemorrhagic stroke: 12%
Causes of haemorrhagic stroke are summarized by a mnemonic 'HAEMATOMA' (Bentley, 2008) (Figures 31.1 through 31.5 and Tables 31.16 and 31.17):

H—hypertension
A—aneurysm

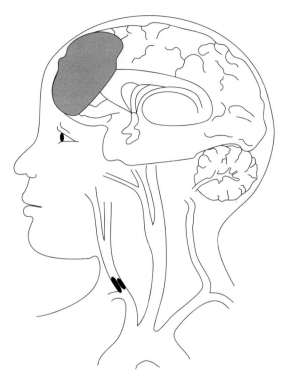

FIGURE 31.1 Anterior cerebral artery infarction.

E—elderly
M—malformations (e.g. arteriovenous malformation)
A—autoimmune causes (e.g. vasculitis)
T—toxins (e.g. cocaine, amphetamine)
O—occlusions (e.g. cerebral venous thrombosis)
M—metastases (e.g. lung, thyroid, and renal cancer)
A—accident (e.g. head injury)

31.11.1.2 Psychiatric Disorders and Cerebrovascular Accident
31.11.1.2.1 Depression
31.11.1.2.1.1 Epidemiology
- The prevalence of major depressive disorder is 30% among patients suffering from cerebrovascular accident (CVA).
- The incidence of depression is lower among patients suffering from an occlusion of the posterior cerebral arteries in comparison to occlusions in anterior and middle cerebral arteries.

31.11.1.2.1.2 Aetiology
- CVA in the left hemisphere (e.g. left lateral frontal lobe) has a stronger association with depression in comparison to CVA in the right hemisphere.

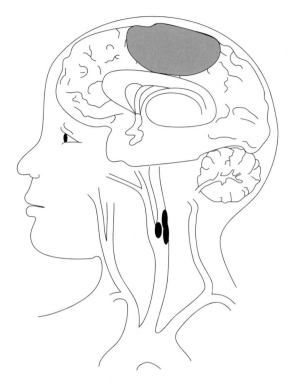

FIGURE 31.2   Middle cerebral artery infarction.

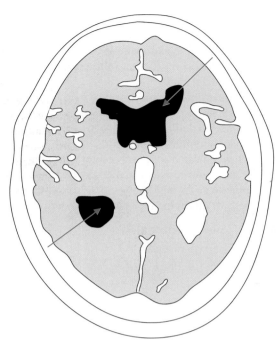

FIGURE 31.4   Subarachnoid haemorrhage with blood in the sulci, third ventricle and the posterior horn of the left lateral ventricle.

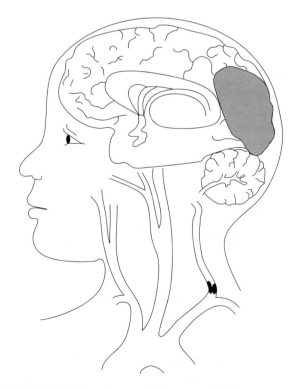

FIGURE 31.3   Posterior cerebral artery occlusion.

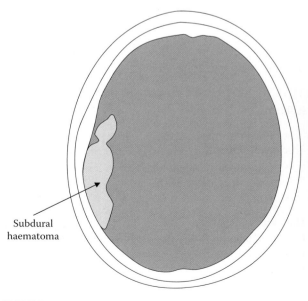

Subdural haematoma

FIGURE 31.5   Subdural haematoma.

TABLE 31.16

Type of CVA, Clinical Example, and Neuropsychiatric Sequelae

Type of CVA	Clinical Example	Neuropsychiatric Sequelae
Anterior cerebral artery infarction. (see Figure 31.1)	A 66-year-old man with history of type II diabetes mellitus presented with a sudden onset of bilateral lower limb weakness and numbness 3 days ago. Physical examination revealed both distal and proximal weakness of both legs with impaired pinprick sensation, which spared the arms and the face. Grasp reflex and sensory neglect were evident on the left side. The patient was extremely emotional when being asked for a physical examination.	*Neuropsychiatric sequelae of anterior cerebral artery infarction:* Occlusion of the anterior cerebral artery may result in global dementia and frontal lobe personality changes.
Middle cerebral artery infarction. (see Figure 31.2)	A 55-year-old woman with history of hypertension presented with an acute onset of left-sided weakness and blurring of vision. Physical examination revealed weakness and sensory loss involving the left half of the face and the left upper and lower limbs. Left homonymous hemianopia and left-sided neglect were also evident.	*Neuropsychiatric sequelae of middle cerebral artery infarction:* Nondominant middle cerebral artery occlusion may cause confusional states, sensory loss, inattention, and anosognosia.
Posterior cerebral artery occlusion. (see Figure 31.3)	A 58-year-old housewife presented with an acute onset of dizziness, nausea, and posterior cranium headache 5 days ago. She sought medical attention before she found that she could not read half of the page of her story book. Physical examination revealed homonymous hemianopia, loss of pinprick sensation in her left face and arm, and severely impaired short-term memory.	*Neuropsychiatric sequelae of posterior cerebral artery infarction:* Posterior cerebral artery occlusion causes cortical blindness and denial of disability and sometimes alexia without agraphia. Occlusion of rostral basilar artery can result in bizarre hallucinations, disorientation, and somnolence.

TABLE 31.17

Type of Hemorrhage, Clinical Example, and Neuropsychiatric Sequelae

Subarachnoid haemorrhage. (see Figure 31.4)	A 40-year-old right-handed man complained of insidious onset of dizziness, nausea, and vomiting for 5 days. He also got generalized headache, which was precipitated by lying down. The headache itself was neither throbbing in nature nor associated with any phobic symptoms, limb weakness, or numbness. Two days before admission, he experienced diplopia, which was more severe on looking downwards, on and off chills, and low-grade fever. The Glasgow coma scale (GCS) was 15/15. Cranial nerves were intact including the range of eye gaze. No focal neurologic sign was elicited. Planter reflex was downgoing on both sides. Fundoscopy did not reveal any papilledema.	*Neuropsychiatric sequelae of subarachnoid haemorrhage:* Persistent memory impairment: 40%. Depression and anxiety: 25%. Severe personality impairment: 20%. Dysphasic disability: 10%. Worsening cognitive sequelae after subarachnoid haemorrhage is caused by normal-pressure hydrocephalus. A severe amnesic syndrome resembling Korsakoff's syndrome may emerge in the days or weeks following subarachnoid haemorrhage.
Subdural haematoma. (see Figure 31.5)	An 87-year-old woman was found lying on the floor unconscious, after a fall. Physical examination revealed unequal pupils, increased tone on her left side, and upgoing plantar reflex on the left side.	*Neuropsychiatric sequelae of subdural haematoma:* *Cause:* Head injury. *Clinical presentation:* 1. Acute presentation with stupor or coma together with some evidence of localizing signs. 2. Chronic presentation with headache, poor concentration memory loss, and fluctuating course.

- Patients who develop depression after right-sided CVA is associated with family history of depression.
- The volume of the lesion is directly proportional to the severity of depression.

31.11.1.2.1.3   Treatment
- SSRI is indicated.

31.11.1.2.2   Mania
31.11.1.2.2.1   Epidemiology
- The prevalence of mania is 0.5%–1% among patients suffering from CVA.

31.11.1.2.3   Aetiology
31.11.1.2.3.1   Biological Factors
- CVA in the right hemisphere (e.g. right orbitofrontal lobe) has a stronger association with mania in comparison to CVA in the left hemisphere.
- Family history of bipolar disorder.
- Post-CVA mania is associated with cortical and subcortical lesions.
- CVA in the thalamus is associated with mania.

31.11.1.2.3.2   Clinical Features
- Post-CVA mania usually occurs 3–9 months after stroke.
- The first episode can be mania or depression.

31.11.1.2.3.3   Treatment
- Mood stabilizer such as lithium is indicated.

31.11.1.2.4   Cognitive Impairment and Dementia
31.11.1.2.4.1   Epidemiology
- 30% of patients suffering CVA develop severe cognitive impairment.

Vascular dementia is considered in Chapter 39.

31.12   NEUROPSYCHIATRIC ASPECTS OF EPILEPSY

31.12.1   INTRODUCTION

31.12.1.1   Classification of Epilepsy (Figure 31.6)

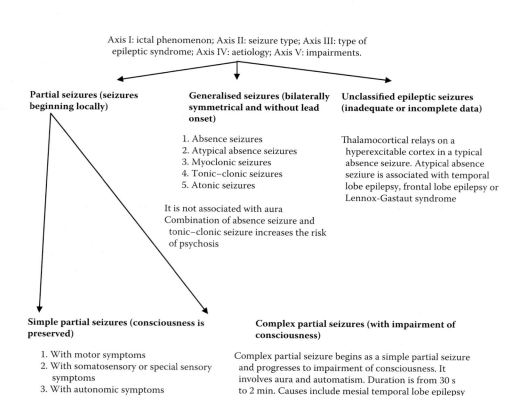

FIGURE 31.6   International league against epilepsy classification.

31.12.1.1.1   Absence Seizure

Characteristics of absence seizure include

- Abrupt onset and offset
- Short duration (usually <10 s)
- Eyes: glazed, blank stare, slight blinking, and eye-rolling
- Normal intelligence, physical examination, and imaging finding
- Clonus and automatism may occur when the duration of seizure increases
- EEG: 3 Hz spike and wave with photosensitivity

Special clinical features associated with epilepsy (5As):

- *Aura*: rising epigastric sensation, déjà vu, and olfactory or auditory hallucinations
- *Autonomic signs*: change in skin colour, temperature, and palpitations
- *Absence seizure*: motor arrest and motionless stare
- *Automatism*: lip-smacking, chewing, swallowing; fumbling, and walking
- *Amnesia*: amnesia of the entire seizure

Frequency of partial seizures according to neuroanatomical areas (Table 31.18):

- Temporal lobe epilepsy: 75%
- Frontal lobe epilepsy: 15%
- Parietal lobe epilepsy: 5%
- Occipital lobe epilepsy: 5%

31.12.1.1.2   Nonepileptic Seizures

Psychiatrists should rule out organic causes of seizure (drug or medication induced, infection, substance misuse/withdrawal) before the diagnosis of nonepileptic seizure.

Classical features of nonepileptic seizure

- Presence of past psychiatric disorders, for example, affective disorders, dissociative states, deliberate self-harm, family history of psychiatric disorders, sexual maladjustment, hysterical personality, and good past health (e.g. absence of head injury, CNS infection, and thromboembolic phenomenon)
- Precipitants including intense current psychosocial stressors
- Characteristics of nonepileptic seizure: occurring in daytime when other people are around, gradual onset, wide range of atypical presentation, pelvic thrusting, lack of tonic and clonic movements, one-sided somatosensory symptoms, and reactive papillary light reflex
- Underlying motives: presence of primary and secondary gains

Investigation

- EEG is normal during and after the seizure. Video telemetry further examines the very stereotyped (and therefore probably epileptic) or the very nonstereotyped (and probably nonepileptic) nature of seizure.

TABLE 31.18

Characteristics of Epilepsy According to Neuroanatomical Locations

Frontal Lobe Epilepsy	Temporal Lobe Epilepsy
Nonspecific 'cephalic' aura.	*Predisposing factors*: history of birth injury and infantile febrile convulsions.
Motor automatisms—'fencing' posture, versive eye and head movement, speech arrest, and bizarre vocalization (e.g. singing). The duration of automatism usually less than 5 min.	*Aura*: complex and varied. It may present as lip-smacking, forced thinking, visual hallucinations, and tinnitus.
Bilaterally coordinated limb movements (e.g. clapping).	*Behaviour*: hyperemotionality and hyposexuality.
Contralateral clonic Jacksonian march when supplementary motor area is involved.	
Brief, frequent, dramatic, nocturnal seizures with immediate recovery.	
Frontal lobe epilepsy is often misdiagnosed as 'hysterical'.	
Prolactin levels remain the same after frontal lobe epilepsy.	
Frontal lobe epilepsy is associated with phonation (i.e. speech during seizure).	

Serum prolactin should be taken within 20 min after the seizure. The interpretation of prolactin levels is listed as follows:

- Generalized seizure: 1000 IU/mL
- Partial seizure: 500 IU/mL
- Pseudo-seizure: 0 IU/mL

Treatment

- If patient stays in the ward, regular nursing monitoring is required.
- Psychotherapeutic exploration (by abreaction: a drug-assisted interview using diazepam or sodium amylobarbitone may be helpful).

31.13   PSYCHIATRIC ASPECTS OF EPILEPSY

31.13.1   EPIDEMIOLOGY

31.13.1.1   Psychiatric Comorbidity of Epilepsy

1. *Depression*: the prevalence of depression is 9%–22% and it is 17 times more likely than general population.
2. *Suicide*: the percentage of death by suicide is 11.5% and the risk of suicide is four to five times higher than general population.
3. *Psychosis or schizophrenia*: patients suffering from epilepsy are two to four times more likely to develop psychosis or schizophrenia. The prevalence of schizophrenia among temporal lobe epilepsy patients is 3%.
4. *Pathological aggression*: 4%–50% of patients suffering from epilepsy exhibit pathological aggression.
5. *Criminal offences*: patients suffering from epilepsy are three times more likely to commit criminal offences in comparison to the general population.

31.13.1.2   Psychiatric Conditions and Epilepsy

31.13.1.2.1   Violence

31.13.1.2.1.1   Aetiology of Violence in Epileptic Patients

31.13.1.2.1.1.1   Biological Factors
- High serum cortisol following seizure
- Sedation and disinhibition
- Presence of neurological signs
- Associated with episodic dyscontrol

31.13.1.2.1.1.2   Psychological Factors
- Cognitive deficits in attention, memory, and motor speed
- Childhood history of impulsive behaviour

31.13.1.2.1.1.3   Clinical Features of Ictal Violence
1. Lack of motivation
2. Sudden paroxysmal onset
3. Nonselective victims including close family member
4. Brief duration
5. Impaired consciousness reported by witness
6. Little attempt to conceal violent act
7. Amnesia for the event
8. Subsequent genuine remorse

31.13.1.2.1.1.4   Investigation and Treatment of Ictal Violence
- Consult a neurologist who is experienced in this field.
- Look for aggression during epileptic automatism during video–EEG telemetry.
- Carbamazepine (400–800 mg/day) is indicated for episodic dyscontrol and violence.

31.13.1.2.1.1.5   Personality Change
- In general, patients with epilepsy are more emotional and irritable.
- Left temporal epilepsy is associated with ruminative tendency.
- Idiopathic generalized epilepsy is not related to any particular personality type.

31.13.1.2.1.1.6   Cognitive Function
- Left temporal epilepsy is associated with verbal memory deficits.
- Other causes include drug intoxication, nonconvulsive status, and hippocampal spike activity.
- Postictal amnesia is common but epileptic dementia is rare.

Ictal and postictal psychiatric phenomenon (Tables 31.19 and 31.20).

31.13.2   PSYCHOTROPIC MEDICATIONS AND EPILEPSY

(See Table 31.21.)

31.14   NEUROPSYCHIATRIC ASPECTS OF HEAD INJURY

31.14.1   EPIDEMIOLOGY

31.14.1.1   Head Injury
- 10% of all visits to the emergency department.
- Incidence of head injury: 1,500 per 100,000.
- 130 per 100,000 suffer from persistent cognitive deficits after head injury.
- Males to females = 2:1.

TABLE 31.19

Summary of Ictal and Postictal Neuropsychiatric Phenomenon

	Ictal	Postictal	Interictal
Confusion or psychosis	*Automatisms* are simple, repetitive movements. It may involve wandering with confusion and clouded consciousness. Automatisms usually last less than 5 min. *Nonconvulsive features*: absence status, myoclonic flickering eyelids. *Complex partial features*: mental confusion, psychosis, fluctuating levels of consciousness, complex automatisms, episodic hallucinations, and marked mood changes. *Underlying cause of ictal phenomenon*: ongoing paroxysmal brain discharges.	Postictal phenomenon may occur immediately upon the occurrence of a fit or within a week. It may occur in a background of clouded consciousness. Two typical postictal phenomenon: 1. *Fugues*: prolonged episode of wandering, altered behaviour, amnesia, and impaired consciousness, which may last for hours or days. 2. *Twilight states*: abnormal subjective experiences (perceptual and affective) and are also associated with cognitive impairment and perseveration. Patients may have paranoid delusions. *EEG*: slow-wave changes that may last up to a few hours. *ECT* may lead to dramatic improvement. Spontaneous remission is common.	Occurs in temporal lobe epilepsy (especially the left temporal lobe). Chronic interictal psychosis is more common than postictal psychosis. Risk factors: • Hamartomas. • An aura of fear. • Left-handed. • Mesial temporal focus. • Onset of epilepsy in adolescence. Classical presentation: Chronic paranoid hallucinatory psychosis with the presence of the first-rank symptoms. Onset: 10–15 years after the first episode of epilepsy. This occurs in 2% of patients with temporal lobe epilepsy. Visual hallucinations or illusions are more common in lesions associated with the right temporal lobe. The person is usually in clear consciousness when psychosis occurs. *Differences from schizophrenia*: 1. No family history of schizophrenia. 2. Good premorbid personality. 3. Less personality deterioration. 4. Warmer affect. 5. Presence of neurological abnormality on examination.
Mood or anxiety symptoms	Fear is the most common anxiety symptom. Sudden severe depression may occur. Elation or mania is rare.	Depression and anxiety are common (15%–45%). Reduced monoaminergic activity causes depression.	Depression is caused by psychosocial factors such as stigma associated with epilepsy.

TABLE 31.20

Acute and Long-Term Management of Epileptic Patients

Acute Management	Long-Term Psychological Management
1. Terminate seizure by IV benzodiazepines or rectal diazepam 2. Remove patients from potential sources of injury 3. Check oxygen saturation to rule out hypoxia	1. Behavioural analysis and conditioning procedures 2. Biofeedback on arousal based on EEG rhythms 3. Self-control strategies 4. Individual psychotherapy

TABLE 31.21

Use of Psychotropic Drugs in Epilepsy

	Antidepressants/Mood Stabilizers	Antipsychotic Drugs
Recommended psychotropic drugs	• SSRIs • Moclobemide • ECT is indicated for severe depression and ECT has anticonvulsant effects	• Haloperidol • Trifluoperazine • Sulpiride
Contraindicated psychotropic drugs	• Amitriptyline (epileptogenic) • Lithium (epileptogenic when patient takes an overdose)	• Chlorpromazine (epileptogenic) • Depot antipsychotics (complex mechanism) • Clozapine (very epileptogenic) • Zotepine (epileptogenic)

Source: Taylor, D. et al., *The Maudsley Prescribing Guidelines*, Informa Healthcare, London, U.K., 2009.

31.14.1.2 Neuropsychiatric Sequelae of Head Injury (Birds and Roger, 2007)

- Postconcussion syndrome (PCS): 50% after 2 months, 12% after 1 year.
- Depression and anxiety are common.
- Secondary mania: 9%.
- Schizophreniform disorder 2.5%.
- Paranoid psychosis: 2%.
- Psychotic depression: 1%.
- Impulsive personality as a result of decreased levels of 5-HIAA after head injury.
- Dementia is usually nonprogressive.
- Memory deficit is the most frequent chronic cognitive disturbance.
- Head injury in children is associated with restlessness, overactivity, disobedience, and temper tantrums.

- Seizure occurs in 5% of head injury victims. If dura mater is penetrated, the risk of epilepsy is 30%.
- Dementia pugilistica (punch-drunk syndrome) is resulted from repeated head injury (e.g. boxer). The underlying pathology is the neurofibrillary tangle and plaque formation. Clinical features include ataxia, dysarthria, tremor, apathy, spasticity, morbid jealousy, irritability, disinhibition, and dementia (Table 31.22).

31.14.1.3 Aetiological Factors and Severity of Head Injury

31.14.1.3.1 Biological Factors

1. Age at the time of injury
2. The extent and location of brain injury
3. Post-traumatic epilepsy

TABLE 31.22

Classification of Head Injury

Primary Head Injury

Primary head injury is a result of either rotational or horizontal acceleration or deceleration.

Rotational acceleration or deceleration results in diffuse shearing of long central fibres and micro-haemorrhages in the corpus callosum and rostral brain stem. This will result in diffuse axonal injury.

The rotational acceleration or deceleration also causes centrifugal pressure waves to spread out so that the brain undergo repeated buffeting against the skull and tentorium where there are sharp bony edges or corners. The frontal poles, orbitofrontal regions, temporal poles, and medial temporal structures are particularly vulnerable.

Secondary Head Injury

Secondary head injury is caused by

1. Haemorrhage (subdural, extradural, and intracerebral).
2. Reactive brain swelling.
3. Acute fluid collections.
4. Raised in intracranial pressure.
5. Coning of brainstem.

31.14.1.3.2 *Psychological Factors*

1. Premorbid personality
2. Premorbid intelligence
3. Psychological reactions to injury

31.14.1.3.3 *Social Factors*

1. Premorbid social functioning
2. Social support
3. Mild head injury

31.14.1.4 Mild Head Injury

Glasgow Coma Scale (GCS): 14–15
Pay attention if the patient

1. Shows neurologic signs
2. Has haematoma
3. Has a history of coagulopathy, drug or alcohol consumption, epilepsy, and past neurosurgery
4. Is aged >60 years

31.14.1.5 Moderate Head Injury

GCS: 9–13
Outcomes

1. Mortality: <20%.
2. Morbidity: 50%.
3. Positive neuroimaging findings: 40%.
4. 8% require neurosurgery.

31.14.1.6 Severe Head Injury

GCS <9
Outcomes

1. 10% of all head injury
2. Mortality: 40%

31.14.2 Postconcussion Syndrome

PCS occurs after minor head injury. PCS is associated with premorbid physical and social problems. It usually lasts from several weeks to 3 months and more likely to be persistent in women. Common physical symptoms include headache, nausea, and sensitivity to light and noise. Common psychological symptoms include cognitive impairment, poor concentration, and irritability.

31.14.3 Posttraumatic Amnesia

Measure of diffuse axonal injury: length of post-traumatic amnesia (PTA) is an index of severity:

- 1–24 h of PTA: moderate (1 h = 1 month of absence from work)
- 24 h of PTA: severe and associated with delirium, permanent disability in cognition, depression, and personality change
- 1 week of PTA: invalidism for 1 year, severe psychiatric and intellectual disability in 5 year follow-up

31.14.3.1 Intracranial Pressure and Head Injury

The intracranial pressure (ICP) increases initially with rise in mean arterial pressure and cerebral blood flow and then decreases (Figure 31.7).

31.14.3.1.1 *Interpretation of ICP*

- Normal ICP: <15 mmHg
- ICP >20–25 mmHg: associated with an increase in morbidity, mortality, neurological deterioration, and unilateral dilation of pupil

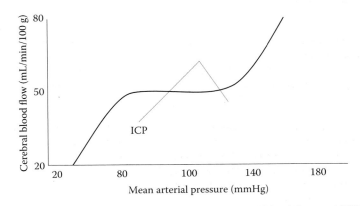

FIGURE 31.7   The relationship between mean arterial blood pressure, cerebral blood flow, and ICP.

31.14.3.2 Imaging and Head Injury

MRI images of diffuse axonal injury: MRI is a better option because CT scan may not show any lesion. MRI scan often shows multiple and diffuse abnormalities in the brain.

31.14.3.3 Neuropsychiatric Sequelae of Frontal Lobe Injury

- Frontal polar damage leads to poor judgement and insight, apathy, and impaired problem solving. There is often no understanding of the impact of the disability on the others.
- Orbitofrontal damage is associated with personality change, impaired social judgement, impulsivity, hyperactivity, disinhibition, lability of mood, excitability, and childishness or moria (childlike interest).
- Dorsolateral damage is associated with executive dysfunction, apathy, psychomotor retardation, preservation, poor initiation of tasks, and memory impairment.
- Dorsolateral damage is associated with akinetic mutism.
- Left frontal lesion is associated with impairment in verbal recall.

31.15 NEUROPSYCHIATRIC SEQUELAE OF HAEMATOMA

Epidural haematoma occurs in 0.5% of patients after head injuries. It results from blunt trauma to temporoparietal region with subsequent arterial tears, resulting in ongoing collection of blood between the dura mater and the skull (Figure 31.8).

Patients may develop symptoms and signs of increased ICP, ranging from headache to coma and death. A lucid interval may be present before the symptoms occur. Around 15%–20% of patients with epidural haematoma die of head injury.

SDH is caused by sudden acceleration–deceleration injury with tearing of bridging veins. SDH is common among old people and alcoholics and classified as acute, subacute, or chronic (Figure 31.9).

Acute SDH carries the worst prognosis and requires urgent surgical decompression. Chronic SDH develops over days to weeks after relatively minor head injury. The bleeding is slow and may not be discovered until months or even years after the

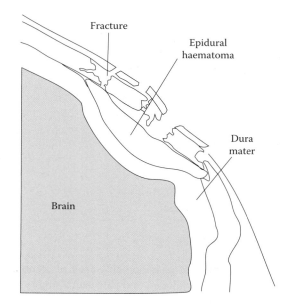

FIGURE 31.8 Epidural haematoma.

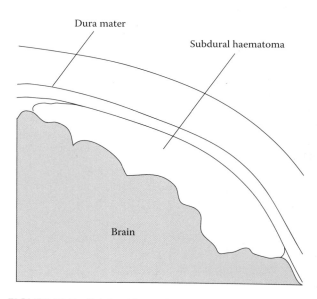

FIGURE 31.9 Subdural haematoma.

initial injury, in which 50% patients cannot recall the details of head injury.

Symptoms mainly result from increase in ICP and depend on the extent and site of bleeding. Other symptoms include loss of consciousness or fluctuating loss of consciousness, irritability, seizures, and ataxia.

TABLE 31.23
Summary of Rehabilitation Strategies in a Multidisciplinary Team

Professionals	Rehabilitation Techniques
Psychiatrists	1. Avoid psychotropic medication if possible. 2. Carbamazepine or valproate is indicated for epilepsy and episodic dyscontrol syndrome. 3. Treat depression by SSRI and psychosis by the second-generation antipsychotics. 4. Methylphenidate may improve attention and concentration.
Neuropsychologist	1. Regular assessment of neuropsychological function. 2. Prepare report for medicolegal purposes.
Nurse or community psychiatric nurse	1. To build rapport and handle emotional aspects and adjustment to head injury. 2. To assist family members to cope with behavioural problems.
Psychologist	1. Token economy or behavioural therapy to reinforce positive behaviours.
Occupational therapist	1. ADL assessment and social skill training. 2. Memory aids and strategies.
Physiotherapist	1. To enhance motor function and improve physical disabilities.

31.15.1 REHABILITATION OF PATIENTS SUFFERING FROM HEAD INJURY

Rehabilitation is offered in a multidisciplinary team (Table 31.23).

31.16 NEUROPSYCHIATRIC ASPECTS OF BRAIN TUMOUR

1. The general effect of brain tumours is a result of the rise in ICP that leads to headache, drowsiness, confusion, and apathy.
2. The local effects of tumour depend on the speed of growth. Rapid-growing tumour is associated with mental disturbances and slow-growing tumour is associated with psychiatric symptoms and personality change.
3. Neuropsychiatric sequelae depend on neuroanatomical locations:
   - *Corpus callosum*: severe cognitive deterioration.
   - *Parietal lobe*: disturbance of body image.
   - *Temporal lobe*: seizures, dysphasia, memory loss, affective disorder, and psychosis.
   - *Frontal lobe*: 80% of patients have psychiatric symptoms including irritability, atypical depression and apathy, cognitive slowing, disinhibition, and childishness.
   - *Tumour* in hypothalamus or third ventricle: dementia and confabulation.
   - *Hypothalamic hamartoma* is a benign tumour. Patients may present with *gelastic* epilepsy. Patients may present with aggressive behaviour such as hypothalamic rage. The onset occurs in the childhood. Patients may develop learning disability and other behaviour problems such as shoplifting.
   - *Thalamus*: worsening intellectual deficit, hypersomnolence, and narcolepsy.
   - *Pituitary*: *mental* slowing, apathy, emotional lability, and paranoid ideation.

31.16.1 MULTIPLE SCLEROSIS

31.16.1.1 Epidemiology

1. Prevalence: 85,000 people suffering from multiple sclerosis (MS) in the United Kingdom
2. Lifetime risk 1:8000
3. Onset: 20–50 years
4. F:M = 2:1
5. Geographical pattern: greater frequency as the distance from the equator increases

31.16.1.2 Pathology

MS is a relapsing and remitting autoimmune disorder with diverse neurological signs as a result of plaques of demyelination and degenerative axonal loss throughout the white matter except the peripheral nerves. MS also involves in focal blood–brain barrier disruption.

31.16.1.3 Clinical Features

Symptoms and signs include hypoesthesia, muscle weakness, muscle spasms and difficulties in coordination and balance, dysarthria, dysphagia, and visual disturbances. In advanced cases, patients may present with sphincter disturbance. Often, the initial attacks are transient, mild, and self-limited. Bilateral internuclear ophthalmoplegia is the pathognomonic eye sign.

31.16.1.4 Psychiatric Manifestations

1. Fatigue: 80%
2. Depression: 14%–27%; associated with interferon treatment
3. Anxiety: 14%–25%
4. Elation: 10%; associated with high dose of steroid therapy or plagues in bilateral temporal horns
5. Mania or hypomania: 2%
6. Pathological laughter and crying: 10%
7. Suicide: 7.5 times higher than general population; 15% of mortality is related to suicide
8. Schizophreniform psychosis: 1%; related to temporal lobe pathology and high-dose steroid therapy

31.16.1.5 Cognitive Impairments

1. 30%–50% have cognitive symptoms and more prominent in the later course of the illness. Memory impairment is common and MS also affects problem solving, abstract reasoning, planning, and organizational skills.
2. The prevalence of dementia is 5%.
3. Subcortical pattern.

31.16.1.6 Management of Neuropsychiatric Conditions Associated with MS (Taylor et al., 2009)

1. *Depression*: SSRIs CBT, combination of SSRI and CBT. Anergia and fatigue may favour more stimulating antidepressants such as fluoxetine, bupropion, or stimulant.
2. *Depression with pain*: SNRIs.
3. *Severe depression*: ECT.
4. *Fatigue*: CBT, amantadine as second-line treatment.

5. *Anxiety*: SSRIs such as paroxetine or sertraline; pregabalin (anticonvulsant that may control anxiety) and CBT.
6. *Steroid-induced mania*: reduction of steroid dose and consider second-generation antipsychotics (e.g. olanzapine or quetiapine to avoid EPSE).
7. *Pathological laughter or crying*: TCAs (e.g. amitriptyline) or SSRI (e.g. fluoxetine, citalopram, and sertraline).
8. *Psychosis*: second-generation antipsychotics (e.g. olanzapine, risperidone).
9. *Cognitive impairment*: treat depression and sleep problems. Donepezil may be useful to treat mild to moderate dementia. Modafinil may be useful to treat cognitive fatigue. Methylphenidate may improve poor attention.

31.17 NEUROPSYCHIATRIC ASPECTS OF LYME DISEASE

Lyme disease is caused by spirochete *Borrelia burgdorferi that is* transmitted by *Ixodes* ticks. The nymph-stage ticks feed on humans and transmit spirochetes.

Lyme disease has three stages:

Stage 1: rash

Stage 2: early neurological signs including lymphocytic meningitis, radicular pains, facial palsy, transverse myelitis, and cranial and peripheral neuropathies

Stage 3 (occurs 7 years after the initial diagnosis): late neurological signs including Bell's palsy, dementia, encephalomyelitis, hemianopsia, hemiplegia, radiculoneuropathy, and seizures

Diagnosis

1. For a positive or equivocal enzyme-linked immunosorbent assay (ELISA) finding, it must be further verified by the Western blot. After treatment, neither IgM nor IgG antibody titers are evidence of recent infection, since antibodies may persist after treatment.
2. CSF examination reveals lymphocytosis, excess protein, IgG, and *B. burgdorferi* antibodies (specific Lyme disease antibodies).
3. Magnetic resonance imaging studies show infarct patterns, white matter disease, and hydrocephalus.

TABLE 31.24

Summary of Clinical Features and Development of Syphilis

Time after Infection	3 Days	2–8 Weeks	1–10 Years	11–20 Years	21–30 Years
Primary syphilis	Painless chancre regional lymphadenopathy				
Secondary syphilis		Skin: maculopapular rash Genitalia: condylomata lata Mouth: snail-track ulcers CNS: headache, meningism			
Tertiary syphilis				Skin: gumma Cardiac: aortitis, aneurysm formation	Argyll Robertson pupil Tabes dorsalis Charcot's joints Psychiatric manifestations
Congenital syphilis	Early signs: rash	Anaemia Hepatosplenomegaly	Osteochondritis	Late signs: saddle nose, frontal bossing, Hutchinson's teeth	

Treatment

Early Lyme disease is treated by

1. Doxycycline, 100 mg BD for 21–28 days
2. Amoxicillin, 500 mg TDS for 21–28 days
3. Cefuroxime, 500 mg BD for 21 days

Late Lyme disease is treated with intravenous benzylpenicillin.

31.17.1 NEUROSYPHILIS

(See Table 31.24)

31.18 PAEDIATRIC AUTOIMMUNE NEUROPSYCHIATRIC DISORDERS ASSOCIATED WITH STREPTOCOCCAL INFECTIONS

31.18.1 EPIDEMIOLOGY (SWEDO ET AL., 1998)

1. 80% of Pediatric Autoimmune Neuropsychiatric Disorders Associated with Streptococcal Infections (PANDAS) patients suffer from tics.
2. 56% of PANDAS patients meet the DSM-IV criteria for OCD.
3. The mean age of onset of OCD is 7.4 years.
4. The mean age of onset of tics is 6.3 years.
5. Comorbidity such as hyperkinetic disorder, oppositional defiant disorder, or major depression is common.

31.18.2 PATHOPHYSIOLOGY

1. PANDAS is caused by the Group A beta-haemolytic streptococcus.
2. There is usually a 6–9 month delay between the first infection and the presentation of the PANDAS symptoms. Recurrences may have shorter time lag, for example, days to weeks.

31.18.3 CLINICAL FEATURES

1. Tic disorder.
2. OCD.
3. Symptoms first become evident between 3 years of age and puberty.
4. Neurological abnormalities such as motor hyperactivity, tics, and choreiform movements are common.
5. The course of illness is episodic with significant improvement and occasional resolution between episodes.

31.18.4 INVESTIGATIONS

1. Children with an explosive OCD or tic exacerbation should have a throat culture. If symptoms are present for more than 1 week, serial antistreptococcal titers should be ordered.
2. Infection is confirmed by a positive throat culture or elevated antistreptococcal antibody titers. In order to meet the diagnosis of PANDAS, the antistreptococcal antibody titers require at least two peak levels after the initial infection. Anti-GAS antibody titers decline with time subsequently.

31.18.5 TREATMENT

Antibiotics should only be used to treat streptococcal infections after a positive throat culture or rapid *streptococcus* test.

Standard psychiatric treatments should be used:

1. SSRIs and CBT for OCD.
2. Alpha agonists and antipsychotics for tics.
3. Intravenous immunoglobulin (IVIG) and plasmapheresis are options for acutely, severely ill children who meet the standard PANDAS criteria.

CASC STATION ON HEAD INJURY

Name: Mr. A
Age: 19
Occupation: student prior to head injury

You are interviewing the mother of Mr. A who has jumped into the river but he denies any suicidal intention. Mr. A suffered from a head injury following a pub fight 2 years ago. His mother reports that his personality has changed since the head injury. She has made this appointment to see you and discuss about his problems.

Task: Elicit information about the psychiatric sequelae and complications of head injury.

CASC Grid

Empathetic statement: I was informed that Mr. A was assaulted 2 years ago and I am very sorry to hear about this. I understand that this has been a difficult time for you since his injury.

(A) Cognitive Impairment	(A1) Injury	(A2) Extent of Injury	(A3) Course of Memory Problem	(A4) Other Neuropsychological Changes	(A5) Current Treatment and Rehabilitation
	'Can you tell me what happened to Mr. A immediately after the injury?' (explore duration of unconsciousness and duration of confusion) 'Did he lose his consciousness? If so, how long did it last?' 'For how long did Mr. A lose his memory?' 'Did he develop fits after the head injury?'	'Can you describe the extent of his injury?' 'Did he require an operation in his head?' 'What did the doctor say about his outcome?'	'Does he often make mistakes after the head injury?' 'What does he do if he cannot remember or recall? Does he make up the answer?' 'What happened in the first one year after the head injury? Did he show any improvement?'	'When you compare Mr. A before and after the head injury, are there any changes in his function and character?' (look for changes in personality, memory, capacity to handle finance, ability to study/ work) 'Can he look after himself?' (assess basic ADL)	'How did Mr. A react to the assault?' 'Did Mr. A go through a treatment programme for people suffering from head injury?' 'Was he given any medication by the doctor or GP? Does it help?'

(B) Impairment of Function Based on Specific Neuroanatomical Areas	(B1) Frontal Lobe Symptoms	(B2) Parietal Lobe Symptoms	(B3) Temporal Lobe Symptoms	(B4) Occipital Lobe Symptoms:	(B5) Postconcussion Syndrome
	'How is his mood at this moment?' 'Can you tell me more about his mood?' (look for liability) 'How about his temper?' 'Does he make jokes very often?' 'Is he motivated to do things?' 'Can he plan? Can he prioritize tasks?' 'How does he interact with women? Has he been overfamiliar?' (look for disinhibition) 'Can you tell me more about his judgement?' 'Does he understand the impact of his behaviours on other people?'	Explore features of Gerstmann's syndrome that involves dominant parietal lobe (e.g. finger agnosia, acalculia, and dysgraphia). Explore nondominant parietal lobe symptoms: apraxia.	'How do you find Mr. A's communication? Does he have difficulty in reading and writing?' 'Does Mr. A hear voices when no one is around?' 'Has Mr. A ever mentioned that someone wanted to harm him?' Explore other features such as trancelike states, hyposexuality, hyperphagia, and temporal lobe epilepsy.	'Does Mr. A have any problems with his vision?' 'If so, is his visual field defect associated with headache?' 'Can he recognize people?'	'Does he have headaches?' 'Does he feel giddy?' 'Is he fearful of light?' 'How about nausea and vomiting?' 'How do you find his concentration?' 'What is his understanding of the current problem?' 'Has he ever had fits?' 'Do the aforementioned symptoms improve in the first 6 months after the injury?'

(C) Risk Assessment	(C1) Danger to Other People	(C2) Self-Harm	(C3) Safety at Home	(C4) Capacity	(C5) Driving
	'Has Mr. A been aggressive to the others?' 'Has he been more violent after the head injury?' 'Is he hyperactive and cannot sit still?'	'Has Mr. A tried to harm himself?' 'Has he ever thought of ending his life?'	'Has there been any accident at home?' (such as fire, fall)	'Can Mr. A handle his finance?'	'Does Mr. A drive after the head injury?'

(D) Other Psychiatric Comorbidity and Com\pensation Issues	(D1) Compensation Issues	(D2) Past Psychiatric History	(D3) PTSD Symptoms	(D4) Substance Abuse	(D5) Closing
	'Did he receive any compensation after head injury? (e.g. insurance or from third party)' 'Is there any unsettled legal matter?'	'Did Mr. A consult a psychiatrist before or after the head injury? If yes, what was the reason?'	'Is he disturbed by nightmare?' 'Does he have flashback of the assault?' 'Does he avoid to go to pub or other places related to the assault?'	'Does Mr. A use any recreational drug? If yes, is it before the head injury or after the head injury?' 'Does he drink very often prior to the head injury?'	Thanks for your information. I am sorry to hear the changes in Mr. A after his head injury and the impact on the family. I would like to meet him and assess him. Then I can formulate a plan to help Mr. A and his family.

REFERENCES

Alim MA, Hossain MS, Arima K et al. 2002: Tubulin seeds alpha-synuclein fibril formation. *The Journal of Biological Chemistry* 277(3):2112–2117.

American Psychiatric Association. 2013: *Desk Reference to the Diagnostic Criteria from DSM-5*. Washington, DC: American Psychiatric Association Press.

Barone P et al. 2006: Pramipexole versus sertraline in the treatment of depression in Parkinson's disease: A national multicenter parallel-group randomized study. *Journal of Neurology* 253:601–607.

Bentley P. 2008: *Memorizing Medicine. A Revision Guide.* London, U.K.: Royal Society of Medicine Press.

Berkman LF, Blumenthal J, Burg M et al. 2003: Effects of treating depression and low-perceived social support on clinical events after myocardial infarction—The enhancing recovery in coronary heart disease patients (ENRICHD) randomized trial. *JAMA* 289:3106–3116.

Bird J and Rogers D. 2007: *Seminars in General Adult Psychiatry*. London, U.K.: Gaskell.

Citron K, Bruillette MJ, Beckett A. 2005: *HIV and Psychiatry: A Training and Resource Manual*, 2nd edn. Cambridge, U.K.: Cambridge University Press.

Cummings J. 1985: *Clinical Neuropsychiatry*. Orlando, FL: Grune & Stratton.

Dougan S, Elford J, Chadborn TR, Brown AE, Roy K, Murphy G, and Gill ON. 2007: Does the recent increase in HIV diagnoses among men who have sex with men in the UK reflect a rise in HIV incidence or increased uptake of HIV testing? *Sexually Transmitted Infection* 83(2):120–125.

Ettinger AB and Kanner AM. 2001: *Psychiatric Issues in Epilepsy—A Practical Guide to Diagnosis and Treatment*. Philadelphia, PA: Lippincott Williams & Wilkins.

Friedman M, Thoreson CE, Gill H et al. 1987: Alteration of type A behavior and its effect on cardiac recurrences in post-myocardial infarction patients: Summary results of the Recurrent Coronary Prevention Project. *American Heart Journal* 114:483–490.

Glassman AH, O'Connor CM, Califf RM et al. 2002: Sertraline treatment of major depression in patients with acute MI or unstable angina. *JAMA* 288:701–709.

Gurnell M. 2001: *Medical Masterclass-Endocrinology*. London, U.K.: Blackwell Science.

Health Protection Agency. 2010: HIV in the United Kingdom: 2010 Report. http://www.hpa.org.uk/web/HPAweb&HPAwebStandard/HPAweb_C/1287145264558 (accessed on 1 May 2012).

Health Protection Agency Centre for Infections, Health Protection Scotland and UCL Institute of Child Health. 2011: United Kingdom new HIV diagnoses to end of December 2010–2011. http://www.hpa.org.uk/web/HPAweb&HPAwebStandard/HPAweb_C/1252660002826 (accessed on 1 May 2012).

Jointed United Nations Programme on HIV/AIDS www.unaids.org (accessed on 1 May 2012).

Low RA Jr et al. 1998: Clozapine induced atrial fibrillation. *Journal of Clinical Psychopharmacology* 18:170.

Lown B. 1987: Sudden cardiac death: Biobehavioral perspective. *Circulation* 76:186–196.

Lishman WA. 1997: *Organic Psychiatry: The Psychological Consequences of Cerebral Disorder*, 3rd edn. Oxford, U.K.: Blackwell Scientific.

Mace C. 1993: Epilepsy and schizophrenia. *British Journal of Psychiatry* 163:439–446.

Marsden CD and Fowler TJ. 1989: *Clinical Neurology*. London, U.K.: Edward Arnold.

Maxwell PH. 2001: *Medical Masterclass—Nephrology*. London, U.K.: Blackwell Science.

Mayou R, Bass C, and Sharpe M. 1995: *Treatment of Functional Somatic Symptoms*. Oxford, U.K.: Oxford University Press.

Olumuyiwa JO and Akim AK. 2005: *Patient Management Problems in Psychiatry*. London, U.K.: Churchill Livingstone.

Van Melle JP, de Jonge P, Honig A et al. 2007: Effects of antidepressant treatment following myocardial infarction. *The British Journal of Psychiatry* 190 (January):460–466.

Rozanski A, Bairey CN, Krantz DS et al. 1988: Mental stress and the induction of silent myocardial ischemia in patients with coronary artery disease. *New England Journal of Medicine* 318:1005–1012.

Sadock BJ and Sadock VA. 2003: *Kaplan and Sadock's Comprehensive Textbook of Psychiatry*, 9th edn. Philadelphia, PA: Lippincott Williams & Wilkins.

Schneider RA et al. 2008: Apparent seizure and atrial fibrillation associated with paliperidone. *American Journal of Health-System Pharmacy* 65:2122–2125.

Sharpe M, Archard L, Banatvala J et al. 1991: Chronic fatigue syndrome: Guidelines for research. *Journal of the Royal Society of Medicine* 84:118–121.

Swedo SE, Leonard HL, Garvey M et al. 1998: PANDAS: Clinical description of the first 50 cases. *American Journal of Psychiatry* 155:264–271.

Taylor D, Paton C, and Kapur S. 2009: *The Maudsley Prescribing Guidelines*. London, U.K.: Informa healthcare.

Trimble M. 2004: *Somatoform Disorders–A Medicolegal Guide*. Cambridge, U.K.: Cambridge University Press.

Treasaden I. 2010: Dissociative (conversion), hypochondriasis and other somatoform disorders. In Puri BK and Treasaden I (eds.) *Psychiatry. An Evidence-Based Test*. London, U.K.: Hodder Arnold.

Verrotti A, Cicconetti A, Scorrano B et al. 2008: Epilepsy and suicide: Pathogenesis, risk factors, and prevention. *Neuropsychiatric Disease and Treatment* 4(2):365–370.

Waters BM et al. 2008: Olanzapine-associated new-onset atrial fibrillation. *Journal of Clinical Psychopharmacology* 28:354–355.

Wessely S, Hotopf M, and Sharpe M. 2003: *Chronic Fatigue and Its Syndrome*. Oxford, U.K.: Oxford University Press.

Wise MG and Rundell JR. 2002: *Textbook of Consultation—Liaison Psychiatry*. Washington, DC: American Psychiatric Publishing Inc.

World Health Organization. 1992: *The ICD-10 Classification of Mental and Behavioural Disorders*. Geneva, Switzerland: World Health Organization.

Yudofsky SC and Hales RE. (eds.) 1992: *The American Psychiatric Press Textbook of Neuropsychiatry*, 2nd edn. Washington, DC: APP.

32 Addiction and Psychoactive Substance Use Disorders

32.1 CLASSIFICATION AND DEFINITIONS

ICD-10 classification of mental and behavioural disorders caused by psychoactive substance use

F10 Mental and behavioural disorders caused by the use of alcohol

F11 ... ... opioids
F12 ... ... cannabinoids
F13 ... ... sedatives or hypnotics
F14 ... ... cocaine
F15 ... ... stimulants, including caffeine
F16 ... ... hallucinogens
F17 ... ... tobacco
F18 ... ... volatile solvents
F19 ... ... multiple drug use and use of other psychoactive substances

Specific clinical conditions are additionally coded as follows:

0 Acute intoxication
1 Harmful use
2 Dependence syndrome
3 Withdrawal state
4 Withdrawal state with delirium
5 Psychotic disorder
6 Amnesic syndrome
7 Residual and late-onset psychotic disorder
8 Other mental and behavioural disorders
9 Unspecified mental and behavioural disorder

32.1.1 DSM-5

The DSM-5 proposes a number of conditions induced by substances:

- Substance-induced anxiety disorder
- Substance-induced bipolar disorder
- Substance-induced depressive disorder
- Substance-induced delirium
- Substance-induced obsessive–compulsive or related disorders
- Substance-induced psychotic disorder
- Substance-induced sleep–wake disorder
- Substance-induced sexual dysfunction
- Substance-induced neurocognitive disorder

32.1.2 ACUTE INTOXICATION

ICD-10: This is a transient condition following the use of a psychoactive substance, resulting in disturbance of one or more of the following:

- Consciousness level
- Cognition
- Perception
- Affect
- Behaviour

Its intensity is closely related to dose and lessening with time, and the effects disappear when following cessation of the intake of the psychoactive substance. Recovery is usually complete.

The DSM-5 criteria state the recent ingestion of substance. The ingestion leads to clinically significant behavioural or psychological changes such as inappropriate sexual or aggressive behaviour, mood lability, impaired judgement, and impaired social or occupational functioning. Each substance is associated with specific intoxication symptoms.

Pathological intoxication applies only to alcohol and refers to sudden aggressive behaviour, out of character, after drinking small amounts, which would not produce intoxication in most people.

32.1.3 HARMFUL USE

This is use that is causing damage to physical or mental health. It does not refer to adverse social consequences.

Use disorder: The DSM-5 proposes a problematic pattern of substance use leading to clinically significant impairment or distress within a 12-month period and requires at least two of the following criteria (APA, 2013):

1. The substance is often taken in large amounts over a long period of time.
2. There is a persistent failure and unsuccessful effort to cut down the substance use.
3. The patient spends a great of time to obtain the substance.
4. Recurrent substance use resulting in a failure to fulfil major role obligations.
5. Continued substance use despite having persistent or recurrent social or interpersonal problems.
6. Abandonment of important occupational, social and recreational activities.
7. Recurrent substance use in dangerous situations (e.g. driving).
8. Continued substance use despite harmful physical and psychological effects.
9. Tolerance: As a result of diminished effect, there is a need for increased amounts of substance to achieve intoxication or desired effect.
10. Withdrawal: Presence of characteristic withdrawal syndrome and relief of withdrawal by the same substance.
11. Craving or strong urge to use the substance.

The DSM-5 proposes the following specifier: early remission (3 months < duration of use < 12 months), sustain remission (no substance use > 12 months), or in a controlled environment where access to substance is limited.

32.1.4   Dependence Syndrome

This is diagnosed if three or more of the following have been present together at some time in the previous year:

- Compulsion to take the substance
- Difficulties in controlling substance-taking behaviour: onset, termination, or levels of use
- Characteristic physiological withdrawal state when substance reduced or withdrawn; use of substance to avoid or relieve withdrawal symptoms
- Increased tolerance, so larger doses are required to achieve effect originally produced by lower doses

- Progressive neglect of other activities with increasing time spent in acquiring, taking, or recovering from the effects of the substance
- Persisting with substance use despite evidence of harmful consequences

The DSM-5 does not propose a dependence syndrome. The dependence syndrome in DSM-IV-TR is replaced by use disorder in DSM-5.

32.1.5   Withdrawal State

ICD-10: Symptoms occur upon withdrawal or reduction of a substance after repeated, usually high dose, and prolonged use. Onset and course are time limited and dose related and differ according to the substance involved. Convulsions may complicate withdrawal.

DSM-5: DSM-5 is similar to ICD-10 and it emphasizes on the significant distress or impairment in social, occupational, or other important areas of functioning as a result of substance withdrawal.

32.1.6   Withdrawal State with Delirium

ICD-10: This is where the withdrawal state is complicated by delirium. Alcohol-induced delirium tremens is a short-lived, sometimes life-threatening, toxic confusional state precipitated by relative or absolute alcohol withdrawal in severely dependent users. Classic symptoms include

- Clouding of consciousness
- Hallucinations and illusions
- Marked tremor

It involves prodromal symptoms of

- Insomnia
- Tremulousness
- Fearful affect

It is usually accompanied by

- Delusions
- Agitation
- Insomnia
- Autonomic overactivity

In addition, convulsions may occur.

DSM-5: This condition is called substance-intoxication or withdrawal delirium, and it requires the evidence from history, physical examination, or laboratory findings that the aforementioned symptoms developed during or shortly after a withdrawal syndrome and not accounted by dementia.

32.1.7 PSYCHOTIC DISORDER

ICD-10: Psychotic symptoms occur during or immediately after psychoactive substance use, in relatively clear sensorium (some clouding of consciousness but not severe confusion). It is not a manifestation of drug withdrawal or a functional psychosis. The characteristics of the psychosis vary according to the substance used, but the following are common:

- Vivid hallucinations in more than one modality
- Delusions
- Psychomotor disturbances
- Abnormal affect

Stimulant-induced psychotic disorders are generally related to prolonged high-dose use. Typically, it resolves at least partially within 1 month and fully within 6 months.

In ICD-10, further subdivisions may be specified:

- Schizophrenia-like
- Predominantly delusional
- Predominantly hallucinatory (includes alcoholic hallucinosis)
- Predominantly polymorphic
- Predominantly depressive symptoms
- Predominantly manic symptoms
- Mixed

The DSM-5 proposes similar criteria as ICD-10 and specifies the onset that is during intoxication or withdrawal.

32.1.8 AMNESIC SYNDROME

ICD-10: This is induced by alcohol or other psychoactive substances. Requirements for diagnosis include

- Chronic prominent impairment of recent memory; remote memory may be impaired; difficulty learning new material; disturbance of time sense.
- Immediate recall preserved; other cognitive functions are usually relatively preserved and consciousness is clear.
- A history of chronic and usually high-dose use of alcohol or drugs.

Confabulation may be present but not invariably so. Korsakov's psychosis is included here.

The DSM-5 proposes a similar condition called substance-induced neurocognitive disorder. The temporal course of the neurocognitive deficits is consistent with the aetiological relationship, and the cognitive domains involved must be consistent with the particular substance misused.

32.1.9 RESIDUAL AND LATE-ONSET PSYCHOTIC DISORDER

ICD-10: Alcohol- or psychoactive substance-induced changes of cognition, affect, personality, or behaviour persist beyond the period during which the substance might reasonably be assumed to be operating. The onset is directly related to substance use.

Residual and late-onset psychotic disorder is further subdivided by ICD-10 into

- Flashbacks—episodic psychotic experiences that duplicate previous drug-related experiences and are usually very short-lived (seconds or minutes)
- Personality or behaviour disorder
- Organic mood disorder
- Dementia—may be reversible after an extended period of abstinence
- Other persisting cognitive impairments

The DSM-5 has one disorder under this category, the hallucinogen persisting perception disorder.

32.2 ALCOHOL: THE CHEMICAL AND PHARMACOLOGICAL PROPERTIES

32.2.1 UNIT OF ALCOHOL

The concentration of alcohol in beverages is stated in terms of 'proof' scales. In the United States, one-degree proof is equal to a concentration of 0.5% by volume (v/v). In the United Kingdom, one-degree proof is equal to 0.5715% by volume (v/v).

One unit of alcohol in the United Kingdom is approximately 8–10 g of ethanol (C_2H_5OH) and is the amount contained in (Figure 32.1)

- A standard measure of spirits
- A standard glass of sherry or fortified wine
- A standard glass of table wine
- One half-pint of beer or lager of standard strength (3%–3.5% by volume)

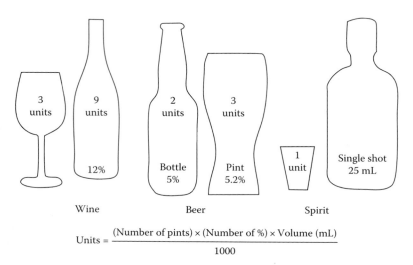

$$\text{Units} = \frac{(\text{Number of pints}) \times (\text{Number of \%}) \times \text{Volume (mL)}}{1000}$$

FIGURE 32.1   Units of alcohol in different forms of beverages.

32.2.2   Levels of Consumption

Up to 21 units of alcohol per week for men and up to 14 units of alcohol per week for women, not consumed in one go and not consumed every day, are considered to be low-risk levels of intake. Women are more susceptible to the harmful effects of alcohol because their lower lean body mass results in higher blood alcohol levels per unit taken.

Table 32.1 classifies the level of consumption based on alcohol units. Hazardous drinking refers to the pattern of alcohol consumption that increases a person's risk of harm in terms of physical, mental, and social consequences (NICE, 2010). Harmful drinking is more serious than hazardous drinking and results in physical or mental damage. It is estimated that around 1/4 of adults drink in a hazardous or harmful way in the United Kingdom (the NHS Information Centre, 2009) and 1/5 of patients admitted to hospital for illnesses unrelated to alcohol are drinking at potentially hazardous levels (Royal College of Physicians, 2001).

Abstinence or minimal alcohol intake is recommended in pregnancy, because of the risk of the development of fetal alcohol syndrome.

32.2.3   Mechanism of Action

GABA$_A$, serotonin, nicotinic, dopamine, and opioid receptors are involved.

GABA receptors: The alcohol enhances neurotransmission, and the interaction between alcohol and the GABA$_A$ receptors leads to *decreased* level of consciousness (stupor or coma if large amount is consumed), reduction of anxiety, disinhibition, and aggression (see Figure 32.2). Its interaction with the GABA$_A$ receptor can lead to

TABLE 32.1

Summary of Safe, Hazardous, and Harmful Levels of Alcohol Consumption and Recommendations from the U.K. Government on Sensible Drinking

	Safer Levels	Hazardous Levels	Harmful Levels	Dependent Levels	Sensible Drinking	Against Heart Disease
Men	21 units per week	21–35 units per week	35–50 units per week	>50 units per week	Max 3–4 units per day	2 units per day for men >40 years
Women	14 units per week	14–21 units per week	21–35 units per week	>35 units per week	Max 2–3 units per day	2 units per day after menopause

Note: Abstinence or minimal alcohol intake is recommended in pregnancy, because of the risk of the development of fetal alcohol syndrome.

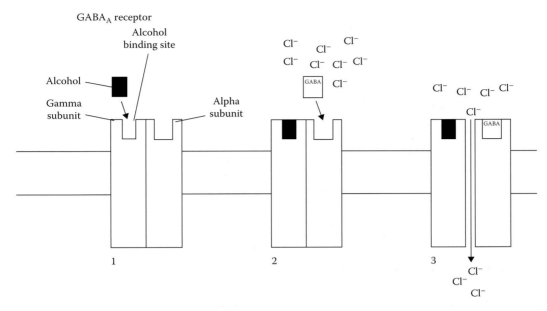

FIGURE 32.2   The binding of alcohol to GABA$_A$ receptor and influx of chloride ions.

delay in reaction time. It also affects the GABA$_A$ transmission in cerebellum and results in unsteady gait and difficulty in standing. Alcohol withdrawal is associated with reduction in GABA function.

Serotonin receptors: Alcohol enhances the action of serotonin at the 5-HT$_3$ receptors (see Figure 32.3). Serotonin plays a role in control of impulse. The change in level of serotonin will result in lability of mood and aggression. Alcohol withdrawal is associated with reduction in 5-HT$_3$ receptor function. Ondansetron, a 5-HT$_3$ antagonist, was

found to reduce drinking in early alcoholics and in combination with naltrexone.

Nicotinic receptors: Alcohol enhances the action of nicotinic receptors and increases the excitatory neurotransmission, resulting in aggression (Figure 32.4).

Dopamine receptors: Alcohol releases dopamine from the ventral tegmental area and nucleus accumbens, leading to euphoria and impaired attention and judgement. Dopamine is involved in reward or novelty seeking, as well as other mesolimbic and cortical projections.

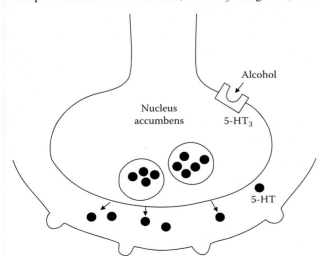

FIGURE 32.3   The binding of alcohol to 5-HT$_3$ receptors and release of serotonin.

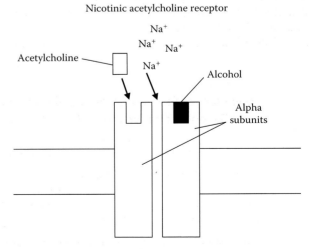

FIGURE 32.4   The binding of alcohol to nicotinic acetylcholine receptors and influx of sodium ions.

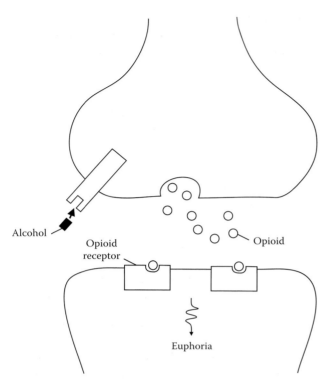

FIGURE 32.5 The binding of alcohol to μ-opioid receptors and subsequent release of opioid.

Alcohol withdrawal is associated with reduced dopaminergic function. Prolonged heavy drinking decreases the number of dopamine transporters, and this may sensitize people with alcohol dependence to dopamine transmission and lead to early relapse after alcohol withdrawal.

Opioid receptors: Alcohol consumption can stimulate the release of opioid in the mesolimbic forebrain and results in euphoria, poor attention, and impaired judgement (see Figure 32.5).

NMDA receptors: Ethanol at low concentrations (5–10 mmol/L) inhibits the action of NMDA–glutamate controlled ion channels and potentiates the actions of GABA type A controlled ion channels. These are the main excitatory and inhibitory systems of the brain; the overall effect of ethanol is therefore as a central nervous depressant. At slightly higher ethanol concentrations, the actions of voltage-sensitive calcium channels and channels controlled by serotonin are affected.

Chronic administration of ethanol produces alterations in the GABA, NMDA, and voltage-sensitive calcium channel systems. The reduction in the production of subunits of the GABA receptors is seen particularly

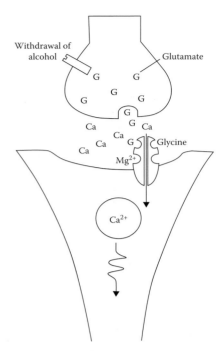

FIGURE 32.6 Alcohol withdrawal and enhancement of glutamate actions at the NMDA receptors.

in mice prone to withdrawal convulsions. Chronic ethanol administration also causes an upregulation of NMDA receptors in mouse hippocampus, more evident in mice prone to withdrawal convulsions. Both of these receptor changes promote central nervous system (CNS) excitability and increase the likelihood of convulsions.

Although ethanol exposure is the cause of increased numbers of NMDA receptors, its presence protects against the neurotoxicity of glutamate overstimulation. Ethanol withdrawal increases glutamate in the brain, which damages neurons. Repeated withdrawal causes increased neuronal death.

On the other hand, the withdrawal of alcohol (see Figure 32.6) enhances the actions of glutamate at the NMDA receptors and the voltage-sensitive Ca^{2+} channels. This will attenuate the action of GABA at inhibitory $GABA_A$ receptors, resulting in agitation during alcohol withdrawal. Intracellular mechanisms (e.g. Ca^{2+} channels) play a role in tension relief reward conditioning with reinstitution of alcohol.

32.2.4 ADVERSE EFFECTS OF ALCOHOL ON PHYSICAL HEALTH

Alcohol accounts for one-fifth to one-third of medical admissions to hospital.

32.2.4.1   Nervous System

Neurological disorders that are associated with excessive drinking include

- Convulsions occurring mainly secondary to alcohol withdrawal, tonic–clonic in nature, within the first 48 h (also secondary to brain damage or hypoglycaemia), occurring in 10% of alcoholics.
- Marchiafava–Bignami disease is a rare fatal demyelinating disease characterized neuropathologically by widespread demyelination affecting the central corpus callosum and often also the middle cerebellar peduncles, the white matter of the cerebral hemispheres, and the optic tracts. It presents clinically with emotional disturbance and cognitive impairment followed by epilepsy, delirium, paralysis, and coma.
- Cerebellar degeneration, affecting mainly the vermis, resulting in ataxia of gait and sensory ataxia (failure in the heel–shin test) with depressed deep tendon reflex.
- Central pontine myelinolysis causing bulbar palsy dysarthria, locked-in syndrome, quadriplegia, loss of pain sensations, and death.
- Optic atrophy due to demyelination.
- Retrobulbar neuropathy resulting in loss of central vision and preventable with vitamin B replacement.
- Peripheral neuropathy resulting in numbness and paraesthesias in glove and stocking distribution, occurring in 45% of alcoholics.
- Coarse tremor (5–7 Hz).

32.2.4.2   Cardiovascular System

Cardiovascular system disorders include

- Hypertension, poorly responsive to conventional treatment but responsive to abstinence
- Coronary artery disease
- Cardiac arrhythmias particularly after binge drinking (holiday heart syndrome)
- Cardiomyopathy, presenting with gradual onset of heart failure (the prognosis is poor with continued drinking)
- Haemorrhagic and thrombotic CVA, even in the young

32.2.4.3   Gastrointestinal Disorders

These include

- Cancer of mouth and pharynx
- Mallory–Weiss tears
- Oesophageal varices
- Nausea and vomiting, particularly in the morning, prevented by drinking more alcohol
- Gastritis
- Peptic ulcers
- Diarrhoea

32.2.4.4   Malnutrition

This may result from

- Poor intake
- Malabsorption
- Impaired metabolism

Results of malnutrition may include

- Thiamine deficiency presenting with Wernicke's encephalopathy acutely, leading in a high proportion of cases to Korsakov's psychosis (may also present with high output heart failure of beriberi)
- Niacin deficiency (vitamin B_3) presenting with pellagra, causing confusion, diarrhoea, and light-sensitive rash
- Vitamin C deficiency presenting with skin haemorrhages and gingivitis

32.2.4.5   Liver

Hepatic damage is another important result of excessive alcohol intake. Fatty infiltration leading to an acute increase in the size of the liver occurs within a few days of excessive intake; it may cause pain in the right hypochondrium, nausea, and vomiting but is usually not detected. It is reversible with abstinence. Alcoholic hepatitis (AST > ALT) may occur secondary to long-term heavy daily drinking.

Liver cell necrosis and inflammation occur, presenting with right hypochondrial pain and jaundice, sometimes accompanied by ascites and encephalopathy.

Cirrhosis with permanent fibrotic changes occurs. This may present with signs of liver failure, including

- Ascites
- Encephalopathy
- Bleeding oesophageal varices

However, cirrhosis may be symptomless initially. Short-acting benzodiazepine such as oxazepam can bed in alcohol withdrawal.

BOX 32.1   NICE GUIDANCE ON ASSESSMENT AND MANAGEMENT OF ALCOHOL-RELATED LIVER DISEASE (NICE, 2010)

1. Exclude alternative causes in alcoholics with abnormal liver function test results.
2. Refer the patients to hepatic specialists for further assessment.
3. For patients with alcohol-related hepatitis, assess nutritional requirements and offer nutritional support (e.g. NG tube feeding).
4. Use the discriminant function (DF) to determine treatment in people with alcohol-related hepatitis.
5. If the score of DF is larger than 32, consider liver biopsy to confirm diagnosis of alcohol-related hepatitis.
6. Corticosteroid (e.g. prednisolone) is used to treat severe alcohol-related hepatitis.
7. Consider liver transplantation in patients who have decompensated liver disease after best management and 3 months' abstinence from alcohol.

32.2.4.6   Pancreas

Acute and chronic pancreatitides lead to food malabsorption and diabetes in some cases.

BOX 32.2   NICE GUIDANCE ON ASSESSMENT AND MANAGEMENT OF ALCOHOL-RELATED PANCREATITIS (NICE, 2010)

1. Diagnosis is established by clinical history, imaging to assess the pancreatic structure (e.g. CT scan), and tests of pancreatic exocrine and endocrine function.
2. Do not offer prophylactic antibiotics to people with mild acute pancreatitis, unless otherwise indicated.
3. Offer pancreatic enzyme supplements to people with steatorrhoea or poor nutritional status.
4. Offer enteral tube feeding rather than parenteral nutritional support if possible.
5. Offer endoscopy surgery to people with obstructive chronic pancreatitis.
6. Offer celiac axis block, splanchnicectomy, or surgery to people with nonobstructive chronic pancreatitis if pain is poorly controlled.

32.2.4.7   Electrolyte Disturbance

Hyponatraemia, hypomagnesaemia, hypophosphataemia, and hypercalcaemia can occur.

32.2.4.8   Endocrine and Sexual Disorders

Endocrine and sexual disorders can occur. There is gonadal atrophy that affects both sexes. Direct toxic effects upon the gonads result in reduced sex hormone synthesis. Liver disease results in oestrogenization in men resulting in gynaecomastia. Fertility may recover with abstinence. Autonomic nervous system dysfunction may result in erectile impotence and central effects cause anorgasmia. There is an increased risk of miscarriage and recurrent abortion in women.

Alcoholic pseudo-Cushing's syndrome may cause

- Obesity
- Hirsutism
- Hypertension

Skin, Muscle, and Skeleton

Dermatological disorders that may occur include acne and rhinophyma.

Musculoskeletal disorders that are associated with excessive drinking include

- Myopathy, presenting acutely with pain and tenderness of swollen muscles (usually symmetrical; if severe, may cause renal failure due to myoglobinuria)
- Proximal muscle weakness and wasting (common in alcoholics)
- Palmar erythema
- Osteoporosis
- Avascular necrosis

32.2.4.9   Blood

Haematological changes may occur, since alcohol is a bone marrow toxin, resulting in the following:

- Macrocytosis (positive predictive value of alcohol misuse is 85%)
- Folate deficiency
- Impaired clotting caused by vitamin K deficiency and/or reduced platelet functioning
- Iron-deficiency anaemia, often as a result of gastrointestinal haemorrhage

32.2.4.10   Infections

There is an increased risk of infections such as tuberculosis and pneumonia, particularly in the homeless.

32.2.4.11 Metabolism

A variety of metabolic abnormalities may occur, including

- Alcohol-induced lactic acidosis.
- Alcoholic ketoacidosis.
- Hyperlipidaemia in one-third of alcohol-dependent subjects (low levels of intake appear protective, however).
- Hypoglycaemia: Alcohol-induced hypoglycaemia occurs in people who are dependent on alcohol after a large drink.
- Hyperuricaemia.
- Haemochromatosis.
- Porphyria cutanea tarda.

32.2.4.12 Neoplasms

There is an increased incidence of the following types of cancer:

- Oropharyngeal
- Oesophageal
- Colorectal
- Pancreatic
- Hepatic
- Lung

32.2.4.13 Early Death

The top four causes of early death among alcoholics

- Heart disease
- Cancer
- Accident
- Suicide

32.2.4.14 Trauma

Accidents and trauma may result from alcohol consumption. These include

- Road accidents
- Assaults (including head injuries)
- Falls (including head injuries)
- Drowning
- Burns
- Death by fire

The most common traumatic injuries include

- Rib fractures
- Head injuries
- Subdural/extradural haematomas
- Long-bone fractures

32.2.4.15 Pregnancy

Excessive alcohol consumption in pregnancy can lead to permanent fetal damage.

Features of the resulting fetal alcohol syndrome include

- Cardiac abnormalities (e.g. atrial septal defect)
- Low-set ears
- Absent philtrum
- Long upper lip with narrow vermilion border
- Depressed bridge of the nose
- Small nose
- Ocular hypertelorism
- Microcephaly
- Strabismus
- Pectus excavatum
- Poor growth
- Increased neonatal mortality

The DSM-5 originally proposed the neurobehavioural disorder associated with prenatal alcohol exposure in its draft. Although this disorder does not appear in the final version, readers may find the criteria useful in clinical practice.

Neurocognitive impairment, as evidenced by one (or more) of the following:

1. Global intellectual impairment (i.e. IQ of 70 or below)
2. Impairment in executive functioning
3. Impairment in learning (e.g. lower academic achievement)
4. Impairment in memory
5. Impairment in visual–spatial reasoning (e.g. disorganized or poorly planned drawings)

Impairment in self-regulation in one (or more) of the following:

1. Impairment in mood or behavioural regulation
2. Attention deficit
3. Impairment in impulse control

Deficits in adaptive functioning as manifested in two (or more) of the following:

1. Communication deficit
2. Social impairment
3. Impairment in daily living
4. Motor impairment

32.2.5 ADVERSE EFFECTS OF ALCOHOL ON MENTAL HEALTH

The major types of psychiatric morbidity that are associated with excessive alcohol intake are

- Organic brain syndromes
- Alcoholic hallucinosis
- Pathological jealousy
- Mood disorders
- Personality disorder
- Neurotic disorders
- Psychosexual disorders

Each of these is now considered in turn.

32.2.5.1 Organic Brain Syndromes

Organic brain syndromes that are associated with excessive alcohol intake may be considered under the headings of

- Acute/subacute syndromes
- Alcoholic blackouts
- Delirium tremens
- Withdrawal fits
- Wernicke's encephalopathy
- Chronic syndromes
- Korsakov's syndrome
- Alcoholic dementia

Each of these is now described.

32.2.5.1.1 Alcoholic Blackouts

Intoxication frequently leads to episodes of short-term amnesia or blackouts. These may occur after just one bout of heavy drinking and are estimated to have been experienced by 15%–20% of those who drink.

Three types of blackout are recognized, which, in order of increasing severity, are as follows:

1. State-dependent memory loss. Memory for events occurring while intoxicated is lost when sober but returns when next intoxicated.
2. Fragmentary blackouts. There is no clear demarcation of memory loss, and islets of memory exist within the gap. Some recovery occurs with time.
3. En bloc blackouts. There is a clearly demarcated total memory loss, with no recovery of this lost memory over time. If this memory loss extends for days, the subject experiences a fugue-like state in which he or she may travel some distance before coming around, with no memory of the events occurring during this time.

32.2.5.1.2 Delirium Tremens

In chronic heavy drinkers, a fall in the blood alcohol concentration leads to withdrawal symptoms including delirium tremens. The peak onset is within 2 days of abstinence, and it usually lasts for about 5 days.

There is a prodromal period with

- Anxiety
- Insomnia
- Tachycardia
- Tremor
- Sweating

The onset of delirium is marked by

- Disorientation
- Fluctuating level of consciousness
- Intensely fearful affect
- Hallucinations
- Misperceptions
- Tremor
- Restlessness
- Autonomic overactivity

The hallucinations are often visual and are commonly Lilliputian in nature. Auditory and tactile hallucinations, and secondary delusions, may also be present. There is a mortality rate of about 5%, associated with cardiovascular collapse or infection. The treatment of delirium tremens is supportive with sedation, fluid and electrolyte replacement, and high-potency vitamins (especially thiamine to prevent an unrecognized Wernicke's encephalopathy progressing to Korsakov's psychosis—see succeeding text).

32.2.5.1.3 Withdrawal Fits

Withdrawal fits may take place within 48 h of stopping drinking.

BOX 32.3   NICE GUIDANCE ON THE MANAGEMENT OF DELIRIUM TREMENS OR SEIZURES (NICE, 2010)

1. Oral lorazepam should be used as first-line treatment for delirium tremens or seizures.
2. If symptoms persist or encountering difficulty to administer oral lorazepam, consider
   a. Parenteral lorazepam.
   b. Parenteral haloperidol (caution in patients suffering from conditions predisposing to convulsions)
   c. Parenteral olanzapine.

3. The aforementioned medications do not have U.K. marketing authorization for treating delirium tremens or seizures. Informed consent should be obtained and documented if possible.
4. Do not use phenytoin to treat alcohol withdrawal seizures.

32.2.5.1.4   Wernicke's Encephalopathy

Wernicke's encephalopathy is caused by severe deficiency of thiamine (vitamin B_1), which is usually caused by alcohol abuse in Western countries. Other causes include

- Lesions of the stomach (e.g. carcinoma) causing malabsorption
- Lesions of the duodenum causing malabsorption
- Lesions of the jejunum causing malabsorption
- Hyperemesis
- Starvation

Important clinical features of Wernicke's encephalopathy include

- Ophthalmoplegia
- Nystagmus
- Ataxia
- Clouding of consciousness

Ten per cent of patients with Wernicke's encephalopathy have the classical triad including ataxia, ophthalmoplegia, and memory disturbance. Peripheral neuropathy may also be present.

Wernicke's encephalopathy and Korsakov's psychosis (see the succeeding text) have overlapping pathology. Eighty per cent of untreated Wernicke's encephalopathy would convert to Korsakov's psychosis if untreated.

Wernicke's encephalopathy is a medical emergency and should be treated with intravenous thiamine plus other B vitamins. Postmortem examination of the brains of those dying of Wernicke's encephalopathy reveals petechial haemorrhages in the

- Mammillary bodies (see Figure 32.7)
- Walls of the third ventricle (less commonly than in the mammillary bodies)
- Periaqueductal grey matter (less commonly than in the mammillary bodies)
- Floor of the fourth ventricle (less commonly than in the mammillary bodies)
- Inferior colliculi (less commonly than in the mammillary bodies)

Nicotinic acid depletion can sometimes give rise to pellagra encephalopathy, a confusional state resembling Wernicke's encephalopathy.

32.2.5.1.5   Korsakov's Syndrome

Korsakov's syndrome is an alcohol-induced amnesic syndrome that, as mentioned earlier, is frequently preceded by Wernicke's encephalopathy. It has been described as being 'an abnormal state in which memory and learning are affected out of all proportion to other cognitive functions in an otherwise alert and responsive patient' (Victor et al., 1971). Clinical features include

- Retrograde amnesia
- Anterograde amnesia
- Sparing of immediate recall
- Disorientation in time
- Inability to recall the temporal sequence of events
- Confabulation
- Peripheral neuropathy

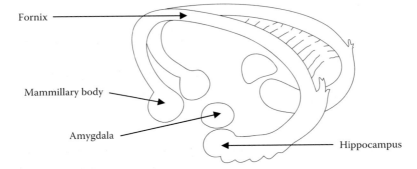

FIGURE 32.7   Neuroanatomical areas involved in Wernicke's encephalopathy.

Neuropathologically, there are scarring and atrophy of the mammillary bodies and anterior thalamus, with substantial frontal lobe dysfunction on neuroimaging. Improvement may occur with abstinence and high-dose thiamine and replacement of other B vitamins, which should be continued for 6 months.

32.2.5.1.6 Alcoholic Dementia

Those who have abused alcohol for some years commonly suffer mild to moderate cognitive impairment, which may improve over a number of years of abstinence. Women, who are known to suffer physical complications of alcohol abuse earlier than men, also develop cognitive impairment earlier in their drinking histories. A CT or structural MRI scan of the brain in alcoholics commonly shows ventricular enlargement and sulcal widening, which does not correlate with the degree of cognitive impairment and largely reverses with abstinence.

Chronic alcoholics show a coarsening of personality, which appears to be related to frontal lobe atrophy.

32.2.5.1.7 Alcoholic Hallucinosis

A rare disorder caused by chronic alcohol intake is alcoholic hallucinosis, characterized by auditory hallucinations in clear consciousness. It is distinguished from schizophrenia by the following features:

- Unpleasant sound or threatening voice
- Association with alcohol abuse
- Lack of family history
- Onset at an older age (40 or 50 years)
- More acute presentation with resolution commonly within a month (if abstinent)
- Absence of thought disorder
- More appropriate affect

It may follow abstinence but can present or recur in those who are still drinking. Alcohol hallucinosis carries good prognosis and shows rapid response to antipsychotics. If it persists for longer than 6 months, the likely diagnosis is schizophrenia.

32.2.5.1.8 Pathological Jealousy

Pathological jealousy is a well-recognized association with alcoholism but may occur with other conditions such as schizophrenia and depression.

32.2.5.1.9 Mood Disorder

Chronic heavy drinking can itself produce severe, usually transient depressive symptoms, which generally improve with abstinence. If symptoms persist with abstinence, antidepressants should be considered. The suicide rate is at least 50 times greater in alcoholics than in the general population. Between one-quarter and one-third of completed suicides occur in alcoholics, and up to four-fifths of those who kill themselves have been drinking.

32.2.5.1.10 Personality Disorder

Those with sociopathic personality disorder engage in excessive drinking, and those who drink heavily often engage in antisocial acts. If antisocial behaviour predates alcoholism by several years, then the primary diagnosis is of personality disorder.

Cloninger (1987) described two types of alcoholic:

- Type 1 (milieu limited). This is the least severe, occurring in men and women and of adult onset (older than 25 years), in dependent, anxious, rigid, less aggressive types, whose biological father or mother may have a mild adult-onset alcohol problem. This type of drinkers has greater ability to abstain from alcohol.
- Type 2. This is severe and of early onset (younger than 25 years), occurring in men who are socially detached and confident, whose biological fathers (but not mothers) often have teenage-onset alcoholism and criminality. This type is thought by some to be alcoholism secondary to sociopathic personality disorder. Genetic predisposition has a powerful aetiological effect, with little contribution from the environment.

There does not appear to be a relationship between schizophrenia and alcoholism other than that occurring by chance. Genetic studies find that people suffering from alcoholism and schizophrenia have a predisposition to each condition separately.

32.2.5.1.11 Neurotic Disorders

Neurotic disorders may predispose to alcoholism in an attempt by the patient to self-medicate. Generalized anxiety, panic attacks, and phobic disorders, particularly agoraphobia and posttraumatic stress disorder, may precede alcoholism. The patient should be reassessed once abstinent, and any underlying condition should be appropriately managed.

32.2.5.1.12 Sleep Disturbance

Alcohol decreases sleep latency and duration of REM sleep. It causes more fragmentation in sleep and longer episodes of awakening.

32.2.5.1.13   *Psychosexual Disorders*

Psychosexual disorders are a common association with excessive alcohol intake. In men, intoxication leads to erectile impotence and delayed ejaculation. Chronic heavy drinking in men can cause

- Loss of libido
- Reduction in the size of the testes
- Reduction in the size of the penis
- Loss of body hair
- Gynaecomastia

In women, chronic heavy drinking can cause

- Menstrual cycle abnormalities
- Loss of breast tissue
- Vaginal dryness

32.2.6   ADVERSE EFFECT OF ALCOHOL ON SOCIAL FUNCTIONS

Heavy drinking is often associated with gambling and the use of other psychoactive substances. The social costs of excessive alcohol consumption are high. They include

- Family breakdown
- Crime
- Road traffic accidents and trauma
- Economic harm

One-third of problem drinkers cite marital discord as one of their problems; one-third of divorce petitions cite alcohol as a contributory factor; three-quarters of battered wives describe their husbands as frequently drunk or subject to heavy drinking. Children of alcoholics often suffer neglect, poverty, or physical violence.

Alcohol misuse is strongly associated with crime, particularly against the person and against property. Half of those committing homicide have been drinking at the time of the offence, and half of victims are intoxicated. Half of rapists were drinking at the time of the offence. One- to two-thirds of burglaries are committed under the influence of alcohol.

It is estimated that 1200 deaths each year, representing one-fifth of all deaths on the roads, result from drink-driving. Alcohol is implicated in one-third of accidents at home and deaths by drowning and 40% of deaths by fire and falling.

Major costs to the country associated with the use of alcohol are incurred through

- Lost productivity and unemployment
- Damage
- Medical costs
- Legal costs
- Social costs

32.3   ALCOHOL CONSUMPTION AND MISUSE

32.3.1   EPIDEMIOLOGY OF ALCOHOL CONSUMPTION AND MISUSE

There is a close association between liver cirrhosis mortality and the national consumption of alcohol. Mortality figures are a useful index of national alcohol consumption. Other indices include the number of arrests for drunkenness, drunken driving, cases of assault and battery, and deaths from alcohol poisoning. Ten per cent of the drinking population drinks half of all the alcohol drunk.

Price greatly affects levels of drinking. Countries with cheap alcohol consume more than countries with more expensive alcohol. As the prices of alcoholic beverages rise, the quantity drunk by even chronic dependent drinkers falls, and the amount of alcohol-related morbidity falls.

It is estimated that of the 55 million U.K. population, 36 million are regular drinkers, 2 million are heavy drinkers (>80 g alcohol daily for men and >40 g for women), 700,000 are problem drinkers, and 200,000 are dependent drinkers.

Men outnumber women, but the sex ratio of alcohol-related problems is falling. About 15 years ago, alcoholic cirrhosis was five times as common in men as in women, but the sex ratio has fallen to about 2:1.

The age of first drinking has fallen to between 12 and 14 years in both sexes. The highest rates of heavy drinking are seen between adolescence and the early twenties.

32.3.2   AETIOLOGY OF ALCOHOL CONSUMPTION AND MISUSE

32.3.2.1   Genetic Factors

There is good evidence that heavy drinking runs in families. The relatives of alcoholics have higher rates of alcoholism than the relatives of controls.

Twin studies indicate that monozygotic twins have a higher concordance rate than dizygotic twins. In normal

TABLE 32.2

Comparison of Monozygotic and Dizygotic Ratio in Alcohol Abuse and Dependence between Men and Women

	Monozygotic:Dizygotic Ratio
Alcohol abuse in men	70%:45%
Alcohol dependence in men	40%:15%
Alcohol abuse in women	50%:40%
Alcohol dependence in women	30%:25%

Source: Caldwell, C.R. and Gottesman, I.I., *Behav. Genet.*, 21, 563, 1991.

twins, approximately one-third of the variance in drinking habits has been estimated to be genetic in origin (Table 32.2).

Adoption studies support the hypothesis of the genetic transmission of alcoholism. The sons of alcoholic parents are three to four times more likely to become alcoholic than the sons of nonalcoholics, irrespective of the home environment.

Strains of rats have been bred, which voluntarily consume large quantities of alcohol. These rats appear to have abnormalities in brain levels of serotonin, noradrenaline, and dopamine.

32.3.2.2 Biological Factors

The EEG of sober, awake alcoholics shows an excess of fast activity and a deficiency of α, θ and δ activity. The sons of alcoholics also show an excess of fast activity when compared to controls, leading to speculation that this may be a specific marker for alcoholism.

Electrically evoked responses show reduced P3 voltage in both abstinent chronic alcoholics and in the young sons of alcoholics when compared to controls.

The metabolism of alcohol is genetically determined and varies between individuals. Over half of Orientals develop an unpleasant flushing response when alcohol is ingested, related to the accumulation of acetaldehyde, caused by the absence of the isoenzyme aldehyde dehydrogenase (ALDH2). It is thought that this intolerance of alcohol protects them from developing alcoholism, since it is much less prevalent in those of Oriental heritage.

32.3.2.3 Psychological Factors

There are three main components to psychological theories of dependence:

- Withdrawal avoidance. Prolonged drug use results in tolerance, with CNS adaptation to allow normal functioning despite the chronic presence of the psychoactive drug. If the drug is suddenly withdrawn, this adaptation results in drug-withdrawal symptoms, which are usually opposite to the effects of the drug. Thus, in terms of this theory, the dependent person continues drug use in order to avoid the adverse effects of drug withdrawal.
- Positive effects of the drug. According to this theory, the pleasant effects of the drug reinforce drug-taking behaviour, despite adverse social and physical consequences.
- Motivational distortion. According to this theory, the repetition of drug-taking behaviour, or the effects of the drugs themselves, changes the motivational system supporting that behaviour. Habit strength is a term describing the strength of the link between stimuli that cues a behaviour. It is possible that it involves habituation at the neuronal level.
- Modelling and social learning from other people who misuse alcohol (e.g. parents, siblings, and peers).

Each of these theories accounts for some but not all aspects of addiction.

32.3.2.4 Psychiatric Illness

This can predispose patients to harmful drinking, particularly anxiety disorders, phobic disorders, depression and bereavement and mania in adulthood, hyperkinetic disorder, conduct disorder, and being a victim of abuse in childhood.

32.3.2.5 Personality Factors

It has been suggested that some problem drinkers are predisposed to harmful drinking by their personality; however, studies in this area give contradictory results. It is known that those with sociopathic personality disorder have a high prevalence of heavy drinking and alcoholism. However, there is no typical pre-alcoholic personality.

32.3.2.6 Social Factors

This can predispose patients to harmful drinking, particularly marital or relationship problems, migration, work-related stress, poor income, low education, and social isolation. Certain occupational groups are at greater risk of drinking problems. Those with jobs in the drink industry are at highest risk, including publicans, bartenders, and brewers. Those whose jobs take them away from home, such as fishermen, armed service personnel, and executives, and those with professional autonomy, such as doctors, are also at higher risk.

32.3.2.7   Cultural Factors

There are high rates of alcoholism in countries where alcohol is drunk routinely with family meals and in places where it is cheap.

32.3.2.8   Religion

There are low rates of alcoholism in certain religions such as conservative Protestantism, Jewish religion, and Islam.

32.3.3   Diagnosis of Alcohol Intoxication and Dependence (Tables 32.3 and 32.4)

32.3.4   Management

32.3.4.1   Clinical Assessment

For screening purposes, the CAGE questionnaire is widely used. Positive answers to two or more of the four questions are indicative of problem drinking. The CAGE questionnaire is as follows:

- Have you ever felt you should cut down on your drinking?
- Have people ever annoyed you by criticizing your drinking?
- Have you ever felt guilty about your drinking?
- Have you ever had a drink first thing in the morning to steady your nerves or get over a hangover? (an eye-opener)

For patients presenting with alcohol withdrawal, consider using an assessment tool such as the Clinical Institute Withdrawal Assessment (CIWA) scale in addition to history taking. CIWA scale is a validated 10-item scale to quantify the severity of the alcohol withdrawal syndrome and to monitor patients throughout detoxification (Stuppaeck et al., 1994).

When alcohol dependence is suspected or diagnosed, it is essential to carry out a full physical examination bearing in mind the multiple-organ systems damaged by this substance.

32.3.4.2   Investigations

- Blood investigations include alcohol levels in the intoxicated (breathalyzers can be useful to give an indication of levels of recent drinking).

TABLE 32.3

Comparison between the ICD-10 and the DSM-5 Criteria Acute Intoxication of Alcohol

	ICD-10 Criteria (WHO, 1992)	**DSM-5 Criteria (APA, 2013)**
Dysfunctional behaviour	At least one of the following	The following changes developed during or shortly after ingestion:
	1. Disinhibition	1. Inappropriate sexual or aggressive behaviour
	3. Aggression	2. Mood lability
	4. Lability of mood	3. Impaired judgement
	5. Impaired attention	4. Impaired social or occupational functioning
	6. Impaired judgement	
	7. Interference with personal functioning	
Other signs	At least one of the following must be present:	One of the following signs after recent ingestion
	1. Unsteady gait	1. Slurred speech
	2. Difficulty in standing	2. Incoordination
	3. Slurred speech	3. Unsteady gait
	4. Nystagmus	4. Nystagmus
	5. Decreases level of consciousness	5. Impaired in attention and memory
	6. Flushed face	6. Stupor or coma
	7. Conjunctive injection	

Note: The DSM-5 does not propose criteria on alcohol dependence. It is called alcohol use disorder.

TABLE 32.4

Comparison between the ICD-10 and DSM-5 Criteria on Alcohol Dependence or Alcohol Use Disorder

Categories	ICD-10 Criteria (WHO, 1992)	DSM-5 Criteria for Alcohol Use Disorder (APA, 2013)
Number of criteria met and duration	Three or more of the following manifestations should have occurred together for at least 1 month. If the manifestations persist for less than 1 month, they should have occurred together repeatedly within a 1-year period	At least two manifestations in a 1-year period
Compulsion	A strong desire or sense of compulsion to consume alcohol	A persistent desire to use alcohol
Control	Impaired capacity to control drinking in terms of its onset, termination, or levels of use. Alcohol is being often taken in larger amounts or over a longer period than intended. There is persistent desire to or unsuccessful efforts to reduce or control alcohol use	Unsuccessful effort to control and cut down
Withdrawal	Physiological withdrawal state: shaky, restless, or excessive perspiration	Characteristic withdrawal symptoms and the same substance is taken to avoid withdrawals
Tolerance	There is a need for significantly increased amounts of alcohol to achieve intoxication or the desired effect or a markedly diminished effect with continued use of the same amount of alcohol	Two components: need to increase the amount and diminished effect with continued use
Preoccupation	Important alternative pleasures or interests being given up or reduced because of drinking or a great deal of time being spent in activities necessary to obtain, take, or recover from the effects of alcohol	Important social, occupational, and recreational activities are reduced
Other criteria	Persistent alcohol use despite clear evidence of harmful consequences even though the person is actually aware of the nature and extent of harm	A great deal of time is spent in activities to obtain the substance and continued consumption despite knowledge
Course specifier	• Currently abstinent (early, partial, and full remission) • Currently abstinent but in a protected environment • Currently on a supervised maintenance or replacement regime • Currently abstinent but receiving treatment with aversive or blocking drugs • Currently using the substance with or without psychotic features • Continuous use • Episodic use	• Early remission (3 months < duration of use <12 months) • Sustained remission (no substance use >12 months) • Controlled environment where access to substance is limited

Note: The DSM-5 proposes the diagnostic criteria for alcohol withdrawal. The cessation of heavy and prolonged alcohol use leads to at least two of the following: anxiety, autonomic hyperactivity hand tremor, insomnia, nausea or vomiting, transient hallucinations or illusions, generalized seizure, and psychomotor agitation. Alcohol withdrawal causes clinically significant distress or impairment in social, occupational, or other important areas of functioning. This withdrawal is not resulted from a general medical condition.

- Alcoholism is the most common cause of raised mean corpuscular volume (MCV), and it is raised in 60% of alcohol abusers. Since the life of a red blood cell is 120 days, the MCV should return to normal 4 months after continued abstinence. Raised g-glutamyl transferase may occur; this is good for screening as an indication of recent alcohol use, but it can be raised after only one heavy drinking session.

- Liver function tests (e.g. aspartate transaminase) may be abnormal, particularly during acute alcoholic hepatitis, less so in fatty liver, and may be normal in cirrhosis.

32.3.5 MANAGEMENT ON WITHDRAWAL AND DETOXIFICATION

- Detoxification can usually be conducted as an outpatient unless severe withdrawal effects such as delirium tremens or convulsions are likely to occur; the patient's mental state causes concern, or there are severe social problems, in which case inpatient care should be organized.
- The score of CIWA scale can be used as a reference to determine treatment setting. If the score of CIWA scale is ≤10 (mild withdrawal), the patient is suitable for home treatment. If the CIWA score is >15 (moderate to severe withdrawal), the patient is suitable for community or hospital treatment.

BOX 32.4 NICE GUIDANCE ON THE MANAGEMENT SETTING IN ACUTE ALCOHOL WITHDRAWAL (NICE, 2010)

Offer admission to hospital:

1. Person at risk of alcohol withdrawal seizures or delirium tremens
2. Young person under 16 years in acute alcohol withdrawal

Consider admission to hospital:

1. Vulnerable people who are frail and have cognitive impairments or multiple comorbidities

Do not offer admission to hospital:

1. Person not at high risk of delirium tremens or seizures
2. Person older than 16 years and not considered vulnerable

Drug treatment for the symptoms of acute alcohol withdrawal should be started.

BOX 32.5 NICE GUIDANCE ON THE TREATMENT FOR ACUTE ALCOHOL WITHDRAWAL (NICE, 2010)

1. Consider offering benzodiazepines: Both diazepam and chlordiazepoxide have U.K. marketing authorization for the management of acute alcohol withdrawal symptoms.
2. Alternatives to benzodiazepines
   a. Carbamazepine can be used in the management of alcohol-related withdrawal symptoms, but it does not have the U.K. marketing authorization for this treatment purpose.
   b. Clomethiazole can be used as in the management of alcohol-related withdrawal symptoms for patients who are determined to discontinue drinking and in the inpatient setting as it can lead to fatal respiratory depression when combined with alcohol in patients with cirrhosis. It has the U.K. marketing authorization.

The dosage of chlordiazepoxide based on Maudsley's guideline recommendations

- *Mild dependence*: Small dose is enough to treat mild perceptual disturbance, and it is safe to be used in pregnancy.
- *Moderate dependence*: Larger dose is required (e.g. 20 mg qid on day 1), and titrate over 5–7 days to 5 mg bid on day 5.
- *Severe dependence*: 40 mg (five times a day) on day 1, and titrate over 10 days to 10 mg nocte on day 10.

Attention should be paid to the state of hydration and nutrition of the patient.

BOX 32.6 NICE GUIDANCE ON PREVENTION OF WERNICKE'S ENCEPHALOPATHY (NICE, 2010)

1. Thiamine should always be given to people at high risk of developing or with suspected Wernicke's encephalopathy.
2. Indications for prophylactic oral thiamine
   a. Malnourishment
   b. Decompensated liver disease
   c. Acute withdrawal

3. Indications for prophylactic parenteral thiamine
   a. Malnourishment or decompensated liver disease
   b. Attendance at emergency department
   c. Admission to hospital with acute illness or injury
   d. Suspected Wernicke's encephalopathy
4. Parenteral thiamine should be given for a minimum of 5 days and followed by oral thiamine

Before thiamine treatment, a glucose load should be avoided as this can precipitate or exacerbate thiamine deficiency. The suicide risk should be assessed.

32.3.6 MAINTENANCE OF ABSTINENCE

Before offering pharmacological and psychological treatment to maintain abstinence, it is important to assess the patient's readiness to change based on a model developed by Prochasaka and DiClemente (see Figure 32.8). If patient is at the precontemplation stage, motivational interviewing can be offered to help the patient to move to contemplation stage.

32.4 PHARMACOLOGICAL TREATMENTS

Medication can be used to help maintain abstinence.

32.4.1 DISULFIRAM

Disulfiram is an aversive agent, and prescribing doctor should ensure that the person has not consumed any alcohol for at least 1 day before starting disulfiram. Patients must be well motivated and aware of the risks of taking alcohol with these agents. Efficacy requires compliance with taking the aversive agent; involving the spouse or partner in administration can improve the success rate.

32.4.1.1 Mechanism of Action
- Disulfiram inhibits ALDH2 (see Figure 32.9) and leads to acetaldehyde accumulation after drinking alcohol, resulting in unpleasant effects.

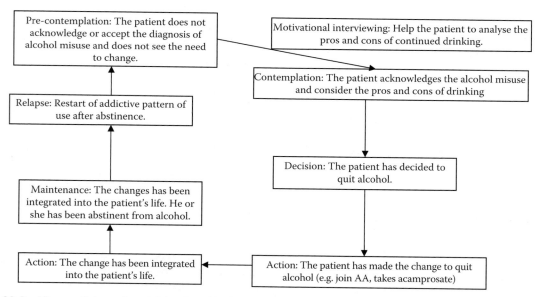

FIGURE 32.8 'Stages of change' model developed by Prochaska and DiClemente.

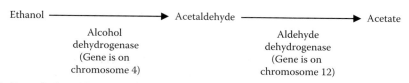

FIGURE 32.9 Metabolism of ethanol by alcohol dehydrogenase and ALDH2.

- Disulfiram blocks dopamine beta-hydroxylase and leads to dopamine accumulation in the CNS, resulting in psychosis in people with underlying schizophrenia when talking disulfiram.

32.4.1.2 Aversive Effects with Ingestion of Alcohol

- Aversive effects include flushing, headache, palpitations, tachycardia, nausea, and vomiting with ingestion of small amounts of alcohol and air hunger, arrhythmias, and severe hypotension with large amounts of alcohol.
- These effects occur 10–30 min after drinking and are dose dependent. The reaction to alcohol discourages the person from drinking and reduces the number of days spent on drinking.
- Doctors need to inform patients that the aversive effects may last for 1 week, and alcohol should be avoided for 1 week after cessation of disulfiram.

32.4.1.3 Dosage

Starting dose of disulfiram is 800 mg and then is reduced to 100–200 mg daily.

32.4.1.4 Side Effects

- Halitosis (common side effect, bad breath from oral cavity).
- Nausea.
- Liver damage.
- Reduction in libido.
- Peripheral neuritis.
- Dangerous side effects include arrhythmia, hypotension, and collapse.

32.4.1.5 Drug Interactions and Contraindication

- Disulfiram increases level of warfarin, diazepam, diazepam, and theophylline.
- Disulfiram is contraindicated in people with cerebrovascular disease, epilepsy, cardiac failure, coronary artery disease, advanced liver diseases, and pregnancy and breast-feeding.

32.4.2 ACAMPROSATE

Acamprosate, in combination with counselling, may also be helpful in maintaining abstinence. It should be initiated as soon as possible after the achievement of abstinence. It should be maintained if a relapse occurs. The patient is allowed to have only one relapse while they are taking acamprosate. If there is more than one relapse, the psychiatrist should advise the patient to stop acamprosate.

32.4.2.1 Mechanism of Action

- The withdrawal of alcohol (see Figure 32.10) enhances the actions of glutamate at the NMDA receptors and the voltage-sensitive calcium channels. This will attenuate the action of GABA at inhibitory $GABA_A$ receptors, resulting in agitation and craving during alcohol withdrawal.
- Acamprosate is a GABA agonist and glutamate antagonist. It inactivates the NMDA receptors and prevents the calcium influx. This will reverse the GABA and glutamate imbalance when abstaining from alcohol and reduce the long-lasting neuronal hyperexcitability.
- Hence, acamprosate blocks increased glutamate in withdrawal and is neuroprotective.

32.4.2.2 Dosage

The starting dose is 666 mg three times a day and indicated for adult with body weight larger than or equal to 60 kg.

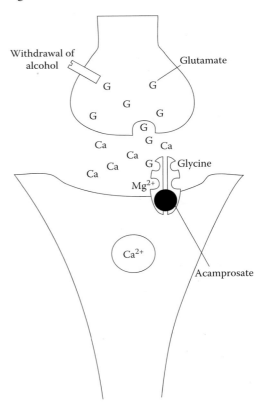

FIGURE 32.10 Acamprosate inactivates the NMDA receptors and prevents the calcium influx during alcohol withdrawal.

32.4.2.3 Side Effects

- Diarrhoea
- Nausea
- Rash
- Pruritus
- Bullous skin reactions
- Fluctuation in libido

32.4.2.4 Drug Interactions and Contraindications

- Acamprosate can be used in combination with disulfiram.
- Contraindications include severe renal or hepatic impairment, pregnancy, and breast-feeding. The use of acamprosate is not licensed for elderly.

32.4.3 NALTREXONE

32.4.3.1 Medical Use

- It is not licensed to treat alcohol dependence in the United Kingdom because of mortality after overdose and potential withdrawal.
- It is only used in people who are in abstinence and highly motivated.
- It is also used to treat violent behaviours among people with learning disability.

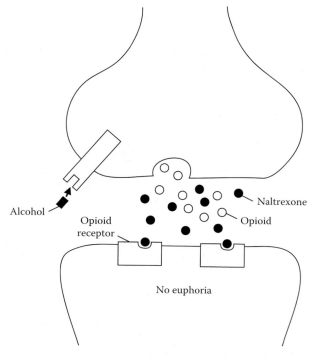

FIGURE 32.11 The mechanism of action of naltrexone on opioid receptors.

32.4.3.2 Mechanism of Action

Opioid receptors are responsible for reward, resulting in craving. Naltrexone is an opioid antagonist (see Figure 32.11). Alcohol becomes less rewarding when opioid receptors are blocked, and the person does not experience euphoric effects.

32.4.3.3 Dosage

The starting dose of naltrexone is 25 mg and then increases to 50 mg per day on weekdays and 100 mg per day on weekend.

32.5 PSYCHOLOGICAL TREATMENTS

32.5.1 ALCOHOLICS ANONYMOUS

- Alcoholics anonymous (AA) is a self-help group, which some alcoholics find helpful.
- AA supports the families of alcoholics, and Alateen the teenage children of alcoholics.
- AA offers the 12-step approach, which emphasizes that addiction damages the whole person and group therapy allows peer pressure to overcome the denial and resistance common in people addicted to alcohol or other substances.
- The AA group usually meets two to three times per week.
- The strongest predictor of the AA group attendance is the severity of alcohol-related problems.

In brief, the 12 steps are summarized as follows:

1. Admission of being powerless over alcohol.
2. Belief that greater power can restore the person back to sanity.
3. Seek help from God.
4. Admit to God their wrongs.
5. Let God remove all the defects in character.
6. Ask God to remove their shortcomings.
7. Searching for moral inventory.
8. Make a list of the people who were harmed (victims).
9. Direct amends to the victims.
10. Continue to take personal inventory.
11. Seek help through prayer and meditation.
12. Finally, a spiritual awakening as the result of the earlier steps.

32.5.2 Other Psychological Treatments

1. Brief intervention known as FRAMES (Miller and Sanchez, 1993)
   a. Feedback about drinking
   b. Responsibility enforcement
   c. Advice to change
   d. Menu of alternatives
   e. Empathetic style
   f. Self-efficacy
2. Cognitive behaviour models appear to be particularly effective in relapse prevention. Such therapies include cue exposure, relapse prevention strategies, contingency management, social skills, and assertiveness training.

32.5.3 Clinical Trials

There are two main trails on the efficacy of psychological treatments for people with alcohol dependence.

- *Project MATCH* (Project MATCH research group, 1993): It is a multicentre clinical trial comparing cognitive behaviour coping skills, 12-step facilitation therapy, and motivational enhancement therapy.
- *Conclusion*: The 12-step facilitation therapy is more effective, and outcome is determined by readiness to change and self-efficacy.

U.K. Alcohol Treatment Trial (UKATT Research Team, 2005)

- *Methodology*: Seven treatment sites around Birmingham, Cardiff, and Leeds were established and involved 742 clients with alcohol problems. Subjects were randomized into the social behaviour and network therapy group versus motivational enhancement therapy group. Outcome measures include alcohol consumption, alcohol dependence, and alcohol-related problems and were compared between the two groups over 12 months.
- *Conclusion*: The novel social behaviour and network therapy for alcohol problems did not differ significantly in effectiveness from the established motivational enhancement therapy.

32.5.3.1 Prognosis

Good prognostic factors include

- Good insight
- Strong motivation
- Good social and family support

Relapse can be precipitated by

- Emotional stress
- Interpersonal conflict
- Social pressures

Long-*term follow-up of alcoholics over a period of 10 years finds that*

- 25% continue troubled drinking.
- 12% are abstinent.

The remainder follow a pattern of intermittent troubled drinking and abstinence.

CASC STATION ON ALCOHOL DEPENDENCE SYNDROME

A 28-year-old homeless man suffers from treatment-resistant schizophrenia and was admitted to the hospital due to relapse of psychotic symptoms. Prior to admission, he was advised to consider clozapine, but he refused. Due to his poor compliance and insight, he is given depot antipsychotic, intramuscular risperidone fortnightly. He is noted to have binge drinking behaviour. His psychotic symptoms have subsided, and he is ready for discharge.

In the first station, take a history from the patient on the alcohol misuse and its relationship to schizophrenia. You will speak to his father in the second station.

Approach to this station

People with schizophrenia are three times more likely than the general population to abuse alcohol and six times more likely to abuse drugs (Ries, 2000):

1. Assess the alcohol dependence syndrome based on the Alcohol Use Disorders Identification Test (AUDIT) (See Box 32.7) (Barbor, 2001).
2. The alcohol consumption history should include information about the evolution of the problem (drinking career, drink-related problems, dependence) and typical recent drinking day (initial, then hourly quantification of alcohol intake, waking nausea, tremor, nightmares, and night sweats).

(continued)

3. Explore the presence of first-rank symptoms of schizophrenia and its relationship with alcohol misuse (e.g. self-medication, relief of anxiety or insomnia).
4. Explore the use of other drugs such as amphetamine, cocaine, cannabis, and hallucinogens and common reasons for misuse (e.g. to relieve dysphoria, depression, and negative symptoms).
5. Explore current living arrangement such as homelessness.
6. Explore the need for detoxification as this is a case of episodic binge drinking.
7. Explore patient's knowledge on previous liver impairment, which may affect the metabolism of antipsychotics
8. Explore the reasons of his refusal of clozapine (e.g. the inconvenience of weekly full blood counts) and the effect on his alcohol consumption if he has taken clozapine for a brief period.

Explore complications associated with concomitant usage of intramuscular risperidone depot injection and drinking (e.g. combination of extrapyramidal side effects and cerebellar signs).

In the second station, his father wants to meet you as he is upset with his son's illness and the discharge plan. Address his father's concerns and explain the management plan. You have the permission from the patient to speak to his father.

Approach to the second station

1. Address the disappointment from his father and explore the source of his anger (e.g. poor control of schizophrenia symptoms, worsening alcohol misuse, poor anger control, and he feels that the addiction service is not doing enough).
2. Explain discharge planning: It will be a planned discharge with the aim to integrate outpatient treatment for both alcohol misuse and schizophrenia. There will be at least one to two contacts per week.
3. Refer the patient to the assertive community treatment (ACT) to increase medication compliance.
4. Refer to social worker for residential accommodation as housing instability is closely related in substance misuse and mental illnesses.
5. Reexplore the option of clozapine as it can reduce the rates of smoking and drinking.
6. Explain long-term treatment (e.g. social and vocational skills training).

BOX 32.7   QUESTIONS USED TO ASSESS ALCOHOL DEPENDENCE BASED ON THE AUDIT

Introduction: Now, I am going to ask you some questions about your use of alcoholic beverages during this past year. Then, candidates need to explain what is meant by 'alcoholic beverages' by using local examples of beer, wine, and vodka.

Hazardous alcohol misuse

1. Frequency of drinking: 'How often do you have a drink containing alcohol?'
2. Average daily quantity: 'How many drinks containing alcohol do you have on a typical day when you are drinking?'
(to estimate the average number of units of alcohol consumed weekly)
3. Frequency of heavy drinking: 'How often do you have six or more drinks on one occasion?'

Dependence symptoms

4. Control over drinking: 'How often have you found that you were not able to stop drinking once you had started?'
5. Increased salience of drinking: 'How often have you failed to do what was normally expected from you because of drinking?'
6. Morning drinking: 'How often have you needed a first drink in the morning to get yourself going after a heavy drinking session?'

Harmful alcohol use

7. Guilt after drinking: 'How often have you had a feeling of guilt or remorse after drinking?'
8. Blackouts: 'How often have you been unable to remember what happened the night before because you had been drinking?'
9. Alcohol-related injuries: 'Have you or someone else been injured as a result of your drinking?'
10. Concerns from significant others: 'Has a relative or friend or a doctor or another health worker been concerned about your drinking or suggested you cutdown?'

A note on AUDIT scores and management (McCloud et al., 2007)
AUDIT score:
0–7: Alcohol education
8–15: Simple advice
16–19: Simple advice, brief counselling, and continued monitoring
20–40: Referral to specialist for diagnostic evaluation and treatment
A high AUDIT score is strongly associated with suicidality.

32.6 NONALCOHOLIC PSYCHOACTIVE SUBSTANCES: LEGAL ASPECTS IN THE UNITED KINGDOM (TABLE 32.5)

32.6.1 MISUSE OF DRUG REGULATIONS 2001

These regulations divide drugs into the following five schedules, which specify the requirements that govern such issues as their supply, possession, prescription, and record keeping:

- Schedule 1 includes drugs such as cannabis and lysergide, which are not used medicinally. Possession and supply are prohibited except in accordance with the authority of the Home Office.
- Schedule 2 includes drugs such as diamorphine (heroin), morphine, remifentanil, pethidine, secobarbital, glutethimide, amfetamine, and cocaine and is subject to the full controlled drug requirements relating to prescriptions, safe custody (except for secobarbital), the need to keep registers, etc. (unless exempted in schedule 5).
- Schedule 3 includes the barbiturates (except secobarbital, which is in schedule 2), buprenorphine, diethylpropion, flunitrazepam, mazindol,

TABLE 32.5

Colloquial Names for Some Abused Drugs and Length of Time to Be Detected in Urine Drug Screen

Drug	Colloquial Name	Length of Time Detected in Urine
Amphetamines	Speed, whizz	48 h
Barbiturates	Downers	24 h (short acting), 3 weeks (long acting)
Cannabinoids	Grass, hash, ganja, pot	3 days to 4 weeks
Cocaine	Snow, coke, girl, lady	6–8 h (metabolites 2–4 days)
Heroin	Smack	36–72 h
LSD	Acid	12–24 h
MDMA	Ecstasy, XTC, Adam, E	48 h
PCP	Angel dust, peace pill	8 days
Temazepam capsules	Jellies	6–48 h

meprobamate, pentazocine, phentermine, and temazepam. They are subject to the special prescription requirements (except for phenobarbital and temazepam) but not to the safe custody requirements (except for buprenorphine, diethylpropion, flunitrazepam, and temazepam) nor to the need to keep registers (although there are requirements for the retention of invoices for 2 years).

- Schedule 4 includes, in Part I, benzodiazepines (except flunitrazepam and temazepam, which are in schedule 3) and zolpidem, which are subject to minimal control. Part II includes androgenic and anabolic steroids, clenbuterol, human chorionic gonadotropin (HCG), non-HCG, somatotropin, somatrem, and somatropin. Controlled drug prescription requirements do not apply, and schedule 4 controlled drugs are not subject to safe custody requirements.
- Schedule 5 includes those preparations that, because of their strength, are exempt from virtually all controlled drug requirements other than retention of invoices for 2 years.

32.6.2 MISUSE OF DRUGS ACT 1971 (MODIFICATION) ORDER 2003 AND MISUSE OF DRUGS REGULATIONS 2003

Changes were made to the legislation on the misuse of drugs by these regulations, which came into force on July 1, 2003. The following eight substances were brought under the control of the Misuse of Drugs Act 1971 and its associated subordinate legislation for the first time:

Remifentanil	4-Androstene-3, 17-dione
Dihydroetorphine	19-Nor-4-androstene-3, 17-dione
Gamma-hydroxybutyrate (GHB)	5-Androstene-3, 17-diol
Zolpidem	19-Nor-5-androstene-3, 17-diol

Remifentanil and dihydroetorphine are controlled as class A drugs. Both are powerful opiates and have similar pharmacological properties to existing class A drugs. Both are listed under schedule 2 of the Misuse of Drugs Regulations 2001.

4-Hydroxy-*n*-butyric acid or GHB and zolpidem are controlled as class C drugs. Both are listed under schedule 4 (Part I) of the 2001 Regulations. GHB has been used as an anaesthetic and to treat alcohol and drug dependence but has also been misused by clubbers. Zolpidem is a prescription medicine (a nonbenzodiazepine hypnotic with a short duration of action) and acts in a similar same way as some sedatives such as benzodiazepines.

The following four anabolic substances are listed in schedule 4 (Part II) of the 2001 Regulations:

4-Androstene-3, 17-dione	5-Androstene-3, 17-diol
19-Nor-4-androstene-3, 17-dione	19-Nor-5-androstene-3, 17-diol

They are now controlled as class C drugs.

Note that schedule 2 drugs are subject to the additional prescription requirements of Regulation 15 (see the following; among other things, prescriptions must be handwritten by doctors). Regulations 14 (documentation), 16 (supply on prescription), 18 (marking of containers), 19, 20, 21, 23 (keeping and preservation of registers), 26 (furnishing of information), and 27 (destruction) also apply to schedule 2 drugs. Most schedule 2 drugs are also subject to the statutory safe custody requirements.

Schedule 4 (Part I) includes benzodiazepines (e.g. diazepam, lorazepam, and nitrazepam). GHB and zolpidem have been added to the list of drugs in schedule 4 (Part I). Persons already authorized by the Regulations (e.g. doctors and pharmacists), or by a written Home Office authority to produce, supply, or possess schedule 4 (Part I) drugs, are automatically so authorized in respect of GHB and zolpidem. In other cases, an appropriate written Home Office authority is required. The Regulation 15 prescription requirements (including handwriting) do not apply to schedule 4 (Part I) drugs. Regulations 22, 23 (keeping and preservation of records), 26 (furnishing of information), and 27 (destruction—holders of written authorities to produce only) also apply to schedule 4 (Part I) drugs. Schedule 4 (Part I) drugs are not subject to the safe custody requirements.

Schedule 4 (Part II) now comprises 54 anabolic substances; examples are nandrolone and testosterone (and the 4 newly added anabolic substances: 4-androstene-3, 17-dione; 19-nor-4-androstene-3, 17-dione; 5-androstene-3, 17-diol; and 19-nor-5-androstene-3, 17-diol). Persons already authorized by the 2001 Regulations (e.g. doctors and pharmacists) or by a written Home Office authority to produce, supply, or possess schedule 4 (Part II) drugs are authorized in respect of the four newly added drugs; in other cases, an appropriate written Home Office authority is required. (Note that possession licences are not required if the substances are in medicinal product form.) The Regulation 15 prescription requirements (including handwriting) do not apply to schedule 4 (Part II drugs). Regulations 22, 23 (keeping and preservation of records), 26 (furnishing of information), and 27 (destruction—holders of written authorities to produce only) also apply to schedule 4 Part II drugs. Schedule 4 Part II drugs are not subject to the statutory safe custody requirements.

32.6.3 PRESCRIBING CONTROLLED DRUGS

The main regulations relating to prescriptions for controlled drugs specified in schedules 2 and 3, under the Misuse of Drugs Regulations 2001, are as follows.

Prescriptions ordering controlled drugs subject to prescription requirements must be signed and dated by the prescriber and specify the prescriber's address. The prescription must always state in the prescriber's own handwriting in ink or otherwise so as to be indelible:

- The name and address of the patient
- In the case of a preparation, the form and where appropriate the strength of the preparation
- The total quantity of the preparation, or the number of dose units, in both words and figures
- The dose
- The words 'for dental treatment only' if issued by a dentist

A prescription may order a controlled drug to be dispensed by instalments. If so, the amount of the instalments and the intervals to be observed must be specified. Prescriptions ordering 'repeats' on the same form are not permitted. A prescription is valid for 13 weeks from the date stated thereon.

It is an offence for a prescriber to issue an incomplete prescription, and a pharmacist is not allowed to dispense a controlled drug unless all the information required by law is given on the prescription.

32.6.4 OPIOIDS

Note: Drugs derived from opium poppies are known as opiates. Synthetically derived opiates are known as opioids.

32.6.4.1 Heroin (Gear, Smack, Scag)

Heroin (3,6-diacetylmorphine) is produced from morphine, which is derived from the sap of the opium poppy. It may be smoked or chased by heating on tin foil and inhaling the sublimate. It is also injected intravenously and much less commonly subcutaneously (skin-popping). Street heroin is usually 30%–60% pure, and 0.25–0.75 g is a common daily consumption for addicts.

32.6.4.2 Epidemiology

The number of addicts notified to the Home Office has increased dramatically over the last 30 years. This is thought to be related to the wider availability of cheap opiates imported from the Middle East. Youth culture has become much more accepting of drug use, and polydrug use is much more common than it used to be. The approximate numbers of notifications have been

1960	500
1980	5,000
1990	15,000

Most heroin users are aged between 20 and 30 years. The steepest increase has occurred in those aged 16–24 years. The male/female ratio is 2:1.

32.6.4.3 Drug Action

The stimulation of opiate receptors produces analgesia, euphoria, miosis, hypotension, bradycardia, and respiratory depression.

Opioid receptors fall into different types, each of which has subtypes. The main types are μ, κ, and δ receptors. The μ receptor is essential for the development of opioid dependence. The μ receptor is potassium channel linked and inhibits adenylate cyclase. The binding of morphine to the μ receptors inhibits the release of GABA from the nerve terminals, reducing the inhibitory effect of GABA on the dopaminergic neurons. The increased activation of dopaminergic neurons in the nucleus accumbens and the ventral tegmental areas that are part of the brain's 'reward pathway' and the release of dopamine into the synaptic result in sustained activation of the postsynaptic membrane. Continued activation of the dopaminergic reward pathway leads to the feelings of euphoria (Figure 32.12).

Euphoria is initially intense and is related in part to the method of administration. Thus, methods delivering a large bolus quickly to the CNS are associated with a greater initial rush. Intravenous and inhalational techniques of heroin fulfil these conditions; oral and subcutaneous methods do not. Dependence may arise within weeks of regular use (Figure 32.13 and Table 32.6).

The DSM-5 proposes the following opioid-induced disorders: major neurocognitive disorder, amnestic disorder, psychotic disorder, depressive or bipolar disorder, anxiety disorder, sexual dysfunction, or sleep disorder.

32.6.4.4 Effects of Opioid Withdrawal

During opioid withdrawal, there is an excessive release of noradrenaline and results in rhinorrhoea or sneezing, lacrimation, muscle cramps or aches, abdominal cramps, nausea or vomiting, diarrhoea, pupillary dilatation (mydriasis), piloerection, recurrent chills, tachycardia, hypertension, yawning, and restless sleep. The ICD-10 criteria (F11.3 opioid withdrawal state) require the presence of any three of the aforementioned symptoms. The DSM-5 criteria are similar to the ICD-10 criteria. Opioid withdrawal is seldom associated with withdrawal fits (Figure 32.14).

These begin within 4–12 h of last heroin use. Peak intensity is at about 48 h, and the main symptoms disappear within a week of abstinence. Although it is unpleasant, opiate withdrawal is not generally dangerous (exceptions include pregnancy, when abortion may result from precipitous withdrawal).

32.6.4.5 Harmful Effects

32.6.4.5.1 Effects of the Drug Itself

Overdose can be caused by the uncertain concentration of street drugs or to reduced tolerance following a period of abstinence (e.g. upon release from prison). The clinical features of opiate overdose include stupor or coma, pinpoint pupils, pallor, severe respiratory depression, and pulmonary oedema. Supportive treatment and administration of an opioid antagonist such as naloxone is indicated. The half-life of opioid antagonists is less than that of most opiate drugs, so the patient must be observed for several hours to ensure that the underlying opiate overdose has passed.

32.6.4.5.2 Intoxication

These include accidents.

32.6.4.5.3 Inhalation

The inhalation of heroin commonly exacerbates or causes lung conditions such as asthma. There are increased rates of pneumonia and tuberculosis in those who are HIV positive.

32.6.4.5.4 Intravenous Use

The hazards of intravenous use are many and include the transmission of infection through the use of shared needles. HIV and hepatitis B, C, and D are commonly transmitted through this route. Those who are HIV positive have a poorer outcome if they continue to inject.

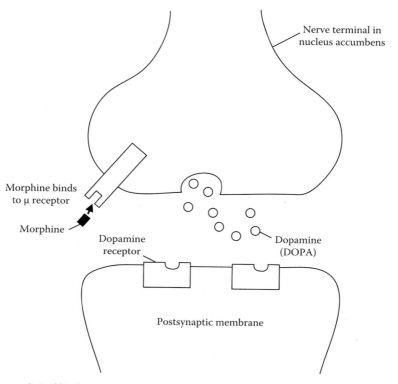

Opioid binding at the μ receptors stimulates release of dopamine into an area called the nucleus accumbens.

This increased dopamine activity in the nucleus accumbens is associated with euphoⅰ and other pleasurable sensations.

FIGURE 32.12　The mechanisms of actions of morphine and the μ receptor.

32.6.4.5.5　Bacterial Infection

Bacterial infection results from the lack of aseptic technique; the risk is not eliminated by using clean needles since the drug itself is not of pharmaceutical quality, has often been adulterated with other substances, and is often not suitable for intravenous administration because of the presence of nonsoluble components.

32.6.4.5.6　Skin Infection

Skin infection at injection sites leads to abscess formation and thrombophlebitis. *Staphylococcus aureus* and *Streptococcus pyogenes* are often responsible.

32.6.4.5.7　Blood Infection

Most injecting results in transient bacteraemia. This can result in septicaemia and/or bacterial endocarditis, even in those with previously normal heart valves. Septic emboli may be carried to distant sites. Septic embolism can result in osteomyelitis.

32.6.4.5.8　Fungal Infection

Systemic fungal infections have been reported, which are difficult to treat and result in death or blindness because of ophthalmic involvement.

32.6.4.5.9　Vascular Complications

Vascular complications include the obliteration of the lung vascular bed with continued prolonged injection of particulate matter. The same effect is seen in the lymphatic system, resulting in puffy hands. Deep vein thrombosis may develop at the site of femoral administration. Arterial administration can result in occlusion caused by spasm or embolism. The loss of a limb may result.

32.6.4.5.10　Long-Term Physical Effects

Long-term users may develop membranous glomerulonephritis or amyloid disease.

32.6.4.5.11　Social Effects

Because of the effects of tolerance and dependence, heroin users usually escalate the dose of drug taken in an

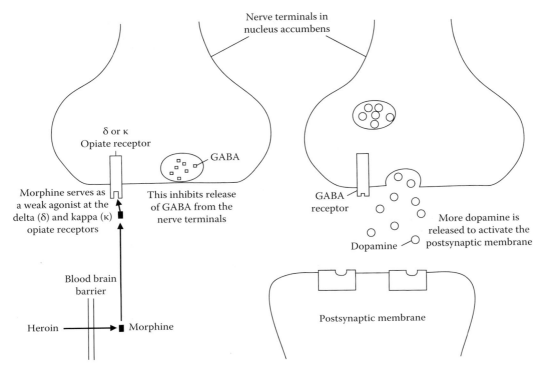

FIGURE 32.13   The mechanism of action of heroin and opioid receptors.

TABLE 32.6

ICD-10 Criteria of Acute Intoxication due to Use of Opioid (F.11)

Dysfunctional Behaviour (At Least One of the Following)	Signs (At Least One of the Following Must Be Present)
1. Apathy and sedation	1. Drowsiness
2. Disinhibition	2. Slurred speech
3. Psychomotor retardation	3. Pupillary constriction
4. Impaired attention	4. Decreased level of consciousness
5. Impaired judgement	
6. Interference with personal functioning	

Note: The DSM-5 only specifies pupillary constriction, drowsiness or coma, slurred speech, and impairment in attention or memory for opioid intoxication.

---

attempt to continue to achieve the euphoriant effects and to keep the unpleasant withdrawal effects of the drug at bay. The result is often that the addict turns to acquisitive crime in order to fund the growing drug habit. It is estimated that the stabilization of heroin addicts on to methadone costs the NHS over £1,000 per year per addict but that this saves society over £30,000 per addict in drug-related crime. Relationships and family commitments usually come second to drug-related activities, and family breakdown often results. It is difficult to continue in employment when seriously addicted to heroin.

32.6.5   CODEINE

Misuse of codeine preparations is common. Preparations include DF118 (dihydrocodeine 30 mg) and codeine linctus (codeine phosphate 15 mg/5 mL).

32.6.5.1   Management of Opiate/Opioid Dependence
32.6.5.1.1   AIMS
The aims of management are to

- Help the person to deal with drug-related problems
- Reduce damage occurring during drug use
- Reduce duration of episodes of drug use
- Reduce the chance of relapse
- Help the person to remain healthy until he or she manages to attain a drug-free state

32.6.5.1.2   History and Examination
Before any treatment is initiated, it is essential to establish that the person is in fact drug dependent. A history

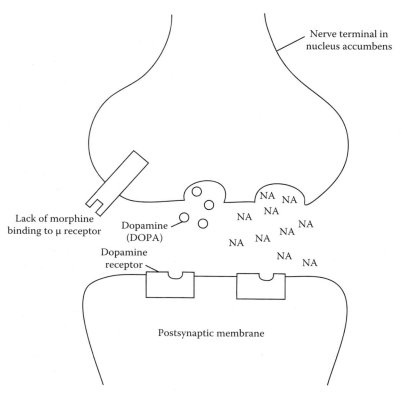

Nerve terminal in
nucleus accumbens

Lack of morphine
binding to μ receptor

Dopamine
(DOPA)

Dopamine
receptor

NA NA
NA
NA
NA
NA NA
NA NA
NA NA
NA
NA NA

Postsynaptic membrane

Repeated use of an opioid causes μ receptors to become tolerant—the first sign of physical
dependence and higher doses of the opioid are needed to produce the intended effect.

FIGURE 32.14   The development of tolerance and withdrawal with chronic opioid misuse.

of drug use, past and current; an account of withdrawal symptoms experienced upon cessation of the drug; a social history including sources of support, accommodation, and employment; the funding of the drug habit; and a medical and psychiatric history are all considered necessary.

Physical examination should seek signs of current drug use and of complications related to the route of administration. It is essential to test urine for a drug screen, to establish that on two separate occasions, the person was taking the drugs claimed. Most drugs will show up on urine screens for at least 24 h after ingestion.

Once it is established that the person is opiate dependent, it is necessary to assess his or her motivation for treatment and to reach an agreement about the aims of treatment.

The Home Office should be notified. The person should be informed that there is a legal obligation upon the doctor to do this but that the information will not be made available to the police.

Patients should receive information about harm minimization, and HIV and hepatitis testing should be arranged after counselling and with the person's consent.

The ultimate aim of treatment is to achieve opiate abstinence. However, this is unacceptable to some patients, in which case the aim is to minimize the harm associated with opiate abuse (harm minimization).

32.6.5.1.3   Harm Minimization

The aims are to stop or reduce the use of contaminated injecting equipment, to prevent the sharing of injecting equipment, to stop or reduce drug use, to stop or reduce unsafe sexual practices, to encourage health consciousness and a more stable lifestyle, and to establish and retain contact with the drug services.

To achieve these aims, education about the potential hazards is important. Sterile injecting equipment and condoms should be provided, nonimmune individuals should be offered hepatitis B vaccination, and substitute oral opiates such as methadone should be prescribed.

32.6.5.1.4 *Detoxification*

Recommendations from the NICE guidelines on opioid detoxification

1. Detoxification should be offered to people who are opioid dependent and have expressed an informed choice to become abstinent after being counselled on the adverse effects of opioid misuse.
2. Methadone or buprenorphine should be offered as the first-line treatment in opioid detoxification.

32.6.5.1.5 *Substitute Prescribing*

32.6.5.1.5.1 *Nonopiate Substitutes*   If dependence is not severe, reassurance, support, and symptomatic treatment with nonopiate drugs may suffice. The following may be used:

1. Clonidine
   a. An α-adrenergic antagonist that inhibits noradrenergic overactivity by acting on the presynaptic autoreceptors.
   b. Provide some symptomatic relief in opiate withdrawal (hypotension can be a problem).
2. Lofexidine
   a. An α_2 agonist, which acts centrally to reduce sympathetic tone (reduction in blood pressure is less marked than that produced by clonidine).
   b. Pharmacodynamics: counteracts the adrenergic hyperactivity during opioid withdrawal.
   c. Indications: (1) detoxification within short period of time (5–7 days) and (2) dependence in young people.
   d. Dosage: start with 800 mcg daily, increase to 2.4 mg in divided daily doses over 3 days, and then reduce in 4 days.
3. Propranolol—for somatic anxiety
4. Thioridazine—relieves anxiety in low doses
5. Promethazine—a sedative antihistamine effective for mild withdrawal
6. Benzodiazepines—for anxiety (do not give for longer than 2 weeks)

32.6.5.1.6 *Substitute Opioids*

32.6.5.1.6.1 *Levo-α-Acetylmethadol*   Levo-α-Acetylmethadol (LAAM) is a synthetic opioid that can block the effects of heroin for up to 72 h. The frequency of usage is three times a week because of its long duration of action. LAAM is associated with torsades de pointes.

32.6.6 METHADONE

32.6.6.1 Indications

1. Opioid drugs are taken on a regular basis.
2. There is convincing evidence of opioid dependence.
3. There is an opportunity to supervise the daily use of methadone for at least 3 months.

32.6.6.2 Contraindications

1. QTc prolongations (consider buprenorphine)
2. Refusal to be supervised

32.6.6.3 Properties of Methadone

- Methadone is a synthetic opiate (opioid) that can be taken orally or intravenously.
- Methadone is a long-acting opioid agonist ($t_{1/2}$ = 24–36 h), allowing once-daily oral prescribing.
- Methadone produces cross-tolerance in opioid misusers because it also blocks μ receptors.
- Methadone is excreted in the urine in a slower pace as compared to heroin.
- Methadone is rapidly absorbed, and the peak levels are achieved within 2–6 h after oral administration.

32.6.6.4 Administration

- Oral methadone mixture 1 mg/mL is the usual choice.
- Any doctor can prescribe methadone to a drug misuser.
- Daily dispensing reduces the risk of overdose and abuse.

32.6.6.5 Dose

- Methadone at 60–100 mg/day is more effective than lower dosages in reducing heroin misuse.
- Methadone at 20–40 mg can attenuate withdrawal symptoms.
- The starting dose of methadone is 10–30 mg per day and increases by 5–10 mg per week to reach therapeutic dose.

32.6.6.6 Duration of Maintenance Treatment

- For maintenance, a substitute opiate is prescribed indefinitely in an effort to stabilize the addict's life and reduce risks of intravenous use.
- For long-term withdrawal, substitute prescribing takes place over a period of months to years with the long-term aim of opiate abstinence.

- For rapid withdrawal, withdrawal takes place over a period of weeks by the use of a substitute drug in decreasing doses.
- For gradual withdrawal, withdrawal takes place over a period of months by the use of a substitute drug in decreasing doses.

32.6.6.7 Treatment Setting

- Treatment should be undertaken initially by the general practitioner (GP), possibly with help from the local community drug team. If these approaches fail, referral to the more specialized drug dependency unit may be required.
- People who are dependent on more than one drug, those with a history of several failed attempts, those with coexisting mental or physical disease, those who are violent or highly manipulative, and those requiring injectable or high doses of substitute drugs should be considered for specialist referral.

32.6.6.8 Management of Methadone Overdose

1. Administer intravenous naloxone (0.4–2 mg over 3 min to a maximum of 10 mg).

32.6.6.9 Cardiovascular Risks

1. Torsades de pointes
2. QTc interval prolongation

32.6.6.10 Management of Pain

1. Nonopioid analgesics such as NSAIDs are preferred.
2. If opioid analgesics are required, titrate up the dose of methadone slowly (Table 32.7).

32.6.7 BUPRENORPHINE

32.6.7.1 Indications

32.6.7.1.1 Chemical Properties

- Buprenorphine is a partial μ-opioid agonist and κ-opioid antagonist.

32.6.7.2 Pharmacodynamics (Figure 32.15)

32.6.7.3 Pharmacokinetics

- Buprenorphine is metabolized in the body by both N-dealkylation and conjugation by the cytochrome P450 enzyme system and excreted principally in faeces and urine.

TABLE 32.7
Advantages and Disadvantages of Methadone Maintenance Programme

Advantages

1. The opportunity to escape from the subculture
2. Relief from the great expenditure of money and time necessary to obtain illicit supplies
3. The possibility of less criminal behaviour that would reflect both upon the addict and the community
4. The avoidance of physical harm derived either from accidental overdose or infections
5. Methadone has longer half-life as compared with the usual agents of addiction
6. The possibility that continuing contact with the methadone programme may permit the use of other forms of treatment

Disadvantages

1. The substitution of one addicting drug for another
2. The need for the most careful structuring or the procedures at the dispensing centres to prevent diversion
3. The fact that polydrug use is common and the psychiatrist is dealing with part of the problem
4. There are very large political difficulties in setting up such a programme and having it accepted in the community
5. It may cause major schisms in the public health authorities
6. There are problems about the safety of methadone itself, for example, children have died from taking their parent's methadone
7. Methadone dispensing facilities become the centres of a social network of addicts in which other drugs are traded and the subculture is preserved or enhanced
8. Methadone can be used merely to tide addicts over the times when illicit drugs are in short supply and reduce their motivation to quit
9. Addicts on programmes find it difficult to get to the appointed places at the proper times particularly if they go to work or if they live in the rural area
10. People who were addicted to nothing at all can get onto a programme and become addicted to methadone

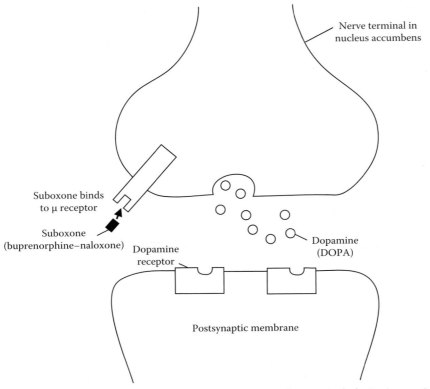

Suboxone binds to the μ receptors, reinitiating opioid activity in the brain. As a partial agonist, buprenorphine produces less euphoria than a full opioid agonist but is sufficient to suppress withdrawal and cravings.

Buprenorphine's high affinity for the μ receptor keeps it from being displaced by other opioids. Once maintenance dosing is established, most μ receptors remain filled and the patient's withdrawal and cravings are controlled.

FIGURE 32.15 The neurochemical effects of buprenorphine/naloxone.

- Peak plasma concentration occurs approximately 3 h after dose administration.
- Buprenorphine has a terminal half-life of about 3–5 h.

32.6.7.4 Dosage

- The titration dosing for induction starts with 2 or 4 mg on the first day.
- The dose can then be increased in 2–4 mg increments to 12–16 mg on the second day.
- Most people can be stabilized on 8–32 mg/day.

32.6.7.5 Side Effects

- The primary side effects of buprenorphine are similar to those of other μ-opioid agonists: nausea, vomiting, and constipation. These side effects may be less intense than those produced by full agonist opioids.

- Hypersensitivity to buprenorphine is rare (fewer than 1% of patients).

32.6.7.6 Contraindications

- Absolute contraindication: hypersensitivity
- Relative contraindication: alcohol or benzodiazepine dependence

32.6.7.7 Withdrawal of Buprenorphine

- Symptoms include yawning, rhinorrhoea, abdominal cramps, nausea, diarrhoea, lacrimation, sweating, insomnia, and irritability.

32.6.7.8 Diversion

- Intravenous misuse of buprenorphine occurs and leads to associated medical complications such as infective endocarditis and cutaneous complications.

- Combination buprenorphine/naloxone (suboxone) rather than buprenorphine alone can avoid diversion because the effects of the opioid antagonist naloxone predominate when people inject suboxone.

32.6.7.9 Antagonist Treatment

Naltrexone, an opioid receptor antagonist, is indicated for people who prefer abstinence programme and are fully informed the risk of withdrawal. Naltrexone is most efficacious in middle-class adults who are highly motivated. Naltrexone has longer half-life than naloxone. Naltrexone cannot be given until all opioids have been cleared from the body. The initial dose is 25 mg and then increases to maintenance dose of 50 mg per day. It is particularly helpful if a partner administers it and if used in conjunction with cognitive behaviour therapy.

Dihydrocodeine is a semisynthetic opioid analgesic. In the United Kingdom dihydrocodeine is a class B drug available in 30 mg tablets. Among GPs in England and Wales, it is the second most commonly prescribed drug (after methadone) for opioid addiction. Dihydrocodeine is much shorter acting than methadone because of its lower affinity of binding to the μ-opioid receptor. Common side effects include constipation, giddiness, hypersensitivity, itching, flushing, and other effects of blood vessel dilation. Tolerance and physical and psychological dependence develop with repeated use. It is not recommended by the NICE guidelines for routine usage.

32.6.7.10 Psychosocial Intervention

The NICE guidelines recommend two types of psychosocial interventions:

1. *Contingency management* (e.g. offering incentives contingent on each drug-negative test such as giving vouchers that can be exchanged for goods or privileges that allow the person taking methadone home) can be offered up to 3–6 months after opioid detoxification.
2. *For people taking naltrexone*: They have to receive contingency management with behavioural family intervention for the person and a nondrug-misusing family member.

32.6.7.11 Psychological Methods

Therapeutic outcome is improved if substitute prescribing is combined with various forms of behaviour therapy.

32.6.7.12 Motivational Interviewing

Motivational interviewing is a cognitive behaviour approach that takes into account the patient's stage of preparedness for change and prompts the patient to consider the favourable reasons to change.

32.6.7.13 Relapse Prevention

Described by Marlatt, this is a short-term intervention with extensive follow-up and preparation of the patient to anticipate urges to return to the drug-taking behaviour for a considerable period after abstinence has been achieved.

People undergoing relapse prevention therapy are more likely to internally attribute change, and are more likely to remain opiate-free during follow-up, or to contain a temporary relapse. The internal attribution of control over drug use maximizes treatment effects.

Naltrexone is a long-acting opioid antagonist that precipitates a withdrawal syndrome in the opiate-dependent person. It is used in the detoxified addict who requires additional help to remain drug-free. The euphoriant effects of opiates are abolished, thus aiding abstinence.

Group therapy and support groups, such as Narcotics Anonymous, often focus on discussions with other people misusing opioid and on sharing experiences and effective coping methods.

32.6.7.14 Prognosis

- The mortality rate for intravenous drug abusers is 20 times that of their nondrug-using peers.
- Since the 1980s, the prevalence of HIV infection among intravenous drug users has increased to approximately 50%–60% in some groups (e.g. New York, Edinburgh), and mortality among this group has increased further.

32.6.8 Cannabis (Grass, Hash, Ganja, Pot)

The major active constituent in cannabis is 9-tetrahydrocannabinol. It is derived from cannabis salve, the Indian hemp plant; the dried leaves contain 1%–10% (marijuana); the resin contains 8%–15% (hashish). It is usually smoked, but it can be eaten, and it is widely used. It is highly lipophilic, so it can be detected in the blood 20 h following a single dose.

32.6.8.1 Mechanism of Actions (Figure 32.16)
32.6.8.2 Cannabinoid Receptors

There are two subtypes of the cannabinoid receptor, CB1 and CB2 receptors. The CB1 receptors are highly expressed in the hippocampus, cortex, basal ganglia, cerebellum, and spinal cord, and this accounts for the effects of cannabis on memory, cognition, and movement. Both CB1 and CB2 cannabinoid receptors are coupled to inhibitory G proteins.

Activation of the cannabinoid receptors causes inhibition of adenylate cyclase and a subsequent decrease in the

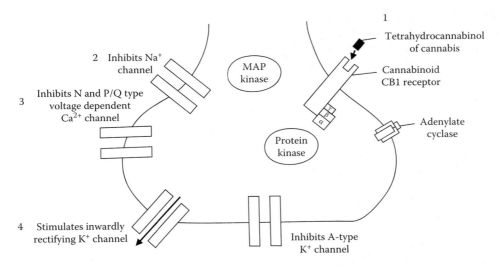

FIGURE 32.16   Neurochemical effects of cannabis.

concentration of cAMP in the cell. This will ultimately result in the inhibition of neurotransmission.

The active ingredient of cannabis is Δ^9-tetrahydrocannabinol (Δ^9-THC), and it is thought to exert its effect by binding to CB1 receptors on presynaptic nerve terminals in the brain. Δ^9-THC binding to CB1 receptors activates G proteins, which causes changes from 2 to 4 as stated in the earlier figure. The changes of these channels will lead to the euphoric feelings associated with cannabis use.

Δ^9-THC has anticholinergic effects, and its action is particularly marked in the hippocampus. It thus has adverse effects on memory, cognition, and other higher mental functions. Δ^9-THC inhibits luteinizing hormone, prolactin, and growth hormone production.

Carriers of the COMT valine (158) allele are most likely to exhibit psychotic symptoms and to develop schizophreniform disorder if they use cannabis (Caspi et al., 2005).

32.6.8.3   Clinical Features

When a patient smokes cannabis, the peak effect occurs at about 30 min, and the effects last for 2–4 h. The motor and cognitive effects may last from 5 to 12 h. Cannabis can also be taken orally when it is mixed with food, but the oral route is less effective as compared to inhalation (Table 32.8).

In high-dosage perceptual distortions, confusion, drowsiness, bradycardia, hypotension, hypothermia, bronchodilatation, and peripheral vasoconstriction can occur. An acute toxic psychosis that resolves with abstinence may occur.

TABLE 32.8

Summary of the ICD-10 Criteria of Acute Intoxication due to Use of Cannabinoids (F.12)

Dysfunctional Behaviour (At Least One of the Following)	Signs (At Least One of the Following Must Be Present)
1. Anxiety or agitation (20% of patients)	1. Conjunctival injection (reddening of eyes)
2. Auditory, visual, or tactile illusions	2. Dry mouth
3. Depersonalization or serialization	3. Increased appetite (cannabis is a well-known appetite suppressant)
4. Euphoria and disinhibition (e.g. giggles)	4. Tachycardia
5. Hallucinations with preserved orientation	
6. Impaired judgement, attention, or reaction time	
7. Interference with personal functioning	
8. Suspiciousness or paranoid ideation	
9. Temporal slowing (a sense that time is passing very slowly or rapid flow of ideas)	

The DSM-5 criteria for cannabis intoxication are less specific than ICD-10. The DSM-5 criteria state that the dysfunctional behaviour and signs (conjunctival injection, increased appetite, dry mouth and tachycardia) occur within 2 h of cannabis use.

32.6.8.4 Drug Withdrawal

In chronic users, cessation of cannabis is often followed by a withdrawal syndrome. The DSM-5 criteria state that the patient should have a least three of the following symptoms within 1 week after withdrawal of cannabis: anxiety, aggression, depression, insomnia, irritability, poor appetite, and weight loss. The patient should have at least one of the following physical symptoms causing significant discomfort: stomach pain, shakiness/tremors, sweating, fever, chills, or headache. Craving and psychological dependence do not occur.

32.6.8.5 Harmful Effects

Chronic cannabis use can lead to a deterioration in personality (a motivational syndrome). An increase in aggressiveness may also occur. Flashbacks, and prolonged depersonalization and derealization, may occur.

Cognitive and psychomotor impairments resulting from even small amounts of cannabis make the performance of skilled tasks (such as driving) hazardous.

32.6.8.6 Treatment

The treatment is abstinence and support.

32.6.9 STIMULANTS

Stimulants considered here are cocaine, amphetamines, and caffeine.

32.6.9.1 Cocaine (Coke, Snow, Crack)

Cocaine is derived from the leaves of the coca shrub. Coca leaves are chewed, and the paste derived from the leaves is smoked.

Cocaine hydrochloride, a white powder usually snorted, may be injected. Crack cocaine (rock or stone) is produced by solvent extraction by using NH_3 to separate cocaine base from hydrochloride salt. Perforated soft drink can, metal foil, and crack pipe are used for consumption. This provides a powerful hit that produces strong psychological dependence.

It is a class A drug, requiring notification.

32.6.9.2 Epidemiology

There has been an epidemic of cocaine use in the United States. Based on the World Health Organization, there are 35 millions of people using amphetamine, 15 millions of people using cocaine, and 10 million of people using opioids. Cocaine remains relatively expensive in the United Kingdom although its use is increasing. Amphetamines tend to be the preferred stimulant of abuse in the United Kingdom. Fewer than 10% of cocaine addicts are notified to the Home Office.

Common psychiatric comorbidity of cocaine users includes dissocial personality disorder (33%), alcoholism (28%), cyclothymia and dysthymia (20%), and schizophrenia (20%).

32.6.9.3 Drug Action

Cocaine blocks dopamine uptake at the dopamine reuptake site. Extracellular levels of dopamine are markedly increased. Dopaminergic activity, particularly at the nucleus accumbens, has been found to have a major role in the pleasurable and reinforcing effects of cocaine, amphetamine, phencyclidine, nicotine, and alcohol. Genetic polymorphisms at the dopamine reuptake site may contribute to an individual's liability to become dependent (Figure 32.17).

The half-life is 50 min. Acute effects last about 20 min and include euphoria, reduced hunger, tirelessness, agitation, tachycardia, raised blood pressure, sweating, nausea, vomiting, dilated pupils, and impairment of judgement

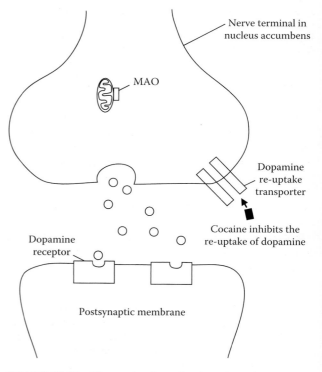

FIGURE 32.17 The mechanism of action of cocaine.

and social functioning. High doses may lead to an acute toxic psychosis with marked agitation, paranoia, and auditory, visual, and tactile hallucinations (cocaine bug).

Chronic use leads to tolerance, withdrawal symptoms, and a chronically anxious state, possibly caused by dopamine depletion.

32.6.9.4 Routes of Administration

- Cocaine can be administered by the intranasal and intravenous routes.
- Intranasal use results in earlier seeking behaviour (after 10–30 min) compared to intravenous route (50 min).
- Injection causes a euphoric rush that lasts for 10–15 min.

32.6.9.5 Clinical Features

Cocaine produces a dose-related increase in arousal, improved performance on tasks of vigilance and alertness, and a sense of self-confidence and well-being (Table 32.9).

TABLE 32.9

Summary of the ICD-10 Criteria of Acute Intoxication due to Use of Cocaine (F.14) or Other Stimulants Including Caffeine (F.15)

Dysfunctional Behaviour (At Least One of the Following)	Signs (At Least One of the Following Must Be Present)
1. Abusiveness or aggression	1. Cardiac arrhythmias
2. Argumentativeness	2. Chest pain
3. Auditory, visual, or tactile illusions	3. Convulsions
4. Euphoria and sensation of increased energy	4. Evidence of weight loss
5. Grandiose beliefs or actions	5. Hypertension (sometimes hypotension)
6. Hallucinations, usually with intact orientation	6. Muscular weakness
7. Hypervigilance	7. Nausea or vomiting
8. Interference with personal functioning	8. Pupillary dilatation
9. Lability of mood	9. Psychomotor agitation (sometimes retardation)
10. Paranoid ideation	10. Sweating and chills
11. Repetitive stereotyped behaviours	11. Tachycardia (sometimes bradycardia)

Note: The DSM-5 criteria for stimulant intoxication are very similar to the ICD-10 criteria. The DSM-5 proposes the following stimulant-induced disorders, which include psychotic disorder, depressive disorder, bipolar disorder, anxiety disorder, sexual dysfunction, or sleep disorder.

32.6.9.6 Cocaine Withdrawal

Following the initial rush of well-being and confidence, when the effects of the drug wear off, there follows a rebound crash. The ICD-10 criteria include lethargy, fatigue, psychomotor retardation or agitation, craving for cocaine, increased appetite, insomnia or hypersomnia, and unpleasant dreams. The crash phase lasts 9 h to 4 days. The withdrawal phase of 1–10 weeks is the period of the greatest risk of relapse. The final phase is of unlimited duration, when stimuli can trigger craving.

32.6.9.7 Harmful Effects

- General effects on the CNS: acute dystonia, tics, migraine-like headaches. 2/3 acute toxic effects occur within 1 h of intoxication.
- Stroke: Nonhaemorrhagic cerebral infarction, subarachnoid, intraparenchymal, and intraventricular haemorrhages. Transient ischaemic attacks have also been associated with cocaine use. The pathophysiological mechanism is vasoconstriction.
- Seizures occur 3%–8% of cocaine users. At high doses, convulsions may occur. The risk of having cocaine-induced seizures is highest in patients using crack cocaine.
- Cardiovascular system: Myocardial infarctions, arrhythmias, and excessive use can also lead to hypertension with cardiac failure.
- Perforation of the nasal septum can follow long-term administration by the nasal route because of the vasoconstriction caused by cocaine. Intravenous use carries with it the risks described earlier.
- Other life-threatening conditions: ischaemic colitis, rhabdomyolysis, hyperthermia, coma, and death.
- Cocaine abusers often take sedatives, including heroin, alcohol, and benzodiazepines. As well as taking the edge off the high produced by cocaine, some of the metabolites of the cocaine–alcohol interaction have been found to have a much longer half-life than cocaine alone. It is possible that this prolongation of the effects of cocaine contributes to its use with alcohol.
- Long-term stimulant abuse results in a stereotyped compulsive repetitive pattern of behaviour and paranoid psychosis resembling schizophrenia.
- Pregnant women who misuse cocaine often have babies (crack babies) with low birth weight, small head circumference, early gestational age, and growth retardation.

32.6.9.8 Pharmacological Treatment

32.6.9.8.1 *Management of Cocaine Intoxication*

- Benzodiazepines: safest drug to be used.
- Alpha-adrenergic blocker (e.g. phentolamine): to treat hypertension.
- Alpha- and beta-blocker (e.g. labetalol): to treat tachycardia.
- Avoid pure beta-blocker (e.g. propranolol), which may lead to cardiac ischaemia.

32.6.9.8.2 *Management of Cocaine Withdrawal*

- Severe withdrawal: amantadine

32.6.9.8.3 *Management of Cocaine Misuse*

1. Abstinence
   a. Complete or partial hospitalization with frequent cocaine misuse
   b. Behavioural contract or contingency management with positive reinforcement for negative urine drug screens
2. Medications for relapse prevention
   a. Dopaminergic medications: amantadine (causes dopamine release) and bromocriptine (dopamine agonist)
   b. Tricyclic antidepressants (e.g. desipramine has been found to reduce the intensity of cocaine craving irrespective of other psychopathology)
   c. SSRI
   d. Bupropion
   e. Modafinil: weak psychostimulant
   f. Methylphenidate: cocaine misuse and ADHD

32.6.9.9 Prognosis

Poor prognostic factors include

- High frequency or intensity of use
- Severe withdrawal symptoms
- Comorbid alcohol misuse
- Comorbid psychiatric conditions (anxiety/depression)
- Poor social support
- Forensic psychiatry

32.6.10 COURSE

- In the early course, the cocaine users experience intense euphoria, alertness, well-being, and self-confidence.
- Chronic use of cocaine is associated with dysphoria and increase in negative effects.
- Repeated cocaine use is associated with psychotic symptoms similar to paranoid schizophrenia.

32.6.10.1 Amphetamines (Speed, Whizz, Sulphate)

Amphetamine is in the form of powder, while methylamphetamine (street name: 'ice') is in the form of large clear crystal. It is a long-acting stimulant and the half life is 10 h. These stimulants are cheap and widely available in the United Kingdom and the United States. The highest rate of amphetamine used is between 18- and 25-year-olds, and amphetamine abuse occurs in all socioeconomic groups and increases among white professionals. They are used clinically in the treatment of narcolepsy, as appetite suppressants and selectively in the hyperkinesis of childhood.

In contrast to cocaine,

- Amphetamine does not have local anaesthetic properties.
- Amphetamine has a longer duration of action.
- Amphetamine has more potent peripheral sympathomimetic effects.

Routes of administration: Amphetamine is administered orally and intravenously.

Mechanism of action: Amphetamines cause excessive release of dopamine. This leads to hyperexcitable state such as tachycardia, arrhythmia, hyperthermia, and irritability. It causes pupil dilation (Figure 32.18).

32.6.10.2 Clinical Features

Psychotic-like state results from acute or chronic ingestion. It leads to paranoia, hallucination, and sometimes a delirium-like state. The effect usually lasts for 3–4 days. In contrast to paranoid schizophrenia, amphetamine-induced psychosis is associated with visual hallucinations, appropriate affect, hyperactivity, hypersexuality, and confusion. Thought disorder and alogia are not found in amphetamine-induced psychosis. It usually resolves with abstinence but may continue for some months.

In the withdrawal state (aka crash), the person will develop fatigue, hypersomnia, hyperphagia, depression, and nightmare.

Following chronic use, profound depression and fatigue occur. Long-term use leads to CNS serotonergic neuronal destruction.

32.6.10.3 Treatment

1. Abstinence: an inpatient setting and combination of psychotherapy techniques
2. Amphetamine-induced psychosis: antipsychotics
3. Agitation and hyperactivity: diazepam
4. Depression: bupropion

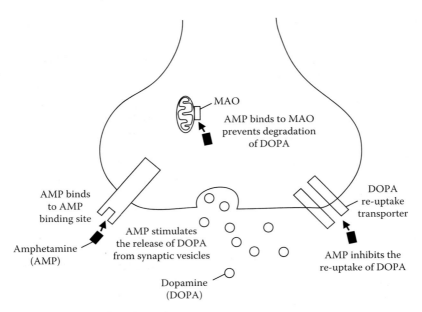

FIGURE 32.18 Mechanisms of actions of amphetamines.

32.6.11 3,4-METHYLENEDIOXYMETHAMPHETAMINE (MDMA, ECSTASY, XTC, E, ADAM)

32.6.11.1 Background
- MDMA is a hallucinogenic amphetamine and was developed by Merck in 1914.
- MDMA is a designer drug and serotonin neurotoxin. It possesses both stimulant and mild hallucinogenic properties.
- This synthetic drug involves combination of amphetamine, ephedrine, or pseudoephedrine with components of lithium batteries. Purity varies depending on the substitutes used, and it is often impure.
- It is widely used at parties or raves by young people, particularly in the 1990s.

32.6.11.2 Chemical Properties
- MDMA causes potent release and reuptake inhibition of serotonin and associated with serotoninergic neurotoxicity in humans.
- MDMA does not cause dependence.

32.6.11.3 Administration
- MDMA is taken orally or intranasally.
- Taken orally in tablet or capsule form, its effects last 4–6 h; multiple dosing is tried, but tolerance develops rapidly, and subsequent doses have less potency.

32.6.11.4 Clinical Effects
- MDMA produces a combination of stimulants and psychedelic effects. The stimulant effects resemble those of amphetamine, and hallucinogenic effects resemble those of LSD.
- MDMA causes a feeling of closeness to other people, altered sensual and emotional overtones, increase in empathy, and extroversion. People taking MDMA report accelerated thinking, impaired decision-making, and memory impairment with chronic use.
- Psychiatric conditions (psychosis, depression, anxiety) in previously vulnerable individuals can occur following MDMA use.
- Acute effects include sweating, tachycardia, dry mouth, jaw clenching, muscle aches, bruxism, jaw clenching, and gait disturbances.
- Physical dependence does not occur.

32.6.11.5 Other Harmful Effects
- Deaths have occurred in those with preexisting cardiac disease caused by cardiac arrhythmias. In the fit user at normal doses, deaths have occurred as a result of hyperpyrexia, resulting in disseminated intravascular coagulation, rhabdomyolysis, and renal failure.
- Convulsions can also occur. Most deaths of this nature occur when the user has been dancing

vigorously for a considerable period, in high ambient temperatures, with inadequate fluid replacement. MDMA has a direct effect upon the thermoregulatory mechanisms that compound these conditions.

- Hypertensive crises may occur leading to CVA in some.
- Toxic hepatitis has been reported in MDMA users possibly related to impurities in the preparation.
- Neurotoxicity is an established fact. Serotonergic nerve terminals are damaged by this drug, and although rat studies indicate that this is reversible, primate studies indicate the opposite. The long-term consequences of MDMA-induced serotonergic neurotoxicity in humans are not known.

32.6.11.6   Management

Abrupt discontinuation is recommended, there being no advantage to gradual withdrawal. Psychiatric disturbance should be treated accordingly.

32.6.12   CAFFEINE

32.6.12.1   Chemical Properties

- Caffeine is a methylxanthine (1,3, 7-trimethylxanthine).
- Caffeine is widely available in coffee, tea, and chocolate and is added to soft drinks and proprietary cold preparations.
- Coffee contains about 80–150 mg of caffeine per cup depending upon the brewing method. Peak blood levels occur 15–45 min following oral administration; the half-life is 6 h. Metabolism is increased by smoking and reduced by oral contraceptives and pregnancy. Neonates cannot metabolize caffeine; therefore, there is a very long half-life.

32.6.12.2   Mechanisms of Actions of Caffeine

- The main action of caffeine is the competitive antagonism of adenosine A_1 and A_2 receptors, which contribute to the neuropsychiatric effects such as psychosis in caffeine intoxication as a result of the release of dopamine.
- Higher doses cause inhibition of phosphodiesterases, blockade of $GABA_A$ receptors, and release of intracellular calcium. It reaches its peak blood levels after 1–2 h and reduces cerebral blood flow although it is a stimulant.

32.6.12.3   Dose and Clinical Effects

- A dose of 80–200 mg produces mood elevation, increased alertness and clarity of thought, increased gastric secretion, tachycardia, raised blood pressure, diuresis, and increased productivity.
- In overdose (greater than 250 mg per day) caffeinism occurs. This results in anxiety, restlessness, nausea, muscle twitching, and facial flushing. Patients may demonstrate rambling thought and speech. The DSM-5 proposes that the minimum amount for caffeine intoxication is 250 mg per day or (e.g. more than two to three cups of brewed coffee).
- At levels of intake in excess of 600 mg per day, dysphoria replaces euphoria, anxiety and mood disturbances become prominent, and insomnia, muscle-twitching, tachycardia, and sometimes cardiac arrhythmias occur.
- The DSM-5 proposes two caffeine-induced disorders (e.g. caffeine-induced anxiety disorder and or caffeine-induced sleep disorder).

32.6.12.4   Other Systemic Effects of Caffeine

1. CNS: migraine.
2. Gastrointestinal system: Caffeine relaxes the lower oesophageal sphincter and can predispose to gastro-oesophageal reflux disease. It also causes hypersecretion of gastric acid and increases the risk of gastric ulcer.
3. Renal system: Caffeine causes diuretic effect, and people are advised to abstain from consuming caffeine in situations where dehydration may be significant.
4. Pregnancy: low birth weight and miscarriage. Caffeine enters amniotic fluid and breast milk. It affects infants because of slow metabolism of caffeine in fetus.

32.6.12.5   Dependence and Withdrawal

1. 10% of caffeine users experience withdrawal effects (e.g. more than six cups per day). Withdrawal starts at 1–2 h post ingestion and becomes worst at 1–2 days and recede with a few days.
2. Common withdrawal effects include headache, irritability, sleeplessness, anxiety, tremor, and impairment of psychomotor performance.

32.6.13   HALLUCINOGENS

Hallucinogens are substances that give rise to marked perceptual disturbances when taken in relatively small quantities.

32.6.13.1   Epidemiology

- The lifetime prevalence is 0.6%.
- Misuse of hallucinogen is common among young white men.
- The peak of hallucinogen misuse was between 1965 and 1969, and it was overtaken by stimulants.

32.6.13.2   Route of Administration

- Most hallucinogens are well absorbed after oral ingestion.
- Tolerance for hallucinogens develops rapidly and takes places after 3 or 4 days of continuous use. Tolerance disappears rapidly, usually in 4–7 days after discontinuation of hallucinogen.

32.6.13.3   Clinical Effects (Table 32.10)

The DSM-5 has similar criteria for hallucinogen intoxication. Additional criteria include synaesthesia shortly after hallucinogen use. The DSM-5 has an additional category called hallucinogen persisting perception disorder, which involves reexperience of false fleeting perceptions in the peripheral fields, flashes of colour, geometric pseudohallucinations, positive afterimages, macropsia, and micropsia after cessation of hallucinogen use.

TABLE 32.10

Summary of the ICD-10 Criteria of Acute Intoxication due to Use of Hallucinogens (F.16)

Dysfunctional Behaviour (At Least One of the Following)	Signs (At Least One of the Following Must Be Present)
1. Anxiety and fearfulness	1. Tachycardia
2. Auditory, visual, or tactile illusions or hallucinations occurring in a state of full wakefulness and alertness (it may lead to accidents and hallucinations are recurrent)	2. Palpitations
	3. Sweating and chills
	4. Tremor
	5. Blurring of vision
	6. Pupillary dilatation
	7. Incoordination
3. Depersonalization	
4. Serialization	
5. Paranoid ideation	
6. Ideas of reference	
7. Lability of mood	
8. Hyperactivity	
9. Impulsive acts	
10. Impaired attention	
11. Interference with personal functioning	

The DSM-5 proposes the following hallucinogen-induced disorders: psychotic disorder, bipolar disorder, depressive disorder, and anxiety disorder.

32.6.13.4   Treatment

1. Severe psychosis: haloperidol and diazepam
2. Hallucinogen persisting perception disorder: clonazepam, valproate, and carbamazepine

32.6.14   Lysergic Acid Diethylamide (LSD, Trips, Acid, Microdots, Supermans)

32.6.14.1   Chemical Properties

LSD is a 5-HT_{2A} agonist and the most potent hallucinogen. LSD suggests the role of serotonin in causing hallucination in schizophrenia.

32.6.14.2   Route of Administration

1. LSD is available in tablets or absorbed onto paper.
2. LSD has been commonly distributed as 'blotter acid', and these are sheets of paper that are soaked with LSD.
3. Then the sheet is dried and perforated into small squares and each square containing 30–75 mg of LSD. Minute amounts (£100 µg) produce marked psychoactive effects.
4. The onset of action of LSD occurs within an hour, peaks in 2–4 h, and lasts 8–12 h.
5. Intravenous use is not common because the onset of the trip is very rapid with oral ingestion (15 min).
6. Tolerance develops rapidly; sensitivity to its effects returns rapidly with abstinence.

32.6.14.3   Drug Action

The substance acts at multiple sites in the CNS, the effects being thought to be related to 5-HT antagonism. The effects are dose related.

Psychic effects include the heightening of perceptions, with perceptual distortion of shape; intensification of colour and sound; apparent movement of stationary objects; and changes in sense of time and place. Hallucinations may occur but are relatively rare. The user usually retains insight into the nature of the experiences. Delusions (e.g. belief in the ability to fly) may occur. Emotional lability, heightened self-awareness, and ecstatic experiences can occur. Synesthaesias in which a stimulus in one sensory modality is experienced in another modality (e.g. hearing colours) are common.

The physical effects are sympathomimetic, with tachycardia, hypertension, and dilated pupils.

Flashback phenomena (posthallucinogen perception disorder) occur, in which aspects of the LSD experience occur spontaneously some time after LSD use. These are usually fleeting.

32.6.14.4 Drug Withdrawal

Physical withdrawal symptoms do not occur following the abrupt discontinuation of LSD or other hallucinogens.

32.6.14.5 Harmful Effects

Accidents may occur while under the influence of hallucinogens, such as jumping from a height because of the delusional belief that the user can fly.

Flashback phenomena occur many months after drug elimination, giving rise to the possibility that these substances may cause permanent neurological changes.

32.6.14.6 Clinical Effects

1. LSD produces psychedelic effects (such as synesthaesia, stimulation of one sense stimulates sensation in the other sense, e.g. intense experience of hearing the colour) as little as 25–50 µg.
2. At 100 mcg, LSD produces perceptual distortions, hallucinations, mood changes (elation or depression), paranoia, and panic.
3. Physical signs include pupillary dilation, increased blood pressure and pulse, facial flushing, salivation, lacrimation, and hyperreflexia. LSD leads to persisting perception disorder even the person is not using LSD. Physical withdrawal is not commonly seen.
4. Death caused by cardiac or cerebrovascular pathology related to hypertension or hyperthermia can occur with hallucinogenic use.
5. The flashbacks: It refers to the spontaneous occurrence of episodic visual disturbances, which resemble to prior LSD trips. Flashbacks may diminish in intensity with time, and psychoeducation should be offered on the nature of the flashbacks.
6. The bad trip: Unpleasant experiences may occur, and these are more likely in the inexperienced or if the ambient mood is disturbed. Users generally avoid being alone, in case of bad trips or dangerous behaviour, while under the influence. The features of adverse experiences include anxiety, depression, dizziness and disorientation, and a short-lived psychotic episode characterized by hallucinations and paranoid delusions. With heavy use, an acute schizophreniform psychosis may persist.

Drug interactions: Chlorpromazine may induce anticholinergic crisis after LSD use.

Treatment: The treatment of bad trip involves diazepam 20 mg. Antipsychotics may worsen the experience.

32.6.15 Hallucinogenic Mushrooms (Magic Mushrooms)

There are a number of fungi growing in the United Kingdom that contain psychoactive substances such as psilocybin and psilocin. Liberty cap and fly agaric mushrooms are the ones most commonly used for their psychoactive effects. Ingestion of these in the raw state is legal, but any attempt to process them, such as by cooking, drying, or freezing, is illegal.

Ingestion causes mild LSD-like effects, with marked euphoria. At high doses, hallucinations, bad trips, and acute psychoses can occur.

32.6.16 Mescaline

Mescaline is the active component of the Mexican peyote cactus. Mescaline is similar to noradrenaline. It is hallucinogenic and is orally administered.

LSD is 200 times as potent as psilocybin, which is 30 times as potent as mescaline.

32.6.17 Phencyclidine (PCP, Angle Dust)

32.6.17.1 Chemical Properties

- PCP is a dissociative anaesthetic agent as the person remains conscious during anaesthetized state.
- PCP is an arylcyclohexylamine related to ketamine. It is taken by smoking, snorting, and injecting.

32.6.17.2 Neurochemical Effects

- PCP blocks NMDA glutamate receptors (Figure 32.19).

32.6.17.3 Clinical Effects

1. It produces stimulant, anaesthetic, analgesic, and hallucinogenic effects. At low doses, it induces euphoria and a feeling of weightlessness. At high doses, visual hallucinations and synesthaesias occur.
2. Psychosis, violence, paranoia, and depression can occur following a single dose.
3. Physical effects include incoordination, slurred speech, blurred vision, convulsions, coma, and respiratory arrest.
4. Prolonged use can result in a withdrawal syndrome upon cessation.

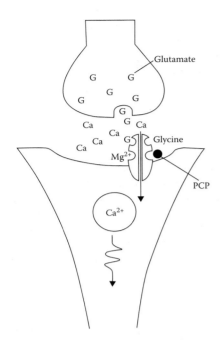

FIGURE 32.19   The mechanism of action of phencyclidine.

32.6.18   KETAMINE (K)

- Ketamine is a shorter-acting derivative of PCP.
- Ketamine is in the form of tablets and it is snorted or injected.
- The action of ketamine is mediated by competitive inhibition from the NMDA receptor complex.
- It leads to cramps, fatigue, depression, and irritability. It may lead to violent reactions (may harm other people) and flashbacks.
- Severe intoxication produces a state of virtual helplessness and lack of coordination.

32.6.19   SEDATIVES

CNS sedatives depress CNS activity with little analgesic effect. They include alcohol (see aforementioned), barbiturates, benzodiazepines, and carbamates. All the CNS depressants have abuse potential and cause both psychological and physical dependence. Cross-tolerance between groups occurs, and the withdrawal syndromes are similar. When taken repeatedly in high doses, all these drugs produce sadness/depression, a worsening of confusional states, and withdrawal syndromes in which anxiety is prominent.

32.6.20   BENZODIAZEPINES

Widely prescribed, these have widespread physical dependence among licit users and are very popular with illicit substance abusers.

The most common route of administration is oral, but some abusers attempt to inject the contents of capsules or ground tablets intravenously.

32.6.20.1   Epidemiology

Over 1 million of the UK population use benzodiazepines continuously for more than 1 year.

32.6.20.2   Drug Action

This group of sedatives potentiates the inhibitory actions of the $GABA_A$ receptor in the limbic areas of the brain. They have anxiolytic, hypnotic, and anticonvulsant properties at normal doses (Table 32.11).

The DSM-5 has similar criteria for sedative/hypnotic intoxication but has less signs and symptoms.

The DSM-5 proposes the following sedative-/hypnotic-induced disorders: major neurocognitive disorder, persisting amnestic disorder, psychotic disorder, depressive or bipolar disorder, anxiety disorder, sexual dysfunction, or sleep disorder.

32.6.20.3   Drug Withdrawal

Tolerance occurs rapidly. There is rebound anxiety after 4 weeks of use; dependence is seen in 45% of users after 3 months.

The onset and intensity of withdrawal symptoms are related in part to the half-life of the drug used (shorter half-lives lead to a more abrupt and intense withdrawal syndrome). The withdrawal syndrome is also related to

---

TABLE 32.11

Summary of the ICD-10 Criteria of Acute Intoxication due to Use of Benzodiazepine (F.13)

Dysfunctional Behaviour (At Least One of the Following)	Signs (At Least One of the Following Must Be Present)
1. Abusiveness or aggression	1. Decreased level of consciousness (e.g. stupor, coma)
2. Apathy and sedation	2. Difficulty in standing
3. Anterograde amnesia	3. Erythematous skin lesions or blisters
4. Euphoria and disinhibition	4. Nystagmus
5. Impaired attention	5. Slurred speech
6. Impaired psychomotor performance	6. Unsteady gait
7. Interference with personal functioning	
8. Lability of mood	

Note: The DSM-5 has similar criteria for sedative/hypnotic intoxication but has less signs and symptoms.

the dose used. Onset is usually within 1–14 days after drug reduction/cessation and may last for months.

Withdrawal symptoms include somatic effects such as autonomic hyperactivity (tachycardia; sweating; anorexia; weight loss; pyrexia; tremor of hands, tongue, and eyelids; GI disturbance; sleep disturbance with vivid dreams due to REM rebound), malaise and weakness, tinnitus, and grand mal convulsions.

There are cognitive effects with impaired memory and concentration. There are also perceptual effects with hypersensitivity to sound, light, and touch; depersonalization; and derealization. Delirium may develop within a week of cessation, associated with visual, auditory, and tactile hallucinations and delusions.

Affective effects such as irritability, anxiety, and phobic symptoms may also occur.

32.6.20.4 Harmful Effects

In a high-dose abuser, severe withdrawal symptoms occur if the person is unable to acquire the usual dose of drug. As in these doses the drugs have usually been acquired illicitly, supply cannot be guaranteed.

Benzodiazepines are relatively safe in overdose but are liable to produce respiratory depression, and in combination with other drugs, they can be lethal.

The injection of street benzodiazepines incurs all the dangers of injecting described earlier but is particularly liable to cause limb ischaemia and gangrene, with resulting amputation.

32.6.20.5 Management

Withdrawal from sedative drugs is potentially lethal and should usually be managed on a medical ward.

32.6.21 Barbiturates

Although the prescribing of barbiturates has largely been superseded by the safer benzodiazepines, they still appear in the form of phenobarbitone, amylobarbitone, and quinalbarbitone (Tuinal) and are widely available.

32.6.21.1 Drug Action

Barbiturates potentiate action at the $GABA_A$ receptor, thus increasing CNS depression. This is particularly marked in the reticular activating system and cerebral cortex.

Clinical effects include impaired concentration, reduced anxiety, and dysphoria. In increasing doses, dysarthria, ataxia, drowsiness, coma, respiratory depression, and death occur.

Chronic use results in tolerance caused by hepatic enzyme induction, cross-tolerance with alcohol, personality change, persistent intoxication, labile affect, poor concentration, impaired judgement, and incoordination.

32.6.21.2 Drug Withdrawal

This causes anxiety, tremor, sweating, insomnia with marked REM rebound, irritability, agitation, twitching, vomiting, nausea, tachycardia, orthostatic hypotension, delirium, and convulsions.

32.6.21.3 Harmful Effects

Barbiturates are dangerous in overdose. Their therapeutic index is low. Tolerance to psychotropic effects exceeds tolerance to respiratory depression.

Parenteral administration of oral preparations is attempted by some addicts, incurring all the risks described.

32.6.21.4 Management

A gradual tapering of the dose is considered to be the most appropriate way to manage barbiturate dependence. Short-acting compounds should first be substituted by long-acting compounds, diazepam being the most commonly used form for the purposes of withdrawal. After stabilizing on diazepam, dose reduction is commenced. At high doses, this can occur quite rapidly (e.g. at 5 mg per week) until the patient starts to complain of unpleasant effects, when the rate of reduction can be reduced. If symptoms of depression are present, an antidepressant is indicated. Propranolol may help with some of the somatic symptoms of anxiety.

Psychological support is very important, with weekly contact initially. The family should be involved in the process.

The withdrawal of barbiturates similarly needs phased withdrawal; inpatient admission is often necessary.

32.6.22 Nicotine

32.6.22.1 Epidemiology

- In the United Kingdom the prevalence of smoking has reduced in the past three decades. Around 20% of male adults are smokers. The highest rates of smoking are people between 20- and 25-year-olds where 30% of these young adults are smokers.
- For people older than 60 years, the prevalence of smoking is around 10%.
- In the United Kingdom analyses of the interactions between smoking, drinking, and cannabis use indicated that the relationship between substance use and psychiatric morbidity was primarily explained by regular smoking and to a lesser extent regular cannabis use.

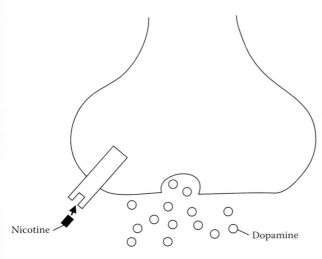

Nicotine

Dopamine

FIGURE 32.20 Mechanism of action of nicotine.

32.6.22.2 Pharmacodynamics (Figure 32.20)

- The nicotinic receptors are found on presynaptic dopaminergic neurons.
- Smoking of tobacco leads to release of dopamine.
- Effects of nicotine include euphoria, enhancing motivation, and sustained vigilance.
- Nicotine also suppresses the insulin production from the pancreas (slight hyperglycaemia).

32.6.22.3 Pharmacokinetics

- Nicotine influences the metabolism of drugs through cytochrome P450 mechanism. For example, nicotine induces P450 1A2 system and enhances metabolism of olanzapine.
- There is a need to reduce the antipsychotic dosage after smoking cessation.
- On the other hand, there are reduced smoking rates in some patients after taking clozapine.

32.6.22.4 Clinical Effects (Table 32.12)

The proposed DSM-5 does not have tobacco intoxication disorder.

32.6.22.5 Tobacco Withdrawal Syndrome

This syndrome may develop if a person stops smoking after 3–10 weeks of tobacco consumption. The onset may be within an hour after the last cigarette. As a result of the reduction in dopamine release, the person feels depressed (lasting for 1 month) and irritable. The DSM-5 proposes other criteria including anxiety, poor concentration, increased appetite, weight again, restlessness, and insomnia. The aforementioned symptoms cause the person to crave for tobacco.

TABLE 32.12

Summary of the ICD-10 Criteria of Acute Intoxication due to Use of Tobacco (F.17)

Dysfunctional Behaviour (At Least One of the Following)	Signs (At Least One of the Following Must Be Present)
1. Bizarre dreams	1. Cardiac arrhythmias
2. Serialization	2. Nausea or vomiting
3. Insomnia	3. Sweating
4. Interference with personal functioning	4. Tachycardia
5. Lability of mood	

Note: The DSM-5 does not have tobacco intoxication disorder.

32.6.22.6 Pharmacological Treatment

32.6.22.6.1 *Varenicline*

Varenicline has high affinity to $\alpha_4\beta_2$ nicotine Ach receptors and prevents tobacco withdrawal syndrome.

Dosage:

Day 1–3: 0.5 mg per day
Day 4–7: 0.5 mg bid
Day 8: Day to quit alcohol
Week 12: 1 mg bid

Contraindication: age < 18 years, pregnancy, end-stage renal failure.

32.6.22.6.2 *Bupropion*

1. Chemical properties: antidepressant with noradrenergic activity that reduces the effect of nicotine withdrawal
2. Dosage: starting dose 150 mg/day and increase to 150 mg bid
3. Side effects: epilepsy (1/1000)
4. Contraindications: history of epilepsy, eating disorders, CNS tumour, and bipolar disorder
5. Side effects: headache (30%), insomnia, and rash (0.1%)

32.6.22.7 Nicotine Replacement Therapy

1. Duration of treatment: 8–12 weeks.
2. Route of administration: sublingual tablets, gum, patch, and nasal spray.
3. Side effects: local irritation, worsen glucose control in diabetes.
4. It is not recommended to administer bupropion and Nicotine Replacement Therapy (NRT) together.

Behavioural treatment is used in nicotine addiction.

32.6.22.8 Prognosis

Among all substances, nicotine causes the highest number of death.

32.6.23 VOLATILE SOLVENTS

Volatile substances are inhaled (glue-sniffing) in order to experience their psychoactive effects. Solvents from glue (such as toluene), correction fluids (e.g. trichloroethane), butane gas, and other aerosol propellants are popular.

Solvents have been tried by 3%–5% of 15-year-olds. Often fumes are rebreathed from a plastic bag with concentrated vapour, but sometimes an aerosol is sprayed directly into the oropharynx (this is particularly dangerous). Rapidly absorbed, its effects last about 30 min.

32.6.23.1 Drug Action (Table 32.13)

The DSM-5 proposes the following inhalant-induced disorders such as mild neurocognitive disorder, major neurocognitive disorder, psychotic disorder, depressive disorder, or anxiety disorder.

Chronic use causes Goodpasture's syndrome, hypokalaemia, and optic neuropathy. High doses cause stupor and death. Aspiration of vomit can occur at any time.

32.6.23.2 Drug Withdrawal

There is no physical withdrawal syndrome.

32.6.23.3 Harmful Effects

Acute intoxication can lead to fatal accidents, particularly through falling or drowning. However, the greatest risk of death is during an episode of sniffing. Butane squirted directly into the mouth can cause cardiac arrest. Propellants squirted directly into the mouth are cooled to −20°C, which can cause burns to the throat and lungs, and may freeze the larynx, causing cardiac arrest through vagal nerve stimulation. Rebreathing from plastic bags can result in asphyxiation.

There are approximately 100 deaths per annum in the United Kingdom with 20% of these occurring in first-time users and the majority in those aged under 20 years.

There are reports of long-term damage to the CNS, heart, liver, and kidneys. Chronic use may cause a persistent cerebellar syndrome and peripheral neuropathy.

32.6.23.4 Management

Abrupt discontinuation is recommended. Advice from social services and/or a child psychiatrist may be needed.

32.6.23.5 Khat

- Khat is a form of fresh leaves that are chewed socially in Arabic and African countries.
- The main constituent is cathinone that has amphetamine-like properties and induces psychosis and hypomania.
- Adverse effects include paralytic ileus.

32.6.23.6 Anabolic Steroid

- People misuse anabolic steroid to increase muscle growth and body bulk.
- It can be swallowed or injected.
- Adverse effects include gynaecomastia in men and clitoral enlargement in women, bone hypertension, cardiac disorders, liver (e.g. drug-induced hepatitis) and renal impairment, shrinking of testicles, and priapism. It also leads to aggression and irritability.
- Death may occur as a result of overdose or severe infection as a result of repeated intramuscular injection.

32.7 ADDICTION WITHOUT SUBSTANCES

32.7.1 PATHOLOGICAL GAMBLING

32.7.1.1 Epidemiology

Findings from the British Gambling Prevalence Survey (2007)

- 67.9% of 8968 respondents (65.2% of female respondents and 70.7% of male respondents) in English, Scotland, and Wales participated in any form of gambling in the past 12 months before the survey.

TABLE 32.13

Summary of the ICD-10 Criteria of Acute Intoxication due to Use of Solvent (F.18)

Dysfunctional Behaviour (At Least One of the Following)	Signs (At Least One of the Following Must Be Present)
1. Apathy and lethargy	1. Blurred vision or diplopia
2. Argumentativeness	2. Decreased level of consciousness
3. Abusiveness or aggression	3. Difficulty in standing
4. Lability of mood	4. Muscle weakness
5. Impaired judgement	5. Nystagmus
6. Impaired attention and memory	6. Slurred speech
7. Psychomotor retardation	7. Unsteady gait
8. Interference with personal functioning	

Note: The DSM-5 calls this inhalant intoxication, which shares similar criteria as ICD-10.

- The prevalence of problem gambling for adults was around 0.8%.
- Internet gamblers were more likely to be young men, single, well educated, and in professional or managerial employment.
- The top five gambling methods in United Kingdom were the national lottery, scratch cards, betting on horses, fruit/slot machines, and 'other' lotteries such as private betting, bingo, and sport betting.
- Men were more common than women to be involved in all gambling activities except playing scratch cards, which has equal gender ratio.
- It is important to note that the prevalence of problem gambling for adolescents was 1.9% and the figure was higher than adults.

McBride et al. (2010) classified British gamblers into three types:

1. Nonproblematic gambler: 88.9%
2. Preoccupied chaser: 9.7%
3. Antisocial impulsivist gambler: 1.4%

32.7.1.2 Aetiology and Risk Factors

32.7.1.2.1 Biological Risk Factors

1. Genetics (Lodo and Kennedy, 2009)
   a. The heritability of pathological gambling is 55%.
   b. Pathological gambling and subclinical pathological gambling are a continuum of the same disorder.
   c. Pathological gambling shares genetic vulnerability factors with antisocial behaviours, alcohol dependence, and major depressive disorder.
   d. Genetic factors underlie the association between exposure to traumatic life events and pathological gambling.
2. Neurochemistry (Potenza et al., 2011)
   a. Serotonin, noradrenaline, and dopamine have been implicated in the aetiology of pathological gambling.
   b. There is an increased level of $5-HT1_B$ receptors in the brain of pathological gamblers.
3. Imaging (van Holst et al., 2010)
   Pathological gambling is consistently associated with blunted mesolimbic–prefrontal cortex activation to nonspecific rewards and increased activation when exposed to gambling-related stimuli in cue exposure paradigms.

5. Psychosocial risk factors
   a. Learning theories: monetary gain and excitement acting as positive reinforcers.
   b. Cognitive theories: cognitive distortions such as magnification of one's gambling skills, superstitious beliefs, and interpretive biases.
   c. Non-Caucasian British men with smoking history were all more likely to be preoccupied chasers or antisocial impulsivist gamblers, rather than nonproblematic gamblers.
   d. Adolescents: male gender, parental gambling, dominated school characteristics, Asian ethnicity, no sibling, and gambling as a source of income (Forrest and McHale, 2011).

32.7.1.3 Clinical Features

The DSM-5 criteria state that there are at least four symptoms for 1-year period:

1. Tolerance: Patient needs to gamble with increasing amounts of money in order to achieve the desired excitement.
2. Withdrawal: Patient is restless or irritable when attempting to cut down or stop gambling.
3. Repeated unsuccessful efforts to control, cut back, or stop gambling.
4. Preoccupation with gambling (e.g. persistent thoughts of reliving past gambling experience).
5. Gambles often when feeling distressed (e.g. helpless, guilty, anxious, depressed).
6. Chasing the loss by gambling more after losing money in gambling.
7. Lying to conceal the extent of involvement with gambling.
8. Loss a significant relationship, job, or educational or career opportunity because of gambling.
9. Relying on others to provide money for gambling as a result of financial problems.

Mania must be excluded, and course specifiers include chronic, episodic, and in remission.

32.7.1.4 Management

32.7.1.4.1 Pharmacological Treatment

- Naltrexone, an opioid antagonist, may reduce urges and thoughts in pathological gamblers.
- SSRIs such as fluvoxamine and paroxetine may reduce of gambling behaviour, urges, and thoughts in pathological gamblers.
- Mood stabilizers such as lithium and valproate may be useful.

32.7.1.4.2 Psychological Treatment

1. Financial counselling, limiting access to money, and restricting admission into gambling venues are simple measures and can be applied to most pathological gamblers.
2. Motivational enhancement therapy (face-to-face or telephone counselling) and self-help workbooks are indicated for patients who are ambivalent about quitting gambling or entering treatment or who are not keen on long-term therapy.
3. Cognitive behaviour therapy
   a. Cognitive therapy aims at correcting gamblers' beliefs about randomness and chance and the false notion that they can control and predict outcome.
   b. Behaviour therapy involves imaginal desensitization, imaginal relaxation, behavioural monitoring, covert sensitization, and spousal contingency contracting.
   c. Relapse prevention follow-up further improves the outcome.
4. Gamblers Anonymous: 12-step recovery programme.

32.8 INTERNET ADDICTION

32.8.1 HISTORICAL DEVELOPMENT

- Ivan Goldberg is the first person to use the term Internet addiction in 1995.

32.8.2 EPIDEMIOLOGY

- The global prevalence rate is between 1.5% and 8.2%.
- The heterogeneity in prevalence is a result of different age groups and different instruments used in the study.

32.8.3 AETIOLOGY AND RISK FACTORS

32.8.3.1 Biological Theories

32.8.3.1.1 Genetics

- The SS genotype of the serotonin transporter gene (5HTTLPR) is associated with Internet addiction in Asians (Lee et al., 2008).
- The nicotinic acetylcholine receptor subunit alpha 4 (CHRNA4) genotype: the CC genotype is associated with Internet addiction in German women (Montag et al., 2008).

32.8.3.1.2 Imaging

1. Structural MRI showed that adolescents with internet addiction had lower grey matter density in the left anterior cingulate cortex and left posterior cingulate cortex compared to normal controls (Zhou et al., 2011).
2. Functional MRI showed that the following areas are activated when patients with Internet addiction are playing online game (Ko et al., 2009):
   a. Right orbitofrontal cortex (compulsion)
   b. Right nucleus accumbens (motivation)
   c. Right dorsolateral prefrontal cortex (impulse control)
   d. Right caudate nucleus (compulsive behaviour)

32.8.3.2 Psychological Theories

- Learning theory emphasizes on the positive reinforcing effects of Internet use, which can induce feelings of well-being and euphoria in the user. The other positive reinforcements include social contact with no real social presence, contact with relative strangers, and immediate gratification.
- Deficient social skill theory: Internet is used by a shy or anxious individual to avoid anxiety-provoking situations such as face-to-face interaction. This reinforces Internet use by avoidance conditioning.
- Internet use is linked to sensation-seeking behaviour and impulsivity.
- Development theory: Erikson crisis that involves identity versus intimacy in young adults.

32.8.4 CLINICAL FEATURES

32.8.4.1 Young's Definition

- The use of the Internet for more than 38 h per week
- Clinically significant impairment or distress

32.8.4.2 Proposed Criteria

1. Preoccupation with Internet gaming
2. Withdrawal symptoms when the Internet is taken away
3. Tolerance: the need to spend increasing amounts of time engaged in Internet gaming
4. Unsuccessful attempts to control Internet gaming use
5. Continued excessive Internet use despite knowledge of negative psychosocial problems

6. Loss of interests, previous hobbies, and enter-tainment as a result of excessive Internet use
7. Use of the Internet gaming to relieve dysphoria
8. Has deceived family members, therapists, or others regarding the amount of Internet use
9. Has jeopardized or lost a significant relation-ship, job, or educational or career opportunity because of excessive Internet use

32.8.5 Subtype of Internet Addiction

Young classifies Internet addiction into four subtypes:

- Net compulsions: online shopping and online gambling addictions
- Online game playing addiction
- Cybersexual addictions
- Cyber-relational addiction (chat rooms, social networking, personal messaging, and email addiction)

32.8.6 Psychiatric Comorbidity

- Anxiety
- Depression
- ADHD
- Alcohol misuse
- Fatigue
- Cognitive impairment in adolescents (Park et al., 2011)

32.8.7 Medical Complications

- Excessive daytime sleepiness
- Repetitive strain injury and backache
- Deep vein thrombosis
- Pulmonary embolus
- Collapse, exhaustion, and death

32.8.8 Management

32.8.8.1 Psychological Treatment

Behaviour therapy (Young et al., 2007; Flisher, 2010)

- Abstinence from Internet use.
- Practising the opposite: identifying the pat-tern of Internet use and replace by other activities.
- External stoppers: for example, an alarm clock to remind the patient that it is time to log off from the Internet.

- Reminder cards—negative consequences of Internet use are written down on a reminder card and carried by the patient all the time.
- Personal inventory—make a list of hobbies to replace Internet use.

32.8.8.2 Pharmacological Treatment

- Stimulants: Methylphenidate can be used to treat attention deficit and hyperkinetic disorder (ADHD) and reduce Internet addiction at the same time.
- Antidepressants: SSRIs (e.g. escitalopram) to reduce obsessions and compulsions associated with Internet use.
- Opioid antagonist: naltrexone.
- Mood stabilizers: lithium and sodium valproate.

32.8.8.3 Prognosis

One-year remission rate is 50%.

Poor prognosis factors include

- High exploratory excitability
- Low reward dependence
- Low self-esteem
- Low family function
- Online game playing

Good prognostic factors include

- Low hostility
- Low interpersonal sensitivity

REFERENCES

Abraham HD and Aldridge A. 1993: Adverse consequences of lysergic acid diethylamide. *Addiction* 88:1327.

Ait-Daoud N, Johnson BA, Prihoda TJ, and Hargita ID. 2001: Combining Ondansetron and Naltrexone treats biological alcoholics: Corroboration of self-reported drinking by serum carbohydrate deficient transferrin, a biomarker. *Alcohol Clinical Experiments and Research* 25:847–849.

Alcohol services for the community. http://www.alcohol-services.co.uk/images/bus-back.jpg (accessed on 31 July 2012).

American Psychiatric Association. 1994: *DSM-IV-TR: Diagnostic & Statistical Manual of Mental Disorders*, 4th edn. Washington, DC: American Psychiatric Association Publishing Inc.

American Psychiatric Association. 2013: *Desk Reference to the Diagnostic Criteria from DSM-5*. Washington, DC: American Psychiatric Association Press.

Babor TF, Higgins-Biddle JC, Saunders JB, and Monteiro MG. 2001: *The Alcohol Use Disorders Identification Test Guidelines for Use in Primary Care*, 2nd edn. Geneva, Switzerland: World Health Organization.

Baigent B, Holme G, and Hafner RJ. 1995: Self reports of the interaction between substance abuse and schizophrenia. *Australia and New Zealand Journal of Psychiatry* 29:6974.

Bebout RR, Drake RE, Xie H et al. 1997: Housing status among formerly homeless dually diagnosed adults. *Psychiatric Services* 48:936–941.

Boys A, Farrell M, Taylor C, Marsden J, Goodman R, Brugha T, Bebbington P, Jenkins R, and Meltzer H. 2003: Psychiatric morbidity and substance use in young people aged 13–15 years: Results from the Child and Adolescent Survey of Mental Health. *British Journal of Psychiatry* 182:509–517.

Brady KT and Sonne SC. 1995: The relationship between substance abuse and bipolar disorder. *Journal of Clinical Psychiatry* 56:19–24.

Buckley PF. 1998: Substance abuse in schizophrenia: A review. *Journal of Clinical Psychiatry* 59:26–30.

Caldwell CR and Gottesman II. 1991: Sex differences in the risk for alcoholism: A twin study. *Behaviour Genetics* 21:563.

Cantwell R and Chick J. 1994: Alcohol misuse: Clinical features and treatment. In Chick J and Cantwell R (eds.) *Seminars in Alcohol and Drug Misuse*, pp. 126–155. London, U.K.: Gaskell.

Caspi A, Moffitt TE, Cannon M et al. 2005: Moderation of the Effect of Adolescent-Onset Cannabis Use on Adult Psychosis by a Functional Polymorphism in the Catechol-O-Methyltransferase Gene: Longitudinal evidence of a gene X environment interaction. *Biological Psychiatry* 57(10):1117–1127.

Chilcoat HD and Breslau B. 1998: Investigation of causal pathways between PTSD and drug use disorders. *Addictive Behaviours* 23:827–840.

Cloninger CR. 1987: Neurogenetic adaptive mechanisms in alcoholism. *Science* 23:410–415.

CNS-forum. http:// www.cnsforum.com (accessed on 31 July 2012).

Cook C. 1994: Aetiology of alcohol misuse. In Chick J and Cantwell R (eds.) *Seminars in Alcohol and Drug Misuse*, pp. 94–125. London, U.K.:Gaskell.

Department of Health, Scottish Office Home and Health Department, Welsh Office. 1991: *Drug Misuse and Dependence: Guidelines on Clinical Management*. London, U.K.: HMSO.

Farrell M, Howes S, Taylor C et al. 1998: Substance misuse and psychiatric comorbidity: An overview of the OPCS national psychiatric comorbidity survey. *Addictive Behaviours* 23:909–918.

Flisher C. 2010: Getting plugged in: An overview of internet addiction. *Journal of Paediatrics and Child Health* 46(10):557–559.

Forrest D and McHale IG. 2011: Gambling and problem gambling among young adolescents in Great Britain. *Journal Gambling Studies* 28(4):607–622.

Fowler JS and Volkow ND. 2004: Neuroimaging in substance abuse research. In Charney DS and Nestler EJ (eds.) *Neurobiology of Mental Illness*. 2nd edn, pp. 740–752. New York: Oxford University Press.

Fu KW, Chan WS, Wong PW, and Yip PS. 2010: Internet addiction: Prevalence, discriminant validity and correlates among adolescents in Hong Kong. *British Journal of Psychiatry* 196(6):486–492.

Gelder M, Mayou R, and Cowen P. 2001: *Shorter Oxford Textbook of Psychiatry*. New York: Oxford University Press.

George S and Murali V. 2005: Pathological gambling: An overview of assessment and treatment. *Advances in Psychiatric Treatment* 11:450–456.

Glass IB. 1991: *The International Handbook of Addiction Behaviour*. London, U.K.: Routledge.

Goodwin DW, Hermansen L, Guze SB et al. 1973: Alcohol problems in adoptees raised apart from alcoholic biological parents. *Archives of General Psychiatry* 28:238–243.

Griffiths M, Wardle H, Orford J, Sproston K, and Erens B. 2009: Socio demographic correlates of internet gambling: Findings from the 2007. British gambling prevalence survey. *Cyberpsychology and Behaviour* 12(2):199–202.

Han DH, Lee YS, Na C, Ahn JY, Chung US, Daniels MA, Haws CA, and Renshaw PF. May–June 2009: The effect of methylphenidate on Internet video game play in children with attention-deficit/hyperactivity disorder. *Comprehensive Psychiatry* 50(3):251–256

Ho RC, Ho EC, and Mak A. 2009a: Cutaneous complications among i.v. buprenorphine users. *Journal of Dermatology* 36:22–29.

Ho RC, Ho EC, Tan CH, and Mak A. 2009b: Pulmonary hypertension in first episode infective endocarditis among intravenous buprenorphine users: Case report. *American Journal of Drug and Alcohol Abuse* 35(3):199–202.

Ho RCM, Chen KY, Broekman B, and Mak A. 2009c: Buprenorphine prescription, misuse and service provision: A global perspective. *Advances in Psychiatric Treatment* 15:354–363.

Home Office, United Kingdom. http://www.homeoffice.gov.uk/drugs/drugs-law/Class-a-b-c/ (accessed on 31 July 2012).

Hulse G. 2004: *Alcohol and Drug Problems*. Melbourne, Victoria, Australia: Oxford University Press.

Jarman CMB and Kellett JM. 1979: Alcoholism in the general hospital. *British Medical Journal* 2(6188):469–471.

Jasinski DR, Fudala PJ, and Johnson RE. 1989: Sublingual versus subcutaneous buprenorphine on opioid abusers. *Clinical Pharmacology and Therapeutics* 45:513–519.

Jaswrilla AG, Adams PH, and Hore BD. 1979: Alcohol and acute general medical admissions. *Health Trends* 11:95–97.

Johns A and Ritson B. 1994: Drug and alcohol-related problems. In Paykel ES and Jenkins R (eds.) *Prevention in Psychiatry*, pp. 103–114. London, U.K.: Gaskell.

Johnson BA, Roache JD, Javors MA et al. 2000: Ondansetron for reduction of drinking among biologically predisposed alcoholic patients: A randomized controlled trial. *Journal of American Medical Association* 284:963–971.

Johnstone EC, Cunningham ODG, Lawrie SM, Sharpe M, and Freeman CPL. 2004: *Companion to Psychiatric Studies*, 7th edn. London, U.K.: Churchill Livingstone.

Jones S and Roberts K. 2007: *Key Topics in Psychiatry*. Edinburgh, Scotland: Churchill Livingstone.

Kampman KM, Volpicelli JR, Mulvaney FD, Rukstalis M et al. 2002: Cocaine withdrawal severity and urine toxicology results from treatment entry predict outcome in medication trials for cocaine dependence. *Addictive Behaviours* 27:251–260.

Kendler KS. 1985: A twin study of individuals with both schizophrenia and alcoholism. *British Journal of Psychiatry* 147:48–53.

Ko CH, Yen JY, Yen CF, Chen CS, and Wang SY. 2008: The association between Internet addiction and belief of frustration intolerance: The gender difference. *Cyberpsychological Behaviour* 11(3):273–278.

Ko CH, Yen JY, Yen CF, Lin HC, and Yang MJ. 2007: Factors predictive for incidence and remission of internet addiction in young adolescents: A prospective study. *Cyberpsychological Behaviour* 10(4):545–551.

Kühlhorn E, Ramstedt M, Hibell B, Larsson S, and Zetterberg HL. 2000: Can the great errors of surveys measuring alcohol consumption be corrected? *Paper presented by Hans L Zetterberg at WAPOR Annual Meeting in Portland.*

LaPlante DA, Nelson SE, LaBrie RA, and Shaffer HJ. 2011: Disordered gambling, type of gambling and gambling involvement in the British Gambling Prevalence Survey 2007. *European Journal of Public Health* 21(4):532–537.

Lee KM, Chan HN, Cheah B, Gentica GF, Guo S, Lim HK, Lim YC et al. 2011: Ministry of Health clinical practice guidelines: Management of gambling disorders. *Singapore Medical Journal* June; 52(6):456–458

Lee YS, Han DH, Yang KC, Daniels MA, Na C, Kee BS, and Renshaw PF. 2008: Depression like characteristics of 5HTTLPR polymorphism and temperament in excessive internet users. *Journal of Affective Disorder* 109(1–2):165–169.

Lejoyeux M and Weinstein A. 2010: Compulsive buying. *American Journal of Drug and Alcohol Abuse* 36(5):248–253.

Li H, Borinskaya S, Yoshimura K, Kal'ina N et al. 2009: Refined geographic distribution of the oriental *ALDH2*504Lys* (nee *487Lys*) variant. *Annals of Human Genetics* 73:335–345.

Lin SC, Tsai KW, Chen MW, and Koo M. 2012: Association between fatigue and Internet addiction in female hospital nurses. *Journal of Advanced Nursing* 69:374383. [Epub ahead of print].

Lobo DS and Kennedy JL. 2009: Genetic aspects of pathological gambling: A complex disorder with shared genetic vulnerabilities. *Addiction* 104(9):1454–1465.

Malhi G and Malhi S. 2006: *Examination Notes in Psychiatry. Basic Sciences*, 2nd edn. London, U.K.: Hodder Arnold.

Marsden J, Gossop M, Stewart D et al. 2000: Psychiatric symptoms among clients seeking treatment for drug dependence intake data from the National Treatment Outcome Research Study. *British Journal of Psychiatry* 176, 285–289.

Mattick RP and Heather N. 1993: Developments in cognitive and behavioural approaches to substance misuse. *Current Opinion in Psychiatry* 6:424–429.

McBride O, Adamson G, and Shevlin M. 2010: A latent class analysis of DSM-IV pathological gambling criteria in a nationally representative British sample. *Psychiatry Research* 30:178(2):401–407.

McCloud A, Barnaby B, Omu N, Drummond C, and Aboud A. 2004: Relationship between alcohol use disorders and suicidality in a psychiatric population: In-patient prevalence study. *British Journal of Psychiatry* 184:439–445.

Miller WR and Sanchez VC. 1993: Motivating young adults for treatment and lifestyle change. In Howard G (ed.) *Issues in Alcohol Use and Misuse in Young Adults*. Notre Dame, IN: University of Notre Dame Press.

Montag C and Reuter M. 2008: Does speed in completing an online questionnaire have an influence on its reliability? *Cyberpsychology Behaviour* 11(6):719–721.

Murali V and George S. 2007: Lost online: An overview of internet addiction. *Advances in Psychiatric Treatment* 13:24–30.

NICE. 2010: *Alcohol—Use Disorders*. London, U.K.: National Collaborating Centre for Chronic Conditions.

NHS Information Centre. 2009. Statistics on alcohol: England. Leeds: The Health and Social Care Information Centre.

NICE. *NICE Guidelines for Drug Misuse.* http://guidance.nice.org.uk/CG51and52 (accessed on 31 July 2012)

O'Brien CP and Cornish JW. 2004: Principles of the pharmacotherapy of substance abuse disorder. In Charney DS and Nestler EJ (eds.) *Neurobiology of Mental Illness*, 2nd edn, pp. 753–770. New York: Oxford University Press.

Olumoroti OJ and Kassim AA. 2005: *Patient Management Problems in Psychiatry*. London, U.K.: Elsevier Churchill Livingstone.

Pallanti S, Quercioli L, Sood E et al. 2002: Lithium and valproate treatment of pathological gambling: A randomised single-blind study. *Journal of Clinical Psychiatry* 63:559–564.

Park MH, Park EJ, Choi J, Chai S, Lee JH, Lee C, and Kim DJ. 2011: Preliminary study of Internet addiction and cognitive function in adolescents based on IQ tests. *Psychiatry Research* 190(2–3):275–281

Paton A. 1988: *ABC of Alcohol*, 2nd edn. London, U.K.: British Medical Journal.

Project MATCH Research Group. 1993: Project MATCH: Rationale and methods for a multisite clinical trial matching patients to alcoholism treatment. Alcoholism. *Clinical and Experimental Research* 17:1130–1145.

Raistrick DS and Davidson R. 1986: *Alcoholism and Drug Addiction*. Edinburgh, Scotland: Churchill Livingstone.

Regier DA, Rae DS, Narrow WE et al. 1998: Prevalence of anxiety disorders and their comorbidity with mood and addictive disorders. *British Journal of Psychiatry* 173:24–28.

Ries RK, Russo J, Wingerson D et al. 2000: Shorter hospital stays and more rapid improvement among patients with schizophrenia and substance use disorders. *Psychiatric Services* 51:210–215.

Royal College of Physicians. 2001: Alcohol—Can the NHS afford it? Recommendations for a coherent alcohol strategy for hospitals. London, U.K.: Royal College of Physicians.

Royal College of Psychiatrists. 1986: *Alcohol: Our Favourite Drug*. London, U.K.: Tavistock.

Sadock BJ and Sadock VA. 2003: *Kaplan and Sadock's Comprehensive Textbook of Psychiatry*, 9th edn. Philadelphia, PA: Lippincott Williams & Wilkins.

Singleton N and Lewis G. 2003: *Better or Worse: A Longitudinal Study of the Mental Health of Adults Living in Private Households in Great Britain*. London, U.K.: The Stationery Office.

Solowij N. 1993: Ecstasy (3,4-methylenedioxymethamphetamine). *Current Opinion in Psychiatry* 6:411–415.

Strang J, Sheridan J, Hunt C et al. 2005: The prescribing of methadone and other opioids to addicts: National survey of GPs in England and Wales. *British Journal of General Practitioners* 55:444–451.

Stuppaeck CH, Barnas C, Falk M, Guenther V, Hummer M et al. 1994: Assessment of the alcohol withdrawal syndrome: Validity and reliability for the translated and modified Clinical Institute Withdrawal Assessment for Alcohol Scale (CIWA-A). *Addiction* 89(10):1287–1292.

Tabakoff B and Hoffman PL. 1993: The neurochemist. *Psychiatry* 6:388–394.

Taylor C, Brown D, Duckitt A et al. 1985: Patterns of outcome: Drinking histories over ten years among a group of alcoholics. *British Journal of Addiction* 80:45–50.

Taylor D, Paton C, and Kapur S. 2009: *The Maudsley Prescribing Guideline*, 10th edn. London, U.K.: Informa healthcare.

Training Centre for Alcohol and Drugs. http://www.alcohol-drugs.co.uk/themes/Cycle%20of%20Change.htm (accessed on 31 July 2012).

U.K. guidelines on clinical management. 2007: *Drug Misuse and Dependence*. London, U.K.: Department of Health.

U.K. ATT Research Team. 2005: Effectiveness of treatment for alcohol problems: Findings of the randomised UK alcohol treatment trial (UKATT). *BMJ* 331:541.

van Holst RJ, van den Brink W, Veltman DJ, and Goudriaan AE. 2010: Brain imaging studies in pathological gambling. *Current Psychiatry Reports* 12(5):418–425.

Victor M, Adams RD, and Collins GH. 1971: *The Wernicke–Korsakoff Syndrome*. Oxford, U.K.: Blackwell.

Winston AP, Hardwick E, and Jaberi N. 2005: Neuropsychiatric effects of caffeine. *Advances in Psychiatric Treatment* 11:432–439.

World Health Organisation. 1992: *ICD-10: The ICD-10 Classification of Mental and Behavioural Disorders: Clinical Descriptions and Diagnostic Guidelines*. Geneva, Switzerland: World Health Organisation.

Wallace P. 1999: *The Psychology of the Internet*. Cambridge, U.K.: Cambridge University Press.

Young KS. 1999: Internet addiction: Symptoms, evaluation and treatment. In VandeCreek L and Jackson T (eds.) *Innovations in Clinical Practice: A Source Book*, pp. 1–17. Sarasota, FL: Professional Resource Exchange.

Young KS. 2007: Cognitive behaviour therapy with Internet addicts: Treatment outcomes and implications. *Cyberpsychology Behaviour* 10(5):671–679.

Zhou Y, Lin FC, Du YS, Qin LD, Zhao ZM, Xu JR, and Lei H. 2011: Gray matter abnormalities in Internet addiction: A voxel-based morphometry study. *European Journal of Radiology* 79(1):92–95.

33 Disorders Specific to Women and Perinatal Psychiatry

33.1 PREMENSTRUAL SYNDROME

33.1.1 EPIDEMIOLOGY OF PMS

Forty per cent of women experience some cyclical premenstrual symptoms; 2%–10% report severe symptoms. There are associations with the following:

- There is a higher prevalence in those around 30 years of age.
- Prevalence increases with increasing parity.
- There is a higher prevalence in those women who have experienced natural menstrual cycles (unmodified by oral contraceptives and uninterrupted by pregnancy) for longer periods of time.
- Women using oral contraceptives, especially if nulliparous, have reduced rates of premenstrual syndrome (PMS).
- Prevalence is increased in those experiencing higher levels of psychosocial stress.

33.1.2 AETIOLOGY OF PMS

33.1.2.1 Genetic Factors

Highly significant correlations between mother and daughter have been reported on a variety of menstrual variables including premenstrual tension.

Condon (1993) reported concordances for global PMS scores:

- 0.28 in dizygotic (DZ) twin pairs
- 0.55 in monozygotic (MZ) twin pairs

Concordances for MZ twins exceeded those of DZ twins on every subscale. The findings support the hypothesis that the familial aggregation of PMS symptoms is determined largely by genetic factors.

33.1.2.2 Neuroendocrine Factors

33.1.2.2.1 Beta-Endorphin

Anxiety, food cravings, and physical discomfort in PMS subjects are associated with a significant decline in β-endorphin (these symptoms are also found in opiate withdrawal).

33.1.2.2.2 Serotonin

Postsynaptic serotonergic responsivity is altered during the late luteal phase of the menstrual cycle. It is thought that gonadal hormones cause changes in the levels of activity of serotonergic systems. Carbohydrate craving and depression are linked to serotonergic brain changes, which are marked in the late luteal phase.

Plasma taken from subjects suffering from PMS inhibits serotonin uptake in rat brain synaptosomes to a greater degree than serum taken from controls.

33.1.2.2.3 Noradrenaline

3-Methoxy-4-hydroxyphenylglycol (MHPG, a metabolite of noradrenaline) in cerebrospinal fluid is elevated in PMS subjects premenstrually.

33.1.2.2.4 Androgens

Serum androgens are higher in women with premenstrual irritability and dysphoria than in controls. Serum-free testosterone levels are significantly higher in PMS subjects than in matched controls around ovulation, and 17-hydroxyprogesterone levels are higher in PMS women in the luteal phase.

33.1.2.2.5 Others

Various hypotheses have been explored, particularly in relation to the balance between oestrogen and progesterone with a relative lack of progesterone and excessive production of prolactin, aldosterone, or antidiuretic hormone. None are conclusive.

33.1.2.3 Neurophysiological Factors

The following have been reported:

- There are consistent cycle-dependent changes in electroencephalographic recordings, most prominent in the α range.
- There are alterations in response to dichotic auditory stimuli premenstrually in comparison with the follicular phase, most markedly in sufferers of PMS.

- There are alterations in skin conductance in response to auditory stimuli premenstrually in comparison with the follicular phase, most markedly in sufferers of PMS.

33.1.2.4 Personality Factors

Neuroticism may be an important determinant of women's experiences and reports of their menstrual cycle and is higher in those reporting PMS.

Women with coronary-prone type A behaviour experience 50% more PMS symptoms than women with noncoronary-prone type B behaviour.

33.1.2.5 Psychological Factors

Psychological views of PMS attribute it to an impoverishment of the ego in relation to feminine self-acceptance and identification with the mother. It is suggested that popular beliefs that derogate femininity are internalized and form part of the socialization of women.

Self-report of PMS is strongly related to psychosocial stress, particularly unusual stress and unhappy relationships.

33.1.3 SYMPTOMS OF PMS

PMS includes emotional and/or physical symptoms occurring premenstrually (late luteal phase) but remitting usually during the week before menstruation (follicular phase).

More than 150 symptoms have been implicated in PMS. There are considerable differences in the patterns of symptoms, but there is strong support for cycle-related variability in most subjects. The existence of PMS as a discrete entity has often been questioned; there is a lack of consensus about its definition.

The common symptoms experienced by those women suffering PMS are listed in Table 33.1.

33.1.4 MANAGEMENT OF PMS

Treatment should be supportive and directed towards symptom relief, psychosocial support, stress reduction, and dietary change.

33.1.4.1 Nonpharmacological Treatment

- Special diets: increasing complex carbohydrates and dietary fibre to 20–40 g/day
- Decrease intake of refined sugar and salt
- Cognitive therapy
- Exercise
- Relaxation

TABLE 33.1

Common Symptoms Experienced by Women Suffering PMS

Mood Symptoms	Other Symptoms
Irritability	Bloated abdomen
Easily angry or upset without good reason	Tender breasts
	Carbohydrate craving
Tension	Disturbed sleep
Emotional lability	Poor concentration
Depressed mood	Clumsiness
Violent feelings	Headaches
	Muscle and joint pain
	Spots

33.1.4.2 Pharmacological Treatment

No single medication has proven effective in the treatment of PMS.

33.1.4.2.1 Antidepressants

Favourable results are sometimes found particularly when a serotonergic antidepressant is used. Psychic, but not somatic, symptoms improve. A 70% reduction in premenstrual irritability and depressed mood is found using clomipramine, compared to a 45% reduction with placebo. Similar results have been obtained using fluoxetine, adding support to the hypothesis that a serotonergic imbalance is involved in premenstrual psychic symptoms.

33.1.4.2.2 Oral Contraceptive Pill

Somatic symptoms are improved but psychic symptoms are not. Oestrogenic effects are thought to exacerbate premenstrual irritability, and progestogenic effects exacerbate premenstrual depression.

Oral contraceptive users report significantly less menstrual pain and premenstrual breast tenderness than controls but also show significantly less improvement in negative mood during the menstrual phase than nonusers.

33.1.4.2.3 Gamma Linolenic Acid

Gamma linolenic acid (GLA), an n-6 essential fatty acid, has been reported to help with several PMS symptoms, such as mastalgia. It is found in products such as evening primrose oil.

33.1.4.2.4 Other Treatments

Other treatments used for which there are conflicting reports of efficacy include

- *Alprazolam*—some reports of usefulness, but double-blind placebo-controlled trial showed absence of any therapeutic benefit.

- *Hysterectomy*—no change in cyclical mood following hysterectomy.
- *Vitamin B6*—produces a reduction in prolactin synthesis; use advocated, but little evidence of improvement in PMS symptoms
- *Progesterones*—use advocated, but little evidence of improvement in PMS symptoms.
- *Diuretics*—produce some relief in symptoms of bloatedness but no improvement in psychic symptoms.
- *Bromocriptine*—effective only in the relief of breast symptoms.

33.2 CYCLIC PSYCHOSIS

A few reports of cyclic psychoses related to menstruation exist in the literature. Psychotic symptoms appear suddenly a few days before menstruation, resolve with the onset of menstrual bleeding, and reappear with the next cycle. Between psychotic episodes, the woman appears largely asymptomatic. Most cases do not show familial psychiatric morbidity. The first psychotic episode usually occurs at a young age.

The psychiatric picture is nonspecific and changes with every menstruation. Some common features include psychomotor retardation, anxiety, perplexity, disorientation, and amnestic features. Transitory EEG abnormalities may occur, not amounting to epileptic activity.

It has been suggested that in some cases menstrual psychoses should be regarded as a specific variant of PMS.

Recommended treatments for menstrual cyclic psychosis include

- Bromocriptine that reduces prolactin
- Progesterone that inhibits ovulation
- Clomiphene citrate
- Acetazolamide, a diuretic
- Psychotropic medications (results inconclusive)

The prognosis is good, and spontaneous remission is usual.

33.3 PREGNANCY

33.3.1 MISCARRIAGE

Miscarriage occurs in 12%–15% of clinically recognized pregnancies. About one-half are associated with chromosomal abnormalities. Other recognized causes include uterine malformation, cervical incompetence, trauma, infection, endocrine disorder, toxins, irradiation, and immune dysfunction.

Animal evidence shows that stress leads to abortion in a number of mammalian species including baboons.

O'Hare and Creed (1995) studied the relationship between life events and miscarriage in 48 case–control pairs matched for known predictors of miscarriage. They found that the miscarriage group was more likely to have experienced

- A severe life event in the 3 months preceding miscarriage
- A major social difficulty
- Life events of severe short-term threat in the fortnight immediately beforehand

Fifty-four per cent of the miscarriage group had experienced some psychosocial stress, compared to only 15% of controls.

Other factors significantly associated with miscarriage include

- Childhood maternal separation
- Poor relationships with partners
- Few social contacts

Stress-induced abortion may involve increased catecholamine levels and α-adrenergic stimulation of the myometrium. Serotonin, implicated in stress responses, promotes abortion. This may be mediated via reduced gonadotropin output.

In the management of recurrent miscarriage, a psychosocial history should be taken in order to ascertain any sources of stress amenable to social intervention.

33.3.1.1 Consequences of Miscarriage

A high percentage of women experience profound loss following miscarriage, reporting symptoms typical of the grief that follows bereavement. Friedman and Gath (1989) found that at 4 weeks after miscarriage 48% of women were psychiatric cases as measured on the PSE, all suffering depressive disorders. Many of the women were already recovering at this time.

Symptoms are increased in women who have experienced a previous miscarriage. Many women are fearful of experiencing loss in a future pregnancy.

Other factors increasing women's vulnerability to developing depressive symptoms are lack of a supportive partner, childlessness, neuroticism, and previous psychiatric consultation.

Psychiatric morbidity can persist for several months. The duration of bereavement reaction is appreciably shortened by support and counselling.

33.3.2　Termination of Pregnancy

Psychological disturbance occurring in association with therapeutic abortion is severe or persistent in only a minority, about 10% of women. Depression and anxiety are most common with psychosis reported very uncommonly, in 0.003% of cases. Of the latter, most have a previous psychiatric history.

Women at greater risk of adverse psychological sequelae include

- Those with a previous psychiatric history
- Younger women
- Those with poor social support
- Those from cultural groups opposed to abortion

About one-third of women experience feelings of loss, guilt, and self-reproach at 6 months after abortion, particularly those ambivalent towards the termination of pregnancy. Those requiring therapeutic abortion because of fetal abnormalities or medical complications have poorer psychological outcomes.

Gilchrist et al. (1995) studied psychiatric morbidity following termination of pregnancy compared with other outcomes of unplanned pregnancy in a large prospective cohort study. They found

- Rates of total psychiatric disorder were no higher after termination of pregnancy than after childbirth.
- Women with a previous psychiatric history were most at risk of disorder after the end of their pregnancy, whatever its outcome.
- Women without a past history of psychosis had a lower risk of psychosis after termination than after childbirth.
- In women without a past psychiatric history, deliberate self-harm was more common in those who were refused a termination (relative risk = 2.9) or who had a termination (relative risk = 1.7).
- There was no overall increase in psychiatric morbidity in those having a termination of pregnancy.

33.3.3　Mental Disorders in Pregnancy

33.3.3.1　Minor Mental Illness

There is an increased risk of minor mental illness in the first trimester. This usually resolves spontaneously by the second trimester, so reassurance and psychological interventions are usually most appropriate.

Benzodiazepines should be avoided particularly in the first and third trimesters.

33.3.3.2　Major Mental Illness

It was previously believed that pregnancy offered protection against mental illness. It is now known that this is not the case. The prevalence of depression in pregnancy is high.

It is always best to avoid drugs in pregnancy if possible. Stable patients may often be withdrawn from medication before conception. In those with great risks of relapse, a judgement has to be made about the relative risk of relapse against the relative risk of taking medication.

If there is a need to prescribe psychotropic drug, the dose should be maintained at a minimum during the first and second trimesters. The dose needs to be increased in the third trimester as a result of expansion of blood volume. It is best to withdraw anticholinergics if possible since the risk of teratogenesis in humans is inconclusive.

The NICE guidelines and Maudsley's guidelines (2012) have made recommendations of psychotropic medications for major psychiatric disorders. The recommendations are summarized as follows.

33.3.3.2.1　*Depressive Disorder and Pregnancy (Table 33.2)*

The NICE and Maudsley's guidelines recommend the following:

1. Consider cognitive behavioural therapy (CBT) or interpersonal therapy (IPT) as first-line treatment.
2. Consider antidepressant if it is preferred by the patient.
3. Consider another monotherapy or electroconvulsive therapy (ECT) before combination of antidepressants.

33.3.3.2.2　*Bipolar Disorder and Pregnancy (Table 33.3)*

The NICE and Maudsley's guidelines recommend the following:

TABLE 33.2

Drug Choices for Depressive Disorder in Pregnancy

Effect on Fetus	TCA	SSRI	Not Recommended
SSRI causes pulmonary hypertension (after 20 weeks) in the newborn The neonates may experience withdrawal (agitation and irritability) especially with paroxetine and venlafaxine	☑ Amitriptyline and imipramine TCAs have been used for many years without causing teratogenic effects The use of TCAs in the third trimester may lead to withdrawal effects and increase the risk of preterm delivery	☑ Fluoxetine has the most data on safety ☒ Paroxetine is associated with fetal heart defects in the first trimester and is less safe as compared to other SSRIs. Sertraline may reduce the Apgar score SSRIs are associated with reduction in the gestational age, reduction in birth weight, and spontaneous abortion	☒ Bupropion Mitrazapine Moclobemide Reboxetine Trazodone Venlafaxine (associated with hypertension in high dose and toxicity in overdose) These drugs are not recommended because of the lack of safety data

Source: Taylor, D. et al., *The Maudsley Prescribing Guidelines*, Wiley-Blackwell, West Sussex, U.K., 2012.
☑, recommended; ☒, not recommended.

TABLE 33.3

Drug Choices for Bipolar Disorder in Pregnancy

Effect on Mother and Fetus	Mania	Bipolar Depression	Not Recommended
The risk of relapse is high if medication is stopped abruptly Lithium: Incidence of the Ebstein's anomaly is between 0.05% and 0.1% after maternal exposure to lithium in the first trimester Valproate: Incidence of fetal birth defect (mainly neural tube defect) is 1 in 100 Carbamazepine: Incidence of fetal birth defect is 3 in 1000	☑ Mood stabilizing antipsychotics • Haloperidol • Olanzapine (increase risk of gestational diabetes) ECT is indicated if antipsychotic fails	☑ CBT for moderate bipolar depression Fluoxetine has the most data on safety and indicated for severe bipolar depression, especially for those patients with very few previous manic episodes	☒ Valproate is the most teratogenic mood stabilizer and should not be combined with other mood stabilizers ☒ Lamotrigine requires further evaluation because it is not routinely prescribed in pregnancy. Lamotrigine causes oral cleft (9 in 1000) and Stevens–Johnson syndrome in infants

Source: Taylor, D. et al., *The Maudsley Prescribing Guidelines*, Wiley-Blackwell, West Sussex, U.K., 2012.
☑, recommended; ☒, not recommended.

1. Treat with an antipsychotic if patient has an acute mania or if she is stable.
2. Consider ECT or mood stabilizer if the patient does not respond to an antipsychotic.
3. If lithium is used, the woman should undergo level 2 ultrasound of the fetus at 6 and 18 weeks' gestation.
4. If carbamazepine is used, prophylactic vitamin K should be administered to the mother and neonate after delivery.
5. The treatment of bipolar depression follows the recommendation of treatment for depression.

33.3.3.2.3 Schizophrenia and Pregnancy (Table 33.4)

The NICE and Maudsley's guidelines recommend the following:

1. Consider switching from an atypical antipsychotic to a low-dose typical antipsychotic.

TABLE 33.4

Drug Choices for Psychosis or Schizophrenia in Pregnancy

Effect on Mother and Fetus/Neonate	Antipsychotics and Other Treatments	Not Recommended
Prior to pregnancy, avoid drugs (e.g. risperidone and sulpiride) that cause hyperprolactinaemia	☑ Chlorpromazine	☒ Depot antipsychotics
Low risk of relapse if antipsychotic is continued with good social support	Trifluoperazine	Anticholinergic drugs
Antipsychotic discontinuation syndrome occurs in the neonate, and mixed breast-/bottle-feeding can minimize withdrawal	Haloperidol	Clozapine (causing agranulocytosis in fetus)
	Olanzapine (gestation DM and weight gain)	
	Quetiapine	

Source: Taylor, D. et al., *The Maudsley Prescribing Guidelines*, Wiley-Blackwell, West Sussex, U.K., 2012.
☑, recommended; ☒, not recommended.

CASC STATION ON PREGNANCY AND USE OF LITHIUM

A 30-year-old lady wants to consult you on the management of bipolar disorder. She is 8-week pregnant. She has history of bipolar disorder, and she takes lithium CR 800 mg every night.

Task: Discuss with the patient on the specific issues that arise in the use of lithium during pregnancy.

Approach to this CASC station

1. The use of psychotropic medication during pregnancy requires careful risk and benefit analysis especially in the first trimester when major organs are formed in the fetus. The psychotropic medication in general plays a role as prophylactic or symptomatic treatment.

2. Candidates need to assess her current mood status (happy or depressed) and inquire whether her pregnancy is planned or unplanned. Past psychiatric history should be explored with special focus on precipitants and severity of previous episodes, previous outcomes of reducing or stopping lithium, past suicide attempts, previous pregnancies and complications, smoking habits, past or current substance abuse, and current social and environmental factors, including support network.

3. There are generally six different approaches:
   a. Continue lithium at current dose if there is high risk of relapse or at the lowest effect dose.
   b. Switch to an antipsychotic gradually such as haloperidol and expose the fetus as few drugs as possible.
   c. Consider ECT if antipsychotics fail.
   d. Stop lithium gradually in the first trimester and resume lithium in the second trimester.
   e. Avoid all psychotropic drugs throughout the pregnancy if the patient is well and at low risk of relapse.
   f. If she is predominantly depressed rather than manic, consider CBT for moderate depression and prescribing an SSRI for more severe depression. The candidate should inform the patient the possible risk to switch to mania. In this station, the candidate is expected to help the patient to make an informed decision.

4. If the patient chooses to continue lithium, the candidate should inform the risk of fetal heart defects (6 in 100) and Ebstein's anomaly (1 in 2000). Stopping lithium at this stage does not remove the risk of malformations.

5. The candidate needs to assess patient's commitment to come back for regular follow-up and monitoring. She needs to check serum levels every 4 weeks, then weekly from the 36th weeks, and within

1 day after childbirth. The regular blood monitoring is important because it will guide the psychiatrist to adjust the dose of lithium and keep the serum lithium levels towards the lower end of the therapeutic range. The candidate should advise the patient to maintain adequate fluid intake.

6. Explore her view on nonpharmacological interventions (e.g. CBT).

7. The candidate needs to find out the current antenatal care and liaise with the obstetrician to ensure adequate fetal screening. The patient needs to undergo level 2 ultrasound of the fetus at 6 and 18 weeks' gestation to screen for Ebstein's anomaly. During delivery, the obstetrician needs to be aware that fetal goitre may press on the fetal trachea and leads to a potential complication during delivery. For patients prescribed with valproate or carbamazepine, they should receive prophylactic folic acid. Prophylactic vitamin K is required to the mother and neonate if carbamazepine is used.

8. If the patient is prescribed with other psychotropic medications, the patient should be given adequate information on the risks and benefits of the particular medication. The psychiatrist needs to obtain an informed consent prior to prescription, and the patient must fully understand the options of other treatments or no treatment. The dose of the medication may need to be increased in the third trimester. There is an increase in blood volume by 30% towards the end of pregnancy, which will affect the distribution of medication. The CYP 1A2 and 2D6 activities increase by more than 50%, and this will affect the metabolism of medication.

9. If lithium is continued or a new medication is started, the psychiatrist needs to monitor adherence and look for factors that may affect adherence. The nurse educator should provide information on the effects of medications on pregnancy, and midwife can help the patient to prepare for delivery.

10. If the patient chooses not to take any medication and she has high risk of relapse, inform her that risk of relapse and potential harm is through poor self-care, poor judgement, and impulsive behaviour. The relapse of mania may affect her fetus.

11. The candidate should advise the patient to quit smoking and drinking. She can switch to nicotine replacement therapy.

12. The candidate should seek permission from the patient to get her partner involved and offer more support to the patient.

13. Reassure the patient that there will be planned intervention to monitor herself and the newborn. During delivery, fluid balance and the risk of lithium toxicity will be monitored especially in prolonged labour. The risk of relapse is 1 in 3 in the first 90 days following childbirth. Additional measures such as augmentation with antipsychotic will be considered to prevent relapse in the postpartum period. The candidate should explore the expectation of the patient on breast-feeding and childcare after delivery.

CASC STATION ON PREGNANCY AND SUBSTANCE ABUSE

You are the psychiatrist working in a local addiction service. You are seeing a 25-year-old woman who is dependent on heroin. She is currently 8-week pregnant.

Task: Take a history to assess the extent of her substance abuse and address her concerns.
     You will speak to her husband in the next station.

Approach to this station
Substance abuse in pregnancy involves the excessive nontherapeutic use of recreational (e.g. alcohol, tobacco, heroin, cannabis, amphetamine) or prescribed drugs (e.g. benzodiazepines and analgesics) resulting in adverse effects on both the mother and her fetus. Such effects also depend on the trimester of pregnancy. Anticipated postnatal problems need to be addressed during the antenatal period.

(continued)

(A) Obtain Information about Current Pregnancy

(A1) Planning of the Pregnancy

'Can you tell me how you got pregnant this time? Was it planned or unplanned?' If it is unplanned, explore the underlying reasons (e.g. failure in contraceptives) 'Who is the father of the fetus? Can you tell me more about him?'

(A2) Assess her Desire to Continue Pregnancy and Assess her View on Motherhood

'How do you feel of being a mother? Are you looking forward to see your baby?'

(A3) Current Antenatal Care

'Do you see a GP? Is your GP aware of this pregnancy? Have you seen by any obstetrician or midwife?'

(A4) Antenatal Care and Outcome of Previous Pregnancies

Explore previous fetal viability and abnormality. Assess her adherence in previous antenatal visits

(B) Substance Abuse History

(B1) Explore the Types of Substances Previously Used

Including opiate and nonopiate (e.g. cannabis, amphetamine), prescribed medication such as benzodiazepine and analgesics, cough medicine, smoking habit, and alcohol misuse.

(B2) Explore Previous Dependence and Withdrawal Symptoms

'In the past few years, is there any change in dosage or pattern of heroin usage?' 'What would happen if you stop using the heroin? Do you experience teary eyes, runny nose, yawning, or tummy pain?'

(B3) Previous Contact with Local Drug Services

'Have you undergone any treatment programme with local drug service? What is the outcome?' (Explore treatment nihilism.) 'Can you tell me the length of the longest period without using heroin?' (abstinence period) 'What was the reason for relapse?' 'Have you heard about methadone? What is your experience with methadone?' 'If methadone is safe for yourself and your fetus, are you keen to try?'

(B4) Current usage of Heroin and other Drugs and Assess Motivation

'Can you tell me when was your last injection of heroin?' 'How often do you inject heroin nowadays?' 'How much do you usually inject?' 'Do you mix heroin with other substances?' 'What is your view of using heroin in pregnancy? Do you have any concern?' 'Do you want to replace heroin with methadone?'

(C) Complications Associated with Heroin Misuse and Risk Assessment

(C1) Physical Complications

Explore the status of blood-borne infections such as HBV, HCV, and HIV and complications associated with intravenous injection such as DVT and endocarditis Explore past medical history and reasons for previous hospitalization

(C2) Psychiatric Complications

Depression, suicide, and psychotic features 'Are you seeing a psychiatrist at this moment?' 'Are you taking any psychotropic medication?'

(C3) Legal or Forensic Complications

Current housing situation Explore previous imprisonment for drug-related offences and history of abusing children

(C4) Risk Assessment

'Have you ever harmed yourself? If so, how many times? What was the reason?' 'Do you still harbour any suicidal thought?' 'Has your partner been aggressive towards you?' 'Did you hurt yourself after taking too much drugs?' (e.g. head injury)

(D) Social Assessment and Address her Concerns	(D1) Assess her Current Support System and her Views about her Partner	(D2) Financial Situation	(D3) Care of other Children	(D4) Address her Concern
	'Is your partner looking forward to seeing your newborn?' 'Besides your partner, are there other people supporting you?'	'Do you work at this moment? How do you get your income? Have you worked as a commercial sex worker in exchange for money? If yes, do you practise safe sex? Are you receiving allowance from social welfare?'	'Do you have other children? Who is looking after them? How is your relationship with your children?'	'Thanks for talking to me. May I know whether you have other concerns?' (e.g. concerns about drug use, her own health, and issues related to the fetus)

After you have spoken to the patient, her partner is very keen to meet you because he is very concerned about her pregnancy.

Task: Explain the management plan to her partner assuming the patient has given you the consent to speak to him.

Approach to this CASC station
First, the candidate needs to seek the partner's view on the pregnancy and his view on fatherhood.

The basic principle is to consider a substitute (e.g. methadone) to minimize harm and manage the patient in a holistic care with the involvement of an addiction specialist, a neonatologist, and an obstetrician. This can take place at any stage of pregnancy and carries a much lower risk than continuing usage of heroin that may lead to withdrawal or overdose as a result of fluctuating opiate level (Table 33.5).

Reassure the partner that physical examination will be performed to assess her nutrition status and look for tattoos, needle marks, and signs of anaemia. Investigations such as full blood count (FBC), liver function test (LFT), renal function test (RFT), and urinary drug screen will be ordered. You will liaise with the obstetrician to perform an ultrasound scan to ensure fetal viability.

Short-term management includes establishing therapeutic alliance and stabilization of heroin intake by referring the patient to a methadone treatment programme. When the patient reaches the second trimester, the addiction specialist will withdraw the methadone over a period of 4 weeks. She will undergo regular monitoring by an obstetrician. The drug prevention worker or counsellor will work with the patient in relapse prevention by motivational interviewing and compliance therapy. Social worker will enhance other supports, and psychologist will offer supportive psychotherapy with focus on pregnancy issues. The psychiatrist will offer treatment for comorbid psychiatric disorders. Education will be offered to her partner and prepare him for the upcoming fatherhood. Prior to discharge, the social worker will be involved if the patient has difficulty to look after the newborn and other children. If there is history of child abuse, it may be necessary to seek a court order to protect the existing children and newborn. The candidate needs to stress to the partner that all decisions will be made in the best interest of the patient and the newborn.

Medium-term management includes establishing a delivery plan with input from all specialties. The psychiatrist will educate the patient on neonatal abstinence syndrome (NAS). Both the patient and the newborn will be transferred to the mother-and-baby unit after delivery. The psychiatrist will monitor her mood and look for signs suggesting postnatal depression and puerperal psychosis. Postnatal education involves advice on breast-feeding. Methadone is compatible with breast-feeding, and the dose should be less than 20 mg/day.

For long-term management, the psychiatrist will assess the patient after delivery and decide whether absolute detoxification or harm minimization technique is appropriate. Her GP will be informed of the outcome of delivery and ensure the well-being of the patient and her newborn in the community.

TABLE 33.5

Summary of the Maudsley's Guideline Recommendation of Detoxification of Opiate during Antenatal and Postpartum Period

First Trimester	Second Trimester	Third Trimester	Delivery and Postpartum
☑ Minimization of drugs that are harmful in the first trimester, for example, benzodiazepines, alcohol, and heroin Optimizing nutrition and supplementation with folate and iron tablets ☒ Detoxification in the first trimester is not recommended because opiate withdrawal in the first trimester may lead to spontaneous abortion	☑ If detoxification is required, it is best done in the second trimester Detoxification is safe and abstinence can be achieved in stable cases The use of methadone is recommended during the antenatal period Buprenorphine needs more data to support its safety in pregnancy	☑ Increase methadone dose because the metabolism will increase towards the end of pregnancy. Patient should be offered divided dose of methadone to prevent withdrawal The main objective during the delivery is to minimize withdrawal in the newborn and ensure assisted breathing for floppy and sedated newborn ☒ Detoxification is not recommended after 32 weeks because it may lead to preterm delivery and stillbirth	☑ Antenatal assessment by an anaesthetist is required to handle potential risks. The anaesthetist needs to decide on the analgesic requirements based on dose of methadone given Management of NAS Newborns who are born with mother dependent on opiate may develop vomiting and diarrhoea leading to dehydration and poor weight gain Other symptoms include • Excessive cry and sucking • Hyperreflexia • Increased in muscle tone • Fever

Source: Taylor, D. et al., *The Maudsley Prescribing Guidelines*, Wiley-Blackwell, West Sussex, U.K., 2012.
☑, recommended; ☒, not recommended.

33.4 PUERPERAL DISORDERS

33.4.1 GENERAL ISSUES

There are associations between the puerperal mental conditions. Severe postnatal blues can progress to postnatal depression; there may also be an association between postnatal blues and puerperal psychosis, since there is an excess of onset of the latter towards the end of the first week postpartum.

ICD-10 does not categorize puerperal mental disorders separately unless they do not meet criteria for disorders classified elsewhere. Thus, under the F50-59 'Behavioural syndromes associated with physiological disturbances and physical factors' is a section (F53) 'Mental and behavioural disorders associated with the puerperium, not elsewhere classified', which includes mild, severe, and other mental and behavioural disorders associated with the puerperium (WHO, 1992).

33.4.2 POSTNATAL BLUES

Postnatal blues is a brief psychological disturbance, characterized by tearfulness, emotional lability, and confusion in mothers occurring in the first few days after childbirth.

33.4.2.1 Epidemiology

It occurs in about 50% of women, peaking at the third to fifth day postpartum.

33.4.2.2 Aetiology

There is some evidence of links with biological factors, including

- A history of premenstrual tension.
- Serum calcium levels.
- Monoamines, serum tryptophan, and platelet a_2-adrenoceptors.
- Progesterone withdrawal postdelivery—women experiencing severe blues have higher antenatal progesterone levels, a steeper rise in the last 2 weeks of pregnancy, a bigger decrement from antenatal levels to the day of peak blues score, and lower progesterone levels on the day of peak blues.

Postnatal blues have also been positively associated with

- Poor social adjustment
- Poor marital relationship

- High scores on Eysenck Personality Inventory (EPI) neuroticism scale
- Fear of labour
- Anxious and depressed mood during pregnancy

There is no association between the development of postnatal blues and life events and demographic and social factors or obstetric factors.

Postnatal women differ significantly from women undergoing elective gynaecological surgery in the frequencies of different symptoms at different times, suggesting that postnatal mood swings are characteristic of the puerperium and are not simply nonspecific reactions to stress.

33.4.2.3 Clinical Features

Postnatal blue is associated with tearfulness, irritability, and anxiety.

33.4.2.4 Management

The woman should receive reassurance. No psychotropic medication is required and prognosis is good.

33.4.3 Postnatal Depression

Postnatal depression is a depressive illness not qualitatively different from nonpsychotic depression in other settings. It is characterized by low mood; reduced self-esteem; tearfulness; anxiety, particularly about the baby's health; and an inability to cope. Mothers may experience reduced affection for their baby and may have difficulty with breast-feeding.

33.4.3.1 Epidemiology

Postnatal depression occurs in 10%–15% of postpartum women usually within 3 months of childbirth. Those women who are emotionally unstable in the first week after childbirth are at an increased risk of developing postnatal depression.

Postnatal depression is not associated with parity.

33.4.3.2 Aetiology

33.4.3.2.1 Environmental Factors

Of the puerperal psychiatric conditions, postnatal depression has the least biological cause. Onset after childbirth is spread over a few months, and studies have repeatedly indicated the importance of social stress in its causation.

Paykel et al. (1980) found the strongest associated factor in mild postpartum depressives was the occurrence of recent stressful life events. Younger age, poor marital relationships, and absent social supports were also notable. Early postpartum blues were associated with postnatal depression in the absence of life events, suggesting a small subgroup of postnatal depression with a hormonal aetiology. A past psychiatric history was a strong risk factor with or without life events.

Murray et al. (1995) found that postnatal depression, but not control depression, was associated with a poor relationship with the woman's own mother.

Postnatal depression is more contingent upon the acute biopsychosocial stresses caused by the arrival of a child, whereas depression not associated with childbirth is more closely related to longer-term social adversity and deprivation.

33.4.3.2.2 Hormonal Factors

Despite the modest association between progesterone levels and postpartum blues, no direct association has been demonstrated between progesterone levels and postnatal depression.

Oestrogens affect dopaminergic transmission in the CNS; their precipitate drop after delivery may be responsible for psychosis and possibly also depression in predisposed women.

Puerperal women, whether depressed or not, are non-suppressors in terms of the dexamethasone-suppression test. However, no associations have been found between postnatal depression and cortisol.

Transient hypothyroidism, sometimes preceded by hyperthyroidism, occurs in up to 5% of women in the postpartum year, peaking at 4–5 months. Such postpartum thyroid dysfunction is associated with depression. It is estimated that 1% of postpartum women in the general population will experience a depressive episode associated with thyroid dysfunction.

33.4.3.3 Clinical Features

Common symptoms seen in the mother

1. Irritability, tearfulness, poor sleep, and tiredness
2. Feeling inadequate as a mother
3. Loss of confidence in mothering

Common symptoms related to the care and safety of the baby

1. Anxieties about the baby's health.
2. Expresses concerns that the baby is malformed and does not belong to her.

3. Reluctance to feed or handle the baby.
4. Forty per cent of patients have thought of harming the baby.

33.4.3.4 Management

The education of health visitors and midwives is necessary to identify cases early. The Edinburgh Postnatal Depression Scale is a 10-item self-report questionnaire, used by health visitors to identify postnatal depression during the course of their normal contacts with new mothers.

Nondirective counselling by health visitors individually or in groups is effective in one-third of cases. Self-help groups and mother-and-baby groups are useful to combat isolation.

In those with more severe symptomatology, or those unresponsive to counselling, antidepressants are required. If depression is severe, admission, preferably with the baby to a mother-and-baby unit, may be required. Suicidal mothers may have thoughts of taking their babies with them, so questions about the safety of the child should form part of the normal assessment of mothers of young children. ECT may be required, particularly if worthlessness, hopelessness, and despair are present.

Breast-feeding should not be routinely suspended. Tricyclic antidepressants are transmitted in reduced quantities in breast milk. They are, however, safe. Lithium is transmitted and should not be given to a breast-feeding mother because of the risk of toxicity to the child.

33.4.3.5 Outcome

If undetected, postnatal depression may last up to 2 years with serious consequences for the marital relationship and the development of the child. There is good evidence for a link between depressive disorders in mothers and emotional disturbance in their children.

The following are more frequent in the children of mothers suffering postnatal depression:

- Insecure attachment
- Behaviour problems
- Difficulties in expressive language
- Fewer positive and more negative facial expressions
- Mild cognitive abnormalities
- Less affective sharing
- Less initial sociability

Social and marital difficulties are often associated with reduced quality of mother–child interactions.

Cooper and Murray (1995) distinguished between those whose postnatal depression was a recurrence of previous affective disturbance and those for whom postnatal depression had arisen *de novo*. Those who were suffering from a recurrence of depression were at raised risk of further non-postpartum episodes but not postpartum episodes. Those for whom the depression had arisen *de novo* were at raised risk for further episodes of postnatal depression but not for non-postpartum episodes.

The relapse rate for subsequent nonpsychotic depression is 1 in 6.

33.4.4 PUERPERAL PSYCHOSIS

The risk of developing a psychotic illness is increased 20-fold in the first postpartum month. Certain symptoms that are distinctive are

- Abrupt onset, within the first 2 weeks after childbirth
- Marked perplexity, but no detectable cognitive impairment
- Rapid fluctuations in mental state, sometimes from hour to hour
- Marked restlessness, fear, and insomnia
- Delusions, hallucinations, and disturbed behaviour, which develop rapidly

33.4.4.1 Epidemiology

Kendell et al. (1987) linked psychiatric and obstetric registers in Edinburgh and found the number of admissions for psychotic disorders to be substantially elevated in the puerperium. This is shown in Table 33.6.

TABLE 33.6

Number of Admissions to Mental Hospitals per Month in the Pre- and Postpartum Periods

	Nonpsychotic	Psychotic
Fifteen months preconception	8	2
During pregnancy	5	2
First postpartum month	17	51
Second postpartum month	14	25
Third postpartum month	10	13
Fourth postpartum month	8	9
Fifth postpartum month	6	6
Mean for next 18 months	9	4

Eighty per cent of puerperal psychoses are affective. Schizophreniform psychoses often have manic features. Those with a previous history of manic–depressive illness have a substantially higher risk than those with a history of schizophrenia or depression.

The following factors are associated with women developing puerperal psychoses:

- Increased rate of Cesarean section
- Higher social class
- Older age at birth of first child
- Primiparae

Psychosis following childbirth is usually of an affective type with a particularly high proportion of manic episodes within the first 2 weeks.

Puerperal psychoses follow 20%–30% of births in those with preexisting bipolar mood disorders.

33.4.4.2 Aetiology

33.4.4.2.1 Genetic Factors

- Family studies of puerperal psychosis point to a familial aggregation of psychiatric disorder, particularly affective illness.
- Children of probands who have had puerperal psychosis have an increased psychiatric morbidity.
- Female relatives of puerperal probands have a higher rate of puerperal illness than the general population, but the majority of illness in the relatives of probands is nonpuerperal.
- The weight of evidence from clinical and family studies suggests that most cases of puerperal psychosis of early onset are closely related to bipolar disorder.

33.4.4.2.2 Environmental Factors

There is no evidence of any excess of life events in puerperal psychotics compared to matched normal puerperal controls. The absence of social stress in this group contrasts with the findings for postpartum depression and disorders with onset in pregnancy. These findings suggest that the aetiology of severe puerperal psychosis is predominantly biological and interactive with previous vulnerability.

33.4.4.2.3 Hormonal Factors

The pathophysiology of puerperal psychosis is not well understood, but it is likely that the precipitous fall in the levels of circulating sex steroid hormones such as oestrogen occurring at the time of parturition plays an important role.

In animals, the administration of oestrogen leads to increased striatal dopamine binding, and oestrogen withdrawal leads to dopamine receptor supersensitivity.

Wieck et al. (1991) have reported increased sensitivity of dopamine receptors in the hypothalamus associated with the onset of affective psychosis following childbirth. It is possible that these changes in sensitivity are mediated by changes in circulating oestrogen levels.

Supersensitivity of dopamine receptors is then thought to precipitate psychosis.

Common symptoms seen in the mother

1. Sleep disturbance in early stage.
2. Mild confusion, disorientation, and perplexity are common.
3. Affective lability often present with marked agitation and mania.
4. The clinical features may resemble affective disorders (70%), schizophreniform disorder (15%), and organic illness (15%).

Common symptoms related to the care and safety of the baby

1. Delusion may involve the baby and her family.
2. Suicidal and infanticidal thoughts may be present.

33.4.4.3 Management

The identification of high-risk patients during pregnancy is important in the planning of postnatal management. Admission to a psychiatric hospital is usually essential, and it is usually preferable to admit mothers with their babies.

The following are some advantages of joint admission:

- Most psychotic mothers are capable of looking after their babies with supervision and support.
- There is evidence suggesting that joint admission may reduce the duration of illness and relapse rates.

The following are some disadvantages of joint admission:

- There is a risk of nonaccidental injury to the child from the mother or fellow patients. A nurse should be dedicated to the care, and supervision of the child and a lockable nursery should be provided.

- Joint admission needs higher staffing levels.
- The long-term effects of admission upon the development of the child are not known.
- The woman's partner needs support and education.

33.4.4.3.1 Treatment

- Phenothiazines and lithium are effective in the treatment of manic episodes. Control of lithium levels in the immediate postpartum period can be difficult because of fluid and electrolyte changes.
- ECT is particularly effective in the treatment of puerperal psychoses and accelerates recovery in all diagnostic categories. It is used generally if the drug treatment has failed.
- In breast-feeding mothers, lithium is contraindicated because it is excreted into breast milk and is toxic to the baby.
- Neuroleptics can be administered to breast-feeding mothers, but high doses should be avoided, and the baby should be observed for signs of drowsiness, such as a failure to feed adequately.
- Neuroleptics should be maintained for at least 3 months following recovery. If there are further manic or depressive episodes, lithium should be considered.

33.4.4.4 Course

Following discharge from hospital, the mother will require close support and follow-up. An assessment of the mother–baby interaction should be made prior to discharge.

The initial prognosis is quite good. Cases often settle within 6 weeks, and most are fully recovered by 6 months. A few, however, have a protracted course.

After one episode of puerperal psychosis, the risk of a further episode in each subsequent pregnancy is between one in three and one in five. For those with a previous psychiatric history or a family history, the risk is higher; for those whose puerperal episode was associated with life events or Cesarean section, the subsequent risk is lower.

33.4.5 Breast-Feeding and Psychotropic Medication

Premature infants, infants with renal, hepatic, cardiac, and neurological impairments, are at a greater risk when they are exposed to psychotropic drugs. Hence, the lowest effective dose should be prescribed, and psychiatrist should avoid polypharmacy.

In order to avoid breast-feeding during the peak drug levels in breast milk, psychotropic drugs should be taken immediately after breast-feeding or before the infant's longest sleep period (Table 33.7).

TABLE 33.7

Summary of the Maudsley's Guideline Recommendation of Psychotropic Medications for Breast-Feeding

☑ Recommended Psychotropic Medications	☒ Psychotropic Medications That Are Not Recommended
Bipolar disorder ☑ Valproate can be used, but advise mother to ensure adequate contraception to prevent pregnancy	Bipolar disorder ☒ Lithium (concentration in breast milk is 50% of serum concentration). If patient is taking lithium during pregnancy, it will be necessary to augment with an antipsychotic during the postpartum period because the risk of relapse is high
Depressive disorder ☑ Paroxetine and sertraline TCA: Imipramine, nortriptyline, and sertraline are present in breast milk at relatively low levels	Depressive disorder ☒ Citalopram and fluoxetine are present in breast milk at relatively high levels
Schizophrenia ☑ Sulpiride and olanzapine	☒ Mirtazapine, venlafaxine
Anxiety and insomnia ☑ Lorazepam for anxiety and zolpidem for insomnia. Advise mother not to sleep with her baby to avoid suffocation accident on the newborn	Schizophrenia ☒ Clozapine, aripiprazole, quetiapine, risperidone, and depot antipsychotic (infants may show extrapyramidal side effects [EPSE])
Substance abuse ☑ Methadone is compatible with breast-feeding, but the dose should be kept as minimum	Bulimia nervosa ☒ No breast-feeding if patient is on high dose of fluoxetine

Source: Taylor, D. et al., *The Maudsley Prescribing Guidelines*, Wiley-Blackwell, West Sussex, U.K., 2012.

CASC STATION ON POSTPARTUM DEPRESSION AND PUERPERAL PSYCHOSIS

You are the psychiatric registrar working in liaison psychiatry. The gynaecologist referred a 30-year-old woman who is a mother of two daughters (a 2-year-old child and 11-month-old baby). She is currently 9-week pregnant and her partner is thrilled. The patient is not able to face another pregnancy, and she requests for an abortion. She has had two previous episodes of severe postnatal depression and managed by her GP. She admits to feeling tired, and the gynaecologist is concerned of her baby's safety.

Task: Take a history from the patient to establish the diagnosis of postpartum psychiatric illness.
    Perform a risk assessment.
    Although this station states that the patient suffers from postpartum depression, candidates will fail this station if they do not explore the symptoms of puerperal psychosis. Candidates are expected to listen in a warm and nonjudgemental manner to what the patient is presenting as the important issues for her. Her distress needs to be acknowledged.

(A) Explore the Issues on Abortion and Obtain More Information about Current Pregnancy	(A1) Clarify the Reason for Abortion	(A2) Explore the Expectation from her Partner	(A3) Issues Related to Abortion and Current Pregnancy	(A4) Risk Assessment Related to her Intention to abort the Fetus	(A5) Chronological History of Current Pregnancy
	'I am sorry to hear that you have gone through two difficult periods after delivery and current stress. Can you elaborate more on your intention to terminate the current pregnancy? Why do you want to go for an abortion?' (Explore transient stress, chronic psychiatric problem, or financial problems.)	'You have told the gynaecologist that your partner is thrilled. Can you tell me more about it? Is he hoping for a boy? Is he supporting you?' 'Does he know about your intention to go for an abortion?'	'Can you tell me more about your background, such as your religion and culture? Does abortion contradict your religious and cultural belief? If so, are you facing a lot of stress?'	'Did you have abortion before? If so, how many times? Was there any complication? How did you feel afterwards?' 'If other people like the gynaecologist or your partner does not support your request, will you do something harmful to the fetus?'	'Was the pregnancy planned or unplanned?' 'How did you know that you have become pregnant this time?' 'How did you feel after knowing the pregnancy test is positive? Do you find yourself in a difficult situation? If so, why?'

(B) Previous Pregnancies and Postpartum Illnesses	(B1) Past Antenatal History	(B2) Past Postnatal History	(B3) Postpartum Depression	(B4) Puerperal Psychosis **Delusions**	(B5) Current Symptoms
	'Can you tell me more about your experience during previous pregnancies?' 'Did you go for regular antenatal checkups? If not, what is the reason?'	'Can you tell me more about the delivery of your two children?' 'How were they delivered?' 'Did they have any complication during delivery?'	'How was your mood in the first 6 weeks after delivery?'	'Have you ever worried that someone wants to harm yourself and your baby?' 'Are you worried that there is something wrong with your baby? If yes, which aspects?'	'Are you still disturbed by the symptoms that you have mentioned? Is there any change in the frequency and severity? Which symptoms are most troubling?'

(continued)

'Did you suffer from any complication such as high blood pressure or diabetes during pregnancy? If so, were you admitted to the hospital?'
'Did you take medication during your previous pregnancy?'
'Did you use any substance including recreational drugs, alcohol, or cigarettes?'

'How did you feel after delivery?'
'Are you breast-feeding your 11-month-old baby at this moment?'

'Did you feel irritable? Did you cry very often? How was your sleep and appetite? Did you feel tired?'
'How do you see yourself as a mother? Are you confident in yourself? Does anyone offer help to look after your baby?'
'Were you admitted to the mother–baby unit? If so, what was the reason and for how long? How did you feel about the service?'

'Have you done something that may be harmful to your baby? If so, what have you done?' 'Have you ever thought that you are superior or special when compared to other people? If so, in what ways?'

Hallucinations
'Have you heard voices after delivery? If so, did the voices give you any instruction, such as telling you to harm your baby?'
'Have you suffered from any episode of confusion after delivery? How do you find your concentration at this moment?'

(Explore current psychotic symptoms, depressive symptoms, and manic symptoms)

(C) Past Psychiatric History and Risk Assessment

(C1) Past Psychiatric History
Explore history of mood disorder (especially bipolar disorder and the use of anticonvulsants).
'How do the others describe yourself as a person?' (Explore personality.)
'Do you know any family member suffering from psychiatric illness. If so, what kind of illness?'

(C2) Treatment of Previous Episodes
'Did the GP prescribe medication to treat postnatal depression?'
'Have you been continuing those medications?'
'Were you admitted to the psychiatric ward before? If so, why? Was the admission voluntary or involuntary?'

(C3) Insight
'What do you think is the cause of the earlier experiences? Do you think you will be unwell again? Do you find medication or talking therapy helpful?'

(C4) Parenting Ability
'Do you feel confident to look after your baby (e.g. feeding and bathing the baby)?'
'Was there any episode when you left your baby unattended? If yes, why did you do so?'
'Are you close to your baby? Do you feel your baby attach to you?'

(C5) Risk Assessment
'How is the health of your children? Do they have any behavioural problems?'
'When you are stressed, do you hit them? If yes, in what ways? Were they injured?'
'Do you have thought of harming yourself at this moment, how about your children?'

(D) Past History and Ending of Interview	(D1) Past Medical History	(D2) History of Contraception	(D3) Social History	(D4) Developmental History	(D5) Ending of Interview
	'Are you seeing your GP? How often do you see your GP?' (If patient is not seeing her GP, explore the underlying reason.) 'May I have your permission to speak to your GP?'	'Do you or your partner use contraception? If so, why did it fail this time? Will you use other contraceptive methods in the future?'	'What is your marital status? Can you tell me more about the quality of your relationship with your partner?' 'Do you hold a job at this moment? Are you on sick leave?' 'How is your financial status?'	'Can you tell me more about your childhood experience?' 'Can you tell me more about your parents? How do feel about them? Is such feeling affecting the way you treat your children?'	'I can imagine that it may be a difficult period for you because you need to make a very major decision. May I suggest that we shall invite your partner in the next session? Would it be alright with you?'

33.5 MENOPAUSE

33.5.1 AETIOLOGY

33.5.1.1 Biological Factors

The biological changes during menopause are summarized as follows:

- Reduction in oestrogen production
- Reduction of serotonin binding sites
- Increase in D_2 receptor sensitivity
- Reduction in the activity of endogenous opioid
- Increase in noradrenaline activity (associated with hot flushes)

33.5.1.2 Psychological Factors

- Negative self-image: dissatisfaction with self
- Premorbid personality: neurotic and dependent personality
- Psychological judgement: negative views towards menopausal symptoms
- Past psychiatric illness: depression and anxiety

33.5.1.3 Social Factors

- Social isolation: living on her own, poor social support, and empty nest syndrome (children leaving home for universities)
- Crisis in psychosocial development: crisis in maturity, leading to despair and disintegration according to Erikson's eight epigenetic stages

33.5.2 CLINICAL FEATURES

General population surveys indicate no major effect of the menopause on a variety of common psychiatric symptoms. If anything, women in the postmenopausal years show less evidence of psychiatric disturbance than younger women.

Hot flush (75%–85%) at night leads to sleep impairment, fatigue, and irritability.

Urogenital atrophy is the second most common manifestation of oestrogen deficiency. The alkaline environment in vagina may lead to vaginitis. Atrophy of vagina also leads to psychosexual problem such as dyspareunia.

33.5.3 MANAGEMENT

Anxiety and depression in postmenopausal women do not respond to oestrogen therapy but may respond to antidepressants such as SSRIs.

REFERENCES

Ashby CR, Carr LA, Cook CL et al. 1992: Inhibition of serotonin uptake in rat brain synaptosomes by plasma from patients with pre-menstrual syndrome. *Biological Psychiatry* 31:1169–1171.

Ballinger CB. 1990: Psychiatric aspects of the menopause. *British Journal of Psychiatry* 156:773–787.

Bancroft J and Rennie D. 1993: The impact of oral contraceptives on the experience of premenstrual mood, clumsiness, food craving and other symptoms. *Journal of Psychosomatic Research* 37:195–202.

Condon JT. 1993: The pre-menstrual syndrome: A twin study. *British Journal of Psychiatry* 162:481–486.

Cooper PJ and Murray L. 1995: Course and recurrence of postnatal depression: Evidence for the specificity of the diagnostic concept. *British Journal of Psychiatry* 166:191–195.

Craddock N, Brockington I, Mant R et al. 1994: Bipolar affective puerperal psychosis associated with consanguinity. *British Journal of Psychiatry* 164:359–364.

Dowlatshahi D and Paykel ES. 1990: Life events and social stress in puerperal psychoses: Absence of effect. *Psychological Medicine* 20:655–662.

Eriksson E, Sundblad C, Lisjo P et al. 1992: Serum levels of androgens are higher in women with pre-menstrual irritability and dysphoria than in controls. *Psychoneuroendocrinology* 17:195–204.

Friedman T and Gath D. 1989: The psychiatric consequences of spontaneous abortion. *British Journal of Psychiatry* 155:810–813.

Giannini AJ, Melemis SM, Martin DM et al. 1994: Symptoms of pre-menstrual syndrome as a function of beta-endorphin: Two subtypes. *Progress in Neuropsychopharmacology and Biological Psychiatry* 18:321–327.

Gilchrist AC, Hannaford PC, Frank P et al. 1995: Termination of pregnancy and psychiatric morbidity. *British Journal of Psychiatry* 167:243–248.

Hannah P, Adams D, Lee A et al. 1992: Links between early post-partum mood and post-natal depression. *British Journal of Psychiatry* 160:777–780.

Harris B. 1994: Biological and hormonal aspects of postpartum depressed mood: Working towards strategies for prophylaxis and treatment. *British Journal of Psychiatry* 164:288–292.

Hicks RA, Olsen C, and Smith Robinson D. 1986: Type A-B behaviour and the pre-menstrual syndrome. *Psychological Reports* 59:353–354.

Iles S, Gath D, and Kennerley H. 1989: Maternity blues: II. A comparison between post-operative women and post-natal women. *British Journal of Psychiatry* 155:363–366.

Jansson LM and Velez M. April 2012: Neonatal abstinence syndrome. *Current Opinion in Pediatrics* 24(2):252–258.

Kantero R and Widholm O. 1971: Correlations of menstrual traits between adolescent girls and their mothers. *Acta Obstetrica and Gynecologica Scandinavica* 14(Suppl. 14):30–36.

Kendell RE, Chalmers JC, and Platz CL. 1987: Epidemiology of puerperal psychoses. *British Journal of Psychiatry* 150:662–673.

Kennerley H and Gath D. 1989: Maternity blues: III. Associations with obstetric psychological and psychiatric factors. *British Journal of Psychiatry* 155:367–373.

Logue CM and Moos RH. 1986: Pre-menstrual symptoms: prevalence and risk factors. *Psychosomatic Medicine* 48:388–414.

Murray D, Cox JL, Chapman G et al. 1995: Childbirth: Life event or start of a long term difficulty? Further data from the Stoke-on-Trent controlled study of postnatal depression. *British Journal of Psychiatry* 166:595–600.

NICE. 2007: *NICE Guidelines for Antenatal and Postnatal Mental Health*. http://guidance.nice.org.uk/CG45 (accessed 22 July 2012).

O'Hare T and Creed F. 1995: Life events and miscarriage. *British Journal of Psychiatry* 167:799–805.

Olumoroti OJ and Kassim AA. 2005: *Patient Management Problems in Psychiatry*. London, U.K.: Elsevier Churchill Livingstone.

Paykel ES, Emms EM, Fletcher J et al. 1980: Life events and social supports in puerperal depression. *British Journal of Psychiatry* 136:339–346.

Pearce J, Hawton K, and Blake F. 1995: Psychological and sexual symptoms associated with the menopause and the effects of hormone replacement therapy. *British Journal of Psychiatry* 167:163–173.

Schmidt P, Grover GN, and Rubinow DR. 1993: Alprazolam in the treatment of pre-menstrual syndrome: A double-blind placebo-controlled trial. *Archives of General Psychiatry* 50:467–473.

Stein A, Gath DH, Bucher J et al. 1991: The relationship between post-natal depression and mother–child interaction. *British Journal of Psychiatry* 158:46–52.

Stein D, Hanukoglu S, Blank S et al. 1993: Cyclic psychosis associated with the menstrual cycle. *British Journal of Psychiatry* 163:824–828.

Sundblad C, Hedberg MA, and Eriksson E. 1993: Clomipramine administered during the luteal phase reduces the symptoms of pre-menstrual syndrome: A placebo controlled trial. *Neuropsychopharmacology* 9:133–145.

Taylor D, Paton C, and Kapur S. 2012: *The Maudsley Prescribing Guidelines in Psychiatry*, 11 edn. West Sussex, U.K.: Wiley-Blackwell.

Warner P and Bancroft J. 1990: Factors related to self-reporting of the pre-menstrual syndrome. *British Journal of Psychiatry* 157:249–260.

Wieck A, Kumar R, Hirst AD et al. 1991: Increased sensitivity of dopamine receptors and recurrence of affective psychosis after childbirth. *British Medical Journal* 303:613–616.

World Health Organization. 1992: *The ICD-10 Classification of Mental and Behavioural Disorders*, pp. 216–217. Geneva: WHO.

Zolese G and Blacker CVR. 1992: The psychological complications of therapeutic abortion. *British Journal of Psychiatry* 160:742–749.

34 Eating Disorders and Metabolic Syndrome

34.1 ANOREXIA NERVOSA

34.1.1 EPIDEMIOLOGY

Incidence and prevalence estimates vary depending on the diagnostic criteria used and the population studied. However, the following can be stated:

- It is rare (prevalence about 1–2 per 1,000 women). The Epidemiological Catchment Area (ECA) study found only 11 cases in 20,000 persons studied.
- The peak age of onset is 15–19 years.
- The incidence is 10 times higher in females compared to males.
- There is a higher prevalence in higher socioeconomic classes and Western Caucasians and a significant association with greater parental education. Rates in private schools are 1%—much higher than in state schools (0.15%). Rates are much higher again in ballet or modelling schools (7%).
- The clinical profile of eating disorders in Hong Kong has increasingly conformed to that of Western countries. Lee et al. (2010) studied eating-disordered patients presented to a tertiary psychiatry clinic between 1987 and 2007 and found that patients were predominantly single (91.8%), female (99.0%), and in their early 20s. The number of patients increased twofold in 20 years. Anorexia nervosa exhibited increasingly fat-phobic patterns, which resemble Western Caucasians.
- The suggestion of increasing prevalence over time is probably not supported, although greater numbers are coming to the attention of services.

34.1.2 AETIOLOGY

34.1.2.1 Genetic Factors

Family studies show an increased incidence of eating disorders among first- and second-degree relatives of those suffering from anorexia nervosa (AN).

Twin studies have shown higher concordance rates for monozygotic (MZ) than for dizygotic (DZ) twins. Holland et al. (1988) found an MZ-to-DZ concordance ratio of 56:5. Fairburn and Harrison (2003) reported that the concordance rates for MZ twins and DZ twins were 38%–55% and 0%–11%, respectively. Five per cent of first-degree relatives are affected. This suggests that genetic factors are significant in the aetiology. This study suggested that the heritability of AN is 80%. Linkage to genes controlling serotonin function on chromosome 1 and AN has been found.

Data suggest a familial component to AN, but the very low prevalence in the general population has prevented determination of whether this is genetic or environmental. There is a chance that genetic predisposition interacts with environmental factors and triggers the onset of AN.

Relatives also have higher rates of obsessive–compulsive disorders, generalized anxiety disorder, panic disorder, and substance misuse. There is an increased risk of mood disorders among first-degree biological relatives, particularly of those with binge-eating/purging type. The morbid risk of affective disorder in families of the eating disordered is similar to that of families of bipolar probands and is significantly greater than that in families of schizophrenics or those with borderline personality disorder. This supports growing evidence that AN and bulimia nervosa (BN) (see following text) are closely related to affective disorder.

34.1.2.2 Biological Factors

34.1.2.2.1 Neurotransmitters

Brain serotonin systems are implicated in the modulation of appetite, mood, personality variables, and neuroendocrine function. An increase in intrasynaptic serotonin reduces food consumption; a reduction in serotonin activity increases food consumption and promotes weight gain.

Kaye et al. (1991) found increased cerebrospinal fluid (CSF) concentrations of major serotonin metabolite 5-HIAA in long-term weight-restored anorectics, which may indicate an increased serotonin activity contributing to pathological feeding behaviour.

It has been suggested that amenorrhoea is caused by primary hypothalamic dysfunction. This is supported by the fact that a return to normal menstruation lags behind the return of body weight, and amenorrhoea sometimes precedes weight loss. This, however, is not proven.

Amenorrhoea is caused by abnormally low levels of oestrogen, because of the diminished pituitary secretion of follicle-stimulating hormone (FSH) and luteinizing hormone (LH). This is usually a consequence of weight loss, but, in a minority of individuals, it may actually precede it. In prepubertal females, menarche may be delayed.

34.1.2.2.2 Other Biological Factors
- Dopamine: A lower level of dopamine is released by striatum and leads to reduction in appetite.
- Brain-derived neutropenic factors (BDNF): The levels of BDNF are reduced in AN.
- Leptin: The levels of leptins are reduced in acute AN and associated with poor appetite.
- Premature birth, small for gestational age, and cephalhaematoma are risk factors for AN.

34.1.2.2.3 Physical Illness
An excess of physical illnesses in childhood has been found in those with AN. Physical illness may be a risk factor for the later development of AN, possibly by inducing pathology in the family dynamics.

Cases of AN have been reported with onset immediately related to a glandular fever-like illness. The disruption of the central corticotropin-releasing hormone (CRH) regulation has been suggested as the mediator of this.

34.1.2.3 Psychological Factors
Psychodynamic theories include fantasies of oral impregnation, dependent relationships with a passive father, and guilt over aggression towards ambivalently regarded mother.

Operant conditioning theories include phobic avoidance of food resulting from sexual and social tensions generated by physical changes associated with puberty.

34.1.2.3.1 Personality
Anorexics have a high prevalence of defined personality disorders and an excess of obsessive, inhibited, and impulsive traits. It is suggested that in an environment that emphasizes thinness as a criterion for self-worth, vulnerable individuals cope with the challenges of

adolescence by repetitive reward-seeking behaviour. Gymnasts, wrestlers, and swimmers have higher risk to develop subclinical AN.

Braun et al. (1994) found that 69% of eating-disordered patients had at least one personality disorder; these were also more likely to have an affective disorder or substance dependence than those without personality disorder.

Anorexics are more likely to suffer from anxious–avoidant personality disorders (cluster C), whereas dramatic–erratic personality disorders (cluster B) are more common in bulimics.

Other psychological factors:

- Childhood obesity and teasing by classmates or teachers
- Failure of identity formation and psychosexual development in adolescence

34.1.2.4 Environmental Factors
34.1.2.4.1 Family
Minuchin et al. (1978) found that relationships in families of anorexics are characterized by overprotection and enmeshment. Kendler found that a typical anorexic came from an inward, often overprotected, and highly controlled family. Young patients with AN may use the illness to gain control and overcome rigidity, enmeshment, and overprotection in the family.

Higher rates of childhood sexual abuse are reported by eating-disordered patients than by controls. Childhood sexual abuse appears to be a vulnerability factor for psychiatric disorder in general, not for eating disorders in particular.

34.1.2.4.2 Sociocultural Factors
There is a cult of thinness. Anorexic and bulimic women viewing fashion images of women show a 25% increase in their body size estimation afterward. The media presentation of idealized women is likely to have some effect upon eating-disordered subjects.

Among 15-year-old schoolgirls, the relative risk of developing AN was eight times greater in those who dieted compared to those who did not in a prospective study.

Immigrants from low-prevalence to high-prevalence cultures may develop AN as thin-body ideals are assimilated. Cultural factors influence the manifestation of the disorder: In some cultures, for example, body-image disturbance may not be prominent, and the expressed motivation for food restriction may have a different content, such as epigastric discomfort or distaste for food.

34.1.3 CLASSIFICATION

34.1.3.1 ICD-10 (F50.0 Anorexia Nervosa)

This condition is characterized by deliberate weight loss resulting in undernutrition with secondary endocrine and metabolic disturbance. It requires the presence of all the following:

1. Body weight maintained at 15% below expected; Quetelet's body mass index (BMI) <17.5 kg/m². (Quetelet's BMI = mass/height²; age 16 or over.)
2. Weight loss self-induced by the avoidance of fattening foods and one or more of the following: self-induced vomiting, self-induced purging, excessive exercise, and the use of appetite suppressants and/or diuretics.
3. Body-image distortion: a specific psychopathology comprising a dread of fatness that persists as an intrusive, overvalued idea; a low weight threshold is imposed on self.
4. Amenorrhoea in women, loss of sexual interest and potency in men, endocrine disorder of hypothalamus–pituitary–gonadal axis (HPA), elevated growth hormone and cortisol levels, abnormal peripheral metabolism of thyroid hormone, and abnormalities of insulin secretion.
5. If onset is prepubertal, the sequence of pubertal events is delayed or arrested; puberty is often completed with recovery, but menarche is late.

34.1.3.2 DSM-5 (Anorexia Nervosa)

34.1.3.2.1 Diagnostic Features

1. Restriction of energy and food intake leading to a significantly low body weight in the context of age, sex, development, and health status. Significantly low weight is defined as a weight that is less than minimally normal. DSM-5 does not specify the percentage of weight loss (i.e. more than 15%) as in DSM-IV-TR.
2. Intense fear of weight gain or persistent behaviour that interferes with weight gain, even though the weight is significantly low.
3. Body image disturbance as a result of repetitive self-evaluation and poor insight of low body weight.

34.1.3.2.2 Subtypes

These are used to specify the presence or absence of regular binge eating or purging during the current episode.

Binge-eating or purging type: The patient has engaged in recurrent episodes of binge-eating or purging behaviour (i.e. self-induced vomiting or the misuse of laxatives, diuretics, or enemas) during the last 3 months.

Restricting type: The patient has not engaged in recurrent episodes of binge-eating or purging behaviour during the last 3 months.

34.1.4 DIFFERENTIAL DIAGNOSIS OF ANOREXIA NERVOSA

Other causes of weight loss should be considered, especially when presenting features are atypical (e.g. an onset of illness after 40 years of age).

In medical conditions such as gastrointestinal disease, brain tumours, occult malignancies, and acquired immunodeficiency syndrome (AIDS), serious weight loss may occur. In these cases, the individuals do not have a distorted body image or a desire for further weight loss.

Superior mesenteric artery syndrome (postprandial vomiting is secondary to intermittent gastric outlet obstruction) should be distinguished from AN, although it may develop in AN because of emaciation.

Depressives do not generally have a desire for excessive weight loss or a morbid fear of gaining weight.

Schizophrenics may exhibit odd eating behaviours and occasionally weight loss. However, they rarely fear weight gain or have body-image disturbance.

34.1.5 CLINICAL FEATURES

34.1.5.1 Psychological Symptoms and Signs

The person may exhibit

- Morbid fear of fatness/excessive pursuit of thinness
- Denial of the problem
- Distorted body image
- Fear of losing control of eating
- Problems with separation and independence
- Depressive feelings—insomnia, lack of concentration, and irritability
- Suicidal ideas
- Obsessional thoughts and rituals that may improve with weight gain
- Preoccupation with thoughts of food (enjoys cooking for others and does not like eating in public)
- Withdrawn

34.1.5.2 Physical Signs and Complications

The person may exhibit the following:

34.1.5.2.1 General Appearance

- Emaciation
- Dehydration
- Hypothermia, cold intolerance
- Pallor (anaemia)
- Peripheral cyanosis
- Purpura secondary to reduced collagen in skin and bone marrow suppression

34.1.5.2.2 Central Nervous System

- Seizures
- Diffuse EEG abnormalities, reflecting metabolic encephalopathy (may result from fluid and electrolyte disturbances)
- Increase in the ventricular/brain ratio secondary to starvation
- Impaired cognition
- Poor concentration

34.1.5.2.3 Cardiovascular System

- Bradycardia (30–40 beats/min)
- Hypotension (systolic BP <70 mmHg)
- Prolonged corrected QT (QTc)
- Cardiac arrhythmias and failure
- Peripheral oedema
- Mitral valve prolapse
- Pericardial effusion
- Cardiomyopathy

34.1.5.2.4 Gastrointestinal System

- Delayed gastric emptying
- Acute gastric dilatation
- Pancreatitis
- Degeneration of myenteric plexus of bowel
- Cathartic colon
- Constipation and abdominal distension
- Impaired liver function

34.1.5.2.5 Urinary System

- Impaired renal function caused by chronic dehydration and hypokalaemia
- Nocturia and renal stones

34.1.5.2.6 Endocrine System

- Amenorrhoea/loss of libido
- Reproductive system atrophy (shrunken uterus and ovaries with cystic multifollicular ovarian changes)
- Hypoglycaemia

34.1.5.2.7 Reproductive System

- Reduced growth, delayed puberty
- Amenorrhoea
- Small ovaries and uterus
- Infertility
- Breast atrophy

34.1.5.2.8 Musculoskeletal System

- Osteoporosis from low calcium intake and absorption, reduced oestrogen, and increased cortisol secretion
- Bone pain and deformity
- Bone density reduction with increasing years of amenorrhoea
- Pathological fractures after about 10 years
- Tetany
- Skeletal muscle wasting
- Proximal myopathy

34.1.5.2.9 Dermatological

- Lanugo hair
- Dry skin
- Brittle nail
- Raynaud's phenomenon: discolouration of fingers and toes

Effects secondary to repeated self-induced vomiting: There may be

- Erosion of tooth enamel
- Dental caries
- Parotid gland enlargement
- Russell's sign (calloused skin over interphalangeal joints)

34.1.6 BASELINE MONITORING AND INVESTIGATIONS

34.1.6.1 Baseline Monitoring

- Blood pressure (BP) and pulse rate.
- BMI.
- Weight.
- Although the weight and BMI are important indicators of severity of AN, the NICE guidelines recommend that BMI and weight should not be considered as sole indicators of physical risk. The nature of the investigations should be adjusted based on the severity of AN.

34.1.6.2 Full Blood Count

- Anaemia: usually normochromic normocytic anaemia.
- Microcytic (iron deficiency) or macrocytic (B12 deficiency) anaemia is possible.

- Leukopenia with relative lymphocytosis.
- Reduced ESR.
- Thrombocytopenia.

34.1.6.3　Electrolyte Disturbances
- Hypokalaemia (cardiac arrhythmias, cardiac arrest, renal damage)
- Hypomagnesaemia
- Hypozincaemia
- Hypophosphataemia

34.1.6.4　Arterial Blood Gas
- Metabolic alkalosis (as a result of self-induced vomiting)

34.1.6.5　Renal Function Tests
- Increase in urea as a result of dehydration
- Renal failure

34.1.6.6　Liver Function Tests
- Reduced albumin
- Raised serum amylase

34.1.6.7　Fasting Blood
- Hypercholesterolaemia as a result of low oestrogen
- Hypoglycaemia

34.1.6.8　Others
- Hypercarotenaemia

34.1.6.9　Hormones
- Decrease in T_3.
- Increase in CRH.
- Increase in cortisol.
- Increase in growth hormone.
- Decrease in FSH.
- Decrease in LH: The 24 h pattern of secretion of LH resembles that normally seen in the prepubertal individual.
- Decrease in oestrogen (in women) or decrease in testosterone (in men).

34.1.6.10　Imaging
- CT brain: brain pseudoatrophy
- Bone scan: reduction in bone mineral density

In summary, most of the parameters are reduced except the following parameters are increased: amylase, carotene, cholesterol, cortisol, CRH, and growth hormone.

34.1.7　MANAGEMENT

34.1.7.1　Treatment Setting
Most people with AN should be treated on an outpatient basis before reaching severe emaciation. If a person is very emaciated, inpatient care may be necessary, and the NICE guidelines recommend the involvement of a physician or paediatrician with expertise in the treatment of medically at-risk patients with AN. Other indications for inpatient treatment are listed as follows:

1. Persistent decline in oral intake or rapid decline in weight (e.g. >1 kg/week) in adults who are already less than 80%–85% of their healthy weights.
2. Vital sign abnormalities: heart rate <40 beats/min and orthostatic hypotension (drop in BP of 20 mmHg from supine to standing position).
3. Low body temperature (less than 36°C).
4. Severe electrolyte imbalance: hyponatraemia or hypokalaemia.
5. Organ failure.
6. Poorly controlled diabetes.
7. Underlying psychiatric disorder (e.g. severe depression and suicidal ideation).
8. Failure of outpatient treatment.
9. Pregnancy: More intensive prenatal care is required to ensure adequate prenatal nutrition and fetal development.

The NICE guidelines provide detailed recommendations on every aspect of management of AN, and the recommendations are summarized as follows:

34.1.7.2　Weight Restoration
1. An average weekly weight gain of 0.5–1 kg in inpatient settings and 0.5 kg in outpatient settings should be an aim of treatment. The weight gain should not be more than 2 kg per week. This requires about 3500–7000 extra calories per week.
2. As a rule of thumb, the premorbid weight, or the weight at which periods stopped plus 5 kg, is a guide to a healthy weight.
3. There may be reduced circulating oestrogens, a shrunken uterus, and small amorphous ovaries. As weight is gained, the uterus increases in size, and the ovaries become multifollicular. At normal weight, the ovaries become follicular; this is detected by pelvic ultrasound and can be used to indicate correct weight.

34.1.7.3   Feeding

1. A dietician should be consulted before the initiation of feeding. There is slowed gastric emptying, so meals must be introduced slowly to reduce the risks of gastric dilatation or rupture.
2. If the patient is very emaciated, liquid feeds may be better initially. Gradually build up from 1000–3500 kcal/day.
3. A multivitamin/multimineral supplement in oral form is recommended for people with AN during both inpatient and outpatient weight restoration.
4. Total parenteral nutrition should not be used unless there is significant gastrointestinal dysfunction.
5. Feeding against the will of the patient should be the last resort option. This should only be done in the context of the Mental Health Act (1983) or Children Act (1989).

34.1.7.4   Managing Risk

1. The frequency of the monitoring is determined by the severity of AN, and the doctor should inform the patient and their carers about the physical risk of AN.
2. Rapid feeding may lead to a life-threatening condition known as refeeding syndrome, which usually occurs in the first 4 days of refeeding. As a result of prolonged starvation and malnourishment, there is an intracellular loss of electrolytes such as phosphates. During feeding, there will be a sudden shift from lipid to carbohydrate metabolism. The carbohydrate metabolism stimulates cellular uptake of phosphate to generate adenosine-5′-triphosphate (ATP). When phosphate is used up for ATP production, this will lead to severe hypophosphataemia (<0.50 mmol/L) and lack of ATP for cardiac muscles. The patient will develop cardiac failure, arrhythmias, and sudden death. Other features include rhabdomyolysis, leukocyte dysfunction, and seizure. Hence, refeeding has to be gradual and should be determined by a dietician.

34.1.7.5   Psychotherapy

1. For outpatients, cognitive analytic therapy (CAT), cognitive–behavioural therapy (CBT), interpersonal therapy (IPT), focal dynamic therapy, and family interventions focused explicitly on eating disorders are the treatment of choice.
2. The aims of psychotherapy should reduce risk, enhance motivation, encourage healthy eating, and reduce other symptoms related to AN.
3. CBT targets at cognitive distortion and behaviours related to body weight, body image, and eating.
4. The minimum duration for outpatient psychological treatment is 6 months.
5. If outpatient psychological treatment fails, the psychiatrist can offer combined individual and family therapy and day-care or inpatient treatment.
6. Psychotherapy is difficult for patients with severe emaciation. Wait until the weight has increased and then offer a structured symptom-focused treatment regimen focusing on eating behaviour and attitude.
7. Rigid inpatient behaviour modification programme should not be used.
8. For inpatients, outpatient psychological treatment should be offered after discharge, and the duration is for at least 12 months.
9. Family therapy is the treatment of choice, particularly for children and adolescents with AN. Individual appointments with a health-care professional should be offered and separate from family members or carers.
10. There are four types of family therapy:
   a. Strategic family therapy developed by Haley (1973) applies paradoxical interventions and reduces family's antagonistic views towards AN.
   b. Structural family therapy developed by Minuchin (1978) focuses on hierarchy and allows patient to have more autonomy in an enmeshed, inflexible, and overprotective family.
   c. Systemic family therapy developed by Milan (1974) views the family as a homeostatic system, and therapist acts as a neutral facilitator and helps family to solve their dilemmas towards AN.
   d. Maudsley family therapy is the first-line treatment for adolescents with AN. This therapy was developed by Dale (1980) and involves 15–20 sessions. Parents play an active role in helping the adolescent to recover, and their participation is crucial for treatment success. The Maudsley's therapy does not support the idea that family is pathological and causes AN. Maudsley's therapy is comprised of three stages: stage 1: weight restoration, stage 2: develop control over eating, and stage 3: establish a healthy identity.

34.1.7.6 Pharmacotherapy

1. Medication should not be used as the sole or primary treatment for AN.
2. Be aware of cardiac side effects such as postural hypotension, prolonged QTc, arrhythmia, and hypothermia. Regular ECG monitoring should be undertaken for drugs that can prolong QTc (e.g. antipsychotics, tricyclic antidepressants).
3. Olanzapine is the most extensively studied antipsychotic in AN (Boachie et al., 2003; Bissada et al., 2008). It is associated with greater weight gain, reduction in obsessive symptoms, reduction in anxiety, and increase in compliance. The mean dose is around 6.6 mg.
4. Risperidone is associated with weight gain and reduction in anxiety when combined with an antidepressant based on a case report (Newman-Toker, 2000).
5. Quetiapine is associated with significant increase in BMI and reduction in Eating Disorder Examination (EDE-12) restraint subscale scores over 8 weeks based on an open label study (Bosanac et al., 2007).
6. Fluoxetine failed to demonstrate any benefit in the treatment of patients with AN following weight restoration based on a randomized controlled trail (Walsh et al., 2006).
7. Oestrogen administration should not be used to treat bone density problems in children and adolescents because this may lead to premature fusion of the epiphyses.

34.1.8 PROGNOSIS

The course and outcome are variable. Some patients recover fully after a single episode. Some exhibit fluctuating

TABLE 34.1
Summary of Good and Poor Prognostic Factors of AN

Good Prognostic Factors	Poor Prognostic Factors
• Onset <15 years of age	• Onset at older age
• Higher weight at onset and at presentation	• Lower weight at onset and at presentation
• Receive treatment within 3 months after the onset of illness	• Very frequent vomiting and presence of bulimia
• Recovery within 2 years after initiation of treatment	• Very severe weight loss
• Outpatient treatment	• Long duration of AN
• Supportive family	• Previous hospitalization
• Good motivation to change	• Extreme resistance to treatment
• Good childhood social adjustment	• Continued family problems
	• Neurotic personality
	• Male gender

patterns of weight gain followed by a relapse. For adolescents with AN, around 80% recover in 5 years and 20% may develop chronic AN. For adults with AN, 50% recover, 25% have intermediate outcome, and 25% have poor outcome. 50% of restrictive AN may develop bulimia after 5 years (Table 34.1).

AN is a serious disorder with substantial mortality (5%–20%). Sullivan (1995) found that the aggregate mortality rate for AN is 5.6% per decade. This is 12 times the annual death rate due to all causes for females aged 15–24. The aggregate mortality rate for AN is substantially greater than that reported for psychiatric inpatients and the general population.

The causes of death were complications of eating disorder in 54% and suicide in 27%. Suicide rates are 200 times greater than in the general population.

CASC STATION ON AN

You are the registrar working in an adolescent psychiatric service. You are seeing a 15-year-old secondary school student with a 2-year history of AN. She is admitted to the hospital following a seizure after prolonged fasting. On admission, her BMI is 10 and her heart rate is 35 beats/min. She has a younger sister aged 13 who has developed AN recently. You are approached by her parents who beg you to save the patient, and they are also very concerned about their younger daughter who is at home at this moment. The patient is not forthcoming, but she has given the consent for you to speak to her mother.

Task:

1. Take a history from her mother to establish the aetiology, diagnosis, and course of AN for the 15-year-old patient.
2. Assess the impact of AN of the two daughters.

(continued)

CASC Grid

(A) Course of AN	(A1) Longitudinal Weight History	(A2) Methods to Lose Weight	(A3) Body-image Distortion and Bingeing	(A4) Psychiatric Complications of AN	(A5) Medical Complications of AN
	'I am sorry to hear that you have two daughters suffering from eating disorders. Can you tell me your views about their conditions?' 'Are they sick at this moment?' 'Can you tell me more about your elder daughter's eating disorder?' 'What is her average weight?' 'What is her lowest weight or highest weight in the past two years?' 'How about her younger sister? What is her lowest weight?'	'What methods does your elder daughter use to lose weight?' 'Does she avoid food? If yes, how?' 'Does she do excessive exercise? If yes, what kind of exercise does she do?' 'Does she induce vomiting? If yes, how does she do it?' 'Does she use laxatives or diuretics to lose weight?' 'What method does your younger daughter use? Do they share the same method?'	'How does your elder daughter feel about her body? Does she think that she is too fat?' 'Have you ever questioned why she feels that she is too fat?' 'How about her sister? Does she share similar belief?' 'Do they compare with each other in their body image?' 'Do they binge? If yes, do they feel guilty? If yes, what would they do?' (Look for self-induced vomiting.)	'How do you find your elder daughter's mental health after developing eating disorder?' 'How do you find her concentration?' 'Does she follow your advice?' 'Is she very rigid and stubborn at this moment?' 'How is her mood?' 'Is she nervous?'	'How do you find your elder daughter's physical health after developing eating disorder?' 'How is her menses? Do her menses come regularly? If not, how long have the menses been absent?' 'Has she ever fainted or had a blackout?' 'Did she have a fit before?' 'Does she look pale?' 'Does she feel weak most of the time?'

(B) Aetiology of AN	(B1) Predisposing Factors in Family	(B2) Common Precipitating Factors—Sibling Rivalry	(B3) Maintaining Factors	(B4) Development	(B5) School and Peers
	'Can you tell me more about your family?' 'Are the family members close to each other? Do you think that you have been too close to each other?' (Look for enmeshment.) 'How do you nurture your children? Are you strict in discipline? Could it be too strict?' 'How is your relationship with your partner? Was there any marital conflict?' 'Did eating disorder run in your family? How about your partner's family?'	'How is the relationship between the two daughters?' 'How does your elder child react to her sister's eating disorder?' 'Are they competing with each other?' 'Was your elder daughter being neglected when her younger sister develops eating disorder?' 'What is your younger daughter's reaction towards her elder sister's eating disorder?'	'How do their illnesses affect the family?' 'Do they get more attention from you and your partner when they suffer from eating disorder?' 'How do you and your partner react when they develop eating disorder?' 'What is the family's view on food and body image? Are you very conscious about weight?'	'Can you tell me more about them when they were young?' 'Did they stay with you and your partner all the time?' 'Was there any unhappy event during their childhood? If yes, what kind of event? Were they being abused before?' 'Does your elder daughter encounter any problem as a teenager?' (e.g. identity problem)	'Do your daughters play any sport? How about ballet dancing or modelling?' 'How are their academic performances? Are they very serious about their academic performances? Do they often compare with each other?' 'Is your elder daughter in a relationship at this moment?' 'Was she bullied in the school? If yes, why? Was she obese in the past?'

(C) Course of Illness, Comorbidity, and Risk	(C1) Previous Treatment	(C2) Outcomes of Previous Treatments	(C3) Assess Insight	(C4) Explore Comorbidity	(C5) Risk Assessment
	'Did your elder daughter receive any treatment before? If yes, what kind of treatment was offered?' 'How about your younger daughter? What kind of treatment did she receive?' 'How did your elder daughter feel when your younger daughter received treatment?'	'What was the outcome of the treatment?' If it fails, please explore the underlying reason. 'How does your elder daughter feel about the treatment for her sister?'	'Does your elder daughter believe that she is ill?' 'Does she see her younger sister suffering from eating disorder?' If patient does not believe that she has eating disorder, explore with the mother the underlying reason and how the elder daughter sees herself different from her younger sister.	'Does your elder daughter suffer other psychiatric problems? For example, does she check things repetitively or is she depressed?' 'How do you describe your elder daughter as a person? Is she perfectionistic?' 'Does she use recreational drugs?' 'Does your younger daughter suffer from other psychiatric illness?'	'Has your elder daughter ever harmed herself? If yes, how did she do it?' 'Did she tell you why she wanted to harm herself?' 'Have she ever thought of harming her younger sister?' 'Did her younger sister harm herself before?'

(D) Explore the Impact and Dynamics of Having Two Daughters with AN	(D1) Explore Her Views on the Current Situation	(D2) Comparison of Her Daughters' Eating Disorder	(D3) Assess Coping Strategies	(D4) Explore the Family's Expectation on the Management	(D5) Explore Her Expectation on the Overlap Between Two Daughters' Treatment
	'Thanks for sharing with me, and we have gone through a lot of details about your daughters' eating disorder. What is your view on the cause of eating disorder in them?'	'How do you feel about their eating disorders? Are they similar? If yes, in what ways? Are they different? How are they different?'	'How do you and your partner cope with their eating disorders?' 'Do you get help from other people?' 'Do you have someone to turn to when you undergo a lot of stress?'	'What is your expectation on the treatment of your elder daughter?' 'She has to be admitted to the hospital. How do you feel about it?' 'The treatment mainly involves psychological treatment aiming at weight restoration and family therapy. How do you feel about that?'	'Where does your younger daughter receiving her treatment? Is she in the same service?' 'Do you want a family therapist to help the family to overcome the eating disorder?'

34.2 BULIMIA NERVOSA

34.2.1 EPIDEMIOLOGY

- The prevalence among adolescent and young adult females is approximately 1%–3%.
- The lifetime prevalence for strictly defined bulimia nervosa (BN) is 1.1% in females and 0.1% in males.
- Kendler et al. (1991) estimate a heritability of liability to BN of 50%.
- The social class distribution is more even than for AN (see preceding text).
- The average age of onset is 18 years, slightly older than in anorectics.
- The female-to-male ratio is 10:1.
- It is reported more frequently in Caucasians in Western Europe, North America, and Australasia.
- There are reports of increasing prevalence with time. Lee et al. (2010) reported that BN became more common in Hong Kong.
- The DSM-IV-TR and DSM-5 have a category known as binge-eating disorder, which has a prevalence of 1%–2%. Onset is 40 years of age. Twenty-five per cent of patients are men.

34.2.2 AETIOLOGY OF BULIMIA NERVOSA

34.2.2.1 Genetic Factors

- In twins, the MZ–DZ concordance rate for narrowly defined BN is 23:9.
- Fairburn and Harrison (2003) reported that the concordance rates were 35% (MZ) versus 30% (DZ).

34.2.2.2 Biological Factors
34.2.2.2.1 Neurotransmitters

Many abnormalities in eating disorders are secondary to dieting, weight loss, and binge/purge behaviour.

Serotonin is involved in the mediation of satiety responses to feeding as well as the regulation of mood, anxiety, and impulsive behaviour. There is evidence in normal-weight bulimics of altered postsynaptic 5-HT$_{1c}$ receptor sensitivity and depression associated with dysregulation of presynaptic 5-HT function.

There is further support for the 5-HT dysregulation hypothesis from findings that CSF concentrations of the serotonin metabolite 5HIAA and dopamine metabolite HVA are inversely correlated with a frequency of binge eating in the month prior to admission.

Beta-endorphin concentration in CSF of bulimics is significantly reduced, possibly related to chronic activation of the HPA axis secondary to dieting.

Cholecystokinin-8 (CCK-8) is involved in regulating satiety and anxiety. It is dependent upon an intact 5HT function. Bulimics have lower CSF CCK-8 concentrations than controls. A central, but not peripheral, CCK dysfunction is implicated in BN.

Arginine–vasopressin (AVP) CSF concentrations are high in bulimics. An increased central AVP may be related to obsessive preoccupation with the aversive consequences of eating and weight gain. It also interacts with 5-HT.

There is a general reduction of sympathetic responsivity and activation of HPA activity in BN, probably as a result of long-term neuroendocrine adaptation to caloric restriction.

34.2.2.3 Psychological Factors
34.2.2.3.1 Personality

- Personality disturbance is more common in patients with eating disorders than in the general population. On the Eysenck Personality Inventory, bulimics score higher for psychoticism and neuroticism than do anorexics and controls. On the MMPI, bulimics have elevated scores for psychopathic deviance.

34.2.2.3.2 Other Psychological Factors

- Low self-esteem, low paternal care, external locus of control, and high neuroticism scores are risk factors for bulimia.
- Bulimics are more likely than anorexics to abuse substances (20%). Lifetime rates of alcohol dependence are high.
- The prevalence of social phobia in eating-disordered subjects, especially in bulimics, far exceeds that in the general population.
- Bulimics have high rates (40%) of major depression. There is significant comorbidity between anorexia and bulimia.

34.2.2.4 Environmental Factors

Prior to illness onset, bulimics are more likely to be overweight than their peers.

Rigid dieting is the most common precipitant of binge eating. Gross bingeing is the most common precipitant for self-induced vomiting. Dieting may affect appetite and satiety mechanisms. Second World War veterans who had been prisoners of war and suffered weight loss report more binge eating afterward than veterans who had not been prisoners. Data are supportive of an aetiological role for eating restraint in promotion of bingeing.

Many normal-weight bulimics are the eldest or only daughters. Lacey et al. (1991) postulate that at times of parental marital discord, the mother can use her daughter as an easily available therapist, burdening the child at an age when she cannot deal with the expressed emotions.

Bulimics report more sexual abuse in childhood than controls.

34.2.3 CLASSIFICATION

34.2.3.1 ICD-10 (F50.2 Bulimia Nervosa)

BN is characterized by repeated bouts of overeating and excessive preoccupation with the control of body weight, leading to extreme measures to mitigate against the fattening effects of food. It shares the same specific psychopathology of fear of fatness as AN.

A diagnosis under ICD-10 requires all of the following:

1. Persistent preoccupation with eating and an irresistible craving for food; episodes of overeating in which large amounts of food are consumed in short periods of time.
2. Attempts to counteract the fattening effects of food by one or more of the following: self-induced vomiting, purgative abuse, alternating periods of starvation, and use of drugs (appetite suppressants, thyroid preparations, diuretics). Diabetic bulimics may neglect insulin treatment.
3. Morbid dread of fatness. Patient sets weight threshold well below healthy weight. Often there is a history previously of AN.

34.2.3.2 DSM-5 (Bulimia Nervosa)

34.2.3.2.1 Diagnostic Features

An episode of binge eating is characterized by both of the following:

1. Recurrent binge eating of large amount of food within short period of time (e.g. 2 h)
2. Lack of self-control over recurrent binge eating.
3. Recurrent inappropriate compensatory behaviours after binge eating (e.g. self-induced vomiting; misuse of laxatives, diuretics, or other

medications; fasting; or excessive exercise) to prevent weight gain.
4. Frequency of binge-eating and compensatory behaviours: at least 1 per week for 3 months.
5. Repetitive self-evaluation as a result of undue influence by distorted body image.
6. The disturbance does not occur exclusively during episodes of AN.

34.2.3.3 DSM-5 (Binge-Eating Disorder)

In this variation, there are recurrent episodes of binge eating in the absence of the regular use of inappropriate compensatory behaviours characteristic of BN. The other criteria listed in BN apply. Furthermore, the DSM-5 requires three of the following criteria: eating much more rapidly than normal, eating until feeling uncomfortably full, eating large amounts of food when not feeling physically hungry, eating alone to avoid embarrassment, feeling disgusted with oneself or very guilty after overeating, and marked distress over binge eating.

34.2.4 DIFFERENTIAL DIAGNOSIS OF BULIMIA NERVOSA

In certain medical conditions, such as the Kleine–Levin syndrome, there is disturbed eating behaviour, but characteristic psychological features of BN such as overconcern with body shape and weight are not present.

Overeating is common in atypical depression, but sufferers do not engage in inappropriate compensatory behaviour or exhibit overconcern with body shape and weight.

Binge eating is included in the impulsive behaviour criterion that is part of the DSM-5 definition of borderline personality disorder. If full criteria for both disorders are met, both diagnoses are given.

34.2.5 CLINICAL FEATURES OF BULIMIA NERVOSA

34.2.5.1 Psychological Symptoms and Signs

The person may exhibit

- Morbid fear of fatness
- Distorted body image—overconcern with shape and weight
- An overwhelming urge to overeat, with subsequent guilt and disgust

- Self-induced vomiting (90%), using fingers and, later, reflex vomiting, which results in relief from physical discomfort and reduction of fear of gaining weight
- Laxative abuse (30%), excessive exercise, and food restriction
- Depression, irritability, poor concentration, and suicidal ideas
- Older than the anorectic, more socially competent, and sexually experienced
- Possibly normal weight or just slightly underweight or overweight
- Menstrual abnormalities (<50%)
- More insight than in AN, often eager for help
- Depressive symptoms (in the majority), anxiety, impulsive and compulsive behaviours, and problems with interpersonal relationships
- Stealing and dependence upon substances

There is also a high prevalence of depression, self-mutilation, attempted suicide, substance abuse, and low self-esteem.

34.2.5.2 Physical Signs and Complications

1. Related to vomiting:
   a. Dental erosion and toothache
   b. Parotid gland enlargement
   c. Callouses on backs of hands: Russell's sign
   d. Oedema
   e. Conjunctival haemorrhages caused by raised intrathoracic pressure
   f. Oesophageal tears
   g. Ipecacuanha intoxication causing cardiomyopathy and cardiac failure, usually fatal
2. Related to purgative abuse:
   a. Rectal prolapse
   b. Constipation
   c. Diarrhoea
   d. Cathartic colon, damaged myenteric plexus
3. Related to binges:
   a. Acute dilatation of stomach (medical emergency)
   b. Hypercarotenaemia: yellowish skin in palm and feet (binge on juices)
4. Other complications:
   a. Epilepsy
   b. Arrhythmia (caused by electrolyte disturbances)
   c. Tetany
   d. Muscle weakness (caused by electrolyte disturbances)

34.2.5.2.1 Common Biochemical Abnormalities

The NICE guidelines recommend that patients with BN who are vomiting frequently or taking large quantities of laxatives should have the following investigations performed:

- Hypokalaemic alkalosis (caused by repeated vomiting).
- Metabolic acidosis with reduced serum bicarbonate in those abusing laxatives.
- Raised serum bicarbonate.
- Hypokalaemia—direct potassium loss from vomiting and indirect renal loss in response to raised aldosterone secondary to volume depletion.
- Hypochloraemia.
- Hypomagnesaemia.
- Raised serum amylase (salivary isoenzyme)—monitoring serum amylase can be used to monitor vomiting behaviour.

34.2.6 Management

Most patients with BN are treated in an outpatient setting. For patients who are at risk of suicide or several medical complications, inpatient treatment is recommended.

34.2.6.1 Psychotherapy

Freeman et al. (1988) conducted a controlled trial of psychotherapy. The controls were left significantly worse than all treatment groups at the end of the trial. Behavioural, cognitive–behavioural, and group therapies were all effective; 77% stopped bingeing. Improvements were maintained at 1 year. Behavioural therapy was the most effective, with the lowest dropout rate and earlier onset of improvement. There seemed to be no advantage in adding a cognitive element. Psychotherapy produces a wider range of changes with more stable maintenance than does drug therapy.

The NICE guidelines provide detailed recommendations on every aspect of management of BN, and the recommendations are summarized as follows:

34.2.6.2 Cognitive–Behavioural Therapy for BN

This includes psychoeducation, self-monitoring, and cognitive restructuring. Eating regular meals is very important. The course of treatment should be aimed at 16–20 sessions over 4–5 months.

The aims of behavioural therapy are to stop bingeing and purging by restricting exposure cues that trigger binge/purge behaviour, developing alternative behaviours, and delaying vomiting.

34.2.6.3 Interpersonal Therapy

If CBT fails, interpersonal therapy (IPT) should be considered, and the duration is between 8 and 12 months.

34.2.6.4 Pharmacotherapy

1. Selective serotonin reuptake inhibitors (SSRIs) (specifically fluoxetine) are the drugs of first choice for the treatment of BN in terms of acceptability, tolerability, and reduction of symptoms.
2. The effective dose of fluoxetine is 60 mg per day.
3. Other psychotropic drugs are not recommended for the treatment of BN.

34.2.7 Prognosis

The outcome for BN improves with time and generally better than AN. The majority of patients make a full recovery or suffer only moderate abnormalities in eating attitudes after 10 years.

There is comorbidity with depression, and prominent anorectic features increase the likelihood of a poor response.

In a 10-year follow-up of treated bulimics, 52% recovered fully, 39% continued to suffer some symptoms, and 9% continued to suffer the full syndrome.

In terms of prognostic factors, there is evidence from a number of studies that the following factors may be associated with poor outcome (Keel and Michell, 1997; Quadflieg and Fichter, 2003):

- Depression
- Personality disturbance
- Greater severity of symptoms
- Longer duration of symptoms
- Low self-esteem
- Substance abuse
- Childhood obesity

Bulimics with multi-impulsive personality disorder do less well than those with bulimia alone.

34.3 METABOLIC SYNDROME

34.3.1 Epidemiology

- In the United Kingdom one in four people are affected by metabolic syndrome (MetS). MetS is more common in certain ethnic groups (such as Asian and Afro-Caribbean people) and among women with polycystic ovary syndrome.

- Wannamethee (2008) studied a total of 5128 British men aged 40–59 years and monitored them for 20 years. The MetS is associated with a significant increase in risk of total coronary heart disease (CHD) (myocardial infarction, angina, or CHD death), stroke, and type 2 diabetes.

34.3.2 Psychiatric Diseases and MetS

34.3.2.1 Schizophrenia

Mitchell et al. (2011) conducted a meta-analysis and reported that the prevalence of MetS was 32.5% in schizophrenia patients.

Findings from the Clinical Antipsychotic Trials in Intervention Effectiveness (CATIE) study (Meyer et al., 2008)

- The prevalence of MetS was increased for olanzapine (from 34.8% to 43.9%) but decreased for ziprasidone (from 37.7% to 29.9%).
- At 3 months, olanzapine and quetiapine had the largest mean increase in waist circumference (0.7 in. for both) followed by risperidone (0.4 in.) compared to no change for ziprasidone.
- Olanzapine demonstrated significantly different changes in fasting triglycerides at 3 months as compared to ziprasidone.

34.3.2.2 Depressive Disorder

Kahl et al. (2012) studied 230 patients with major depressive disorder in Germany and found that the age-standardized prevalence of MetS was 2.4 times higher than controls (41.0% vs. 17.0%).

Pyykkönen et al. (2012) reported that depressive symptoms were related with the MetS and the individual components of MetS. Such associations were not driven by the use of antidepressant medication.

34.3.2.3 Bipolar Disorder

The prevalence of MetS was between 22.4% and 26.5% in European patients with bipolar disorder (Garcia-Portilla et al., 2008; Salvi et al., 2011). Young male patients and lack of exercise are important risk factors.

Elmslie et al. (2009) found that the frequency of MetS was 50% in bipolar disorder patients treated with sodium valproate. Dyslipidaemia is a major concern.

34.3.3 CLASSIFICATION

The U.S. National Cholesterol Education Program Adult Treatment Panel III (ATP-III) (2001) requires at least three of the following:

- Dyslipidaemia: triglycerides (TG) ≥150 mg/dL (1.7 mmol/L)
- BP: ≥130/85 mmHg
- Fasting plasma glucose: ≥110 mg/dL (6.1 mmol/L)
- Central obesity: waist circumference ≥102 cm (male), ≥88 cm (female)
- Dyslipidaemia: high-density lipoprotein cholesterol (HDL-C) <40 mg/dL (male), <50 mg/dL (female)

The World Health Organization criteria (1999) require the presence of any two of diabetes mellitus, impaired glucose tolerance, impaired fasting glucose or insulin resistance, and one of the following:

- BP: ≥140/90 mmHg
- Dyslipidaemia: TG: ≥1.695 mmol/L and HDL-C ≤0.9 mmol/L (male), ≤1.0 mmol/L (female)
- Central obesity: waist/hip ratio >0.90 (male), >0.85 (female), or BMI >30 kg/m²
- Microalbuminuria: urinary albumin excretion ratio ≥20 μg/min or albumin/creatinine ratio ≥30 mg/g

The International Diabetes Federation criteria (2006) require the presence of central obesity (defined as waist circumference with ethnicity-specific values) and any two of the following:

- Raised TG: >150 mg/dL (1.7 mmol/L) or specific treatment for this lipid abnormality
- Reduced HDL-C: <40 mg/dL (1.03 mmol/L) in males, <50 mg/dL (1.29 mmol/L) in females, or specific treatment for this lipid abnormality
- Raised BP: systolic BP >130 or diastolic BP >85 mmHg or treatment of previously diagnosed hypertension
- Raised fasting plasma glucose: >100 mg/dL (5.6 mmol/L) or previously diagnosed type 2 diabetes
- If BMI is >30 kg/m², central obesity can be assumed and waist circumference does not need to be measured

34.3.4 MANAGEMENT

See Table 34.2.

TABLE 34.2

Summary of Recommendations from the NICE Guidelines and Maudsley's Guidelines (2012) on the Management of MetS in Schizophrenia

Impaired glucose control	• Monitoring: oral glucose tolerance test (OGTT) or fasting glucose at baseline, 1 month and 6 months for patients taking clozapine and olanzapine. Urine glucose or rapid blood glucose at baseline and annually for other antipsychotics
	• ☑ Aripiprazole, amisulpride, asenapine, and ziprasidone
	• ☒ Clozapine and olanzapine
	• Prevention: lifestyle interventions aimed at changing an individual's diet (starchy foods or fibre-rich foods) and increasing the amount of physical activity (at least 30 min of physical activities for 5 days per week) may prevent impaired glucose tolerance to type 2 from developing into diabetes.
Dyslipidaemia	• Monitoring: fasting lipids at baseline, at 3 months and annually
	• ☑ Haloperidol and risperidone
	• ☒ Clozapine and olanzapine
	• Prevention: cardioprotective diet (total fat intake is ≤30% of total energy intake, saturated fats are ≤10% of total energy intake, or dietary cholesterol is less than 300 mg/day), regular exercise, weight management, reduction of alcohol consumption, and smoking cessation
	• Offer 40 mg simvastatin for patients who are older than 40 years and have history of CHD, angina, stroke, peripheral vascular disease, diabetes, and dyslipidaemia.
Weight gain	• Measurement of BMI and waist circumference at baseline and each outpatient visit
	• ☑ Aripiprazole, amisulpride, asenapine, haloperidol, sulpiride, and ziprasidone
	• ☒ Clozapine and olanzapine
	• Bupropion, metformin, and topiramate may reduce body weight.
	• Refer patient to the weight management programme. The patient should aim to lose 5%–10% of original weight with maximum weekly weight loss of 0.5–1 kg.

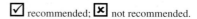 ☑ recommended; ☒ not recommended.

34.4 DSM-5

Feeding and eating disorders (APA, 2013):

307.53 Rumination disorder: repeated regurgitation of food for at least 1 month.

307.59 Avoidant or Restrictive Food Intake Disorder: lack of interest in food and results in significant weight loss and nutritional deficiency.

307.59 Atypical anorexia nervosa: no significant weight loss but other criteria are met.

307.59 Bulimia nervosa (of low frequency or limited duration): no or infrequent binge eating but other criteria are met.

307.59 Purging disorder: recurrent purging.

307.59 Night eating syndrome: recurrent episodes of night eating.

REFERENCES

American Psychiatric Association. 2013: *Desk Reference to the Diagnostic Criteria from DSM-5*. Washington, DC: American Psychiatric Association Press.

Bissada H, Tasca GA, Barber AM, and Bradwejn J. 2008: Olanzapine in the treatment of low body weight and obsessive thinking in women with anorexia nervosa: A randomized, double-blind, placebo-controlled trial. *American Journal of Psychiatry* 165(10):1281–1288.

Boachie A, Goldfield GS, and Spettigue W. 2003: Olanzapine use as an adjunctive treatment for hospitalized children with anorexia nervosa: Case reports. *International Journal of Eating Disorder* 33(1):98–103.

Braun DL, Sunday SR, and Halmi KA. 1994: Psychiatric comorbidity in patients with eating disorders. *Psychological Medicine* 24:859–867.

Brewerton TD and Ballenger JC. 1994: Biological correlates of eating disorders. *Current Opinion in Psychiatry* 7:150–153.

Collings S and King M. 1994: Ten-year follow-up of 50 patients with bulimia nervosa. *British Journal of Psychiatry* 164:80–87.

Elmslie JL, Porter RJ, Joyce PR, Hunt PJ, Shand BI, and Scott RS. 2009: Comparison of insulin resistance, metabolic syndrome and adiponectin in overweight bipolar patients taking sodium valproate and controls. *Australian and New Zealand Journal of Psychiatry* 43(1):53–60.

Expert Panel on Detection, Evaluation, and Treatment of High Blood Cholesterol in Adults. May 2001: Executive summary of the third report of the National Cholesterol Education Program (NCEP) expert panel on detection, evaluation, and treatment of high blood cholesterol in adults (Adult Treatment Panel III). *The Journal of the American Medical Association* 285(19):2486–2497.

Fahy TA, Eisler I, and Russell GFM. 1993: Personality disorder and treatment response in bulimia nervosa. *British Journal of Psychiatry* 162:765–770.

Fairburn CG. 1993: Eating disorders. In Kendell RE and Zealley AK (eds.), *Companion to Psychiatric Studies*. Edinburgh, Scotland: Churchill Livingstone.

Fairburn CG and Harrison PJ. 2003: Eating disorders. *Lancet* 361(9355):407–416.

Fombonne E. 1995: Anorexia nervosa: No evidence of an increase. *British Journal of Psychiatry* 166:462–471.

Freeman CPL, Barry F, Dunkeld-Turnbull J, and Henderson A. 1988: Controlled trial of psychotherapy for bulimia nervosa. *British Medical Journal* 296:521–525.

Garcia-Portilla MP, Saiz PA, Benabarre A et al. (2008) The prevalence of metabolic syndrome in patients with bipolar disorder. *Journal of Affective Disorders* 106(1–2):197–201.

Garfinkel PE, Lin E, Goering P et al. 1995: Bulimia nervosa in a Canadian community sample: Prevalence and comparison of subgroups. *American Journal of Psychiatry* 152:1052–1058.

Gillies CL, Abrams KR, Lambert PC et al. 2007: Pharmacological and lifestyle interventions to prevent or delay type 2 diabetes in people with impaired glucose tolerance: Systematic review and meta-analysis. *British Medical Journal* 334:299–307.

Hamilton K and Waller G. 1993: Media influences on body size estimation in anorexia and bulimia: An experimental study. *British Journal of Psychiatry* 162:837–8340.

Holland AJ, Sicotte N, and Treasure JL. 1988: Anorexia nervosa: Evidence for a genetic basis. *Journal of Psychosomatic Research* 32:561–571.

Hsu LKG, Crisp AH, and Harding B. 1979: Outcome of anorexia nervosa. *Lancet* 313:61–65.

Hudson J, Pope HG, Jenas JM et al. 1983: Family history of anorexia nervosa and bulimia nervosa. *British Journal of Psychiatry* 142:133–138.

International Diabetes Foundation. http://www.idf.org/webdata/docs/IDF_Meta_def_final.pdf (accessed on 25 July 2012).

Kahl KG, Greggersen W, Schweiger U, Cordes J, Balijepalli C, Lösch C, and Moebus S. June 2012: Prevalence of the metabolic syndrome in unipolar major depression. *European Archives of Psychiatry and Clinical Neuroscience* 262(4):313–320.

Kaye WH, Gwirtsman HE, George DT et al. 1991: Altered serotonin activity in anorexia nervosa after long-term weight restoration. *Archives of General Psychiatry* 48:556–562.

Keel PK and Mitchell JE. 1997: Outcome in bulimia nervosa. *American Journal of Psychiatry* 154:313–321.

Kendler KS, Maclean C, Neale M et al. 1991: The genetic epidemiology of bulimia nervosa. *American Journal of Psychiatry* 148:1627–1637.

Lacey HJ, Gowers SG, and Bhat AV. 1991: Bulimia nervosa: Family size, sibling sex and birth order. A catchment area study. *British Journal of Psychiatry* 158:491–494.

Lee S, Ng KL, Kwok K, and Fung C. 2010 The changing profile of eating disorders at a tertiary psychiatric clinic in Hong Kong (1987–2007). *International Journal of Eating Disorders* 43(4):307–314.

Metabolic syndrome. http://www.bbc.co.uk/health/physical_health/conditions/metabolicsyndrome1.shtml (accessed on 25 July 2012)

Meyer JM, Davis VG, Goff DC et al. 2008: Change in metabolic syndrome parameters with antipsychotic treatment in the CATIE Schizophrenia Trial: Prospective data from phase 1. *Schizophr Research* 101(1–3):273–286.

Minuchin S, Rosman BC, and Baker L. 1978: *Psychosomatic Families: Anorexia Nervosa in Context.* Cambridge, MA: Harvard University Press.

Mitchell AJ, Vancampfort D, Sweers K, van Winkel R, Yu W, and De Hert M. December 2011: Prevalence of metabolic syndrome and metabolic abnormalities in schizophrenia and related disorders—A systematic review and meta-analysis. *Schizophr Bulletin* 39(2):295–305.

Newman-Toker J. 2000: Risperidone in anorexia nervosa. *Journal of the American Academy of Child and Adolescent Psychiatry* 39(8):941–942.

NICE. *NICE Guidelines for Eating Disorders.* http://guidance.nice.org.uk/CG9 (accessed on 22 July 2012).

NICE. *NICE Guidelines for Lipid Modification.* http://publications.nice.org.uk/lipid-modification-cg67 (accessed on 22 July 2012).

NICE. *NICE Guidelines for Obesity.* http://www.nice.org.uk/nicemedia/live/11000/30364/30364.pdf (accessed on 22 July 2012).

NICE. *NICE Guidelines for Prevention of Diabetes.* http://publications.nice.org.uk/preventing-type-2-diabetes-population-and community-level-interventions-ph35 (accessed on 22 July 2012).

Palmer RL and Robertson DN. 1995: Outcome in anorexia nervosa and bulimia nervosa. *Current Opinion in Psychiatry* 8:90–92.

Park RJ, Lawrie SM, and Freeman CP. 1995: Post-viral onset of anorexia nervosa. *British Journal of Psychiatry* 166:386–389.

Patton GC, Johnson-Sabine E, Wood K et al. 1990: Abnormal eating attitudes in London schoolgirls (a prospective epidemiological study): Outcome at twelve months follow-up. *Psychological Medicine* 20:383–394.

Patton GC, Wood K, and Johnson-Sabine E. 1986: Physical illness and anorexia nervosa. *British Journal of Psychiatry* 149:756–759.

Piran N. 2005: Prevention of eating disorders: A review of outcome evaluation research. *The Israel Journal of Psychiatry and Related Sciences* 42(3):172–177.

Pyykkönen AJ, Räikkönen K, Tuomi T, Eriksson JG, Groop L, and Isomaa B. 2012: Association between depressive symptoms and metabolic syndrome is not explained by antidepressant medication: Results from the PPP-Botnia Study. *Annals of Medicine* 44(3):279–288.

Quadflieg N and Fichter MM. 2003: The course and outcome of bulimia nervosa. *European Journal of Child and Adolescent Psychiatry* 12(Suppl. 1):99–109.

Robins LN and Regier DA (eds). 1991: *Psychiatric Disorders in America: The Epidemiologic Catchment Area Study.* New York: Free Press.

Salvi V, D'Ambrosio V, Rosso G, Bogetto F, and Maina G. 2011: Age-specific prevalence of metabolic syndrome in Italian patients with bipolar disorder. *Psychiatry and Clinical Neurosciences* 65(1):47–54.

Sohlberg S and Strober M. 1994: Personality in anorexia nervosa: An update and a theoretical integration. *Acta Psychiatrica Scandinavica* 89(Suppl. 378):1–15.

Sullivan PF. 1995: Mortality in anorexia nervosa. *American Journal of Psychiatry* 152:1073–1074.

Taylor D, Paton C, and Kapur S. 2012: *The Maudsley Prescribing Guidelines in Psychiatry,* 11th edn. West Sussex, U.K.: Wiley-Blackwell.

Treasure JL. 2007a: Getting beneath the phenotype of anorexia nervosa: The search for viable endophenotypes and genotypes. *Canadian Journal of Psychiatry* 52(4):212–219.

Treasure J. 2007b: Anorexia nervosa and bulimia nervosa. In Stein G and Wilkinson G (eds.) *Seminars in General Adult Psychiatry,* pp. 616–634. London, U.K.: Gaskell.

Vize CM and Cooper PJ. 1995: Sexual abuse in patients with eating disorders, patients with depression and normal controls: A comparative study. *British Journal of Psychiatry* 167:80–85.

Walsh T, Casadei S, Coats KH et al. 2006: Spectrum of mutations in BRCA1, BRCA2, CHEK2, and TP53 in families at high risk of breast cancer. *The Journal of American Medical Association* 295(12):1379–1388.

Wannamethee SG. May 2008: The metabolic syndrome and cardiovascular risk in the British Regional Heart Study. *International Journal of Obesity (London)* 32(Suppl. 2):S25–S29.

35 Sexual Disorders

35.1 HISTORY

- In 1910, Havelock Ellis, a British pioneer, was the first to subject normal as well as pathological sexuality to scientific investigation (Ellis, 2010).
- Starting in 1948, Kinsey and associates conducted landmark research into human sexual experience in thousands of men and women. A wide range of human sexual expression was noted. Methodological problems included non-random sampling. Volunteers were recruited from a variety of sources, with a nonrepresentative excess of college-educated people, criminals, and sex offenders (Kinsey et al., 1953).
- In 1957, William H. Masters and Virginia E. Johnson studied human sexual response cycle in the United States and established the principles of sensate-focus therapy (Masters and Johnson, 1966).
- In 1981, acquired immune deficiency syndrome (AIDS) was first described in the United States. It was initially believed to be confined to a small group of promiscuous homosexual men. Subsequently, a primarily heterosexual worldwide epidemic of major proportions has developed and the awareness of safe sex was raised globally (Sepkowitz, 2001).

35.1.1 BRITISH SEXUAL BEHAVIOUR AND ATTITUDES

A major survey of British sexual attitudes and lifestyle (Johnson et al., 1994) has provided the most comprehensive evaluation of sexual behaviour in the British public in the 1980s and 1990s. The survey involved 18,876 British men and women in a random population sample aged 16–59. The following statistics were among many that emerged. Kupek (2001) studied the sexual attitudes of 550 young heterosexual British men.

35.1.2 FIRST HETEROSEXUAL INTERCOURSE

- Age at occurrence is decreasing over time. In the past four decades, the median age of first heterosexual intercourse has fallen from 21 to 17 for women and from 20 to 17 for men.

- The proportion occurring before age 16 has increased over time. Fewer than 1% of women aged 55 or over report heterosexual intercourse before the age of 16, compared to 20% of those in their teens.
- People today are more likely to use contraception (usually condoms) than those of a previous generation. However, the earlier first intercourse occurs, the less likely it is that contraception is used.
- It is very rare for men's first sexual intercourse to be with a prostitute.

35.1.3 HETEROSEXUAL PARTNERSHIPS

- Age and marital status are associated with multiple partnerships. The young and those previously married or single (including cohabitees) are most likely to report high partner numbers.
- There is increasing partner change with increasing social class.
- For young heterosexual British men, the main predictor of the number of sexual partners in the last 5 years was the time since the first sexual intercourse.
- Serial monogamy is more common in those aged 16–24. Concurrent partnerships are more common in those over the age of 35.
- Raised odds of ever using a prostitute are associated with age, previous marriage or current cohabitation, working away from home, and a history of having a homosexual partner.

35.1.4 HETEROSEXUAL PRACTICES

- Frequency of heterosexual sex (oral, vaginal, or anal intercourse) shows wide variability, with a small proportion of the population reporting a very high frequency of sexual contact.
- Age is closely related to the number of acts, frequency peaking in mid-twenties, then gradually declining.
- Frequency is affected by partner availability, being highest in married and cohabiting groups of all ages.

- There is a strong association in all age groups between length of relationship and frequency of sex: a much lower frequency in longer relationships.
- Vaginal intercourse predominates. Seventy-five per cent have experience of nonpenetrative sex and 70% have some experience of oral sex. Any experience of anal intercourse is reported by 14% of men and 13% of women.
- Those not married have a wider repertoire of sexual practice. Prevalence of oral, anal, and nonpenetrative sex increases with increasing numbers of partners.

35.1.5 SEXUAL DIVERSITY AND HOMOSEXUAL BEHAVIOUR

- No sexual attraction or experience of any kind is reported by 0.4% of men and 0.5% of women.
- Some form of homosexual experience is reported by 6% of men and 3% of women.
- Lifetime experience of homosexual orientation is higher in higher social classes.
- Recent homosexual experience is strongly associated with region. Greater London has more than twice the proportion of men reporting homosexual experience and current practice than anywhere else in Britain.
- Those who had a boarding-school education are more likely to report any homosexual contact; this has little or no effect on homosexual practice in later life.
- Exclusively homosexual behaviour is rare. The majority of those with homosexual experience have had sex with both men and women. Ninety per cent of men and 95% of women reporting same-gender sexual partners in their lifetime have also had an opposite-gender partner.
- Men reporting anal sex do so usually (60%) as both the receptive and insertive partner.
- Highest levels of homosexual activity are reported by 25–34 year olds, nearly a decade later than heterosexual partnerships, consistent with later age at first experience.

35.1.6 SEXUAL ATTITUDES

- Acceptance of premarital sex is now nearly universal, as is its practice.
- Disapproval of infidelity extends to all age groups, the young being marginally more tolerant than older people.

- Sex is not considered the most important part of a relationship; a monogamous relationship is considered more likely to lead to greater sexual satisfaction.

35.1.7 PHYSICAL HEALTH

- Multiple sexual partnerships are significantly associated with smoking and increasing levels of alcohol consumption.
- Attendance at a clinic for sexually transmitted diseases (STDs) is strongly associated with the number of heterosexual partners and a history of homosexual partnerships.
- The likelihood of termination of pregnancy increases markedly with the numbers of heterosexual partners.

35.1.8 PERCEIVED RISK

- The use of oral contraception declines steeply with age; condom use is most prevalent in the young; sterilization increases with age.
- The message to use condoms to prevent the risks of STD has been more acceptable than the message to restrict numbers of partners.
- The perceived risk of HIV infection is higher among those reporting higher risk behaviours.

35.2 SEXUAL RESPONSE CYCLE

The normal sexual response cycle consists of desire; arousal, mediated by the parasympathetic nervous system; plateau; orgasm, mediated by the sympathetic and central nervous system; and resolution (longer in males and increases with age):

1. Sexual desire is determined by cognitive process, mood, neurophysiological mechanisms (e.g. hormones), personal preferences, and cultural practices. There is a spontaneous occurrence of sexual thoughts and awareness of an interest in initiating sexual activity.
2. Sexual excitement is signified by erection in men and vaginal lubrication in women. Genital response is caused by vasocongestion in both men and women. Peripheral responses include raised blood pressure, altered heart rate, skin temperature, and skin colour changes.
3. Plateau is the maintenance of sexual arousal state.
4. Orgasm is the peak of sexual arousal with explosive discharge of physical, emotional, and psychological

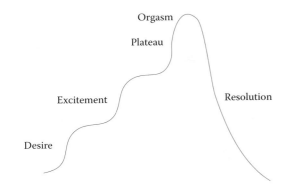

FIGURE 35.1   Sexual response cycle.

buildup. In men, there is an ejaculatory inevitability and ejaculation follows within 1–3 s. In woman, orgasm usually include vaginal contractions, heightened feeling of excitement, or somatic sensations. Small proportions of women produce fluid from the glandular structures along the urethra. The rhythmic muscle contractions may lead to ejaculation of fluid observed in some women.

5. Resolution refers to the return to an unarousal state. In men, there is a refractory period that may last from minutes to hours when the person remains unresponsive to further sexual stimuli. This helps men to replenish the sperm number. In contrast, women are able to experience repeated multiple orgasms in a short period (Figure 35.1).

35.3   SEXUAL DYSFUNCTION

With sexual dysfunctioning the individual is unable to participate in a sexual relationship as he or she would wish. Both psychological and somatic processes are usually involved in the causation of sexual dysfunction. Women present more commonly with complaints about the subjective quality of sexual experience; men present with a failure of specific sexual response.

35.3.1   ICD-10 CLASSIFICATION (WHO, 1992)

ICD-10 categorizes *Sexual dysfunction not caused by organic disorder or disease* under 'Behavioural syndromes associated with physiological disturbances and physical factors', as follows:

- *Lack or loss of sexual desire*: This is not secondary to other sexual difficulties. It does not preclude sexual enjoyment or arousal, but makes initiation of sexual activity less likely.

- *Sexual aversion*: Sexual interaction is associated with strong negative feelings of sufficient intensity that sexual activity is avoided.
- *Lack of sexual enjoyment*: Sexual responses and orgasm occur normally but there is a lack of pleasure. This is much more common in women.
- *Failure of genital response*: In men, this is primarily erectile dysfunction (ED). In women, it is primarily due to vaginal dryness.
- *Orgasmic dysfunction*: Orgasm does not occur or is delayed. It is more common in women than men.
- *Premature ejaculation*: This is the inability to control ejaculation sufficiently for both partners to enjoy the sex act.
- *Nonorganic vaginismus*: This is occlusion of the vaginal opening caused by spasm of the surrounding muscles. Penile entry is either impossible or painful.
- *Nonorganic dyspareunia*: Pain during intercourse may occur in both sexes. The term is used only if an organic cause is not present and if there is no other primary sexual dysfunction.
- *Excessive sexual drive*: This usually occurs in men or women during late teenage or early adult years. If it is secondary to mental illness (e.g. mania), the underlying disorder is coded.

35.3.2   DSM-5 CLASSIFICATION

302.72 Erectile disorder
302.73 Female orgasmic disorder
302.74 Delayed ejaculation
302.75 Early ejaculation
302.73 Female orgasmic disorder
302.72 Female sexual interest/arousal disorder
302.71 Male hypoactive sexual desire disorder
302.76   Genito-pelvic   pain/penetration   disorder
    Substance/medication-induced sexual dysfunction
302.80 Sexual dysfunction not elsewhere classified

35.3.3   SENSATE-FOCUS THERAPY

Masters and Johnson (1970) described behavioural psychotherapy involving a couple in graded assignments that may be modified according to the particular problem presenting. The process is used extensively in the treatment of sexual disorders affecting both men and women.

It consists of a combination of specified homework tasks together with setting specific limits to the extent of sexual contact allowed:

- Stage 1: Touching partner without genital contact for subject's own pleasure.
- Stage 2: Touching partner without genital contact for subject's and partner's pleasure.
- Stage 3: Touching partner with genital contact, but intercourse not permitted.
- Stage 4: Simultaneous touching of partner and being touched by partner with genital contact, but intercourse not permitted.
- Stage 5: If both feel ready, the female invites the male to put his penis into her vagina. Female in the top position heightens female control and allows the male to relax. No thrusting is allowed. Initial containment is brief, being lengthened with each session.
- Stage 6: Vaginal containment with movement is allowed. Different positions are encouraged. This does not inevitably lead to climax. The couple should practice stopping before climax. Provided physical contact is pleasurable, orgasm is not necessary.

35.4 ERECTILE DYSFUNCTION

35.4.1 NORMAL PHYSIOLOGY

Erection is a neurovascular phenomenon requiring an intact arterial supply and intact venous valves, allowing cavernosal pressures to rise to those approaching systolic blood pressures. Vascular changes are brought about by the parasympathetic autonomic nervous system (S2, 3, 4) influenced by tactile stimuli and central limbic and cognitive mechanisms. Psychic erections are mediated by thoracic sympathetic outflow, whereas reflex erections result from sacral parasympathetic outflow. Androgens also influence erection, particularly those occurring in sleep, via the limbic system.

35.4.2 EPIDEMIOLOGY OF ERECTILE DYSFUNCTION

- In the United Kingdom, Dunn et al. (1998) reported that men aged 18–75 showed a rate of 26% and 39% for current and lifetime prevalence of ED, respectively.
- ED comprises about 50% of male cases presenting to a psychosexual disorder service.
- The incidence rises with age, from about 1.3% at 35 years to 55% at 75 years.

35.4.3 AETIOLOGY OF ERECTILE DYSFUNCTION

The aetiology can be organic (in about 50%), psychological, or a combination.

35.4.3.1 Organic Causes

35.4.3.1.1 Local Organic Causes

- *Peyronie's disease*: There is progressive fibrosis in the tunica albuginea and sometimes also in the cavernosa, resulting in curvature of the penis on erection. The cause is unknown.
- *Congenital deformities*: Examples are hypospadias and epispadias, or the absence of suspensory ligaments.
- *Priapism*: Although rare, priapism may result in impotence if not treated adequately within 24 h.

35.4.3.1.2 Endocrine Causes

- Diabetes causes a combination of arteriopathy and neuropathy. Two-thirds of diabetic males have ED. Of these, it is complete in two-thirds and partial in the remaining third. A few also complain of other difficulties such as premature ejaculation. Onset is insidious, the course progressive with marked decline in sexual activity and desire.
- Nocturnal erections are androgen dependent. Studies are conflicting on the role of androgens in ED. Effects are probably mediated through lowered sexual interest.
- Hyperprolactinaemia may be secondary to hypothalamic/pituitary disease. It occurs in those on phenothiazines, and sometimes in alcoholics.
- Naltrexone (endorphin) therapy significantly improves ED in males with an apparent nonorganic cause. Alteration in central opioid tone may be responsible.

35.4.3.1.3 Neurological Causes

- There may be peripheral or autonomic neuropathy (e.g. in diabetes, alcoholism).
- Radical pelvic surgery may cause autonomic neurological disruption.
- There may be a spinal cord lesion (e.g. transection, multiple sclerosis).

35.4.3.1.4 Vascular Causes

- Arterial disease can interfere with the blood supply to pelvic organs.
- Venous valves may be incompetent.

35.4.3.2 Pharmacological Factors

Alcohol has complex effects, including neuropathy and indirect effects on sex steroids and gonadotropins. Oestrogen levels are raised causing gynaecomastia and testicular atrophy in advanced liver disease. Raised blood alcohol levels inhibit sexual responses through central inhibitory effects. Psychosocial factors are also prominent in these patients.

Ganglion blockers (*antihypertensives*) interfere with both sympathetic and parasympathetic postganglionic transmission and cause both ED and ejaculatory failure. Propranolol crosses the blood–brain barrier and may exert its effect centrally. Alpha-adrenergic blockers are not associated with erectile failure, but cause ejaculatory failure.

35.4.3.3 Psychological Factors

The classical history of ED that is suggestive of a psychological cause comprises lack of sexual interest but continued morning erections.

35.4.3.3.1 Psychoanalytic Concepts

Sexual physiological changes result from the interplay between conscious and unconscious thoughts and feelings and interpersonal relationships. Anxiety and fear, whether conscious or unconscious, can interfere with vascular changes required for erection. Arousal phase disorders of ED in men are common. Interference with abandonment to erotic feelings can impair arousal in men and lead to difficulties with erection.

Psychoanalytic formulations of ED recognize anxiety about the persecutory object and unresolved Oedipal conflicts. Deep ambivalence about intimate involvement leading to fear of sexual failure is common.

In younger men with primary ED, Oedipal conflicts are said to predominate, whereas in secondary impotence, neurotic partnership conflicts at a pre-Oedipal level, and narcissistic crises in middle age are said to predominate.

35.4.3.3.2 Cognitive Concepts

ED is considered to be a sign of negative self-image within a depressive view of the relationship and is linked to abandonment fear.

Subjects with psychogenic ED have a situational sexual disorder in which sexual anxiety plays an important role. Compared to those with organic impotence or to controls, they view themselves as more insecure and tend to overidealize their partners and their mothers.

Consideration should also be given to the following:

- Fear of hurting the female
- Fear of pregnancy
- Distaste for female genitalia
- Placing the partner on a pedestal
- Nonsexual stress
- Unsympathetic or angry partner
- Trying too hard

35.4.4 ASSESSMENT OF ERECTILE DYSFUNCTION

The assessment of ED includes the following:

- A full history is needed, including the nature of the current ED and previous erectile capacity, detailed sexual history, history of physical trauma to genitalia or spine, medical and psychiatric histories, medication and substance use, past investigation, and treatment.
- Assessment of the couple's relationship is essential. Difficulties such as hostility, lack of communication, and unresponsive or unerotic partner may be important.
- Identify predisposing factors such as poor past sexual experience, religious or cultural beliefs, restrictive upbringing, unclear sexual preference, and previous sexual abuse.
- Identify precipitating factors such as family pressures, partner menopause, and acute physical or mental problems.
- Identify maintaining factors such as relationship problems and ongoing physical or mental illnesses.
- Physical examination includes the assessment of testes or penis; laboratory investigations including blood glucose and tests of renal and hepatic function.
- The use of International Index of Erectile Function (IIEF) is helpful to assess severity of ED.

35.4.5 DIAGNOSTIC CRITERIA

ICD-10 classifies ED under the F52.2 Failure of genital response. ED is defined as erection insufficient for intercourse when intercourse is attempted. There are four types of ED:

1. Full erection occurs during the early stages of sexual activity but disappears or declines before ejaculation.
2. Erection does occur, but only at times when intercourse is not being considered.
3. Partial erection, insufficient for intercourse, occurs, but not full erection.
4. No penile tumescence occurs at all.

35.4.5.1 DSM-5 Criteria: 302.72 Erectile Disorder

35.4.5.1.1 General Criteria (Apply to Most Sexual Dysfunctions)

- The sexual dysfunction must have been present for at least 6 months and occur for at least for 75% of sexual activity.
- The sexual dysfunction causes clinically significant distress or impairment.
- The sexual dysfunction is not attributable to a primary nonsexual psychiatric disorder, by the effects of a substance/medication, by an underlying medical condition, and by partner violence or other significant stressors.
- Subtype includes acquired or lifelong type.
- Specifier include situational versus generalized, partner's factors, relationship factors, individual vulnerability, cultural/religious factors, and medical factors.

35.4.5.1.2 Specific Criteria

- ED is defined as marked difficulty in obtaining and maintaining erection during sexual activity.
- There is marked decrease in erectile rigidity that interferes with sexual activity.

35.4.6 INVESTIGATIONS

The doctor needs to consider the background history in deciding the choice of investigations:

- As metabolic syndrome is a risk factor for ED, fasting lipids and glucose should be measured in most patients.
- Thyroid function tests and prolactin levels can rule out hyperthyroidism and hyperprolactinaemia, respectively.
- If a man is suspected to have hypogonadism, serum testosterone should be measured between 8:00 to 11:00 a.m.
- A penile–brachial artery pressure index of less than 0.6 is indicative of arterial disease to the penis. Angiography may be necessary, especially in younger patients.
- Nocturnal penile tumescence and rigidity (NPTR) can be used to measure circumference change in REM sleep erections. This can help distinguish organic from psychogenic; if the cause is organic, erections at night are abolished.

NPTR is a noninvasive investigation but requires overnight measurement in hospital.

- Intracorporeal injection of a prostaglandin E inhibitor (papaverine or phentolamine) can be diagnostic to establish the capacity for erection and hence reduce the likelihood of a primarily arterial cause.
- Duplex ultrasound of penile arteries is a radiological investigation that measures blood flow. This investigation provides an excellent assessment of penile vasculature in response to an injection of a prostaglandin E inhibitor.
- Arteriography is a highly specialized procedure and only be performed when an arterial lesion has been found on Duplex ultrasound investigation.
- Dynamic cavernosometry, in which normal saline is infused into the corpus cavernosum, may detect venous incompetence.

35.4.7 MANAGEMENT OF ERECTILE DYSFUNCTION

35.4.7.1 Objectives

The primary goals of management include

1. Identify and treat reversible causes of ED (e.g. testosterone for hypogonadism, treatment of hyperthyroidism)
2. Initiate lifestyle change (e.g. regular exercise) and risk factor modification
3. Provide psychoeducation to patient and his partner

The British Society for Sexual Medicine classifies ED treatment as follows:

35.4.7.2 First-Line Treatment

35.4.7.2.1 Phosphodiesterase Type 5 (PDE 5) Inhibitors

Orally administered phosphodiesterase type 5 inhibitors that are licenced for treatment of ED include sildenafil, tadalafil, and vardenafil.

35.4.7.2.2 Pharmacodynamics

1. The mechanism of erection of the penis involves release of nitric oxide (NO) in the corpus cavernosum during sexual stimulation. NO then activates the enzyme guanylate cyclase, which results in increased levels of cyclic guanosine monophosphate (cGMP), producing smooth muscle relaxation in the corpus cavernosum that allows the blood inflow.

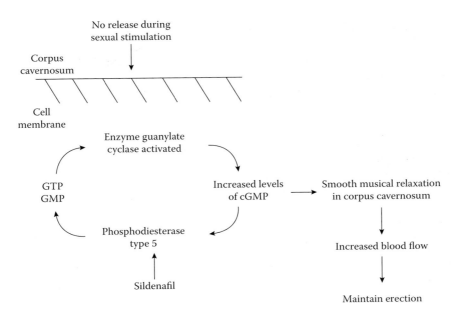

FIGURE 35.2   Pharmacodynamics of sildenafil.

2. Sildenafil citrate is ingested orally prior to sexual intercourse and enhances the effect of NO by inhibiting phosphodiesterase type 5 (PDE5), which is responsible for degradation of cGMP in the corpus cavernosum.
3. The increase in cGMP resulting in smooth muscle relaxation and inflow of blood to the corpus cavernosum (Figure 35.2).

The drugs are contraindicated in patients:

- Receiving nitrates
- In whom vasodilation is inadvisable
- In whom sexual activity is inadvisable
- With hypotension
- With a history of recent stroke
- With unstable angina
- With myocardial infarction

35.4.7.2.3   Drug Interactions

These drugs should not be administered with other pharmacological treatments for ED. They should be used with caution in cardiovascular disease, anatomical deformation of the penis (e.g. angulation, cavernosal fibrosis, Peyronie's disease), and in those with a predisposition to prolonged erection (e.g. in sickle-cell anaemia, multiple myeloma, or leukaemia).

35.4.7.2.4   Side Effects

The side effects of these drugs include dyspepsia, vomiting, headache, flushing, dizziness, visual disturbances, raised intraocular pressure, and nasal congestion. Hypersensitivity reactions (including rash), priapism, and painful red eyes have also been reported.

35.4.7.2.5   Nonresponders to PDE5 Inhibitors

- Approximately 25% of ED patients do not respond to PED5 inhibitors.
- Re-counsel on proper use and reevaluate for new risk factors.
- Treat concurrent hypogonadism by apomorphine or testosterone.

35.4.7.2.6   Apomorphine

Apomorphine hydrochloride is administered sublingually and stimulates dopamine receptors in the hypothalamus and midbrain regions. Once the sexual stimulation has occurred, apomorphine hydrochloride enhances the excitatory signal that is transmitted via the spinal cord to stimulate the parasympathetic activity in the pelvic region (Figure 35.3).

Although apomorphine is licenced for the treatment of ED, it is more effective in patients with sexual desire disorder rather than ED. Vasovagal symptoms (including sweating and syncope) can occur infrequently.

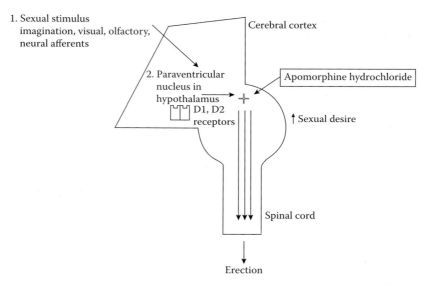

FIGURE 35.3 Pharmacodynamics of apomorphine.

35.4.7.2.7 Psychotherapy

Psychotherapy can be combined with medication.

Cognitive behavioural methods report success rates of 70% for erectile impotence. Couple therapy appears to be superior to surrogate or individual therapies. Factors associated with successful outcome include the state of the marriage, better pretreatment communication, better general sexual adjustment, female partner's interest and enjoyment of sex, absence of psychiatric history in the female partner, and early engagement in homework assignments.

Sensate focus therapy may need to be combined with other methods, such as improvement in communication skills. Once erections are starting to occur, a form of 'paradoxical intent' may be used, in which the couple is instructed to get rid of the erection as soon as it occurs, and then to resume touching. The purpose is to demonstrate that erections do not need to be used as soon as they arise.

Psychodynamic therapists challenge disturbing fantasies and prevent their reenactment. The patient is offered a psychotherapeutic 'holding' to counteract the unsafe internal world. Gradually he becomes freed from his sexually disempowering psychic reality to respond to the external reality of erotic stimulation. Behavioural interventions may also be incorporated into the treatment.

35.4.7.2.8 Vacuum Suction Devices

- Vacuum tumescence constriction therapy is efficacious and useful in those with organic as well as psychogenic impotence.

- These devices provide a safe method of obtaining an erection adequate for penetration in up to 90% of patients.
- Many couples derive substantial benefit from their use, but the disadvantages of a not fully rigid erection, lack of spontaneity, decreased sensation, and delayed or absent ejaculation in some limit their acceptability.
- Adverse effects include bruising, local pain, and feeling cold in penis.

35.4.7.3 Second-Line Treatment

35.4.7.3.1 Intracavernosal Injection of Vasoactive Drugs

Papaverine is commonly used to treat impotence. Self-injected, it gives an erection lasting about an hour and may be used up to twice a week. Half those presenting to a sexual dysfunction clinic benefit from intracorporeal papaverine. Many decline the treatment because of the perception that injection is cumbersome and interrupts sexual foreplay or because of objection to the use of needles. Intracorporeal pharmacotherapy provides a useful treatment option in the management of impotence but it is limited by the method of administration.

Complications include priapism that should be treated promptly by the withdrawal of 20–60 mL of blood and injection of an α-adrenergic agent such as phenylephrine 1–5 mg, or metaraminol 2 mg. Fibrosis is associated with prolonged use and rises in proportion to the total numbers of injections given. Hematomas and bruising are relatively common but of little significance.

35.4.7.3.2 *Intraurethral Alprostadil*

Alprostadil (prostaglandin E_1) is administered by intracavernosal injection or intraurethral application for the management of ED (after exclusion of treatable medical causes); it is also used as a diagnostic test.

35.4.7.3.3 *Alpha-Adrenergic Blocking Agents*

Phenoxybenzamine or phentolamine may also be used to give more prolonged erection.

35.4.7.4 Third-Line Treatment

35.4.7.4.1 *Penile Prosthetic Implants*

Surgically implanted penile prostheses are inserted into the corpus cavernosa. Three types are available: malleable, constructed of silastic with a malleable metal core giving permanent rigidity; self-contained inflatable; and multipart inflatable prostheses.

The psychological outcome of penile prosthesis implantation appears to be mediated by the nature of the marital relationship. Follow-up of recipients of penile implants 2.5 years following surgery found that those with organogenic impotence had no adverse sequelae, but some of those with psychogenic impotence had an exacerbation of preexisting relationship difficulties. Ideally couple therapy should be offered as well as mechanical treatments, especially in those with a psychogenic cause.

35.4.7.4.2 *Vascular Surgery*

Correction of venous leak may be successful if a specific leak is detected. Arterial surgery is less successful. Large vessel reconstruction for proximal arterial obstruction generally gives poor results, as most patients also have distal arterial disease.

35.5 FAILURE OF GENITAL RESPONSES FOR WOMEN

The ICD-10 defines that there is a failure of genital response, experienced as failure of vaginal lubrication and inadequate tumescence of the labia. There are three different types:

1. General: lubrication fails in all relevant circumstances.
2. Lubrication may occur initially but fails to persist for long enough to allow comfortable penile entry.
3. Situational: lubrication occurs only in some situations (e.g. with one partner but not another, or during masturbation).

35.6 LACK OF SEXUAL DRIVE OR SEXUAL ENJOYMENT

35.6.1 Aetiology and Risk Factors

- Ageing
- Anticonvulsant
- Depression
- Hyperprolactinaemia
- Multiple sclerosis
- Malignancy
- Relationship problem
- Restrictive upbringing on the issues of sex

35.6.2 Diagnostic Criteria

35.6.2.1 ICD-10 Criteria (WHO, 1992)

35.6.2.1.1 *F52.0 Lack or Loss of Sexual Desire*

1. Lack or loss of sexual desire as manifested by diminution of seeking out sexual cues and of thinking about sex or of sexual fantasies.
2. Lack of interest in initiating sexual activity either with a partner or during masturbation. Sexual activities become less frequent compared to the norms or previous level.

35.6.2.1.2 *F52.10/F52.11 Sexual Aversion and Lack of Sexual Enjoyment*

1. The sexual interaction with a partner produces sufficient aversion or anxiety. As a result, sexual activity is avoided. It is also associated with strong negative feelings and an inability to experience any pleasure.
2. Genital response (e.g. orgasm or ejaculation) may occur but is not accompanied by any pleasurable sensations or feelings of excitement.

35.6.2.2 DSM-5 Criteria (APA, 2013)

35.6.2.2.1 *302.72 Female Sexual Interest/ Arousal Disorder*

1. The general criteria (6-month duration, frequency of 75%, subtype, specifier, and functional impairment) for sexual dysfunctions apply.
2. Absence or reduced frequency in at least three of the following criteria: interest in sexual activity, sexual/erotic thoughts or fantasies, initiation of sexual activity, sexual excitement/sexual pleasure, and sexual interest/arousal in response to any internal or external sexual/erotic cues.

35.6.2.2.2 302.71 Male Hypoactive Sexual Desire Disorder

1. The general criteria (6-month duration, frequency of 75%, subtype, specifier, and functional impairment) for sexual dysfunctions apply.
2. Persistently or recurrently deficient (or absent) sexual/erotic thoughts or fantasies and desire for sexual activity. The judgement of deficiency is made by the doctor taking into account of background factors such as age or sociocultural background.

35.6.3 TREATMENT

1. Treat the underlying psychiatric or medical disorders.
2. Couple therapy, cognitive therapy, or counselling may be useful.
3. Apomorphine hydrochloride may improve sexual desire.

35.7 PREMATURE EJACULATION

35.7.1 NORMAL PHYSIOLOGY

Orgasm, seminal emission, and ejaculation are physiologically distinct processes and are potentially separable.

Ejaculation is the forceful expulsion of semen from the urethra. If semen is released from the urethra without force, it is emission. Before orgasm the male becomes aware that ejaculation is imminent and it follows within 1–3 s—'ejaculatory inevitability'. Ejaculation and emission are mediated by the α-adrenergic sympathetic nervous system. Androgens have a role, since the first sexual consequence of castration is the inability to ejaculate, which is rapidly restored with androgen replacement.

In severe premature ejaculation, emission alone may occur with no ejaculatory component, minimal or absent orgasm, and a long refractory period.

In youth, males have a tendency to ejaculate quickly. This usually diminishes with increasing age because of increasing control with experience, an ability to recognize the approach of ejaculatory inevitability, the dampening in responsiveness with age, and the lessening of novelty that arises in a stable relationship.

35.7.2 EPIDEMIOLOGY OF PREMATURE EJACULATION

Studies with community samples indicate the prevalence of 36%–38% for premature ejaculation. Thirteen per cent of attendees at a sexual disorders clinic present primarily with this problem.

35.7.3 AETIOLOGY OF PREMATURE EJACULATION

35.7.3.1 Nonphysical Factors

- Anxiety promotes emission but inhibits orgasm and thus plays a crucial role in premature ejaculation.
- Primary premature ejaculation is always present. Secondary premature ejaculation develops after a period of satisfactory sexual functioning.
- Those with primary premature ejaculation are more impaired in sexual functioning and are more anxious. Those with secondary premature ejaculation are more likely to have coexisting erectile disorder, a reduction in sex drive, and a reduction in arousal.
- In psychological terms, whereas erectile disorder seems to belong to a depressive organization, premature ejaculation belongs to a phobic one.
- A variety of psychological factors may interfere with the learning process, impairing the ability to identify the point of impending ejaculation.

35.7.3.2 Physical Factors

There are few physical causes. Drugs do not cause premature ejaculation. It is possible that the autonomic control of ejaculation is very sensitive and therefore more difficult to control in some individuals.

Those with premature ejaculation do not have penile hypersensitivity compared to controls.

No differences in the pituitary gonadal system are found between those with erectile impotence, premature ejaculation, and normal controls.

35.7.4 DIAGNOSTIC CRITERIA

35.7.4.1 ICD-10 Criteria: F52.4 (WHO, 1992) Premature Ejaculation

There is an inability to delay ejaculation sufficiently to enjoy sexual intercourse. Ejaculation occurs very soon after the beginning of intercourse (before or within 15 s). Ejaculation may occur in the absence of sufficient erection to make intercourse possible.

35.7.4.2 DSM-5 Criteria: 302.75 Early Ejaculation

The general criteria (6-month duration, frequency of 75%, subtype, specifier, and functional impairment) for sexual dysfunctions apply.

Persistent or recurrent pattern of ejaculation occurring during individual or partnered sexual activity (vaginal or nonvaginal) within approximately 1 min from the beginning.

35.7.5 Management of Premature Ejaculation

Education in ejaculatory control using the 'pause' technique is the treatment of choice. During sensate-focus exercises, the male, when he predicts that he will ejaculate shortly, asks his partner to stop, allow his arousal level to subside slightly, and then return to being caressed, repeating the process again when arousal increases.

If difficulty is experienced using this method, then the 'squeeze technique' is used. Just before ejaculation becomes inevitable, stimulation is stopped and the tip of the penis is grasped firmly for about 10 s, reducing the reflex ejaculatory response.

At therapeutic doses, some antidepressants (e.g. fluoxetine) have a beneficial effect in men with premature ejaculation.

35.8 ANORGASMIA

35.8.1 Normal Physiology

The final stage of sexual excitement may be orgasm. In both sexes, if no orgasm occurs, there is a slow resolution of physical and psychological changes associated with sexual excitement. Apart from ejaculation for which there is no female counterpart, the correlates of orgasm are similar in the sexes. Heart rate and blood pressure increase, there is a sudden increase in skeletal muscle activity involving almost all parts of the body. Rhythmic muscle contractions in the male genital tract expel semen; in females, there is transient rhythmical contraction of the uterus and vagina. Psychologically there is an instant sense of relief; at its most extreme, there can be a virtual loss of consciousness, and relaxation ensues.

The exact mechanism of orgasm is not known. In addition to local spinal mechanisms, the central nervous activity is also involved. EEG recordings during intense orgasm show changes that have been likened to those occurring during epileptic fits.

35.8.2 Epidemiology of Anorgasmia

The prevalence in community samples is around 5%–10% for inhibited female orgasm, and 4%–10% for inhibited male orgasm. Among attendees at a sexual disorders clinic, 5% of males and 7% of females present primarily with orgasmic dysfunction. In females, the prevalence of anorgasmia reduces with increasing age.

35.8.3 Aetiology of Anorgasmia

Little is known.

35.8.3.1 Physical Factors

- In primary complete anorgasmia in both sexes, the bulbocavernosus reflex has been reported to be absent in a proportion; this is strongly correlated with the failure of treatment.
- Sometimes local pain, possibly secondary to muscle spasm, or in local viscera (uterus, rectum), can create fear of orgasm.
- Opiates appear to have a direct inhibitory effect, and antiserotonergic drugs inhibit orgasm.
- Female anorgasmia has been reported in association with tricyclic, MAOI, and SSRI antidepressants and neuroleptic drugs.

35.8.3.2 Psychological Factors

The aetiology of anorgasmia is usually psychological. Anxiety inhibits orgasm in women but can hasten emission in men. Sex may be viewed as bad, disgusting, or threatening the need to remain in control at all times. There may be a fear of pregnancy or venereal disease.

35.8.4 Diagnostic Criteria

35.8.4.1 ICD-10 Criteria: F52.3 (WHO, 1992) Orgasmic Dysfunction

There is orgasmic dysfunction that involves either absence or delay of orgasm. There are three forms:

1. Orgasm has never been experienced in any situation.
2. Orgasmic dysfunction occurs in all situations and with any partner.
3. Orgasmic dysfunction is situational.

For women: Orgasm may occur in certain situations (e.g. when masturbating or with certain partners).

For men: Orgasm may only occur during sleep and never during waking state.

35.8.4.2 DSM-5 Criteria (APA, 2013)

The general criteria (6-month duration, frequency of 75%, subtype, specifier, and functional impairment) for sexual dysfunctions apply.

302.73 Female orgasmic disorder: Marked delay in orgasm, marked infrequency, or absence of orgasm and markedly reduced intensity of orgasmic sensation.

302.74 Delayed ejaculation: Marked delay in ejaculation or marked infrequency or absence of ejaculation.

35.8.5 Management of Anorgasmia

Sociocultural expectations and deficits in skills and sexual techniques are the two most important factors present in most cases. Direct masturbation training is the treatment of choice.

Treatment may take place in individual, couple, or group settings. Tasks include relaxation, fantasizing, and masturbation. Treatment is often successful, but the generalization of orgasm induced by masturbation to that induced by intercourse does not always occur.

For men with delayed ejaculation, yohimbine may assist ejaculation. Side effects include anxiety, agitation, diarrhoea, and flu-like symptoms.

35.9 VAGINISMUS AND DYSPAREUNIA

35.9.1 Normal Physiology

When sexually aroused, the upper two-thirds of the vagina are lax and capacious, whereas the lower third is closely invested by the surrounding musculature of the pelvic floor. The strongest of these muscles is the levator ani that forms a U-shaped sling around the posterior and lateral vaginal wall. Intense spasm in a nulliparous woman can virtually occlude the vagina. If these muscles are too tense, vaginal entry is impaired and painful—a condition known as vaginismus. A vicious circle ensues; pain or anticipation of pain causes further muscle contraction thereby increasing the likelihood of experiencing pain.

35.9.2 Epidemiology of Vaginismus

Ten per cent of women presenting to a sexual disorders clinic have a primary presentation of vaginismus.

35.9.3 Aetiology of Vaginismus

The majority of cases are primary. The problem was evident at first attempt at intercourse, and usually the woman has been reluctant to introduce anything to her vagina previously.

Occasionally onset can be related to a traumatic episode such as a painful vaginal examination or rape.

Sometimes vaginismus results from ambivalence about the relationship, or it may be secondary to reluctance to assume the mature adult's role. Irrational fears may also underlie the condition.

35.9.4 Diagnostic Criteria

35.9.4.1 ICD-10 Criteria (WHO, 1992)

35.9.4.1.1 F52.5 Nonorganic Vaginismus

There is a spasm of the perivaginal muscles preventing entry of penis into vagina or make intercourse uncomfortable. There are two types:

1. Primary vaginismus: the patient has never been experienced normal response.
2. Secondary vaginismus: the patient develops vaginismus after a period of relatively normal response. The patient may either have a normal sexual response when vaginal entry is not attempted or any attempt at sexual contact can lead to generalized fear and efforts be made to avoid vaginal entry.

35.9.4.1.2 F52.6 Nonorganic Dyspareunia

For women:

1. Pain is experienced at the entry of the vagina, either throughout sexual intercourse or only when deep thrusting of the penis occurs.
2. This disorder is either a result of vaginismus or failure of lubrication.

For men:

1. Pain or discomfort is experienced during sexual response. The timing of pain and the exact location should be carefully recorded.
2. The discomfort is not the result of local physical factors or organic causes.

35.9.4.1.3 DSM-5 Criteria: 302.76 Genito-Pelvic Pain or Penetration Disorder (APA, 2013)

The general criteria (6-month duration, frequency of 75%, subtype, specifier, and functional impairment) for sexual dysfunctions apply.

Persistent or recurrent difficulties with one or more of the following during vaginal intercourse or penetration:

1. Marked vulvovaginal or pelvic pain
2. Marked fear or anxiety about vulvovaginal or pelvic pain
3. Marked tensing or tightening of the pelvic floor muscles

35.9.5 Management of Vaginismus

Emphasis is upon helping the woman to gain comfort in exploring her own genitalia and inserting her finger. Finger insertion may be all that is required, combined with sensate-focus techniques. Additional dilatation may be required using graded dilators. Initially carried out on her own, the partner is included when her confidence has increased.

35.10 DISORDERS OF GENDER IDENTITY

35.10.1 Classification

The ICD-10 classification codes *Gender identity disorders* under 'Disorders of adult personality and behaviour'.

35.10.1.1 Transsexualism

There is the desire to live as a member of the opposite sex, discomfort with anatomic sex, and a wish to change body into that of the preferred sex.

It must have been persistently present for 2 years; it must not be a symptom of another mental disorder such as schizophrenia, or be associated with an intersex, genetic, or sex-chromosomal abnormality.

35.10.1.2 Dual-Role Transvestism

This includes the wearing of clothes of the opposite sex for part of the time to enjoy the temporary experience of membership of the opposite sex, without the desire for a more permanent sex change. No sexual excitement accompanies this cross-dressing, distinguishing it from fetishistic transvestism.

35.10.1.3 Gender Identity Disorder of Childhood

This is persistent, intense distress about assigned sex, together with desire to be of the other sex, usually manifest during early childhood, and always before puberty. It is relatively uncommon. There is a profound disturbance of the sense of maleness or femaleness.

Between one- and two-thirds of boys with gender identity disorder of childhood show homosexual orientation during and after adolescence. However, very few exhibit transsexualism in later life, although most adults with transsexualism report having had a gender identity problem in childhood. Some girls retain male gender identification in adolescence and some go on to homosexual orientation. Most, however, do not.

It is more common in boys than girls in clinic samples.

35.10.2 Diagnostic Criteria

35.10.2.1 ICD-10 (WHO, 1992)

35.10.2.1.1 *F64.2 Gender Identity Disorder of Childhood*

For girls:

1. The child shows persistent and intense distress about being a girl and has a stated desire to be a boy.
2. Either of the following must be present:
   a. Persistent marked aversion to feminine clothing and insistence on wearing stereotypical masculine clothing, for example, boys' underwear and other accessories.
   b. Persistent rejection of female anatomical structures, as evidenced an assertion that (i) she wants to have a penis, (ii) refuse to urinate in a sitting position, and (iii) assertion that she does not want to grow breasts or have menses.
3. The girl has not yet reached puberty.
4. Duration of symptoms: at least 6 months.

For boys, the symptoms are very similar to girls. The prepubertal child shows persistent and intense distress about being a boy and has a desire to be a girl. The child prefers female activities and clothing and rejects male anatomical structure.

35.10.2.1.2 *F64.0 Transsexualism*

The individual desires to live and be accepted as a member of the opposite sex, usually accompanied by the wish to make his or her body as congruent as possible with the preferred sex through surgery and hormonal treatment. Duration required for persistent transsexual identity for at least 2 years.

35.10.2.1.3 *DSM-5 (APA, 2013)*

302.6 Gender dysphoria (in children): The proposed DSM-5 criteria are very similar to the ICD-10 criteria with additional characteristics such as a strong preference for playmates of the other gender and functional impairment. The DSM-5 further classifies this condition as with or without a disorder of sex development.

302.85 Gender dysphoria (in adolescents or adults): Marked incongruence between one's gender and primary and/or secondary sex characteristics, a strong desire to be rid of one's primary and/or secondary sex characteristics, a stronger desire to be of and be treated as the other gender, displaying the typical feelings and reactions of the other gender, and functional impairment for at least 6 months. The DSM-5 further classifies this condition as with or without a disorder of sex development.

35.10.3 TREATMENT OF DISORDERS OF GENDER IDENTITY

Sex-reassignment treatment for transsexuals is a process of active rehabilitation into the new gender role, the provision and monitoring of opposite-sex hormones, and after a reasonable period of successful cross-gender living, sex-reassignment surgery is performed. The majority of transsexuals do experience a successful outcome in terms of subjective well-being and personal happiness.

35.11 SEXUAL DEVIATION

35.11.1 CLASSIFICATION

The ICD-10 classification codes sexual deviation as *Disorders of sexual preference* under 'Disorders of adult personality and behaviour'. The proposed DSM-5 classifies these disorders as paraphilic disorders.

35.11.1.1 ICD-10 F 65.0 Fetishism/DSM-5 302.81 Fetishistic Disorder

Definition: Fetishism is the reliance on some nonliving object as a stimulus for sexual arousal and gratification. It is often an extension of the human body such as clothing or footwear. It is often characterized by texture such as plastic, rubber, or leather.

Epidemiology: Fetishism is more common in men and 20% are homosexuals.

Aetiology: Fetishism is caused by classical conditioning between an object and sexual arousal during masturbation. It is associated with temporal lobe dysfunction.

Clinical features: Fetishism is diagnosed only if the fetish is the most important source of sexual stimulation. Fantasies are common but do not amount to disorder unless they are so compelling that they interfere with sexual intercourse and lead to distress.

The DSM-5 criteria specify minimum 6 month duration and further classify fetishistic disorder as body part, nonliving part, in a controlled environment or in remission.

Treatment: Behavioural therapy focusing masturbatory reconditioning and response prevention.

Course and prognosis: Onset is often during adolescence. Most fetishism diminishes after developing a satisfying heterosexual relationship. The prognosis is worse in single man or those with forensic history related to fetishism.

35.11.1.2 ICD-10 F65.1 Fetishistic Transvestism/ DSM-5 302.3 Transvestic Disorder

Definition: Fetishistic transvestism is the wearing of clothes of the opposite sex to obtain sexual excitement. More than a single item is worn, often an entire outfit. It is clearly associated with sexual arousal; there is no wish to continue cross-dressing once orgasm occurs, distinguishing this from dual-role transvestism.

Epidemiology: Fetishistic transvestism is more common in men and most patients are heterosexual.

Aetiology: Fetishistic transvestism is caused by classical conditioning between the clothes and sexual arousal during masturbation. It is associated with temporal lobe dysfunction.

35.11.1.3 F64.1 Dual-Role Transvestism

1. The individual wears clothes of the opposite sex in order to experience temporarily membership of the opposite sex. There is no sexual motivation for the cross-dressing.
2. The individual has no desire for a permanent change of gender.
3. Age of onset: puberty and the behaviour is concealed without guilt.

The DSM-5 specify minimum 6 month duration and further classify transvestic disorder into three types:

1. With fetishism (sexually aroused by fabrics, materials, or garments)
2. With autogynephilia (sexually aroused by thought or image of self as a woman)

Treatment: No specific treatment is required for dual-role transvestism but allowing the person to ventilate their feelings may help to reduce the frequency of cross-dressing. For fetishistic transvestism, behavioural therapy focusing masturbatory reconditioning and response prevention may reduce.

Prognosis: The condition becomes less severe as sexual drive declines. Some patients with dual-role transvestism convert to fetishistic transvestism.

35.11.1.4 ICD-10 F65.2 Exhibitionism/DSM-5 302.4 Exhibitionistic Disorder

Definition: Exhibitionism is the recurrent or persistent tendency to expose the genitalia to strangers or people (usually of the opposite sex) in public places. There is usually sexual excitement at the time, often followed by masturbation. The tendency may only manifest at times of emotional stress or crisis, without such behaviour between.

Clinical features: It is almost entirely limited to heterosexual males, exhibiting to adult or adolescent females, usually from a safe distance in a public place. For some, it is their only sexual outlet; for others, they may also continue a normal sex life. A reaction in the victim heightens the excitement in the perpetrator and the patient usually has no intention to have sexual intercourse with the victim.

The DSM-5 criteria specify minimum 6 month duration and further classify exhibitionistic disorder into three types:

1. Sexually attracted to exposing genitals to pubescent or prepubescent persons younger than 15 years of age
2. Sexually attracted to exposing genitals to physically mature older than 15 years of age
3. Equally sexually attracted to exposing genitals to both age groups

35.11.1.5 ICD-10 F65.3 Voyeurism/DSM-5 302.82 Voyeuristic Disorder

Definition: Voyeurism is the persistent tendency to look at people engaging in sexual behaviour or undressing. It usually leads to sexual excitement and masturbation. The victim is usually unaware. The voyeur has no intention of sexual involvement with the person observed.

Clinical features: The voyeur is usually a man who is shy, socially awkward with girls, and has difficulty with normal sexual expression.

35.11.1.6 ICD-10 F65.4 Paedophilia/DSM-5 302.2 Paedophilic Disorder

Definition: Paedophilia is the sexual preference for children, usually prepubertal or pubertal. Some are attracted to either one or both sexes.

Epidemiology: The overall prevalence is less than 3%. More than 90% of paedophiles are men and it is rare in women. Ninety-five per cent of paedophiles are heterosexual. Fifty per cent of paedophiles consumed alcohol at the time of the offence.

Clinical features: Included in this diagnosis are those men who retain a preference for adult sex partners, but when frustrated in their efforts turn to children as substitutes. Paedophiles may have previously committed exhibitionism and voyeurism. They have low self-esteem and feel more accepted by young children. The ICD-10 specifies that the individual is at least 16 years old and at least 5 years older than the child victim.

The DSM-5 criteria specify minimum 6 month duration and the individual is at least 18 years old and at least 5 years older than the child victim. The DSM-5 further specifies if the patient is sexually attracted to boys, girls or both. Other classification include:

1. Classic type—sexually attracted to prepubescent children (Tanner stage 1)
2. Hebephilic type—sexually attracted to early pubescent children (Tanner stages 2–3)
3. Paedohebephilic type—sexually attracted to both groups of young people

35.11.1.7 ICD-10 F65.5 Sadomasochism/DSM-5 302.83 Sexual Masochism Disorder and 302.84 Sexual Sadism Disorder

Definition: Sadomasochism is the preference for sexual activity that involves the infliction of pain or humiliation. It is diagnosed only if this is the most important source of sexual stimulation. The sadomasochistic activity involves a recipient (masochist) and a provider (sadist).

The DSM-5 criteria specify minimum 6 month duration and specify a subtype of asphyxiophilia (i.e. sexually aroused by asphyxiation).

35.11.1.8 DSM-5 302.89 Frotteuristic Disorder

Froutteuristic disorder involves recurrent and intense sexual arousal from touching or rubbing against a nonconsenting person, as manifested by fantasies, urges, or behaviours.

35.11.2 MULTIPLE DISORDERS OF SEXUAL PREFERENCE

This is when more than one disorder of sexual preference occurs in one person and none is predominant.

35.11.3 OTHER DISORDERS OF SEXUAL PREFERENCE

This includes obscene telephone calls (telephone scatologia), sexual activity with animals (bestiality), the use of anoxia to heighten sexual pleasure (anoxophilia), and necrophilia.

35.12   SEXUAL ORIENTATION

Sexual disorientation alone is no longer classed as a disorder. ICD-10 allows for variations of sexual development or orientation that are problematic for the individual:

- Heterosexual
- Homosexual
- Bisexual
- Other, including prepubertal

Evidence suggestive of a genetic basis to sexual orientation is provided in twin studies with 52% MZ to 22% DZ concordance in homosexual males, and 48% MZ to 16% DZ concordance in female homosexuals. Hamer et al. (1993) carried out a family pedigree study in which the distribution of homosexuality in the male relatives suggested a sex-linked inheritance. They found convincing evidence in this family of a correlation between homosexual orientation and the inheritance of polymorphous markers at the Xq28 region of the X chromosome.

35.13   ANTISOCIAL SEXUAL BEHAVIOUR

The acceptability of sexual behaviour is determined by society and is incorporated into the law. What constitutes unacceptable behaviour varies largely between cultures and within the same culture over time.

Antisocial sexual behaviours can be divided into two groups:

1. 'Normal' activities carried out inappropriately, without consent or with the wrong age group
2. Sexual activity that is morally perverse

35.13.1   SPECIFIC ANTISOCIAL SEXUAL BEHAVIOURS

35.13.1.1   Rape

Rape is unlawful sexual intercourse with a person by force or against the person's will. Rapists are not a homogeneous group.
Classification of Rapists (Trick and Tennant, 1981)

- *Situational stress rapist.* Otherwise sexually normal, these individuals commit rape when under extreme situational stress. There is much guilt and remorse afterwards.
- *Sociopathic rapist.* These have poor social adjustment with criminality, a poor work record, involve substance abuse, and have unstable relationships. Rape is often impulsive, with

immediate gratification and little regard to the consequences. Threats of violence are common.
- *Sexually inadequate rapist.* These are shy, timid, and insecure, lacking social skills. They often plan a rape against an attractive or sexually threatening woman.
- *Sadistic rapist.* These have a deep-rooted hatred of women arising from early relationships. The object of the rape is the infliction of humiliation and suffering; intercourse may be trivial in comparison to humiliating acts and the serious injuries inflicted. The rape is often carefully planned; precautions are taken to avoid detection.
- *Psychotic rapist.* These constitute a very small proportion of rapists. The rape is often bizarre, violent, and terrifying for the victim.

35.13.1.2   Paedophilia

Paedophilia is the sexual attraction and preference for partners who are physically immature. Offenders are mostly men. Some prefer child victims of the opposite sex, some of the same sex. About 10% are bisexual in their preference.

Adolescent offenders have a better prognosis than older offenders.

The mentally immature offender with poor social skills may prefer child sexual partners because they are the only people with whom the person can relate at a general level.

The persistent middle-aged offender often has evidence of personality problems with poor relationships and unstable work patterns. These offenders usually have low rather than high sex drives. There is often an emotional bond between them and their child victims.

Some paedophiles are more dangerous than those described earlier. This offender has evidence of a serious personality disturbance affecting more aspects of his or her life than choice of sexual outlet.

Killing a child as part of a sexual offence is rare. It usually results from a state of panic or from a desire to dispose of the evidence.

35.13.1.3   Incest

Incest is generally forbidden across cultures. In law it is an offence for a man to have sexual intercourse with a woman he knows to be his daughter, granddaughter, mother, sister, or half-sister and for a woman over 16 to allow a man whom she knows to be her son, father, grandfather, brother, or half-brother to have sexual intercourse with her.

Sibling incest relationships are the most common, but father–daughter relationships are most commonly seen in court. They often reflect some breakdown in the marital relationship.

Incestuous families are characterized by alienation, disorganization, and disintegration. They are rarely reported to the police.

Sibling incest is often the result of experimentation. It is more likely if there is a lack of parental control. Youngest sisters are the most vulnerable.

35.13.1.4 Indecent Exposure

Indecent exposure is an offence under the 1824 Vagrancy Act: 'openly, lewdly and obscenely exposing his person with intent to insult any female' (British Government, 1824). It is one of the most common sexual offences.

Exhibitionism, the exposing of genitals to the opposite sex, is categorized into the following two main groups:

- Type I—Inhibited young men of relatively normal personality and good character who struggle against the impulse but find it irresistible. They expose with a flaccid penis and do not masturbate. They expose to individuals, not seeking a particular response. The frequency of exposure is often related to other sexual stresses and anxieties, such as marital conflict or pregnancy in the spouse.
- Type II—Less inhibited, more sociopathic men. Individuals expose with erect penis in a state of excitement and may masturbate. Pleasure is obtained and little guilt is shown. The person is more likely to expose to a group of women or girls and may return repeatedly to the same place. The person seeks a response from the victim, either shock or disgust. There are fewer attempts to resist the urge to expose. The behaviour is associated with other psychosexual disorders and other types of offences. This may lead on to more serious sexual offences.

Eighty per cent do not reoffend if they are charged with a first offence. The chances of reconviction rise dramatically with the second offence. There is a small group of recidivists who persist, but these tend to reduce in their forties. It is generally a harmless nonviolent offence, except in a minority who may progress to more violent offences.

There is a good prognosis associated with being married, good social relationships, and work record.

35.13.1.5 Others
- Fetishism may come to the attention of the police if articles used are stolen (e.g. women's underwear).
- Sadomasochism may result in conviction for assault if extreme injury results, even if both parties consent.

- Transvestites may be charged with behaviour likely to cause a breach of the peace if they cross-dress in public.
- Frotteurism is the practice of rubbing the penis against another person in a clandestine way in a public place. It is liable to charges of either indecent assault or offence against public order.

35.13.2 TREATMENT OF ANTISOCIAL SEXUAL BEHAVIOUR

In a critical review of the literature, Marshall et al. (1991) concluded that some treatment programmes have been effective with paedophiles and exhibitionists but not with rapists. In examining the value of the various treatment approaches, they concluded that comprehensive cognitive behavioural therapy (CBT) were most likely to be effective with paedophiles and exhibitionists. There was also a clear value in the use of antiandrogens in those offenders who engage in excessively high rates of sexual activity.

35.14 SEX OFFENDER TREATMENT PROGRAMME

- The Sex Offender Treatment Programme (SOTP) aims at increasing the responsibility and motivation of the sexual offender to change.
- SOTP involves anger management, CBT, relationship skill training, relapse prevention, sex education, social skill training, stress management, and thinking skill programme.
- Sex offenders are encouraged to develop victim empathy by understanding the consequences of their actions and minimize denial.
- Behaviour treatments include aversion, sensitization, and biofeedback with penile plethysmography that measures the penile blood flow with thoughts of illegal sexual practices.

35.15 PHARMACOLOGICAL TREATMENT

- The aim of the pharmacological treatment is to reduce sexual drives and prevent future sexual offences especially in sex offenders who fail to response to SOTP.

Baseline investigations:
- Blood investigations: FBC, LFT, RFT, and glucose
- Hormonal investigations: LH, FSH, and serum testosterone

- ECG and bone scan
- Baseline weight and blood pressure

Subsequent monitoring after initiation of treatment:

- Weight and blood pressure during each visit
- Monthly testosterone for the first 4 months and every 6 months afterwards
- LFT, RFT, and prolactin levels every 6 months
- Bone scan for patients being prescribed with leuprolide

SSRI: Commonly prescribed with less side effects; no consent is required but consent is required for following drugs.

Cyproterone is a testosterone antagonist. The range dose is between 100 and 500 mg/day (oral) or 100 and 600 mg/week (intramuscular injection). Cyproterone is contraindicated in patients with chronic liver diseases and thromboembolic diseases. Side effects include depression, fatigue, gynaecomastia (15%), and weight gain.

Medroxyprogesterone provides negative feedbacks to the production of FSH and LH and reduce testosterone production. The range of dose is between 100 and 600 mg/day (oral) or 100 and 700 mg/week (intramuscular). Medroxyprogesterone is contraindicated in patients suffering from chronic liver diseases and thromboembolic disorders. Side effects include anxiety, depression, excessive sweating, fatigue, hypertension, insomnia, oedema, and weight gain.

Leuprolide is a GnRH analogue that controls the release of LH and FSH and subsequently reduces the testosterone production. The intramuscular dose is between 3.75 and 7.5 mg/month IM or 11.5 and 22.5 mg every 3 months. Leuprolide is contraindicated in patients suffering from osteopenia. Side effects include excessive sweating, hot flushes, myalgia, oedema, and osteopenia.

Finasteride is a 5α-reductase inhibitor and reduces sexual drive by inhibiting the peripheral conversion of testosterone to dihydrotestosterone.

CASC STATION ON EXHIBITIONISM

You are a registrar receiving forensic psychiatry training and are asked to carry out a risk assessment on a 30-year-old man, Mr. C. He has an 8-year history of multiple instances of flashing his genitalia to women in the park. He has been referred to your outpatient clinic by his GP. He appears very anxious about being caught by the police.

Tasks:

1. Perform an assessment of exhibitionism and related psychopathology.
2. Perform a risk assessment.

CASC Grid

Seek permission and opening statement: 'Hello Mr. C, I am Dr. Lucas. I am trying to understand what has happened to you. I need to ask you some questions. They may involve sensitive issues. Is it alright with you? I was informed that you have exposed your genitals to ladies recently. Can you tell me more about your behaviour?'

(A) Index Offence: Exposure	(A1) Onset of the Problem	(A2) Precipitants	(A3) Details of the Exposure	(A4) Previous Exposure	(A5) Impact of Exposure
	'How old were you when it started?' 'Can you tell me what happened at that time?' 'What kind of people do you choose to expose to? May I know why? Do you feel an emotional attachment to them?'	'What is your view on the causes of your behaviour?' (explore attribution by patient) 'What makes you do it?' 'Do you have a strong urge or mounting tension?' 'Was it part of your fantasy?'	'Did you plan beforehand?' 'Where did you do it?' 'What kind of people (gender, age) were you looking for? Did you know them?' 'Did you do it alone?' (look for organized crime)	'How many times did you flash your penis?' 'How did you manage to escape?' 'Have the police or legal system ever been involved?' If yes, were you sent to prison? If so, how many times?	'How is your mood?' 'Do you feel depressed?' 'Do you feel guilty over your act?' 'How do you feel about the victims? Do you feel sorry for them?' (explore victim empathy)

(A) Index Offence: Exposure	(A1) Onset of the Problem	(A2) Precipitants	(A3) Details of the Exposure	(A4) Previous Exposure	(A5) Impact of Exposure
	Explore emotional congruence with victims (especially children) as patient may be fixated at the child's level of emotional development and relate better to the young victims.	'Do you use pornography?' If so, what kind (related to paedophilia) and what form (Internet or book)	'Did you carry any weapon with you?' 'Was your penis hard or soft when you flashed to them?' 'What did you do next after flashing your genitalia? Did you masturbate?' 'Can you control your urge to expose?' 'What is the worst thing that might happen?'		If patient does not feel guilty, then ask him, 'Do you feel excited by exposing your genitals? Are you concerned about the fact that more women will face sexual assault?'
(B) Risk Assessment	(B1) Other Avenues for Exhibitionism	(B2) Other Sexual Offences	(B3) Assessment of Denial	(B4) Acute and Chronic Dynamic Risk Factors	(B5) Self-harm and Other Harms
	'Are you working at present? What do you do for a living?' (e.g. postman or teacher who may expose to children in the neighbourhood or school) 'Do you have contact with young children in your daily life?'	'Do you make obscene phone calls? If so, do you masturbate at the same time?' 'Have you ever touched other ladies?' 'Have you ever tried to impose sex on someone?' 'Were you ever sent to prison for other sexual offences? If yes, after you were released from prison, did you reoffend again?'	'Do you acknowledge that your behaviour, like flashing your genitalia, is an offence?' 'Do you think the problem is serious?' 'Do you feel that you need treatment at this moment?' Assess levels of denial and classify in the following: (1) absolute denial, (2) denial of seriousness, (3) denial of the need for treatment.	Acute risk factors: isolation, unemployment, chaotic life style, relapse of depression, intoxicated by substances Chronic risk factors: low self-esteem, poor impulse control, substance abuse	'Have you ever thought of harming yourself?' 'How about harming the others?' 'Have you ever been violent to others?' 'Have you ever damaged any property?'

(continued)

(C) Other Comorbidity	(C1) Other Psychosexual Disorders?	(C2) Delusions or Abnormal Beliefs	(C3) Psychotic Experience	(C4) Personality	(C5) Drug and Substance Abuse
	'Do you have other sexual preferences (explore paraphilia, voyeurism)?' 'What is your sexual orientation?' 'Do you have any sexual problem such as erectile dysfunction?'	'How do you compare yourself with the others?' (explore grandiosity) 'Have you ever thought that you are entitled to expose yourself to the ladies? If so, what is your rationale?'	'Do you hear voices talking to you when nobody is around?' 'If yes, what do they say?' (look for command hallucinations) Assess threat/control and overcome (TCO) 'Do you feel Threatened by the voices?' 'Can you exercise Control over the voices?' 'Are you Overcome by the voices?'	'Can you describe your personality?' 'How do you feel about authoritative figures?' (look for resentment) Look for sociopathic trait (impulsiveness, hatred, not caring safety of others), and social incompetence. Look for avoidant personality.	'Have you consumed any alcohol or drug prior to exposing yourself?'

(D) Family, Personal and Psychosexual History	(D1) Family	(D2) Psychosexual Development	(D3) Learning Disability	(D4) Relationship and Marital History	(D5) Social Adequacy
	'Can you tell me about your family?' 'How do you feel about your parents? Did you separate from them when you were young? Do you feel angry about them?' 'How did they treat you? Have you ever experienced any abuse?' (sexual, physical, and emotional)	'How old were you when you first learn about sex?' 'Have you ever encountered difficulty with intimacy?' 'Do you feel that you need to suppress sexual feelings?'	'What is your highest level of education?' 'Have you encountered learning difficulty? Were you in a special school? Do you have any difficulty to understand the other people?'	If the patient is single, ask, 'How is your dating experience?' If patient is married, ask, 'How's your relationship with your spouse or partner?' 'Can you tell me more about your sexual life with her?' 'Does she know about your behaviour?'	'Can you tell me about your relationship with other people?' 'Can you comment on your self-esteem?'

REFERENCES

American Psychiatric Association. 2013: *Desk Reference to the Diagnostic Criteria from DSM-5*. Washington, DC: American Psychiatric Association Press.

Bancroft J. 1983: *Human Sexuality and Its Problems*. Edinburgh, Scotland: Churchill Livingstone.

Bancroft J. 1994: Homosexual orientation: The search for a biological basis. *British Journal of Psychiatry* 164:437–440.

Bancroft J. 1995: Sexual disorders. In Kendell RE and Zealley AK (eds.) *Companion to Psychiatric Studies*, 5th edn, pp. 754–771. Edinburgh, Scotland: Churchill Livingstone.

Brindley GS and Gillian P. 1982: Men and women who do not have orgasms. *British Journal of Psychiatry* 140:351–356.

British Government. 1824: *Vagrancy Act*. London, U.K.: George Edward Eyre and William Spottiswood.

British Society for Sexual Medicine. 2007: Guidelines on management of erectile dysfunction. http://www.bssm.org.uk/downloads//BSSM_ED_Management_Guidelines_2007.pdf (accessed on 22 July 2012).

Cooper AJ, Cernovsky ZZ, and Colussi K. 1993: Some clinical and psychometric characteristics of primary and secondary premature ejaculators. *Journal of Sex and Marital Therapy* 19:276–288.

Derogatis LR, Schmidt CW, Fagan PJ et al. 1989: Subtypes of anorgasmia via mathematical taxonomy. *Psychosomatics* 30:166–173.

Dunn KM, Croft PR, and Hackett GI. 1998: Sexual problems: A study of the prevalence and need for health care in the general population. *Family Practice* 15:519–524.

Ellis H. 2010: *My Life: Autobiography of Havelock Ellis*. Whitefish, MT: Kessinger Publication for Rare Reprint.

Fabbri A, Jannini EA, Gnessi L et al. 1989: Endorphins in male impotence: Evidence for naltrexone stimulation of erectile activity in patient therapy. *Psychoneuroendocrinology* 14:103–111.

Gelder M, Mayou R, and Cowen P. 2001: *Shorter Oxford Textbook of Psychiatry*. Oxford, U.K.: Oxford University Press.

Gilbert HW and Gingell JC. 1991: The results of an intracorporeal papaverine clinic. *Sex and Marital Therapy* 6:49–56.

Goldbeck-Wood S. 2010: Psychosexual medicine. In Puri BK and Treasaden IH (eds.) *Psychiatry: An Evidence-Based Text*. London, U.K.: Hodder Arnold.

Gregoire A. 1992: New treatments for erectile impotence. *British Journal of Psychiatry* 160:315–326.

Hamer DH, Hu S, Magnuson VL et al. 1993: A linkage between DNA markers on the X chromosome and male sexual orientation. *Science* 261:321–327.

Hawton K, Catalan J, and Fagg J. 1992: Sex therapy for erectile dysfunction: Characteristics of couples, treatment outcome and prognostic factors. *Archives of Sexual Behavior* 21:161–175.

Hiller J. 1993: Psychoanalytic concepts and psychosexual therapy: A suggested integration. *Sex and Marital Therapy* 8:9–26.

Janssen PL. 1985: Psychodynamic study of male potency disorders: An overview. *Psychotherapy and Psychosomatics* 44:6–17.

Johnson AM, Wadsworth J, Wellings K et al. 1994: *Sexual Attitudes and Lifestyles*. Oxford, U.K.: Blackwell Scientific.

Kinsey AC, Pomeroy WB, and Martin CE. 1948: *Sexual Behavior in the Human Male*. Philadelphia, PA: W.B. Saunders.

Kinsey AC, Pomeroy WB, Martin, CE et al. 1953: *Sexual Behavior in the Human Female*. Philadelphia, PA: W.B. Saunders.

Kupek E. 2001: Sexual attitudes and number of partners in young British men. *Archives of Sexual Behavior* 30(1):13–27.

Kockett G. 1980: Symptomatology and psychological aspects of male sexual inadequacy: Results of an experimental study. *Archives of Sexual Behavior* 9:457–475.

Marshall WL, Jones R, Ward T et al. 1991: Treatment outcome with sex offenders. *Clinical Psychology Review* 11:465–485.

Masters WH. 1959: The sexual response cycle of the human female: Vaginal lubrication. *Annals of the New York Academy of Science* 83:301–317.

Masters WH. 1960: The sexual response cycle of the human female. I. Gross anatomic considerations. *Western Journal Surgery, Obstetrics and Gynecology* 68:57–72.

Masters WH and Johnson VE. 1966: *Human Sexual Response*. New York: Bantam Books.

Masters WH and Johnson VE. 1970: *Human Sexual Inadequacy*. London, U.K.: Churchill Livingstone.

Master WH and Johnson VE. 1976: Principles of the new sex therapy. *The American Journal of Psychiatry* 133(5):548–554.

Mishra DN and Shulka GD. 1988: Sexual disturbances in male diabetics: Phenomenological and clinical aspects. *Indian Journal of Psychiatry* 30:135–143.

Olumoroti OJ and Kassim AA. 2005: *Patient Management Problems in Psychiatry*. London, U.K.: Churchill Livingstone.

Pena LE. 1987: An analysis of female primary orgasmic dysfunction. *Revista de Análisis del Comportamiento* 3:151–163.

Perry GP and Orchard J. 1992: *Assessment and Treatment of Adolescent Sex Offenders*. Sarasota, FL: Professional Resource Press.

Pirke KM et al. 1979: Pituitary gonadal system function in patients with erectile impotence and premature ejaculation. *Archives of Sexual Behavior* 8:41–48.

Rowland DL, Haensel SM, Blom JH et al. 1993: Penile sensitivity in men with premature ejaculation and erectile dysfunction. *Journal of Sex and Marital Therapy* 19:189–197.

Segraves RT, Taylor R, and Schoenberg HW et al. 1982: Psychosexual adjustment after penile prosthesis surgery. *Sexuality and Disability* 5:222–229.

Sepkowitz KA. 2001: AIDS—The first 20 years. *New England Journal of Medicine* 344(23):1764-1772.

Snaith P, Tarsh MJ, and Reid R. 1993: Sex reassignment surgery. *British Journal of Psychiatry* 162:681–685.

Spector IP and Carey MP. 1990: Incidence and prevalence of the sexual dysfunctions: A critical review of the empirical literature. *Archives of Sexual Behavior* 19:389–408.

Stone JH, Roberts M, O'Grady J et al. 2000: *Faulk's Black Forensic Psychiatry*, 3rd edn. Oxford, U.K.: Blackwell Science.

Tondo L, Cantone M, and Carta M et al. 1991: An MMPI evaluation of male sexual dysfunction. *Journal of Clinical Psychology* 47:391–396.

Trick RL and Tennant TG. 1981: *Forensic Psychiatry: An Introductory Text*. London, U.K.: Pitman Medical.

World Health Organization. 1992: *ICD-10: The ICD-10 Classification of Mental and Behavioural Disorders: Clinical Descriptions and Diagnostic Guidelines*. Geneva, Switzerland: World Health Organization.

36 Sleep Disorders

36.1 CLASSIFICATION

The ICD-10 classification of nonorganic sleep disorders is

F51.0 Nonorganic insomnia
F51.1 Nonorganic hypersomnia
F51.2 Nonorganic disorder of the sleep–wake schedule
F51.3 Sleepwalking
F51.4 Sleep terrors
F51.5 Nightmares

The DSM-5 classifies sleep–wake disorders as follows:

780.52 Insomnia disorder
780.54 Hypersomnolence disorders
347.00 Narcolepsy/hypocretin deficiency
327.23 Obstructive sleep apnoea hypopnoea syndrome
Central sleep apnoea
Sleep-related hypoventilation
Circadian rhythm sleep-wake disorder
307.46 Sleepwalking disorder
307.46 Sleep terror disorder
307.47 Nightmare disorder
327.42 Rapid eye movement sleep behaviour disorder
333.94 Restless legs syndrome
Substance-induced sleep disorder

36.2 DYSSOMNIAS

36.2.1 INSOMNIA

Insomnia is the disturbance of normal sleep pattern and characterized by an insufficient quantity or quality of sleep.

36.2.1.1 Epidemiology

- The prevalence of insomnia is between 1% and 10% in general population.
- The estimated 1-year prevalence in adults ranges from 15% to over 40%.
- Prevalence is particularly high in the elderly (up to 25%).
- Gender ratio: F > M.

36.2.1.2 Aetiology

Table 36.1 gives the main causes of insomnia.

36.2.1.3 Clinical Features

- The patient has history of being a 'light' sleeper with easily disturbed sleep.
- The patient usually concerns about sleep duration and quality. This often leads to increased cognitive, physiological, and emotional arousal prior to sleep. Their over-concerns and poor sleep often form a viscous cycle.
- The main result of insomnia is daytime tiredness or napping, low mood, decreased attention and concentration, low energy level, and fatigue.

36.2.1.4 Diagnostic Criteria

36.2.1.4.1 Nonorganic Insomnia (ICD-10)

- The sleep disturbance occurs nearly every day for at least 1 month and causes marked distress or interference with personal functioning in daily living.
- A complaint of excessive daytime sleepiness or prolonged transition to the fully aroused state upon awakening (sleep drunkenness).
- Absence of narcolepsy or sleep apnoea (nocturnal breath cessation).
- Absence of any organic factor, psychoactive substance use disorder, or effect of medication.

36.2.1.4.2 Insomnia Disorder (DSM-5)

- The sleep difficulty occurs at least three nights per week and is present for at least 3 months. The sleep difficulty occurs despite adequate opportunity for sleep.
- Specific insomnia symptoms such as difficulty initiating and maintaining sleep, early-morning awakening with inability to return to sleep, and nonrestorative sleep.
- Significant distress and impairments such as fatigue, cognitive impairment, mood disturbance, behavioural problems, and impaired functioning.
- For children, insomnia can be manifested as prolonged resistance to going to bed and/or bedtime struggles.

TABLE 36.1
Causes of Insomnia

Environmental	Poor Sleep Hygiene
	Change in time zone
	Change in sleeping habits
	Shiftwork
Physiological	Natural short sleeper
	Pregnancy
	Middle age
Life stress	Bereavement
	Exams
	House move, etc.
Psychiatric	Acute anxiety
	Depression
	Mania
	Organic brain syndrome
Physical	Pain
	Cardiorespiratory distress
	Arthritis
	Nocturia
	GI disorders
	Thyrotoxicosis
Pharmacological	Caffeine
	Alcohol
	Stimulants
	Chronic hypnotic use
Parasomnias	Sleep apnoea
	Sleep myoclonus
Primary sleep disorders	

Source: Reproduced from Puri, B.K. et al., *Textbook of Psychiatry*, 2nd edn., Churchill Livingstone, Edinburgh, Scotland, 2002. With permission.

36.2.1.5 Differential Diagnosis

Important disorders that may cause insomnia, and that should therefore be excluded, include

- Depressive disorders
- Mania
- Anxiety disorders
- Substance misuse and dependence
- Organic disorders (see Table 36.1)

36.2.1.6 Management
36.2.1.6.1 *Nonpharmacological Treatment*

1. Sleep hygiene education: a moderate intake of easily digested warm food; a comfortable bed; avoid caffeine, nicotine, alcohol, and excessive fluid intake in the evening; keep a regular sleep schedule and regular daytime exercise; limit time in bed; and remove clock from bedroom to avoid excessive monitoring.
2. Sleep restriction therapy: the patient should keep a sleep log that records the total sleep duration, bedtime, and wake-up time. The time allowed in bed is reduced to the total sleep duration and the patient is advised to increase the time in bed by 15 min on a weekly basis by adjusting the bedtime.
3. Stimulus control therapy: arise at the same time every morning, avoid daytime napping, go to bed only when sleepy, use the bed only for sleep, leave the bed when unable to sleep, and reduce lighting and level of noise in bedroom.
4. Cognitive therapy aims at correcting cognitive distortions (e.g. being catastrophic after insomnia) and unrealistic expectations (e.g. must have 10 h uninterrupted sleep).
5. Behaviour therapy: progressive muscle relaxation techniques for any associated anxiety.

36.2.1.6.2 *Pharmacological Treatment*

1. The NICE guidelines recommend that doctors should consider offering nonpharmacological treatments first. If they think that pharmacological treatment is the appropriate way to treat severe insomnia that is interfering with normal functioning, they should prescribe one hypnotic agent for only short periods of time and strictly according to the licence for the drug.
2. Doctors are advised to consider nonbenzodiazepine hypnotic agents such as
   a. Antihistamines: hydroxyzine.
   b. Melatonin receptor agonists: agomelatine and ramelton.
   c. Sedating antidepressants: amitriptyline, mirtazapine, and trazodone.
   d. Antipsychotics: low-dose quetiapine.
   e. Melatonin: the Maudsley guidelines recommend the use of melatonin for the treatment of insomnia in children and adolescents.
3. Benzodiazepines are only indicated for short-term use (<4 weeks). Benzodiazepine hypnotic agents include
   a. Benzodiazepines: temazepam, oxazepam, lorazepam, and diazepam
   b. Benzodiazepine receptor agonists: zaleplon, zolpidem, and zopiclone

4. Treatment should only be changed from one of these hypnotics to another if side effects occur that are directly related to the medicine. If treatment with one of the benzodiazepines or benzodiazepine receptor agonist does not work, the doctor should not prescribe one of the others.

36.2.1.7 Course and Prognosis

- Insomnia typically occurs in young or middle adulthood. Chronic insomnia may last through to old age.
- Previous insomnia is the most significant predictor for future insomnia.
- 50%–75% of patients have insomnia that lasts for more than 1 year.
- Insomnia caused by life event or stressor usually has a limited course to a period of less than 1 year.

36.2.2 HYPERSOMNIA

36.2.2.1 Epidemiology

- Daytime drowsiness occurs in 0.3%–4% of the population.
- Incidence over 5-year period: 8%.
- Lifetime prevalence: 15%.

36.2.2.2 Aetiology

The common causes of hypersomnia are

- Family history of hypersomnia and association with autonomic dysfunction
- As an early symptom of depressive disorder
- Unknown cause: idiopathic

36.2.2.3 Clinical Features

- Long duration of major sleep episode (8–12 h) with rapid onset of sleep and good sleep efficiency
- Excessive daytime sleepiness and unrefreshing naps during normal waking hours causing a disturbance of social or occupational functioning
- Sleep drunkenness with prolonged impairment of alertness at sleep–wake transition and results in difficulty waking in the morning

36.2.2.4 Diagnostic Criteria

36.2.2.4.1 *Nonorganic Hypersomnia (ICD-10)*

- Excessive daytime sleepiness, sleep attacks, and sleep drunkenness.
- Frequency and duration: sleep disturbance occurs nearly every day for at least 1 month.

- No symptoms of narcolepsy and evidence for sleep apnoea.
- No other causative factors.

36.2.2.4.2 *Hypersomnolence Disorder (DSM-5)*

- Frequency and duration: hypersomnolence occurs at least three times per week and for at least 3 months. The patient has a main sleep period lasting at least 7 h per day.
- Symptoms of excessive sleepiness such as recurrent periods of sleep and naps within the same day, a prolonged and nonrestorative main sleep episode (>9 h), and sleep inertia with difficulty in waking up.
- The hypersomnolence causes significant impairments in functioning and is not accounted for by another sleep disorder.
- Specify if:
  - With mental disorder/medical condition
  - Acute/subacute/persistent
  - Mild/moderate/severe

36.2.2.5 Differential Diagnosis

Important differential diagnoses include

- Narcolepsy
- Sleep apnoea
- Organic disorders
- Fatigue states
- Kleine–Levin syndrome (M/F = 3:1, begins in adolescence and resolves by middle age, recurrent sleepiness, indiscriminate hypersexuality, compulsive overeating, and weight gain)

36.2.2.6 Assessment and Investigations

- Epworth Sleepiness Scale: cutoff score for men >11 and cutoff score for women >9.
- Multiple Sleep Latency Test (MSLT) involves asking the patient to nap for 20 min and then being awaken. EEG, heart rates, and other physiological parameters are recorded. The MSLT measures sleep latency, which is the time elapsed from the start of the nap to the first signs of sleep (sleep latency = 0–5 min [severe sleepiness], 5–10 min [troublesome sleepiness], 10–15 min [manageable sleepiness], 15–20 min [mild sleepiness]). The naps are repeated for four to five times.
- Polysomnography is an overnight procedure that records the cardiac rhythm (ECG), brain activity (EEG), muscular activity (EMG), eye

movement (EOG), and oxygen saturation (pulse oximetry) during sleep. Polysomnography provides information on sleep onset latency, the proportion of REM and non-REM sleep. Such information allows specialists to establish the diagnosis of breathing-related sleep disorders, narcolepsy, and periodic limb movement disorder.

36.2.2.7   Management
- Treat any identified underlying cause.
- In idiopathic hypersomnia, stimulants are occasionally used.
- Methylphenidate has potential for misuse and associated with excessive sweating and insomnia.
- Modafinil is a stimulant with less potential for misuse and less peripheral sympathomimetic effects.

36.2.2.8   Course and Prognosis
- The onset is usually gradual.
- The course is that of the underlying disorder and often chronic but stable.
- Idiopathic hypersomnia typically begins between the age of 15 and 30 years and may improve with age.

36.2.3   NARCOLEPSY (HYPOCRETIN DEFICIENCY)

36.2.3.1   Epidemiology
- Prevalence: 3–6/100,000.
- Gender ratio: M = F.

36.2.3.2   Aetiology
- Genetics: The genotype HLA-DQB1*0602 is present in nearly 99% of patients suffering from narcolepsy with cataplexy and 40% of patients suffering from narcolepsy without cataplexy. Around 5%–15% of first degree relatives of probands develop narcolepsy.
- Loss of hypocretin cells in hypothalamus. Hypocretin (aka orexin) is a neurotransmitter regulating arousal and wakefulness.

36.2.3.3   Clinical Features
- *Onset*: first symptom is almost always daytime sleepiness and occurs during adolescence.
- *Hypersomnia*: sleepiness in between sleep attacks.

- *Sleep attacks*: two to five episodes of sleep attacks per day. Sleep attacks are irresistible and last for 10–20 min with dreaming. The attacks cause functional impairments.
- *Cataplexy* (70%): sudden loss of muscle tone with consciousness lasting for a few seconds to minutes. The hypotonia causes spontaneous grimaces and jaw opening with tongue thrusting. Eye and respiratory muscles are spared. Cataplexy can be precipitated by laughter. Cataplexy increases the risk of fall and accident.
- *Hypnagogic hallucinations* (20%–40%): usually visual hallucinations or dreamlike imagery. Hypnopompic hallucinations are less common than hypnagogic hallucinations.
- *Sleep paralysis*: mainly affecting ability to speak and movement of four limbs. Diaphragm is spared in sleep paralysis.
- *Common psychiatric comorbidity*: depression, anxiety, substance misuse, and parasomnia.

36.2.3.3.1   DSM-5 Criteria (APA, 2013)
- Hypersomnia and recurrent sleep attacks have been occurring at least three times per week over the last 3 months.
- Cataplexy occurs at least a few times per month.
- Evidence of hypocretin deficiency, as measured using cerebrospinal fluid hypocretin-1 immunoreactivity measurements (<1/3 of values obtained in healthy subjects tested during the same assay, or ≤110 pg/mL). Low cerebrospinal fluid hypocretin-1 must not be observed in the context of acute brain injury, inflammation, or infection.
- Nocturnal sleep polysomnography showing rapid eye movement (REM) sleep latency less than or equal to 15 min.
- MSLT showing a mean sleep latency less than or equal to 8 min and two or more sleep onset REM periods.

Investigation: The diagnosis is confirmed with overnight polysomnography.

36.2.3.4   Management
36.2.3.4.1   Nonpharmacological Treatment
- Lifestyle adjustment
- Scheduled napping

36.2.3.4.2 *Pharmacological Treatment*

- Stimulants such as methylphenidate and modafinil can reduce daytime sleepiness.
- REM suppressants such as SSRIs can treat hypnagogic hallucinations, cataplexy, and sleep paralysis.

36.2.3.5 Course

- Hypersomnia and cataplexy have stable course over time.

36.3 BREATHING-RELATED SLEEP DISORDER

36.3.1 Obstructive Sleep Apnoea

36.3.1.1 Epidemiology

- Obstructive sleep apnoea (OSA) is the most common breathing-related sleep disorder.
- Prevalence: 1%–10% of adult population.
- Higher prevalence of OSA is found in older people.

36.3.1.2 Risk Factors

- Obesity
- Increase in neck size (>43 cm in men and >41 cm in women)
- Structural abnormality such as adenotonsillar enlargement and nasal airway obstruction

36.3.1.2.1 *DSM-5 Criteria (APA, 2013)*

The following criteria must be present:

- Nocturnal breathing disturbances (e.g. snoring, breathing pauses)
- Daytime sleepiness and fatigue
- At least five obstructive apnoeas or hypopnoeas per hour of sleep during polysomnography
- No other sleep disorders

36.3.1.3 Other Clinical Features

- Daytime naps are unrefreshing.
- Patients may complain of dull headache upon awakening, low mood, poor concentration, and memory disturbance.
- For children, they usually present with irritability, behavioural problems, and chest retractions during sleep. The number of apnoeas/hypopnoeas supportive is expected to be lower (<5).

Investigation: The diagnosis is confirmed with overnight polysomnography.

36.3.1.4 Management

- Psychiatrists or GPs should avoid prescribing benzodiazepines or sedative drugs.
- Refer patient to a weight management programme to lose weight.
- Refer patient to see a sleep specialist, respiratory specialist, or otolaryngologist for nasal continuous positive airway pressure (CPAP), nasal surgery, and uvulopalatoplasty.
- Advise patient not to sleep supine.
- Advise patient to avoid alcohol.

36.3.2 Central Sleep Apnoea

36.3.2.1 Epidemiology

- Prevalence: 0.1%–1% of adult population

36.3.2.2 Risk Factors

- Old age
- Cardiac diseases: congestive heart failure
- Neurological diseases: Parkinson's disease, stroke, brainstem lesion, and encephalitis
- Skeletal diseases: cervical spine degeneration

36.3.2.2.1 *DSM-5 Criteria (APA, 2013)*

The following criteria must be present:

- At least five central apnoeas per hour of sleep during polysomnography
- No other sleep disorders

36.3.2.3 Other Clinical Features

- There is no evidence of airway obstruction
- Less likely to be overweight

Investigation: The diagnosis is confirmed with overnight polysomnography.

36.3.2.4 Management

- Treat underlying medical conditions.
- Psychiatrists or GPs should avoid prescribing benzodiazepines or sedative drugs.
- Refer to a respiratory specialist for CPAP or bilevel positive airway pressure (BiPAP).
- Advise patient to avoid alcohol.

36.3.3   Disorders of the Sleep–Wake Cycle

Disorders of the sleep–wake cycle are characterized by sleep occurring out of phase with environmental and social cues (zeitgebers).

36.3.3.1   Epidemiology
- The prevalence of delayed sleep phase type is between 0.1% and 4% in the general population.
- The prevalence of shift work type can be as high as 50% among night shift workers.

36.3.3.2   Aetiology
- Genetics: 40% of delayed sleep phase type have a family history.

36.3.3.3   Diagnostic Criteria
The circadian rhythm sleep–wake disorder (DSM-5 criteria):

- A persistent or recurrent pattern of sleep disruption leading to excessive sleepiness, insomnia, or both. This is caused by a change in the circadian system, leading to a misalignment between the endogenous circadian rhythm and the sleep–wake schedule required by the patient.
- The sleep disturbance causes clinically significant distress or impairment in functioning.
- There are five subtypes:
  1. Advanced sleep phase: advanced sleep onset and awakening times as compared to the norms
  2. Delayed sleep phase: delayed sleep onset and awakening times as compared to the norms
  3. Irregular sleep–wake type: a temporally disorganized and various sleep and wake patterns in 24 h
  4. Non-24-h sleep–wake type: a pattern of sleep and wake cycles that is not synchronized to the 24-h environment, with a delayed sleep phase
  5. Shift work type: insomnia during the major sleep period and/or excessive sleepiness during the major awake period as a result of shift work

36.3.3.4   Management
- Treat any primary disorder.
- Advanced sleep phase: bright light therapy in the morning.
- Delayed sleep phase: advancing sleep in small increments may help in cases of delayed sleep phase syndrome; offer bright light and melatonin in the morning.

- Irregular or non-24-h sleep–wake type (entrainment failure): if entrainment failure is secondary to a lack of sleep–wake cues in a modality such as vision (because of poor vision, say), then cues from other modalities and a careful routine may be employed.
- Shift work type: advise patient to take a nap before work, schedule a nap on break, avoid light during the day, and receive bright light at night.

36.3.3.5   Course and Prognosis
- Delayed sleep phase: onset is between adolescence and early adulthood. The course may last for years if without treatment.
- Shift work type: reversal of pattern in 2 weeks after termination of shift work.

36.3.4   Restless Leg Syndrome

36.3.4.1   Epidemiology
- The prevalence is between 2% and 10% of the general population and up to 30% in people with chronic medical illness.
- The prevalence increases with age.
- Gender ratio: M = F.

36.3.4.2   Aetiology
Restless leg syndrome is associated with the following medical conditions:

- Autoimmune thyroid disorders
- Iron deficiency or microcytic anaemia
- Diabetes mellitus
- Pregnancy
- Renal failure
- Rheumatoid arthritis

36.3.4.3   DSM-5 Criteria (APA, 2013)
The DSM-5 criteria have two components:

- Compulsory criteria include an urge to move the legs as a result of unpleasant sensations, worsening of symptoms during periods of rest and at night, and no relief of symptoms by movement.
- Sequelae include clinical sleep disturbance, cognitive impairments, daytime sleepiness, fatigue, hyperactivity, impulsivity, mood disturbance, and impaired in functioning.
- The minimum duration of restless leg syndrome is 3 months.

36.3.4.4   Other Clinical Features

- Patients have a frequent desire to move arms and legs to relieve uncomfortable sensations such as burning, crawling, and tingling sensations.
- Uncomfortable sensations and desires to move are getting worse in the evening.
- Restless leg syndrome is associated with delayed sleep phase, nocturnal awakenings, and daytime fatigue.

36.3.4.5   Management

36.3.4.5.1   Nonpharmacological Treatment

- Apply hot compresses to legs
- Encourage sleep hygiene
- Reduce alcohol, caffeine, and nicotine consumption

36.3.4.5.2   Pharmacological Treatment

- Treat any primary disorder, for example, iron deficiency.
- Psychopharmacological treatment is indicated if symptoms impairing sleep for more than two nights per week. For example, benzodiazepine such as clonazepam, anticonvulsants such as gabapentin, and dopamine agonists such as levodopa.

36.3.5   Parasomnias

Parasomnias are phenomena occurring as part of or alongside sleep; they are shown in Table 36.2.

TABLE 36.2

Parasomnias

Sleepwalking (somnambulism)

Night terrors (pavor nocturnus)

Nightmares or dream anxiety

Bruxism (teeth grinding)

Nocturnal enuresis

Headbanging (jactatio capitis nocturna)

Sleep paralysis

Nocturnal painful erections

Cluster headache

Physical symptomatology occurring at night,
  e.g. paroxysmal nocturnal dyspnoea, sleep epilepsy

Sleep myoclonus

Source: Reproduced from Puri, B.K. et al., *Textbook of Psychiatry*, 2nd edn., Churchill Livingstone, Edinburgh, Scotland. With permission.

36.4   NON-REM PARASOMNIAS

36.4.1   Somnambulism (Sleepwalking)

In this disorder, there occurs a state of altered consciousness in which, while asleep, the individual arises and walks.

36.4.1.1   Epidemiology

- Sleepwalking occurs at least once in 15% of children aged 5–12 years and in 0.5% of adults.
- Women are more affected than men (sex ratio [F/M] = 4:3).

36.4.1.2   Aetiology and Risk Factors

- Somnambulism is familial in up to 20% of cases.
- If both parents suffer from somnambulism, the risk for somnambulism is 60%.
- There are no characteristic EEG changes.
- Sleep laboratory studies do not lend credence to the view that somnambulism represents the acting out of dreams.
- Risk factors include alcohol misuse, benzodiazepine use, fever, and sleep deprivation.

36.4.1.3   ICD-10 Criteria

- Repeated (two or more) episodes of arising from bed during the first third of nocturnal sleep and walking for several minutes to 30 min.
- During the sleepwalking, the person exhibits a blank staring face, unresponsive to others, and can be awaken only with considerable difficulty.
- The person has amnesia after sleepwalking.
- No impairment of mental activity or behaviour after awakening.
- No evidence of organic mental disorder.

36.4.1.4   DSM-5 Criteria (APA, 2013)

- Sleepwalking is listed under non-rapid eye movement sleep arousal disorder. The criteria are similar to ICD-10 with emphasis on impairment in functioning.

36.4.1.5   Other Clinical Features

- Majority of episodes begin with first few hours of sleep, during NREM stage 3 or 4 sleep.
- The sufferer is difficult to awaken during an episode and may suffer injury if sleeping in an unfamiliar setting.
- Somnambulism in adults may be associated with anxiety disorder, depressive disorder, and personality disorder. Somnambulism in children is not associated with other psychiatric disorders.

- Although complex behaviours, including attempted homicide, have been described as occurring during somnambulism, in general, this is not common.

36.4.1.6 Differential Diagnosis

Important differential diagnoses include

- Psychomotor epilepsy during sleep
- Fugue states
- Sleep drunkenness

36.4.1.7 Management

- The person's nighttime surroundings should be made safe in order to reduce the risk of injury during episodes.
- Reassurance, anxiety-reduction techniques, and offering psychoeducation to patient and family.
- Small doses of benzodiazepines, tricyclic antidepressants, and SSRIs may help in severe cases.

36.4.2 SLEEP TERRORS (NIGHT TERRORS)

36.4.2.1 Epidemiology

- In children, night terrors are common and occur on a frequent basis in 1%–4%. M > F.
- They are far less common in adulthood (<1%). M = F.

36.4.2.2 Aetiology

Aetiological factors that have been suggested include

- Stress
- Previous loss of sleep
- Familial: 10-fold increase in prevalence in first degree relatives
- Induction by benzodiazepine antagonists (hence the theories about benzodiazepine receptor changes or endogenous substances acting on benzodiazepine receptors)
- Upper airway obstruction in children

36.4.2.3 ICD-10 Criteria

- Repeated (two or more) episodes of arising from bed during the first third of nocturnal sleep and presents with panicky scream, intense anxiety, body mobility, and autonomic hyperactivity.
- The duration of the episode is less than 10 min.
- There is a lack of response followed by disorientation and preservative movements.
- The individual has limited recall for the event.
- There is no known causative factor.

36.4.2.4 DSM-5 Criteria (APA, 2013)

- Sleep terrors are listed under non-rapid eye movement sleep arousal disorder. The criteria are similar to ICD-10 with emphasis on impairment in functioning.

36.4.2.5 Other Clinical Features

- Sleep terrors occur during sleep stages 3–4 and therefore usually 1–2 h after sleep starts.
- Enuresis may occur during an episode.
- In children, there is no increase in rate of psychopathology of mental disorders.
- In adults, sleep terrors are associated with generalized anxiety disorder, post-traumatic stress disorder, and personality disorders.

36.4.2.6 Differential Diagnosis

- The main differential diagnosis is nightmares.

36.4.2.7 Management

Methods that may be tried include

- Reassurance—of the child and the parents
- Changing the settling routine
- Keeping a diary and then waking the child just before each episode is expected
- Small doses of benzodiazepines, tricyclic antidepressants, and SSRIs may help in severe cases

36.4.2.8 Course and Prognosis

- The onset is usually between 4 and 12 years and sleep terrors often resolve spontaneously by adolescence.
- Frequency of sleep terrors can range from every night to once per few weeks.
- Adulthood sleep terrors often run a chronic course.

36.5 REM PARASOMNIAS

36.5.1 NIGHTMARES

Nightmares are 'bad' (i.e. frightening) dreams. They occur universally.

36.5.1.1 Epidemiology

- Young children (3–5 years old): 10%–50% have nightmares.
- Adults: 3% report frequent nightmares and 50% report occasional nightmares.
- F/M = 2–4:1.

36.5.1.2 Aetiology

Aetiological factors that have been suggested include

- Negative dreams associated with
  - Daytime depression
  - Daytime anxiety
  - Daytime stress
- Hypnotic withdrawal
- Alcohol withdrawal
- Medications:
  - β-adrenoceptor antagonists
  - Reserpine

36.5.1.3 ICD-10 Criteria

- Awakenings during the second half of sleep and patient presents with detailed and vivid recall of intensely frightening dreams, involving threats to survival, security, or self-esteem.
- The person is orientated and alert after awakening from a frightening dream.
- The dream experience cause marked distress to the individual.
- There is no known causative organic factor or substance misuse.

36.5.1.4 DSM-5 Criteria (APA, 2013)

- The diagnostic criteria for nightmare disorder listed in DSM-5 are very similar to ICD-10 with the emphasis on impairment in functioning.

36.5.1.5 Other Clinical Features

- Nightmares tend to occur during middle and late sleep; they usually occur during REM sleep but occasionally during stages 1–2.
- The dream is remembered and patients may have difficulties falling asleep again as a result of anxiety.
- Nightmares are not associated with violent body movements and vocalization because of low muscle tone in REM sleep.
- Depression and anxiety symptoms are common in people with frequent nightmares since childhood.

36.5.1.6 Differential Diagnosis

The main differential diagnosis is sleep terrors.

36.5.1.7 Management

- Any underlying disorder (e.g. PTSD) may require treatment.
- Nonpharmacological treatment: reassurance, conflict resolution, image rehearsal therapy, and progressive muscle relaxation therapy.
- Pharmacological treatment is indicated for severe cases. REM suppressants such as SSRIs are indicated.
- Prazosin, a sympatholytic agent, can treat PTSD-associated nightmares.

36.5.2 REM Sleep Behaviour Disorder

36.5.2.1 Epidemiology

- REM sleep behaviour disorder is more common in old men.

36.5.2.2 Aetiology

Aetiological factors that have been suggested include
- Alcohol withdrawal
- Early signs of Parkinson's disease, Lewy body dementia, and multisystem atrophy
- Precipitation by antidepressants and beta-blockers

36.5.2.3 DSM-5 Criteria (APA, 2013)

- Behaviours include repeated episodes of arousal during sleep associated with vocalization and complex motor behaviours that may cause injury to bed partner or self.
- The vocalization and complex behaviours correlated with dream mentation simultaneously and is often described as acting out of dreams.
- The duration of behavioural disturbance is longer than 90 min after sleep onset with more frequent episodes during the later part of the nocturnal sleep.
- The person is orientated and alert after awakening.
- Loss of REM atonia.
- Polysomnographic evidence of abnormal REM behaviours or an established synucleinopathy diagnosis if polysomnographic evidence is absent.
- Significant functional and occupational impairment.
- No organic causative factor or substance abuse.

Investigation: The diagnosis is confirmed with overnight polysomnography.

36.5.2.4 Management

- Ensure safety of patient and his or her bed partner.
- Prescribe clonazepam in severe case.

REFERENCES

American Psychiatric Association. 2013: *Desk Reference to the Diagnostic Criteria from DSM-5*. Washington, DC: American Psychiatric Association Press.

Avidan AY. 2009: Parasomnias and movement disorders of sleep. *Seminars in Neurology* 29(4):372–392.

Barion A and Zee PC. 2007: A clinical approach to circadian rhythm sleep disorders. *Sleep Medicine* 8(8):566–577.

DeMartinis NA and Winokur A. 2007: Effects of psychiatric medications on sleep and sleep disorders. *CNS and Neurological Disorders–Drug Targets* 6:17–29.

Edinger JD and Means MK. 2005: Cognitive behavioral therapy for primary insomnia. *Clinical Psychology Review* 25:539–558.

Ekbom K and Ulfberg J. 2009: Restless legs syndrome. *Journal of Internal Medicine* 266:419–431.

Golbin AZ, Kravitz HM, and Keith LG. 2004: *Sleep Psychiatry*. London, U.K.: Taylor & Francis Group.

Laking PJ. 2002: Sleep disorders. In Puri BK, Laking PJ, and Treasaden IH (eds.) *Textbook of Psychiatry*, 2nd edn, pp. 844–853. Edinburgh, U.K.: Churchill Livingstone.

NICE. *NICE Guidelines on Zaleplon, Zolpidem and Zopiclone for Insomnia*. http://www.nice.org.uk/nicemedia/pdf/TA077publicinfoenglish.pdf (accessed on 17 July 2012).

Parkes JD. 1985: *Sleep and Its Disorders*. London, U.K.: WB Saunders.

Sadock BJ and Sadock VA. 2007: *Kaplan & Sadock's Synopsis of Psychiatry. Behavioral Sciences/Clinical Psychiatry*, 10th edn. Philadelphia, PA: Lippincott Williams & Wilkins.

Taylor D, Paton C, and Kapur S. 2012: *The Maudsley Prescribing Guidelines in Psychiatry*, 11th edn. West Sussex, U.K.: Wiley-Blackwell.

Thorpy MJ, Westbrook P, Ferber R, Fredrickson P, Mahowald M, Perez-Guerra F, Reite M, and Smith P. 1992: The clinical use of the multiple sleep latency test. *Sleep* 15:268–276.

Wise MS, Arand DL, Auger RR, Brooks SN, and Watson NF. 2007: Treatment of narcolepsy and other hypersomnias of central origin. *Sleep* 30(12):1712–1717.

World Health Organization. 1992: *ICD-10: The ICD-10 Classification of Mental and Behavioural Disorders: Clinical Descriptions and Diagnostic Guidelines*. Geneva, Switzerland: World Health Organization.

37 Child and Adolescent Psychiatry

37.1 EPIDEMIOLOGY

37.1.1 PRESCHOOL

The main epidemiological study is the Waltham Forest Study (Richman et al., 1982) in the early 1970s of 3-year-olds, carried out in the London borough of that name. The Vineyard study (Martha) essentially confirmed its findings. The main findings included

1. 7% prevalence of moderate to severe behavioural and emotional problems, slightly greater in boys than girls
2. 15% prevalence of mild behavioural and emotional problems
3. Strong associations found with
   a. Maternal depression
   b. Poor parental marriage
   c. Delayed development of language
4. Strong continuities of behaviour and language disorders over the early school years

37.1.2 MIDDLE CHILDHOOD

The main epidemiological studies are the Isle of Wight and inner London borough studies (by Rutter and colleagues) in the 1960s, of 10- and 11-year-olds. Recent studies in Norway and Puerto Rico essentially confirmed the findings. The main findings included

- 6.8% overall point prevalence of child psychiatric disorder in the Isle of Wight
- 4% prevalence of conduct disorder
- 2.5% prevalence of emotional disorder
- Male to female sex ratio of 1.9:1
- An overall point prevalence of child psychiatric disorder in inner London twice that in the Isle of Wight

37.1.3 ADOLESCENCE

- 10%–20% prevalence of psychiatric disorder
- A male to female sex ratio of approximately 1:1.5

37.2 ASSESSMENT

The information to be obtained in a child psychiatric interview is shown in Table 37.1.

37.3 PERVASIVE DEVELOPMENTAL DISORDERS

37.3.1 CHILDHOOD AUTISM (ICD-10 F84.0)/ AUTISTIC DISORDER (DSM-5 299.0)

37.3.1.1 Historical Development
- The term 'autism' was coined by Leo Kanner in 1943. Childhood autism is also known as Kanner's syndrome.

37.3.1.2 Epidemiology
- Prevalence: 7–28/10,000.
- Male/female ratio = 4:1.
- Autism accounts for 25%–60% of all autistic disorders.
- No epidemiological studies have demonstrated an association between autistic disorder and any socioeconomic status.

37.3.1.3 Aetiology
1. Genetic causes:
   a. Heritability is over 90%.
   b. Monozygotic twins/dizygotic twins: 36%:0%.
   c. The recurrence rate in siblings is roughly 3% for narrowly defined autism but is about 10%–20% for milder variants.
   d. The loci may involve chromosome 2q and 7q.
   e. Family history of schizophrenia-like psychosis or affective disorder.
2. Neurodevelopmental theory:
   a. Perinatal injuries (e.g. maternal bleeding after the first trimester or meconium in the amniotic fluid).
   b. Antenatal infections (e.g. congenital rubella, cytomegalovirus).
   c. Maternal use of sodium valproate in pregnancy.
   d. Gestational age less than 35 weeks.
   e. Birth defects associated with central nervous system malformation (e.g. cerebral palsy).

TABLE 37.1

Information to Be Assessed in a Child Psychiatric Interview

Source and nature of referral
Who made referral?
Who initiated referral?
Family attitudes to referral
Description of presenting complaints
Onset, frequency, intensity, duration, location (home, school, etc.)
Antecedents and consequences
Ameliorating and exacerbating factors
Specific examples
Parental and family beliefs about causation
Past attempts to solve problem
Description of child's current general functioning
School
    Behaviour and emotions
    Academic performance
    Peer and staff relationships
Peer relationships generally
Family relationships
Personal/developmental history
Pregnancy, labour, delivery
Early developmental milestones
Separations/disruptions
Physical illnesses and their meaning for parents
Reactions to school
Puberty
Temperamental style
Family history
Personal and social histories of both parents, especially
    History of mental illness
    Their experience of being parented
History of family development
    How parents came together
    History of pregnancies
    Separations and effects on children
Who lives at home currently
Strengths/weaknesses of all at home
Current social stresses and supports
Information from observation of family interaction
Structure, organization, communication, sensitivity
Information from observation of child at interview
Motor, sensory, speech, language, social relating skills
Mental state, concerns, and spontaneous account if age appropriate
Results of physical examination
Plan for future investigation and management

Source: Reproduced from Puri, B.K. and Treasaden, I.H., *Textbook of Psychiatry*, 3rd edn., Churchill Livingstone, Edinburgh, U.K., 2011. With permission.

f. Presence of minor congenital abnormalities (e.g. ear abnormalities, dermatoglyphics) as a result of abnormal neuroectodermal development within the first trimester of pregnancy.

g. Hypoplasia of cerebellar vermal lobules and cortical abnormalities particularly polymicrogyria that reflect abnormal cell migrations in the first 6 months of gestation.

h. Immunological incompatibility (e.g. maternal antibodies directed at the fetus) may contribute to autistic disorder.

i. Respiratory distress syndrome, anaemia, encephalopathy in neonatal period.

j. Exaggerated growth of the brain in the first 2 years of life and 20% of patients have head circumference above 97th percentile.

3. Association with learning disability.
4. Fragile X syndrome.
5. Tuberous sclerosis.
6. Phenylketonuria.
7. Neurofibromatosis.
8. Infantile spasms are recognized causes.

37.3.1.4 Pathogenesis and Neurobiology

- High serotonin and 5-HIAA levels
- Hypodopaminergic activity
- Hypoplasia of cerebellar vermis
- Underactivation of fusiform gyrus
- Abnormality in the medial temporal lobe

37.3.1.5 Theory of Mind

- This refers to the capacity to attribute independent mental states to oneself and to others, thereby allowing one to predict and explain actions.
- People with autism have an impaired ability to understand other people's thought process, motivations, intentions, and feelings and to make inferences about the thoughts of others. As a result, they have impaired empathy and social reciprocation.

37.3.1.6 ICD-10 Diagnostic Criteria and Clinical Characteristics

1. *The presence of abnormal development that is manifested before the age of 3 years* including abnormal receptive or expressive language, abnormal selective or reciprocal social interaction, and abnormal functional or symbolic play. Children with autism are often attached to odd objects and have relative lack of creativity and fantasy in thoughts.

2. *Abnormal reciprocal social interactions* include failure in eye gaze and body language, failure in development of peer relationship, lack of socio-emotional reciprocity, and lack of spontaneous sharing with other people.

3. *Abnormal communication* include lack of development of spoken language, lack of social imitative play, failure to initiate or sustain conversational interchange, and stereotyped and repetitive use of language. Their languages are frequently associated with pronoun reversals. A child with child autism may say, 'You want the pencil' when he means he wants it. Echolalia (repetition of spoken words by others) and palilalia (repetitions of one's spoken words) are common.

4. *Restricted, stereotyped, and repetitive behaviour* include preoccupation with stereotyped interest, compulsive adherence to rituals, motor mannerisms, and preoccupation with part-objects or nonfunctional elements of play materials. Some children with autism enjoy vestibular stimulations such as spinning and swinging.

5. Other nonspecific problems include phobias, sleeping and eating disturbances, temper tantrums, self-directed aggression, and self-injury (e.g. wrist biting).

6. There should be an absence of other causes of pervasive developmental disorders, socio-emotional problems, and schizophrenia-like symptoms.

37.3.1.7 Differences between the ICD-10 and DSM-5 Criteria

1. The DSM-5 criteria on autism spectrum disorder emphasize two main symptom clusters:
   a. Persistent deficits in social communication, social interaction across contexts and maintain relationships
   b. Restricted, repetitive patterns of behaviour, interests, or activities

2. There are no major differences between ICD-10 and DSM-IV-TR in diagnostic criteria for autism. A total of five symptoms are required (At least three symptoms from the social domain and the communication domain and one symptom from the repetitive behaviour domain.).

3. In ICD-10, atypical autism is a stand-alone disorder under pervasive developmental disorder.

4. ICD-10 also specifies that atypical autism differs from autism in *either* the age of onset (after 3 years) *or* not meeting all the diagnostic criteria for autism.

5. DSM-5 has other specifiers: with intellectual impairment, known medical or genetic condition, catatonia and associated with another neurodevelopmental disorder.

37.3.2 NICE GUIDELINES

The NICE guidelines summarize the signs and symptoms of possible autism in preschool children, primary school children, and secondary school adolescents.

Consider the possibility of autism

The NICE guidelines advise psychiatrists to not rule out autism because of

- Good eye contact, smiling, and showing affection to family members
- Reported pretend play or normal language milestones
- Difficulties appearing to resolve after an intervention
- A previous assessment that concluded that there was no autism especially when new information becomes available

Differential diagnosis

The NICE guidelines recommend that psychiatrists should consider the following differential diagnoses.

37.3.2.1 Neurodevelopmental Disorders
- Atypical autism (onset after 3 years without full-blown symptoms)
- Asperger's syndrome (no impairment in verbal communication and higher verbal IQ than non-verbal IQ)
- Rett's disorder (predominantly in girls, microcephaly, loss of previously acquired abilities after 6 months of normal development and earlier onset of seizure)
- Childhood disintegrative disorder (a developmental regression that follows at least 2 years of normal development and better language development)
- Epileptic encephalopathy

37.3.2.2 Mental and Behavioural Disorders
Children with the following disorders show normal communication and social interaction:

- Attention-deficit hyperactivity disorder (ADHD)
- Mood disorder
- Anxiety disorder
- Attachment disorder

- Oppositional defiant disorder
- Conduct disorder
- Obsessive–compulsive disorder
- Childhood-onset schizophrenia (later age of onset, equal gender ratio, family history of schizophrenia, normal intelligence, and presence of psychotic features)

37.3.2.3 Other Conditions

- Selective mutism: lack of communication is not consistent
- Deafness: usually respond to loud noises and abnormal audiogram
- Severe visual impairment
- Maltreatment
- Schizotypal disorder (more social awareness and emotional reciprocity but less stereotyped behaviours and interests)

37.3.2.4 Physical Examination

The NICE guidelines recommend that the psychiatrist should perform a general physical examination and look specifically for

- Microcephaly or macrocephaly
- Dysmorphic features (genetic evaluation may be necessary)
- Skin stigmata of neurofibromatosis or tuberous sclerosis using a Wood's light
- Signs of injury, for example, self-harm or child maltreatment
- Congenital anomalies and dysmorphic features including macrocephaly or microcephaly

37.3.2.5 Investigations

Instruments that require training

- Autism Diagnostic Observation Schedule (ADOS) is a semi-structured instrument that aims to assess patients aged from toddlers to adults.
- Autism Diagnostic Interview (ADI) is a semi-structured instrument and assesses caregivers.
- Childhood Autism Rating Scale (CARS) is a scale that differentiates children with autism from other pervasive developmental disorders. (Schopler et al., 1980)

Instruments that do not require training

- Autism Behaviour Checklist (ABC): This questionnaire was developed with behaviours selected from a variety of checklists and instruments used

to identify autism. It has 57 questions divided into five categories: (1) sensory functions, (2) relationship, (3) use of body parts and objects, (4) language, and (5) social function and self-help (Krug et al., 1980).
- Social Communication Questionnaire (SCQ): A questionnaire completed by parents with 40 'yes-or-no' items.
- Social Responsiveness Questionnaire (SRQ): A 15 min questionnaire that measures the severity of autistic social impairment across the entire range of the autism spectrum, from nonexistent to severe.
- Pervasive Developmental Disorder Behaviour Inventory (PDDBI): PDDBI is used to evaluate children with the age range from 6 months to 12 years who have been diagnosed with a pervasive developmental disorder as defined by the DSM-IV. Rating forms completed by parents and teachers yield age-standardized scores that are helpful in planning treatment, monitoring progress, assessing outcome, and making placement decisions.

Multidisciplinary assessment

- Audiological examination to differentiate autism from deafness.
- Speech therapist assessment.
- IQ test: children with autistic disorder are more skilled in visual–spatial tasks than in tasks requiring skill in verbal reasoning.
- A Developmental NEuroPSYchological Assessment (NEPSY) is a neurological test for children aged 3–16 years, and assessment is classified into six domains: executive functions, language, sensorimotor functions, visuospatial functions, memory, and social perception. Other standardized neuropsychological tests including Halstead–Reitan Battery and Luria–Nebraska Battery.
- EEG: 30% have nonspecific EEG abnormalities. EEG is indicated if there is history of clinical seizures, subclinical seizures (e.g. staring spells), and developmental regression.
- MRI is not routinely recommended. Ventricular enlargement is found in 20%–25% of people with autism.
- Metabolic testing: phenylketonuria.

37.3.2.6 Comorbidity

Medical comorbidity

- Epilepsy (30%)
- Motor coordination problems

- Visual or hearing impairment
- Respiratory infections
- Feeding problems: including restricted diets
- Constipation, altered bowel habit, faecal incontinence, or encopresis
- Loose bowel movements
- Urinary incontinence or enuresis

Psychiatric comorbidity

- Learning disability: 70% of children with autism have mental retardation, mild to moderate mental retardation (30%), and severe to profound mental retardation (50%).
- Academic learning problems in literacy or numeracy.
- ADHD (50%).
- Obsessive–compulsive disorder (10%).
- Tics or Tourette's syndrome.
- Anxiety disorders.
- Depression: irritability and social withdrawal.
- Temper tantrums.
- Oppositional defiant disorder.
- Self-injurious behaviour.

37.3.2.7 Treatment
Psychological treatment

- *Applied behaviour analysis (ABA)*: operant conditioning helps to develop specific social, communication and behavioural skills by reinforcing positive behaviour. The triggers for problematic behaviour are analysed.
- *Intensive behavioural intervention (IBI)*: the design, implementation, and evaluation of environmental modifications that aim to produce socially meaningful changes in behaviour.
- *Sensory integration therapy*: for example, brushing of the skin or swinging to stimulate vestibular responses that will help to reduce the hypersensitivity to stimuli.
- *Facilitated communication*: training on reading and writing.

Pharmacological treatment

- Risperidone: reduce repetition and aggression and improve behaviour
- Fluoxetine: reduce the levels of ritualistic behaviours and improved mood and anxiety
- Anticonvulsants: reduce self-injurious behaviour

- Naltrexone: reduce self-injurious behaviour
- Atomoxetine: reduce inattention, hyperactivity, and aggression

Multidisciplinary treatment

The NICE guidelines recommend patients with autism to be treated by a multidisciplinary team that include paediatrician and/or child and adolescent psychiatrist, speech therapist, clinical and/or educational psychologist, and occupational therapist.

- *Education programme*: Autistic children often do well in a well-structured educational setting with experienced teachers and educational psychologists.
- *Behaviour therapy* establishes underlying reasons for disruptive behaviour and provides alternative and more socially acceptable ways of indicating needs. Behaviour therapy also aims at reducing behavioural problems such as temper tantrums, feeding and toilet problems, aggression, rituals, and obsessions.
- *Social skill training* helps the child to understand beliefs and emotions of the others based on the theory of mind. Teaching a child to 'mind read' by first helping a child understand his own thoughts or feelings and thus eventually be able to deduce actions from other people.
- *Speech therapy*: Speech therapist can help the child to facilitate communication and the parents to understand echolalic speech and consider alternative mode of communication.
- *Occupational therapy*: Occupational therapist can assess a child's behaviour from the sensory processing and self-regulation perspectives and help the child to develop more adaptive ways to self-regulate.
- *Parent education and support* is provided for parents and family members about childhood autism and refer them to community resources for further support (e.g. autism advocacy and support organizations).

Alternative treatment

- Casein- and gluten-free diet: requires further study
- Highly unsaturated fatty acid supplements: some success
- Secretin: no improvement in language
- Vitamins A and C

37.3.2.8   Course of Illness

- In the first 3 years of life, 70% of children with autism do not achieve normal development.
- Peak age of seizure is between 11 and 14 years old.
- Inappropriate sexual behaviour may emerge in adolescence and early adulthood.
- Most children with autism show improvement in social relation and communication but not in rituals or repetitive behaviour.
- Childhood autism often causes lifelong disability. 10% of people with autism will ultimately lose language skills with intellectual deterioration.

37.3.2.9   Prognosis

- The most important predictor is childhood IQ and presence of speech by 5 years.
- Nonverbal IQ<60 is associated with severe social impairment and lack of independent living.
- 50% do not develop useful speech.
- Only 10% are able to work.

37.4   ASPERGER'S SYNDROME (ICD-10 F84.5)

37.4.1   HISTORICAL DEVELOPMENT

- Asperger's syndrome was coined by Hans Asperger in 1944 and reappraised by Wing in 1981.

37.4.2   EPIDEMIOLOGY

- 3–4 per 1000 children
- Male to female ratio is 9:1

37.4.3   CLINICAL FEATURES

- The DSM-5 criteria suggest merging Asperger's syndrome into autistic spectrum disorder.
- People with Asperger's syndrome usually do not have delay in language development (e.g. be able to speak single words by age of 2 years and communicate by age of 3 years) and cognitive development. Speech is characterized by poor prosody (stress, rhythm, intonation of speech), unusual rate, poorly modulated volume, tangentiality, circumstantiality, and verbosity.
- People usually have intense circumscribed interests and this may develop into isolated special skills. Classic interests include scientific fields (e.g. trains, weather, and dinosaurs) or interest in other fields such as arts and music.
- Impairment in social interactions:
  - Marked impairment in the use of multiple non-verbal behaviours (eye gaze, facial expression)
  - Failure to develop peer relationship
  - Lack of spontaneous seeking to share enjoyment, interests, achievements
  - Lack of social or emotional reciprocity
- Restricted repetitive and stereotyped patterns of behaviour:
  - Inflexible adherence to routines and rituals
  - Stereotyped and repetitive mannerism (e.g. hand or finger flapping)
  - Persistent preoccupation with parts of objects

37.4.4   DIFFERENCES BETWEEN CHILDHOOD AUTISM AND ASPERGER'S SYNDROME (TABLE 37.2)

37.4.5   COMORBIDITY

- ADHD (most common comorbidity in children).
- Depression (most common comorbidity in adults).
- Anxiety.
- Obsessive–compulsive disorder.
- Possible development of schizophrenia.
- Criminal offending is related to lack of concern of outcome, impulsivity, social naivety, overriding compulsion to steal, and misinterpretation of actions from others.

37.4.6   TREATMENT

- Psychoeducation should be offered to parents to enhance acceptance and maintain routines at home and school.
- As the child gets older, he will be helped by verbally mediated treatment, supportive counselling, and self-sufficiency training.
- He will be encouraged to obtain employment in jobs with regular routines. Sheltered employment and sheltered residence are reserved for severe cases.

37.4.7   PROGNOSIS

- Good prognostic features include normal intelligence and high level of social skills.
- There is a strong tendency for the abnormalities to persist into adolescence and adult life.
- Psychotic episodes occasionally occur in early adult life.

TABLE 37.2
Compare and Contrast Autism and Asperger's Syndrome

	Autism	Asperger's Syndrome
Gender ratio	Male to female ratio is 3:1	Male to female ratio is 9:1
Neuropathology	Lesions in amygdala, corpus callosum, and cerebellum	Right hemisphere lesions Association with aminoacidurias
Development	Abnormal early development Onset is younger than 3 years There is a delay in language development	Relatively normal early development The child is noted to have lack of warmth and interest in social relationships around the third year of life Language development is not delayed and single word should have developed by age of 2 and communicate phrases by age of 3 Motor milestones are delayed
Salient clinical features	Restricted, stereotyped, and repetitive behaviours such as motor mannerisms are more common than Asperger's syndrome Preoccupation with part-objects or nonfunctional elements of play materials is more common than Asperger's syndrome	Preoccupation with restricted, stereotyped, and repetitive interests. Extensive information is often acquired in a mechanical fashion Patients are good with logics, rules, and routines. They tend to see the details and argue over minor details without seeing the whole picture
Intelligence quotient (IQ)	Performance IQ is higher than verbal IQ	Reasonably preserved IQ Verbal IQ is higher than performance IQ
Speech	Severe expressive speech disorder	Fluent but monotonous, staccato, and pedantic speech

37.5 RETT'S SYNDROME (ICD-10 F84.2)

37.5.1 Historical Development

- Rett's syndrome was coined by Andreas Rett in 1966.

37.5.2 Epidemiology

- Prevalence rate is between 1 in 15,000 and 1 in 22,000 females.
- The incidence of sudden and unexpected death is around 2%.
- It is predominantly a female disorder but men with clinical features similar to Rett's syndrome have been described.

37.5.3 Inheritance

- Mutation in the transcription regulatory gene MECP2 at chromosome Xq28
- X-linked dominant mutation with lethality in hemizygous males

37.5.4 Clinical Features and Course of Illness

1. Age: 0–6 months:
   a. Normal prenatal and perinatal development
   b. Normal head circumference at birth
   c. Normal psychomotor development in the first 5 months of life
   d. Plateau in social skill development by 6 months
2. 7–24 months:
   a. Deceleration in head growth.
   b. Loss of speech.
   c. Loss of skills in locomotion.
   d. Loss of purposive hand movements and replaced by hand-wringing stereotypies.
   e. Hyperventilation.
   f. Social and play development are arrested by 24 months.
   g. Severe impairment in expressive and receptive language.
3. 4 years:
   a. Trunk ataxia and apraxia: poorly coordinated trunk movements.

b. Development of choreoathetoid movements: poorly coordinated gait.

c. Breathing dysfunction: irregular respiration, episodes of hyperventilation, and apnoea.

d. Seizures (75%).

e. Scoliosis.

f. Spasticity.

g. Growth retardation.

h. Hypotrophic small feet are supportive diagnostic criteria.

i. Profound mental retardation: mental deterioration precedes motor deterioration.

j. Patients are usually in wheelchairs by their late teens and die before the age of 30.

37.5.5 TREATMENT

- Anticonvulsant treatment: seizure control
- Behaviour therapy: control self-injurious behaviour
- Physiotherapy: prevent muscular dysfunction and regulate breathing

37.6 CHILDHOOD DISINTEGRATIVE DISORDER (ICD-10 F84.3)

37.6.1 EPIDEMIOLOGY

- Prevalence: 1.7 per 10,000
- Age of onset: 3–4 years old
- Male predominance

37.6.2 CLINICAL FEATURES

- Normal development for at least 2 years after birth
- Loss of previously acquired skills before age of 10 in the following areas: language, social skills, bowel control, bladder control, motor skills, and play
- Qualitative impairments in social interactions involving nonverbal behaviour, communications involving spoken language, and stereotyped behaviour (e.g. stereotypies or mannerism)

37.6.3 COMORBIDITY

- Seizure disorders: 50% have EEG abnormalities
- Tuberous sclerosis
- Metachromatic leukodystrophy
- Schilder's leukoencephalopathy
- Landau–Kleffner syndrome (acquired aphasia with epilepsy): preserved social interest and nonverbal communicative skills

37.6.4 COURSE OF ILLNESS

- Three-fourths of patients do not have further deterioration in behaviour and reach stabilization. Life expectancy is normal.
- Some children show recovery of previous developmental skills and few children have very good recovery.
- Progressive deterioration occurs in one-fourth of children, especially in those associated with a progressive neuropathological process and death may result.
- Most patients suffer from moderate mental retardation.

37.7 HYPERKINETIC DISORDER (ICD-10 F90)

37.7.1 ATTENTION DEFICIT AND HYPERACTIVITY DISORDER (DSM-5 314)

37.7.1.1 Terminology

- ADHD is an American term. In the United Kingdom, it is often known as 'hyperkinetic disorder'.

37.7.1.2 Epidemiology

- In the United Kingdom, 1.7% of school-aged children suffer from hyperkinetic disorder based on ICD-10 criteria and are more stringent and require both hyperactivity and inattention to be present.
- In the United States, 3%–10% of school-aged children suffer from ADHD. Increased prevalence in the United States is a result of better recognition, psychosocial adversity, and the change of DSM-III–DSM-IV criteria that classifies ADHD into three subtypes. The DSM-5 requires either hyperactivity or inattention to be present.
- Male to female gender ratio: 3:1.
- Peak age of onset: 3–8 years.

37.7.1.3 Aetiology

37.7.1.4 Genetics

- ADHD is a heritable disorder. Siblings of ADHD children have twice the risk of ADHD when compared to the general population.
- Biological parents of children with the disorder have a higher risk for ADHD than adoptive parents. The parents of children with ADHD show an increased incidence of hyperkinesis, sociopathy, alcohol use disorders, and conversion disorder.

- Genes related to dopaminergic function are implicated (e.g. dopamine receptor D4 gene, dopamine transporter (DAT1) gene, alpha 2A gene, norepinephrine transporter gene, catechol-O-methyltransferase (COMT) gene).
- First-degree biological relatives of ADHD children are at high risk to develop ADHD and other disorders such as disruptive behaviour disorders, anxiety disorders, and depressive disorders.

37.7.1.5   Neurodevelopment

- September is the peak month for births of children with ADHD with and without comorbid learning disorders.
- Early infection, inflammation, toxins, and trauma cause circulatory, metabolic, and physical brain damage and lead to ADHD in adulthood.
- Psychosocial adversity (e.g. maternal psychopathology, large family size, parental conflict, and emotional deprivation) is associated with ADHD in childhood.

37.7.1.6   Neurochemistry

- Noradrenaline: A dysfunction in peripheral noradrenaline leads to negative feedback to the locus coeruleus and results in reduction of noradrenaline in the central nervous system.
- Evidence: Stimulants and tricyclic antidepressants increase catecholamine concentrations by promoting their release and blocking their uptake. Clonidine, a noradrenaline agonist, may reduce hyperactivity in ADHD.

37.7.1.7   Clinical Features

1. Persistent pattern of inattention, hyperactivity, and impulsivity across two different settings and result in significant functional impairments. The behaviours are maladaptive and inconsistent with developmental level.
2. The onset is before the age of 7 years.
3. Symptoms of inattention include *(Mnemonic: SOLID)*
   a. *Starts tasks or activities but not able to follow through and finish.*
   b. *Organization of tasks or activities is impaired.*
   c. *Loses things necessary for tasks and activities such as school assignments or stationary.*
   d. *Instructions are not followed.*
   e. *Distraction by external stimuli.*
   f. *Other features: careless mistakes and forgetfulness in daily activities.*
4. Symptoms of hyperactivity and impulsivity include *(Mnemonic: WORST FAIL)*
   a. *Waiting for in lines or await turns in game cause frustration (impulsivity).*
   b. *On the move most of the time such as running and climbing (hyperactivity).*
   c. *Restlessness and jitteriness (hyperactivity).*
   d. *Squirms on seat (hyperactivity).*
   e. *Talk excessively without appropriate response to social constraints (impulsivity).*
   f. *Fidgets with hands and feet (hyperactivity).*
   g. *Answers are blurted out before questions (impulsivity).*
   h. *Interruption of other people's conversations (impulsivity).*
   i. *Loud noise in playing (hyperactivity).*
5. The DSM-5 classifies ADHD into three subtypes:
   a. Inattentive type: at least six symptoms of inattention but not hyperactivity and impulsivity symptoms for 6 months.
   b. Hyperactivity type: at least six symptoms of hyperactivity and impulsivity but no symptoms of inattention for 6 months.
   c. Combined type: at least six symptoms from both inattention and hyperactivity/impulsivity for 6 months.
6. The DSM-5 has raised the upper limit of age of onset to 12 year olds (previously 7 year olds).
7. The ICD-10 criteria require at least six symptoms of inattention, three symptoms of hyperactivity, and one symptom of inattention for duration of 6 months. ICD-10 criteria do not classify ADHD into three subtypes.
8. Adult ADHD: the symptoms of ADHD focus more on inattentive symptoms. Symptoms of hyperactivity tend to improve with time. The following are symptoms of adult ADHD:
   a. Irritability
   b. Impatience
   c. Forgetfulness
   d. Inattention
   e. Impulsivity
   f. Disorganization
   g. Distractibility
   h. Chronic procrastination with many projects underway simultaneously and trouble in completing them
   i. Difficulty in tolerating boredom

9. Mental state examination may reveal hyperactivity, anxiety, distractibility, perservation, and concrete thinking.
10. Neurological examination may reveal visual, auditory, motor impairments, and reflex asymmetries.
11. Cognitive assessment may reveal difficulty in copying age-appropriate figures and performing rapidly alternative movements and left–right differentiation.

37.7.1.8 Rating Scales and Cognitive Assessment

- Connors' rating scale: Connors' rating scale is a diagnostic scale for ADHD using the DSM-IV criteria. This scale includes measures of behaviour described by parents and teachers. The behaviour scale includes the following: (1) ADHD symptoms, (2) anxiety, (3) cognitive problems, (4) oppositional behaviour, (5) perfectionism, and (6) social problems (Gladman and Lancaster, 2003).
- Child Global Assessment Scale (CGAS): a score 60/100 is the cutoff that requires treatment.
- Swanson, Nolan, and Pelham (SNAP) Questionnaire: this teacher and parent rating scale is composed of 18 items and determines if symptoms of ADHD are present.
- Arrange direct school observation by a member of Child and Adolescent Mental Health Service (CAMHS).
- Psychometric testing such as IQ assessment or academic assessment if there is evidence of learning disability.

37.7.1.9 Further Investigations

1. *EEG*: increased beta waves and decreased delta waves are associated with arousal and hyperactivity.
2. MRI brain:
   a. Reduction in size in corpus callosum and cerebellum
   b. Decreased activities in the anterior cingulated gyrus
   c. Decreased activities in the thalamus, hippocampus, globus pallidus, and caudate

37.7.1.10 Differential diagnosis

- Early-onset bipolar disorder: mania is more goal-orientated and episodic.

37.7.1.11 Comorbidity

- Speech or language impairment: 50%
- Oppositional defiant disorder (40% of children meet the diagnostic criteria of oppositional defiant

disorder. About 75% of children with ADHD show behavioural symptoms of aggression)
- Conduct disorder (30%–50%)
- Anxiety disorders (25%)
- Tics (11%)
- Substance abuse (e.g. cannabis, alcohol, nicotine, and cocaine)

37.7.1.12 Treatment

Pharmacological treatment

1. Prior to initiation of medication, the psychiatrist is advised to
   a. Look for exercise syncope, undue breathlessness, and other cardiovascular symptoms in the history
   b. Perform physical examination including measurement of heart rate and blood pressure and examination of the cardiovascular system
   c. Measure baseline height and weight
   d. Order an electrocardiogram (ECG) if history of cardiac disease is present

Stimulants

- Examples of stimulants include methylphenidate and dexamfetamine.
- The stimulant inhibits dopamine reuptake and causes direct release of dopamine.
- Stimulant is indicated for ADHD without comorbidity or ADHD with comorbid conduct disorder.
- Beneficial effects of methylphenidate: improve attention span and hyperactivity for a certain number of hours while in the school setting.
- Dosing: Regular Ritalin requires 5–10 mg TID. Consider modified release preparations (e.g. long acting Ritalin or Concerta XL) that allows single-day dosage and promotes adherence. Starting dose is 18 mg OM and slowly titrates up to 54 mg/day.
- Common side effects include reduction in appetite, gastric discomfort, insomnia, headache, elevation of blood pressure, tics, dysphoria, and irritability.
- Serious and rare side effects include liver impairment, leukopenia, and sudden cardiac death.
- Continuous monitoring for height and weight (every 6 months), cardiovascular status (every 3 months), seizure, tics, psychotic symptoms, anxiety symptoms, and drug diversion is required.

- There is a risk of misuse in patients with history of stimulant misuse.
- Dexamfetamine is not the first-line stimulant because it is associated with higher risk of side effects in comparison to methylphenidate. Begin with low doses and offer divided doses up to 20 mg/day. Children from age 6–18 years require up to 40 mg/day. Side effect profile is similar to methylphenidate.
- Continue treatment for as long as it is effective with regular review of clinical need, benefits, and side effects.

Nonstimulants

1. Examples of nonstimulants include:
   a. Atomoxetine (a noradrenaline reuptake inhibitor)
   b. Imipramine or nortriptyline (a tricyclic antidepressant)
   c. Bupropion (a dopamine–noradrenaline reuptake inhibitor)
   d. Clonidine: (an alpha adrenergic agonist)
2. Indications for nonstimulants:
   a. Inability to tolerate side effects (e.g. high blood pressure) associated with stimulant
   b. Unsatisfactory treatment response to two types of stimulant
   c. History of stimulant misuse
   d. Comorbid condition (e.g. childhood-onset schizophrenia, Tourette's syndrome) that makes the prescription of stimulant contraindicated
   e. Comorbid condition (e.g. depression or anxiety) that requires tricyclic antidepressant and avoid polypharmacy in a child
3. Atomoxetine:
   a. The starting dose of atomoxetine is 0.5 mg/kg/day and increase the dose to 1.2 mg/kg/day.
   b. Common side effects include agitation, irritability, appetite suppression, gastrointestinal discomfort, suicidal thinking, self-harming behaviour, and unusual changes in behaviour such as psychosis or mania.
   c. Rare side effect: liver damage, abdominal pain, unexplained nausea, malaise, and darkening of the urine or jaundice.
   d. Monitoring on height, weight, cardiac function, blood pressure, seizure, and self-harm is required on a regular basis.

4. Nortriptyline or imipramine:
   a. Tricyclic antidepressants have weaker evidence in treating ADHD.
   b. Beware of anticholinergic side effects.
   c. Effects of imipramine tend to wear off and cause dysrhythmias.
   d. It is not advisable to combine methylphenidate and imipramine because of cardiovascular stimulation.
5. Clonidine:
   a. Clonidine is a centrally acting α-2 agonist.
   b. Indications:
      i. More effective in controlling the aggression or hyperarousal
      ii. Less effective for inattention
      iii. Comorbidity of ADHD and Tourette's syndrome
      iv. Dose of clonidine: 0.2–0.6 mg/day in divided doses
      v. Monitor for hypotension
   c. Common side effects include hypotension, sedation, tachycardia, constipation, dizziness, dry mouth, weakness, loss of libido, agitation, and depression.
   d. Dangerous side effects associated with high doses include sinus bradycardia and atrioventricular block.
6. Omega-3 fatty acids and diet:
   a. Except in situations when dietary deficiency is known, NICE guidelines do not recommend any particular dietary supplements (such as omega-3 fatty acids) in the treatment of ADHD.
   b. NICE guidelines do not recommend elimination of artificial colouring and additives from the diet but advise parents to keep a diary if there are foods or drinks that appear to affect behaviour.

37.7.1.13 Psychosocial Treatment

1. *Parent-training/education programmes*
   a. Offer referral to educational programmes to learn about ADHD, the management, and coping strategies.
   b. Individual or group-based parent-training or education programmes for parents.
   c. Individual-based or group CBT or social skill training for children and adolescents suffering from ADHD.
   d. Training for applying behavioural interventions for teachers.
   e. Academic remediation.

2. *Behaviour therapy*
   a. Positive reinforcement (e.g. reward system and praises to promote positive behaviour).
   b. Time-out skills include planned ignoring to reduce negative behaviour.
   c. Environmental modifications (e.g. placing the child in the front row in class may reduce distractions).
   d. Combination of behaviour therapy and medication is better than medication alone.
3. *Social interventions*
   a. Working closely with school and parents in monitoring the child's behaviour.

b. The CAMHS team can provide support to parents and teachers.
c. Consider referral to a special school if the child has low IQ or learning disability (Table 37.3).

37.7.2 MULTIMODAL TREATMENT STUDY

1. In the Multimodal Treatment Study, 485 children took part in a 3-year follow-up study. Their mean age was 12 years. The primary outcome measures were severity of ADHD and oppositional defiant disorder, reading scores, social skills, level of impairment, and diagnosis. At the

TABLE 37.3
Summary of Treatment Recommendations for ADHD from the NICE Guidelines

Interventions	Preschool Children	School-Age Children and Young People with Moderate ADHD	School-Age Children and Young People with Severe ADHD	Adults with ADHD
Pharmacological treatment	Pharmacological treatment is not recommended	Pharmacological treatment is not indicated as first-line treatment. Reserve drug treatment to children • With moderate impairment • Non-pharmacological interventions have been refused • Persistence of significant impairment after psychosocial treatment	Offer drug treatment as first-line treatment and part of comprehensive treatment programme. If patient and parents do not accept pharmacological treatment, provide information about the benefits and superiority of pharmacological treatment. If patient and parents are still not keen, offer a group parent-training or education programme	Methylphenidate is first-line treatment. Dose: 5 mg TID and increase to a maximum of 100 mg/day. Target dosage is usually 1mg/kg/daily. Consider atomoxetine if drug diversion is a problem. Maintenance dose is 80–100 mg/day. Maximum dose of dexamfetamine is up to 60 mg/day
Parent-training and education programme	Offer parents or carers referral to a parent-training or education programme as first-line treatment	Offer parents or carers referral to a parent-training or education programme as first-line treatment	Offer the parents a group-based parent-training or education programme with medication	Not applicable
Interventions for the patient and family	Before discharge from secondary care, review the child with their parents and siblings for residual coexisting conditions. Monitor for recurrence of ADHD symptoms and associated impairment after the child returns to school	Offer group CBT or social skill training for the child and young person. Offer individual CBT or social skill training for older adolescents. If the child has learning disability, refer to either individual or group setting based on preference of the child	If psychological intervention is ineffective, discuss the possibility of pharmacological treatment and highlight the benefits and superiority of pharmacological treatment in severe ADHD	Offer a comprehensive treatment programme (group or individual CBT) addressing psychological, behavioural, and occupational needs

end of the first year, the research protocol was dropped and allowed for more naturalistic and personalized treatment.

2. The Multimodal Treatment Study is composed of four treatment groups:
   a. Medication only
   b. Psychoeducation
   c. Combined medication and psychosocial treatment
   d. Community control group

3. The four treatment groups demonstrated reduction in ADHD symptoms. The combined medication and psychosocial treatment group demonstrated significant improvement. At 24 and 36 months, the magnitude of differences among the four groups reduced but the combination group still demonstrated superior outcomes.

4. Good prognostic factors include strong response to initial treatment, high IQ, and strong social network.

5. This study shows that children with ADHD continue to show higher than normal rates of delinquency (4 times) and substance use (2 times).

37.7.2.1 Prognosis

1. ADHD symptoms persist at the age of 30 in one-quarter of ADHD children. Most patients do not require medications when they get older. Nevertheless, it is appropriate to continue treatment in adults whose ADHD symptoms remain disabling.

2. Although symptoms of hyperactivity often improve as the child grows older, inattention is likely to persist.

3. Remission is unlikely before the age of 12 years. When remission does occur, it usually takes place between the ages from 12 to 20 years. Overactivity is usually the first symptom to remit. Distractibility is the last symptom to remit.

4. Predictors for persistence of ADHD symptoms into adulthood:
   a. Family history of ADHD
   b. Psychosocial adversity
   c. Comorbid conduct disorder
   d. Comorbid depressive disorder
   e. Comorbid anxiety disorder

5. 20% of children with ADHD develop antisocial personality disorder in adulthood. 15% develop substance misuse in adulthood.

37.8 CONDUCT DISORDER (ICD-10 F91.0-F91.2/DSM-5 312) AND OPPOSITIONAL DEFIANT DISORDER (ICD-10 F91.3/DSM-5 313)

37.8.1 EPIDEMIOLOGY

- Conduct disorder was diagnosed in 4% of children in the Isle of Wight study. The prevalence of oppositional defiant disorder is between 6% and 16%.
- The prevalence is higher in socially deprived inner city areas and large families.
- The male to female gender ratio for conduct disorder is 3:1. The male to female gender ratio for oppositional defiant disorder is 3:1 before puberty but approaching 1:1 after puberty.
- The age of onset of conduct disorder begins earlier in boys (10–12 years) as compared to girls (14–16 years). The comorbidity of ADHD and aggressive behaviour is associated with early onset of conduct disorder. The age of onset of oppositional defiant disorder is before the age of 8 years.
- In the United Kingdom, the peak age of offending is between 14 and 17 years and the age of criminal responsibility is 10 years.
- 5%–10% of children suffer from problems with a mixture of oppositional defiant disorder and conduct disorder symptoms.

37.8.2 AETIOLOGY

1. Genetic factors: conduct disorder is associated with inheritance of antisocial trait from parents who demonstrate criminal behaviours.

2. Biological factors:
   a. Low plasma serotonin level.
   b. Low plasma dopamine level.
   c. Low cholesterol.
   d. Low skin tolerance.
   e. Excess testosterone excess.
   f. Greater right frontal EEG activity.
   g. Abnormal prefrontal cortex.
   h. History of head injury.
   i. Neurological impairment.
   j. Maternal alcohol and smoking during pregnancy.

3. Psychological factors:
   a. Fearlessness theory states that children with conduct disorder exhibit a lack of anxiety and fear.
   b. Stimulation-seeking theory states that children with conduct disorder often have low arousal level and need to engage in antisocial behaviour to increase arousal levels.
   c. Difficult temperament and a poor fit between temperament and emotional needs.
   d. Impulsivity.
   e. Poor social skills.
   f. Failure to take responsibility for actions.
   g. Education retardation: for example, reading problems.
   h. Low IQ.
   i. Substance misuse before the age of 12 years.
4. Parental factors:
   a. Failure to set rules and monitor.
   b. Inconsistency.
   c. Negativism.
   d. Harsh, punitive parenting with severe physical and verbal aggression.
   e. Hostility, resentment, and bitterness between parents with marital discord.
   f. Parental psychopathology (associated with early-onset conduct disorder).
   g. Father with antisocial personality disorder and alcohol dependence.
   h. Maternal depression.
   i. Parental criminality.
   j. Repeated physical and sexual abuse.
   k. Rejection from parents.
   l. Low income (associated with early-onset conduct disorder).
   m. Unemployment.
   n. Single parent and death of parent of the same gender.
   o. Attention seeking from parents by inducing antisocial behaviour.
5. Social factors:
   a. Family dysfunction (associated with early-onset conduct disorder).
   b. Lack of supportive social network.
   c. Lack of participation in community activities.
   d. Uncaring and hostile school environment.
   e. Gang involvement and aberrant peer group.
   f. Overcrowding environment with more than 4 children.

6. Protective factors:
   a. Economics stability in family.
   b. Family commitment to normal social values.
   c. Female gender.
   d. Good coping strategies.
   e. High IQ.
   f. Positive social interaction.
   g. Prepubertal anxiety such as separation anxiety.
   h. Resilience.
   i. Stable social organization in the community.
   j. Warm supportive family.

37.8.3 Clinical Features

See Table 37.4.

37.8.4 DSM-5 Criteria (APA, 2013)

1. The DSM-5 criteria suggest three symptom clusters for oppositional defiant disorder:
   a. Angry or irritable mood.
   b. Defiant or headstrong behaviour.
   c. Vindictiveness.
2. Conduct disorder involves repetitive and persistent pattern of behaviours in which the basic rights of others or major age-appropriate societal norms or rules are violated, as manifested by the presence of three or more of the following symptoms (aggression, destruction, deceitfulness, serious violation of rules) in the past 12 months, with at least one criterion present in the past 6 months.
3. Oppositional defiant disorder is defined as a recurrent pattern of negativistic, hostile, and disobedient behaviour towards authority figures for 6 months. The child should have at least four symptoms: losing temper, arguing with adults, refusing to comply with adult's requests, annoying the others, being angry, actively defiant, blaming the others for personal mistakes, and showing spiteful behaviour. In contrast to ICD-10 criteria, the child should not meet the general diagnostic criteria for conduct disorder.
4. The DSM-5 further divides conduct disorder into two subtypes: childhood-onset and adolescent-onset. Childhood-onset conduct disorder carries a poor prognosis if left untreated.

TABLE 37.4

Compare and Contrast the Conduct Disorder and Opposition Defiant Disorder

	Conduct Disorder	Oppositional Defiant Disorder
General criteria	According to the ICD-10, there is a repetitive and persistent pattern of behaviour in which either the basic rights of the others or major age-appropriate societal rules are violated. The minimum duration of symptoms last for at least 6 months.	According to the ICD-10, the general criteria for conduct disorder are met.
Individual symptoms	The child often displays severe temper tantrums, being angry and spiteful, often telling lies, and breaking promises. To adults: frequent argument, refusing adults' requests or defying rules, and staying out after dark against parental prohibition (onset earlier than age 13 years). To other people: annoying other people deliberately, blaming them for his mistakes, initiating fights with the others, using weapons to harm the others, exhibiting physical cruelty (also to animals), confronting victims during a crime, forcing another person into sexual activity, and frequently bullying the others. To objects or properties: deliberately destroying properties, setting fire, stealing objects of value within home or outside, and breaking into someone's house. Running away from school (truancy occurs at the age younger than 13 years) or from parental surrogate home (at least twice).	At least four symptoms from conduct disorder and must have been present for 6 months. Children with oppositional defiant disorder tend to have temper tantrums, being angry and spiteful, argument with adults, defying rules, and blaming the others. Children with oppositional defiant disorder should not have more than two symptoms related to physical assault, damage of property, and running away from school and home.
Type of conduct disorder	The ICD-10 criteria classify conduct disorder into mild, moderate, and severe. The ICD-10 criteria recommend specifying the age of onset as childhood-onset (younger than 10 years) and adolescent-onset (older than 10 years). Substance abuse is not a diagnostic criterion for conduct disorder. F90.0: Conduct disorder confined to the family context. F91.1: Unsocialized conduct disorder: poor relationships with the individual's peer group, as evidenced by isolation, rejection, unpopularity, and lack of lasting reciprocal relationship. F91.2: Socialized conduct disorder: normal peer relationship F92.0: Depressive conduct disorder: both criteria of CD and mood disorders are met. F92.8: Other mixed disorders of conduct and emotions. Criteria of conduct disorder and one of the neurotic, stress-related, somatoform disorders or childhood emotional disorders are met. F93: Mixed disorders and emotions, unspecified	No sub-category. Although the ICD-10 criteria do not specific the age, children with oppositional defiant disorder are usually younger than 10 years old with onset at age 3–8 years. The minimum duration of oppositional defiant disorder is 6 months. Defiant behaviours usually occur at home with familiar people.

5. In the DSM-5, the ICD-10 category 'mixed disorders of conduct and emotion' does not exist (APA, 2013).

6. The DSM-5 proposed a new specifier, the limited prosocial emotions for conduct disorder that has four components ((1) lack of remorse/guilt, (2) Callous–lack of empathy, (3) unconcerned about performance, and (4) shallow or deficient affect).

7. 90% of patient fulfil the DSM-IV-TR criteria conduct disorder also meet the diagnostic criteria of oppositional defiant disorder.

37.8.5 Sex Differences

- Girls with conduct disorder are more likely to engage in covert behaviours and prostitution. Boys are more concrete and egocentric.
- Girls with conduct disorder are more verbal and use indirect and relational aggression. Boys use physical aggression.
- Girls with conduct disorder are more likely to develop depression, anxiety, and somatization.
- Both boys and girls with conduct disorder demonstrate low empathy and ability to identify interpersonal issues.

37.8.6 Differential Diagnosis

Differential diagnosis for conduct disorder

- Oppositional defiant disorder
- ADHD (more inattention and hyperactivity)
- Mild mental retardation
- Pervasive developmental disorder
- Mental retardation
- Intermittent explosive disorder
- Childhood-onset bipolar disorder
- Somatization disorder
- Borderline personality trait in adolescence
- Substance misuse
- Childhood-onset schizophrenia
- Organic brain disorder

Differential diagnosis for oppositional defiant disorder

- Transient oppositional behaviours often occur during the preschool and adolescent years.
- Conduct disorder.
- ADHD (more inattention and hyperactivity).
- Mild mental retardation.
- Anxiety disorders (e.g. post-traumatic stress disorder, separation anxiety, and panic disorder. Behavioural problems often limited to situations in which fear occur).
- Depressive disorder.
- Bipolar disorder.
- Dissociative disorder.

37.8.7 Comorbidities

Comorbidities for conduct disorder

- ADHD: 50% of children with conduct disorder
- Mood disorders (e.g. depressive/bipolar disorder): 5%–31% of patients

- Anxiety disorders (30% of children with anxiety disorders also suffer from conduct disorder)

Comorbidities for oppositional defiant disorder

- Anxiety disorders (14% of children with anxiety disorder also suffer from oppositional defiant disorder).
- ADHD (5%–10% of preschoolers with oppositional defiant disorder will end up with ADHD).
- Depressive disorder (9%).
- Learning disabilities and language disorders are common.

37.8.8 Management of Conduct Disorder

Pharmacological treatment

- *Aggression and acute behavioural problems:* Antipsychotics such as risperidone, olanzapine, and haloperidol reduce physical aggression and assault. Side effects include sedation and extrapyramidal side effects (e.g. acute dystonia or pseudoparkinsonism).
- *Depression and impulsivity:* SSRIs such as fluoxetine, sertraline, paroxetine, and citalopram reduce impulsivity, irritability, and depression.
- *Conduct disorder and ADHD:* Stimulants reduce behavioural problems associated with hyperactivity and improve attention.

Multimodal treatment

1. Multimodal and multidisciplinary treatment.
2. Parent management training:
   a. The NICE guidelines recommend group-based parent-training and education programmes.
   b. When there are particular difficulties in engaging with the parents or family's needs are too complex, individual-based parent-training or education programmes are recommended.
   c. Training should be structured and have a curriculum informed by principles of social learning theory.
   d. Include relationship-enhancing strategies and role-playing sessions.
   e. Enable parents to identify their own parenting objectives.
   f. 8–12 sessions to maximize the possible benefits for participants.

3. Family therapy.
4. Individual psychotherapy:
   a. Problem solving
   b. Impulse control
   c. Anger management
   d. Social skill training
5. Environmental interventions: consistent and structured environment (e.g. boy's home).

37.8.9 Management of Oppositional Defiant Disorder

- Behaviour therapy: discourage oppositional defiant behaviour and encourage appropriate and adaptive behaviour. Parents can couch them to develop adaptive responses.
- Individual psychotherapy: restoration of self-esteem may lead to positive responses to external control.
- Parental training: eliminating harsh and punitive parenting; increasing positive parent–child interactions.

37.8.10 Prognosis

Conduct disorder

- 40% of young people with conduct disorder develop dissocial personality disorder in adulthood. Borderline IQ, mental retardation, and family history of dissocial personality disorder are predictive factors.
- 35%–75% of patients have comorbid ADHD and the presence of ADHD predicts worse outcome for boys with conduct disorder.
- Callous unemotional trait predict a more severe and persistent course of conduct disorder.
- Adolescent-onset conduct disorder carries a better diagnosis and those with adolescent-onset are less likely to show antisocial behaviour and commit a crime.

Oppositional defiant disorder

- Two-thirds of children with oppositional defiant disorder no longer meet the diagnostic criteria after 3 years. One-third of children will develop conduct disorder.
- Children with early onset, more severe symptoms, and comorbidity of ADHD are three times more likely to progress to a diagnosis of conduct disorder.

- Being argumentative, noncompliant, rule breaking, and demonstrating spiteful hurtful behaviour predict aggressive conduct disorder.
- Children with oppositional defiant disorder have higher chance of developing mood disorders, anxiety disorders, impulse control disorders, and substance abuse disorders in adolescence and adulthood.

37.9 ELECTIVE MUTISM (ICD-10 F94.0)

37.9.1 Epidemiology

Elective mutism usually manifests in early childhood (peak age 6–10 years), and boys and girls are equally represented. The prevalence is below 0.8 per 1000 children.

37.9.2 Aetiology

- Overprotective mother
- Distant father
- Trauma
- No association with social adversity

37.9.3 Diagnosis

According to ICD-10, elective mutism is characterized by a marked, emotionally determined selectivity in speaking, such that the child demonstrates language competence in some situations but fails to speak in other (definable) ones. The mutism lasts at least for 4 weeks.

37.9.4 Clinical Features

In addition to the features given earlier, elective mutism tends to be associated with personality features such as

- Social anxiety
- Withdrawal
- Sensitivity
- Resistance

37.9.5 Management

Management approaches include

- Excluding any speech abnormalities
- Behavioural approaches
- Use of tape recordings or the telephone
- Play therapy
- Art therapy
- Family therapy

37.9.6   Course and Prognosis

In general, in the long term, the prognosis is good unless other disorders are also present. Poor prognosis is associated with duration of elective mutism longer than 12 months.

37.10   TIC DISORDERS AND GILLES DE LA TOURETTE'S SYNDROME (ICD-10F 95.2; DSM-5 A11)

37.10.1   Epidemiology

Between 10% and 24% of children manifest tics during development. Tourette's syndrome (combined vocal and multiple motor tic disorder) is rare, with a prevalence rate of about 4.5 per 10,000 among 16 and 17 year olds, with a male to female ratio of about 2:1.

37.10.2   Age of Onset

- The average age of onset is 7 years (range 2–15 years).
- Mean age of onset of motor tics is 7 years.
- Mean age of onset of vocal tics is 11 years.

37.10.3   Aetiology (Table 37.5)

37.10.4   Pathophysiology

1. Neurotransmitter dysregulation:
   a. Increase in D_2 receptor sensitivity
   b. Reduction in noradrenaline
   c. Reduction in choline in the left putamen
   d. Abnormalities in the basal ganglia and caudate nucleus

37.10.5   Clinical Features

- Onset is before 18 years of age.
- Tics are sudden, rapid, and involuntary movements of circumscribed muscles without any purpose.
- Presence of multiple motor tics and at least one vocal tic.
- Eye blinking is the most common initial presenting sign and tics occur in a downward progression along the human body.
- Tics occur many times per day, most days for over 12 months without remission period being longer than 2 months based on the ICD-10 criteria.

Common simple motor tics include (ICD-10)

- Eye blinking
- Shoulder shrugging
- Neck jerking
- Facial grimacing

TABLE 37.5
Aetiology of Tics

Family	Individual
Family clusters reported, especially Tourette's	No gross neurological abnormalities
Prevalence of multiple tics in 14%–24% of first-degree relatives of patients with Tourette's	Increased incidence of 'soft' neurological signs and 'nonspecific' EEG changes
Increased family psychopathology in families of ticqueurs, although may be cause or effect	Some verbal–performance discrepancies in functioning
Monozygotic/dizygotic ratio: 50%:10%	Some neuroleptic medications effective in controlling tics
The mode of inheritance varies from autosomal dominance to an intermediate of autosomal dominance and autosomal recessive	Tics exacerbated by dopamine agonists or stimulants
	Wide range of psychological mechanisms proposed for tic disorders, from the psychoanalytic to the classically behavioural
	Tic movement have been shown to mimic involuntary startle responses to sudden stimulus
	Paediatric Autoimmune Neuropsychiatric Disorders Associated with Streptococcal infections (PANDAS)

Source: Reproduced from Puri, B.K. and Treasaden, I.H., *Textbook of Psychiatry*, 3rd edn., Churchill Livingstone, Edinburgh, U.K., 2011. With permission.

Common simple vocal tics include (ICD-10)

- Throat-clearing
- Sniffing
- Barking
- Hissing

Common complex motor tics include (ICD-10)

- Hitting oneself
- Hopping
- Jumping

Common complex vocal tics include (ICD-10)

- Coprolalia.
- Repeating certain words.
- Palilalia.
- DSM-IV-TR requires the tic-free period to be less than 3 consecutive months.
- The DSM-5 requires that the tics may wax and wane in frequency but have persisted for more than 1 year since first tic onset.
- Associated features include obsessions, compulsions, learning difficulties, impulsivity, inattention, and emotional disturbance.

37.10.6   Investigations

- Two-thirds of children with Tourette's syndrome demonstrate EEG abnormalities.

37.10.7   Differential Diagnosis

- Transient tic disorder (ICD-10 F95.0) affects 10%–20% of children. The age of onset is less than 18 years. Tics involving blinks, frowns, grimaces, head flicks, grunts, throat clearing, and sniffing from 4 weeks to 1 year. Prognosis is good.
- Chronic motor or vocal tic disorder (ICD-10 F95.1) is rare and does not require the presence of both motor and vocal tics. The age of onset is less than 18 years. The duration is longer than 1 year with remission of less than 2 months.
- Movement disorders: athetoid, choreiform, dystonia hemibalismic movements, mannerisms, myoclonia, and stereotypic movements.
- Neurological disorders include Huntington's disease, Parkinson's disease, Sydenham's chorea, and Wilson's disease.
- Obsessive–compulsive disorder.

37.10.8   Comorbidity

- ADHD: up to 50% of children with Tourette's syndrome
- OCD: up 40% of children with Tourette's syndrome
- Depression
- Disruptive behaviour

37.10.9   Management

Transient tics resolve spontaneously and thus require no further treatment.

Pharmacological treatment for Tourette's syndrome

1. Indications for pharmacological treatment:
   a. Disruptive behaviour at school or at home
   b. Very poor academic performance
   c. Rejection by peers
2. Haloperidol (0.5–5 mg/day): up to 80% with satisfactory response. Haloperidol is associated with extrapyramidal side effects.
3. Risperidone (1–4 mg/day) and sulpiride (100–400 mg/day) are effective and better tolerated than haloperidol.
4. Pimozide (1–2 mg/day): the child requires ECG monitoring. There is little experience in children younger than 12 years.
5. Clonidine (0.05 mg TDS) improves attention. 40%–70% of patients benefit from clonidine. Antipsychotics may be more effective than clonidine.
6. Tricyclic antidepressant such as imipramine may decrease disruptive behaviour.
7. 20%–30% of patients may require long-term pharmacological therapy.

Psychological treatment for Tourette's syndrome

- Habit reversal involves performing simultaneous incompatible movements to reduce unwanted movements.
- Behaviour therapy targets at replacing the tic behaviour by a desired behaviour in premonitory urge.
- Massed practise involves repeating tics for many times as an attempt to reduce the frequency of tics.
- Other behaviour therapies include self-monitoring, incompatible response training, and removal of positive reinforcement.
- Self-esteem building and social skill training may be helpful.

37.10.10 COURSE OF ILLNESS

- Transient tic disorder is not chronic or recurs during periods of stress. There may be a progression from simple tics to Tourette's syndrome in a minority of cases.
- Tourette's syndrome is a chronic disease with remissions and exacerbations.
- People with severe syndrome may develop severe depressive episode and suicide attempt.
- Chronic motor or vocal tic disorder usually lasts for 4–6 years and stops in early adolescence.

37.11 PICA (ICD-10 F98.3)

- Persistent eating of nonnutritive substances for at least twice per week for duration of 1 month.
- Chronological and mental age is above the age of 2 years.
- Associated with learning disability, psychosis, and social deprivation.

37.12 STAMMERING (ICD-10 F98.5)

- A disturbance of rhythm and fluency of speech by frequent repetition or prolongation of sounds or syllables, leading to hesitation.
- The duration of stammering is longer than 3 months.
- Affecting 1% of children at school entry.
- The peak age of onset is 5 years.
- Treatment: speech therapy.
- Prognosis: 50%–80% of children recover from stammering.

37.13 CLUTTERING (ICD-10 F98.6)

- A rapid rate of speech with breakdown in fluency
- No repetitions or hesitations
- Reduction in speech intelligibility

37.14 COMMUNICATION DISORDERS (DSM-5)

The DSM-5 includes the following seven communication disorders:

- Language impairment
- Late language emergence
- Specific language impairment
- Social communication disorder
- Speech sound disorder
- Childhood-onset fluency disorder
- Voice disorder

37.15 NONORGANIC ENURESIS (ICD-10 F98.0; DSM-5 307.6)

37.15.1 DEFINITION

According to ICD-10, nonorganic enuresis is characterized by the involuntary voiding of urine, by day and/or by night, which is abnormal in relation to the individual's mental age and which is not a consequence of a lack of bladder control resulting from any neurological disorder, epilepsy, or a structural urinary tract abnormality. The minimum duration of enuresis is 3 months. It is generally not diagnosed before the age of 5 years and may be subdivided into

- Primary: urinary continence never achieved.
- Secondary: urinary continence has been achieved in the past.

The DSM-5 criteria are similar to ICD 10 and further subdivide enuresis into

- Nocturnal only: passage of urine only during nighttime sleep
- Diurnal only: passage of urine during waking hours
- Nocturnal and diurnal: a combination of the two aforementioned subtypes

37.15.2 EPIDEMIOLOGY

1. Prevalence. The prevalence at different ages has been found to be
   a. 7 years—6.7% in boys and 3.3% in girls
   b. 9–10 years—2.9% in boys and 2.2% in girls
   c. 14 years—1.1% in boys and 0.5% in girls
2. Sex ratio:
   a. Male to female = 1:1 at the age of 5 years; approximately 2:1 in adolescence.
   b. Secondary enuresis is more common in boys.

37.15.3 CLINICAL FEATURES

Nonorganic enuresis may be associated with emotional problems, although it should be noted that the latter may be secondary to the enuresis itself.

37.15.4 Aetiology

Possible causes that have been proposed include

- Genetic—70% have a first-degree relative with late attainment of continence.
- Stressful life events—a doubling of frequency.
- Delayed toilet training.
- Developmental delay—twice as common in enuretic children as in controls.
- Bladder structure—enuretic children are more likely than non-enuretics to have a different shape of bladder baseplate and to have a reduced functional bladder volume.

37.15.5 Management

Points in the management include

1. A full assessment including a physical assessment to exclude a physical cause; look for evidence of:
   a. Urinary frequency
   b. Haematuria
   c. Dysuria
   d. Urgency
2. Urinary microscopy and microbiological analysis
3. Urodynamic study if the patient is older than 15 years
4. Observation period
5. Fluid restriction at night
6. Star chart—relapse rate of approximately 40%
7. Pad and buzzer or, in older children, a pants alarm—relapse rate of approximately 40%
8. Low-dose tricyclic antidepressants—but there are side effects and there is a high rate of relapse on discontinuation—can be useful for short time periods (e.g. school trips)
9. Nasal desmopressin—should not be continued for more than 3 months without stopping for a week for full reassessment
10. Exercises to increase the functional capacity of the bladder
11. Habit training

37.15.6 Course and Prognosis

In general, the prognosis is very good.

37.16 NONORGANIC ENCOPRESIS (ICD-10 F98.1) (DSM 5 307.7)

37.16.1 Definition

According to ICD-10, nonorganic encopresis is the repeated voluntary or involuntary passage of faeces, usually of normal or near-normal consistency, in places not appropriate for that purpose in the individual's own sociocultural setting. It is generally not diagnosed before the age of 4 years and there should be at least one episode per month for 6 months. It may be subdivided into

1. Continuous encopresis: bowel control has never been achieved.
2. Discontinuous encopresis: there has been a period of normal bowel control in the past.

DSM-5 criteria are similar to the ICD-10 except the minimum duration is 3 months.

37.16.2 Epidemiology

- Prevalence. At the age of 5 years, the prevalence is 1.5%. In 12 year olds, the Isle of Wight study found a prevalence of 1.3% in boys and 0.3% in girls.
- The male to female sex ratio is between 3:1 and 4:1.

37.16.3 Clinical Features

The presentation of this disorder is summarized in Table 37.6.

37.16.4 Aetiology

Causes of nonorganic encopresis are shown in Table 37.7.

37.16.5 Management

Points in the management include

- A full assessment, but take care in carrying out an anal and rectal examination as informed consent is required from the child who may have been sexually abused (if there is evidence of sexual abuse, the appropriate procedures should be brought into play)
- Assessment of family relationships and the home circumstances

TABLE 37.6

Presentation of Faecal Soiling (Encopresis)

Consistency of Faeces	Normal, Loose, or Constipated
Place deposited	In pants, hidden, or in 'significant' places (e.g. in a particular person's cupboard)
Development	Never continent (continuous), after period of continence (discontinuous), or regression (in various contexts—see succeeding text)
Activity	Smearing, anal fingering, or masturbation
Context	Power battle, upsetting life events (e.g. sexual abuse, divorce), and/or other psychiatric disorder
Physical	With soreness, anal fissures, etc., or with normal anus

Source: Reproduced from Puri, B.K. and Treasaden, I.H., *Textbook of Psychiatry*, 3rd edn., Churchill Livingstone, Edinburgh, U.K., 2011. With permission.

TABLE 37.7

Causes of Encopresis

Congenital	Constitutional Variability Can Include Bowel Control
Individual	Developmental delay
	Physical trigger—anal fissure—constipation (low-roughage diet)
	Other bowel disorders
	Chronic constipation
	Hirschsprung's disease
	Anxiety (fear of soiling)
Parent–child	Coercive toilet training
	Emotional abuse or neglect
	'Battleground' for relationship problems
	Anger (protect against parents)
Wider environment	Sexual abuse
	Family disharmony

Source: Reproduced from Puri, B.K. and Treasaden, I.H., *Textbook of Psychiatry*, 3rd edn., Churchill Livingstone, Edinburgh, U.K., 2011. With permission.

- Investigations: thyroid function test, barium enema if suspected obstructive lesions in bowels
- Education of the carers with respect to the mechanics of defaecation
- Improving the child's self-esteem
- Individual therapy
- Family therapy
- Pharmacotherapy to soften the stools or to promote gastrointestinal motility
- Behaviour therapy, for example, star chart

If the aforementioned procedures fail, an intense behavioural programme in hospital may be required

37.16.6 COURSE AND PROGNOSIS

In general, the prognosis is very good.

37.17 SCHOOL REFUSAL

School refusal is refusal to attend or stay at school because of anxiety and in spite of parental or other pressure.

37.17.1 EPIDEMIOLOGY

Boys and girls are equally represented. There are three main incidence peak ages:

1. Separation anxiety at age of 5 years
2. At age of 11 years, which may be precipitated by the change from junior to secondary schooling
3. At age of 14–16 years, which may be a symptom of a psychiatric disorder:
   a. Depressive disorder
   b. A phobia (e.g. social phobia)

The most common presentation is the one at 11 years.

37.17.2 DIFFERENCES FROM TRUANCY

Truancy is an important differential diagnosis. Truancy differs from school refusal in the following aspects (Table 37.8):

37.17.3 MANAGEMENT

The mechanisms underlying the school refusal should be identified. If the condition is acute, a return to school should be arranged as soon as possible (the Kennedy approach), whereas if the condition is chronic, a graded return to school should be arranged. Any specific problems (e.g. social phobia) should be addressed. If the individual does not return to school, then inpatient treatment may be necessary.

37.17.4 COURSE AND PROGNOSIS

Younger children have a better prognosis. Most children and adolescents do return to school, but approximately one-third of older patients seen in clinics develop neurotic difficulties or social impairment or social withdrawal in adulthood.

TABLE 37.8
Compare and Contrast School Refusal and Truancy

	School Refusal	Truancy
Ego	Ego-dystonic	Ego-syntonic and intended
Family history of psychiatric disorders	Anxiety disorders and failure of parents to separate from own families of origin	Antisocial personality disorder or forensic history
Family size	Small family and the patient is the youngest child	Large family size
Parenting style	Overprotective parenting or unassertive parents (ineffective father, overanxious mother)	Inconsistent discipline
Age of child and aetiology	Three peaks: Age 5 years: manifestation of separation anxiety at school entry Age 11 years: triggering by transfer to secondary school or avoidance character Age 14–16 years: manifestation of depression or phobia such as agoraphobia or social phobia	More common in adolescents than younger children
Symptoms	Overt anxiety at the time of going to school with 'somatic disguise' such as abdominal pain (aka Masquerade syndrome)	Not associated with psychiatric symptoms but wilful intention to skip classes
Location when absent from school	Usually at home with parental permission. Parents are aware of their whereabouts	Usually outside home, engage in alternative activities without parental permission and awareness
Academic performance	Satisfactory academic performance	Poor academic performance

37.17.5 DISORDERS IN SCHOLASTIC SKILLS

See Table 37.9.

37.18 OTHER PSYCHIATRIC DISORDERS IN CHILDHOOD (0–11 YEARS) AND ADOLESCENCE (12–17 YEARS)

See Tables 37.10 through 37.17.

37.19 SUBSTANCE MISUSE IN ADOLESCENCE

37.19.1 TYPE OF SUBSTANCE MISUSE

- Experimental use (e.g. initial use as a result of curiosity)
- Recreational use (e.g. under peer pressure)
- Dependent (e.g. strong compulsion to take illicit drugs)

TABLE 37.9

Summary of the ICD-10 Classifications

ICD-10 Classification	ICD-10 Criteria
	Common exclusion criteria include sensory impairment, IQ < 70, and extreme inadequacies in education.
F80.0 Specific speech articulation disorder	Articulation skills are 2 standard deviation (SD) below the lower limit of child's age and 1 SD below the nonverbal IQ. Language expression and comprehension are within expected limit of child's age.
F80.1 Expressive language disorder	Expressive language skills are 2 SD below the lower limit of child's age and 1 SD below the nonverbal IQ. Receptive language skills, nonverbal communication, and imaginative language functions are within expected limit of child's age.
F80.2 Receptive language disorder	Language comprehension are 2 SD below the lower limit of child's age and receptive language skills are 1 SD below the nonverbal IQ.
F80.3 Acquired aphasia with epilepsy (Landau–Kleffner Syndrome)	Severe loss of expressive and receptive language skills occur over a period of time not exceeding 6 months. Language development was normal before the loss. Paroxysmal EEG abnormalities affecting one or both temporal lobes become apparent within a time span within 2 years after the initial loss of language. Hearing and nonverbal intelligence are within normal range.
F81.0 Specific reading disorder	Prevalence is 4% among 9–10 year olds. Male to female ratio is 3:1. A score on reading and/or under comprehension that is 2 SE below the level expected on the basis of the children's chronological age and intelligence. A history of serious reading difficulty at earlier age, spelling test score being at least 2 SE below expected level, and the reading impairment significantly interferes with academic achievement or ADL.
F81.1 Specific spelling disorder	The score on a standardized test is at least 2 SE below the expected level but scores on reading accuracy and comprehension are within normal range. In spelling disorder, arithmetical skill is normal and vice versa.
F81.2 Specific disorder of arithmetical skills	The difficulties have been present from the early stages of learning and lead to significant interferences of academic achievement and activities of daily living (ADL). Epidemiological studies show that this disorder is more common in females.
F82 Specific developmental disorder of motor function	The score on a standardized test of motor function is at least 2 SE below the expected level with no diagnosable neurological disorder. Common exclusion criteria: IQ is less than 70.
Other disorders	F81.3 Mixed disorder of scholastic skills (combination of arithmetical, reading, and spelling disorders). F81.8 Other developmental disorders of scholastic skills. F81.9 Developmental disorder of scholastic skills, unspecified.

Source: WHO, *ICD-10: The ICD-10 Classification of Mental and Behavioural Disorders: Clinical Descriptions and Diagnostic Guidelines*, World Health Organization, Geneva, Switzerland, 1992.

TABLE 37.10

Compare and Contrast Childhood- and Adolescence-Onset Schizophrenia

Childhood-Onset Schizophrenia	Adolescence-Onset Schizophrenia
Epidemiology	Epidemiology
Psychosis is extremely rare before 13 years of age.	• Prevalence is 2–3/1000.
	• The prevalence of very early-onset schizophrenia (age 13 years) is around 1/100,000.
	• The prevalence of early-onset schizophrenia (age 18 years) is 18/100,000.
	• Slight excess in boys.
Aetiology	Aetiology
Strong family history of schizophrenia.	• Genetic predisposition.
	• Neurodevelopmental hypothesis with reduction in cortical volumes and increase in ventricular size.
	• Drug-induced psychosis.
	• Organic causes (e.g. central nervous system infection).
	• Tuberous sclerosis.
	• Partial complex seizures.
	• Leukodystrophies.
Clinical features	Clinical features
• Uneven development with delay in language and social behaviour.	• Deterioration in scholastic ability and self-care may be the first sign.
• Cognitive impairment and behavioural abnormalities in childhood.	• Visual hallucinations and anxiety symptoms are common.
• Gradual onset.	• Mood disturbance.
• Common features include visual hallucinations ideas of reference and negative symptoms.	• Persecutory ideation.
• Paranoid symptoms are less frequent compared to adults.	• Abnormal perceptual experience.
	• Cognitive and social impairment.
	• Negative symptoms, passivity, well-formed delusions, thought disorders, and first rank symptoms are not common.
Differential diagnosis	Differential diagnosis
• Disintegrative disorder in childhood.	• Conduct disorder
• Obsessive–compulsive disorder.	• Severe emotional disorder
	• Subacute sclerosing panencephalitis
Treatment	Treatment
• Risperidone is effective.	• Similar to the treatment used in childhood schizophrenia.
• Children are more prone to the metabolic side effects and weight gain associated with olanzapine.	• Lorazepam assists stabilization of acutely disturbed patients.
• Avoid first-generation antipsychotic that associate with high rate of extrapyramidal side effects.	• Clozapine can be used in adolescents with treatment resistant schizophrenia.
	• Close liaison with paediatrician is necessary if the psychosis is a result of organic causes.
Prognosis	Prognosis
• Childhood psychosis carries the worst prognosis among all psychiatric disorders in childhood.	• 80% of adolescent diagnosed with schizophrenia still suffer from schizophrenia in early adulthood.

37.19.2 AETIOLOGY

- Community factors include widespread drug availability, high crime rate, poverty, and cultural acceptance of drugs.
- School factors include peer rejection, lack of interest in studies, and academic failures.
- Family factors include parental substance abuse and family conflict.

- Individual risk factors include low self-esteem, high sensation seeking, and self-destruction.

37.19.3 SMOKING

- Two-thirds of 15- and 16-year-old adolescents smoke cigarettes.

TABLE 37.11

Compare and Contrast Childhood- and Adolescence-Onset Depressive Disorder

Childhood-Onset Depressive Disorder	Adolescent-Onset Depressive Disorder

Childhood-Onset Depressive Disorder

Epidemiology

- Prevalence is 1% (rare).
- Boys and girls have equal frequency until the age of 14 years.
- Childhood depression is less common than childhood dysthymia.

Aetiology

- Genetic causes (50%).
- Adverse parenting and maltreatment.
- Conduct disorders in childhood carry an increased risk for depressive symptoms in early adult life.
- Impair neurogenesis in hippocampus.

Clinical features

- Boredom.
- Growth impairment.
- Low motivation to play.
- Poor academic performance.
- Poor feeding.
- Somatic complaints.
- Mood symptoms are similar to adults and severe cases may present with mood congruent psychotic features.
- More anxiety and anger but fewer vegetative symptoms when compared with adults.

Diagnostic instrument

- Children Depression Inventory (CDI).

Treatment

- Psychotherapy (e.g. CBT, family therapies) is the first-line treatment.
- For children at age 5–11 years, cautiously consider the addition of fluoxetine if psychotherapy fails after 3 months. There is no doubt that antidepressants increase the risk of suicidal behaviours in children.
- TCA is not effective in prepubertal children.
- ECT is not recommended in children at age between 5 and 11 years.

Adolescent-Onset Depressive Disorder

Epidemiology

- 6.6% at 15 years and 22.1% at 18 years.
- Similar to adult depression with female dominance (35% for girls, 19% for boys).
- Mean duration of illness is 7–9 months.

Aetiology

- 60–70% of patients are caused by adverse life events.
- Arguments with parents.
- Multiple family disadvantages.
- Positive family history of depression is common.

Clinical features

- Symptoms similar to adult with a minimum of 2 week period if sadness, irritability, loss of interest, and loss of pleasure.
- Impairment in social and role functions.
- Promiscuity may be the presenting feature.
- Anxiety symptoms and conduct disorders are most commonly associated disorders.
- Less likely to have psychomotor retardation in comparison to adults.

Diagnostic interview K-SADS-PL

- Kiddie-Sads-Present and Lifetime Version (K-SADS-PL).

Treatment (NICE guidelines)

- Mild depression.
- Watchful waiting for 2 weeks.
- Offer supportive psychotherapy, group-based CBT or guided self-help for 2–3 months.
- No antidepressant is required.

Moderate to severe depression (including psychotic depression)

- Individual CBT, IPT, and short-term family therapy may be helpful.
- If the adolescent does not respond, consider alternative psychotherapy or augment with fluoxetine after multidisciplinary review.
- If patient is unresponsive after combination treatment, arrange another multidisciplinary review and consider either systemic family therapy (at least 15 fortnightly sessions) or individual child psychotherapy (30 weekly sessions).

Use of antidepressants

- Fluoxetine 10 mg/day is the first-line treatment for those who need antidepressant.
- Citalopram and sertraline can be used if there is clear evidence after a trial of fluoxetine and psychotherapy.
- Antidepressants should be discontinued slowly over 6–12 weeks to reduce discontinuation symptoms.
- Avoid TCA, paroxetine, venlafaxine, and St John's wort.

TABLE 37.11 (continued)

Compare and Contrast Childhood- and Adolescence-Onset Depressive Disorder

Childhood-Onset Depressive Disorder	Adolescent-Onset Depressive Disorder
Prognosis	Prognosis
• Most children have good prognosis.	• High remission rate: 90% by 2 years.
• Very early-onset depression is associated with poor prognosis.	• High recurrence rate: 40% by 2 years.
	• High rate of conversion to bipolar disorder: 40% by 2 years.
	• Depression and conduct disorder is associated with an increased risk of suicide, alcoholism, substance misuse, and antisocial personality disorder.

37.19.4 ALCOHOL ABUSE IN ADOLESCENCE

- Equal sex incidence.
- 50% of adolescents taste the first alcohol at home.
- 50% of 16- to 19-year-olds are regular drinkers.
- Alcohol dependence is associated with adolescent suicide.

37.19.5 VOLATILE SUBSTANCES

- Common volatile substances include solvent and glue.
- 21% of adolescents have tried volatile substances.
- The effects include euphoria, disinhibition, impulsiveness, giddiness, nausea, vomiting, slurred speech, visual hallucination, and paranoid delusion.
- Students prefer this method because they can be intoxicated in school.
- Chronic use leads to tolerance and withdrawal symptoms.

37.19.6 CANNABIS

- Most adolescents in the United Kingdom, United States, and Australia have tried cannabis in their life.
- Most adolescents will stop using cannabis in their 20s.
- About one-tenth will use it on a daily basis.
- Regular use of cannabis may precipitate acute schizophrenia.

37.19.7 OTHER SUBSTANCES

- Amphetamine, benzodiazepine, and hallucinogen are commonly used by adolescents.
- The use of cocaine and opiate misuse is less common.

37.19.8 TREATMENT

- Refer the child or adolescent to the young people's substance misuse service.
- The service should be user-friendly and promote self-referral.
- Strategies include harm reduction, needle exchange, motivational enhancement, detox regimes, and family therapy.

37.19.9 PROGNOSIS

1. Substance misuse in adolescence is associated with
   a. Accidental deaths
   b. Delinquency
   c. Suicide

37.19.10 LEGAL ASPECTS OF THE CHILD AND ADOLESCENT PSYCHIATRY

- Gillick competence states that a child below the age of 16 years can give consent to treatment without parental agreement (e.g. contraception) provided that the child have achieved sufficient maturity to understand fully the treatment proposed. The child has no right to refuse treatment that is in his or her best interests.
- In the United Kingdom, parents have parental responsibility under the Children Act (2004) to give consent on the child's behalf, especially when the child is refusing treatment in the best interest of the child.
- If both child and parents refuse treatment and the child is at high psychiatric risk, the Mental Health Act can be applied.
- If the child is in danger, the clinician can make the best medical decision for the child based on the Common Law.

TABLE 37.12

Compare and Contrast Childhood- and Adolescence-Onset Suicide and Self-Harm

Childhood-Onset Suicide and Self-Harm	Adolescent-Onset Suicide and Self-Harm

Childhood-Onset Suicide and Self-Harm

Epidemiology

- Suicide is very rare in prepubertal children.

Aetiology

- It may be caused by accident (e.g. accidental hanging by playing with curtain string).
- The child may exhibit stereotyped movements to an extent that either causes physical injury or marked interference with normal activities for at least 1 month.

Adolescent-Onset Suicide and Self-Harm

Epidemiology

- 20,000 young people in England and Wales are referred to hospital for assessment of self-harm each year.
- Rate of attempted suicide: 8%–9% in western countries.
- Rate of suicidal ideation: 15%–20%.
- Suicide is common among young people at age between 14 and 16 years.
- Male to female ratio for self-harm is 1:6.
- Male to female ratio for suicide = 4:1.
- Suicide is the third commonest cause of death for young people after accident and homicide.
- Self-harm is the most common cause of admission to a general hospital.

Aetiology

Psychiatric disorders (e.g. depression, psychosis, substance abuse, conduct disorder, isolation, low self-esteem, and physical illness). For girls, self-harm is strongly predicted by depressive disorder. For boys, self-harm is strongly predicted by previous suicide attempt.

Family issues like loss of parent in childhood, family dysfunction, abuse, and neglect.

Increase in adolescence suicide is a result of

1. *Factors influencing reporting* ('copycat' suicides resulting from media coverage; the fostering of illusions and ideals through internet suicide groups and pop culture).
2. *Factors influencing the incidence of psychiatric problems* (e.g. problems with identify formation, depression, substance abuse, and teenage pregnancy).
3. *Social factors* (e.g. bullying, the impact of unemployment for older adolescents, poverty, loosening of family structures, living away from home, migration, parental separation, and divorce).

Common Self-harm and suicide methods

Self-harm: Cutting and scratching are common impulsive gestures. Cutting often has a dysphoric-reducing effect.

Suicide: Self-poisoning is a common method used by British adolescents. The use of firearms is more common in the United States.

Management of Self-harm and suicide (NICE guidelines)

Management of Self-laceration

- Offer physical treatment with adequate anaesthesia.
- Do not delay psychosocial assessment.
- Explain the care process.
- For those who repeatedly self-poison, do not offer minimization advice on self-poisoning because there is no safe limit.
- For those who self-injure repeatedly, teach self-management strategies on superficial injuries, harm minimization techniques, and alternative coping strategies.

TABLE 37.12 (continued)

Compare and Contrast Childhood- and Adolescence-Onset Suicide and Self-Harm

Childhood-Onset Suicide and Self-Harm	Adolescent-Onset Suicide and Self-Harm
	Management of suicidal adolescent
	• Consider inpatient treatment after balancing the benefits against loss of family support.
	• Involve the young person in the admission process.
	• ECT may be used in adolescents with very severe depression and suicidal behaviour not responding to other treatments.
	Prognosis
	Self-harm
	• 10% will repeat in 1 year.
	• Higher risk of repetition in older male adolescents, history of suicide attempts, persistent suicide ideation, psychotic symptoms, substance misuse, and use of methods other than overdose or self-laceration.
	Suicide
	• 4% of girls and 11% of boys will kill themselves in 5 years after first episode of suicide attempt.

TABLE 37.13

Compare and Contrast Childhood- and Adolescence-Onset Bipolar Disorder

Childhood-Onset Bipolar Disorder	Adolescent-Onset Bipolar Disorder
Epidemiology	Epidemiology
• Rare.	• 20% of adult bipolar patients experience their first episode of mania before the age of 20.
• Associated with ADHD.	• The prevalence of bipolar disorder in adolescences is 0.5–1.0%.
Clinical Features	Aetiology
• Reduction of sleep is often the first indicator for childhood bipolar disorder.	• Genetic predisposition.
Treatment	• Drug induced (e.g. illicit [amphetamine] and therapeutic [e.g. steroid] drugs).
• First line of treatment is olanzapine.	Clinical Features
Prognosis	• Similar to adults.
• Childhood bipolar disorder is ranked as having the second worst prognosis among all psychiatric disorders in childhood.	• First rank symptoms present in 20% cases.
	Diagnostic Interview: K-SADS-PL
	Treatment
	• First line of treatment is olanzapine although valproate and lithium are effective.
	• For ADHD children with manic symptoms, stimulants can be prescribed.
	• Adjunctive family therapy is useful in stabilizing symptomatology.

TABLE 37.14

Compare and Contrast Childhood- and Adolescence-Onset Anxiety Disorders

Childhood-Onset Anxiety Disorders

Epidemiology
- Prevalence for separation anxiety disorder is 3.6%.
- At least 50% of adult cases of anxiety symptoms had their onset in childhood.
- 2% of children have phobia.

Aetiology
- In infancy, fear and anxiety are provoked by sensory stimuli.
- In early childhood, fear is evoked by stranger and separation anxiety.
- In late childhood, it is caused by fear of dark, animals (more common in girls), and imaginary creatures.

Comparison with older patients
- Sleeping difficulties and somatic complaints such as headache are common.
- Panic attacks are less common.

Separation anxiety disorders of childhood (ICD-10 F93.0)
- Onset is before 6 years.
- Unrealistic persistent worry: possible harm befalling major attachment figures or about loss of such figures. The child will have anticipatory anxiety of separation (e.g. tantrums, persistent reluctance to leave home, excessive need to talk with parents, and desire to return home when going out).
- Symptoms in the day: persistent reluctance or refusal to go to school because of the fear over separation from a major attachment figure in order to stay at home. Repeated occurrence of physical symptoms (e.g. nausea, stomachache, headache, and vomiting).
- Symptoms at night: difficulty in separating at night as manifested by persistent reluctance or refusal to go to sleep without being near to the attachment figure. The child also has repeated nightmares on the theme of separation.
- Minimum duration is 4 weeks.

Phobic anxiety disorder of childhood (ICD-10 F93.1)
- The individual manifests a persistent or recurrent fear that is developmentally phase—appropriate but is abnormal in degree.
- It is associated with significant social impairment.
- Minimum duration of symptoms is 4 weeks.

Social anxiety disorder of childhood (ICD-10 F93.2)
- Persistent anxiety in social situations where the child is exposed to unfamiliar people including peers.
- The child exhibits self-consciousness, embarrassment, and over-concern about the appropriateness of his or her behaviour.
- The child has satisfying social relationship with familiar people but there is significant interference with peer relationships.
- Onset of the disorder coincides with the developmental phase.
- Minimum duration of symptoms is 4 weeks.

Childhood emotional disorder
- Prevalence is 2.5%.
- More common in girls.
- It presents as anxiety and somatic complaints with good prognosis.

Post-traumatic stress disorder
- Compulsive repetitive play representing part of the trauma, failing to relieve anxiety, and loss of acquired developmental skills in language and toilet training.
- Emergence of new separation anxiety.

Adolescent-Onset Anxiety Disorders

Epidemiology
- Prevalence rate for generalized anxiety disorder in adolescents is 3.7%.

Aetiology
- In adolescence, anxiety is caused by performance anxiety and fear of social situations.
- 30% of patients have family history of phobia and anxiety disorder.

Clinical features
- Clinical features are similar to adult.
- Somatic complaints are common.

Social phobia
- Common in adolescents.
- This is a fear centred on scrutiny by other people when in small social groups, e.g. when the patient is in a restaurant.
- It is often associated with low self-esteem.

Panic disorder
- Panic attacks are associated with agoraphobia.

Separation anxiety
- Patients may present as a case of school refusal.

PTSD
- Occur in young people exposing to a traumatic event, e.g. physical or sexual abuse and fatal accident happens to friends or relatives.
- Depression is common among older children and adolescents.
- New aggression may emerge.
- Other symptoms such as nightmares, social withdrawal, and numbing are common.

Differential diagnosis
- Hyperthyroidism.

Treatment
- CBT should be the first-line treatment.
- If CBT fails, the child and adolescent psychiatrist can consider prescribing fluoxetine or fluvoxamine.
- Psychoeducation.
- Benzodiazepine and buspirone should be avoided in adolescents because this will cause disinhibition syndrome.

TABLE 37.14 (continued)

Compare and Contrast Childhood- and Adolescence-Onset Anxiety Disorders

Childhood-Onset Anxiety Disorders	Adolescent-Onset Anxiety Disorders
Treatment • Behavioural therapy for the child. • Psychoeducation for the parents. Prognosis • There is a potential link between separation anxiety in childhood and panic disorder in adult.	Prognosis • Majority have good prognosis. • Increase in risk of anxiety disorder and substance misuse. • Phobic disorder may persist into adulthood as phobic disorder has its origin in adolescence.

• In the United Kingdom, the Mental Capacity Act (2005) is only applicable to people above the age of 16 and over.

• The Mental Health Act can be applied to provide involuntary psychiatric treatment for patients (regardless of age) who are at high psychiatric risk and refusing treatment.

37.20 PHYSICAL AND SEXUAL ABUSE IN CHILDREN AND ADOLESCENTS

37.20.1 EPIDEMIOLOGY

• In the United Kingdom, 7% of children were rated as experiencing serious physical abuse and 6% had serious emotional maltreatment.

• 3/1000 children are on the official Child Protection Register for the ages between 0 and 18 years.

• 10% of children have been victims of sexual abuse if a loose definition of sexual abuse including exhibitionism, lascivious talk, and being sexually active at the age of 15 is applied.

• The male to female ratio is 1: 2.5.

• Each year, 3% of children up to the age of 13 years are brought to the attention of professional agencies because of suspected abuse.

37.20.2 ASSESSMENT

1. There are four types of abuse: physical abuse, sexual abuse, emotion abuse, and neglect.

2. The assessment should include the following:

   a. Evaluate and validate the claim of abuse from the child's perspectives.

   b. Assess the impact of abuse on the physical and emotional conditions.

   c. Look for further evidence to support the claim of abuse and consistency in the child's accounts.

   d. Explore other types of abuse and family members being involved.

   e. Assess cognitive and language competence of the child.

   f. Identify emotional and behavioural disturbance in the child (e.g. conduct disorder and truancy).

   g. Recognize the emotional, physical, and therapeutic needs of the child.

   h. Seek the child's view on staying in a safe and protective environment (e.g. staying in a shelter administered by the social agency).

   i. Assess family dynamics, family members involved, and parental psychopathology.

3. For young children, special techniques of interviewing such as drawing and using anatomically correct dolls may facilitate disclosure of sensitive information from the child's perspectives.

4. It is important of not asking leading questions that may suggest certain answers.

5. Psychiatrist should use age-appropriate language and ask one question at a time.

6. After the initial assessment, further interview may be videotaped with the parental consent and permission from the child. This will avoid the child to mention the traumatic experience repeatedly to different professionals.

7. Address the dilemma whether other family members shall be involved in the assessment of child. Psychiatrist should always seek the child's view on this issue.

TABLE 37.15

Compare and Contrast Childhood- and Adolescence-Onset Obsessive–Compulsive Disorder

Childhood-Onset Obsessive–Compulsive Disorder (OCD)	Adolescent-Onset OCD
Epidemiology	Epidemiology
• One-third of OCD patients have their onset in childhood.	• Two-thirds of OCD patients have their onset in adolescence.
• Prevalence is 0.25%.	• Prevalence is 0.6%.
• Boys have earlier onset than girls.	• No predomination by male adolescents.
• Boys predominate childhood OCD.	
Aetiology	Aetiology
• 5% of parents have OCD.	• Similar aetiology as childhood OCD.
• Four times increase in risk of OCD among relatives.	
• PANDAS is caused by haemolytic streptococcal infection and associated with OCD.	
• The association between OCD and tics suggests the role of basal ganglia lesions.	
Clinical features	Clinical features
• Insidious onset.	• Similar to adult-onset OCD.
• Symptoms include contamination, checking rituals, and worry about harm to self.	• Adolescents usually demonstrate internal resistance to obsessions.
• Mild obsessions and rituals (e.g. magical number of repetition to get good exam result) is part of the normal development.	
Comorbidity	Comorbidity
• Tourette's syndrome.	• Tourette's syndrome.
• ADHD.	• Conduct disorder.
• Anxiety.	• Trichotillomania.
• Depression.	• Nail biting.
• Bedwetting.	• Body dysmorphic disorder.
• Sleep disturbance.	• Depression.
• Psychomotor changes.	• Anxiety.
• Joint pain.	• Eating disorders.
Management	Management
Investigations for PANDAS	• Treatment is similar to treatment in childhood OCD.
• Measure *streptococcus* titer.	• Treatment-resistant OCD requires further assessment at specialist centre.
• The antistreptolysin O (ASO) titer rises 3–6 weeks after a *streptococcus* infection.	• Consider clomipramine and low-dose risperidone.
• The *antistreptococcal* DNAse B (anti-DNAse B) titer rises 6–8 weeks after a *streptococcus* infection.	
Treatment	
• CBT and exposure response prevention (ERP) is the first-line treatment.	
• Train parents to supervise ERP.	
• Sertraline has the licence to treat OCD from the age of 6 years onwards.	
• Fluvoxamine has the licence to treat OCD.	
• From the age of 8 years onwards.	
• Fluoxetine is indicated for OCD with significant comorbid depression.	
• Avoid TCA (except clomipramine), SNRIs, and MAOIs.	
• If antipsychotic drug is required, do not prescribe antidepressant concurrently.	

TABLE 37.15 (continued)

Compare and Contrast Childhood- and Adolescence-Onset Obsessive–Compulsive Disorder

Childhood-Onset Obsessive–Compulsive Disorder (OCD)	Adolescent-Onset OCD
• There is a delayed onset of action up to 4 weeks and full therapeutic effect up to 8–12 weeks. • Duration of treatment is at least for 6 months. • In childhood body dysmorphic disorder, fluoxetine is the drug of choice.	
Prognosis • 50% of children with OCD continue to suffer from OCD in adulthood. • Some of them develop anankastic personality disorder. • 25% of children with OCD have remission. • Short duration is a positive prognostic sign.	Prognosis • Remission in one-third of patients. • There is a strong continuity into adulthood in two-thirds of patients.

TABLE 37.16

Compare and Contrast Childhood- and Adolescence-Onset Somatization Disorders

Childhood-Onset Somatization Disorders	Adolescent-Onset Somatization Disorders
Epidemiology • Recurrent abdominal pain occurs in 10%–25% of children between the ages of 3–9 years. • Hysteria in childhood is rare with equal gender ratio.	Epidemiology • About 10% of adolescents report multiple physical symptoms. • Prevalence of somatization disorder is less than 0.1%.
Aetiology • Stress (e.g. bullying) and anxiety can initiate and amplify somatic symptoms. • Somatic symptoms are commonly associated with school refusal. • Factors in the child include obsessional, sensitive, insecure, or anxious personality. • Factors in the family include over-involved parent, parental disharmony and overprotection, rigid rules, and communication problems.	Aetiology • Recent-onset somatization disorder is associated with anxiety, depression, learning difficulty, and obsessional personality trait. • Chronic somatization disorder is associated with early adverse experience, seeking attention from parents, and failure to recognize the connection between somatic complaints and emotion. • Family factors include difficulty to express emotion and abnormal parental beliefs on somatic complaints.
Clinical features • Recurrent localized abdominal pain lasting for few hours is commonly associated with emotional disorder. • For hysteria, the child may present with disorders of gait or loss of limb function. • Secondary gain is often implicated.	Clinical features • Headache. • Low energy. • Stomach pain. • Joint pain. • Some adolescents meet the ICD-10 diagnostic criteria for somatization disorder.
Treatment • Medical reassurance. • Psychoeducation. • Behaviour therapy.	Treatment • Work with family to facilitate expression of emotion and change maintaining factors. • Medical reassurance. • CBT.
	Prognosis • Most adolescents with somatization disorder have good prognosis. • Poor prognostic factors include chronic disorders, multiple physical complaints, neurasthenic presentations, and onset in late adolescence.

TABLE 37.17

Compare and Contrast Childhood- and Adolescence-Onset Eating Disorders

Childhood-Onset Eating Disorders (Fox and Carol, 2001)

Epidemiology

- One-third of British children have mild to moderate eating difficulties at age 5 years

Aetiology

- Male gender
- Low birth weight
- Developmental delay
- Early onset of the feeding problem
- History of vomiting for long duration
- High social class

Type of childhood-onset eating disorders:

- *Childhood-onset anorexia nervosa*: weight loss and abnormal cognitions on weight and shape
- *Childhood-onset bulimia nervosa*: recurrent binges, lack of control, and abnormal cognition
- *Food avoidance emotional disorder*: weight loss, mood disturbance, and no features of anorexia nervosa
- *Selective eating:* narrow range of food and unwilling to try new food
- *Restrictive eating*: smaller amount than expected and normal diet in terms of nutritional content
- *Food refusal*: episodic, intermittent, or situational food refusal
- *Functional dysphagia*: fear of swallowing, choking, and vomiting
- *Pervasive refusal syndrome*: refusal to eat, drink, walk, talk, or self-care

Treatment

- Behaviour therapy can enhance the child's motivation to eat and reduce maladaptive behaviour such as expelling food
- Social skill training
- Family therapy

Adolescent-Onset Eating Disorders

Epidemiology

- Anorexia nervosa
  - Prevalence is 0.5%
  - Male adolescents account for 5% of anorexia nervosa
- Bulimia nervosa
  - Prevalence: 1%
  - Peak age is around 17 years

Aetiology

- Heritability is high in anorexia nervosa but not in bulimia nervosa
- Neurotic personality
- Family adopts critical attitude
- Cultural pressure to pursue thinness
- Perfectionism

Clinical features

The clinical features for adolescent anorexia nervosa and bulimia nervosa are similar to the criteria used in adult patients

Anorexia nervosa:

- Self-induced weight loss leading to low weight (typically below 85% expected weight)
- Body mass index (BMI) of less than 17.5
- Fear of fatness or weight gain
- Disturbed body image
- Amenorrhoea

Bulimia nervosa:

- Recurrent episodes of binge eating
- A preoccupation with eating including compulsions to eat
- Compensatory behaviours to reduce weight (e.g. dietary restriction between binges and self-induced vomiting)
- Excessive exercise
- Laxative abuse

Treatment

Anorexia nervosa:

- CBT
- Referral to a dietician
- Aim at gaining 0.5–1 kg/week
- Some patients require hospitalization if they have medical risk (e.g. bradycardia)
- Mortality: 2.16%

Bulimia nervosa:

- CBT
- Fluoxetine will reduce the impulse to binge

TABLE 37.17 (continued)

Compare and Contrast Childhood- and Adolescence-Onset Eating Disorders

Childhood-Onset Eating Disorders (Fox and Carol, 2001)	Adolescent-Onset Eating Disorders
Prognosis	Prognosis
For childhood-onset anorexia nervosa, two-thirds of patients make good recovery	Anorexia nervosa
	• Good outcome in 50% of patients
	• Intermediate outcome in 30% of patients
	• Poor outcome in 20% of patients
	• Younger onset is associated with better outcomes
	• Poor prognostic factors include achievement of body weight < 65% of expected weight and admission to the hospital
	• Long-term suicidal rate in adolescent anorexia nervosa is 5%
	Bulimia nervosa
	• Better outcome than anorexia nervosa
	• Complete remission is more likely than anorexia nervosa
	• Poor prognostic signs include borderline personality disorder and impulsivity

8. Physical examination must be carried out by an appropriately experienced paediatrician or gynaecologist.
9. If abuse is confirmed, the psychiatrist needs to assess the child to determine the effects of abuse, safety issues, and recommend further treatment.

37.20.3 MANAGEMENT

• The safety of the child is the most important and the psychiatrist needs to discuss with the paediatrician and social worker to notify the authority and remove the child from danger.

• Recognize the physical and emotional consequences of abuse (e.g. anxiety, guilt, psychiatric morbidity secondary to sexual abuse and fears about the consequences of disclosure, regression to an earlier developmental stage) and make appropriate referrals.
• Evaluate the continuing risk to the child and siblings.
• Evaluate the therapeutic needs of child and parents.
• Individual psychotherapy may help the child to overcome symptoms of post-traumatic stress disorder and poor self-esteem.
• Family therapy may be useful to restore the roles and boundaries in family.

CASC STATION IN CHILD AND ADOLESCENT PSYCHIATRY

Assessment of ADHD

Name: John Smith **Age:** 10

You are a specialist trainee in Child and Adolescent Psychiatry. John was referred to you as he has been very active and disruptive in school. The school is considering suspending him because of his behaviour. Developmental milestones are known to be normal.

Task: You are asked to talk to John's mother to take a history of his problem. Full developmental history is not required. The NICE guidelines suggest that the diagnostic process for ADHD involves an assessment of the person's needs, coexisting conditions, social, familial, educational or occupational circumstances, and physical health. For children and young people, there should also be an assessment of their parents' or carers' mental health.

(continued)

(A) Core Symptoms of ADHD	(A1) Hyperactivity	(A2) Inattention	(A3) Impulsiveness and Other Behaviour
	'In school, do the teachers ever say he has trouble sitting still or staying in his seat?' 'Compared to other kids, do you find John more hyperactive?' 'Can you give me some examples?' 'Does he often climb excessively?' 'If so, since when have you noticed this?'	'In school, does he often fail to follow through instructions or to finish school work?' 'In schoolwork, does he often fail to give close attention to details? Does he make careless mistakes easily? Does he dislike homework?' 'Does he appear to have difficulty to sustain attention in tasks? Is he easily distracted by external stimuli?' 'Does he have difficulty in listening to what is being said to him?' 'How good is he in organizing tasks? Does he easily misplace his belongings? Does he often lose thing?' 'Does he finish one activity before moving to the next? Does he tend to start one thing and go on to the next before finishing?'	'Does he tend to act before thinking?' 'Can you give me some examples?' 'Does he seem to be impatient and have difficulty waiting for his turn?' 'Does he interrupt often into conversations? How about blurting out answers before questions have been completed?' 'Do you find that he talks excessively and you have difficulty to stop him?' 'Does he have twitching movement on his face?' (Candidates must be considered for Tourette's syndrome and make stimulants contraindicated.) If the child is a girl, candidate is advised to focus more on mood swings because girls with ADHD are less aggressive and impulsive.
(B) Other Aspects of History to Establish the Diagnosis	(B1) Age of Onset and Duration of Symptoms	(B2) Pervasiveness	(B3) Impairments in Social Functioning
	'At what age did you notice problems with hyperactivity or inattention?' (Age of onset is expected to be before 7 years old.) 'How long has he been hyperactive and inattentive?' (Duration is expected to be at least for 6 months.)	'Do these problems happen at both at home and school?' 'Does he have the same problems at other places? (e.g. going to a shopping mall)' Hyperactivity, inattention, and impulsivity are present for more than one situation.	'Does he have any problem in making or keeping friends?' 'Does he get invited over to see friends or to birthday parties?' 'Does he have friends in school?' 'What do you think stops him from being able to keep friends?' 'Does his behaviour affect his relationships with his siblings or family members? How does the family cope with him?'

(C) Current Academic Function and Developmental History

(C1) Behavioural Problems in School

'Do the teachers complain about him?'

'Does he display any conduct problem?'

(C2) Academic Background

'Is he doing well in school?'

'Has his studies been affected by his symptoms?'

'Is he in a mainstream school or special school? Did the teacher say he has special education need?'

(C3) Developmental History

Although the question states that you do not need to take a full developmental history, the candidate is expected to take a brief history.

'Was there any delay in his development?'

'How old did he start walking?'

'How old did he start to say simple words?'

(D) Family Background and Home Environment

(D1) Family History of ADHD

'Is there any family member who is also diagnosed with ADHD?'

(D2) Parental Relationship

'How are you getting along with your husband or partner?'

'Do both of you have any disagreement over John's problems?'

(D3) Major Changes in Social Circumstances

Explore:

- Financial problems
- Recent birth of young sibling
- Recent changes in home environment

'Are you in contact with the social service?'

(E) Risk Assessment and Background History

(E1) Risk Assessment

'I am very sorry to hear what has happened to John and your family. I would like to inquire safety issues. Has John ever done anything impulsive that may harm himself or the others? If yes, how do you keep him safe?'

'Does John think before he acts? Has he ever involved in any road traffic accident?'

'Have you or your partner ever become angry with John? If so, what would you do? Did you punish him physically?'

(E2) Past Medical History and aetiology

'Did you smoke or drink when you were pregnant?'

'Did he have low birth weight when he was born?'

'Does John have any medical problems such as having a fit?'

'Does he have any hearing problems or suffer from a genetic disease?' (to rule out fragile X syndrome)

'Is John currently taking any other medications such as inhaler for asthma?' (e.g. ventolin may cause hyperactivity in some children)

(E3) Past Psychiatric History and Family History of Psychiatric Illness

'Was John previously seen by a psychiatrist before? How about yourself or your husband? What advice did the psychiatrist offer?'

Note: autism, mental retardation, or mood disorders can be causative factors for hyperactivity and inattention.

Explore other psychiatric comorbidity:

- 'Does he feel sad recently?'
- 'Is he more nervous lately?'
- 'Does he use recreational drugs?'

REFERENCES

Academy of Medicine Singapore-Ministry of Health Clinical Practice Guidelines Workgroup on Autism Spectrum Disorders. 2010: Academy of Medicine Singapore-Ministry of Health clinical practice guidelines: Autism Spectrum Disorders in pre-school children. *Singapore Medical Journal* 51(3):255–263.

American Psychiatric Association. 1994: *DSM-IV-TR: Diagnostic and Statistical Manual of Mental Disorders (Diagnostic & Statistical Manual of Mental Disorders)*, 4th edn. Washington, DC: American Psychiatric Association Publishing, Inc.

American Psychiatric Association. 2013: *Desk Reference to the Diagnostic Criteria from DSM-5*. Washington, DC: American Psychiatric Association Press.

Apter A, Pauls D, Bleich A et al. 1993: An epidemiological study of Gilles de la Tourette syndrome in Israel. *Archives of General Psychiatry* 50:734–738.

Baker P. 2004: *Basic Child Psychiatry*, 7th edn. London, U.K.: Blackwell.

Bates G. 2009: Drug treatments for attention-deficit hyperactivity disorder in young people. *Advances in Psychiatric Treatment* 15:162–171.

Black D and Cottrell D. (eds.) 1993: *Seminars in Child and Adolescent Psychiatry*. London, U.K.: Gaskell.

Biederman J, Newcom J, and Sprich S. 1991: Comorbidity of attention deficit hyperactivity disorder with conduct, depressive, anxiety and other disorders. *American Journal of Psychiatry* 148: 564–577.

Centres for Disease Control. 1999: Youth risk behaviour surveillance: United States 1999. *Morbidity and Mortality Weekly Report* 49:1–96.

Dickinson M and Singh I. 2010: Learning disability psychiatry. In Puri BK and Treasaden IH (eds.) *Psychiatry: An Evidence-Based Text*. London, U.K.: Hodder Arnold.

Dunnachie B. 2007: *Evidence-Based Age-Appropriate Interventions: A Guide for Child and Adolescent Mental Health Services (CAMHS)*. Auckland, New Zealand: The Workforce Development.

Fonagy P, Target M, Cottrell D, Phillips J, and Kurtz Z. 2002: *What Works for Whom? A Critical Review of Treatments for Children and Adolescents*. New York: Guilford Press.

Fergusson D, Horwood J, and Lynsky M. 1997: Children and adolescents. In Ellis PM and Collings SC (eds.) *Mental Health in New Zealand from a Public Health Perspective*. Wellington, New Zealand: Ministry of Health.

Fombonne E. 1995: Eating disorders: Time trends and possible explanatory mechanisms. In Rutter M and Smith D (eds.) *Psychosocial Disorders in Young People: Time Trends and Their Causes*, pp. 544–615. Chichester, U.K.: John Wiley & Sons.

Fombonne E, Wostear G, Cooper V et al. 2001: The Maudsley long-term follow-up of child and adolescent depression 2: Suicide, criminality and social dysfunction in adulthood. *British Journal of Psychiatry* 179:218–223.

Fox C and Carol J. 2001: *Childhood-Onset Eating Problems*. London, U.K.: Gaskell.

Gelder M, Mayou R, and Cowen P. 2001: *Shorter Oxford Textbook of Psychiatry*. Oxford, U.K.: Oxford University Press.

Gladman M and Lancaster S. 2003: A review of the behavior assessment system for children. *School Psychology International* 24:276–291.

Golubchik P, Mozes T, Vered Y, and Weizman A. 2009: Late let poor plasma serotonin level in delinquent dolescents diagnosed with conduct disorder. *Progress in Neuropsychopharmacology and Biological Psychiatry* 33:1223–1225.

Goodman R and Scott S. 2005: *Child Psychiatry*, 2nd edn. Oxford, U.K.: Blackwell Publishing.

Graham P. 1986: *Child Psychiatry: A Development Approach*. Oxford, U.K.: Oxford University Press.

Hoare, P. 1993: *Essential Child Psychiatry*. Edinburgh, Scotland: Churchill Livingstone.

Hollis C. 2000: Adult outcomes of child and adolescent onset schizophrenia: Diagnostic stability and predictive validity. *American Journal of Psychiatry* 157:1652–1659.

Jensen PS, Hinshaw SP, Kraemer He et al. 2001: ADHD comorbidity findings from the MTA study: Comparing comorbid sub groups. *Journal of the American Academy of Child and Adolescent Psychiatry* 43:792–801.

Johnstone EC, Cunningham ODG, Lawrie SM, Sharpe M, and Freeman CPL. 2004: *Companion to Psychiatric Studies*, 7th edn. London, U.K.: Churchill Livingstone.

Krug DA, Arick J, and Almond P. 1980: Behavior checklist for identifying severely handicapped individuals with high levels of autistic behavior. *Journal of Child Psychology and Psychiatry* 21(3):221–229.

Lewinsohn PM, Hops H, Roberts RE et al. 1993: Adolescent psychopathology: I. Prevalence and incidence of depression and other DSM-III-R disorders in high school students. *Journal of Abnormal Psychology* 102:133–144.

Lewinsohn PM, Rohde P, Klein D, and Seeley JR. 1999: Natural course of adolescent major depressive disorder: 1. Continuity into young adulthood. *Journal of the American Academy of Child and Adolescent Psychiatry* 38:56–63.

Maskey S. 2003a: Schizophrenia. In Skuse D (ed.) *Child Psychology and Psychiatry: An Introduction*, pp. 115–120. Abingdon, U.K.: Medicine Publishing Company.

Maskey S. 2003b: Obsessive-compulsive disorder. In Skuse D (ed.) *Child Psychology and Psychiatry: An Introduction*, pp. 95–100. Abingdon, U.K.: Medicine Publishing Company.

NICE. *NICE Guidelines for Attention Deficit Hyperactivity Disorder*. http://guidance.nice.org.uk/CG72 (accessed on 12 March 2012).

NICE. *NICE Guidelines for Autism*. http://guidance.nice.org.uk/CG128 (accessed on 5 March 2012).

NICE. *NICE Guidelines for Parental Management Training*. http://guidance.nice.org.uk/TA102 (accessed on 5 March 2012).

NICE. *NICE Guidelines for Depression in Children and Young People*. http://guidance.nice.org.uk/CG28 (accessed on 19 March 2012).

NICE. *NICE Guidelines for Self Harm.* http://guidance.nice. org.uk/CG16 (accessed on 19 March 2012).

Offord DR, Boyle ME, and Racine YA. 1991: The epidemiology of antisocial behaviour in childhood and adolescence. In Pepler DJ and Rubin KH (eds.) *The Development and Treatment of Childhood Aggression*, pp. 31–52. Hillsdale, NJ: Lawrence Erlbaum Associates.

Puri BK and Treasaden IH. 2011: *Textbook of Psychiatry*, 3rd edn. Edinburgh, U.K.: Churchill Livingstone.

Richman N, Stevenson J and Graham P. 1982: *Preschool to School: A Behavioural Study*. London, U.K.: Academic Press.

Sadock BJ and Sadock VA. 2007: *Kaplan & Sadock's Synopsis of Psychiatry. Behavioral Sciences/Clinical psychiatry*, 10th edn. Philadelphia, PA: Lippincott Williams & Wilkins.

Schopler E, Reichler RJ, DeVellis RF, and Daly K. 1980: Toward objective classification of childhood autism: Childhood Autism Rating Scale (CARS). *Journal of Autism and Developmental Disorders* 10(1): 91–103.

Shaffer D and Gutstein J. 2002: Suicide and attempted suicide. In Rutter M and Taylor E (eds.) *Child and Adolescent Psychiatry*, 4th edn, pp. 529–554. Oxford, U.K.: Blackwell.

Sweda SC, Rapoport JL, Leonard HI, and Lenane M. 1989: Obsessive-compulsive disorder in children and adolescents: Clinical phenomenology of 70 consecutive cases. *Archives of General Psychiatry* 46:335–341.

Taylor D, Paton C, and Kapur S. 2009: *The Maudsley Prescribing Guidelines*, 10th edn. London, U.K.: Informa Healthcare.

Timmi S and Dwivedi K. 2010: Child and adolescent psychiatry. In Puri BK and Treasaden IH (eds.) *Psychiatry: An Evidence-Based Text*, pp. 1047–1078. London, U.K.: Hodder Arnold.

Weinberg WA, Harper CR, and Brumback RA. 2002: Substance use and abuse: Epidemiology, pharmacological considerations, identification and suggestions towards management. In Rutter M and Taylor E (eds.) *Child and Adolescent Psychiatry*, 4th edn, pp. 455–462. Oxford, U.K.: Blackwell.

World Health Organization. 1992: *ICD-10: The ICD-10 Classification of Mental and Behavioural Disorders: Clinical Descriptions and Diagnostic Guidelines*. Geneva, Switzerland: World Health Organization.

38 Learning Disability

38.1 CLASSIFICATION OF MENTAL RETARDATION

ICD-10 defines mental retardation as being a condition of arrested or incomplete development of the mind, which is especially characterized by impairment of skills manifested during the developmental period, which contribute to the overall level of intelligence, that is, cognitive, language, motor, and social abilities.

The following is a summary of the ICD-10 classification of mental retardation:

- **F70 Mild mental retardation**
  - Intelligence quotient (IQ) range 50–69
  - 85% of all learning disability
  - Delayed understanding and use of language
  - Possible difficulties in gaining independence
  - Work possible in practical occupations
  - Any behavioural, social, and emotional difficulties are similar to the 'normal'

- **F71 Moderate mental retardation**
  - IQ range 35–49
  - 10% of all learning disability
  - Varying profiles of abilities
  - Language use and development variable (may be absent)
  - Often associated with epilepsy and neurological and other disabilities
  - Delay in achievement of self-care
  - Simple practical work possible
  - Independent living rarely achieved

- **F72 Severe mental retardation**
  - IQ range 20–34
  - 3% of all learning disability
  - More marked motor impairment than F71 often found
  - Achievements at lower end of F71

- **F73 Profound mental retardation**
  - IQ difficult to measure but <20
  - 2% of all learning disability

- Severe limitation in ability to understand or comply with requests or instructions
- Little or no self-care
- Mostly severe mobility restriction
- Basic or simple tasks may be acquired (e.g. sorting and matching)

38.1.1 DSM-5 ADOPTS SIMILAR CLASSIFICATION

Mild mental retardation: able to maintain age-appropriate personal care

Moderate mental retardation: extended period of teaching and time is needed to teach the patient to become independent.

Severe mental retardation: require full support for basic activities of daily living.

Profound mental retardation: dependent on other people for daily living.

The onset of age is before the age of 18.

38.2 EPIDEMIOLOGY OF LEARNING DISABILITY

The prevalence of learning disability—defined as having an IQ of less than 70—is 3.7%, which is considerably higher than would be expected from the normal distribution of IQ. The prevalence of self-injurious behaviour among people with learning disability is 20% and 50% for those in institutions. The peak age of self-harm is between 15 and 20 years and associated with male gender.

The levels of coexistence of different impairments are shown in Table 38.1.

38.3 AETIOLOGY OF LEARNING DISABILITY

The causes of learning disability are summarized in Table 38.2.

38.4 DOWN SYNDROME

38.4.1 CLINICAL CASE

A 6-year-old boy is referred to you. On mental state examination, he is pleasant and cooperative. On physical examination, he has a small mouth, small teeth, and a

TABLE 38.1
Levels of Coexistence of Different Impairments

	Severe Mental Retardation	Mild Mental Retardation
Cerebral palsy	Approx. 20%	Approx. 8%
Epilepsy	30%–37%	12%–18%
Hydrocephalus	5%–6%	2%
Severe visual impairment	6%–10%	1%–9%
Severe hearing impairment	3%–15%	2%–7%
One or more major impairments	40%–52%	24%–30%

Reproduced from Puri, B.K. and Treasaden, I.H., *Textbook of Psychiatry*, 3rd edn., Churchill Livingstone, Edinburgh, U.K., 2011. With permission.

TABLE 38.2
Aetiology of Learning Disability

Prenatal	Perinatal	Postnatal
Inborn errors of metabolism	*Asphyxia/hypoxia at birth*	*Meningitis/ encephalitis*
Chromosomal abnormalities: Numerical abnormalities (e.g. Turner's syndrome), partial chromosomal duplications or deletions (e.g. cri du chat syndrome), translocation (e.g. Down syndrome), mosaicism (e.g. Down syndrome), and microdeletion (e.g. Prader–Willi syndrome)	*Mechanical birth trauma*	*Head injury* (e.g. accidental or inflicted)
Congenital infections (rubella, measles, influenza [type B], Japanese encephalitis, cytomegalovirus, syphilis, HIV, toxoplasmosis)	*Small babies* (20% of low birth weight babies develop learning disabilities)	*Lead poisoning* (and other heavy metals)
Irradiation	*Hyperbilirubinaemia* (kernicterus)	*Environmental chemicals*
Drugs (e.g. thalidomide, valproate, and lithium)	*Hyperoxia* (iatrogenic)	*Malnutrition*
Maternal alcohol, opioid intake, and smoking	*Hypoglycaemia*	*Other infections* (e.g. whooping cough)
Malnutrition (including vitamin and iodine deficiencies)	*Prematurity* (e.g. intraventricular haemorrhage)	

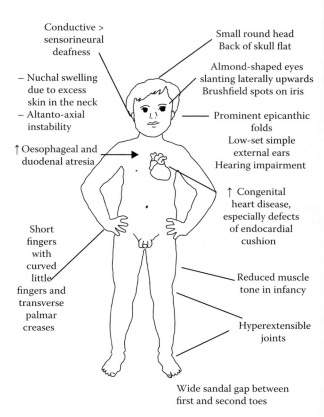

FIGURE 38.1   Clinical features of Down syndrome.

high arched palate. His palpebral fissure is oblique and he has epicanthic folds. He has short broad hands and hyperextensible joints (Figure 38.1).

38.4.2   Epidemiology

- Down syndrome is the most common cytogenic cause of learning disability.
- It accounts for 30% of all children with mental retardation.
- The prevalence is 1 in 800 live births (1 in 2500 if the mother is younger than 30 years and 1 in 80 if the mother is older than 40 years). Paternal age is not an important factor.

38.4.3   Genetic Mechanism

- 94% of cases are caused by meiotic nondisjunction or trisomy 21 (47 chromosomes).
- 5% of cases are caused by translocation that refers to a fusion between chromosome 21 and 14 (46 chromosomes).

- 1% of cases are caused by mosaicism that refers to nondisjunction occurring after fertilization in any cell division.
- Robertsonian translocations are caused by fusion of chromosome 14 and 21. The extra chromosome is usually of maternal origin (90%), and most maternal errors occur during the first meiotic division. The risk of recurrence of translocation is around 10%.
- Defect at 21q21.1 leads to overexpression of genes encoding amyloid precursor protein, but other enzymes such as superoxide dismutase are underactive.
- *Screening for Down syndrome*: Maternal serum markers at 16 weeks of gestation show raised human chorionic gonadotropin (HCG), lowered α-fetoprotein, and lowered unconjugated estriol.

38.4.4 Intelligence

- The IQ of people with Down syndrome is between 40 and 45. IQ < 50 is found in approximately 85% of cases.
- Verbal processing is better than auditory processing.
- Their social skills are more advanced than intellectual skills.
- Defects in the scanning environment tend to focus on a single stimulus.

38.4.5 Growth

- People with Down syndrome have stunted growth with an average adult height of 141 cm in women and 151 cm in men.

38.4.6 Behavioural Features

- Passive and affable
- Obsessional and stubborn
- 25% have attention deficit and hyperactivity

38.4.7 Comorbidity

- People with Down syndrome are at higher risk to develop Alzheimer's disease (50–59-year-olds = 36%–40%; 60–69-year-olds = 55%). Over the age of 40, there is high incidence of neurofibrillary tangles and plaques with increase in P300 latency.
- Hearing loss occurs in 50% of people with Down syndrome.
- Immune system is often impaired, and they are at high risk to develop diabetes mellitus.

- Hypothyroidism is also common.
- 10% of people with Down syndrome suffer from leukaemia.
- Psychiatric comorbidity includes obsessive–compulsive disorder (2% of patients, especially presenting with a need for excessive order or tidiness), depression, autism, bipolar disorder, psychosis, and sleep apnoea.
- The average life expectancy of people with Down syndrome is between 58 and 66 years. The most common cause of death is chest infection.

38.5 LEARNING DISABILITY AND GENETIC DEFECTS IN SEX CHROMOSOMES

38.6 FRAGILE X (MARTIN-BELL) SYNDROME

38.6.1 Clinical Case

A 4-year-old child is referred to you for delayed speech and language. He was initially suspected to suffer from autism. He has gaze aversion and social avoidance. His IQ is 60. He also has attention deficit. Physical examination shows enlarged testes, large ears, long face, and flat feet. Mental state examination reveals limited eye contact, preservation of words, echolalia, and stereotypical behaviour such as hand flapping.

38.6.2 Epidemiology

- Fragile X syndrome is the most common inherited cause of learning disability. It accounts for 10%–12% of mental retardation in men.
- Fragile X syndrome affects 1 in 4000 men and 1 in 8000 women. 1 in 700 women is a carrier for fragile X syndrome.
- The prevalence is less common in women because only 1 in 5 women affected by mutation at fragile site is phenotypically and intellectually unaffected.

38.6.3 Mode of Inheritance

- Fragile X syndrome is an X-linked dominant genetic disorder with low penetrance.
- The fragile site is located at band q27.3 on the X chromosome. Examination of karyotype in performed in the folate-depleted and thymidine-depleted medium.
- The trinucleotide repeats CGG (cytosine, guanine, and guanine) are found on the long arm of X chromosome. Normal number of

repeats is 30, and the repeats for carriers range from 55 to 200. Full mutation with more than 200 repeats leads to hypermethylation at fragile X mental retardation (FMR)—one gene and underexpression of FMR protein.

38.6.4 INTELLIGENCE

- Women with fragile X syndrome suffer from mild learning disability, and men with fragile X syndrome suffer from moderate to severe learning disability (in 80% of male patients, IQ is less than 70).
- Verbal IQ > performance IQ.
- The length of trinucleotide repeats is inversely related to IQ because shorter length (<200 triplets) may not cause methylation, and hence, it results in higher IQ scores.

38.6.5 CLINICAL FEATURES

In general, men with fragile X syndrome are more likely than women (only 50%) to exhibit the typical physical features (Figure 38.2).

38.6.6 OTHER CLINICAL FEATURES

- Short stature.
- Seizure: 20% of patients.
- Strabismus.
- Mitral valve prolapse in 80% of cases.
- Single transverse palmar crease.

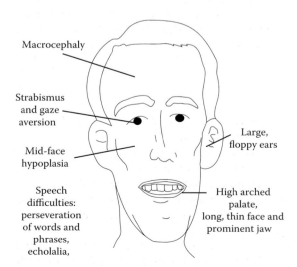

FIGURE 38.2   Facial features of fragile X syndrome.

- Soft velvety skin.
- Boys with fragile X syndrome are often tall in childhood, but their heights become average in adulthood.
- Macroorchidism (70% after puberty).
- Increased incidence of connective tissue disorders.
- Hyperextensible joints.
- Flat feet.

38.6.7 PSYCHIATRIC FEATURES

- Autism-like behaviour
- Speech and language delays
- Idiosyncratic linguistic and interpersonal styles
- Attention deficit and hyperactivity
- Delay in language acquisition with cluttering speech
- Hypersensitivity to social and sensory stimuli
- Self-injury
- Social anxiety and gaze aversion
- Idiosyncratic linguistic and interpersonal styles

38.6.8 MANAGEMENT

- Anticonvulsant for treating seizures.
- Educational package designed to meet the needs of individual, family support, and social care.
- Genetic counselling should be offered to parents and other family members at risk of producing a child with fragile X syndrome.
- Self-help group (e.g. Fragile X Society).

38.7 TURNER'S (XO) SYNDROME

38.7.1 EPIDEMIOLOGY

- Prevalence: 1 in 3300 live births

38.7.2 MODE OF INHERITANCE

- Nondisjunction of paternal XY results in sex chromosomal monosomy.
- 50% of patients have a karyotype consisting of 45X or 46XX mosaicism.
- 50% of patients have 46 chromosomes with one normal X chromosome and the other X chromosome, which is abnormal in the form of a ring, a long arm isochromosome, or a partially deleted X chromosome.

38.7.3 CLINICAL FEATURES (FIGURE 38.3)

- Most fetuses with Turner's syndrome develop hydrops fetalis due to delayed maturation of the lymphatic drainage system.

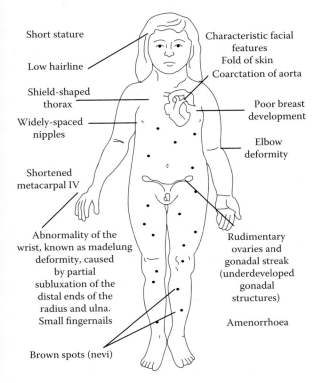

Short stature

Low hairline

Shield-shaped thorax

Widely-spaced nipples

Shortened metacarpal IV

Abnormality of the wrist, known as madelung deformity, caused by partial subluxation of the distal ends of the radius and ulna. Small fingernails

Brown spots (nevi)

Characteristic facial features
Fold of skin
Coarctation of aorta

Poor breast development

Elbow deformity

Rudimentary ovaries and gonadal streak (underdeveloped gonadal structures)

Amenorrhoea

FIGURE 38.3   Clinical features of Turner's syndrome.

- At birth, the neonate always has a normal female feature with residue of intrauterine oedema in the form of neck webbing and puffy extremities.
- Short stature becomes apparent in early childhood, and average adult height is 140–145 cm without hormone therapy.

38.7.4   INTELLIGENCE

- Normal IQ
- Mild learning disability
- Subtle defects in visuospatial perception and fine motor skills

38.7.5   COMORBIDITY

- Infertility is very common in women with full Turner's syndrome as a result of ovarian dysgenesis.
- Pregnancy has been achieved in a small number of female patients by embryo transplantation following in vitro fertilization using their partner's sperm and a donor egg.

38.7.6   TREATMENT

- Oestrogen replacement therapy should be introduced from the age of 12 years onwards to promote pubertal development and prevent the onset of osteoporosis.

38.8   KLINEFELTER'S SYNDROME (XXY)

38.8.1   CASE EXAMPLE

A 25-year-old married man with history of mild learning disability is referred to you. His history suggests possible fertility problems. Physical examination shows gynaecomastia and small testes. There is no family history of similar problems.

38.8.2   EPIDEMIOLOGY

- The incidence is between 1 in 500 and 1 in 1000 live male births.

38.8.3   GENETIC MECHANISMS

- 50% due to maternal and 50% due to paternal nondisjunction.
- Paternal nondisjunction is paternally derived and associated with advanced paternal age.
- 80% of males with Klinefelter's syndrome have a 47XXY karyotype with an additional X chromosome being derived equally from meiotic errors in each parent.
- Other karyotypes include 47XXY or 46XY mosaicism and severe X chromosome aneuploidy such as 48XXXY and 49XXXXY. These karyotypes usually occur as sporadic events in a family.

38.8.4   CLINICAL FEATURES (FIGURE 38.4)

- Newborn boys with Klinefelter's syndrome are clinically normal.
- Sexual orientation is usually normal and results in heterosexual marriage.
- Passive and compliant in childhood.
- Aggressive and antisocial past puberty.

38.8.5   INTELLIGENCE

- Mild learning disability with some difficulty in acquiring verbal skills.

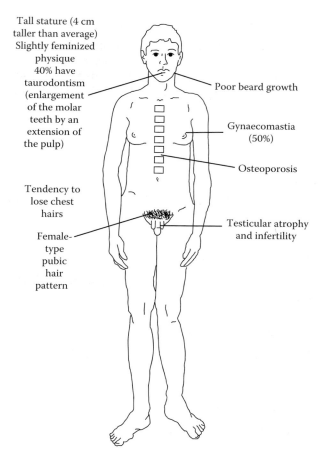

Tall stature (4 cm taller than average)
Slightly feminized physique
40% have taurodontism (enlargement of the molar teeth by an extension of the pulp)

Poor beard growth

Gynaecomastia (50%)

Osteoporosis

Tendency to lose chest hairs

Female-type pubic hair pattern

Testicular atrophy and infertility

FIGURE 38.4   Clinical features of Klinefelter's syndrome.

- 48XXXY and 49XXXXY are associated with severe learning disability and marked hypogonadism.

38.8.6   TREATMENT

- Fertility can be achieved using haploid spermatocytes obtained by testicular biopsy.

38.9   OTHER X-LINKED SYNDROMES

- *Hunter syndrome* is an X-linked recessive mucopolysaccharide disorder. There are two forms. Type A presents with progressive learning disability leading to death between 10 and 20 years, and type B affected individuals usually present with normal intelligence and survival.
- *Duchenne muscular dystrophy* is an X-linked recessive disorder. Abnormalities at Xp21 lead to failure to produce dystrophin, resulting in a progressive muscular deterioration over 20 years, and the patients become wheelchair bound at the end of childhood. 20% have learning disability with impairment of verbal IQ. Depression is common.
- *Rett syndrome* is an X-linked dominant disorder (refer to Chapter 37 for details).

38.10   XYY SYNDROME

38.10.1   EPIDEMIOLOGY

- It affects approximately 1 in 1000 male neonates.
- Up to 3% of patients in maximum security hospitals have XYY karyotype.
- Men with 47, XYY karyotype show an increased rate of petty crime (an average three times more common than in the general population). This is a result of impulsiveness, and there is no propensity towards severe aggression or violent crime.

38.10.2   MODE OF INHERITANCE

- Primary nondisjunction of the Y chromosome.
- About 10% have mosaic, that is, 46, XY and 47, XYY chromosome complement.

38.10.3   CLINICAL FEATURES

- Mild physical abnormalities
- Proportionate tall stature
- Enlarged teeth
- Increased susceptibility to develop acne
- Muscle weakness and poor coordination
- Normal sexual development and fertility

38.10.4   INTELLIGENCE

- Mild learning disability.
- Verbal skills are delayed.

38.11   LEARNING DISABILITY AND INBORN ERROR OF METABOLISM

38.12   LESCH–NYHAN SYNDROME

38.12.1   CLINICAL HISTORY

A 16-year-old boy is referred to you because of severe self-mutilation including biting of lips, inside of mouth, and fingers. There is a failure of secondary sexual development. His maternal grandfather and maternal uncle also suffer from the same disorder.

38.12.2 Epidemiology

- Incidence 1/10,000–1/38,000
- Exclusive to men

38.12.3 Mode of Inheritance

- X-linked recessive
- CAG trinucleotide repeats

38.12.4 Error in Metabolism

- Defect in hypoxanthine guanine phosphoribosyl-transferase resulting in accumulation of uric acid

38.12.5 Clinical Features

- Microcephaly.
- During infancy, orange uricosuric acid sand is found in the nappy.
- Then patient develops hypotonia followed by spastic choreoathetosis, dysphagia, and dysarthria.
- The age of onset of self-injurious behaviours is usually before the age of 3. Lips and fingers are often bitten.

38.12.6 Behavioural Features

- Generalized aggression with tantrums directed against objects and people

38.12.7 Intelligence

- Mild to moderate learning disability

38.12.8 Medical Comorbidity

- Gout
- Epilepsy (50%)
- Respiratory or renal failure (often the cause of death)

38.12.9 Treatment

- Well planned behavioural intervention may reduce self-injurious behaviour.
- Allopurinol reduces uric acid levels but offers no therapeutic benefits in behavioural symptoms.

38.13 HURLER'S SYNDROME

38.13.1 Case History

A 3-year-old child presents with hepatosplenomegaly, hirsutism, corneal clouding, and recurrent respiratory infections.

38.13.2 Epidemiology

One in 100,000

38.13.3 Mode of Inheritance

Autosomal recessive

38.13.4 Error in Metabolism

Deficiency in L-iduronidase mucopolysaccharidosis type I

38.13.5 Clinical Features

Short stature, hepatosplenomegaly, and hirsutism (Figure 38.5)

38.13.6 Psychiatric Features

Anxiety and fearful feelings

38.13.7 Intelligence

Moderate to severe learning disability

38.13.8 Causes of Death

Recurrent respiratory infections and death before the age of 10 years

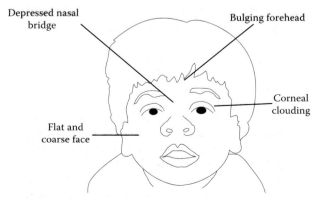

FIGURE 38.5 Facial features of Hurler's syndrome.

38.13.9 TREATMENT

Allogeneic bone marrow transplantation

38.14 PHENYLKETONURIA

38.14.1 EPIDEMIOLOGY

- Incidence: 1 in 4,500–15,000
- Frequency among institutionalized retarded patients: 1%
- Predominantly in people of North European origin

38.14.2 MODE OF INHERITANCE

- Autosomal recessive
- Phenylalanine hydroxylase gene on chromosome 12 (12q22–24.1)

38.14.3 ERROR IN METABOLISM

- Defects in phenylalanine hydroxylase or cofactor (biopterin)
- Accumulation of phenylalanine

38.14.4 CLINICAL FEATURES

- Symptoms absent neonatally
- Blond hair
- Fair skin
- Blue eyes
- Triad: eczema, epilepsy, and vomiting (30%)

38.14.5 BEHAVIOURAL FEATURES

- Autistic features
- Stereotyped behaviour destructiveness
- Self-injury
- Hyperactivity
- Psychotic symptoms that resemble childhood-onset schizophrenia

38.14.6 INTELLIGENCE

- Mild to profound learning disability
- Language delay

38.14.7 SCREENING TEST

- Guthrie immunoassay detects phenylalanine in the blood soon after birth.

38.14.8 TREATMENT

- The neonates are required to take a low-phenylalanine diet before 6 months of age.
- Initiation of low-phenylalanine diet before 3 months of age may preserve normal intelligence. Other benefits include reduction of irritability and abnormal EEG and enhanced social responsiveness and attention span.
- Side effects of low-phenylalanine diet include anaemia, hypoglycaemia, and oedema.

38.15 SANFILIPPO SYNDROME

38.15.1 CASE HISTORY

A 6-year-old child presents with developmental delay, claw hand, hypertrichosis, deafness, hepatosplenomegaly, biconvex lumbar vertebrae, and joint stiffness. He has claw hands. His parents mention that he is often restless with sleep problems and challenging behaviour.

38.15.2 METABOLIC PROBLEMS

Dysfunction in the breakdown of heparan sulphate

38.15.3 INTELLIGENCE

Severe learning disability

38.15.4 CAUSE OF DEATH

Respiratory tract infections (between the age of 10 and 20 years)

38.15.5 GALACTOSAEMIA

38.15.6 EPIDEMIOLOGY

One in 60,000

38.15.7 MODE OF INHERITANCE

Autosomal recessive

38.15.8 METABOLIC PROBLEMS

Absence of galactose-1-phosphate uridyl transferase and results in intracellular accumulation of galactose-1-phosphate (toxic)

38.15.9   CLINICAL FEATURES

- Jaundice, vomiting, and diarrhoea after exposure to galactose
- Fanconi syndromes (growth failure, renal tubular dysfunction, acidosis, hypokalaemia, galactosaemia)
- Increased intracranial pressure
- Ovarian failure
- Failure to thrive

38.15.10   BEHAVIOURAL FEATURES

Increased behavioural problems, anxiety, social withdrawal, and shyness

38.15.11   INTELLIGENCE

Learning disability with visuospatial deficits and language disorders

38.16   METACHROMATIC LEUKODYSTROPHY

38.16.1   MODE OF INHERITANCE

Autosomal recessive

38.16.2   ERROR OF METABOLISM

Lysosomal storage disease with problems in lipid metabolism resulting in accumulation of galactosyl sulphatide affecting myelin

38.16.3   CLINICAL FEATURES

- *Infantile form*: before the age of 3 and progresses to severe motor retardation and learning disability
- *Juvenile form*: motor retardation and learning disability
- *Adult form*: presents with dementia or psychosis

38.17   TAY–SACHS DISEASE

38.17.1   MODE OF INHERITANCE

Autosomal recessive and mainly occur in people with Jewish origin

38.17.2   ERROR OF METABOLISM

Increase in lipid storage (accumulation of gangliosides in neurons).

38.17.3   COURSE OF ILLNESS

Infants initially develop normally in the first few months of life followed by subsequent relentless deterioration of physical and mental abilities.

38.18   LEARNING DISABILITY AND NEUROCUTANEOUS SYNDROMES

38.19   TUBEROUS SCLEROSIS

38.19.1   CASE HISTORY

A 20-year-old woman presents with white skin patches and gingival fibromata. She has history of epilepsy. A whole-body scan shows tumours in kidney, spleen, and lungs.

38.19.2   EPIDEMIOLOGY

- Men and women are equally affected.
- One in 7000 population.

38.19.3   MODE OF INHERITANCE

- Autosomal dominant with 100% penetrance.
- Spontaneous mutation in 70% of cases.
- Two tumour suppressor genes are involved: TSC1 (on 9q34, which codes for hamartin) and TSC2 (on 16p13.3, which codes for tuberin).

38.19.4   CLINICAL FEATURES (FIGURE 38.6)

- Most common feature is skin depigmentation that is especially noted under ultraviolet light.
- Hypomelanotic macules.
- Intractable epilepsy.
- Classical diagnostic triad of epilepsy, learning disability, and characteristic facial skin lesions seen in 30% of people with tuberous sclerosis.

38.19.5   PSYCHIATRIC FEATURES

- Autism (75%)
- Hyperactivity
- Impulsivity
- Aggression
- Self-injurious behaviours
- Sleep disturbance

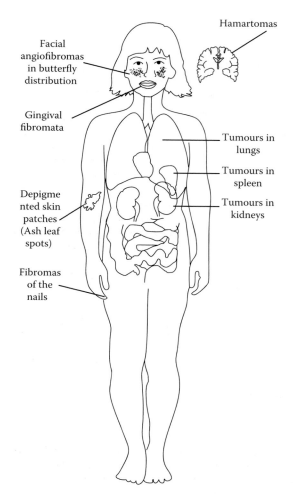

Facial
angiofibromas
in butterfly
distribution

Gingival
fibromata

Depigme
nted skin
patches
(Ash leaf
spots)

Fibromas
of the
nails

Hamartomas

Tumours in
lungs

Tumours in
spleen

Tumours in
kidneys

FIGURE 38.6   Clinical features of tuberosus sclerosis.

38.19.6   Intelligence

- 30% of people with tuberous sclerosis have normal IQ.
- If learning disability is present, it is usually profound.

38.19.7   Comorbidity

- Seizures are common (90%).
- The initial presentation is usually infantile spasms.

38.20   NEUROFIBROMATOSIS TYPE 1 (VON RECKLINGHAUSEN DISEASE)

38.20.1   Epidemiology

- Male = female
- One in 1/2500–4000 live births

38.20.2   Mode of Inheritance

- Autosomal dominant.
- 50% are caused by sporadic mutations.
- Mutation in neurofibromatosis (NF) allele at chromosome 17q11.2.
- Abnormal in production of neurofibromin.

38.20.3   Intelligence

- 30% have mild learning disability.
- 10% have severe to profound learning disability.
- Verbal IQ is better than performance IQ.

38.20.4   Clinical Features

- Short stature.
- Macrocephaly (30%–45%).
- Optic nerve glioma.
- Hypertension.
- Tumours arise from the connective tissue of nerve sheaths.
- Café au lait spots.
- Cutaneous neurofibromas.
- Freckling of groin or armpit.
- Skeletal deformities.
- Lisch nodules.

38.20.5   Psychiatric Features

- Depression
- Anxiety
- Speech and language difficulties (50%)
- Distractibility
- Impulsiveness
- Hyperactivity

38.21   LEARNING DISABILITY AND MICRODELETION SYNDROMES

See Tables 38.3 through 38.6.

38.22   PRADER–WILLI SYNDROME

38.22.1   Case History

A 13-year-old obese boy with learning disability is referred. He presents with irresistible hunger drive and incessant skin picking with compulsion and anxiety. He tends to talk to himself (Figure 38.7).

TABLE 38.3
Other Microdeletion Syndromes

Syndromes	Epidemiology	Chromosome Abnormalities	Clinical Features
Wolf–Hirschhorn syndrome	Incidence: 1 in 90,000	Short arm of chromosome 4 80% arise as de novo deletions. 20% is a result of parentally transmitted unbalanced translocations.	• Severe mental retardation • Microcephaly • High incidence of congenital heart defects • Severe psychomotor and growth retardation • 70% survive beyond early childhood.
Cri du chat syndrome	Incidence: 1 in 50,000	Short arm of chromosome 5 A de novo deletion is present in 85% of cases. 10%–15% of cases are familial. More than 90% is a result of parental translocation. 5% is resulted from an inversion of chromosome 5.	• A round face with microcephaly • Slanting palpebral fissures • Broad flat nose • Low set ears • Cardiac abnormality (50%) • Gastrointestinal abnormalities • Severe mental retardation • Infantile cat cry • Severe psychomotor retardation • Hyperactivity • Stereotypies • Rate of survival is low

TABLE 38.4
Summary of Clinical and Psychiatric Features and Related Syndromes

Clinical and Psychiatric Features	Syndromes
Hyperactivity and aggression	(1) Hurler syndrome, (2) Soto syndrome, (3) fragile X syndrome, (4) phenylketonuria (PKU), and (5) tuberous sclerosis
Autism	(1) Fragile X syndrome, (2) rubella, (3) tuberous sclerosis, (4) PKU, and (5) Cornelia de Lange syndrome
Short stature	(1) Prader–Willi syndrome, (2) Williams syndrome, (3) fetal alcohol syndrome, (4) Cornelia de Lange syndrome, (5) Rubinstein syndrome, and (6) Sanfillipo syndrome
Tall stature	(1) XYY syndrome, (2) Klinefelter's syndrome, and (3) homocystinuria (mild learning disability, ectopia lentis, fine and fair hair, and history of thromboembolic episodes)
Microcephaly	(1) Wolf–Hirschhorn syndrome, (2) cri du chat syndrome, (3) DiGeorge syndrome, (4) Rubinstein syndrome, (5) Cornelia de Lange syndrome, and (6) Angelman syndrome
Macrocephaly	NF
Obesity	(1) Prader–Willi syndrome and (2) Laurence–Moon–Biedl syndrome (mild–moderate LD, short stature, polydactyly, spastic paraparesis, hypogenitalism, night blindness, diabetes, and renal failure) In general, 30% of people with learning disability are overweight and 25% are obese

38.22.2   EPIDEMIOLOGY

- 1/10,000 live births.
- 90% of cases are sporadic.

38.22.3   MODE OF INHERITANCE

- Autosomal dominant transmission.
- Deletion of chromosome 15q11–13 of paternal origin.
- Uniparental disomy (sporadic with no risk or recurrence): 25%.

- Imprinting error (can have a recurrence rate up to 50%).
- The main gene implicated is small nuclear ribonucleoprotein polypeptide N (SNRPN).

38.22.4   CLINICAL FEATURES

- *Infancy*: Hypotonia leads to feeding difficulties and failure to thrive. Triangular mouth also causes feeding and swallowing problems.

TABLE 38.5

Psychiatric Comorbidity Associated with Learning Disability and the Use of Psychopharmacological Agents

Psychiatric Comorbidity

Schizophrenia
1. People with learning disability have higher prevalence of schizophrenia (3%).
2. The prevalence of schizophrenia is inversely related to IQ.
3. Schizophrenia cannot be diagnosed reliably if IQ is less than 45.

Depressive disorder
1. Can be easily missed.
2. Biological symptoms (e.g. anhedonia, changes in activity level, changes in appetite) are more useful for diagnosis.
3. Negative cognition and suicidal ideation are rare.

Bipolar disorder
1. Mania should be differentiated from other causes of overactivity.
2. For cyclical disorders, individualized recording schedules may be useful.

Anxiety disorders
1. The patient may present repeated somatic complaints. Facial expression and physiological signs such as tachycardia are more reliable in diagnosis.
2. Phobia may manifest as avoidance of feared situation.
3. PTSD: sudden and unexplainable changes in arousal, avoidance of certain activities, fear, and evidence of trauma.

Attention deficit and hyperactivity

Severely challenging behaviour
1. The intensity and frequency of certain behaviour put the safety of the patient or others in serious jeopardy.
2. This behaviour limits or denies access to the use of ordinary community facilities.

Stereotypical motor movements
Repetitive ritualized behaviour is common among people with learning disability.

Recommended Psychopharmacological Agents

Antipsychotics are useful for
1. Comorbid psychiatric disorders (e.g. schizophrenia and related psychosis).
2. Behavioural disturbances.
3. Stereotypies that may benefit from low-dose antipsychotics.

Antidepressants are useful for
1. Depression or anxiety disorder.
2. Self-injurious behaviour.
3. Obsessions and compulsions.

SSRIs
Fluoxetine, paroxetine, and sertraline are used.

Lithium and other mood stabilizers
1. Control of aggression or intentional self-harm.
2. Mania.
3. Augmentation therapy for depression.
4. Valproate is used for rapid cycling bipolar disorder.

SSRIs
Fluoxetine, fluvoxamine, paroxetine, and sertraline can reduce obsessive–compulsive symptoms.

Benzodiazepines
1. For short-term use.
2. Avoid long-term usage of benzodiazepine.

Psychological treatment
1. Acknowledge the patient's fear of the trauma.
2. Drawings may facilitate expression in people with learning disability.
3. Relaxation techniques may be helpful.

Antipsychotic
1. Risperidone can reduce attention deficit and hyperactivity.

Stimulant
1. Methylphenidate improves attention and focus on tasks.

Anticonvulsants/mood stabilizer
1. Carbamazepine is useful in the treatment of episodic dyscontrol.
2. Valproate can reduce aggression.
3. Lithium can reduce aggression and self-injurious behaviour.

β-adrenergic receptor antagonists
Propranolol can reduce explosive rages.

Behaviour therapy
Shaping social behaviours and minimizing destructive behaviours.

Opiate antagonist
Naltrexone is used in the treatment of repetitive self-injury.

Antilibidinal medication
Cyproterone acetate and medroxyprogesterone reduce testosterone levels and can be used in the treatment of sexual offending. Side effects include liver toxicity and hyperglycaemia.

SSRIs
SSRIs such as fluoxetine or fluvoxamine can reduce repetitive behaviours.

TABLE 38.6
Prevention of Learning Disability

Primary prevention	1. Population screening, carrier detection, and prenatal diagnosis have been improved by the advances in molecular genetics and used to prevent diseases like fragile X syndrome. 2. Prevention of Down syndrome by genetic counselling is limited to potential cases with translocation abnormality inherited from the parent. 3. Prevention of exposure to ionizing radiation and teratogenic drugs. 4. Reduction of birth trauma by positive family planning, better obstetric care, hospital deliveries, and regular maternal and fetal monitoring. 5. Vaccination to reduce infection such as measles, mumps, and rubella (MMR). 6. Prevention of neural tube defect by taking folate during pregnancy. 7. Smoking cessation and avoiding alcohol and opioid misuse during pregnancy. 8. Prevention of head injury by wearing bicycle hamlet and enforcing the use of safety car seat for children.
Secondary prevention	1. Advances in molecular genetics, amniocentesis, ultrasonic imaging, and chorionic villous sampling allow prenatal diagnosis of fetuses affected by genetic diseases in the first trimester. 2. Maternal serum alpha-fetoprotein level is a reliable indicator of neural tube defect. 3. Triple tests: HCG, estriol, and alpha-fetoprotein as well as the nuchal translucency scan allow detection of Down syndrome in the first trimester. 4. Metabolic diseases like PKU, galactosaemia, Lesch–Nyhan syndrome, maple syrup urine disease, Hunter's syndrome, Hurler's syndrome, and Tay–Sachs disease are identified prenatally. 5. Neonatal screening may detect endocrine diseases like congenital hypothyroidism and metabolic diseases like PKU and maple syrup urine disease in newborns.
Tertiary prevention	1. At the community level, active resettlement programmes with expansion of support networks, special educational services, training placements, and day and residential services can prevent long-term hospital care. 2. At the individual level, the use of computer and electronic aids can promote independence and provide opportunity for alternative methods of communication may improve the quality of life of people with learning disability. 3. Education for the child that addresses adaptive skills, social skills, and communication skills. 4. Family interventions such as family education about the condition and family therapy to enhance self-esteem and allow expression of feelings (e.g. guilt).

Source: Day, K., Mental handicap, in Paykel, E.S. and Jenkins, R. (eds.) *Prevention in Psychiatry*, London, U.K., Gaskell, 1994, pp. 130–147.

- *Childhood*: Orthopaedic problems such as congenital dislocation of hip and scoliosis are common.
- *Adolescence*: Behavioural disorders such as overeating and obesity, self-injurious behaviour, compulsive behaviour, aggression, excessive daytime sleepiness, skin picking, hoarding, and anxiety. Insatiable appetite is diagnostic.

38.22.5 INTELLIGENCE

- Mild to moderate learning disability
- Speech abnormalities

38.22.6 COMORBIDITY

- Obsessive–compulsive disorder

38.22.7 TREATMENT

- Dietary restriction to reduce obesity

38.23 ANGELMAN SYNDROME

38.23.1 CASE HISTORY

A 10-year-old boy presents with severe learning disability, frequent hand flapping, happy disposition, paroxysmal laughter, and microcephaly. He has history of epilepsy.

38.23.2 EPIDEMIOLOGY

- Prevalence is 1/20,000–1/30,000.

38.23.3 MODE OF INHERITANCE

- Autosomal dominant transmission
- Deletion on chromosome 15q11–13 of the maternal origin
- Frequent deletion of GABA B-3 receptor subunit
- Mutations in ubiquitin–protein ligase E3A (UBE 3A) and associated with severe psychomotor retardation

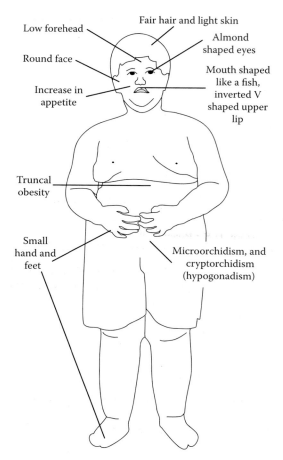

FIGURE 38.7   Prader–Willi syndrome.

38.23.4   INTELLIGENCE

- Severe or profound learning disability

38.23.5   CLINICAL FEATURES (FIGURE 38.8)

- Angelman syndrome is known as happy puppet syndrome characterized by paroxysms of laughter, cheerful disposition, and ataxia.
- Axial hypotonia.
- Jerky movements.
- Epilepsy (90%): EEG changes develop during the first year of life.
- Gastrointestinal problems (reflux, rumination, pica).

38.23.6   PSYCHIATRIC FEATURES

- Autism
- Attention deficit syndrome
- Sleep disturbance
- Nightmares

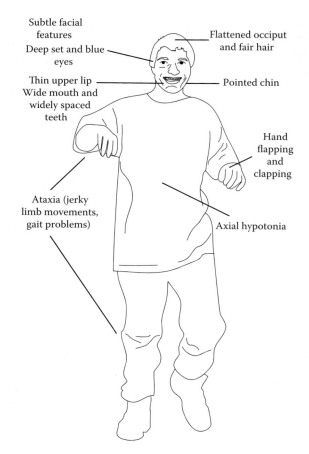

FIGURE 38.8   Clinical features of Angelman syndrome.

38.24   WILLIAMS SYNDROME

38.24.1   CASE SCENARIO

A 13-year-old girl with an 'elfin' facial appearance presents with obsessions, compulsions, impulsive behaviour including hyperphagia, aggression, and skin picking. Mental state examination reveals a talkative and over-friendly child. Echocardiogram shows pulmonary stenosis and mitral valve regurgitation. Blood tests show hypercalcaemia. She was born at full term. She has developmental delay and retarded growth.

38.24.2   EPIDEMIOLOGY

- 1 in 20,000 live births

38.24.3   MODE OF INHERITANCE

- Autosomal dominant transmission
- Small deletion of one elastin allele at chromosome 7q11.23

38.24.4 PHYSICAL FEATURES (FIGURE 38.9)

- Short stature
- Hypercalcaemia (50%)
- Microcephaly (30%)
- Supravalvular aortic stenosis
- Kidney and bladder complications

38.24.5 PSYCHIATRIC FEATURES

- Cocktail-party and hyperverbal speech characterized by fluent and well-articulated speech with overfamiliar manner
- Anxiety
- Fears
- Poor peer relationships
- Hypersensitivity to sound
- Outgoing, sociable, and disinhibited character
- Excessive friendliness

38.24.6 INTELLIGENCE

- Moderate to severe learning disability
- Verbal skills often better than motor and visual–spatial skills

38.24.7 ASSOCIATION

- Anxiety disorder
- Phobia

38.25 DIGEORGE (VELO–CARDIO–FACIAL) SYNDROME

38.25.1 EPIDEMIOLOGY

Incidence: one in 4000 live births

38.25.2 GENETIC DEFECT

Microdeletion in chromosome 22q11.2

38.25.3 INTELLIGENCE

More than 50% of patients have mild to moderate learning disability.

38.25.4 CLINICAL FEATURES (FIGURE 38.10)

- Cardiac abnormalities include tetralogy of Fallot, ventricular septal defect, interrupted aortic arch, and pulmonary atresia.
- Hypocalcaemia.
- Seizures (60%).
- Short stature.

38.25.5 PSYCHIATRIC FEATURES

- There is an increased incidence of schizophrenia.

38.26 RUBINSTEIN—TAYBI SYNDROME

38.26.1 EPIDEMIOLOGY

- Male = female
- Incidence: one in 125,000

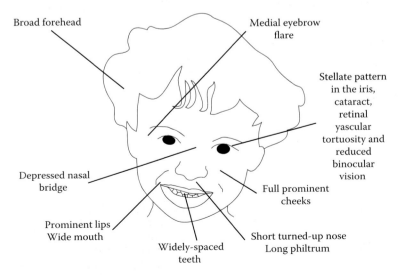

FIGURE 38.9 Facial features (elfin face) of Williams syndrome.

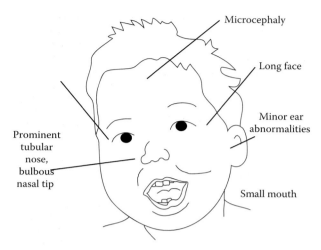

FIGURE 38.10   Facial features of DiGeorge (velo–cardio–facial) syndrome.

38.26.2   MODE OF INHERITANCE

- Autosomal dominant transmission
- Microdeletions in chromosome 16p13.3

38.26.3   CLINICAL FEATURES (FIGURE 38.11)

- Feeding difficulties in infancy
- Congenital heart disease
- EEG abnormalities and seizure

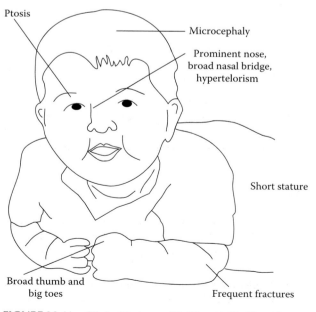

FIGURE 38.11   Clinical features of Rubinstein–Taybi syndrome.

38.26.4   PSYCHIATRIC FEATURES

- Happy, loving, and sociable personality in childhood
- Mood lability and temper tantrums when patient gets older
- Poor concentration
- Distractibility
- Expressive language difficulties
- Self-stimulating behaviour
- Obsessive–compulsive disorder

38.26.5   INTELLIGENCE

- Performance IQ > verbal IQ

38.27   SMITH–MAGENIS SYNDROME

38.27.1   CASE HISTORY

A 4-year-old boy presents with poor attention, over-activity, and bruxism. He has history of chronic otitis media and conductive and sensorineural deafness. He also exhibits stereotyped self-hugging and self-injurious behaviour including skin picking, pulling out nails, biting, and slapping. During the interview, he licks his fingers initially. Then he finds a book in the consultation room and repeatedly licks and flips the pages (lick and flip). His mother reports that he has insomnia at night and feeling sleepy in the day time.

38.27.2   EPIDEMIOLOGY

1/25,000

38.27.3   GENETIC DEFECT

Complete or partial deletion of chromosome 17p11.2

38.27.4   CLINICAL FEATURES (FIGURE 38.12)

- Hearing problems
- Hoarse and deep voice
- Renal problems
- Inguinal/umbilical hernia
- Hypospadias (10% of male patients)
- Short, broad hands and small toes
- Hypotonia
- Hyperextensible fingers

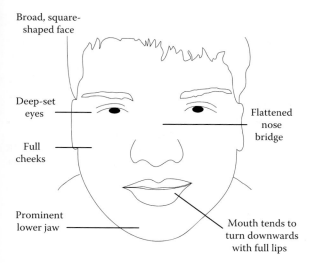

FIGURE 38.12   Facial features of Smith–Magenis syndrome.

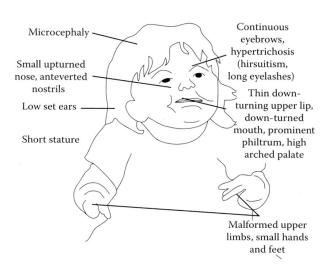

FIGURE 38.13   Facial features of Cornelia de Lange syndrome.

38.27.5   PSYCHIATRIC FEATURES

- Schizophrenia like psychosis
- Inappropriate affect
- Aggression
- Seep disturbance (decreased REM sleep)
- Self-harm (pulling out finger and toenails)

38.27.6   INTELLIGENCE

Moderate to severe learning disability

38.27.7   TREATMENT

Naltrexone is useful in reducing self-injurious behaviour.

38.28   CORNELIA DE LANGE SYNDROME

38.28.1   EPIDEMIOLOGY

One in 40,000 to 1 in 100,000; males = females

38.28.2   GENETIC MECHANISM

Mutations in chromosome 5p; production of plasma protein A (PAPPA) and associated with infertility

38.28.3   CLINICAL FEATURES (FIGURE 38.13)

38.28.4   PSYCHIATRIC FEATURES

Autistic behaviour, self-injury, language delays, limited speech in severe cases, feeding difficulties, avoidance of being held, stereotypic movements, temper tantrums, and mood disorders

38.28.5   INTELLIGENCE

Severe to profound learning disability

38.28.6   COMORBIDITY

Obsessive–compulsive disorder, gastrointestinal problems, congenital heart defects, visual and hearing problems, skin problems, epilepsy, and death in infancy

38.29   FETAL ALCOHOL SYNDROME

38.29.1   EPIDEMIOLOGY

- Variable incidence
- Leading cause of learning disability in Western countries
- One in 3000 live births in Western countries

38.29.2   PATHOGENESIS

- It is not known whether the amount, frequency, or timing of alcohol consumption during pregnancy causes a difference in the degree of damage.
- Mothers consuming more than 100 g/week (>10 Units/week) in early pregnancy associated with low birth weight.

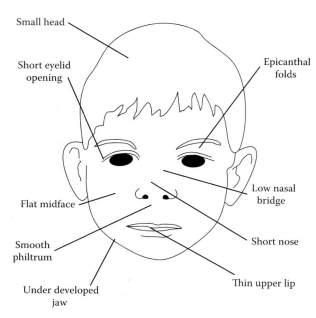

Small head

Short eyelid opening

Epicanthal folds

Flat midface

Low nasal bridge

Smooth philtrum

Short nose

Under developed jaw

Thin upper lip

FIGURE 38.14 Facial features of fetal alcohol syndrome.

38.29.3 CLINICAL FEATURES (FIGURE 38.14)

- Prenatal and postnatal growth retardation
- Retrognathia in infancy
- Micrognathia in adolescence

38.29.4 PSYCHIATRIC FEATURES

- Infants show withdrawal symptoms from birth.
- Irritability during infancy.
- Hyperactivity, hypotonia and poor coordination, distractibility, and poor attention during childhood.
- Memory impairment.

38.29.5 INTELLIGENCE

- Mild to moderate learning disability

BIBLIOGRAPHY

Besler RC and Sudhalter V. 2001: Conversational characteristics of children with fragile X syndrome: Repetitive speech. *American Journal of Mental Retardation* 106:28–38.

Braddock D. 1999: Aging and developmental disabilities: Demographic and policy issues affecting American families. *Mental Retardation* 37:155–161.

Clarke AM, Clarke ADB, and Berg JB (eds.) 1985: *Mental Handicap: The Changing Outlook.* London, U.K.: Methuen.

Day K. 1994: Mental handicap. In Paykel ES and Jenkins R (eds.) *Prevention in Psychiatry*, pp. 130–147. London, U.K.: Gaskell.

Dickinson M and Singh I. 2010: Learning disability psychiatry. In Puri BK and Treasaden IH (eds.) *Psychiatry: An Evidence-Based Text*, pp. 1079–1099. London, U.K.: Hodder Arnold.

Emerson E. 1995: *Challenging Behaviour: Analysis and Intervention in People with Learning Disabilities.* Cambridge, U.K.: Cambridge University Press.

Fraser W. and Kerr M. 2003: *Seminars in the Psychiatry of Learning Disabilities,* 2nd edn. London, U.K.: Gaskell.

Gasson EJ, Sullivan SG, Hussain R. et al. 2002: The changing survival profile of people with Down's syndrome: Implications for genetic counselling. *Clinical Genetics* 62:390–393.

Hangerman RJ, Ono MY, and Hangerman PJ. 2005: Recent advances in fragile X: A model for autism and neurodegeneration. *Current Opinion in Psychiatry* 18:490–496.

Laking PJ. 2002: Psychiatry of disability. In Puri BK, Laking PJ, and Treasaden IH (eds.) *Textbook of Psychiatry*, 2nd edn, pp. 347–362. Edinburgh, Scotland: Churchill Livingstone.

McGuffin P, Owen MJ, O'Donovan MC, Thapar A, and Gottesman II. 1994. *Seminars in Psychiatric Genetics.* London, U.K.: Gaskell.

Roth MP, Feingold J, Baumgarten A et al. 1983: Reexamination of paternal age effect in Down's syndrome. *Human Genetics* 63:149–152.

Russell O. 1985: *Mental Handicap.* Edinburgh, Scotland: Churchill Livingstone.

Sadock BJ and Sadock VA. 2007: *Kaplan & Sadock's Synopsis of Psychiatry. Behavioural Sciences/Clinical Psychiatry*, 10th edn. Philadelphia, PA: Lippincott Williams & Wilkins.

Young ID. 2005: *Medical Genetics.* Oxford, U.K.: Oxford University Press.

39 Old-Age Psychiatry

39.1 EPIDEMIOLOGY

In 2010, 17% of the population was aged 65 and over in the United Kingdom, and the size of ageing population has increased by 20% since 1985. The number of people aged 85 and over is the fastest growing segment of population, and the size has doubled in the past years. By 2035, the number of people aged 85 and over is projected to be almost 2.5 times larger than in 2010, reaching 3.5 million and accounting for 5% of the total population. In 2006, the life expectancies of British at birth were 77.2 years for men and 81.6 years for women. The shorter life expectancy in men is caused by male-predominant risk factors such as alcohol dependence, cardiovascular diseases, motor vehicle accidents, and suicide. Within the elderly population, disability rises steeply with age, from 16 per 1000 who are in their 60s to 133 per 1000 who are aged over 80 (Table 39.1) (Office for National Statistics, 2011).

39.2 PHYSICAL PROCESSES OF AGEING

39.2.1 THEORIES OF AGEING

There are two theories of ageing, Hayflick limit and stochastic damage. The mechanisms and outcomes are summarized in Table 39.2.

39.2.2 GENETIC FACTORS

It is speculated that this effect is caused by the progressive loss of DNA sequences in the telomere involved in the maintenance of DNA stability and replication. Changes in ageing may involve errors in the control of DNA expression, and this is known as epigenetic defects.

39.2.3 NONGENETIC THEORIES

Age-related decline in organ function is no longer thought tenable as a central cause of ageing; it is probably secondary to ageing.

Mitochondrial decline
Across species, mitochondria show a reduction in number, an increase in size, and structural changes in old organisms. Damage to mitochondrial membranes caused by free radicals is thought to contribute to these changes.

Free radical theories
Free radicals commonly result from oxidative reactions in normal cellular processes, particularly in the inner membranes of mitochondria and during phagocytosis. The resulting damage includes lipid peroxidation, which can result in cell death. In animal experiments, antioxidants (free radical scavengers) have been shown to increase life expectancy but not to increase maximum life span, raising doubt about the role of free radicals in the primary ageing process.

The only method proven to increase the maximum life span in experimental animals is calorie restriction. This mechanism is unknown, but it may involve the delayed maturation of the immune system or reduced free-radical damage secondary to reduced metabolic rate.

39.2.4 NEUROBIOLOGY OF AGEING

In normal ageing, there is a slow reduction in weight and volume of the human brain (reduction by 5% by the age of 70, 10% by the age of 80, and 20% by the age of 90), with a proportionate increase in the size of the ventricles and subarachnoid space after the age of 50 years.

The brain is overprovided with neurons, so a loss of neurons does not necessarily result in a loss of function. Some parts of the brain show no loss in the number of neurons with normal ageing (e.g. dentate nucleus of cerebellum). Great losses in neurons and neuron connection are found in the frontal cortex (executive function), hippocampus (memory), locus coeruleus (sleep), and substantia nigra (gait). In normal ageing, especially after the age of 85, a shrinkage of nerve cells is known to occur in the cerebral cortex and putamen.

The rate of loss of nerve cells is around 1% per year after the age of 60. Nerve-cell connections are reduced in some cells with compensatory increases seen in others in normal ageing.

Lipofuscin accumulates in the cytoplasm of nerve cells from childhood.

Tau protein, involved in linking neurofilaments and microtubules, accumulates in a small proportion of ageing nerve cells particularly in the hippocampus and entorhinal cortex, resulting in neurofibrillary tangles (NFTs). NFTs are composed of paired helical filaments with no amyloid. NFTs are found in Alzheimer's

TABLE 39.1

Summary of the Prevalence of Psychiatric Morbidity in Those Aged 65 and Over

Dementia	Delirium	Other Psychiatric Disorders
The prevalence of dementia rises exponentially with age, doubling every 5 years • 1.5% (65–69 years) • 3% (70–74 years) • 6% (75–79 years) • 12% (80–84 years) • 24% (85–89 years) • 48% (90–94 years)	• The 3 year incidence is 13%. • 5%–10% incidence during hospitalization • 6%–14% long-term care home residents • 10%–15% general surgical patients • 10%–20% prevalence at time of admission to a medical unit • 30% cardiac surgery patients • 50% hip fracture patients • 70% intensive care unit patients • 80% palliative patients with advanced cancer	• Depression 13.5% • Phobic disorders 10% • Generalized anxiety 4% • Personality disorder 1% • Paranoid states 0.5% • Panic disorder—rare

TABLE 39.2

Compare and Contrast the Hayflick Limit and Stochastic Damage

	Hayflick Limit	Stochastic Damage
Concept	Programmed ageing	Wear and tear as a result of ageing
Mechanism	1. Human diploid cells cultured in vitro have a finite life span. Upon repeated subculture of normal cells, mitosis ceases independently of culture conditions. 2. This finding suggests that there is a finite number (the Hayflick limit) of subcultivations and the cells cannot divide further. 3. Cells derived from tumour tissue do not display this limit.	1. There is a decline in basic metabolic rate when a person gets older. 2. There is an accumulation of toxic substances (e.g. lipofuscin), leading to free-radical damages in the processing of ageing. 3. The macromolecules distort the physical and chemical properties of a normal human body.
Outcome	• The Hayflick limit causes irreversible cessation of mitosis and, ultimately, the death of an organism. • The Hayflick limit supports the theories of genetically programmed ageing.	• The accumulation of the earlier adverse events in the process of ageing ultimately leads to the end of survival.

disease (AD), normal ageing, progressive supranuclear palsy (PSP), Pick's disease, punch-drunk syndrome (dementia pugilistica), Parkinson's disease, dementia of Lewy bodies (DLB), and Down syndrome. Senile plaques are made up of a core of extracellular amyloid surrounded by abnormal collections of neuritic processes. Senile plaques are formed from an aggregation of beta A4 amyloid. In the normal ageing brain, these are found in the neocortex, amygdala, hippocampus, and entorhinal cortex.

Rod-shaped Hirano bodies are intracellular crystalline deposits and found near the hippocampal pyramidal cells. These comprise the microfilament actin. Accompanying their presence is a granulovacuolar degeneration in the pyramidal nerve cells.

Pick bodies consist of a hyaline eosinophilic mass of neurofilaments, paired helical filaments, endoplasmic reticulum, and microtubules that distend the cytoplasm of affected neurons and displace the nucleus to the periphery. Pick bodies are argyrophilic.

Lewy bodies are hyaline, eosinophilic concentrically laminated inclusions. Lewy bodies are found characteristically in the substantial nigra and locus coeruleus in patients with idiopathic parkinsonism and normal old people. They comprise a spherical body in the cytoplasm of a nerve cell. They have a laminated appearance with a dense granular core and fibrillary material radiating to the periphery, creating a pale peripheral rim.

In normal old brains, amyloid can be found deposited in the walls of blood vessels. Deposits are usually small, widespread, and in superficial cortical and leptomeningeal vessels overlying the cerebral lobes. Amyloid and senile plaques are deposited in irregular patches in the normal ageing cerebral cortex (Table 39.3).

TABLE 39.3

Summary of Histological Changes in Various Types of Dementia

Dementia	AD	Pick's Disease	DLB
Neuro-pathological features	Granulo-vacuolar degeneration (vacuoles in the cytoplasm in the pyramidal cells in hippocampus) Hirano bodies NFTs Senile plaques	Pick bodies Hirano bodies Amyloid deposition NFTs Granulovacuolar degeneration	Lewy bodies DLB is the only dementia that is characterized by inclusion bodies in its pathology

TABLE 39.4

Summary of Changes in Sleep Architecture in Ageing

Sleep Parameters That Increase among Old People	Sleep Parameters That Decrease among Old People
↑ Sleep latency or the time to fall asleep	↓ Duration of slow-wave sleep
↑ Frequency of awakenings at night	↓ Sleep efficiency
↑ Episodes and fragmentation of REM sleep	↓ Total sleep time

39.2.5 CHANGES IN SLEEP ARCHITECTURE

The changes in sleep architecture as a result of ageing are summarized in Table 39.4.

39.3 PSYCHOLOGY OF AGEING

39.3.1 COGNITION

39.3.1.1 Intellectual Functioning

Intelligence peaks at the age of 25 years. It levels off until the age of 60–70 and declines thereafter. Many studies have demonstrated an accelerated decline in cognitive functioning in those who are closest to their death. This has been referred to as the *terminal drop*, and poor health may be the cause.

Using the WAIS-R, a classic pattern of intellectual decline is seen, with performance IQ declining more rapidly than verbal IQ. Factors thought to account for this pattern include the following:

- *Speed of processing.* This makes some contribution to the age-related decline but is not the whole explanation.
- *Familiarity/novelty.* Tasks that have been learnt over a lifetime, relying on overlearned abilities, are most resistant to age-related changes (*crystallized intelligence*). Tasks requiring the less-practised processing of new information are the most sensitive to age-related decline (*fluid intelligence*).

Although intelligence declines with age, there are considerable individual differences.

- *Problem-solving.* The ability to abstract a concept and apply it to a new situation declines with age, most prominently after the age of 70.
- *Creativity.* Scientific creativity peaks in the 30s, whereas artistic creativity peaks in the 50s. Humans seem to be most creative when they are producing the greatest volume of work: intellectual vigour.

39.3.2 PSYCHOMOTOR SPEED

Reaction time increases with age, with most slowing occurring in the central processing of information. Older people are less able to maintain a state of readiness and less likely to choose flexible active information processing than younger people.

39.3.3 MEMORY

- *Short-term memory.* Short-term memory as tested by the digit span does not change with age.
- *Working memory.* Memory tasks requiring monitoring or complex decision-making are performed more poorly in the elderly than in the young. Decline is increased with the complexity of the task or increased memory load.
- *Long-term memory.* The retrieval of information in the elderly is impaired; thus, uncued recall shows an age-related decrement, but cued recall reduces the extent of the decrement. Memory is more durable if it is encoded at a semantic level, rather than at a phonological or orthographic level. Older subjects are less likely to code at the semantic level. Memory performance in the elderly is best if the meaning is easily extracted.

TABLE 39.5

Summary of Changes in Neuropsychological Functions in Elderly

Neuropsychological Functions That Are Preserved in Old People	Neuropsychological Functions That Are Declined in Old People
• Implicit or procedural memory (e.g. riding a bicycle) • Registration • Semantic memory (e.g. crystallized intelligence or factual knowledge) • Short-term recall	• Acquisition of new information • Problem-solving • Fluid intelligence • Retrieval of new information

Memory of source is impaired in the elderly, which is thought to be related to deficits in frontal lobe functioning.

The poorer the memory of distant events becomes, the more remote the patient is from the event.

Retention of knowledge is retained with age. Knowledge-based skills are relatively preserved into old age (Table 39.5).

39.3.4 IMPORTANCE OF LOSS

After the age of 65, the ageing individual increasingly suffers the loss of physical strength, employment, and grief as a result of loss of loved ones through death.

Erikson describes the psychosocial changes that individuals negotiate as they develop. The last of these—*integrity versus despair*—is concerned with the way the individual approaches death. A well-lived life is more likely to result in a sense of integrity and wholeness at this time of reflection upon life achievements. Those with regrets and thoughts of opportunities missed are more likely to approach death with a sense of despair.

39.3.5 PERSONALITY CHANGES

Most studies of personality in older age support the concept of the stability of personality with age.

Adjustment to ageing can be explained by different models, which may apply in different individuals. The activity theory entails the successfully adjusted individual as being fully engaged with life, with interests, and with social contact. The disengagement theory suggests that the individual focuses increasingly on his or her inner world as adjustment is made to diminished family and social roles.

High anxiety levels in the elderly are correlated with physical ill-health, but most chronic neurotic conditions improve in old age. Anxiety-prone personalities arise from a more biological origin, whereas insecure personalities arise more from early environmental events. Dysthymic personalities seem to persist into old age.

39.4 SOCIAL AND ECONOMIC FACTORS IN OLD AGE

39.4.1 ATTITUDES

Western culture and young-/middle-aged adults in Western countries devalue old age, with women perceived more negatively than men. Old women are more likely to live alone and are more likely to be poor.

The majority of old people cope well with ageing, reporting high life satisfaction, good cognitive skills, and openness to new experience. These are considered to display an integrated personality. Those that cope less will display either passive–dependent or disintegrated personalities.

Deviance from social norms generally decreases with age, while the prevalence of stigmatizing conditions increases.

39.4.2 STATUS

As people age, the number of social roles they occupy decreases. This may reduce their social worth. Much of the decline in the status of the elderly is associated with their reduced socioeconomic circumstances.

The status of elderly people is high in preliterate societies and low in modern societies. The factors thought to contribute to this effect include the reduction in the usefulness of the elderly as repositories of knowledge, the breakup of the extended family, and the reduced importance of land inheritance.

39.4.3 RETIREMENT

Retirement in itself is not a cause of increased morbidity. The main problem experienced in retirement is substantial income reduction: the relative value of pensions today has fallen compared with 50 years ago. In 1997, a retiree who had paid £200 a month into a personal pension for 20 years received a typical annuity of £20,500 per year. In 2007, a retiree making the same amount of contributions only received £4,613 per year. The pension received in 2007 was 78% less as compared to 1997 (Barrow, 2007).

39.4.4 ACCOMMODATION

The likelihood that elderly people will live alone and away from their families is relatively common in Britain. The ageing population is living longer and is thus more likely to live alone at some stage in their later years.

For health reasons, large proportions of the very old live in institutional care or with relatives or friends. Old people living alone make more use of statutory services than those living with others.

Disengagement theories hold that older people gradually withdraw from society in preparation for death have now lost favour. Instead, activity theories encourage the maintenance of social interaction and role. Elderly people do maintain a high level of social contact with others. Unhappiness is associated with a lack of friends in a social network.

39.4.5   Sociocultural Differences

39.4.5.1   Social Class

Almost half of pensioners from social classes I and II have money in addition to the state pension, from private pension schemes and savings, compared to only 5% of those in social classes IV and V.

39.4.5.2   Ethnicity

There are competing theories about the effect of ethnicity and ageing:

- The age as leveller hypothesis argues that, because all old people are socially disadvantaged, the relative disadvantage experienced by ethnic minorities reduces in old age.
- The double jeopardy hypothesis argues that disadvantages are exacerbated with age.

Language difficulties are common in ethnic minority groups, and lack of income is most common in Asian people who have travelled from abroad to join their families and lack pension entitlement.

39.5   PSYCHOPHARMACOLOGY OF OLD AGE

39.5.1   Pharmacokinetics and Pharmacodynamics

Age-related changes in drug handling

Changes with ageing that may affect pharmacokinetics include

- ↓ Total body mass
- ↓ Proportion of body mass that is composed of water
- ↓ Proportion of body mass that is composed of muscle

- ↑ Proportion of body mass that is composed of adipose tissue
- ↑ First-pass availability
- ↑ Gastric pH
- ↓ Gastric acid secretion and intrinsic factor (associated with increased risk of vitamin B_{12} deficiency)
- ↓ Rate of gastric emptying
- ↓ Blood flow in splanchnic circulation
- ↓ Gastrointestinal absorptive surface
- Changes in plasma-protein concentration: this may be the result of illness
- ↓ Metabolically active tissue
- ↓ Hepatic mass and blood flow
- ↓ Demethylation
- ↓ Hydroxylation
- ↓ Renal blood flow
- ↓ Glomerular filtration rate and rate of elimination
- ↓ Tubular secretion

39.5.1.1   Absorption

There is no evidence that the rate or extent of absorption of orally administered psychotropic medications is changed in the elderly.

39.5.1.2   Clearance

Reduction in clearance may increase the steady-state plasma drug concentration in old people. Because of lowered renal clearance, lithium doses in the elderly should be approximately 50% lower than in the young. Diuretics may reduce renal clearance even further, increasing the risk of lithium toxicity.

39.5.1.3   Metabolism

All other psychotropic drugs are cleared by hepatic biotransformation, which is variably reduced with age. As a result, the half-life of psychotropic medications (e.g. clonazepam) can be markedly prolonged, having residual effects for weeks after discontinuation.

39.5.1.4   Distribution

This is determined by the drug's relative solubility in lipid as opposed to water, proclivity for various body tissues, and plasma–protein binding. Most psychotropic drugs, being lipophilic, have a relatively small plasma concentration compared to the total amount of drug in the body. Nevertheless, the increased fat over muscle ratio causes lipophilic drugs to have increased distribution volume and risk of accumulation.

39.5.2 Drug Interactions

The incidence of side effects and adverse drug reactions increases with age. For example, the combination of lithium and NSAIDS increases the lithium level in elderly markedly. The causes that may contribute to this include underlying physical illnesses, polypharmacy in old people, poor compliance, reduction of hepatic metabolism, and renal clearance.

39.5.3 Side Effects

Old people are more sensitive to side effects as a result of altered receptor and neurotransmitter function. For example, tricyclic antidepressants are more likely to cause orthostatic hypotension as a result of blocking α_2 adrenergic receptor in elderly. Furthermore, the presence of medical comorbidity may affect their ability to metabolize or tolerate side effects of medications. For example, an old person with chronic obstructive lung disease is less able to tolerate respiratory depression associated with benzodiazepine.

39.5.4 Practical Considerations

Antipsychotics
The elderly are more sensitive to anticholinergic side effects. Parkinsonian side effects are more likely in the elderly, in women, and in those with organic brain disease. The prevalence of tardive dyskinesia increases with age and is more common in women. The length of treatment is more strongly related than the absolute dose. Acute dystonias, although common in the young, are rare in the elderly.

An alert has been issued on the use of antipsychotics in dementia-related psychosis and dementia-related behavioural disturbance because of the increase in mortality and cerebrovascular adverse events compared to placebo.

Prescribers should consider carefully the risk of cerebrovascular events before treating any patient with a previous history of stroke or TIA, hypertension, diabetes, current smoking, and atrial fibrillation.

Tricyclic antidepressants
Heart disease is a relative contraindication. Again, the elderly are particularly prone to postural hypotension and anticholinergic side effects, which may result in acute brain syndromes, urinary retention, and glaucoma.

MAOIs
Extreme caution is needed if considering prescribing these to patients with hypertension and cardiovascular disease.

Benzodiazepines
Accumulation in the elderly is not more likely to occur than in the young. The elderly are at an increased risk of delirium and falls.

39.6 DISTRICT SERVICE PROVISION

39.6.1 Principles of Service Provision

The planning of services for the elderly must take into account the age distribution of the population, including the numbers of the very elderly who are most likely to need the most costly institutional care.

The elderly require accurate medical, psychological, social, and functional assessment; specialist knowledge; least disruptive solutions; and prompt interventions. Informal carers should be considered and supported, and liaison between all aspects of service is paramount.

39.6.2 Needs of Carers

Community care of the mentally ill, especially dementia sufferers, results in significant strain on an informal carer or a very close relative, such as a spouse or a child. Female carers outnumber males 2:1. The carers of demented elderly people have more problems than others, which increase with the degree of dementia.

The sources of stress include

- Practical—for example, elderly person requiring help with personal and household tasks and care
- Behavioural—for example, nocturnal disturbance, incontinence, wandering, and aggression
- Interpersonal
- Social—for example, restrictions on the carer's personal life

39.7 ASSESSMENT OF A REFERRAL

39.7.1 Psychiatric Assessment

The most informative setting for the initial assessment is within the person's home. Coordination is required to ensure that informants are available, and that is essential in those with organic brain syndromes. The interview should be unhurried, allowing the patient to relate a full family and personal history. An assessment of how the patient deals with questioning is made throughout.

The psychiatrist should be vigilant for unrecognized physical illness presenting with psychiatric symptoms and

TABLE 39.6

Information to Be Assessed in a Psychiatric Interview for an Old Person

Source and nature of referral

Who made the referral?

What the referrer wishes to know?

What the patient and the carers have been told to expect?

Description of presenting complaints

Onset, frequency, intensity, duration, location (home, nursing home, etc.)

Antecedents and consequences

Ameliorating and exacerbating factors

---

if this is suspected should ensure that the patient receives the appropriate medical interventions. Examination at home allows an assessment of the patient's coping in the immediate environment, including visuospatial orientation and the ability to manage independently. It also allows assessment of local resources such as neighbours' and relatives' availability and any evidence of the unwise use of alcohol.

If the first assessment occurs on a medical ward as a liaison visit, the medical notes should be read and the medical and nursing staff should be interviewed before the patient is seen. Carers should be contacted to supplement the information gathered on the ward. The patient interview should take place in the most private conditions available (Table 39.6).

Supporting features to suggest underlying medical causes for a psychiatric or cognitive symptom

- History of trauma or exposure to toxic substance
- Presence of focal neurological symptoms
- Rapid onset and progression
- Recent illness or history of chronic illnesses
- Younger age of onset than expected

Description of the elderly current interpersonal relationship and activities of daily living (ADL)

- Behaviours that can jeopardize placement in the community (e.g. day/night reversal, wandering, aggression, sliding or throwing themselves to the floor, stripping off their clothes, and the smearing of faeces)
- Emotions: negative and positive
- Peer and staff relationships for old person who stays in a nursing home facility
- Family relationships for old person who stays at home

- Basic activities of daily livings (BADLs) (mnemonics: DEATH): dressing, eating, ambulation, toileting, and hygiene (Bookman et al., 2007)
- Instrumental activities of daily livings (IADLs) (mnemonics: SHAFT): shopping, housework, accounting, food preparation, and transportation (Bookman et al., 2007).

Past psychiatric history

- Past psychiatric disorders (e.g. schizophrenia, mood disorders, anxiety disorders)
- Current psychiatric medications
- History of heavy drinking, alcohol misuse, substance misuse, and smoking
- Premorbid personality

Past medical history

- The history of chronic medical illnesses, for example, diabetes, cardiovascular diseases, and metabolic syndrome
- The history of neurological disorders, for example, Parkinson's disease, multiple sclerosis, epilepsy, and cerebrovascular accidents (CVAs)
- The history of head injury and related operations
- Current medications

39.7.1.1 Mental State Examination

Appearance and behaviour

- Careful observation is important in a person with difficulties with verbal exchange (e.g. severe dementia, delirium, aphasia, severe hearing and/or visual impairments).
- Observe for signs of psychomotor retardation or agitation, perplexity, or behavioural disturbance.
- Poor hygiene, incontinence, or inadequate nutrition gives an indication of the patient's ability to live independently.
- An inability to focus or sustain attention appropriately may be a sign of clouded consciousness.

Speech: Cognitive impairment may result in circumlocution, paraphrasia, and polite evasions hiding a lack of depth and detail in speech.

Thought patterns of early dementia include a repetition of themes, a lack of internal logic, and a limitation of discussion inconsistent with the level of intelligence.

Mood: Depression or mania that can be easily missed.

Hallucinations and delusions

- Auditory hallucinations are less descriptive and contain less details when compared to those reported by young schizophrenia patients.
- Visual hallucinations may suggest dementia with Lewy bodies (DLB).
- Paranoid delusion is common among old people.

Physical examination

- Check the person's temperature (using a low-reading thermometer).
- Check the state of hydration if clouding of consciousness is suspected.
- The presence of hemiparesis may suggest large-vessel infarct.
- The presence of parkinsonism may suggest DLB.
- Pseudobulbar palsy is found in patients with human immunodeficiency virus (HIV)-associated dementia, PSP, vascular dementia (VaD), and Parkinson's disease.
- Tremors and involuntary movements (e.g. be alert to the possibility of a cerebrovascular event, the onset of Huntington's or Wilson's disease, or, more commonly, L-dopa for Parkinson's disease).
- Check gait that may indicate fall risk. Gait changes occur in chronic alcoholism, DLB, normal-pressure hydrocephalus, multiple sclerosis, Parkinson's disease dementia, tertiary syphilis, and VaD.
- Myoclonus is found in HIV-associated dementia and Creutzfeldt–Jakob disease (CJD).
- Primitive reflexes and frontal release signs are found in patients with frontotemporal lobe dementia (FTD). Examples include the palmomental reflex, grasp reflex, pout reflex, sucking reflex, and glabellar tap.
- Check visual or hearing impairments.

The NICE guidelines recommend that clinical cognitive assessment should include the examination on attention, concentration, orientation, short- and long-term memory, praxis, language, and executive function (Table 39.7). Standardized instruments for formal cognitive testing include the mini-mental state examination (MMSE), Addenbrooke's Cognitive Examination Revised (ACE-R), Montreal Cognitive Assessment (MoCA), Clinical Dementia Rating Scale (CDRS), General Practitioner Assessment of Cognition (GPCOG), 6-Item Cognitive Impairment Test (6-CIT), and 7 Minute Screen. Patients with learning disability require different tests such as dementia questionnaire for mentally retarded person or dementia scale for Down

---

TABLE 39.7

Information to Be Assessed during Cognitive Examination

- Orientation—to time, place, and person
- Attention and concentration—assessed using 'serial sevens' or naming months of the year backward if numerical abilities are not good
- Immediate memory—assessed using digit span
- Short-term verbal memory—assessed using name and address with six parts, repeated immediately to assess registration, then again after 5 min with intervening distraction to prevent rehearsal, also using Babcock sentence
- Short-term nonverbal memory—assessed by immediate recall (registration) of a geometric shape, then recall after 5 min with intervening distraction to prevent rehearsal
- Long-term memory—assessed during history taking (ask date and place of birth)
- General knowledge—assessed by asking historical and recent commonly known facts (e.g. the current prime minister, monarch and family, the President of the United States, the colours of the Union Jack, the names of capital cities)
- Verbal fluency—number of words beginning with T in 1 min or the number of four-legged animals in 1 min
- Calculation—assessed by asking a simple calculation such as a subtraction
- Writing
- Spatial—including bodily awareness
- Recognition—of objects and faces
- Appropriate use of everyday objects
- Naming things—to detect nominal dysphasia
- Receptive and expressive use of written and spoken language
- Perseveration—suggestive of frontal lobe dysfunction
- Tests of praxis—such as drawing a square or a clock face (constructional apraxia) and asking the patient to make a fist, oppose thumb and little finger, fold a piece of paper, and place it in an envelope
- Tests of gnosis—such as picture recognition, tactile recognition

---

syndrome. Cambridge Cognition Examination (CAMCOG) is a neuropsychological screening instrument used in the United Kingdom. CAMCOG is part of Cambridge Mental Disorders of the Elderly Examination (CAMDEX). CAMDEX incorporates the MMSE, Blessed Dementia Rating Scale and Hachinski Ischaemic Score, National Adult Reading Test (NART), Kendrick Object Learning Test for memory, and Wisconsin Card Sorting Test for executive function. Detailed psychometrics may be necessary if screening tests are positive (Table 39.8).

39.7.2   Investigations

Routine investigations in the hospitalized elderly should include full blood count (FBC) with differential white

TABLE 39.8

Compare and Contrast MMSE, ACE-R, MoCA, and Clinical Dementia Rating Scale

	MMSE (Folstein et al., 1975)	ACE-R (Mioshi et al., 2006)	MoCA (Nasreddine et al., 2005)	Clinical Dementia Rating Scale (CDRS) (Morris, 1993)
Person(s) assessed	Patient only	Patient only	Patient only	Patient and carer
Components and domains	1. Orientation	1. Orientation	1. Orientation	1. Memory
	2. Registration and recall	2. Registration	2. Attention	2. Orientation
	3. Attention and calculation	3. Attention	3. Memory	3. Judgement
	4. Language	4. Recall	4. Executive function (verbal fluency, abstract thinking)	4. Community affairs
	5. Visuospatial ability	5. Anterograde and retrograde memory	5. Visuospatial abilities	5. Home and hobbies
	6. Praxis	6. Verbal fluency	6. Attention and calculation	6. Personal care
	MMSE is lack of frontal lobe assessment	7. Language (writing, comprehension, reading, naming)	7. Language	
		8. Visuospatial ability		
		9. Perceptual abilities		
		10. Recognition		
Time required	10–15 min	10–15 min	10–15 min	30 min
Scoring	Normal score >24 (sensitivity = 0.44–1; specificity = 0.46–1) Score is determined by education. For patients with only primary school education, the following cutoffs are used: Ages 18–69: median MMSE score 22–25; ages 70–79: median MMSE score 21–22; age over 79: median MMSE score 19–20	Two cutoffs were defined: 88: sensitivity = 0.94, specificity = 0.89 and 82: sensitivity = 0.84, specificity = 1.0	Normal score >26 (sensitivity = 1, specificity = 0.87) AD: 11–21	The score is calculated based on an algorithm. Normal: 0 Possible dementia: 0.5 Mild dementia: 1 Moderate dementia: 2 Severe dementia: 3
Mild cognitive impairment (MCI)	Normal score >24	MCI patients to be impaired in areas (e.g. attention/orientation, verbal fluency, and language) other than memory	Score between 21 and 26	Not applicable

cell count (WCC), erythrocyte sedimentation rate (ESR), urea and electrolytes (U&E), creatinine, liver function tests (LFTs) with calcium and proteins, glucose, TSH, electrocardiogram (ECG), chest x-ray (CXR), and a midstream urine examination.

The prevalence of thyroid disease increases in old age. Physical signs are often unreliable in the elderly, so TSH screening should be performed in all. Hyperthyroidism can be mistaken for anxiety states, hypomania, or delirium. Hypothyroidism can present as depression with psychomotor retardation, dementia, or delirium.

A CXR is required in all sick elderly people, even if the chest is apparently clear on physical examination. Pneumonia, tuberculosis, and carcinoma can all present with acute confusional states or depression. An ECG is also required because some psychotropic medications may prolong the corrected QT (QTc) interval.

39.7.3 STRUCTURAL IMAGING

In normal ageing, there is progressive cortical atrophy and increasing ventricular size. Imaging can identify potentially treatable intracranial lesions. The indications for imaging in a person present with cognitive impairment are summarized as follows (Clair and Seitz, 2011):

- Age of patient: younger than 60 years
- Duration of cognitive impairment: short duration
- Focal neurological sign: urinary incontinence and gait disorder
- History of anticoagulant use, bleeding disorders, head injury, and cancer
- Onset of cognitive impairment: rapid decline (e.g. 1–2 months)
- Specific symptoms: frontal lobe signs, progressive aphasia, new onset headache, and seizure

Conventional structural imaging is helpful in discovering the aetiology of dementia, although it does not establish the diagnosis, which is determined clinically. The distribution of cerebral atrophy helps to distinguish different types of dementia.

Recently, fludeoxyglucose 18F (FDG) is one of the most commonly used radiotracers in imaging. It is an analogue of glucose and concentrated in metabolically active tissue such as the brain. After absorbed in cells, phosphorylation prevents the glucose from being released from the cell. Fluoro-2-deoxy-D-glucose-positron emission tomography (FDG-PET) is more sensitive than SPECT in separating normal elderly individuals from dementia patients when areas in the temporoparietal and posterior cingulate are scanned. Changes on FDG-PET scans appear closely related to histopathological changes (Table 39.9).

39.7.4 ELECTROENCEPHALOGRAPHY

In normal ageing (after the age of 60), the following changes occur in the Electroencephalography (EEG):

- Slowing of α rhythm
- Increased θ activity particularly in the left temporal region
- Increased δ activity particularly in the anterior regions
- Diminished β activity (only in those aged over 80)

39.7.4.1 Dementias

In Alzheimers disease (AD), the EEG may be normal (6%) or show minor nonspecific changes. The following changes may occur:

- Diffuse slowing in early stages
- Reduced α and β activity, plus increased θ and δ activity as the disease progresses
- Paroxysmal bifrontal δ waves (more common than in normal ageing)

TABLE 39.9

Comparison of Different Imaging Modalities in Old-Age Psychiatry

Imaging Targets	Brain Volume and Structural Changes	Oxidative Metabolism	Glucose Metabolism
Clinical examples	• Normal-pressure hydrocephalus: enlarged ventricles without cortical atrophy • Huntington's disease: gross shrinkage of the caudate nucleus • Lacunes • White matter hyperintensities	• Differentiating AD, VaD, and FTD • Assessing synaptic strength (e.g. protein synthesis, axonal transport, and synaptogenesis)	• Detecting changes in radioligands in specific areas of the brain affected by AD
Imaging methods	• CT and MRI are useful in detecting clinically significant structural lesions • MRI has better resolution than CT	• SPECT is 85% accurate in differentiating AD, FTD, and VaD	• FDG-PET

In Pick's disease, the EEG is more likely than in AD to be normal and shows less slowing of the a waves.

In VaD, the tracing shows asymmetry and localized slow waves, with a sparing of background activity.

In CJD, a slow background rhythm with paroxysmal sharp waves is characteristic.

In Huntington's disease, a low-voltage pattern may be seen.

39.7.4.2 Delirium

Most conditions causing delirium cause slowing of the EEG tracing:

1. Metabolic causes
   a. Hepatic encephalopathy—slowing of rhythm with posterior preservation; triphasic waves are highly indicative.
   b. Acute renal failure—low-voltage activity with posterior slowing.
   c. Bursts of θ activity.

d. Hypocalcaemia—slowing with bursts of spikes.

e. Hypercalcaemia—runs of 1–2 s waves.

f. Hyperthyroidism—acceleration of a rhythm.

g. Hypothyroidism—low-voltage EEG.

2. Drugs

a. Phenothiazines increase voltage, slow α activity, and reduce β activity; in overdose, paroxysmal slow waves are characteristic.

b. Antidepressants increase EEG activity but reduce a rhythm; in overdose, widespread a activity and spikes.

c. Benzodiazepines—increase β waves, especially frontal; in overdose, prominent fast activity unresponsive to stimuli.

d. Lithium—slow α rhythm with occasional, sometimes focal, spikes; in overdose, diffuse slowing, triphasic waves, and paroxysmal abnormalities.

Of those with delirium, 90% of patients have abnormal traces. Delta activity, asymmetry in δ waves, and localized spike and sharp wave complexes occur more frequently in those with intracranial pathology. Alpha activity correlates with cognitive functioning, and δ activity correlates with the length of illness.

39.7.5   Psychological Assessment

39.7.5.1   Psychometric Testing and Measures of Function

Psychometric testing quantifies the level and range of ability. Serial measures can be used to monitor the effect of interventions or to measure progress of the patient's condition over time. It is essential, when any particular test is used in the elderly, that both the test itself and its predictions have been validated in the local elderly population.

Psychometric measures of function are used to clarify the diagnosis, to predict outcome, to predict need, and to monitor change:

- *Clarifying the diagnosis*: Batteries of tests have been devised to distinguish between different diagnostic groups: the Kendrick Battery was developed to distinguish normal, functionally impaired, and demented elderly groups. The Geriatric Depression Scale (GDS) is a 30-item self-administered rating scale, with cut-off score determining whether depressed (extensively validated and highly discriminant).

- *Predicting outcome*: Various scales, such as the Clifton Assessment Procedures for the Elderly (CAPE), can predict survival, placement, and decline in elderly subjects. The Kew Cognitive Map assesses parietal lobe function and language functions in the dementing patient. This successfully predicts 6 month survival (McDonald, 1969).

- *Predicting need*: The CAPE assesses the level of disability and thus allows for prediction of need for support services. Identification of impairments allows for interventions that may overcome the problems posed by the impairment. Assessments can be used to provide objective evidence for allocation of resources.

- *Monitoring change*: The NART is used to determine premorbid IQ, thus aiding in the initial assessment of apparent cognitive impairment. Premorbid function is compared to current functioning using the Wechsler Adult Intelligence Scale (WAIS).

Repeating tests over time can give an estimate of deterioration, but this can be unreliable since even the elderly with dementia can show practise effects with repeated testing.

39.7.5.2   Experiential Assessment and Analysis of Function

Experimental assessment tries to clarify the nature of impairment. By understanding the nature of the impairment, it is possible to develop interventions that ameliorate the impairment.

Experiential analysis of function is used to explain dysfunction and to develop strategies for intervention.

- *Explaining dysfunction*. A finding in a psychometric test may conclude that a patient is unable to carry out a task but does not try to establish why. The decomposition of impaired performance is used to establish which ability is impaired. A hypothesis of what the disability comprises is tested before a conclusion is reached.

- *Developing strategies for interventions*. A behavioural approach may be used with an ABC (antecedents, behaviour, and consequences) analysis before attempting an intervention.

39.7.5.2.1   Social Assessment

Assessment is usually conducted by a social worker. This involves a detailed assessment of living conditions, personal care, dynamics of family/carer, support network, financial situation, family structure, level of independence, and physical functioning in the person's environment.

39.7.5.2.2 Occupational Therapy Assessment

Occupational therapy assessment provides a baseline of functioning in areas of basic and instrumental ADLs. An important part of the assessment is to identify strengths that can be built on to overcome deficits. The best place to conduct ADL assessments is within the person's own home, as early in the illness as possible in order to establish baselines. ADL assessment is invaluable in helping to establish the most appropriate placement on discharge and to determine those packages of care that are most likely to enable ongoing independent living.

39.8 PSYCHOLOGICAL REACTIONS TO PHYSICAL DISEASE

Theories of 'successful ageing' maintain that elderly people select a range of activities they want or need to do, then optimize their performance of these activities, and compensate for losses of physical or mental abilities.

39.8.1 Adjusting to Physical Illness

Several factors contribute to the experience of a physical illness:

- The meaning of the illness, both generally and specifically to that patient
- The response of those close to the patient
- Physical symptoms
- Social consequences of the illness
- Coincidental life events and difficulties

39.8.2 Responses to Physical Illness

There are three components to coping style:

- The exercise of autonomy and independence
- The sense of personal responsibility or locus of control
- Activity versus passivity

Psychiatric disorder may arise as a consequence of the stresses imposed by the physical condition, but it may also arise as a direct physical consequence of the pathological process. For example,

- Hyperthyroidism may give rise to an anxiety state.
- Hypercalcemia, infection, hypoxia, or organ failure may give rise to delirium.
- Steroids may give rise to depression, elation, or emotionalism.
- Frontal lobe lesions are likely to result in apathy.

39.8.3 Psychiatric Consequences of Specific Physical Disorders

39.8.3.1 Cerebrovascular Disease

Mood disorders may follow a stroke. These are mixed and affect different patients differently. General dysphoria and worry are common. Poststroke depression and anxiety are recognized. Mania following stroke is described but uncommon. Apathy and social withdrawal are seen in the absence of depression.

Syndromes more characteristic of stroke include emotional lability and the denial of handicap (anosognosia).

39.8.3.2 Sensory Impairment

Most commonly seen are impairments of hearing and/or vision. These have a dramatic impact upon the individual's ability to communicate with others, which may cause social withdrawal, reduced activity, and apparent cognitive decline. They may increase the risks of depression and paraphrenia in the elderly although this is not proven.

39.9 MILD COGNITIVE IMPAIRMENT (MCI)

39.9.1 Epidemiology

- The conversion rate from normal ageing to Mild cognitive impairment (MCI) is around 15%.
- The conversion rate from MCI to dementia is around 5%–10% per year.

39.9.2 Pathology

- Atrophy of hippocampus
- Beta-amyloid deposition
- Depression
- Vascular atherosclerotic changes

39.9.3 Clinical Features

- MMSE: 24–30.
- Subjective complaint of memory loss.
- Objective evidence of cognitive impairment.
- Decline from previously normal level of function.
- Preserve basic ADL.
- No underlying medical or surgical conditions causing reversible dementia.
- Cognitive impairments are not severe to meet the diagnostic criteria for dementia (Table 39.10).

TABLE 39.10

Classification of MCI

MCI (Amnesic Type)	MCI (Nonamnestic Type)
This is the most common form and manifests as preclinical manifestation of AD. Patients present with impaired performance on delayed recall. There is objective evidence of impairment of short-term memory, but general cognitive functions are normal. There is no substantial interference with work, usual social activities, or other ADLs. There is absence of the diagnosis of dementia. Amnestic MCI has higher chance to convert to dementia compared to nonamnestic MCI.	Nonamnestic MCI may involve multiple cognitive domains (e.g. executive function) rather than amnesia. This type of MCI manifests as localized impairment of other cognitive domains rather than memory. Nonamnestic MCI may develop into non-Alzheimer's dementias.

Source: Loewenstein, D.A. et al., *Dementia and Geriatric Cognitive Disorders*, 27, 418, 2009.

39.9.4 TREATMENT

- Cognitive rehabilitation
- Physical exercise and healthy lifestyle
- Treat underlying vascular risk factors (e.g. hypertension, hyperlipidaemia)
- Treat underlying depression
- Yearly follow-up on instrumental ADL and cognition

39.10 DEMENTIA IN OLD AGE

Dementia is defined as a global deterioration in brain functions in clear consciousness, which is usually progressive and irreversible. It results in the deterioration of all higher brain functions including memory, thinking, orientation, comprehension, calculation, the capacity to learn, language, and judgement and is accompanied by deterioration in emotional control, behaviour, and motivation.

The dementias become more prevalent with increasing age. The most common dementia in the elderly is AD (50%), followed by mixed AD and VaD (15%), VaD (5%), frontotemporal dementia (FTD) (10%), DLB (2%), and other types of dementia (18%).

Dementia can be broadly classified into cortical and subcortical dementia. Cortical dementias arise from the cerebral cortex, which plays a key role in memory and language. AD, frontal lobe dementia, and CJD are examples of cortical dementia. Subcortical dementias result from dysfunction in neuroanatomical structures that are beneath the cortex. Memory impairments and language difficulties are not the early signs of subcortical dementias. Examples of subcortical dementias include HIV-related dementia, Huntington's chorea, and Parkinson's disease. Examples of mixed cortical and subcortical dementias include VaD, DLB, and neuropsychiatric sequelae after carbon monoxide poisoning (Table 39.11).

The DSM-5 (APA 2013) classifies dementia into major and minor neurocognitive disorders. Major neurocognitive disorder involves significant decline from previous level of cognitive performance and

TABLE 39.11

Compare and Contrast Cortical and Subcortical Dementia

	Cortical Dementia	Subcortical Dementia
Classical symptoms	• The 'A's': amnesia, agnosia, acalculia, apraxia, and aphasia	• The 'D's': dysexecutive function, dysarthria, and depression
Memory deficits	• Primarily a storage and recall deficit	• Forgetfulness or failure of retrieval is initially amenable to prompting
Executive dysfunction	• Late executive function impairment (except FTD)	• Early executive function impairment
Gnostic–practic abilities	• Agnosia, acalculia, and apraxia are common	• Agnosia, acalculia, and apraxia are less common
Language	• Aphasia	• Dysarthria
Movement	• Fine and gross movements are generally preserved until later in the course of dementia	• Abnormal movements are common and manifest as a slowing or as chorea or tremor early in the course of dementia
Personality	• Personality often remains intact or displays minor variations (except FTD)	• Personality change is often marked
Affective expression	• Affective expression is generally preserved	• Major depression or mania occurs frequently

interference with ADL. Minor neurocognitive disorder is associated with mild cognitive decline and no interference with ADL.

39.10.1 Risk and Protective Factors for Dementia

See Table 39.12.

39.10.2 Alzheimer's Disease

39.10.2.1 Aetiology

39.10.2.1.1 Neurotransmitter Abnormalities

Of most interest is the loss of cholinergic neurons in basal forebrain, low cortical cholinergic activity, and reduced choline acetyltransferase especially in the temporal cortex. This is thought to be secondary to the degeneration of neurons in the nucleus basalis of Meynert, which provides the cortex with its cholinergic projection.

Other neurochemical changes in AD include

- ↓ Dopamine beta-hydroxylase.
- ↓ Dopamine.
- ↓ Noradrenaline and serotonin in the cortex.
- ↓ Cortico-neuropeptides such as somatostatin.
- ↑ Glutamate and hyperexcitation leads to neuronal toxicity and impair learning.

39.10.2.1.2 Genetic Factors

Genetic factors must account for the disease in some patients. It is familial in some families, especially those in which the onset is early (under 65, presenile dementia). The finding of AD in many patients with Down syndrome who reach middle age has focused interest on chromosome 21 on which is located the amyloid precursor protein (APP) gene. The following genes are involved:

- APP gene on chromosome 21 (accounting for 20% early-onset AD)
- Presenilin 1 (PS 1) gene on chromosome 14 (presenilin is implicated in β-amyloid production and accounting for 70% early-onset AD)
- Presenilin 2 (PS2) gene on chromosome 1

It is also hypothesized that late-onset AD is an autosomal-dominant trait with age-dependent expression and low penetrance, resulting in apparent sporadic cases.

39.10.2.1.3 Environmental Factors

Aluminium. The brains of those with AD contain more total aluminium than those of controls. Aluminium is found in the areas of the brain most affected in AD, particularly in the neurons containing tangles and in the core of senile plaques. Those receiving haemodialysis accumulate aluminium from the dialysate. Before this was recognized, patients developed severe dementia. Steps are now taken to reduce the burden of aluminium accumulation in those receiving haemodialysis. Aluminium probably accumulates in the brains of those with AD secondary to the disease process rather than being directly causative. It remains possible that aluminium is a contributory factor in some cases of AD.

Head injury. In sporadic AD, there is an increased risk in those who have experienced head injury within the preceding 10 years.

Infection. It is hypothesized that an infectious agent entering via the transolfactory route may be responsible for some cases of AD. Herpes simplex type 1 is known to have a predilection for those brain areas particularly affected in AD and is suspected by some as a possible cause. However, this remains speculative.

39.10.2.2 Neuropathology

The neuropathological findings in AD include (Graham et al., 2006)

- *Amyloid deposition*: Amyloid deposition is predisposed by apolipoprotein E e4 allele on chromosome 19. Amyloid is deposited as extracellular

---

TABLE 39.12

Classification of Risk and Protective Factors of Dementia

Modifiable Risk Factors	Nonmodifiable Risk Factors	Protective Factors
Endocrine: history of diabetes	Demographics: advanced age and female gender	Bilingualism
Lifestyle: exposure to pesticides, lack of physical activity, repetitive head injury, and smoking	Genetics: Apolipoprotein E4 on chromosome 19; abnormalities in chromosomes 1, 14, and 21; and family history of dementia	Cognitive engagement and late retirement
Psychiatric: history of depressive disorder		Fish intake (more than once a week)
Vascular: hypertension, hyperlipidaemia, high homocysteine levels, and stroke	Intelligence: low intelligence and limited education	High level of education (longer than 15 years)
	History of MCI	High level of physical activities (more than three times a week)
		Use of NSAIDs and statin

plaques that comprise a central core of amyloid, silica, and aluminium. These plaques are found in the neocortex (layer 3 and 4), amygdala, hippocampus, and entorhinal cortex. The amyloid deposition in the walls of blood vessels leads to amyloid angiopathy. The brain of a patient with AD has more than 10 plaques/mm^2.

- *NFTs*: Intracytoplasmic NFTs are found in the cortex, hippocampus, substantia nigra, and locus coeruleus. The diagnostic significance of amyloid plaques is greater than that of the tangles.
- Granulovacuolar degeneration of the neurons is caused by inflammation.
- *Hirano bodies*: Rod-shaped actin found in hippocampal pyramidal cells.
- *Neuronal losses*: There is significant loss of neurons in the brains of AD patients compared to controls. Most neuronal loss is found in the superior, middle, and inferior frontal gyri; superior and middle temporal gyri; and the cingulate gyrus.

39.10.2.3   Clinical Features

AD is a diagnosis that can be made with accuracy only at postmortem. However, it is possible to make a reasonably accurate diagnosis on the basis of clinical findings (Table 39.13).

39.10.2.4   Diagnostic Criteria (Table 39.14)

Behavioural and psychiatric symptoms (BPSDs) associated with AD (Butler and Pit, 1998):

- *Psychiatric symptoms*: paranoid delusions (15% of AD patients), hallucinations (10%–15% of AD patients, with visual hallucinations being more common than auditory hallucinations).
- *Behavioural disturbances*: aggression, wandering, explosive temper, sexual disinhibition, and searching behaviour.
- *Personality changes*: exaggeration of premorbid personality.

TABLE 39.13
Summary of Clinical Features of AD in Different Stage of the Illness

Early Stage—Until About 2 Years	Intermediate Stage	Late Stage	Final Stage
• Impaired concentration • Memory impairment • Fatigue and anxiety • Fleeting depression of mood • Exaggeration of preexisting personality traits • Unusual incidents cause increasing concern • Occasional difficulty with word finding • Altered handwriting • Perseveration of words and phrases	• Further deterioration in the aforementioned • Neurological abnormalities start to appear • 5%–10% develop epilepsy • Apraxias and agnosias develop • Disorientation in time and space • Get lost in familiar surroundings • Speech problems with nominal dysphasia, receptive dysphasia, expressive dysphasia, dysarthria, and reduced vocabulary • Groping for words, mispronunciation, reiteration of parts of words (logoclonia), and echolalia • Reduced ability to read and write • Concurrent progressive memory loss involving recent and past events • Misidentification (e.g. mirror sign) • Emotional lability • Catastrophic reaction (extreme anxiety and tearfulness when unable to complete a task) • Motor restlessness or inertia	• All intellectual functions grossly impaired • Considerable neurological disability • Increased muscle tone • Wide-based unsteady gait • Personality changes, often with fatuous gross euphoria • No communication • Failure to recognize self or family • Speech replaced by jargon dysphasia	• No personality • No communication • Emaciated • Incontinent • Limb contractures • Death often from pneumonia and inanition

TABLE 39.14

Compare and Contrast the ICD-10 and NINCDS–ADRDA Criteria

ICD-10 Criteria for Dementia in AD (F00) (WHO, 1992)	NINCDS–ADRDA Criteria for AD (Blacker et al., 1994)
1. A decline in memory that is most evident of learning new information Recall of learnt information is affected in severe cases. This impairment applies to both verbal and nonverbal materials.	1. Cognitive deficits are affected in more than two areas: amnesia plus one or more additional features (aphasia, apraxia, agnosia, executive dysfunction).
2. A decline in judgement, thinking, planning, and organizing.	2. No disturbance of consciousness.
3. Awareness of environment and consciousness are preserved.	3. Resultant disability.
4. Decline in emotional control and motivation (emotional lability, irritability, apathy, and coarsening of social behaviour).	4. Gradual onset and progressive deterioration.
5. Dementia is classified as mild (able to live independently), moderate (dependent on others in ADL), and severe (unable to retain information and absence of intelligence).	5. No systemic disorders or exclusion of other general medical conditions.
6. Exclude other causes of dementia.	6. Dementia does not occur exclusively during delirium.
7. ICD-10 classifies DAT as early onset (<65 years old) and late onset (>65 years old).	7. Exclude other mental disorders.
	The age of the patient is expected to be between 40 and 90 years.

NINCDS–ADRDA: National Institute of Neurological and Communicative Disorders and Stroke and the Alzheimer's Disease and Related Disorders Association.

- *Orientation:* if disorientation occurs, it is more common for time than for place.
- *Neurological features*: epilepsy (75%) and extrapyramidal symptoms (60%).
- *Sleep disturbance*: reduction of REM sleep, frequent nocturnal waking periods, and shortened sleep periods.

39.10.2.5 Investigations

Memory assessment service should be the single point of referral for all people with a possible diagnosis of AD. Routine blood tests should include FBC, C-reactive protein, ESR, vitamin B_{12}, folate, fasting lipid and glucose, calcium, LFTs, renal function tests (RFTs), and thyroid function tests (TFTs). These tests would help to identify reversible causes of dementia. Clinicians are advised not to routinely order VDRL, HIV, and cerebrospinal fluid (CSF) analysis unless there are indications. A midstream urine test should be ordered if delirium is a possibility. CXR and ECG are ordered if there are indications.

Imaging (McMahon et al., 2003; Petrella et al., 2003)

- CT scans of brain do not reliably differentiate normals from those with AD, with approximately 20% overlap between these groups. Generally, cortical atrophy and ventricular enlargement are greater than in controls, with increasing cognitive dysfunction correlating with increasing cerebral atrophy, but more so with increasing ventricular size. An increase in ventricular size over a span of 1 year is suggestive of AD.
- The clinical usefulness of neuroimaging can be improved by using a temporal lobe orientation in CT scanning, which allows an accurate measurement of the medial temporal lobe. In AD, a dramatic thinning of the width of the medial temporal lobe in the region of the brain stem is seen.
- Magnetic resonance imaging (MRI) scan may reveal atrophy of the hippocampus. MRI is the preferred modality to assist with early diagnosis or detect subcortical vascular changes.
- PET scan may show reduced O_2 and glucose uptake in parietal and temporal lobes.
- SPECT scans also reveal significantly reduced parietotemporal perfusion in these subjects. Combining SPECT scans with temporal-lobe-oriented CT scans improves the diagnostic accuracy of AD.
- The NICE guidelines recommend the use of perfusion hexamethylpropyleneamine oxime (HMPAO) SPECT to differentiate AD, VaD, and FTD. If HMPAO SPECT is not available, consider 2[^{18}F] FDG-PET as an alternative.

39.10.2.6 Management

A multidisciplinary team is essential, as are close links with physicians, general practitioners (GPs), social services, and the voluntary sector. The Alzheimer's Disease

Society can provide carers with valuable information about local facilities and often run local counselling and sitting services. Driving should cease as soon as there is any evidence that it may be unsafe. The patient should be asked to inform the Driver and Vehicle Licensing Authority (DVLA), but if they fail to do so, the doctor has a duty to inform them.

For patients suffering from mild to moderate AD (MMSE > 20), the NICE guidelines recommend to offer them the chance to participate in a structured group cognitive stimulation programme irrespective of the prescription of drug treatment for cognitive symptoms.

For patients suffering from moderate AD (MMSE score of 10–20 points or score >20 with significant impairment in functions or learning disability), the NICE guidelines recommend the specialist to prescribe the acetylcholinesterase inhibitors (AChEIs) including donepezil, galantamine, and rivastigmine. The three major benefits of AChEIs include stabilization of cognitive decline, improvement of the ADL, and reduction of behavioural problems. Treatment should be started in the specialist dementia clinic. The NICE guidelines recommend patient-centred care, and the specialist has to consider issues relating to informed consent to pharmacological treatment.

The specialist should also seek carer's view on the patient's functions at baseline. AChEIs are broadly similar in efficacy, and they are chosen based on their costs, side effect profiles, and patients' preferences. The specialist should consider an alternative AChEI if adverse events or drug interaction occurs. MMSE and global, functional, and behavioural assessment should be performed every 6 months. Treatment will be continued if either the MMSE score remains at or above 10 points or global, functional, and behavioural conditions indicate worthwhile effects (Table 39.15).

Common side effects of AChEIs include excessive cholinergic effects such as nausea, diarrhoea, dizziness, urinary incontinence, and insomnia. Other side effects include headache, parasympathetic stimulation, and bradycardia. Pretreatment ECG is required. Donepezil is contraindicated in people suffering from asthma, but rivastigmine is safe in asthma and chronic obstructive pulmonary disease.

For patients suffering from severe AD (MMSE score <10 points), memantine is indicated in a well-established clinical setting based on recommendations from the NICE guidelines. Memantine is a NMDA receptor antagonist, and it has neuroprotective properties (Figure 39.1). Memantine may be useful in patients suffering from VaD. The usual treatment dose of memantine is 10 mg B.D., and its half-life is 60–100 h. Memantine is available in oral tablets and droplets. It metabolism is nonhepatic.

TABLE 39.15
Comparison of the Pharmacokinetics and Pharmacodynamics of AChEIs

	Donepezil	Rivastigmine	Galantamine
Indications	AD, VaD	AD, DLB (improve hallucinations and delusions), and dementia related to Parkinson's disease	AD
Pharmacokinetics			
Preparation	Oral tablets	Oral capsules, solution, and patches	Oral tablets and solution
Plasma half-life	70 h	10 h	6 h
Frequency of administration	Once per day	Twice per day	Twice per day
Daily dose	5–10 mg/day	3–6 mg/day	8–12 mg/day
Metabolism	P450CYP 2D6 P450CYP 3A4	Not by P450 system	P450CYP 2D6 P450CYP 3A4
Organ of elimination	Liver	Kidney	Both liver and kidney
Pharmacodynamics			
Specific for CNS	Selective	Selective	Selective
Reversibility	Reversible	Pseudoirreversible	Reversible
Enzymes inhibited	AChE	AChE and BChE	AChE
Nicotine receptor modulation	No	No	Yes

Source: Taylor, D. et al., *The Maudsley Prescribing Guidelines*, 10th edn., Informa Healthcare, London, U.K., 2009.

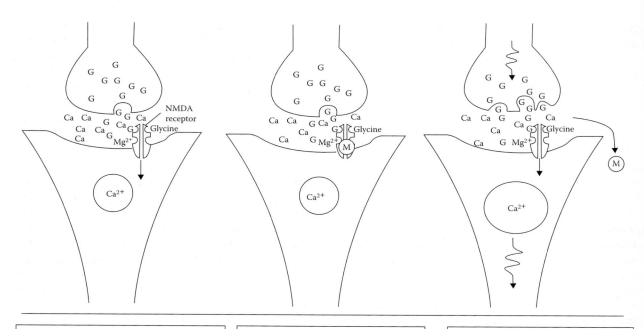

Neuronal excitotoxicity: The release of glutamate (G) from presynaptic neuron stimulates *N*-Methyl-D-aspartic acid(NMDA) receptors which have high affinity for Mg^{2+} ions and leads to prolonged influx of Ca^{2+} ions.

Memantine (M) is a low-affinity voltage-dependent uncompetitive antagonist at the NMDA receptors. It may be neuroprotective and disease modifying.

Its low affinity to the NMDA receptors with rapid off-rate kinetics allows NMDA receptors to be activated by the relatively high concentrations of glutamate released following depolarization of the presynatic neurons.

FIGURE 39.1 Pharmacodynamics of memantine.

39.10.2.7 Management of Behavioural and Psychological Symptoms of Dementia

Small of antipsychotic medication may be needed in those patients who are agitated, distressed, and aggressive or who have sleep reversal. If antipsychotic drug is ineffective, you may consider giving him or her AChEIs. According to the NICE guidelines, intramuscular lorazepam can be used as a single agent (not diazepam or chlorpromazine). Those with AD are predisposed to developing depression, which may require treatment with antidepressant medication, preferably using preparations with few antiadrenergic and anticholinergic (antimuscarinic) side effects (e.g. SSRIs).

The following nonpharmacological treatments may be useful:

- Reality orientation involves consistent use of orientation devices such as signposts, notices, and other memory aids to remind the patients and environment.
- Resolution therapy is a companion to reality orientation and looks for meaning in the 'here and now' in the behaviour and confused talk of the patient.
- Reminiscent therapy involves reliving the past experiences with old TV set, radio, and home environment.
- Validation therapy empathizes with the feelings and meanings hidden behind their confused speech and behaviour.
- Snoezelen involves the utilization of specially designed room with soothing and stimulating environment.
- Art therapy (painting and drawing), aromatherapy (lavender and Melissa balm), and music therapy (singing or playing an instrument) may be useful.

39.10.2.8 Prognosis

Disease progression varies considerably from subject to subject. The younger the age of onset, the more rapid the decline. In those aged under 50, the mean survival time is about 7 years, whereas in those aged between 55 and 74, the mean survival is increased to about 9 years.

Poor prognostic factors include

- Significant language impairment
- Poor cognitive functioning
- Clinical evidence of parietal lobe involvement
- CT scan showing reduced density of left parietal region

39.10.3 VASCULAR DEMENTIA

39.10.3.1 Aetiology

There is an excess of VaD in males, which is probably caused by an increased prevalence of cardiovascular disease in men. Hypertension is the most frequent risk factor among those with VaD (contributing to 50% of VaD). Risk factors known to increase the risk of stroke also increase the risk of VaD, for example, cigarette smoking, heart disease, homocystinuria, hyperlipidaemia, metabolic syndrome, low levels of high-density lipoprotein, moderate alcohol consumption, polycythaemia, and sickle cell anaemia.

Cerebral **a**utosomal-**d**ominant **a**rteriopathy with **s**ubcortical **i**nfarcts and **l**eukoencephalopathy (CADASIL) is a genetic disease with Notch 3 mutations in chromosome 19 and results in recurrent subcortical CVAs (80%), cognitive deterioration (50%), mood changes (30%), epilepsy (10%), and gait abnormalities.

39.10.3.2 Clinical Features

VaD is characterized by a stepwise deteriorating course with a patchy distribution of neurological and neuropsychological deficits. There is evidence of vascular diseases on physical examination (hypertension, hypertensive changes on fundoscopy, carotid bruits, enlarged heart, focal neurological signs suggestive of CVA).

Three presentations occur:

- Dementia follows a stroke.
- Dementia gradually develops following multiple asymptomatic cerebral infarcts.
- Neuropsychiatric symptoms gradually become evident.

Distinguishing between VaD and AD can be difficult; indeed, in a certain proportion of cases, both coexist. A more insidious onset with a continuous rather than stepwise course, less insight, fewer affective symptoms, and lack of hypertension or neurological signs is more suggestive of AD. VaD is more likely than AD to produce coexistent depression, persecutory delusions, anxiety, and emotional disturbance.

Based on clinical presentation, history and CT scan findings of VaDs have been subdivided into Binswanger's disease, leukoaraiosis, and multiple lacunar states.

39.10.3.2.1 Binswanger's Disease

This is a progressive subcortical vascular encephalopathy with CT scan revealing markedly enlarged ventricles secondary to infarction in hemispheric white matter. Infarcts are observed to affect periventricular and central white matter. The age of onset is 50–65, with a gradual accumulation of neurological signs, dementia, and disturbances in motor function including pseudobulbar palsy. There is often a history of severe hypertension, systemic vascular disease, and stroke.

39.10.3.2.2 Leukoaraiosis

This was used by Hachinski to describe CT scan appearances of reduced density of white matter. It differs from infarcts in that it affects only white matter, is patchy and diffuse, and does not result in the enlargement of cerebral sulci or ventricles. It is found in nondemented subjects as well as those with degenerative and vascular dementia.

39.10.3.2.3 Multiple Lacunar States

These are CT scan appearances of small well-localized subcortical infarcts. It is associated with dementia characterized by dysarthria, incontinence, and explosive laughing, secondary to frontal lobe disturbance.

39.10.3.3 Diagnostic Criteria

National Institute of Neurological and Communicative Disorders and Stroke and the Alzheimer's Disease and Related Disorders Association (NINCDS–ADRDA) (Table 39.16).

The ICD-10 criteria (WHO, 1992) emphasize on unevenly distributed cognitive impairment and signs of focal brain damage (unilateral spastic weakness, unilaterally increased tendon reflexes, an extended plantar response, and pseudobulbar palsy). In multi-infarct dementia, the onset is gradual with minor ischaemic episodes. In acute onset VaD, the onset of dementia is within 1 month of CVA. In subcortical VaD, there is evidence of deep white matter lesions.

TABLE 39.16
Comparison of NINDS-AIREN Criteria and Hachinski Ischaemic Score

NINDS-AIREN Criteria (Roman et al., 1993)	Hachinski Ischaemic Score (Moroney, 1997)
A relationship between the aforementioned dementia and CVAs manifested or inferred by the presence of one or more of the following	*Course of the illness* 1. Abrupt onset of symptoms (two points) 2. Stepwise deterioration (one point) 3. Fluctuating course (two points)
1. Amnesia and cognitive impairment in at least 1 domain with resultant disability 2. Focal sign and image findings 3. Onset of dementia within 3 months following a recognized stroke 4. Abrupt deterioration in cognitive functions (fluctuating and stepwise)	*Symptoms* 1. Nocturnal confusion (one point) 2. Personality relatively preserved (one point) 3. Depression (one point) 4. Somatic complaints (tingling, clumsy) (one point) 5. Emotional lability (one point)
Clinical features consistent with the diagnosis of probable VaD	*History* 1. Presence of hypertension (one point) 2. Stroke (two points) 3. Atherosclerosis (one point)
1. Early presence of a gait disturbance 2. History of unsteadiness and frequent unprovoked falls 3. Early urinary symptoms not explained by urologic disease 4. Pseudobulbar palsy 5. Mood changes or abulia	*Focal neurological symptoms*: hemiparesis, hemianopia, aphasia (two points) *Focal neurological signs*: unilateral weakness, sensory loss, asymmetric reflexes, Babinski's sign (two points)
Note that the early presence of gait disturbance and early urinary symptoms are not included in Hachinski Ischaemic Scale	A total score > 7 suggests of VaD and score < 4 suggests DAT

39.10.3.4 Investigation
- CT and MRI may show infarcts, lacunes, and leukoaraiosis.
- SPECT and PET scans may show patchy hypoperfusion.

39.10.3.5 Management
- The NICE guidelines do not recommend the use of AChEIs or memantine for cognitive decline in VaD except in properly constructed clinical studies. Donepezil may be beneficial but not licenced in VaD.
- It is worth attempting to treat the underlying cardiovascular condition in order to slow or halt the progression of VaD. The treatment of hypertension is important.
- Depression may respond to an antidepressant.

39.10.3.6 Prognosis
Prognosis of VaD is worse than that of AD. The mean survival of AD is 6 years, while the mean survival of VaD is only 3 years.

Poor prognostic factors include

- Severity of dementia
- Being bedridden
- Urinary incontinence

39.10.4 FRONTOTEMPORAL LOBE DEMENTIAS

39.10.4.1 Epidemiology
Dementia of frontal lobe type and Pick's disease both mainly affect the frontal and anterior temporal areas of the brain. In a large-scale neuropathological study over 20 years, 10% of dementia cases had dementia of the frontal lobe type, and a further 2.5% had Pick's disease (the Lund study, 1987).

39.10.4.2 Aetiology and Classification
See Figure 39.2.

39.10.4.3 Neurochemistry
FTD is associated with cortical and striatal serotoninergic deficits but not cholinergic deficit.

39.10.4.4 Diagnostic Criteria (Table 39.17)
The similarities and differences between AD and Frontotemporal lobe dementias (FTD) (Orrell and Sahakian., 1991)

- Patients with FTD have younger age of onset, more severe apathy, disinhibition, reduction in speech output, loss of insight, and coarsening of social behaviour but less spatial disorientation as compared to patients with AD. Primitive reflexes such as grasp, pour, and palm mental reflexes often reappear in FTD.
- Patients who suffer from AD have more impairment in calculation and constructions,

FTD

Semantic dementia

Semantic dementia involved impairment in understanding of word meaning or object identity with lesions in the temporal lobe. Other clinical features include:

1. Anomia: loss ability to recognize or understand words.

2. Dominant temporal lobe lesion: fluent aphasia or semantic paraphasia. For example, a patient names 'elephant' as 'cat'.

3. Nondominant temporal lobe dementia: associative agnosia and prosopagnosia.

4. Memory is better for recent events than remote events. Episodic memory is not affected.

5. Onset age is 50–65 years.

6. Orientation is normal.

Progressive non-fluent aphasia

Patients suffering from progressive nonfluent aphasia have difficulty with initiation but not comprehension of speech due to the lesions in dorsolateral pre-frontal cortex. Other clinical features include:

1. Hesitant, effortful speech.

2. Speech apraxia.

3. Stutter (including return of a childhood stutter).

4. Anomia.

5. Phonemic paraphasia (sound errors in speech, e.g. 'gat' for 'cat').

6. Agrammatism (using the wrong tense or word order).

7. As the disease develops, speech quantity decreases and many patients will become mute.

Frontotemporal lobe degeneration

1. Pathology: neuronal loss and reactive astrocytosis.

2. Characterized primarily by personality change and disordered social conduct.

Pick's disease
1. Age of onset: 45–65 years; F:M = 2:1

2. 50% of patients are caused by autosomal-dominant inheritance of tau gene on chromosome 17. This results in abnormal insoluble tau isoforms which accumulate in neurons and glia.

3. Pathology: atrophy of frontotemporal lobe, swollen achromatic neurons (balloon cells), pick bodies with tau and ubiquitin positive neurons.

4. ICD-10 criteria: slow onset, steady deterioration, frontal lobe symptoms (emotional blunting, coarsening of social behaviour, disinhibition, apathy, aphasia), sparing of memory and parietal lobe in the beginning stage.

5. Seizure and apraxia are uncommon.

6. CT brain shows knife-blade atrophy in frontotemporal lobe.

7. SSRIs or trazodone are beneficial for behavioural symptoms.

FIGURE 39.2 Classification of frontotemporal lobe dementia (FTD).

lower MMSE scores, and higher prevalence of depression (20%) as compared to patients with FTD.
- Both AD and FTD have insidious onset.
- Kluver–Bucy syndrome consisting of emotional placidity, hyperorality (bulimia and pica), hypersexuality, and tendency to place things in the mouth may occur concurrently with AD or FTD.

39.10.4.5   Investigations

- Psychometry will show characteristic impairments in higher executive function, verbal fluency, and agnosia.
- Structural imaging may not show characteristic lesion in early stage, and functional imaging shows anterior hypoperfusion. EEG is usually normal in FTD.

39.10.4.6   Management

- There is no specific pharmacological intervention for cognitive impairments in FTD. SSRIs or trazodone is indicated for noncognitive features.
- Psychosocial interventions is often useful.

39.10.4.7   Prognosis

The mean duration of dementia of frontal lobe type is 8 years, and of Pick's disease 11 years.

39.10.4.8   Diogenes Syndrome

Diogenes syndrome or senile squalor is associated with frontal lobe dysfunction and compulsive collecting (syllogomania or hoarding rubbish). Thus, it is usually inappropriate to invoke the Mental Health Act; instead, Section 47 of the Public Health Act is usually used to deal with these situations if required. The prognosis is poor with almost inevitable relapse. Day care may help, and institutional care is often required.

TABLE 39.17

Summary of the Lund–Manchester Consensus on Diagnosis of FTD

Frontotemporal Lobe Features	Affective Features	Supporting Features
1. High executive functions: loss of interest, preservation, disinhibition (jocularity and hypersexuality), inflexibility and impulsiveness, and lack of personal and social awareness	1. Depression 2. Anxiety 3. Hypochondriasis 4. Emotionally unconcerned	1. Age of onset <65 years 2. Family history of FTD 3. Bulbar palsy 4. Akinesia, rigidity, and tremor 5. Early incontinence
2. Premotor cortex: primitive reflex and stereotypies (compulsion without obsessions) and strange eating habits		
3. Broca's area: progressive reduction in speech, poor verbal fluency, and echolalia		
4. Preserved visuospatial ability		

Source: Miller, B.L. et al., *British Journal of Psychiatry*, 158, 76, 1991.

39.11   DEMENTIA WITH MOVEMENT DISORDERS

39.11.1   DEMENTIA WITH LEWY BODIES

39.11.1.1   Epidemiology

- Dementia with Lewy bodies (DLB) is the third most common cause of late-onset dementia and less common cause of early-onset dementia.
- DLB occurs frequently in combination with AD.
- DLB more commonly affects men than women.

39.11.1.2   Neuropathology

- There is little atrophy in the early stage of DLB. The neuroanatomical areas affected in DLB include hippocampus, temporal lobes, and neocortex.
- Lewy bodies are located in cingulated gyrus, cortex, and substantia nigra. They contain eosinophilic inclusion with high amyloid content but absence of tau pathology. Lewy bodies are α-synuclein and ubiquitin positive. α-Synuclein is aggregated and insoluble protein, which is pathognomonic of LBD and idiopathic Parkinson's disease.

39.11.1.3   Neurochemistry

The cholinergic deficits are more pronounced in DLB than DAT:

- The dopaminergic deficits are more pronounced in idiopathic Parkinson's disease than DLB.

39.11.1.4   Clinical Features (McKeith's Criteria) (Barber et al., 2001)

- *Differences between DLB and Parkinson's disease dementia*: The cognitive and extrapyramidal signs develop concurrently in DLB, but cognitive symptoms occur at least 1 year after the development of extrapyramidal signs in Parkinson's disease dementia.
- *Cognitive symptoms*: Enduring and progressive cognitive impairment with impairments in consciousness, alertness, and attention. Cognition is fluctuating and short-term memory is not affected in early stage. Patients suffering from DLB have less episodic amnesia, more executive dysfunction, and more apraxagnosia as compared patients suffering from AD.
- *Common noncognitive features*: Apathy, depression, hallucinations (complex visual hallucinations: 80%, auditory hallucinations: 20%), and delusions (paranoid delusions: 65%).
- *Extrapyramidal signs and parkinsonism*: Loss of facial expression, changes in the strength and tone of the voice, slowness, muscle stiffness, trembling of the limbs, a tendency to shuffle when walking (mild parkinsonism: 70%, no parkinsonism: 25%).
- *Serious clinical events*: Neuroleptic sensitivity (60%), falls, syncope, and spontaneous loss of consciousness.

39.11.1.5   Investigations

- Psychometry will be useful with more impairments in visuospatial tests.

There are two scans that can help to establish the diagnosis of DLB as recommended by the NICE guidelines:

- Dopaminergic iodine-123-radiolabelled 2β-carbomethoxy-3β-(4-iodophenyl)-N-(3-fluoropropyl) nortropane (FP-CIT) SPECT is be used to help establish the diagnosis in those with suspected DLB if the diagnosis is in doubt.

- DaTSCAN is a radiopharmacological drug composed of ioflupane (^{123}I) 74 MBq/mL and is used in SPECT to detect loss of functional dopaminergic neuron terminals in the striatum. DaTSCAN is able to differentiate probable DLB from AD. DaTSCAN is unable to discriminate between DLB and Parkinson's disease dementia.
- 90% of DLB patients have EEG abnormalities.

39.11.1.6 Management

- Antipsychotics are not indicated for mild-to-moderate noncognitive symptoms in DLB because of the risk of severe adverse reactions. If it needs to be used, consider quetiapine and monitor for extrapyramidal side effects.
- *AChEIs*: Consider for people with DLB who have noncognitive symptoms causing significant distress or leading to behaviour that challenges. Rivastigmine has the best research evidence for improvement of cognitive functions in DLB. It may also improve cognitive symptoms, delusions, and hallucinations.
- Chlormethiazole is used for night sedation.

39.11.2 PARKINSON'S DISEASE DEMENTIA

It is difficult to distinguish dementia specifically associated with Parkinson's disease from other causes of dementia, which are likely to occur coincidentally in elderly people suffering from Parkinson's disease. It is estimated that dementia occurs in 15%–20% of those with Parkinson's disease, compared to 5%–10% of the normal population, corrected for age.

39.11.2.1 Aetiology

This is not known. It is known that in Parkinson's disease, there is damage to the ascending monoaminergic system affecting central dopamine, serotonin, and noradrenaline systems. There is also damage to substantia innominata, causing cortical cholinergic disruption.

All patients with Parkinson's disease have Lewy bodies in their cerebral cortex, with a subset having more Lewy bodies than most. Not all of these have dementia, although it appears that all have some evidence of cognitive decline.

39.11.2.2 Clinical Features

Cognitive deficits seem to occur in most subjects with Parkinson's disease; it is possible that those considered to be suffering from dementia are simply those at the extreme end of cognitive decline in this condition.

Cognitive deficits in Parkinson's disease include

- Slowness in comprehension and response (bradyphrenia)
- Impaired abstract reasoning
- Memory impairment, including poor retrieval and poor short-term memory, especially frontal lobe working memory
- Impaired remote memory (only in the late stages)

Patients with typical extrapyramidal signs of Parkinson's disease who later develop cognitive impairment, especially of a subcortical type, are given a diagnosis of dementia of Parkinson's disease.

39.11.2.3 Management

Exclude treatable pathology, such as depression or acute brain syndrome.

Treatment with anti-parkinsonian drugs does not improve the cognitive manifestations of the disease. Avoid anticholinergic drugs if possible.

Transplants of fetal nerve cells are experimental and may improve the outlook for those with Parkinson's disease. It is not known how helpful this will be in the treatment of dementia of Parkinson's disease.

39.11.2.3.1 Corticobasal Degeneration

Clinical features include extrapyramidal signs such as poor coordination, akinesia, rigidity, disequilibrium, and limb dystonia. Other symptoms include cognitive impairments, visual–spatial disturbance, apraxia, hesitant and halting speech, myoclonus, and dysphagia. The patient may lose their ability to walk.

The pathology involves large swollen achromatic neurons in the cortex, and tau positive glial inclusions are found in the frontal and parietal lobes. Neuronal inclusions are also found in the substantia nigra and basal ganglia.

Drugs used to treat Parkinson's disease do not produce any significant or sustained improvement in corticobasal degeneration. Clonazepam may reduce the myoclonus.

39.11.2.3.2 Progressive Supranuclear Palsy

Patients suffering from Progressive supranuclear palsy (PSP) present with mild cognitive deficits, apathy, slowing of cognitive processing, and memory deficits. It is distinguished from AD and DLB by prominent parkinsonism, gait and poor balance, and brain stem abnormalities (ophthalmoplegia and pseudobulbar palsy).

The pathology is located in neocortex and cerebral cortex (e.g. frontal lobe). Microscopic lesions include neuronal loss astrocytosis, tau positive NFTs, and glial inclusions.

39.11.3   Normal-Pressure Hydrocephalus

39.11.3.1   Clinical Features

There is insidious onset of dementia with psychomotor retardation, unsteady gait, and urinary incontinence. Onset is usually in the 60 or 70s. Behavioural disturbance, hallucinations, and paranoia are uncommon.

The diagnosis is made on the basis of clinical presentation, with a CT scan of the brain revealing dilated ventricles (especially the third ventricle) without cortical atrophy, with normal CSF pressures.

39.11.3.2   Aetiology

There is obstruction to outflow of CSF from the subarachnoid space, but the ventricular system remains in communication with the subarachnoid space, thus allowing CSF to flow out of the ventricular system. This scenario is associated with

- Subarachnoid haemorrhage
- Cerebrovascular disease
- Meningoencephalitis
- Post-intracranial surgery

39.11.3.3   Management

Insertion of a shunt will allow the drainage of CSF from the ventricles to the heart.

39.11.3.4   Prognosis

The best results are seen in those with a full clinical syndrome, a short history, and an obvious cause for their condition. Mental and physical improvement is likely after surgery.

One-third of those undergoing surgery will develop complications such as

- Shunt infection and malfunction
- Epilepsy
- Subdural haematoma

39.11.4   Creutzfeldt–Jakob Disease

39.11.4.1   Epidemiology

- Creutzfeldt–Jakob disease (CJD) is extremely rare and affects only 1–2 per million.
- CJD is most common in Libyan and Tunisian Jews.

39.11.4.2   Aetiology

- CJD is transmissible to laboratory animals by intracerebral inoculation, with symptoms developing years later. The effect is similar to spongiform encephalopathies observed in animals (scrapie in sheep, bovine spongiform encephalopathy [BSE] in cows).
- A form of CJD known as the BSE variant has been identified in humans. It has a slightly different clinical presentation. There can be onset in younger people. It is rapidly progressive and is thought to be associated with eating or being otherwise exposed to cattle infected with BSE.
- The aetiology of CJD is classified into familial and environmental causes (Figure 39.3):

CJD

Familial causes

Familiar CJD: about 10% of cases appear to be familial.

Gerstmann–Straussler–Scheinker syndrome is characterized by neuronal loss, astrocytosis, spongiform degeneration, and extensive multicentric amyloid plaques. Cerebellar ataxia forming is a prominent clinical feature. This syndrome is rare.

Familial fatal insomnia is characterized by lesions in the thalamus. Patients have early onset at the age of 20–40 and the course of disease is slow progression.

Environmental causes

Sporadic CJD

Iatrogenic CJD is related to pituitary-derived growth hormone, through cross contamination from instruments used in brain biopsy or through dural grafts with 2 years of incubation period.

Kuru is caused by ritual cannibalism in New Guinea with prion plague formation in cerebellum. Kuru is rare.

New variant CJD is characterized by extensive prion plaque formation in cerebellum.

FIGURE 39.3   Classification of the aetiologies of Creutzfeldt–Jakob disease.

39.11.4.3 Pathology

- The prion protein (PrP) is responsible for transmission. This is an unusual infective agent since it does not appear to contain nucleic acid, being made up entirely of protein.
- PrP differs from normal cell-membrane-derived proteins in that it is highly resistant to degradation by cellular proteases, heat, or conventional chemical disinfectants.
- The PrP gene mutations are located on chromosome 20, and this mutation produces protein with conformational change into PrP^{CJD}, which are cytotoxic, insoluble, and often deposit in cerebellum.
- Microscopy of brain material reveals vacuolar changes in grey matter particularly in cerebral and cerebellar cortex, creating characteristic spongiform appearances.
- There is a loss of nerve cells and reactive astrocytosis.
- In CJD, there is rapid brain shrinkage and reduction in size due to diffuse and focal atrophy and neuronal loss.

39.11.4.4 Clinical Features

CJD is a very rare cause of a rapidly progressive dementia.

There may be a brief prodromal period of anxiety, depression, or hallucinations. Sudden onset and rapid progression of dementia, pyramidal, and extrapyramidal deficits present usually in the 50–60-year age group.

Physical features include limb spasticity, muscular wasting and fasciculation, tremor, rigidity, choreoathetoid movements, myoclonus, dysarthria, and dysphagia. Convulsions may occur.

In addition to the previously mentioned classic form, three variant forms are described:

- *Heidenhain form.* Prominent visual defects may result in cortical blindness. Extrapyramidal symptoms and myoclonus occur.
- *Ataxic form.* There is rapidly progressive cerebellar ataxia, with involuntary movements and myoclonic jerks. Finally, muteness and generalized rigidity occur.
- *Cortical form.* This includes parietal lobe symptoms.

39.11.4.5 Investigations

The EEG is always abnormal in CJD, showing an increase in slow-wave activity and a reduction in a rhythm; as the disease progresses, bilateral slow spike wave discharges may accompany myoclonic jerks.

Gross atrophy is seen in the frontotemporal regions (knife-blade atrophy) in Pick's disease, but the diagnosis cannot be made on this evidence alone.

39.11.4.6 Management

There is no specific pharmacological intervention for CJD.

39.11.4.7 Prognosis

There is terminal decline.

39.11.5 HUMAN IMMUNODEFICIENCY VIRUS DEMENTIA

39.11.5.1 Epidemiology

- This is one of the most prominent features of Human immunodeficiency virus (HIV) encephalopathy.
- Prevalence of dementia is 30% among HIV-infected patients.

39.11.5.2 Aetiology

The encephalopathy of HIV is thought to be directly caused by HIV, which is a neurotropic virus.

39.11.5.3 Pathology

Pathology is found in the white matter of cerebral and cerebellar hemispheres and in deep grey matter. Multinucleated giant cells deriving from macrophages are found in the affected brain tissue.

39.11.5.4 Clinical Features

- The onset of HIV dementia is usually insidious and occurs later in the course with significant immunosuppression. There is initial lethargy, apathy, cognitive disturbance, reduced libido, and general withdrawal. As the condition progresses, evidence of dementia becomes apparent with cognitive disturbance, incontinence, ataxia, hyperreflexia, and increased muscle tone. Clinical features can be classified into cognitive, behavioural, and motor symptoms.
- Cognitive symptoms include memory, concentration impairment, and mental slowing. The patient may need a written reminder to help them to recall.
- Behavioural symptoms include apathy, reduced spontaneity, and social withdrawal. Depression, irritability or emotional lability, agitation, and psychotic symptoms may occur.
- Motor symptoms include loss of balance and coordination and clumsiness and leg weakness.

- At a later stage, HIV dementia results in a global deterioration of cognitive functions as manifested by word finding difficulties. Patients may exhibit psychomotor retardation and mutism. Speech becomes slow and monotonous.
- Neurological examination reveals that patients become unable to walk as a result of paraparesis. Patients usually lie in bed indifferent to their illness and to their surroundings. Bladder incontinence and bowel incontinence are common findings. Myoclonus and seizures may occur.

39.11.5.5   Classification
See Table 39.18.

39.11.5.6   Differential Diagnosis
The presentation of the following differential diagnosis may be more acute as compared to AIDS-associated dementia:

- *Opportunistic infections*: cerebral *toxoplasmosis*, *Cryptococcal* meningitis, *CMV* encephalitis, and *herpes simplex* encephalitis
- Neoplasms and cerebral lymphoma
- Metabolic encephalopathies
- HIV encephalitis or leukoencephalopathy

TABLE 39.18

Comparison of Diagnostic Criteria of HIV-Associated Cognitive Motor Disorder and AIDS Dementia Complex

HIV-Associated Cognitive Disorder (Grant et al., 2005)	AIDS Dementia Complex (Brew, 2004)
Two or more of the following for >1 month	Acquired abnormality in at least two of the following cognitive abilities for at least 1 month
• Impaired attention or concentration	• Attention/concentration
• Mental slowing	• Speed of information processing
• Impaired memory	• Abstraction/reasoning
• Slowed movements	• Visuospatial skill
• Incoordination	• Memory/learning
• Personality change, irritability, and symptoms must be verified by neurological examination or neuropsychological testing	• Speech/language
	At least one of the following
• Accompanied by mild impairment of functional status (e.g. work or ADL)	• Acquired abnormality in motor function
• Emotional lability	• Decline in motivation or emotional control or change in behaviour
	Absence of clouding of consciousness (delirium)
	No evidence of other aetiology

39.11.5.7   Investigations
MRI and CT scans usually show the cerebral atrophy and white matter abnormalities in HIV dementia.

39.11.5.8   Management and Prognosis
Therapeutic trials of antiviral treatment suggest that improvement in HIV dementia may occur, but the prognosis is poor.

39.11.6   HUNTINGTON'S DISEASE (CHOREA)

39.11.6.1   Epidemiology
This is a genetic disorder resulting in a condition characterized by continuous involuntary movements and a slowly progressive dementia. There are 5 cases per 100,000 in the United Kingdom.

39.11.6.2   Aetiology
Transmission is mostly by a fully penetrant single autosomal-dominant gene (located on chromosome 4), affecting 50% of offspring (see Chapter 19 for more details). Occasionally sporadic cases occur.

Pathological appearances include a marked atrophy of head of caudate nucleus and putamen and severe generalized neuronal loss resulting in cortical atrophy, which is most marked over the frontal lobes, with ventricular dilatation.

39.11.6.3   Clinical Features
The onset is usually between the ages of 35 and 45, but childhood onset accounts for 10%–20% of cases. The onset is insidious, with fidgety movements or nonspecific psychiatric symptoms in the early stages.

Movement disorder consists of choreiform movements in the head, face, and arms; ill-sustained and jerky voluntary and involuntary movements affecting all muscles; and a distinctive wide-based gait with sudden lurching.

Psychiatric disturbance is variable but common. Initial insight may result in depression. Prodromal personality changes, antisocial behaviour with substance misuse, and affective and schizophreniform disorders are sometimes seen. Insight gives way to mild euphoria with explosive outbursts, irritability, and rage. There is a slowly progressive intellectual impairment, with some patients profoundly demented in the final stages, whereas others remain reasonably aware.

39.11.6.4   Investigation

- In Huntington's disease, the EEG consists of an absence of rhythmic background activity, along with low-voltage intermittent random activities (θ and δ wave).
- CT scan may show a characteristic shrinkage of caudate nuclei.

39.11.6.5 Management

Tetrabenazine helps to reduce the movement disorder. The main side effect of tetrabenazine is depression. Antidepressants, ECT, and minor tranquillizers may be helpful in the early stages, with phenothiazines in low dose in later stages to control behavioural disturbance.

Genetic counselling for family members should be offered.

39.11.6.6 Prognosis

The duration to death is 12–16 years.

39.11.7 General Paralysis of the Insane

This is a rare condition and can be missed.

39.11.7.1 Aetiology

The disease is a terminal consequence of syphilis. There is marked cerebral atrophy with meningeal thickening, resulting from neuronal loss and astrocyte proliferation. The presence of iron pigment in microglia and perivascular spaces is specific for the disease. Spirochetes are found in the cortex in 50% of cases.

39.11.7.2 Clinical Features

The condition develops 5–25 years after primary infection with Treponema pallidum. The onset is usually gradual with depression as a dominant symptom. There is then slowly progressive memory and intellectual impairment. Frontal lobes are particularly involved, resulting in characteristic personality change with disinhibition, uncontrolled excitement, and overactivity, which may be mistaken for hypomania. Grandiose delusions are present in only 10%.

Physically there is slurred speech, a tremor of lips and tongue, and Argyll Robertson pupil in 50%. As the condition progresses, there is increasing leg weakness leading to spastic paralysis.

The Wassermann reaction on CSF examination is always positive, with lymphocytosis, raised protein, and raised globulin.

39.11.7.3 Management and Prognosis

Treatment is with high-dose penicillin under steroid cover to prevent Herxheimer reaction. Following treatment, mental symptoms may diminish.

39.12 DELIRIUM IN OLD AGE

This is a state of fluctuating global disturbance of the cerebral function, abrupt in onset and of short duration, arising as a consequence of physical illness or toxic effects.

It is most common at the extremes of life both in the very young and the elderly. This may be caused by reduced cerebral reserve, a concurrence of multiple physical problems, and a higher prevalence of polypharmacy in the elderly.

It affects 10%–25% of the over-65s admitted to medical wards. Those with dementia are particularly vulnerable to developing superimposed delirium.

39.12.1 Aetiology

Although delirium presents with global disturbance of cognitive function, certain neurological pathways seem to be specifically involved. Autonomic disturbance implicates the brain stem. Cholinergic and adrenergic pathways are also thought to mediate delirium.

Any physical insult can result in delirium particularly in a predisposed individual. In the elderly, the following causes are the most common:

- Hypoxia
- Infection
- Metabolic disturbance
- Iatrogenic
- CNS disease
- Epilepsy

39.12.2 Clinical Features

- There is rapid onset with a fluctuating course. Lucid intervals occur.
- The delirium tends to be more marked at night particularly in conditions of poor illumination.
- Awareness is always impaired. Alertness tends to fluctuate and can be both increased and decreased.
- Orientation is always impaired, particularly for time.
- Recent and immediate memory is impaired with poor new learning and lack of recall for events occurring during the delirious period. However, the knowledge base remains intact.
- Thinking may be slowed or accelerated.
- Misperceptions, particularly visual, are common.
- Hallucinations and delusions may occur.
- Heightened anxiety and fear are often prominent.
- The sleep–wake cycle is always disturbed, with daytime drowsiness and nocturnal insomnia.
- Physical illness or drug intoxication is usually present (Table 39.19).

TABLE 39.19
Comparison between Dementia and Delirium

Clinical Features	Dementia	Delirium
Presence of acute physical illness	Usually absent	Usually present (e.g. infection, electrolyte disturbance)
Onset	Insidious	Acute
Attention	Normal attention	Poor attention and distractible
Memory	Impairment in immediate recall and recent memory	Impairment in recent and remote memory
Perceptual disturbances	Usually no hallucination	Visual hallucinations are common.
Duration	Long, months to years	Short, hours to weeks
Course of illness	Stable	Fluctuation

39.12.3   Classification

There are three types of delirium:

- Hyperactive delirium (30%), which is characterized by agitation, aggression, autonomic arousal, hyperactivity, and restlessness.
- Hypoactive delirium (40%), which is characterized by apathy, drowsiness, confusion, and lethargy. Hypoactive delirium is often mistaken for depression.
- Mixed hyperactive and hypoactive delirium (30%).

39.12.4   Investigation

Delirious patients should be fully investigated physically:

- Laboratory investigations include FBC (raised white blood cells may indicate infection), electrolytes (sodium, potassium, calcium, magnesium, phosphate), RFTs, LFTs, TFTs, and arterial blood gases.
- Infection screen includes syphilis, blood culture, and urinalysis.
- ECG.
- Imaging include CXR, CT (space occupying lesions, cerebral haemorrhage), or MRI scan (white matter lesions).
- Electroencephalogram: diffuse slowing of brain activity.
- Lumbar puncture and CSF analysis (if signs of meningitis or encephalitis).

39.12.5   Management

The treatment of delirium is the treatment of the underlying condition.

39.12.5.1   Nonpharmacological Treatment
- Avoid physical restraints.
- Avoid sensory deprivation and overload.
- Adequate oxygenation.
- Correct sensory deficits.
- Encourage normal sleep pattern.
- Environmental cues such as signposting.
- Family involvement.
- Maintain hydration and electrolyte balance.
- Mobilization of the patient.
- Pain management.
- Presence of familiar objects.
- Psychoeducation on delirium.
- Reorientation strategies (clock, access to window).
- Repetition of information in a slow and regular manner.
- Staff consistency.
- Well-illuminated environment.

39.12.5.2   Pharmacological Treatment
- Vitamin supplements, particularly thiamine, should be administered if there is any possibility of previous alcohol abuse or malnutrition.
- Drugs known to exacerbate delirium should be avoided if possible. Benzodiazepine should be avoided because it can exacerbate delirium. The use of benzodiazepine is only indicated in delirium tremens.
- Behaviour not amenable to other interventions, such as gentle reassurance, may respond to treatment with an antipsychotic.
- Haloperidol is the most frequently used in this situation because it is generally effective and safe. A baseline ECG is required to check QTc interval. Side effects include QTc prolongation, extrapyramidal side effects, orthostatic hypotension, and sedation.
- Second-generation antipsychotics such as risperidone, olanzapine, and quetiapine are indicated for patients who are prone to extrapyramidal side effects (e.g. DLB, Parkinson's disease). Side effects include sedation, orthostatic hypotension, and metabolic syndrome if used for a long duration.

- General principles of prescription in delirium include monotherapy, prescription with the lowest dose, and tapering off the medication when delirium resolves.
- Treatment of hypoactive delirium with psychotropic medications is not recommended.

39.12.6 Prognosis

- Delirium is associated with an increase in mortality. 1 month after delirium, the mortality rate is 16%. 6 months after delirium, the mortality rate is 26%.
- Between 30% and 50% of delirious patients on medical wards die of the underlying condition in 6 months.
- Those who recover have a good prognosis, and only 5% go on to develop dementia.

39.13 DEPRESSION IN OLD AGE

39.13.1 Epidemiology

Depressive symptoms affect 11%–16% of the over-65s. About 3% suffer major depression.

Female first admissions for affective illness peak at age 80, then fall off. Male first admissions continue to climb until the end of life, overtaking women at the age of 85.

The prevalence of depression declines with advancing age despite the earlier findings. This may be because of a survivor effect with fewer young depressed surviving to old age, or it may imply that depression in older age is more likely to require inpatient admission.

39.13.2 Aetiology

39.13.2.1 Genetic Factors

The genetic contribution to depressive illness reduces with age. The risk of depression in first-degree relatives is lowered with the increasing age of onset of depression in the proband. The risks to relatives are also lower if there has been only a single episode, whereas they are increased with recurrent depression in the proband.

39.13.2.2 Neurobiological Factors

Felix Post (1968) suggested that subtle cerebral changes may make ageing persons increasingly liable to affective disorders.

A subgroup of elderly depressives has ventricular enlargement on a CT scan of the brain. They are characterized as being older, with a later age of onset, more neurovegetative symptoms, and a higher death rate at 2 years than elderly depressives without ventricular enlargement. CT scan appearances in late-onset depressives are more comparable to those with AD than to those with early-onset depression or normal controls. Thus, early- and late-onset depression may be different disorders, and the late-onset type may have a stronger association with neurological dementing disorders than the early-onset type.

Depressed patients with ischaemic brain lesions have more vascular risk factors and less family history of mood disorders than those without.

In a proportion of elderly depressives, subtle brain disease is a risk factor.

39.13.2.3 Physical Illness

Depression can present secondary to a variety of physical conditions and may sometimes be the first indication of ill-health. The following are the main causes of secondary depression, which is more common in the elderly:

- Occult carcinoma, particularly of lung and pancreas
- Chronic obstructive airway disease (COAD)
- CVA
- Myocardial infarction (MI)
- Hypercalcaemia
- Cushing's disease
- Hypo- and hyperthyroidism
- Alcoholism
- Pernicious anaemia
- Iatrogenic—steroids, β-blockers, methyl-dopa, reserpine, clonidine, nifedipine, digitalis, L-dopa, and tetrabenazine
- Infections—brucellosis, neurosyphilis, and influenza

39.13.2.4 Personality

It is suggested that personality dysfunction is associated with some late-life depression.

39.13.2.5 Environmental Factors

Murphy (1982) found an association between the onset of depression and severe life events occurring significantly more commonly in the previous year compared to healthy controls. These included physical illness, separation, bereavement, financial loss, and enforced change of residence.

39.13.3 Clinical Features

Elderly depressives present with much the same features of depression as younger people, but some features may be more common in the elderly (Tables 39.20 and 39.21).

TABLE 39.20
Summary of Similarities and Differences in Depression between Young and Old People

Similarities	Differences
The following features are similar between young and old people: • Sleep disturbance (e.g. early morning awakening, frequent awakening, and subjective poor sleep quality) • Poor appetite • Weight loss	The following features may be more common in old people: • Behavioural disturbance (e.g. food refusal, aggressive behaviour, shoplifting, alcohol abuse) • Complaints of loneliness • Complaints disproportionate to organic pathology and pain of unknown origin • Depressive pseudodementia (e.g. poor concentration and memory) • Hypochondriacal preoccupations • Irritability or anger • Loss of interest often replaces depressed mood in elderly • Minimization/denial of low mood • Neurovegetative symptoms • Onset of neurotic symptoms (e.g. excessive worry) • Psychomotor retardation or agitation • Paranoid and delusional ideation

39.13.4 DIAGNOSIS

Because the elderly commonly suffer from coexistent physical disorders affecting neurovegetative functioning, the diagnosis of depression can prove more difficult than in the young. A careful history usually suffices to address this difficulty. The GDS is helpful since it focuses almost entirely on cognitive rather than physical symptoms of depressive disorder. The GDS-30 score > 11 or GDS-15 score > 5 indicates depression (Sheikh and Yesavage, 1986). The Cornell Scale for Depression in Dementia (CSDD) was developed to assess signs and symptoms of depression in patients with dementia (Alexopoulos et al., 1988). The CSDD uses an interviewing approach that derives information from the patient and the informant. Scores below 6 as a rule are associated with absence of significant depressive symptoms.

TABLE 39.21
Comparison between Dementia and Depression/Pseudodementia in Old People

Clinical Features	Dementia	Depression/Pseudodementia
Personal or family history of mood disorder	Usually absent	Usually present
Onset	Insidious	Acute
Response to memory assessment	Cooperative and attempt to answer questions with incorrect answers (e.g. confabulation)	Lack of motivation and does not attempt to answer the questions. Answer 'don't know' for most of the questions.
	Memory deficits are reported by relatives or caregivers.	Memory deficits are often reported by patients.
Mood	Labile mood or no mood changes	Low mood and irritability
Anhedonia	Capacity to enjoy things in life maintained	Cannot enjoy things in life and preoccupied with somatic complaints
Aphasia	May be present (e.g. word finding difficulties)	Absent
Perceptual disturbance	No hallucinations	Mood congruent hallucinations (e.g. auditory hallucinations with negative content)
Other neuropsychological findings	Acalculia Agnosia Impaired in visual–spatial organization	Intact arithmetic skills Intact paired associate learning (e.g. shape and name of objects) Intact visual–spatial organization
Suicidal ideation	Absent	Present
Course of illness	Slow progression	Rapid progression

39.13.5 MANAGEMENT

The depressed elderly person should be treated in much the same way as a depressed younger person, with antidepressants in an adequate dose for an adequate duration. The choice of antidepressant will depend on concurrent physical morbidity, and the dose is generally lower, particularly when commencing a new drug.

Newer antidepressants such as SSRIs and SNRIs are better tolerated than TCAs because SSRIs have low anticholinergic activity. Examples of antidepressants and daily starting dose for old people are listed as follows: escitalopram (5 mg), mirtazapine (7.5–15 mg), sertraline (25 mg), and venlafaxine (37.5 mg). Old people are prone to hyponatraemia. Baseline and regular blood pressure measurement, ECG, and sodium level are required for old people. If a TCA is required, lofepramine is the treatment of choice.

Deluded depressed patients require the addition of an antipsychotic.

ECT remains the most effective treatment for depression and is the treatment of choice in those with life-threatening depression. It is generally well tolerated, although memory problems may follow, so unilateral electrode placement is sometimes considered preferable. The seizure threshold increases with age, and older people have shorter seizure duration. It is contraindicated in those with raised intracranial pressure and is inadvisable within 3–6 months of a CVA, pulmonary embolus, or MI. However, the anaesthetist's views should be sought in any patient over whom there is particular concern. The liable consequences of inadequately treated or resistant depression should be weighed against the potential adverse effects of a general anaesthetic and ECT. Monoamine oxidase inhibitors should be discontinued at least 10 days prior to giving ECT.

About two-thirds of cases resistant to first-line therapy show an improvement with lithium augmentation. Generally, this is well tolerated, although the levels need careful monitoring in those with impaired renal function or those on diuretics.

Psychotherapy can be considered, although this should usually be in addition to drug therapy. The focus of psychotherapy should support self-esteem, instil hope, and encourage adequate nutrition and healthy lifestyle. Problem-solving may be useful and advise the elderly depressed patient to postpone major life decisions.

Socially isolated elderly depressed patients are at a high risk of committing suicide, so it is important that they be treated energetically.

39.13.6 Prognosis

Depression in old age is a heterogeneous condition and therefore has a heterogeneous outcome. Seventy per cent of elderly depressives recover within a year, but 20%

relapse. Only 10%–15% are considered to suffer from treatment-resistant depression. The death rate is higher for late-life depressives than for nondepressed patients.

Chronicity in late-life depression is more common in those with

- Male sex
- Active medical illness or poor physical health
- High severity and frequent episodes of depression
- Atypical features of depression
- History of dysthymia
- Delusions
- Cognitive impairment
- Morphologic brain abnormalities

The development of a transient dementia syndrome during a depressive episode, the onset of the first depressive episode in very old age, and abnormalities in brain morphology may be predictors of dementia in an elderly person with major depression.

39.14 MANIA IN OLD AGE

In most elderly people suffering from mania, the age of onset was usually in their young adult life. However, in the elderly population, the onset of the first manic episode is bimodally distributed with peaks at ages 37 and 73. Mania in the elderly is relatively uncommon, comprising about 5% of elderly psychiatric admissions.

39.14.1 Aetiology

39.14.1.1 Genetic Factors

Late-onset cases appear to have less genetic loading than younger-onset cases, with fewer of the former giving a family history of affective disorder.

39.14.1.2 Organic Factors

Secondary mania is that arising in a patient with no previous history of affective disorder, soon after a physical illness such as cerebral tumour or infection. However, evidence suggests that this is more likely to arise in those genetically predisposed to a bipolar affective disorder by virtue of a family history of such.

People with late-onset mania have a greater number of large subcortical hyperintensities on brain MRI compared to controls. It is thought that some cases of late-onset mania are a subtype of secondary mania attributable to changes in the brain's deep white matter.

39.14.2 CLINICAL FEATURES

These are similar to the features in younger adults, but it is thought that the following are more common in elderly manic patients:

- Garrulousness
- Slow flight of ideas
- Speech more circumstantial and less disorganized
- More paranoid delusions
- Less hyperactivity
- Cognitive impairment
- Irritable surliness, anger, and less euphoria
- Mixed affective states
- Depression following soon after mania recovers
- Longer duration and higher frequency of acute episodes
- Presence of neurological abnormalities especially old male patients

39.14.3 MANAGEMENT

Acute manic episodes may require treatment in hospital. Old-age psychiatrists need to rule out underlying medical causes and order RFT, TFT, and ECG and measure baseline body weight. The old-age psychiatrist needs to check potential drug interactions from existing medications such as diuretics and NSAIDS. Treatment is with antipsychotics and/or lithium. Lithium should be started at 150 mg daily if the old person is frail or 300 mg/day if the old person is physically fit. The dose is increased by 150 mg on a weekly basis. The maximum total daily dose is recommended to be less than 600 mg/day. The blood lithium level is aimed between 0.6 and 0.9 mmol/L during acute mania and 0.4–0.6 mmol/L during the maintenance period. The old person requires monthly monitoring of blood lithium levels in the initial period and regular monitoring of thyroid, renal, and cardiac status and measurement of body weight. The response rate for lithium is similar between young and old people. Addition of carbamazepine is recommended if the combination of lithium and antipsychotics is not fully effective.

If the person is unresponsive or intolerant to this combination, ECT can be effective for manic or mixed affective states. Lithium prophylaxis is advisable in the longer term.

39.14.4 PROGNOSIS

The outlook is the same as in bipolar disorder. Recurrence is usual, and therefore mood stabilizers are advisable in the longer term.

39.15 PARAPHRENIA OR PSYCHOSIS IN OLD AGE

39.15.1 EXPLANATORY NOTE

Paraphrenia is a term introduced originally by Kraepelin in 1909 to describe a psychotic condition characterized by the relatively late age of first onset, chronic delusions and hallucinations, the preservation of volition, and a lack of personality deterioration. The term quickly lost favour until Roth reintroduced it in 1955 to describe late paraphrenia, a condition with age of first onset after 60 years, well-organized delusions with or without hallucinations, and a well-preserved personality and affective response.

In ICD-10 (WHO, 1992), late-onset disorders are not differentiated from early-onset disorders, so most paraphrenias are coded in ICD-10 under schizophrenia or delusional disorders. Nevertheless, evidence suggests that some late-onset delusional disorders are distinct from schizophrenia, and the use of the term late paraphrenia therefore persists.

39.15.2 EPIDEMIOLOGY

Good epidemiological studies in this area have not been completed. It is estimated that in Camberwell (London), there is an annual incidence of late paraphrenia of 17–26 per 100,000. There is a well-established preponderance of females over males in late paraphrenia. Late paraphrenics are more likely to be unmarried and have a lower fecundity than controls.

39.15.3 AETIOLOGY

39.15.3.1 Genetic Factors

There is an increased risk of schizophrenia in the first-degree relatives of paraphrenics, but it is less than the risk to the relatives of younger-onset schizophrenics.

Paraphrenia is partly genetically determined, but the part played by inheritance requires further study.

39.15.3.2 Personality

In a subset of paraphrenic patients, there is a history of those who have long-standing paranoid personalities, which are thought to predispose to the development of paraphrenia in old age.

39.15.3.3 Sensory Impairment

Hearing impairment is associated with the development of paranoid symptoms. The characteristics most strongly associated with late paraphrenia are the early age of onset of hearing impairment and long-duration and profound hearing loss. Auditory hallucinations are most consistently associated with hearing loss. It is thought that deafness may exert its action through increased social isolation, withdrawal, and suspiciousness. Late paraphrenia has also been associated with visual impairment.

39.15.3.4 Brain Disease

Compared to normal controls, late paraphrenics have significantly larger cerebral ventricles and are more cognitively impaired.

Miller et al. (1991), in an MRI study of nondemented late paraphrenics, found that organic brain pathology was common. In a group selected to exclude obvious organic pathology, the following abnormalities were found:

- Forty-two per cent had structural brain abnormalities, with white matter lesions particularly evident in temporal, occipital, and frontal areas.
- Fifty-eight per cent had neuromedical illness, such as tumours and metabolic disorders.
- Twenty-five per cent had evidence of silent cerebral vascular disease, most commonly associated with hypertension.
- Neuropsychological testing revealed deficits in intellectual, frontal lobe, and verbal memory functions.

39.15.4 CLINICAL FEATURES

Osvaldo et al. (1995) studied the psychopathology of late paraphrenics and found the following:

- All had at least one type of delusion. These most frequently involved persecution and self-reference; delusions of thought broadcast, sin, guilt, and grandiosity were also present.
- Forty-six per cent had at least one Schneiderian first-rank symptom.
- Eighty-three per cent had some hallucinatory experience, most commonly auditory, but also visual, somatic, and olfactory.
- Thought disorder and catatonic symptoms were almost never seen.
- Inappropriate affect was not seen.
- Negative symptoms were seen frequently but were mild.
- Other psychiatric symptoms such as worry, irritability, poor concentration, self-neglect, and obsessive features were all seen more commonly in late paraphrenics than in controls.

39.15.5 MANAGEMENT

Assessment and management are usually best undertaken in the patient's home where the psychopathology is most likely to be evident. Time must be spent developing a rapport and trying to engage with the patient.

39.15.5.1 Pharmacological Treatment

The treatment of metabolic disorders or other physical conditions may bring about an improvement in the mental state. The treatment of hypertension may prevent a deterioration if this is caused by silent cerebrovascular disease.

Antipsychotic medication may bring about an improvement. Antipsychotics with low anticholinergic, low hypotensive potential are recommended for old people. First-line treatment includes risperidone (1–3 mg/day). Second-line treatment includes olanzapine (2.5–7.5 mg/day) and quetiapine (50–300 mg/day). A substantial minority show no significant response, and about one-quarter show a full response to treatment. Treatment response is associated with improved compliance, the use of depot medication, an involvement of a CPN, and lower medication doses.

39.15.5.2 Nonpharmacological Treatment

- Day-care centre attendance may be helpful in increasing socialization.
- If sensory impairment is present, there is evidence that the condition can improve upon treatment of the deficit (e.g. a hearing aid for the deaf person).

39.15.6 PROGNOSIS

Some patients make little or no response to treatment, while others make a full response. Long-term contact with psychiatric services is required.

39.16 ANXIETY IN OLD AGE

39.16.1 EPIDEMIOLOGY

Anxiety disorders are often chronic, but about one-third of cases in the elderly have an onset after the age of 65 years.

39.16.1.1 Phobias

Phobias are quite evenly distributed across the age groups, with lower rates in the over-75s compared to the 65–75-year group. Phobias are the most common psychiatric disorder in elderly women in a community sample. Specific phobias are more common than agoraphobia or social phobia. The 1 month prevalence for phobic disorders is approximately 10%.

39.16.1.2   Generalized Anxiety Disorder

Prevalence increases with age and is more common in women. The 1-month prevalence for generalized anxiety disorder (GAD) is approximately 4%.

39.16.1.3   Panic Disorder

This is rarely encountered in the elderly. The 1 month prevalence for panic disorder is <1%.

39.16.2   AETIOLOGY

39.16.2.1   Environmental Factors

Early parental loss is associated with phobic disorders in younger and older adults.

39.16.2.2   Physical Illness

Anxiety disorders and neuroses are associated with increased mortality and increased cardiovascular, respiratory, and gastrointestinal morbidity.

The onset of agoraphobia after the age of 65 is often associated with a physical insult such as an MI, a surgery, or a fracture.

Anxiety symptoms can be caused by a number of physical disorders, and a full physical examination should form a part of the assessment of the elderly anxious patient. Causes include

- Cardiovascular (e.g. MI, cardiac arrhythmia, postural hypotension)
- Respiratory (e.g. pulmonary embolism, asthma, hypoxia, COAD)
- Endocrine (e.g. hyper-/hypothyroidism, hypoglycaemia, phaeochromocytoma)
- Neurological (e.g. epilepsy, cerebral tumour, vestibular disease)
- Drug induced (e.g. caffeine, sympathomimetics, sedative withdrawal)

39.16.2.3   Comorbidity

There are high levels of comorbidity with other psychiatric conditions, particularly depression. Late-onset cases of anxiety are almost always associated with depression, which may be either a primary or secondary association.

39.16.3   CLINICAL FEATURES

Features are generally similar to those seen in younger adults, but the following are more common in the elderly:

- Anxious preoccupation with physical illness, finance, crime, and family.
- Subjectively impaired sleep, which may be a normal part of ageing.
- Somatic symptoms of anxiety may be misattributed to physical causes.
- Abuse and overprescription of sedative drugs.

39.16.4   MANAGEMENT

Although there is less formal evaluation of therapies for anxiety disorders in the elderly, there is evidence that they do respond to psychological interventions including behavioural, cognitive, and anxiety-management training.

Benzodiazepines and other sedatives are not generally indicated in the treatment of persistent anxiety disorders, particularly not in the elderly because of the problems of tolerance, dependence, confusion, and falls.

Some anxiety disorders will respond to treatment with an antidepressant, particularly the SSRIs, which are specifically helpful in depression associated with anxiety and panic disorder.

Antipsychotics (e.g. quetiapine) are sometimes helpful for their anxiolytic properties, but caution is required in the elderly (e.g. orthostatic hypotension).

39.17   FURTHER CONSIDERATIONS IN OLD-AGE PSYCHIATRY

39.17.1   SUICIDE AND ATTEMPTED SUICIDE

Suicide is overrepresented in the elderly. The elderly comprise 15% of the U.K. population, yet they account for 25% of all completed suicides and only 5% of attempted suicides. Ninety per cent of those completing suicide in old age were depressed, and two-thirds of those attempting suicide in old age had a psychiatric disorder. Suicide rates increase with age until very old age, when they seem to tail off, more so for women.

The suicide rate is greater in men than in women; men are more likely to use a violent method and to use alcohol.

The depressed elderly who complete suicide tend to suffer from a moderate, often first-episode depression with the clinical picture often comprising severe agitation, hopelessness, guilt, insomnia, hypochondriasis, and delusion of guilt. Prior to suicide attempt, the old person may have an increase in alcohol intake, giving away possessions, reviewing will, and taking risk. The times of highest risk include

- Bereavement and their anniversaries
- The first few weeks after antidepressant treatment when the person develops the ability to enact his or her thoughts prior to full recovery
- In the first few weeks after discharge from hospital

Eighty per cent of those completing suicide had seen their GP before their death.

The incidence of physical illnesses in completed elderly suicides is higher than expected. Chronic pain is often a contributory factor, particularly postherpetic neuralgia. Living alone, a widowed or separated status, and alcohol abuse are also risk factors.

Cultural factors probably play a role since suicide rates among some elderly populations, such as elderly Indian people, are extremely low.

Thus, suicidal elderly patients should always be taken seriously. Depression should be adequately treated, isolation should be ameliorated if possible, and pain should be properly managed.

39.17.2 Alcohol and Drug Abuse

39.17.2.1 Alcohol
Alcohol abuse reduces with ageing, especially in men. However, about 3% of the over-75s in a general practise survey drank above the safe limits.

The reasons for this apparent decline in alcohol abuse with age include the selective death of early-onset alcoholics, reduced tolerance to the effects of alcohol secondary to reduced liver enzymes, increased sensitivity of the ageing brain to sedatives, increased poverty in old age, and reduced opportunities to drink in elderly social circles.

New cases of alcoholism in old age tend to be more neurotic with less evidence of personality disorder than in younger-onset cases. Physical ill-health and psychiatric illness may be a trigger to excessive alcohol use in old age.

39.17.2.2 Drugs
Illicit drug abuse is not a great problem in the elderly, but addiction to prescribed benzodiazepines, opiates and other analgesics, barbiturates, cough syrups, and laxatives is problematic. In the United States where the very elderly comprise 12% of the population, they are responsible for the consumption of 50% of prescribed hypnotics.

Doctors need to take care in their prescribing, to prevent the initiation of prescribed drug addiction. It is often worth attempting to wean even elderly persons from their drug of addiction, since abstinence can greatly improve the quality of life. However, there is a group, particularly the very elderly, who are better left on the drug if they strongly object to withdrawal.

39.17.3 Somatization and Somatoform Disorders

Five per cent of old people suffer from somatoform disorders. The most common somatic complaints in elderly include pain, constipation, fatigue, headache, impaired balance, dry mouth, nausea, change in appetite, and difficulty in urinating. Somatic complaints may be a presentation of underlying depressive (masked depression) and anxiety disorders. Three-quarters of old people suffering from psychiatric disorders also present with somatic complaints. The presentation of somatoform disorders (e.g. somatization disorder, pain disorder, conversion disorder, and hypochondriasis) in old people is similar to young adults. Management includes reducing unnecessary visits and assigning the care to one GP. Medical reassurance is important and avoids unnecessary investigations. Modified cognitive behavioural therapy with shorter session may be useful for old people.

39.17.4 Sexual Activity

39.17.4.1 Normal Sexual Behaviour in Old Age
Sixty per cent of married couples aged 60–75 and 25% of those over 75 are sexually active. One-fifth of men aged over 80 have sexual intercourse at least once a month. Thus, sexual activity and sexual interest continue into old age.

The determinants of sexual activity in old age include

- Age
- Sex—men are more sexually active than age-matched women
- Married status
- Own physical health
- Physical health of partner
- Enjoyment of sex

Loss of, or illness in, a partner is a common reason for the cessation of sexual activity in the elderly.

39.17.4.2 Physiological Changes with Ageing
The female genitalia atrophy with age particularly after the menopause. Blood flow is also reduced during arousal, resulting in reduced vaginal lubrication. However, regular sexual intercourse or masturbation protects the female genitalia from these changes. Clitoral sensitivity and orgasm do not change with ageing.

In the male, erections are slower to develop and require more tactile stimulation than in youth. The erection is less firm and persistent than in youth. The plateau phase can be prolonged longer, and, although ejaculation is less forceful, orgasm remains unaltered. The refractory period is much longer than in youth.

39.17.4.3   Sexual Problems in Old Age

Physical illness may impair sexual activity because of

- Fear of the risk involved in sexual intercourse (e.g. MI)
- Difficult or painful intercourse (e.g. arthritis)
- Impaired responsiveness of genitalia (e.g. neuropathy)
- Reduced feelings of sexual attractiveness (e.g. after mastectomy or colostomy)
- Reduced sexual desire (e.g. dementia)
- Drug effects (e.g. antidepressants, antipsychotics, antihypertensives, thiazide diuretics, benzodiazepines)

Elderly people in residential homes or hospitals should be provided with the privacy required to continue sexual expression with a consenting partner or by masturbation if they wish. The attitudes of staff and family may need to change through a process of education and discussion.

39.17.5   Sleep Disorders

Forty per cent of older adults complain of chronic sleep problems and use a disproportionate amount of nighttime sedation, often on a long-term basis.

The cause of sleep disturbance in the elderly is multifactorial. Assessment therefore requires a careful history, with selective investigation.

39.17.5.1   Primary Sleep Disorders

These include sleep apnoea and nocturnal myoclonus, both of which are age related.

39.17.5.1.1   Sleep Apnoea

Sleep apnoea is an extremely common disorder affecting a quarter of independently living old people and higher proportions of those in institutional care. However, the presence of sleep-related breathing disturbance in the absence of daytime sleepiness or impaired daytime functioning is probably not clinically significant.

Sleep apnoea is associated with increased morbidity and mortality. It is associated with daytime fatigue, memory problems, hypertension, and cardiac arrhythmias. It is further associated with the increased risk of a stroke, even after controlling for other risk factors such as hypertension, cardiac arrhythmia, and obesity.

39.17.5.1.2   Circadian Rhythms

Some sleep disturbance in old age is associated with changes in the systems that regulate circadian rhythm.

In older age, the body's circadian rhythms lose strength, with a breakdown in timing and amplitude. Proposed interventions include

- Fitness training
- Evening bright-light exposure
- Melatonin supplementation in those deficient

All these methods have brought about an improvement but are of only limited usefulness. Fitness training and bright-light exposure require a lot of time and effort and are continued after trials in only a minority of subjects. Melatonin is not commercially available in reliable formulations and in some can cause depression.

39.17.5.2   Secondary Sleep Disorders

The significant numbers of complaints of disturbed sleep are secondary to other conditions such as medical or psychiatric illness, drug and alcohol use, and behavioural and environmental factors. It is essential that the primary problem be identified and treated, rather than treating the secondary sleep disturbance. The use of hypnotics should be avoided whenever possible. Sleep disturbance is typically associated with poor physical health and depression.

In some elderly people, the apparent sleep disturbance is simply the unrealistic expectation that they should sleep for as long and as soundly as when they were younger. This often responds well to reassurance. In other patients, attention to issues of sleep hygiene is required. This involves addressing behaviour such as the excessive use of caffeine-containing drugs and environmental conditions improving the conduciveness to sleep, such as ensuring the bedroom is peaceful and dark, without stimulation, and keeping regular sleep hours without daytime napping.

39.17.6 BEREAVEMENT

Mood disorders associated with bereavement are prevalent in later life and are associated with morbidity and chronicity similar to other late-life depression. In a study of late-life widows, 24% were depressed at 2 months after the loss, 23% at 7 months, and 16% at 13 months. Risk factors for depression at 13 months included a past history of mood disorder, intense grief or depression early after the loss, and few social supports (Zisook et al., 1993).

It is important to understand the differences between depression and bereavement. Based on clinical experience, the following features are more common in depression but not in bereavement:

- Active suicidal ideation
- Depressive symptoms 'out of proportion' with loss
- Feelings of guilt not related to deceased
- Marked functional impairment for long period
- Marked psychomotor changes lasting for long period
- Preoccupation with worthlessness

39.18 PSYCHOTHERAPY WITH OLDER ADULTS

39.18.1 INDIVIDUAL PSYCHODYNAMIC THERAPY

Older adults can be treated with psychodynamic therapy. Conditions suitable for treatment include neurotic and personality disorders rooted in unconscious, unresolved childhood conflict.

39.18.2 ADAPTATIONS IN THERAPY

Patients treated include those suffering from depression, phobias, anxiety neurosis, and hysteria. Psychosomatic disorders in patients over the age of 60 are not considered treatable with psychotherapy.

It is suggested that the treatment of choice for neurotic disorders in the 55–75-year age group is one to two 50 min sessions per week for between several months to 2 years. In those with reactive crises, short-term low-frequency dynamic therapy of 5–20 sessions is indicated until the age of about 80.

Older adults have completed their psychosexual and psychosocial development but still have to cope with psychosocial tasks such as retirement, loss of partner,

ill-health, and impending death. They also have to struggle with unresolved unconscious psychological conflict and intergenerational difficulties.

With age, the ego adapts by deploying increasingly mature defence mechanisms. The superego similarly adapts. However, the unconscious id is largely unchanged with time. Inner psychological conflict can persist from childhood.

39.18.3 TRANSFERENCE AND COUNTERTRANSFERENCE

Early in therapy with elderly patients, the transference and countertransference are likely to be reversed compared to therapy with younger patients. With the younger patient, the therapist unconsciously assumes the position of a powerful parent. With the elderly patient, the transference is likely to be reversed whereby the therapist experiences the unconscious transference of their own parental relationships. It is essential that supervision be provided such that the therapist is aware of these issues as they arise in therapy. Similarly, early in therapy, the patient is likely to transfer past experiences with younger people, such as his or her own children, but as the therapy progresses, the patient will develop the more classical transference relationships.

39.18.4 COMMON THEMES

In older age, an increasing number of threatening and loss events occur. The therapist must work with the patient to mourn the losses, thus freeing the patient to continue to take up new opportunities and relationships. Decreasing independence and increasing dependence are often central themes in therapy. Coming to terms with the past and changed relationships and power structures is also relevant.

For the isolated elderly person, group work may be more appropriate than individual therapy.

39.19 MEDICOLEGAL ISSUES IN OLD-AGE PSYCHIATRY

39.19.1 ELDER ABUSE

The abuse of elderly people by their carers has received increasing attention since the 1970s. Its prevalence is difficult to estimate and depends on the definition of abuse—which can range from irritability and verbal abuse to sexual and physical abuse.

Among patients referred for respite care to geriatric wards in London, there was a high morbidity for dementia. Almost half of the carers admitted to some form of abuse, verbal more commonly than physical. Verbal abuse was associated with poor premorbid relations between patient and carer and depression and anxiety in the carer. Physical abuse was associated with poor communication by the patient and high alcohol consumption in the carer. Few patients admitted to any abuse by their carers.

39.19.2   MANAGEMENT OF FINANCIAL AFFAIRS

Mental disorder from whatever cause can restrict a person's ability to handle financial affairs and is more common in the elderly, particularly among those suffering from dementing conditions. Various options exist to help deal with the financial affairs of people unable to do so themselves because of mental disorder. See Chapter 11 in which mental capacity, the powers of attorney, the Court of Protection, and testamentary capacity are considered. The effect of psychiatric disorders on driving capability is also considered in that chapter.

CASC GRID: ESTABLISH THE DIAGNOSIS OF DEMENTIA

An 80-year-old man is brought by his children because they are concerned about his memory. They worry that he suffers from dementia and seeks your assessment.

Task: Take a history from his son to establish the type of dementia.

(A) AD/cortical Dementia	(A1) Amnesia	(A2) Alogia	(A3) Apathy	(A4) Apraxia	(A5) Acalculia and Family History
	'How do you find his memory?' 'Can he recall recent events? How about remote events?' 'Did he forget where he put his items? If yes, how did he react? Did he accuse someone stealing his item?' 'Does he make up story to fill the memory gaps?'	'How do you find his command of language?' 'Does he have word finding difficulty?'	'How do you find his expression of emotion?' 'Does he express a full range of emotion?' 'How does he spend his time in the daytime? Does he have motivation or initiative to do the things he used to do?'	'Does he show any difficulty to using a household tool (e.g. comb or toothbrush)?' 'Can he wear a shirt or jacket by himself?' 'Can he follow instructions to accomplish a simple motor task (e.g. collecting his laundry)?'	'Does he have difficulty to perform simple arithmetic (e.g. adding up the prices of several items from the supermarket)?' 'Does the memory problem run in the family? If so, at what age did they start to have memory loss?'
(B) VaD	(B1) The History of CVAs	(B2) Course of the Illness	(B3) Focal Neurological Symptoms	(B4) Focal Neurological Signs	(B5) Other Clinical Features
	'Did he have a stroke before?' 'If yes, did his memory impairment start within 3 months of a stroke?' 'Did he suffer from hypertension or high cholesterol?'	'Did his memory problems come abruptly or gradually?' 'Is his memory problems fluctuating or being consistent?'	'Does he show weakness on one side of his body?' 'Does his face show asymmetry?'	'Does he have incontinence (e.g. passing urine or motion involuntarily?' 'Can you comment on his walking? Does he walk steadily?'	'Do you find him becoming more emotional after the stroke?' 'Does he laugh or cry excessively?'

	(C1) Personality Change	(C2) Progressive Nonfluent Aphasia	(C3) Orbitofrontal Syndrome	(C4) Assess Dorsolateral Prefrontal Syndrome	(C5) Temporal Lobe Symptoms/ Semantic Dementia
(C) FTD	'Do you find that there is a change in his personality or character?' 'Can you tell me which component changes first, his memory or his personality?'	'How do you find the way he speaks?' 'Is his speech becoming more effortful and halting?'	'Do you find that he is overfamiliar with other people (e.g. women)?' Does he display any inappropriate sexual behaviour?' 'Is he becoming more irritable?' 'How do you find his judgement?' 'Is he easily distractible?'	'How do you find his planning nowadays?' 'How do you find his flexibility?' 'Does he have difficulty in changing topics in his conversation?' 'How do you find his attention and concentration?'	'Can he name objects correctly?' 'Does he have difficulty to recognize items, for example, tools or common household items?' 'Does he have difficulty to recognize a person (e.g. a friend, a relative, or a family member)?'

	(D1) Extrapyramidal Symptoms and Cognitive Impairment	(D2) Diagnosis of Parkinson's Disease	(D3) Visual Hallucination	(D4) Delusion	(D5) Sensitivity to Antipsychotic Medications
(D) DLB	'Is he slow in his movement?' 'Do you find his hands become shaky?' 'Does he fall easily?' 'If he has movement problems, does his memory problem start at the same time or one year after the movement problem?'	'Was he given a diagnosis? If so, did the doctor say he suffers from a condition called Parkinson's disease?' 'If yes, was he given any medication to treat his motor problems (e.g. carbidopa or levodopa)?'	'Does he see things that others cannot see?' Explore the nature, content, source, timing, and his sense of reality.	'Has he become more suspicious?' 'Does he say someone wanted to harm him?' 'How certain is he in his belief?'	'Has he ever taken any medication that worsens his movements? If yes, do you know the nature of the medication? What is the name of the drug? Was it called haloperidol?'

	(E1) Onset and Family History of Depression	(E2) Memory Problems	(E3) Poor Task Performance and Island of Normality	(E4) Insight	(E5) Treatment of Depression
(E) Pseudodementia	'Did he suffer from depression before?' 'Does he have any family members who suffer from depression?'	'Did he notice that he has memory problems?' 'If he suffers from depression, did the memory problem start before or after depression?'	'Does he have the tendency to give 'don't know' answers to questions?' 'Is there a time when his memory is perfectly normal?'	'Is he aware about his memory problems?' 'Does he seek help on his own?' 'Is he very worried that his memory is not well?'	'Was he treated by his GP for depression?' 'If yes, what kind of treatment was offered?' 'Did his memory improve with antidepressant treatment?'

(continued)

(F) Risk Assessment	(F1) Risk of Wandering and Self-Neglect	(F2) Safety at Home and Fall	(F3) Risk of Self-Harm, Suicide, and Machinery	(F4) Risk to Others	(F5) Risk of Exploitation and Abuse
	'Does he lose his way home? Was he ever found wandering by the police?' 'Was he searching for someone, for example, his spouse or a friend?'	'Has he ever left the cooker or fire on?' 'Has he been a victim of burglary?' 'What kind of medication does he take at home (e.g. water tablets or diuretics, sleeping pills, or heart medication such as digoxin and warfarin)?'	'Has he ever attempted suicide before?' 'Does he drive? Has he ever been involved in road traffic accident?'	'Has he been aggressive to other people?' 'How do the other family members react to his aggressive behaviour?'	'Has he ever been being taken advantages in sexual, financial, or emotional ways?' 'Was he ill-treated in the family?'

REFERENCES

Alexopoulos GA, Abrams RC, Young RC, and Shamoian CA. 1988: Cornell scale for depression in dementia. *Biological Psychiatry* 23:271–284.

American Psychiatric Association. http:// www.psych.org/aids (accessed on 12 April 2012).

American Psychiatric Association. 2013: *Desk Reference to the Diagnostic Criteria from DSM-5*. Washington, DC: American Psychiatric Association Press.

Ballard CG, O'Brien J, James I, and Swann A. 2001: *Dementia: Management of Behavioural and Psychological Symptoms*. Oxford, U.K.: Oxford University Press.

Barber R, Panikkar A, and McKeith IG. 2001: Dementia with Lewy bodies: Diagnosis and management. *International Journal of Geriatric Psychiatry* 16(Suppl 1):S12–S18.

Barrow B. 2007: Pension payouts have fallen 78% in ten years. London, U.K.: Daily Mail, http://www.dailymail. co.uk/news/article-440246/Pension-payouts-fallen-78-years.html (accessed on 7 July 2013).

Blacker D, Albert MS, Bassett SS, Go RC, Harrell LE, and Folstein MF. 1994: Reliability and validity of NINCDS-ADRDA criteria for Alzheimer's disease. The National Institute of Mental Health Genetics Initiative. *Archives of Neurology* 51(12):1198–1204.

Bookman A, Harrington M, Pass L, and Reisner E. 2007: *Family Caregiver Handbook*. Cambridge, MA: Massachusetts Institute of Technology.

Brew BJ. 2004: Evidence for a change in AIDS dementia complex in the era of highly active antiretroviral therapy and the possibility of new forms of AIDS dementia complex. *AIDS* 18(Suppl 1):S75 -S78.

Brun A. 1987: Frontal lobe degeneration of the non-Alzheimer type: I. Neuropathology. *Archives of Gerontology and Geriatrics* 6:193–208.

Buchsbaum MS and Hazlett EA. 2004: Functional brain imaging studies in dementia. In Charney DS and Nestler EJ (eds.) *Neurobiology of Mental Illness,* 2nd edn, pp. 849–862. New York: Oxford University Press.

Butler R and Pit B. 1998: *Seminars in Old Age Psychiatry*. London, U.K.: Gaskell.

Clair KL and Seitz D 2011: The patient with dementia. In Goldbloom DS, Davine J (eds.) *Psychiatry in Primary Care*. Ottawa, Canada: Centre for Addiction and Mental Health.

Danysz W et al. 2000: Neuroprotective and symptomatological action of memantine relevant for Alzheimer's disease— A unified glutamatergic hypothesis on the mechanism of action. *Neurotoxicity Research* 2:8–97.

DATSCAN. http://www.datscan.com/downloads/DaTSCAN_SPC_April%202007.pdf (accessed on 5 April 2012).

Department of Health. 1991: *Epidemiological Overview of the Health of Elderly People*. London, U.K.: Central Health Monitoring Unit.

Douglas S, James I, and Ballard C. 2004: Non-pharmacological interventions in dementia. *Advance in Psychiatric Treatment* 10:171–177.

Folstein MF, Folstein SE, and McHugh PR. 1975: "Mini-mental state". A practical method for grading the cognitive state of patients for the clinician. *Journal of Psychiatric Research* 12(3):189–198.

Graham DI, Nicoll JAR, and Bone I. 2006: *Introduction to Neuropathology*, 3rd edn. London, U.K.: Hodder Arnold.

Grant I, Sacktor H, and McArthur J. 2005: HIV neurocognitive disorders. In Gendelman HE, Grant I, Everall I, Lipton SA, and Swindells S (eds.). *The Neurology of AIDS*, 2nd edn, pp. 357-373. London, UK: Oxford University Press.

Herholz K. 1995: FDG PET and differential diagnosis of dementia. *Alzheimer Disease and Association Disorders* 9:6–16.

Mioshi E, Dawson K, Mitchell J, Arnold R, and Hodges JR. 2006: The Addenbrooke's Cognitive Examination Revised (ACE-R): A brief cognitive test battery for dementia screening. *International Journal of Geriatric Psychiatry* 21(11):1078–1085.

Huppert FA, Brayne C, Gill C, Paykel ES, and Beardsall L. 1995: CAMCOG—A concise neuropsychological test to assist dementia diagnosis: Socio-demographic determinants in an elderly population sample. *British Journal of Clinical Psychology* 34(4):529–541.

Jacoby R and Oppenheimer C. (eds.) 1991: *Psychiatry in the Elderly*. London, U.K.: Oxford University Press.

Kay DWK, Beamish P, and Roth M. 1964: Old age mental disorders in Newcastle upon Tyne: I. A study of prevalence. *British Journal of Psychiatry* 110:146–158.

Lindesay J, Briggs K, and Murphy E. 1989: The guy's/age concern survey: Prevalence rates of cognitive impairment, depression and anxiety in an urban elderly community. *British Journal of Psychiatry* 155:317–329.

Loewenstein DA, Acevedo A, Small BJ, Agron J, Crocco E, and Duara R. 2009: Stability of different subtypes of mild cognitive impairment among the elderly over a 2- to 3-year follow-up period. *Dementia and Geriatric Cognitive Disorders* 27(5):418–423.

McDonald C. 1969: Clinical heterogeneity in senile dementia. *British Journal of Psychiatry* 115:267–271.

McMahon PM, Araki SS, Sandberg EA, Neumann PJ, and Gazelle GS. 2003: Cost-effectiveness of PET in the diagnosis of Alzheimer disease. *Radiology* 228(2):515–522.

Murphy E. 1982: Social origins of depression in old age. *British Journal of Psychiatry* 141:135–142.

McKeith IG, Galasko D, Wilcock GK et al. 1995: Lewy body dementia-diagnosis and treatment. *British Journal of Psychiatry* 167:709–718.

Miller BL, Lesser IM, Boone KB et al. 1991: Brain lesions and cognitive function in late-life psychosis. *British Journal of Psychiatry* 158:76–82.

Miller BL, Iknote C, and Ponton M. 1997: A study of Lund-Manchester research criteria for frontal-temporal lobe dementia: Clinical and single—Photon emission of CT correlation. *Neurology* 48:937–942.

Moroney JT. 1997: Meta-analysis of the Hachinski Ischaemic Score in pathologically verified dementias. *Neurology* 49:1096–1105.

Morgan G and Butler S. 1993: *Seminars in Basic Neurosciences*. London, U.K.: Gaskell.

Morris JC. 1993: The Clinical Dementia Rating (CDR): Current version and scoring rules. *Neurology* 43(11):2412–2414.

Nasreddine ZS, Phillips NA, Bédirian V et al. 2005: The montreal cognitive assessment (moca): A brief screening tool for mild cognitive impairment. *Journal of American Geriatric Society* 53:695–699.

National Institute of Neurological Disorders and Stroke. http://www.ninds.nih.gov/disorders/corticobasal_degeneration/corticobasal_degeneration.htm (accessed on 11 April 2012).

NICE. *NICE Guidelines for Dementia*. http://www.nice.org.uk/nicemedia/pdf/CG042NICEGuideline.pdf (accessed on 5 April 2012).

Office for National Statistics. 2011: Data from Office for National Statistics Longitudinal Study; National Records of Ireland; Northern Ireland Statistics and Research Agency. http://www.statistics.gov.uk/hub/population/ageing/older-people (accessed on 5 April 2012).

Orrell MW and Sahakian B. 1991: Dementia of the frontal lobe type. *Psychological Medicine* 21:553–556.

Osvaldo P, Almeida R, Howard RJ et al. 1995: Psychotic states arising in late life (late paraphrenia): Psychopathology and nosology. *British Journal of Psychiatry* 166:205–214.

Osvaldo P, Almeida R, Howard RJ et al. 1995: Psychotic states arising in late life (late paraphrenia): The role of risk factors. *British Journal of Psychiatry* 166:215–228.

Petersen RC, Smith GE, Waring SC, Ivnik RJ, Tangalos EG, and Kokmen E. 1999: Mild cognitive impairment: Clinical characterization and outcome. *Archives of Neurology* 56(3):303–308.

Petrella JR, Coleman RE, and Doraiswamy PM. 2003: Neuroimaging and early diagnosis of Alzheimer disease: a look to the future. *Radiology* 226(2):315–336.

Post F. 1968: The factor of ageing in affective illness. In Coppen A and Walk A (eds.) *Recent Developments in Affective Disorders*. Ashford, Kent: Headley Brothers, pp. 105–116.

Roman GC, Tatemichi TK, Erkinjuntti T et al. 1993: Vascular dementia: Diagnostic criteria for research studies. Report of the NINDS-AIREN International Workshop. *Neurology* 43:250–260.

Rogawski MA. 2000: Low affinity channel blocking (uncompetitive) NMDA receptor antagonists as therapeutic agents—Toward an understanding of their favorable tolerability. *Amino Acids* 19(1):133–149.

Rogawski MA and Wenk GL. 2003: The neuropharmacological basis for the use of memantine in the treatment of Alzheimer's disease. *CNS Drug Reviews* 9(3):275–308.

Sadock BJ and Sadock VA. 2007: *Kaplan & Sadock's Synopsis of Psychiatry. Behavioural Sciences/Clinical Psychiatry*, 10th edn. Philadelphia, PA: Lippincott Williams & Wilkins.

Schneider LS. 1993: Treatment of depression, psychosis, and other conditions in geriatric patients. *Current Opinion in Psychiatry* 6:562–567.

Sheikh JI and Yesavage JA. 1986: Geriatric depression scale (GDS): Recent evidence and development of a shorter version. *Clinical Gerontologist* 5:165–173.

Snowden JS, Goulding PJ, and Neary D. 1989: Semantic dementia: A form of circumscribed cerebral atrophy. *Behavioural Neurology* 2:167–182.

Taylor D, Paton C, and Kapur S. 2009: *The Maudsley Prescribing Guidelines*, 10th edn. London, U.K.: Informa Healthcare.

World Health Organisation (WHO). 1992: *ICD-10: The ICD-10 Classification of Mental and Behavioural Disorders: Clinical Descriptions and Diagnostic Guidelines*. Geneva, Switzerland: World Health Organisation.

United Nations World Population Prospects. 2006 revision. http://www.un.org/esa/population/publications/wpp2006/WPP2006_Highlights_rev.pdf (accessed on 5 April 2012).

Zisook S and Peterkin JJ. 1993: Mood disorders and bereavement in late life. *Current Opinion in Psychiatry* 6:568–573.

Zisook S, Shuchter SR, Sledge P, and Mulvihill M. 1993: Aging and bereavement. *Journal of Geriatric Psychiatry and Neurology* 6(3):137–143.

40 Forensic Psychiatry

40.1 EPIDEMIOLOGY OF OFFENDING

40.1.1 RELATIONSHIP WITH AGE

In the United Kingdom, the peak age of offending is 14 years in girls and 17–18 years in boys. Half of all indictable crimes are committed by people aged under 21 years. By the age of 30 years, 30% of males in the United Kingdom have been convicted of an indictable offence.

40.1.2 SEX RATIO

The sex ratio of convicted males to females in the United Kingdom is approximately 5:1.

40.2 JUVENILE DELINQUENCY

Juvenile delinquency is defined as law-breaking behaviour by 10- to 21-year-olds.

40.2.1 AETIOLOGY

The aetiology is multifactorial and is not associated with an established psychiatric disorder. Factors associated with the development of delinquency include the following:

- Unsatisfactory child rearing
- Low IQ
- Conduct disorder in childhood
- Parental criminality
- Large family size

40.2.2 MANAGEMENT AND PROGNOSIS

Factors that may improve the prognosis with respect to adult criminality include the following:
Counselling

- Establishing a good relationship with a parent or counsellor
- Improvement in the home environment
- A good experience in school
- A good peer group
- Successful employment
- A good relationship or marriage

Approximately 50% have stopped their delinquent behaviour by the age of 19 years.

40.3 MENTALLY ABNORMAL OFFENDERS

40.3.1 EPIDEMIOLOGY

The prevalence of mental abnormality in all offenders is estimated to be 1%. The prevalence of mental abnormality in those in prison in the United Kingdom is estimated to be up to 33%.

40.3.2 MENTAL DISORDERS

Mental disorders that may be associated with offending include (see Table 40.1).

40.4 PSYCHIATRIC ASPECTS OF OFFENCES

40.4.1 SHOPLIFTING

Most shoplifting is a conscious and goal-directed activity without the presence of a psychiatric disorder. Possible contributing factors include personal gain, organized criminal activity, poverty, low self-esteem, frustration, boredom, and thrill seeking.

Sixty per cent of the total number of shoplifting is committed by women, but convictions are more common for men. Only 2% are referred for psychiatric assessment. There are two peaks in terms of age groups: adolescence and adults who are 50–60 years old (Chiswick and Cope, 1995).

Among shoplifters with associated psychiatric disorders, 33% suffer from psychiatric illnesses. Acute situational crises and adjustment disorder are the most common psychiatric illnesses. About 5% of shoplifters are depressed middle-aged women. Shoplifters with a depressive illness make little effort to conceal their actions. Absentmindedness is an acceptable defence.

Other psychiatric disorders include personality disorder (17%), acting on delusions (15%), learning disability (LD; 11%), dementia and delirium (5%), mania, influence from drugs (3%), and dissociative state (Sims, 2002). Organic disorder such as epilepsy is a recognized cause (Chiswick and Cope, 1995).

Distressed children steal for self-comfort. Conduct disorder or antisocial personality traits are associated with criminal stealing and the peak age of onset is 15 years.

TABLE 40.1

The Relationship between Psychiatric Disorders and Criminal Behaviour

Psychiatric Disorders	Criminal Behaviour
Affective disorder	• Shoplifting in middle-aged offenders may be associated with depression. • Violent offending during mild or moderate depressive episode is rare. If a candidate encounters a case of severe depression in the CASC exam, inquiry should be made about homicidal ideation. Family members are the usual victims of altruistic homicides. • Offending is more common in mania and hypomania than in depression.
Schizophrenia	• Schizophrenic patients have similar rate of offending as compared to the general population. • Schizophrenia is mostly associated with minor offending secondary to deterioration in personality and social functioning. • Schizophrenic patients are more likely to commit violent offences as compared to the general population, but most of the violent offences are not committed by schizophrenic patients. • Violence is a common precipitant prior to the first admission to a psychiatric ward.
Personality disorder	• The term psychopathic disorder should only be used as a legal category. • Personality disorders in forensic psychiatry are usually mixed in types. • A wide range of personality traits such as immaturity, inadequacy, hostility, and aggression contribute to offending behaviour.
LD	• Offending is more common in people with mild to moderate LD. • Property offences are committed with a lack of forethought. • Offences committed by people with LD are generally similar to offenders without LD although there have been reports for increase in rates for sex offending and fire setting in patients with LD.
Organic state	• Personality change is an early feature of frontal lobe dementia and associated with impulsivity. • In general, offending by patients with dementia is uncommon. The most common offence is theft. • In patients with Huntington's disease, antisocial behaviour may appear before any sign of neurological or psychiatric disturbance. • For patients with epilepsy, the rate and type of offending is similar to those of offenders in general. There is no excess of violent crimes in epileptic prisoners. Offending in epileptics is rarely ictal. The increase of prevalence of epilepsy in prisoners (about two times of the general population) is a result of common social and biological adversity leading to both epilepsy and crime (Whitman et al., 1984).
Substance abuse	• Alcohol misuse is commonly seen in the more than 50% of perpetrators and victims of violence and rape (Coid, 1986). • Substance misuse is common in offenders with antisocial personality disorder. • Alcohol and drugs that have been taken voluntarily do not, in general, lessen the individual's full legal responsibility. While amnesia is not a legal offence, its underlying cause may well be.
Morbid delusional jealousy (Othello syndrome)	• This is associated with repetitive and serious injury to the spouse/partner (refer to CASC grid for further details).

Source: Chiswick, D. and Cope, R., *Seminars in Forensic Psychiatry*, Gaskell, London, U.K., 1995.

40.4.2 KLEPTOMANIA

Kleptomania (ICD-10 F63.2) is an impulse control disorder characterized by repeated failure to resist the impulse to steal in which tension is relieved by stealing (Cooper, 2001). The sex ratio of F/M is 4:1.

Classically, the compulsion is characterized by a feeling of tension associated with an urge to steal. The person feels excited during the theft and feels relieved after the act. At the same time, the urge is recognized as senseless and wrong and the act is followed by guilt. The stealing is not an expression of anger or a part of dissocial personality trait.

Pure kleptomania is extremely rare (Sims, 2002). Such compulsions are associated with depression, anxiety, bulimia nervosa, sexual dysfunction, and fetishistic stealing of women's underwear (Cooper, 2001).

Stolen items are usually not acquired for personal use (e.g. same set of T-shirts) or monetary gain. The person may discard the objects, give them away, or hoard the items.

40.4.3 FIRE SETTING

There are about 30,000 episodes in England and Wales per year. The most common motives are revenge and fraud insurance claims (Johnstone et al., 2004). The other causes include anger and the need to relieve tension by fire setting (Chiswick and Cope, 1995).

There is a higher representation of men with LD (IQ 70–79) because they display passive aggression and a sense of power or excitement during arson. Twenty to thirty per cent of arsonists have psychiatric disorders (e.g. alcohol misuse, schizophrenia) (Gelder et al., 2001). Pyromania is a rare condition when the arsonist derives sexual satisfaction through fire setting.

Most cases of arson (80%) do not lead to criminal conviction and only a tiny proportion lead to psychiatric disposal (more common in women) (Chiswick and Cope, 1995). The recidivism rate for arson is 10%. If it is a gang crime, the recidivism rate is low for the gang members but high for the gang leader.

40.5 DANGEROUSNESS

Dangerous individuals are people who have caused or who might cause serious harm to others. Its features include

- Repetition
- Incorrigibility
- Unpredictability
- Untreatability
- Infectiousness

The best predictor of future dangerous behaviour is the individual's past behaviour. Shorter-term prediction is better than longer-term prediction. Dangerousness is associated with the availability of weapons, morbid jealousy, and the sadistic murder syndrome.

Schizophrenic patients usually assault a known person, but if they assaulted a stranger, the arresting police officer is the most common target. The delusional ideas often motivate the violent behaviours and the patients usually admit experiencing command hallucinations after the violent offences. Schizophrenic patients with negative symptoms commit violent offences inadvertently and neglectfully. In clinical practice, psychiatrists should be aware that schizophrenic patients may display persistence of their normal selves especially in patients without past history of violence (Chiswick and Cope, 1995).

40.5.1 MULTIAGENCY PUBLIC PROTECTION ARRANGEMENTS

1. Multi-Agency Public Protection Arrangements (MAPPA) is a collaboration of different responsible authorities in the United Kingdom aiming at public protection, and its main focus is on sex offenders or violent offenders and offenders who pose a serious risk of harm to the public.
2. The role of MAPPA involves sharing information on offenders being referred, deciding on the level of risk, setting up an action plan, monitoring of the action plan, reviewing current risk level, and considering the need of disclosure to relevant persons.
3. MAPPA has major differences from mental health services because it deals with its targets as offenders rather than patients.
4. Offenders are not informed about the discussion by MAPPA and they have no right to appeal.

CASC STATION ON MORBID JEALOUSY

A GP asks you to see a 55-year-old man who has history of alcohol misuse from when he lost his job 7 years ago. He has accused his wife of infidelity. He was diagnosed with type II diabetes six years ago and the GP reports he is depressed.

Task:

1. Take a history to establish diagnosis of morbid jealousy.
2. Perform a risk assessment.

CASC Grid

(A) Assess Morbid Jealousy Symptoms	(A1) Onset	(A2) Precipitants	(A3) Evidence to Support his Beliefs	(A4) Degree of Conviction	(A5) Consequences
	'Hello, I am Dr. Wilson. I can imagine that you have gone through a difficult period. Can you share with me when you started to suspect your wife is having an affair?' Explore the temporal relationship between the morbid jealousy, alcohol misuse, and diabetes.	'Can you describe your recent relationship with your wife?' 'Is there any event which triggers off your suspicion?'	'How did you arrive at the conclusion that your wife is unfaithful? Can you share with me your evidence?' 'Do you know the identity of the third party?' 'Do you follow your wife? If yes, how often?' 'How often do you call your wife?' 'Do you search her belongings? (e.g. hand phone, text messages, underwear, handbag, credit card bill)?'	'Could there be other possible explanations for her infidelity?' 'If I give you a scale from 1–10, 1 means that you do not believe and 10 means that you firmly believe that your wife is unfaithful, how do you rate your belief?'	'I can imagine that you have gone through a tough time. What is your plan on your marriage? Are you going to divorce your wife?' 'Are you going to confront her?' 'How do you cope with the current situation?'

(B) Risk Assessment	(B1) Self	(B2) Partner or Spouse	(B3) The Third Party	(B4) Children	(B5) Access to Weapons
	'Have you thought of harming yourself? If yes, how would you do it?'	'What would you do to your wife if she still denies of the affair? Will you be more aggressive?'	'Are you going to take any action against the third party? If yes, how would you do it?'	'Do you have any children? How old are they? What is their views on the current situation?' 'Have you ever thought of harming them?'	'Do you have access to weapons? If yes, what kind of weapons do you have?' 'Do you carry the weapon with you?' 'When will you use it?'

(C) Psychiatry Comorbidity	(C1) Alcohol and Drug History	(C2) Psychosexual History	(C3) Assess Mood	(C4) Assess Psychotic Experience	(C5) Personality
	'Can you take me through how much you drink in a day?' 'Has there been an increase in alcohol intake recently?' 'Have you developed further problems as a result of drinking? (e.g. liver problems, fits, or head injury)' 'When people are stressed, they turn into recreational drugs, have you tried those drugs?'	'Do you encounter any sexual problem? (e.g. cannot maintain erection during sex?) If yes, how long did you have this problem? Was it related to diabetes?' 'Can you tell me more about your past relationship? Did you suspect your partners or girl friends in the past?' 'Have you been unfaithful to your partners in the past?'	'How is your mood at this moment? Do you feel sad? Can you tell me more about your sleep, appetite and energy?' 'How do you see your future? Do you feel guilty? How is your confidence level?' 'Do you experience anxiety? Can you tell me more about your fear?' (e.g. losing his wife)	'Do you have unusual experience such as hearing voices when no one is around? Do the voices give you instructions?' 'Do you feel that someone wants to harm you at this moment? Do you think there is plot behind your wife's infidelity?'	'How do other people describe you as a person? Do they say that you are more suspicious? Do you have problems with your friends or neighbours? Do you trust them?'

(D) Past History	(D1) Forensic History	(D2) Medical History	(D3) Marital History	(D4) Family History	(D5) Insight
	'Do you have any encounter with the police? If yes, for what reason?' 'What was the consequence?' 'Have you ever appeared in court? If yes, were you sentenced to the correctional service?'	'Can you tell me more about your diabetes? Which kinds of medication do you take? Do you take them regularly? Have you ever experienced low sugar level and felt very giddy? Were you violent at that time?' 'Do you feel that there is a change in your sensation?' (Look for peripheral neuropathy that may be related to erectile dysfunction.)	'Is this your first marriage? If not, how did it end last time?'	'Can you tell me more about your family? Is there any family history of violence?'	'I understand that you are very affected by what had happened.' (Demonstrate empathy.) 'I have seen patients who presented with similar problems. You are not alone. They seem to have an illness in their belief system. Do you think you have a similar problem?' 'If yes, do you think you need treatment? What kind of treatment would you prefer?'

5. Psychiatrists can advise the police, probation officers, and other social agencies in MAPPA on the appropriateness of mental health interventions with offenders suffering from psychiatric illnesses who may present some level of risk. Confidentiality remains the important challenge.

6. Based on the good psychiatric practice guidelines (Royal College of Psychiatrists, 2006), a psychiatrist needs to consider the following before disclosure of any information to MAPPA:

   a. The crime must be sufficiently serious for the public interest to prevail.

   b. Without the disclosure, the prevention of crime would be seriously prejudiced or delayed.

   c. Inform the offenders before the disclosure and seek his or her consent unless obtaining consent would enhance the risk of harm or inhibit effective investigation.

   d. Reveal only minimum information necessary to achieve the objective.

BOX 40.1   FORENSIC PSYCHIATRIC ASSESSMENT

1. Full history and mental state of the patient, including fantasies and impulses to offend
2. Objective account of offence, e.g. from arresting police officer or from statements (depositions) in Crown Court cases
3. Objective accounts of past offences, if any, e.g. obtain list of previous convictions
4. Additional information gathering, e.g. interviews with informants (e.g. relatives), reading a social inquiry report from a probation officer (if prepared)
5. Review of previous psychiatric records, e.g. to ascertain relationship of mental disorder to previous behaviour and to psychiatric treatment and need for security

Source: Puri, B.K. and Treasaden, I.H., *Psychiatry: An Evidence-Based Text*, Hodder Arnold, London, U.K., 2011.

BOX 40.2 CLINICAL RISK ASSESSMENT AND RISK MANAGEMENT PLANNING

The aim is to get an understanding of the risk from a detailed historical longitudinal overview, obtaining information not only from the patient, who may minimize his or her past history, but also from informants. Ideally it should not be a one-off single interview assessment.

Reconstruct in detail what happened at the time of the offence or behaviour causing concern.

Independent information from statements of victims or witnesses or police records should be obtained where available. Do not rely on what the offender tells you or the legal offence category—for example, arson may be of a wastepaper bin in a busy ward or with intent to kill. Possession of an offensive weapon may have been prelude to homicide.

$$\text{Offence} = \text{offender} \times \text{victim} \times \text{circumstances/environment}$$

Risk factors associated with violence to be sought in a forensic assessment have been usefully summarized and are detailed later in the CASC Station On the Assessment of Dangerousness.

Consider also protective factors:

Practical risk assessment (history × mental state × environment) can be supplemented by standardized instruments of risk, including actuarial risk instruments based on static risk factors, such as the Violence Risk Appraisal Guide (VRAG), and dynamic risk instruments, such as the Historical, Clinical, Risk Management-20 (HCR-20), based on factors that can change or be managed, for example, symptoms of mental illness and noncompliance.

In conclusion:

1. Aim to answer how serious the risk is (i.e. its nature and magnitude): is it specific or general, conditional or unconditional, immediate, long-term, or volatile? Have the individuals or situational risk factors changed? Who might be at risk?
2. From such a risk assessment, a risk management plan should be developed to modify the risk factors and specify response triggers. This should ideally be agreed with the individual. Is there a need for more frequent follow-up appointments, an urgent care programme approach meeting or admission to hospital, detention under the Mental Health Act, physical security, observation, or medication? If the optimum plan cannot be undertaken, then reasons for this should be documented and a backup plan specified.
3. Risk assessments and risk management plans should be communicated to others on a 'need to know' basis. On occasions, patient confidentiality will need to be breached if there is immediate grave danger to others. The police can often do little unless there is a specific threat to an individual, whereupon they may warn or charge the subject. Very careful consideration needs to be given before informing potential victims to avoid their unnecessary anxiety. Their safety is often best ensured by management of those at risk.

Source: Puri, B.K. and Treasaden, I.H., *Psychiatry: An Evidence-Based Text*, Hodder Arnold, London, U.K., 2011.

40.6 RISK ASSESSMENT

40.6.1 ACTUARIAL AND CLINICAL RISK ASSESSMENT

In general, actuarial risk assessment requires the collection of a large amount of historical data that can indicate whether the offender is likely to reoffend.

Risk factors measured by actuarial tools can be static (unchangeable) or dynamic (changeable). For example, an actuarial risk prediction tool may measure a number of static factors such as prior convictions, age at the time of the offence and childhood factors, as well as dynamic factors such as substance abuse, access to weapons, and insight.

Clinical risk assessment is based on the professional opinions of the clinician, who take a more holistic approach to predicting whether an offender will reoffend. Clinicians may consider personality traits, presence of psychiatric illness, as well as biological, social, and psychological factors that are related to offending.

CASC STATION ON ASSESSMENT OF DANGEROUSNESS

You are the psychiatric registrar on call and being asked to carry out a risk assessment for a 25-year-old man who suffers from schizophrenia. He was remanded for an offence that he is reluctant to talk about. He has just assaulted a nurse in the forensic ward. He is calm at this moment.

Tasks:

1. Assess the causes of his aggression and violence.
2. Perform a risk assessment and explore the index offence.

Approach to this station: The candidate should establish rapport, show concern, maintain a supportive non-threatening stance, and avoid confrontation.

(A) Assess Contextual Factors in the Ward	(A1) Patient's View on the Event	(A2) Precipitants and Aftermath	(A3) Staff Factors	(A4) Ward Factors	(A5) Visitors
	'Hello. I am Dr. Patten and I am here to help you. Can you tell me what has happened tonight?' 'I can imagine that it may be stressful for you. Why did you attack the nurse?'	'Was there any event which upset you in the ward?' 'Do you have difficulty in controlling your impulses?' 'How do you feel about the nurse who is injured? Do you feel sorry for the nurse?' 'If you are going to harm someone again, are you going to inform us before you carry out your attack?'	'Can you share with me your experience with the staff on the ward?' 'Is there a rapid turnover of staff recently? How do you feel about the new staff? Is the nurse attacked by you is a new staff on the ward? Do you feel comfortable with the new staff? If not, why?' 'How do the staff react to you when you are angry? How do you feel the way they are handling you?' 'Is there enough staff to respond to you promptly?'	'From your views, is the ward overcrowded?' 'Do you feel that the ward is too custodial?' 'How do you feel about the other patients in the ward? Do you feel comfortable with them?' 'Do you find the ward too noisy?' 'How do you find the ward programme? Is it too boring or stimulating?'	'Have your friends or relatives visited you here? If yes, can you tell me more about them?' 'Did they pass you alcohol/or recreational drugs? If yes, which drugs?' 'Did they pass you sharp objects like razor blades?'

(B) Risk Assessment and Historical Factors	(B1) Assess Aggression	(B2) Past History of Violence	(B3) Access to Weapons	(B4) Forensic History	(B5) Suicide
	'May I know what kind events make you aggressive?'	'Did you assault other people before admission?'	'Do you have access to knives or other weapons in the ward?'	'Did you have any trouble with the police or the legal system? If yes, how did you get into the trouble?'	'Do you have any current thought of harming yourself? If yes, how would you do it?'

(continued)

(B) Risk Assessment and Historical Factors	(B1) Assess Aggression	(B2) Past History of Violence	(B3) Access to Weapons	(B4) Forensic History	(B5) Suicide
	'Did you feel aroused after assaulting the victim?' 'Did you plan for the assault beforehand?' 'Is there any goal you can achieve by being violent?' 'Are you hostile to the victim?'	'Can you tell me under what circumstances you would attack the others?' 'Were you under supervision in the community by the public protection panel?'	'If yes, where are those weapons at this moment?' 'Do other patients know about it?' 'Do you own those weapons? Do you share weapons with other patients?'	(Look for vandalism, sexual offences, and drug trafficking offences.) 'What happened after the court hearing? Were you sentenced to the correctional services? If yes, for how long?'	(Look for dangerous methods such as hanging.) 'Did you attempt suicide in the past? If yes, how many times?' 'What made you to attempt suicide in the past? Did you attempt suicide in the prison?'

(C) Clinical Factors Leading to the Violence	(C1) Auditory Hallucinations	(C2) Paranoid Misinterpretation of Staff	(C3) Motor Agitation Accompanied by Poor Concentration	(C4) Depression or Mania	(C5) Substance Abuse
	'Do you have any unusual experience such as hearing voices when no one is around? If yes, what do the voices say?' 'Do the voices give you any instruction? Do they ask you to attack the nurse?'	'Do you feel that the staff are doing something behind you? Do you feel that they want to harm you? If yes, what is their motive?' 'Do you feel that the staff or other patients are talking behind you?' 'How certain you are about your suspicion? Could it be a misunderstanding?'	'Have you been feeling restless lately?' 'What has caused that? Could it be related to psychiatric medications?' 'How do you find your attention or concentration?'	'How do you feel about yourself at present?' 'How's your sleep and appetite?' 'Do you feel low in your mood?' 'How about feeling high? Have you ever felt as if you are on top of the world or as if you have special powers?'	'Have you ever used any drug or alcohol prior to admission to the ward? 'How do you feel if you do not have those drugs? Do you feel shaky?' 'Do you want to go out of the ward to get those drugs?'

(D) Background History	(D1) Childhood and Family	(D2) Socioeconomic Status	(D3) Personality	(D4) Past Medical History	(D5) Insight
	'Were you bought up in a violent environment?' 'How do you feel about your parents? Is your father an alcoholic? Does he have trouble with the law?' 'Were you cruel to animals?' 'Did you set fire in the past?' 'Did you have difficulty to follow school rules?'	'Can you tell me your employment status prior to admission?' (Look for occupations that have access to firearms.) 'Do you have difficulty to stay in one job?'	'Can you tell me more about your character?' 'Are you concerned about the safety of other people?' 'Are you an honest person? Do you tend to tell lies?' 'How often do you feel frustrated? What would you do if you are frustrated?'	'Did you suffer from any head injury?' 'Did you have fit before?'	'In general, do you feel that you are aggressive?' 'Do you think your violent or aggressive behaviour is acceptable?' 'Could it be related to an underlying psychiatric condition? If yes, do you want treatment?'

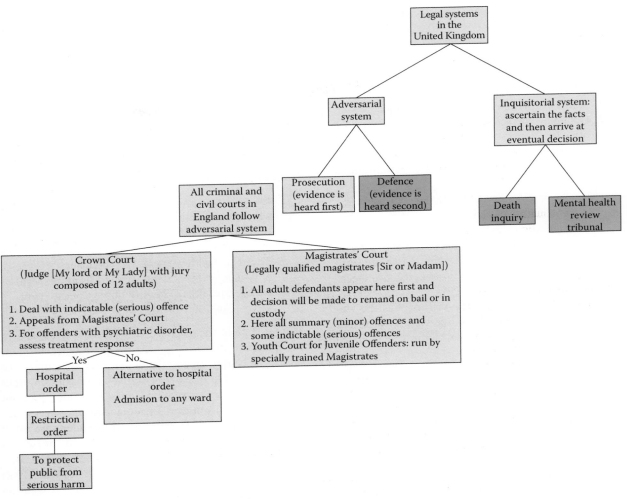

FIGURE 40.1   Legal systems in the United Kingdom.

40.7   LEGAL SYSTEMS IN THE UNITED KINGDOM

See Figure 40.1.

40.8   CRIMINAL RESPONSIBILITY IN THE UNITED KINGDOM

In England and Wales, criminal responsibility starts at the age of 10 years. In Scotland it starts at the age of 8 years.

40.8.1   DEFINITIONS

1. *Doli incapax.* Criminal responsibility is partial between the ages of 10 and 14 years. After the age of 14 years, an individual is legally responsible for his or her actions unless caused by
   a. A mistake
   b. An accident
   c. Duress
   d. Necessity
   e. Mental disorder
2. *Actus reus.* This is an unlawful act.
3. *Mens rea.* This is guilty intent and is required in addition to an unlawful act for certain offences, such as murder and rape.

40.8.2   FORENSIC PSYCHIATRIC ASSESSMENT AND COURT REPORTS

Before the assessment, the psychiatrist needs to emphasize to the offender that his or her role is to write a medical report to the court. The psychiatrist needs to state that the assessment is similar to other clinical interviews except that he or she has to share the information with the court.

These should include the following:

1. A full history and mental state examination
2. Obtaining an account of the offence from the offender
   a. Assess mental state during the offence and explore the possible influences of substances on mood and perception.
   b. Explore details of the offence such as degree and quality of violence, use of weapons, premeditation, and planning.
   c. Aftermath of the offence: Did the offender offer any help to the victim? Explore guilt and victim's empathy. Assess defence mechanisms and insight.
   d. Relationship with the victim: Was the victim provocative? (e.g. the victim was drunk and violent). Was the victim the intended target?
3. Obtaining an objective account of the offence from police statements
4. Obtaining an objective account of previous offences
5. Additional information from relatives, friends, social workers, probation officers, etc.
6. Assessing the current circumstances
   a. Assess current impulse control.
   b. Assess his or her relationship with other offenders in the custody.
   c. Assess his or her views towards custody officers and other mental health professionals.
   d. Explore current stressors.
   e. Assess risk to self and others.
7. A review of previous psychiatric and other relevant records
8. Assessing fitness to plead
   a. Understanding of the charge and its implication: 'Do you understand what the police say you have done wrong?'
   b. Understanding and appreciating the importance of entering a plea: 'Do you know the difference between saying guilty and not guilty?'
   c. Ability to instruct counsel: 'Can you tell your solicitor your side of story?'

d. Ability to challenge the juror: 'Do you know what it means if they say you can object to some of the members of the jury in your case?'
e. Ability to challenge a witness: 'If you disagree with what a witness is saying in court, what could you do about it?'
f. Ability to follow the course of the trial and understand the evidence: 'Will you be able to follow the procedures in the court?'

There are instruments to assess fitness to stand trial:

1. Fitness Interview Test—Revised (FIT-R): a reliable and sensitive semistructured instrument to screen for fitness to stand trial (McDonald et al., 1991).
2. The Nussbaum Fitness Questionnaire (NFQ): a 19-item self-report measure focusing on legal issues typically addressed during fitness interviews (Nussbaum et al., 2008).

Mental state at the time of the offence is irrelevant to the fitness to plead. Although the prevalence of mental illness is high among the defendants, the number of cases found unfit to plead and given a restriction order is less than 50 per year in the United Kingdom. Rates of mental illness are higher in remanded prisoners compared to sentenced prisoners as ill offenders are often diverted. Among those on remand, female prisoners show more behavioural disorder than male prisoners.

In criminal cases, medical report (Table 40.2) requested by the court or the Crown Prosecution Service will be disclosed in the court to the defendants and prosecutors. On the other hand, the medical report requested by the defence solicitor may be retained by the solicitor if the report does not help his or her client. In civil cases, the medical report is always the property of the person who requests it.

40.8.3 CLASSIFICATION OF HOMICIDE (STONE ET AL., 2000)

In the United Kingdom, there are 600–700 homicides per year. There are around 220 manslaughter verdicts per year with a wide discretion in sentencing. Homicides are divided into normal and abnormal homicides based on the legal outcome. Normal homicides include a conviction for murder or manslaughter. Abnormal homicides include a conviction of diminished responsibility or infanticide (Figure 40.2).

TABLE 40.2
Psychiatric Court Report Model

Para 1	Introduction: Inform the court of when and where the patient was seen; at whose request; what information was available, e.g. statements related to the case; who were the informants; and sometimes what information was not available. State the current offence(s) with date for which it is charged.
Para 2	Inform the court of his or her past medical history and of the result of medical examination, e.g. 'Physical examination revealed no abnormality'.
Para 3	Report the important, relevant points of the family history, including family psychiatric disorder and criminality.
Para 4	Personal history: Report the important points of his or her personal history, i.e. physical development, e.g. birth, milestones, bedwetting (enuresis), schooling (e.g. bully/bullied, truancy), and occupational history (which will include difficulties sustaining employment or with colleagues at work).
Para 5	Report his or her sexual and marital history: Be reasonably discreet as the report may be read in open court.
Para 6	Report details of his or her personality in terms of social interaction, emotions, and habits, e.g. drinking, gambling, and drugs.
Para 7	Report past forensic history, e.g. past convictions. This is, however, inadmissible.
Para 8	Report past psychiatric history (dates, diagnoses, relevant details, and relationship of mental disorder and treatment to offending).
Para 9	Report circumstances leading to current offence(s) and the defendant's state of mind at the time of the offence. Restrict discussion to the phenomena observed, e.g. 'For the time of the offence he gives a history of tearfulness, loss of hope, poor sleeping' and 'These are symptoms of the mental illness of depressive disorder'.
Para 10	Report the result of the interview: 'He showed/did not show evidence of mental illness or mental impairment.' Then give a brief outline of the evidence, e.g. 'He muttered to himself, looked around the room as though hallucinating', or list symptoms detected and say 'These are symptoms of the severe mental illness of schizophrenia'.

Information in paragraphs 1–10 should be factual, verifiable, and ideally agreed by all, even if others' opinions of these facts differ from your own.

Para 11	The final paragraph should express your opinion. The court will be interested particularly in your opinion regarding the following: (a) Is the defendant fit to plead and stand his or her trial? (b) Is he or she suffering from a mental disorder, i.e. mental illness, a form of mental impairment, or psychopathic disorder? (c) Where appropriate, comment on issues of responsibility, e.g. not guilty by reason of insanity; diminished responsibility in cases of homicide. (d) If suffering from mental disorder, can arrangements be made for his or her treatment in the National Health Service? (Arrange this if you think they can.)

Make suggestions to the court about which Mental Health Act order would be appropriate, e.g. Sections 37/41 in England and Wales, or suggest treatment as a condition of a Probation Order, e.g. 'In my opinion this man suffers from the severe mental illness schizophrenia, characterized by delusions (false beliefs) and hallucinations (voices, or visions). I consider he would benefit from treatment in a psychiatric hospital. I have made arrangements for a bed to be reserved for him at X hospital under Section 37 of the Mental Health Act 1983 if the court considers that this would be appropriate. I additionally recommend, if the court so agrees, that he be made subject to restrictions under Section 41 of the Mental Health Act 1983 to protect the public from serious harm and to facilitate his long-term psychiatric management, including specifying the conditions of his discharge from hospital, e.g. of residence and compliance with out-patient psychiatric treatment'. As an alternative: 'In my opinion this man does not suffer from mental illness, mental impairment nor psychopathic disorder and is not detainable in hospital under the Mental Health Act 1983. He has an anxious and dependent personality disorder, requires considerable support and would benefit from group psychotherapy as an out-patient. The court may consider that it would be an appropriate disposal to help this man if he were to attend an out-patient group under my direction at X Health Centre as a condition of probation'.

Comment should be made on any mitigating circumstances, e.g. marital/work stress, and on the prognosis. Express any doubts you may have as to the likelihood of benefit from treatment.

If you have no psychiatric recommendation, say so, e.g. 'I have no psychiatric recommendation to make in this case'.

Finally, if essential information is lacking or if time is not sufficient to make the necessary arrangements for a hospital bed, then do not hesitate to state your findings up to date, state what you would like to do, and ask for a further period of remand.

Source: Reproduced from Puri, B.K. and Treasaden, I.H., *Textbook of Psychiatry*, 3rd edn., Churchill Livingstone, Edinburgh, U.K., 2011. With permission.

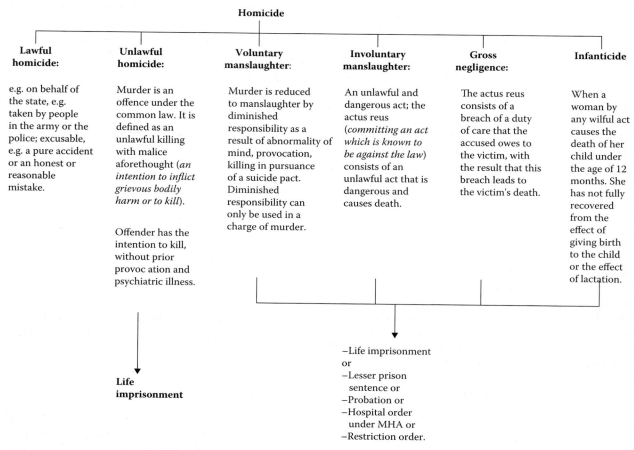

FIGURE 40.2   Classification of homicide.

40.8.4   McNaughton Rules (Puri et al., 2012)

In this defence, the offender is arguing that he or she is not guilty by reason of his or her insanity. The offender meets the McNaughton Rules if he or she fulfils the following criteria:

1. That by reason of such defect from disease of the mind, the person did not know the nature or quality of his or her act.
2. The person did not know that what he or she was doing was wrong (forbidden by law).
3. If the person was suffering from a delusion, then his or her actions would be judged by the relationship to the delusion, that is, if he or she believed his or her life to be immediately threatened, then he or she would be justified in striking out, but not otherwise.

In the legal concepts, the term 'disease of mind' is divided into two parts. Mind refers to 'mind for reason, memory and understanding' and disease refers to 'organic/functional, permanent/temporary, treatable/not treatable', and is 'internal'. Criticisms of the McNaughton Rules include a small number of offenders meeting the rigid criteria and ignoring the linkage with other higher mental functions (e.g. emotion and cognition).

40.8.4.1   Diminished Responsibility (Puri et al., 2012)

In the case of a charge of murder, a defence of diminished responsibility (Homicide Act 1957) may be brought in, whereupon it has to be shown that, at the time of the offence, the offender suffered from:

such abnormality of mind, whether caused from a condition of arrested or retarded development of mind or any inherent causes or induced by disease or injury, as substantially impai red [the individual's] mental responsibility for [his or her] act.

Diminished responsibility is determined by the court (usually by the jury or by the judge if both prosecution and defence agree on plea). Examples of diminished responsibility include killing a spouse in a state of depression. The abnormality of mind substantially impairs criminal responsibility of the person's acts. If a person is found to have diminished responsibility, it may imply that the court will return such a person to society earlier than a 'responsible' offender. In England and Wales, 7% of homicides result in diminished responsibility or infanticide and 50% of these cases result in hospital disposal. Criticisms of diminished responsibility include the problem of balancing the concept of responsibility with 'determinism'.

40.8.5 AUTOMATISM (JOHNSTONE ET AL., 2004; PURI ET AL., 2012)

Under the British law, automatism is a legal concept. Automatism is different from automatic behaviour, which is a clinical concept, and there is no relationship between these two terms. The defendant pleads that his or her behaviour was automatic at the time of the offence (i.e. no mens rea/guilty mind or no decision making). Automatism refers to unconscious, involuntary, non-purposeful acts where the mind is not conscious of what the body is doing. There is a separation between the mind and the act. Sane automatism is a once-only event, resulting from external causes, for example, hypoglycaemia caused by insulin. Insane automatism is caused by diseases of the mind such as mental illness or brain disease (intrinsic factors), for example, epilepsy, dissociative fugue states, and sleepwalking and night terrors in slow-wave sleep. Insane automatism tends to recur. Voluntary intoxication by itself does not constitute a defence.

40.8.6 OUTCOME OF SENTENCING

The outcome of sentencing of mentally abnormal offenders in England and Wales is shown in Tables 40.3 and 40.4.

40.9 CIVIL ASPECTS

40.9.1 TESTAMENTARY CAPACITY

This is considered in Chapter 11.

40.9.2 TORT

A mentally disordered person is considered incapable of committing a tort (a civil wrong to an individual or to the reputation or estate of an individual) unless the disorder did not preclude an understanding of the nature or probable consequences of the act.

TABLE 40.3

Outcome of Sentencing of Mentally Abnormal Offenders

(a) The law takes its course, e.g. a fine and prison

(b) Conditional or absolute discharge, possibly with voluntary psychiatric treatment

(c) Probation order, with or without condition of psychiatric treatment (e.g. under Section 3 of the Powers of the Criminal Courts Act 1973 in England and Wales)

(d) Detention under the Mental Health Act, e.g. under Section 37 with or without a Section 41 Restriction order under the Mental Health Act 1983 of England and Wales

Source: Reproduced from Puri, B.K. and Treasaden, I.H., *Textbook of Psychiatry*, 3rd edn., Churchill Livingstone, Edinburgh, U.K., 2011. With permission.

40.9.3 CONTRACTS

A contract requires free full consent and is void if an individual was of unsound mind at the time of making the contract.

40.9.4 MARRIAGE

Being a contract, marriage is void if an individual had a mental disorder at the time of marriage such that the nature of the contract was not appreciated at that time. A marriage may be annulled for any of the following reasons:

- The partner has a mental disorder at the time of marriage so as not to appreciate the nature of the contract.
- One partner did not disclose that he or she suffered from epilepsy or a communicable venereal disease.
- Either party was under 16 years at the time of marriage.
- Pregnancy by another male at the time of marriage was not disclosed.
- There was non-consummation.
- One of the partners was forced to agree to the marriage by duress.

Readers are advised to refer to Table 76.10 in Treasaden (2011a). The table provides an excellent summary on the civil treatment orders under the Mental Health Act (1983).

TABLE 40.4

Forensic Treatment Orders for Mentally Abnormal Offenders

	Grounds	Made by	Medical Recommendation	Maximum Duration	Eligibility for Appeal to Mental Health Review Tribunal
Section 35—Remand to hospital for report	Mental disorder	Magistrate's or Crown Court	Any doctor	28 days; renewable at 28 day intervals; maximum 12 weeks	
Section 36—Remand to hospital for treatment	Mental disorder (not if charged with murder)	Crown Court	Two doctors: one approved under Section 12	28 days; renewable at 28 day intervals; maximum 12 weeks	
Section 37—Hospital and guardianship orders (Section 37(3) without conviction)	Mental disorder— accused or convicted of an imprisonable offence	Magistrate's or Crown Court	Two doctors: one approved under Section 12	6 months; renewable for further 6 months and then annually	During second 6 months; then every year; mandatory every 3 years
Section 41— Restriction order	Added to Section 37 to protect public from serious harm	Crown Court	Oral evidence from one doctor	Usually without limit of time; effect— leave, transfer, or discharge only with consent from the Justice Secretary	As Section 37
Section 38—Interim hospital order	Mental disorder— for trial of treatment	Magistrate's or Crown Court	Two doctors: one approved under Section 12	12 weeks; renewable at 28 day intervals; maximum 12 months	None
Section 47—Transfer of sentenced prisoner to hospital	Mental disorder	Justice Secretary	Two doctors: one approved under Section 12	Until earliest date of release (EDR) from sentence	Once in the first 6 months; then once in the next 6 months; thereafter, once a year
Section 48—Urgent transfer to hospital of remand prisoner	Mental disorder	Justice Secretary	Two doctors: one approved under Section 12	Until date of trial or sentence	Once in the first 6 months; then once in the next 6 months; thereafter, once a year
Section 49— Restriction direction	Added to Section 47 or Section 48	Justice Secretary		Until end of Section 47 or 48; effect—leave, transfer, or discharge only with consent of Justice Secretary	As for Sections 47 and 48 to which it is applied

Source: Puri, B.K. and Treasaden, I.H., *Psychiatry: An Evidence-Based Text*, Hodder Arnold, London, U.K., 2011.

CASC STATION ON STALKING

You are the registrar in forensic psychiatric service. The police has asked you to see a 35-year-old man who was arrested for stalking on a female nurse with threats to harm her.

Task:

1. Assess his stalking behaviour
2. Perform a risk assessment
3. Explain your management

(A) Assess Stalking Behaviour	(A1) Ask the Person to Describe Stalking Behaviour	(A2) Unsolicited Telephone Calls	(A3) Electronic Mail	(A4) Gifts	(A5) Assess Motive
	'Hello, I am Dr. Trench. Can you tell me why you are under the police custody at this moment?' 'What is your relationship with the nurse? What have you done to her so far?' 'What is her name?' 'Do you feel desperate for her?' 'Did she encourage you to follow her?'	'Do you know her phone number? How often do you call her?' 'Do you call her constantly even though she does not respond to your call?' 'Do you usually leave a voice mail? Would you mind to tell me the content of the message?'	'Do you know her email address? How often do you send her an email?' 'Did she respond to your email? How do you feel if she does not respond? Do you continue to send emails if she does not respond?' 'Would you mind to tell me the content of the message?'	'Have you sent any gift to her? If yes, what kinds of gifts did you send? How often do you send her a gift?' 'Has she rejected your gift? How do you feel after that? Were you upset? If you were upset, what would you do next?'	'Why do you need to take the above actions? Do you want to be close to her?' 'From your views, how does your behaviour affect her life?' 'Do you feel sorry for her?'
(B) Risk Assessment	(B1) Plan	(B2) Threats	(B3) Violence	(B4) Self-Harm	(B5) Harm on Others
	'Are you planning to do something to the nurse? If yes, would you mind to tell me the details?'	'Do you plan to harm her? If yes, what would you do?' 'Is this part of your fantasy?'	'Have you ever applied force on her? What was her reaction? Did she defend herself? Will you do it again in the future?'	'Have you ever thought of harming yourself? Have you ever thought of ending your life?'	'Has anyone tried to stop you following her? If yes, what did you do? Do you carry a weapon? Will you use it to harm those who try to stop you?'

(continued)

(C) Four Types of Stalkers	(C1) Incompetent Stalker	(C2) Rejected Stalker	(C3) Intimacy Seekers and Erotomania	(C4) Resentful Stalker	(C5) Insight of Current Problem
	'Did you encounter any difficulty in having a relationship in the past?' 'Does the nurse remind you of the unpleasant past?'	'When you are ignored or rejected by the nurse, how do you feel?' 'Do you feel that both of you were in a relationship?' 'Do you hope to reconcile by following her?'	'Are you in love with her?' 'Do you think she is love with you? How about the future? Do you think she will love you?' 'How certain you are that she is in love with you? Could it be a misunderstanding?' 'Do you have sexual feelings towards her?'	'Have you tried to frighten her?' 'Are you taking revenge on her'	'You have done a lot in following her. Do you feel stressed?' 'Do you want to continue this behaviour? Have you thought of changing yourself?' 'Do you think that you need treatment?'
(D) Background History	(D1) Forensic History	(D2) Past Psychiatric History	(D3) Substance Misuse	(D4) Personality	(D5) Organic Causes
	'Did you have trouble with the police in the past? If yes, what was the reason? Were you charged subsequently?' (Explore past history of violent behaviour and sexual offences.) 'Did you break any court order in the past?'	'How is your mood at this moment?' 'Have you ever felt high in the past? If yes, did have high sexual drive? Were you more impulsive?' 'Do you have any unusual experience such as hearing voices in the past? If yes, what did the voices say to say? Do they give you instruction to follow her?' 'Did you receive any psychiatric treatment?'	'How often do you drink?' 'What kind of alcohol do you drink?' 'What would you do if you are drunk?' 'What would happen if you do not drink for a day?' 'Do you use any recreational drug before?'	'How do your friends describe you as a person?' 'Are you concerned about safety of other people in general?' 'Are you a honest person?' 'How do you compare yourself with other people? Are you entitled to be treated specially? Was it a blow to your ego when the nurse rejected you?' (narcissistic personality and narcissistic injury)	'Have you ever had a head injury? If yes, which part of the brain was affected?' 'Did you have fits before?' 'Do you have other medical problems such as diabetes?'

(E) Explain Management	(E1) Biological Treatment	(E2) Psychological Treatment	(E3) Social Management	(E4) Legal	(E5) Victim
'Thanks for sharing with me. I understand that you have gone through a lot of stress. I would like to share with you some of the treatment which I can offer to you. Are you interested to hear about it? There are medications like antidepressants, mood stabilizers or antipsychotic which could help you'.	'I can refer you to see a psychologist for psychotherapy. I would recommend cognitive behavioural therapy (CBT). It will help you to change your behaviour and you will be more sympathetic to the nurse'.	'I will also refer you to see a social worker who will address your social and occupational needs in long run'.	'Do you have a lawyer representing you at this moment? The court will decide whether the treatment will take place in a hospital or in the community'.	'Will you look for her again if you are released from here? She is also under tremendous stress. Would you mind to cancel your plan to visit her? Do you have other concerns?'

40.10 PRISON PSYCHIATRY

Readers are advised to refer to Treasaden (2011a). This chapter provides an excellent summary of prison psychiatry.

REFERENCES

Chiswick D and Cope R. 1995: *Seminars in Forensic Psychiatry*. London, U.K.: Gaskell.

Coid J. 1986: Alcohol, rape and sexual assault: Socioculture in alcohol related agression. In *Brain PF. Alcohol and aggression*. London, U.K.: Croom Helm.

Cooper JE. 2001: *ICD – 10 Classification of Mental and Behavioural Disorders with Glossary and Diagnostic Criteria for Research*. London, U.K.: Churchill Livingstone.

Faulk M. 1988: *Basic Forensic Psychiatry*. Oxford, U.K.: Blackwell.

Gelder M, Mayou R, and Cowen P. 2001: *Shorter Oxford Textbook of Psychiatry*. Oxford, U.K.: Oxford University Press.

Johnstone EC, Cunningham ODG, Lawrie SM, Sharpe M, and Freeman CPL. 2004: *Companion to Psychiatric Studies*, 7th edn. London, U.K.: Churchill Livingstone.

Kingham M and Gordon H. 2004: Aspects of morbid jealousy. *Advances in Psychiatric Treatment* 10:207–215.

McDonald DA, Nussbaum DS, and Bagby RM. 1991: Reliability, validity and utility of the Fitness Interview Test. *Canadian Journal Psychiatry* 36(7):480–484.

Mullen PE, Pathé M, and Purcell R. 2001: The management of stalkers. *Advances in Psychiatric Treatment* 7:335–342.

Nussbaum D, Hancock M, Turner I, Arrowood J, and Melodick S. 2008: Instruments, and cross-validation of the Nussbaum fitness questionnaire fitness/competency to stand trial: A conceptual overview, review of existing. *Brief Treatment and Crisis Intervention* 8(1):43–72.

Puri BK, Brown R, McKee H, and Treasaden, IH. 2012: *Mental Health Law Handbook*, 2nd edn. London, U.K.: Hodder Arnold.

Puri BK and Treasaden IH. 2011: *Psychiatry: An Evidence-Based Text*. London, U.K.: Hodder Arnold.

Royal College of Psychiatrists. 2006: Good psychiatric practice: Confidentiality and information sharing. Council Report CR133.

Sims A. 2002: *Symptoms in the Mind: An Introduction to Descriptive Psychopathology*, 3rd edn. London, U.K.: Saunders.

Stone JH, Roberts M, O'Grady J, Taylor AV, and O'Shea K. 2000: *Faulk's Black Forensic Psychiatry*, 3rd edn. Oxford, U.K.: Blackwell Science.

Taylor PJ and Gunn J. 1984: Violence and psychosis. I: Risk of violence among psychotic men. *British Medical Journal* 288:1945–1949.

Treasaden I, 2011a: Forensic psychiatry. In Puri BK and Treasaden I (eds.) *Psychiatry: An Evidence-Based Text*, pp. 1153–1213. London, U.K.: Hodder Arnold.

Treasaden IH. 2011b: Forensic psychiatry. In Puri BK and Treasaden IH (eds.) *Textbook of Psychiatry*, 3rd edn, pp. 391–426. Edinburgh, U.K.: Churchill Livingstone.

Whitman S, Coleman TE, Patmon C et al. 1984: Epilepsy in prisons: Elevated prevalence and no relationship to violence. *Neurology* 34:775–782.

41 Preparation for Psychiatric Examinations

Preparation for the various parts of the MRCPsych examination or similar psychiatric examinations should ideally begin early during one's psychiatric higher training. This brief chapter mentions some important key points that should enable a candidate to perform well in these examinations:

- Familiarize yourself with the format of the examinations. Always check the latest version of the examination regulations.
- Particularly early on during your training, it is invaluable to clerk as many patients as you can, including in the psychiatric subspecialties. Try to find suitable opportunities to present such cases, for example, in ward rounds and at case conferences.
- Being on call in a busy psychiatric rotation can offer an excellent opportunity to see a wide variety of different patients and to make numerous clinical decisions that cause you to learn about or revise your knowledge of different conditions and different treatments. Rather than avoiding the busiest jobs on the rotation, you might wish to consider volunteering for those placements, seeing them as valuable learning opportunities.
- Try to begin your study of suitable textbooks as early as possible during your training.
- There may be good courses available locally. You should supplement the course material with detailed textbook learning.

- Try to keep up with a good selection of journals. Try to make a habit of at least skimming the titles and abstracts of relevant papers published in journals such as
  - *American Journal of Psychiatry*
  - *JAMA Psychiatry*
  - *British Journal of Psychiatry*
  - *Lancet*
  - *New England Journal of Medicine*

If you are interested in biological psychiatry, then *Nature Neuroscience Reviews* is an excellent source of high-quality up-to-date erudite review papers.

- Make it a regular habit to attend (and present at) journal clubs and relevant research meetings.
- There are many books and online sources of multiple-choice questions, extended matched items, etc. Obtain those of a high quality, preferably sources that give explanations to the answers, and try to work through these diligently. Whenever you make a mistake, go back and reread the corresponding textbook material until you understand the relevant subject matter.
- In the 6 months leading up to a clinical examination, try to find the opportunity to see and present cases under examination conditions to senior colleagues.

Index